MEDICAL MICROBIOLOGY

MEDICAL MICROBIOLOGY

K. Rajeshwar Reddy
M.Sc. (Med. Micro); M.Ed; PGDEM; PGDCA; Ph.D.
Associate Professor
Department of Microbiology
Prathima Institute of Medical Sciences
Nagunur, Karim Nagar, AP-505417

PUBLISHING FOR ONE WORLD

NEW AGE INTERNATIONAL (P) LIMITED, PUBLISHERS
New Delhi • Bangalore • Chennai • Cochin • Guwahati • Hyderabad
Jalandhar • Kolkata • Lucknow • Mumbai • Ranchi
Visit us at **www.newagepublishers.com**

Published by New Age International (P) Ltd., Publishers
First Edition: 2009

Branches:

- 36, Malikarjuna Temple Street, Opp. ICWA, Basavanagudi, **Bangalore**. ✆ (080) 26677815
- 26, Damodaran Street, T. Nagar, **Chennai**. ✆ (044) 24353401
- Hemsen Complex, Mohd. Shah Road, Paltan Bazar, Near Starline Hotel, **Guwahati**. ✆ (0361) 2543669
- No. 105, 1st Floor, Madhiray Kaveri Tower, 3-2-19, Azam Jahi Road, Nimboliadda, **Hyderabad**. ✆ (040) 24652456
- RDB Chambers (Formerly Lotus Cinema) 106A, 1st Floor, S.N. Banerjee Road, **Kolkata**. ✆ (033) 22275247
- 16-A, Jopling Road, **Lucknow**. ✆ (0522) 2209578
- 142C, Victor House, Ground Floor, N.M. Joshi Marg, Lower Parel, **Mumbai**. ✆ (022) 24927869
- 22, Golden House, Daryaganj, **New Delhi**. ✆ (011) 23262370, 23262368

ISBN: 978-81-224-2579-6

Rs. 525.00

C-09-03-3515

Printed in Ramprintographs, Delhi.
Typeset at Kalyani Computer Services, Delhi.

PUBLISHING FOR ONE WORLD
NEW AGE INTERNATIONAL (P) LIMITED, PUBLISHERS
4835/24, Ansari Road, Daryaganj, New Delhi-110002
Visit us at **www.newagepublishers.com**

Dedicated

to

Lord Sri Raja Rajeshwara Swamy

Vemulawada, A.P.

Dedicated

to

Lord Sri Raja Rajeshwara Swamy

Vemulawada

PREFACE

This book has originated from my lecture notes which have been compiled over the last 20 years of my teaching Medial Microbiology. It presents the essential information in a novel, readable, interesting, enjoyable and varied format. This book is a concise review of the medically important aspects of Bacteriology, Immunology, Virology, Mycology and Parasitology.

Undertaking this job was an incredible task, because any text book to remain useful, must keep up with advances in knowledge and with changes in teaching patterns. The contents were reorganised, particularly in General Microbiology and Applied Clinical Diagnostic Microbiology to expand the scope of the book.

This book is primarily intended for undergraduate and postgraduate medical students. It is also extremely useful for clinicians as a comprehensive text in applying microbiological knowledge to the clinical management of infections. In addition, this book is also useful for students of dental, nursing, veterinary, home sciences and biological sciences.

This comprehensive text book has been compiled, edited and prepared as per the curriculum devised by Medical Council of India, New Delhi. Therefore, this book will be immensely useful for medical teachers as a ready reference.

I hope that students, teachers, microbiologists will find this book as a worthy successor to previous books in Microbiology. I request the readers to give their constructive criticism and valuable suggestions to improve this book further.

Kasarla Rajeshwar Reddy
Thurkapally; *via*: Hakimpet
Secunderabad A.P.

CONTENTS

PART-IV : MEDICAL VIROLOGY 587—768

PART-I

GENERAL MICROBIOLOGY

1

History of Microbiology

- *Antony Van Leeuwenhoek*
- *The theory of spontaneous generation (abiogenesis)*
- *La Zaro Spallanzani and Biogenesis*
- *Edward Jenner*
- *Louis Pasteur*
- *Robert Koch/ Koch's Postulates*
- *Joseph Lister*
- *Iwanowsky*
- *Metchnikoff*
- *Alexander Flemming*
- *Paul Ehrlich*
- *Mac Farlane Burnet*

ANTONY VAN LEEUWENHOEK (1632-1723)

He was the first Person, who invented the microscope and discovered the microbial world. He was a draper (Merchant) from Delft, Holland. He used to grind lenses and made microscopes as a hobby. The microscopes of Leeuwenhoek could magnify objects about 200-300 times.

With his microscopes, Leeuwenhoek observed a variety of things like rain water, pond water and scrapings from his own teeth. He saw minute moving objects and called them as **"Little animalcules"**, which we now know them as protozoa, yeasts and bacteria. He made accurate sketches and communicated his findings to "Royal Society of London".

Thus, Leeuwenhoek was the first person to discover microscope and the presence of bacteria and spirochetes in mouth.

THE THEORY OF SPONTANEOUS GENERATION (ABIOGENESIS)

After the discovery of microorganisms by Leeuwenhoek, scientists began investigations about the origin of microbes. Since organic matter decomposes quickly outside the living body, it was assumed that microorganisms were arising by spontaneous generation. John Needham (1749), an Irish priest, observed the appearance of microorganisms in putrefying meat and interpreted this as spontaneous generation.

LA ZARO SPALLANZANI (1729-1799) - THEORY OF BIOGENESIS

Spallanzani, an Italian priest, boiled beef broth for an hour, sealed the flasks and observed no appearance of microorganisms and disproved the theory of spontaneous generation or abiotic origin of life and proposed the theory of biogenesis. He said that every form of life takes its origin from their parents, germ cells or seeds. This theory of biogenesis was later proved and supported by Louis Pasteur.

EDWARD JENNER (1749-1823)

Jenner was an English country physician, who discovered a safe and efficient vaccination against small pox. which ultimately led to the eradication of small pox (**Variola**).

Jenner observed that dairy workers, exposed to occupational cowpox infection were immune to small pox. He proved experimentally that resistance to small pox can be induced by injecting cow pox material (**Vaccinia**) from disease pustules in to man (in 1796).

Pasteur gave the general term "**Vaccine**" (Vacca = cow) in honour of Jenner's cow pox vaccine, to various materials used to induce active immunity. Jenner published his findings in 1798 in a pamphlet "*An inquiry into the cause and effect of variole vaccine*".

LOUIS PASTEUR (1822-1895)

He was a Professor of Chemistry at the University of Lille, France. He is considered as "**Father of Microbiology**", as his contribution led to the development of Microbiology as a separate scientific discipline.

He proved the theory of "Biogenesis" and disproved the "Theory of spontaneous generation" (Abiogenesis), experimentally by using swan-necked flasks.

He worked on souring of wine and beer and found that this alcohol spoilage is due to the growth of undesirable organisms, while the desirable microorganisms produce alcohol by a chemical process called "**Fermentation**". He showed that wine did not spoil, if it is heated to 50-60°C for a few minutes. This method is called **"Pasteurization"**, now widely used in dairy units, to kill pathogenic microorganisms in milk.

He is a founder of **"Germ theory of disease"** as he visualized that diseases are caused by microorganisms. In course of his research, he discovered the importance of sterilization and discovered steam steri-lizer, autoclave and hot air oven. He also established the importance of cotton wool plugs for protection of culture media from aerial contamination. He differentiated between aerobic and anaerobic bacteria and coined the term "**anaerobic**" to refer to the organisms that do not require oxygen for growth.

He worked on "Pebrine", a silk-worm disease caused by a protozoan and showed that infection can be controlled by choosing worms free from the parasite for breeding.

He developed the process of **"attenuation"** during his work on "chicken cholera" in fowls. He found that cultures which had been stored in the laboratory for sometime would not kill the animals as fresh cultures did. This attenuation is now used in protective vaccination against diseases.

Pasteur showed that the anthrax disease in cattle and sheep is caused by a bacterium. He cultivated anthrax organisms in sterile yeast water, and showed that these cultures can produce disease when inoculated in to healthy animals. He developed a live attenuated **anthrax vaccine**, by incubation at 40-42°C, which proved to be useful in protecting animals against anthrax. He also worked on swine erysipelas.

Pasteur developed a **vaccine against rabies** (Hydrophobia), which made a greatest impact in medicine. He obtained the causative agent of rabies by serial intracerebral passage in rabbits and the vaccine was prepared by drying pieces of spinal chord. In 1888, Pasteur institute was established for mass antirabic treatment.

Pasteur gave the general term **"Vaccine"** (Vacca=cow) in honour of Jenner's cow pox vaccine, to various materials used to induce active immunity.

ROBERT KOCH (1843-1912)/KOCH'S POSTULATES

He was a German country Doctor who later became the Professor of hygiene and Director of institute of infective diseases at Berlin. He perfected many bacteriological techniques and known as **"Father of Practical Bacteriology"**.

He discovered rod shaped organisms in the blood of animals, that died of anthrax. He experimentally obtained the anthrax organisms in pure culture on a depression slide by inoculation of infected blood into the aqueous humour of a bullock's eye. He observed multiplication of bacteria and spore formation. He injected these spores into mice and reproduced the disease.

He found that in certain conditions, the anthrax bacillus forms spores, that can survive on earth for years. He passed anthrax bacilli, from the blood of an infected animal, from one mouse to another through twenty generations, and found that they bred true. He worked out its life-history.

He introduced staining techniques. He prepared dried bacterial films (Smears) on glass slides and stained them with aniline dyes for producing a better contrast under microscope. He discovered tubercle bacillus (*Mycobacterium tuberculosis*) which is popularly called as **Koch's bacillus**. He injected tubercle bacilli into laboratory animals and reproduced the disease, satisfying all Koch's postulates.

He discovered *Vibrio cholerae*, the causative agent of cholera disease.

He developed pure culture techniques by introducing solid media. The use of agar-agar obtained from dried sea weeds (*Gelidium Sp.*) in the preparation of solid bacteriological media was first suggested by Frau Hesse, the wife of Koch' student. This agar-agar is totally inert with no nutritive value, solidifies at 45°C and melts at 90°C, and was found to be most suitable solidifying agent in the preparation of culture media. Koch isolated bacteria in pure cultures on these solid media. It revolutionized bacteriology.

He discovered "Old **Tuberculin**". Koch noted that when tubercle bacilli or its protein extract was injected into a Guinea-pig already infected with the bacillus, an exaggerated reaction took place and the reaction remain localized. This is popularly called **"Koch Phenomenon"** and it is a demostration of cell mediated immunity. The tuberculin test is based on Koch's phenomenon. He erroneously thought that protein extracted from tubercle bacilli, called "Old tuberculin", could be used in the treatment of tuberculosis. Koch did a series of experiments to fulfill the criteria laid by his teacher Henle to establish the causative role between a particular microorganism and a particular disease. They are popularly known as **Koch's postulates** (Henle-Koch's Posulates). They are :

1. A specific organism should be found constantly in association with the disease.
2. The organism should be isolated and grown in a pure culture in the laboratory.
3. The pure culture when inoculated into a healthy susceptible animal should produce symptoms/ lesions of the same disease.
4. From the inoculated animal, the microorganism should be isolated in pure culture.
5. An additional criterion introduced is that specific anitbodies to the causative organism should be demonstrable in patient's serum.

JOSEPH LISTER (1827-1912)

He is popularly known as **"Father of antiseptic surgery"**. He was a professor of surgey at University of Glasgow and Edinburg and later at King's College, London.

He was deeply interested in the prevention of post-operative sepsis. He was attracted by Pasteur's germ theory of disease and concluded that sepsis or wound infection may be due to microbial growth, derived from the atmosphere.

He successfully prevented post-operative sepsis by introducing antiseptic techniques. He chose carbolic acid (Phenol) and used as spray on the wound or during surgery. He applied dressings soaked in carbolic acid on wounds. As a result, there was a marked reduction of post-operative sepsis, wound inflammation and suppuraton. It saved millions of lives from the jaws of death due to wound infections.

Lister's antiseptic surgery later led to the development of aspetic surgery. He suffered many criticism but never lose courage and followed his own ideas and revolutionzed the science of surgery by introducing antiseptic system in 1867.

IWANOWSKY (1892)

Dmitri Iwanowsky, a Russian botanist, occupies a pivotal position in the history of virology.

In 1866, Adeolf E. Meyer, a Dutch agricultural chemist described a disease of tobacco called "Mosaic" and showed that the disease could be transmitted to healthy plants through the sap of the diseased plant.

Iwanowsky (1892) demonstrated that this disease was caused by an agent which could pass through the filter, which withholds bacteria. He obtained the sap from infected leaves and passed it through a bacterial filter, called chamberland candle filter, which retained all bacteria and the filtered sap still retained infectivity when applied to healthy leaves.

Beijerinck (1898), a Dutch Microbiologist, showed that this infectious agent could diffuse through an agar gel and that it was a non-corpuscular "*Contagion vivum fluidum*" which he called **"Virus"**.

Stanley (1935), a British Mycologist was able to obtain the infectious agent of tobacco mosaic in a crystalline form.

METCHNIKOFF (1845-1916)

Elie Metchnikoff, the Russian-French biologist, discovered the phenomenon of phagocytosis, the cellular concept of immunity.

In Italy, where he had gone on a research visit, he studied the transparent larvae of starfish and noticed some of their cells could engulf and digest foreign protein particles. These cell eaters are called **"Phagocytes"**.

He continued his work on phagocytic action, at Pasteur Institure, Paris and found that in human blood a large proportion of the leucocytes (White blood cells) are phagocytic and attack invading bacteria. This, in turn, results in increased numbers of leucocytes in the infected areas followed by the inflamed area becoming hot, red, swelled and painful due to dead phagocytes forming pus.

He spent his last two decades on the study of human aging, since he believed that phagocytes eventually begin to digest the host cells aided by the effects of intestinal bacteria and that effectively combating them would increase the life span of human being.

ALEXANDER FLEMMING (1881-1955)

He was an English scientist worked at St. Mary's hospital in London.

Flemming was associated with two major discoveries-**lysozyme** and **penicillin**. In 1922, he doscovered lysozyme by demonstrating that the nasal secretion has the power of dissolving or lysing certain kinds of bacteria. Subsequently, he showed that lysozyme was present in many tissues of the body.

In 1929, Flemming made an accidental discovery that the fungus *Penicillium notatum* produces an antibacterial substance which he called penicillin. Flemming was culturing Staphylococci in petridishes and some of his cultures were contaminated with a mold, subsquently indetified as *Penicillium notatum.* Around the mold colony, there were clear zones, where Staphylococci disappeared. Flemming attributed this to the production of an antibacterial susbstance by the mold. Flemming cultured the fungus *Penicilium notatum* in broth cultures, filtered the fungal mat and obtained the penicillin in soluble form in the culture filtrate.

In 1940, Howard Florey and Ernst Chain demonstrated its antibacterial action *in vivo.* Working in U.S.A., they were able to produce large quantities of penicillin in pure form. In 1945, Flemming, Florey and Chain shared the nobel prize in physiology and medicine for the discovery of penicillin.

PAUL EHRLICH (1854-1915)

He was a German Bacteriologist, who pioneered the technique of chemotheraphy in medicine.

From his discovery that certain tissues have a specific affinity, he reasoned that organisms causing diseases could be selectively killed with chemical drugs. This led him to produce "arsphenamine" (an arsenic compound), the first synthetic drug, which destroyed the syphilis microbe in the body.

Ehrlich observed that organic arsenicals killed trypanosomes in an infected animal, but, if smaller doses were administered, the trypanosomes acquired tolerance to the drug. Therefore, he aimed at "*therapia magna sterilans*" *i.e.,* the introduction into the blood of a single dose of chemotherapeutic agent sufficient to kill the parasite. He also observed that drug would undergo certain changes in the body after it would produce the desired action.

SIR FRANK MAC FARLANE BURNET (1967)

Burnet is an Australian scientist, won nobel prize for the discoery of acquired immunological tolerance. He proposed clonal selection theory to explain antibody synthesis.

His work on bacteriophages and method for culturing some viruses in live chick embryo, led him to the view that an animal's ability is not inborn, but is developed during fetal life.

Burnet (1967) developed concept of **"immunological surveillance",** according to which the primary function of the immune system is to preserve the integrity of the body, seeking and destroying all "foreign" antigens, whether autogenous or external in origin.

Burnet's work also included the mode of action and the epidemiology of influenza virus, polio, Q fever and the cholera vibrio.

QUESTIONS

Short Notes:

1. Louis Pasteur.
2. Robert Koch.
3. Koch's Postulates.
4. Burnet.
5. Iwanowsky.
6. Joseph Lister.
7. Leeuwenhoek.
8. Jenner.
9. Flemming.
10. Metchnikoff.
11. Paul Ehrlich.

2

Microscopy

- *Introduction*
- *Compound microscope*
- *Magnification*
- *Numerical aperture*
- *Resolution/Resolving power*
- *Definition and Aberrations*
- *Objectives*
- *Oil-immersion objective*
- *Eye-pieces (oculars)*
- *Condensers*
- *Care and use of microscope*
- *Phase-contrast microscope*
- *Dark-field microscope*
- *Interference microscope (Stereo microscope)-NDIC microscope*
- *Fluorescent (UV) microscope*
- *Electron microscope*
- *Immune electron microscopy*
- *Micrometry*

INTRODUCTION

Microscope is an optical instrument used to magnify (enlarge) minute objects or microorganisms which cannot be seen by naked eye.

The morphological study of bacteria requires the use of microscopes. It provides the magnification wich enables one to see the organism and structures invisible to the naked eye. A microscope, therefore, is the most important tool for a microbiologist. Microscopes are of several types:

COMPOUND MICROSCOPE/LIGHT MICROSCOPE/BRIGHT-FIELD MICROSCOPE

The microscope essentially consists of following parts:

1. The supporting system in the form of a base, body and stage.
2. The illuminating system consists of a plano-concave mirror and condenser with the iris diaphragm.
3. The magnifying system consists of optical lenses. The objectives on the rotating nose piece, the mechanical tube and the ocular or eye-piece.
4. The adjustment system consists of coarse and fine adjustment knobs and the rack and pinion system on the stage to move slide either laterally or forward or backward.

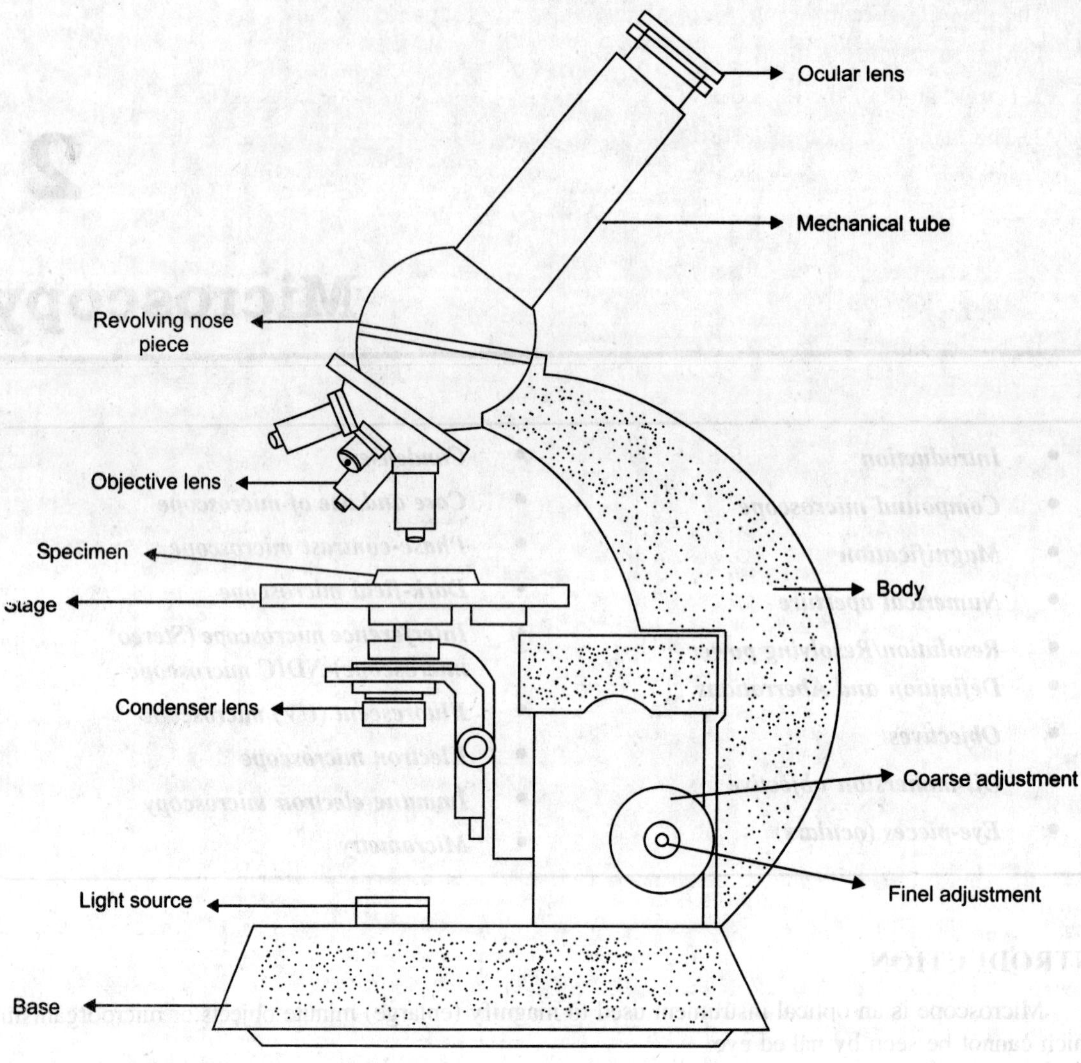

Fig. 2.1 The compound microscope

MAGNIFICATION

Magnification is defined as the degree of enlargement of object achieved by a microscope. Magnification through a microscope is achieved by a series of two lens systems. The lens system nearest the object called **"objective"** magnifies the specimen and produces a **"real image"** inside the mechanical **tube**. The eye-piece lens system magnifies the real image further yielding **"virtual image"** which is seen by the eye.

Hence, there is magnification at two levels. The final magnification achieved by a microscope is a product of the magnifying power of the eye-piece and the magnifying power of the objectives.

$$\text{The total magnification of microscope} = \text{Objective magnification} \times \text{Eye-piece magnification}$$

The magnification of a microscope depends on the following factors:

1. Mechanical tube length
2. Focal length of the objective
3. The magnifying power of eye-piece.

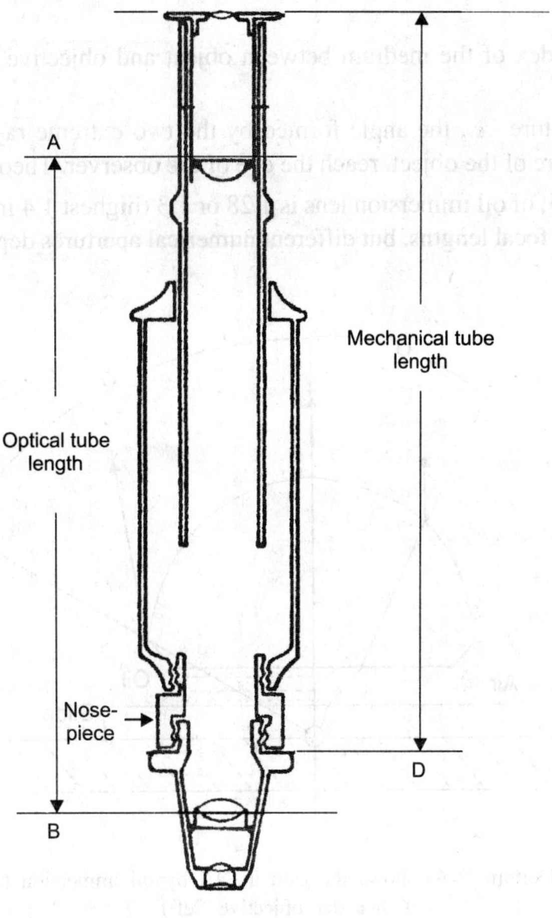

Fig. 2.2 Mechanical tube length and optical tube length

The **mechanical tube length** is the distance between the point where the objective fits in to the lower end of the body or the nose-piece and eye lens of the eye-piece; a measurement easily made with a ruler. Most modern microscopes have a mechanical tube length of 160 mm; but a few manufacturers employ 170 mm.

$$\text{The magnification of an objective} = \frac{\text{Mechanical tube length}}{\text{Focal length of objective}}$$

The magnification of eye piece is clearly engraved on the mount.

Since the total magnification of the compound microscope is the product of the magnification of the two lens systems, one might expect that the total magnification would be indefinitely increased by the use of additional lenses. However, this is not so, owing to the property of the lenses called **"Resolving power"**.

NUMERICAL APERTURE (NA)

The numerical aperture may be defined as the ratio of the diameter of the lens to its focal length. In other words, NA is the product of the refractive index of the medium between the object and objective lens, and sine of half of the angle formed by the light rays entering the lens from a point on the object.

NA is expressed mathematically as follows:

NA = n sin U

Where n = Refractive index of the medium between object and objective (1.0 for air, 1.5 for cedar wood oil)

U = angle of aperture *i.e.*, the angle formed by the two extreme rays of light, which starting from the centre of the object, reach the eye of the observer. Theoretical limit of 2U = 180°.

NA of dry lens is 0.65; of oil immersion lens is 1.28 or 1.3 (highest 1.4 in apochromatic objective). Objectives may have equal focal lengths, but different numerical apertures depending on the diameter of the front lens.

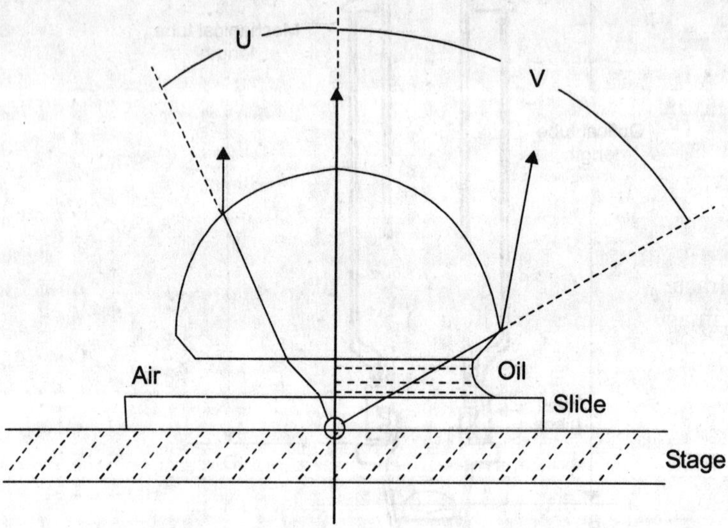

Fig. 2.3 Numerical aperture (NA) shows the gain in NA by oil immersion (right) as compared with a dry objective (left)

RESOLUTION/RESOLVING POWER

The resolving power of a microscope is its ability to reveal closely adjacent structural details as separate and distinct. Expressed, quantitatively, resolution is its capacity to distinguish two neighboring points as separate entities. For example, the human eye has a resolving power of 0.25 mm, which means that two dots placed 0.25 mm apart can be distinguished as two separate dots. If the distance between the two dots is less than 0.25 mm, only one dot will be seen. Thus, the **"limit of resolution"** may be defined as the shortest distance between two objects, where they can be distinguished as two separate entities.

$$\text{Resolution (R)} = \frac{0.61 \times \lambda}{\text{NA}}$$

Where, λ = Wavelength of light used for illumination
NA = Numerical aperture

Therefore, resolving power of a microscope depends upon two factors :

1. Wavelength of light used for illumination
2. Numerical aperture.

The shortest wavelength of light will give the maximum resolution. Similarly, the higher the numerical aperture, the finer will be the detail (high resolution) revealed by the objective.

Resolving power of normal eye = 0.25 mm

Resolving power of compound microscope = 0.25 µm

Resolving power of electron microscope = 5 Å.

DEFINITION AND ABERRATIONS

"Definition" is the capacity of an objective to render the outline of the image of the object clear and distinct.

Lens systems are made up of lenses having spherical surfaces, and such surfaces do not form perfect images. This is because of inequalities of refraction and focus by peripheral portions of the objective lenses. This phenomenon is known as **"Aberrations"**. They are of two types :

Spherical aberration : It is due to light rays passing through the edge of lens will never be brought to same focus as those passing nearer the center, resulting in serious distortion of the image.

Chromatic aberration. White light while passing through a lens is diffracted as it would be in a prism, to its various component colors, each with its own wavelength. The light rays of different wavelengths are refracted by the lens to varying extents and may not be recombined in the same focus, resulting in a hazy image fringed with colors of the spectrum.

OBJECTIVES

The objective is the most important lens in a microscope. The main functions of objective lens are :

1. to gather light rays coming from any point of the object
2. to unite the light rays in a point of the image
3. to magnify the image.

An objective capable of utilizing a large angular cone of light coming from the specimen will have better resolving power than an objective limited to a smaller cone of light.

In microbiology, three objectives are generally adequate, 1. low power (10X), 2. high dry power (45X), 3. oil immersion objective (100X). If we employ 10X ocular, we get magnifications of 100, 450, 1000 times respectively.

OIL IMMERSION OBJECTIVES

Oil immersion objectives are most frequently used in microbiology, because of their greater magnification and resolution. It is so named because the medium between slide (object) and objective is occupied by oil.

When a dry objective is used, the space between objective and object is occupied by air (refractive index 1.0). When light rays pass from a dense medium (glass of slide and cover slip; Refractive index 1.5) to a less dense medium (air; Refractive index 1.0) are refracted obliquely outwards so that many light rays cannot enter the objective lens. Since the brightness of the image depends upon the amount of light entering the objective, and the resolution depends on the effective numerical aperture, this refraction of light outwards diminishes brightness and clarity of the image.

If the space between slide (object) and objective is filled with some transparent oil, with same refractive index as glass, then the light rays do not undergo refraction and pass directly into the objective. Usually cedar wood oil (R.I. = 1.515) is used. Castor oil can also be used. As a result, the NA of the lens is increased. The lens can be brought much closer to the object, admitting most of divergent rays into the objective lens, and thus resolution is increased.

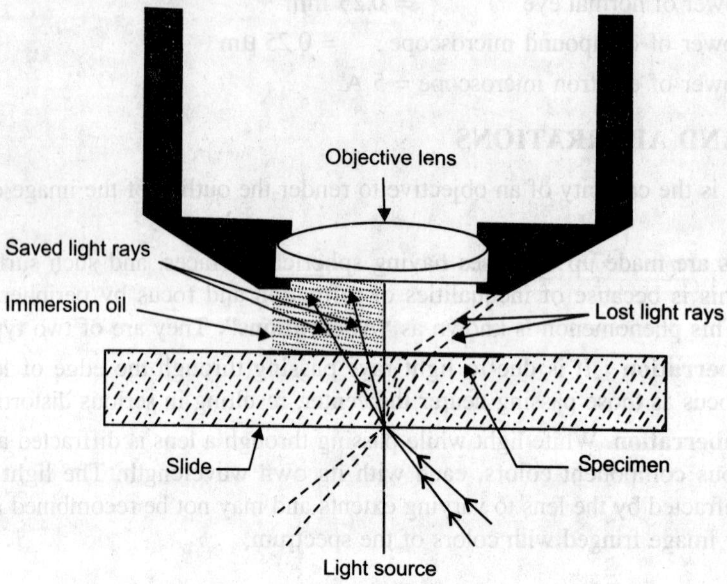

Fig. 2.4 How the oil immersion objective increases the amount of light passing from the specimen into the objective lens

EYE-PIECES (OCULARS)

Eye-piece is a short tube consisting of two lenses and fits into the upper part of the mechanical tube. Eye-pieces are available with 5X, 10X, 15X magnifications, engraved on the mount. The functions of the eye-pieces are :

1. the magnification of the real image
2. the formation of a virtual image of the real image produced by the objective
3. carries markers, measurement scales, cross-hairs etc.

CONDENSERS

A condenser may be defined as a series of lenses for illuminating the object; located under the stage of the microscope, hence, referred to as substage condenser.

CARE AND USE OF A MICROSCOPE

Clean the microscope with a clean soft cloth. The objectives and eye-pieces must be cleaned with a lens paper and xylol or benzol. Alcohol and acetone should not be used as it dissolves cement that binds the lenses. Set up the microscope in a convenient position, facing the source of light. Place the object (slide with smear) on the stage and adjust the mirror to the illuminant. Always tilt the mirror towards blue sky, if artificial light is not available. Direct sunlight should not fall on the mirror. For prolonged work, it is advisable to use artificial light of a particular wavelength.

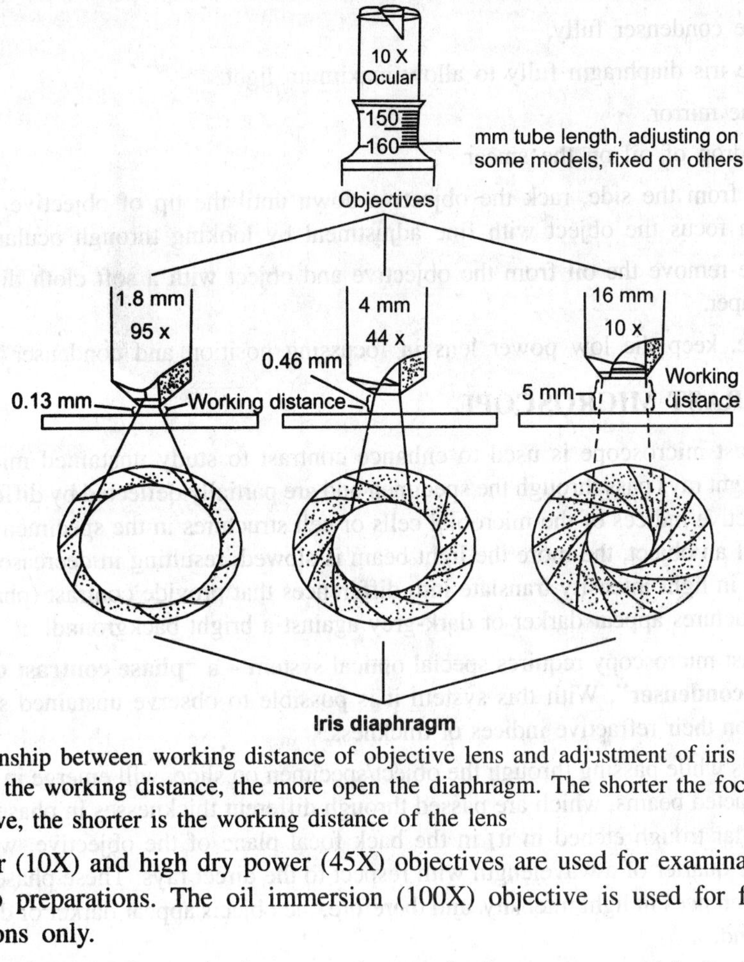

Fig. 2.5 Relationship between working distance of objective lens and adjustment of iris diaphragm. The shorter the working distance, the more open the diaphragm. The shorter the focal length of the objective, the shorter is the working distance of the lens

Low power (10X) and high dry power (45X) objectives are used for examination of wet films or hanging drop preparations. The oil immersion (100X) objective is used for fixed and stained smears or sections only.

For the examination of unstained preparations under low power or high dry power objectives, following adjustments have to be made :

1. Lower the condenser.
2. Close the iris diaphragm partially to reduce the light intensity.
3. Use concave mirror.
4. Lower the objective to near about the working distance by looking from the side. Never attempt to bring the object into focus by lowering the body tube while looking through the eye-piece.

5. Focus under low power and then turn on to high dry power objective. Focussing is achieved by movement of coarse or fine adjustment slightly.

For the examination of stained smears under oil-immersion objective, following adjustments have to be made (Fig. 2.5) :

1. Raise the condenser fully.
2. Open the iris diaphragm fully to allow maximum light.
3. Use plane mirror.
4. Place a drop of oil on the smear.
5. Looking from the side, rack the objective down until the tip of objective lens touches the oil. Then focus the object with fine adjustment by looking through ocular.
6. After use remove the oil from the objective and object with a soft cloth dipped in xylol or tissue paper.
7. After use, keep the low power lens in focussing position and condenser lowered down.

PHASE-CONTRAST MICROSCOPE

Phase contrast microscope is used to enhance contrast to study unstained microorganisms in living state. The light rays pass through the specimen and are partially deflected by different densities or thickness or refractive indices of the microbial cells or cell structures in the specimen. The greater the refractive index of an object, the more the light beam is slowed, resulting in decreased light intensity. These differences in light intensity translate into differences that provide contrast (phase contrast). As a result, some structures appear darker or dark-grey against a bright background.

Phase contrast microscopy requires special optical system – a **"phase contrast objective"** and a **"phase contrast condenser"**. With this system it is possible to observe unstained structures within cells, based only on their refractive indices or thickness.

The light rays while passing through the object/specimen on slide, will emerge in different phases as direct and diffracted beams, which are passed through different thicknesses in phase plate (a disk of glass with a circular trough etched in it) in the back focal plane of the objective, which retards the diffracted rays one quarter of a wavelength with respect to the direct rays. These phase differences are converted into differences in light intensity, and therefore, the objects appear darker or dark-grey against a bright background.

The special phase condenser consists of annular diaphragms on a rotating disk fitted to the bottom of the condenser. A different size of annulus is required for use with each objective of different NA.

Phase contrast microscope is more valuable in general biology. It is useful

1. to study unstained living cells
2. to differentiate internal structures in living cells
3. to study flagellar movements and motility of bacteria and protozoans
4. to study intestinal and other live protozoa such as amoebae and *Trichomonas*
5. to examine fungi grown in culture.

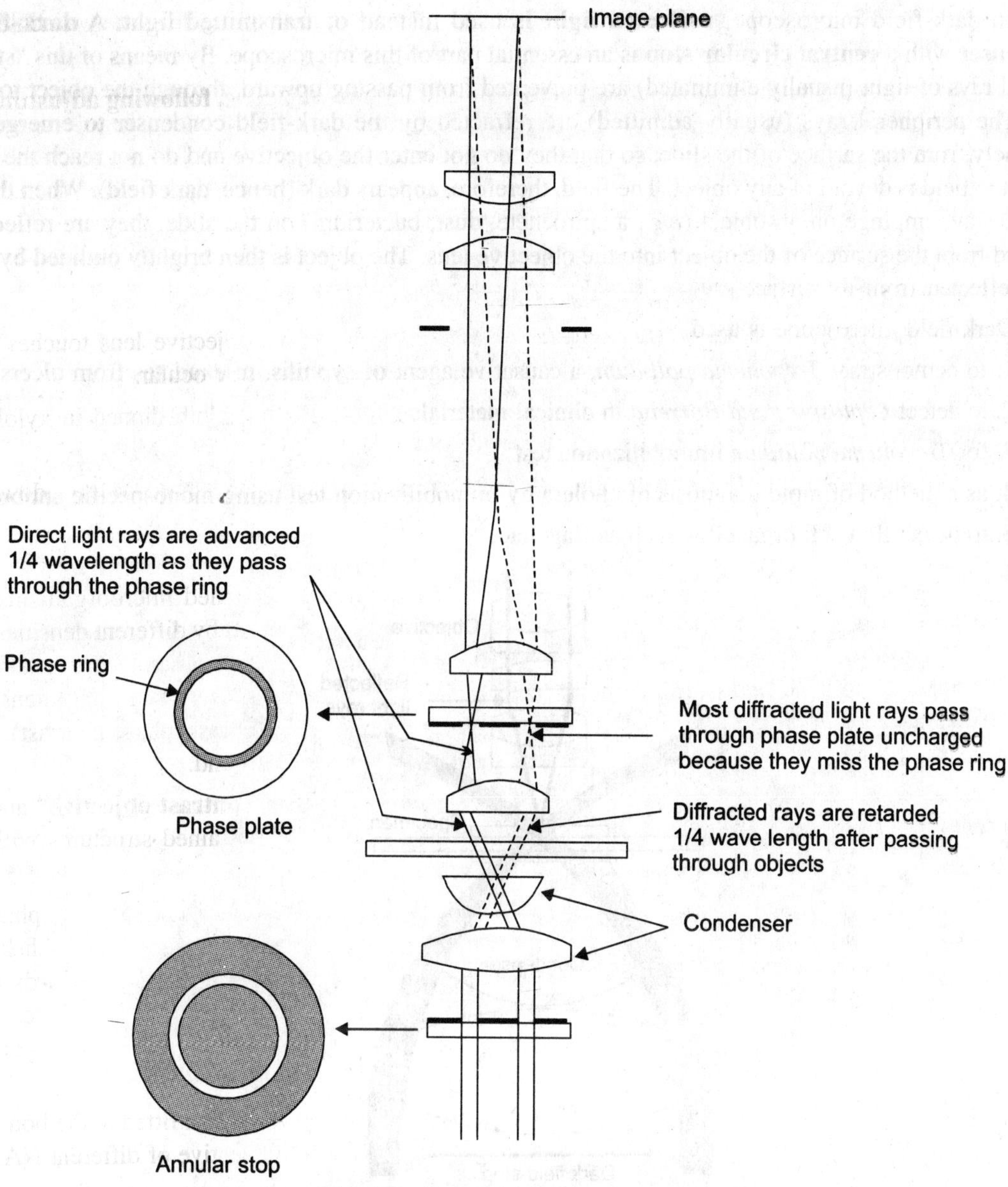

Fig. 2.6 Phase-contrast microscope

DARK-FIELD (GROUND) MICROSCOPE

In dark-field microscope, objects are seen brightly illuminated against a dark background. It gives an increased resolution and is used to observe microorganisms that cannot be resolved by ordinary microscope. It is used to observe very slender microorganisms such as spirochetes.

Dark field microscope is based on the principle that when a beam of light enters a dark room, it renders minute dust particles floating in the air, which cannot be seen ordinarily in a room with light.

In dark-field microscope, **reflected light** is used instead of transmitted light. A **dark-field condenser** with a **central circular stop** is an essential part of this microscope. By means of this "stop" central rays of light (usually eliminated) are prevented from passing upward, through the object to the eye. The peripheral rays (usually admitted) are refracted by the dark-field condenser to emerge so obliquely from the surface of the slide, so that they do not enter the objective and do not reach the eye when the field is devoid of any object. The field, therefore, appears dark (hence, dark field). When these oblique rays impinge on an object (*e.g.*, a spirochete, dust, bacterium) on the slide, they are reflected upward from the surface of the object into the objective lens. The object is then brightly outlined by the rays reflected from its surface.

Dark field microscope is used

1. to demonstrate *Treponema pallidum*, a causative agent of syphilis, in exudates from ulcers
2. to detect *Leptospira and Borrelia* in clinical materials
3. for *Treponema pallidum* immobilization test
4. as a method of rapid diagnosis of cholera by immobilization test using monospecific antibody
5. to detect thin cell organelles such as flagellae.

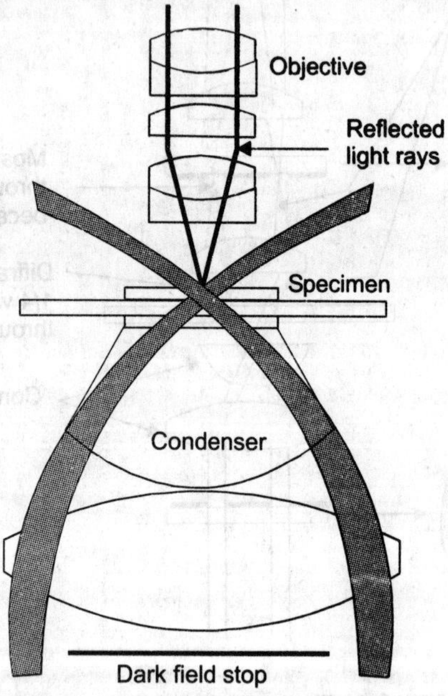

Fig. 2.7 Dark-field microscope

FLUORESCENT MICROSCOPE (ULTRAVIOLET MICROSCOPE)

When certain dyes and minerals are exposed to invisible light such as ultra-violet or blue-violet light, they absorb radiant energy, and become excited and release their trapped energy as light, and so become luminous (fluorescent). This phenomenon is known as **Fluorescence,** and it provides a good contrast, which is exploited in fluorescence microscope.

In fluorescence microscope, the specimen is exposed to ultraviolet, violet or blue light and forms an image of the object with the resulting fluorescent light. A mercury vapour arc lamp produces an intense beam of UV light. A special infrared filter or heat filter filters out infrared rays produced by

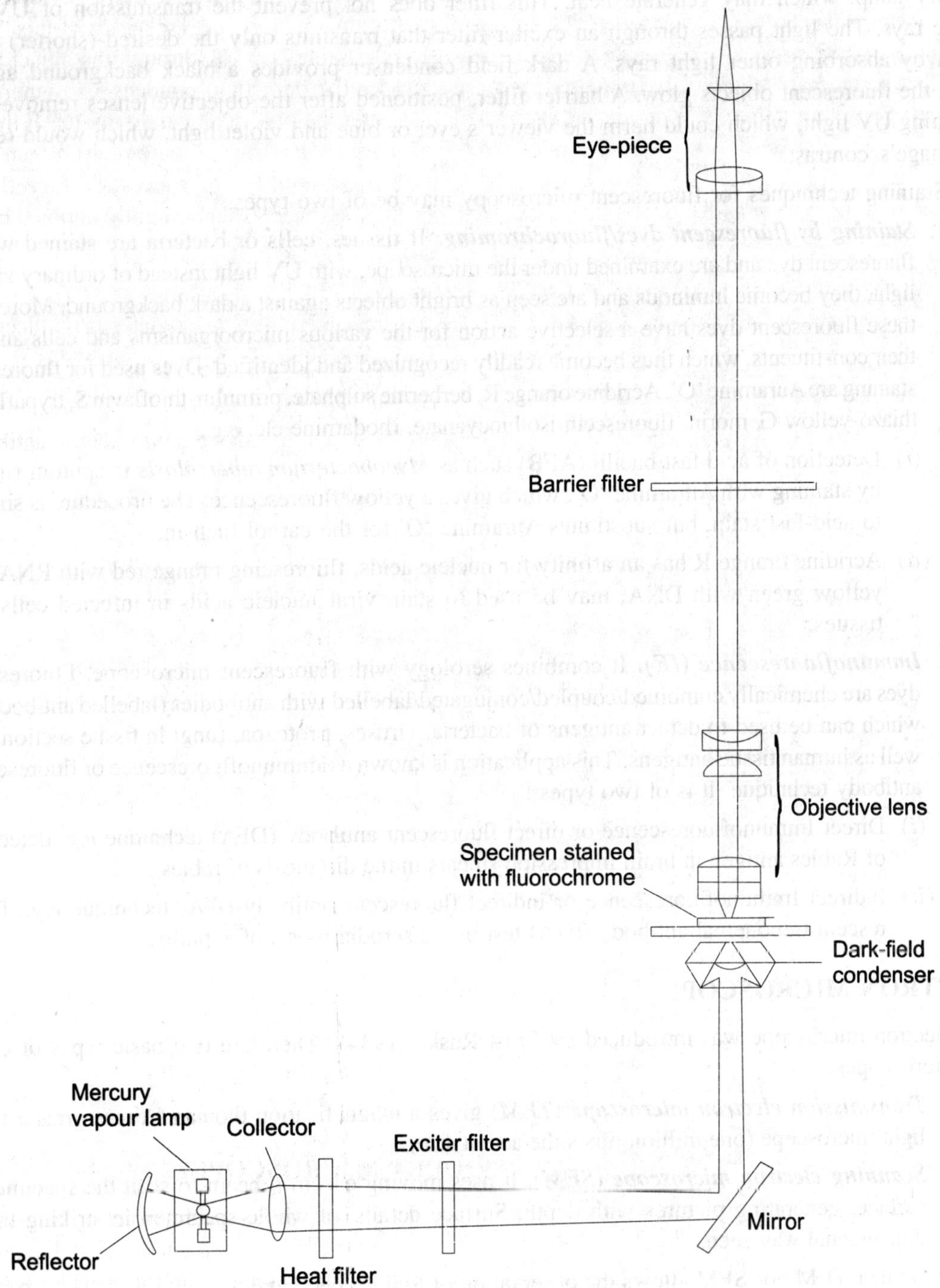

Fig. 2.8 Fluorescence microscopy

mercury lamp, which may generate heat. This filter does not prevent the transmission of UV and visible rays. The light passes through an exciter filter that transmits only the desired (shorter) wave length by absorbing other light rays. A dark field condenser provides a black background against which the fluorescent objects glow. A barrier filter, positioned after the objective lenses removes any remaining UV light, which could harm the viewer's eye; or blue and violet light, which would reduce the image's contrast.

Staining techniques for fluorescent microscopy may be of two types.

1. ***Staining by fluorescent dyes/fluorochroming.*** If tissues, cells or bacteria are stained with a fluorescent dye and are examined under the microscope, with UV light instead of ordinary visible light, they become luminous and are seen as bright objects against a dark background. Moreover, these fluorescent dyes have a selective action for the various microorganisms and cells and for their constituents, which thus become readily recognized and identified. Dyes used for fluorescent staining are Auramine 'O', Acridine orange R, berberine sulphate, primulin, thioflavin S, trypaflavin, thiazo-yellow G, morin, fluorescein isothiocyanate, rhodamine etc. *e.g.,*
   (*i*) Detection of acid fast bacilli (AFB) such as *Mycobacterium tuberculosis* in sputum smears by staining with Auramine 'O', which gives a yellow fluorescence. The procedure is similar to acid-fast stain, but substitutes Auramine 'O' for the carbol fuchsin.
   (*ii*) Acridine orange R has an affinity for nucleic acids, fluorescing orange red with RNA and yellow green with DNA, may be used to stain viral nucleic acids in infected cells and tissues.
2. ***Immunofluorescence (IF).*** It combines serology with fluorescent microscope. Fluorescent dyes are chemically combined/coupled/conjugated/labelled with antibodies (labelled antibodies), which can be used to detect antigens of bacteria, viruses, protozoa, fungi in tissue sections, as well as human tissue antigens. This application is known as immunofluorescence or fluorescent-antibody technique. It is of two types :
   (*i*) Direct Immunofluorescence or direct fluorescent antibody (DFA) technique *e.g*, detection of Rabies antigen in brain impression smears in the diagnosis of rabies
   (*ii*) Indirect Immunofluorescence or indirect fluorescent antibody (IFA) technique *e.g.*, fluorescent treponemal antibody (FTA) test in the serodiagnosis of syphilis.

ELECTRON MICROSCOPE

Electron microscope was introduced by Ernst Ruska (1934). There are two basic types of electron microscopes.

1. ***Transmission electron microscope (TEM)*** gives a magnification thousand times greater than light microscope (one million times the actual size).
2. ***Scanning electron microscope (SEM).*** It uses moving electron beam to scan the specimen's surface, generating pictures with depth. Surface details of whole specimen in striking three dimensional way seen.

   Neither TEM nor SEM allows the observation of living specimens.

TRANSMISSION ELECTRON MICROSCOPE (TEM)

In electron microscope, an electron beam is used instead of light to visualize objects. Because of the relatively long wavelength of visible light (about 500 nm), objects than a certain distance (0.2 μm) apart cannot be differentiated (or resolved) by ordinary microscope. Electrons have a much shorter wavelength than ordinary light (about 0.5 nm). Therefore, a microscope utilising electron beams, instead of visible light has a much greater resolving power and is capable of giving distinct images at magnifications of 1,00,000 (one lakh) or more.

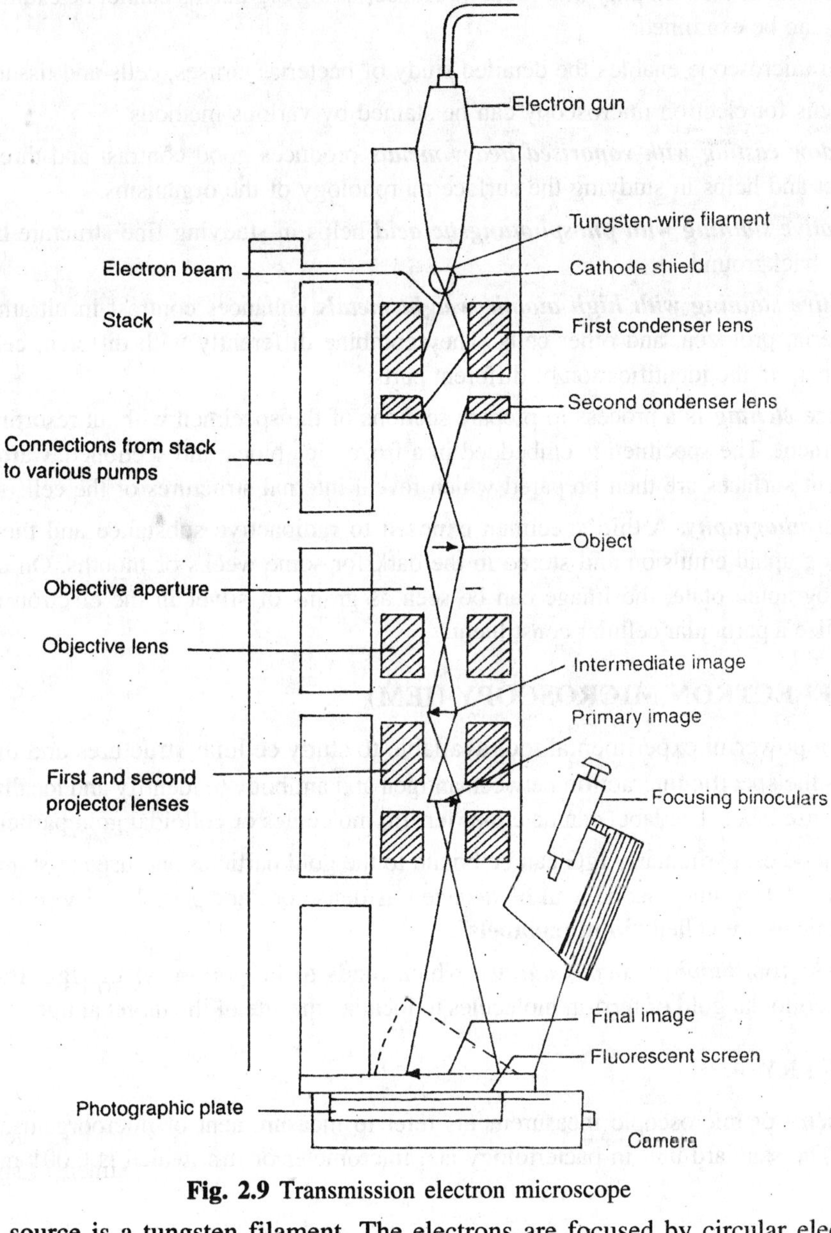

Fig. 2.9 Transmission electron microscope

Electron source is a tungsten filament. The electrons are focused by circular electromagnets, which take the place of glass lenses, since glass is opaque to electrons. Electrons are focused by varying the strength of the magnetic fields. Three major magnet-lens systems are used, each having a function analogous to its counterpart in an ordinary microscope. The specimen to be examined is placed in a special holder and then introduced into electron microscope between the condenser and objective lenses. Because electron images are not directly visible to the eye, they are viewed on a fluorescent screen or are recorded on photographic plates. Like X-ray pictures, they are electron-shadow graphs (electron micrographs).

Since gas molecules scatter electrons, the interior of electron microscope must be maintained at vacuum. Electrons travel well only in a vacuum. Hence, living organisms cannot be examined; dead and dried objects can be examined.

Electron microscope enables the detailed study of bacteria, viruses, cells and tissues.

Specimens for electron microscopy can be stained by various methods :

1. ***Shadow casting with vaporised heavy metals*** produces good contrast and three dimensional effect and helps in studying the surface morphology of the organisms.
2. ***Negative staining with phosphotungstic acid*** helps in studying fine structure by providing a dark background.
3. ***Positive staining with high atomic weight metals*** enhances contrast in ultrathin sections of bacteria, protozoa, and other cells. They combine differently with different cell components and help in the identification of different parts.
4. ***Freeze-etching*** is a process to prepare sections of the specimen without resorting to chemical treatment. The specimen is embedded in a frozen ice block and sectioned. Carbon replicas of the cut surfaces are then prepared which reveal internal structures of the cell.
5. ***Autoradiography.*** A thin specimen exposed to radioactive substance and then coated with photographic emulsion and stored in the dark for some weeks or months. On developing the photographic plate, the image can be seen as grains of silver in the electron microscope to localize a particular cellular constituent.

IMMUNE ELECTRON MICROSCOPY (IEM)

IEM is a powerful experimental tool available to study cellular structures and their functions. IEM exploits the specific interaction between antigen and antibody to identify and localize proteins via an electron dense label. The label can be either ferritin molecules or colloidal gold particles.

The antibodies, particularly IgG can be bound to the gold particles and used to stain the specimen processed for electron microscope, can be detected as dense or dark particles. These IgG bound gold or ferritin particles are called "**immunolabels**".

Protein-A from *Staphylococcus aureus*, which binds to Fc portion of the IgG fraction may be labelled with colloidal gold or ferritin molecules to localize the site of the target antigen.

MICROMETRY

Micrometry or microscopic measurements refer to measurement of microorganisms under light microscope. The standard unit in bacteriology is a micrometer or µm, which is 0.001 mm.

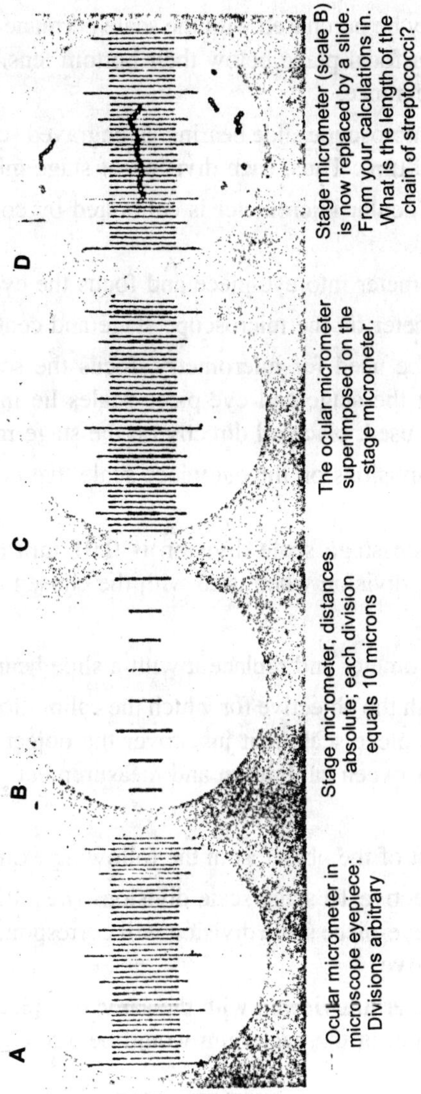

Fig. 2.10 Microscopic measurements.

Standardization of the ocular micrometer and its use in measuring bacterial cells. In measuring a microscopic object an **ocular micrometer** serves as a scale or ruler. This is simply a disc of glass upon which are etched equally spaced divisions. When placed in the ocular, these ruled lines superimpose certain distance markers on the microscope field. The actual distance superimposed may be calibrated by using a stage micrometer at the focal plane of the microscopic field on which parallel lines exactly 0.01 mm apart are etched.

To measure microscopic objects ocular micrometer and stage micrometer are used in conjunction.

Ocular micrometer. It is a small, circular, glass disc on which a graduated scale is engraved. This scale is arbitrary and do not indicate any measurement of length. It usually contains 100 equally spaced divisions, marked 0 to 10 equally. This occular micrometer is placed inside the eye piece.

Eye piece micrometers may be purchased with the scale permanently in position. These are usually kellner eye pieces which have a focal plane below their bottom lens. They give a sharp image on the scale and have a greater eye clearance.

Stage micrometer. It is a microscope slide bearing an engraved scale 1 mm in length and graduated at intervals of 0.01 mm (*i.e.*, 10 μm). Thus, each division of stage micrometer is equal to 10 μm.

Calibration. The scale of ocular micrometer is calibrated by comparison with stage micrometer, under different objectives :

1. Insert the ocular micrometer into eye-piece and focus the eye-piece scale.
2. Place the stage micrometer on the microscope stage and centre the scale in the field.
3. With the objective to be used for micrometry, focus the scale of the stage micrometer and move the stage so that the stage and eye-piece scales lie in parallel, side-by-side. When oil immersion objective is used, place oil directly on the stage-micrometer scale.
4. Count the number of divisions on the eye-piece scale that correspond to a definite number in the stage scale.

From knowledge, that each stage scale division is 0.01 mm (or 10 μm), calculate the length measured by an eye-piece scale division when used with the chosen objective.

Measurement

1. Remove the stage micrometer and replace it with a slide bearing the specimen to be studied.
2. Focus the specimen with the objective for which the calibration was done and count the number of divisions of the eye-piece scale that just cover the object to be measured. The tube length should not be altered between calibration and measurement.

Calculation

Calculate the measurement of the object as in the following example.

If with oil immersion objective 10 stage scale divisions (*i.e.*, 10 × 10 μm) are found equal to 91 eye-piece scale divisions, each eye-piece scale division will correspond to 100/90 μm *i.e.*, 1.1 μm, in the field of the oil immersion objective.

If then, the length of a bacterium viewed with the same eye-piece and objective is found to equal 3.5 eye-piece divisions, the length of the bacterium would be 3.5 × 1.1 μm = 3.85 μm.

QUESTIONS

Essay Type Questions

1. Give a list of microscopes used in microbiology and explain with a neat sketch the working principle of fluorescence microscope.
2. Briefly describe the working principles of operation and importance of electron microscope.
3. Describe the working principles of light microscope and phase-contrast microscope.
4. Bring out the differences between the working principles of a light microscope and an electron microscope.
5. Describe the principles involved in the phase-contrast microscope and electron microscope.

Short Notes

1. Compound microscope/bright-field microscope.
2. Magnification.
3. Numerical aperture/NA.
4. Resolution.
5. Limit of resolution.
6. Definition.
7. Aberrations.
8. Spherical aberration.
9. Chromatic aberration.
10. Oil immersion lens.
11. Care and use of a microscope.
12. Dark field microscope.
13. Transmission electron microscope (TEM).
14. Immune electron microscopy (IEM).
15. Micrometry.
16. Phase contrast microscope.

3

Staining Methods

- *Introduction*
- *Examination of living bacteria in unstained condition*
  - *Wet coverslip preparation*
  - *Hanging drop experiment*
- *Terms used in staining*
- *Smear preparation*
- *Bacteriological staining methods*
  - *Simple staining*
  - *Differential stains*
    - *Gram's staining*
    - *Acid-fast (Ziehl-Neelsen's) staining*
  - *Fluorochrome staining for tubercle bacilli*
  - *Silver impregnation methods*
  - *Negative staining (background staining)*
- *Stains to demonstrate volutin granules*
  - *Albert's stain*
  - *Neisser's stain*
  - *Ponder's stain*
  - *Pugh's stain*
- *Vital staining and supravital staining*

INTRODUCTION

The morphological features of an organism can be studied by examining them under microscope by using unstained and stained preparations.

EXAMINATION OF LIVING BACTERIA IN UNSTAINED CONDITION

The unstained preparations of living organisms can be studied by any one of the following methods :

1. Wet coverslip preparation
2. Hanging drop preparation
3. Phase contrast microscope
4. Dark ground microscope.

Wet coverslip preparation

A small drop of material to be examined is taken on a clear glass slide and covered with a coverslip, without allowing air bubbles to form. Examined under low and high dry power objectives.

Uses : 1. Examination of urinary sediment, cerebrospinal fluid (CSF), other body fluids etc., for pus cells, crystals, casts and bacteria.

2. Examination of vaginal secretions for presence of motile protozoan parasites like *Trichomonas vaginalis*.

3. Examination of feces in saline and iodine preparations for protozoans and helminthic eggs.

Hanging drop preparation

This experiment is done to demonstrate motility and to study morphology of bacteria.

Requirements : 1. A clean cavity (depression) slide
2. A clean coverslip
3. Young broth culture
4. Wire loop
5. Bunsen burner/spirit lamp
6. Microscope.

Procedure :

1. Apply a small amount of vaseline/grease on four corners of the coverslip.
2. Place drop of culture using the sterile wire loop on the centre of the coverslip.
3. Invert the cavity slide over the coverslip so that the drop of the culture is in the center of the cavity; press it lightly, so that the coverslip adheres to the vaseline ring.
4. Quickly and carefully turn the slide over, so that the coverslip is upper most, and a drop hanging from the coverslip into the cavity.
5. Focus the edge of the drop under dry low power objective, after reducing the light intensity (by partial closing of iris diaphragm), so that the edge of the drop is exactly in the center of the microscopic field. Then turnover to high dry power objective (45X) to observe the motility and morphology of bacteria. Their shape, approximate size and general structure can be observed (Fig. 3.1).

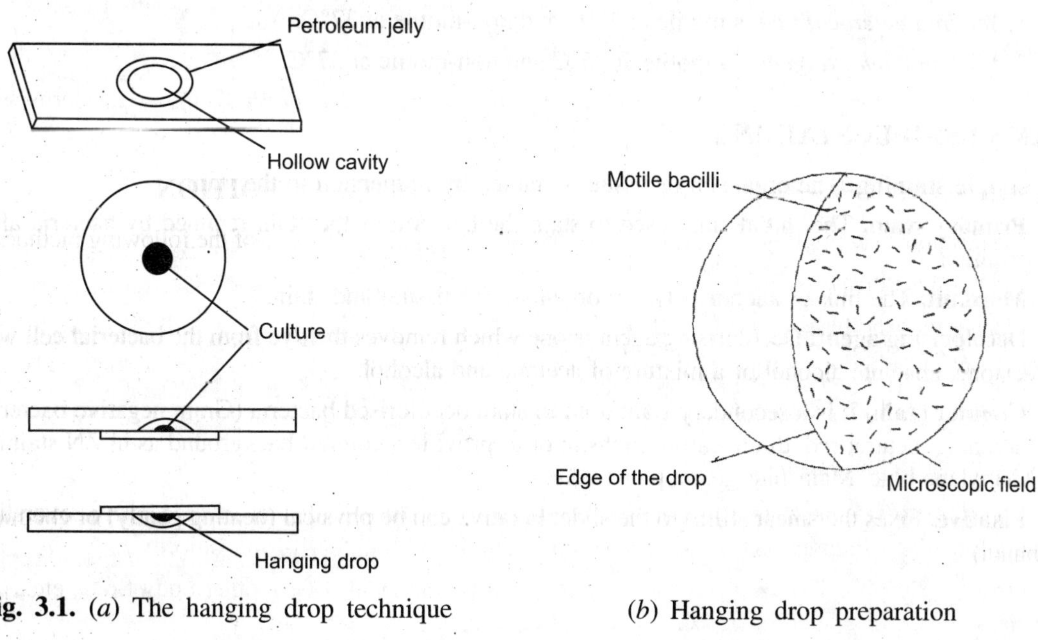

Fig. 3.1. (*a*) The hanging drop technique (*b*) Hanging drop preparation

The edge of the drop is focussed to observe motility and morphology for the following reasons :

1. The concentration of the organisms is more at the edge, because – (*a*) aerobic organisms tend to move towards the edge, (*b*) surface tension is less at the edge, hence the concentration of organisms is more.

2. Density is less at the edge of the drop, hence the contrast is better, so that organisms are clearly visible. The differences in refractive index of light rays that pass through glass slide and liquid gives a better contrast at the edge.

It is essential to differentiate between true motility and false motility. In **true motility**, there is a displacement of position *i.e.,* the organism moves from one place to another in different directions. The **false motility**, also known as **brownian movement** is an oscillatory vibration, exhibited by both living and non-living bodies, due to water convection currents.

Apart from hanging drop experiment, motility can also be demonstrated by :

(*i*) Macroscopic methods :

1. Noting swarming growth on agar medium
2. Use of semi-solid agar (0.2 % agar) medium
3. Craigie's tube or 'U' shaped tube

(*ii*) Microscopic methods :

1. Dark ground microscopy
2. Phase contrast microscopy

(*iii*) Demonstration of flagellae.

Motile bacilli: *E. coli, Vibrio cholerae, Pseudomonas, Proteus, Clostridium tetani, Salmonella, Helicobacter, Campylobacter, Enterobacter*

Nonmotile bacilli: *Klebsiella, Shigella*

Some organisms are motile at one temperature and nonmotile at another temperature *e.g.,*

1. *Yersinia enterocolitica* is motile at 22°C and non-motile at 37°C.
2. *Listeria monocytogenes* is motile at 25°C and non-motile at 37°C.

TERMS USED IN STAINING

simple staining. The organism or tissue is stained by immersion in the stain.

Primary stain. The initial stain used to stain the bacteria or the stain retained by bacteria after decolorisation.

Mordant. The link or anchor between organism (or tissue) and stain.

Decolorising agent. Decolorising agent is one which removes the dye from the bacterial cell wall *e.g.,* acetone, absolute alcohol or a mixture of acetone and alcohol.

Counter stain. It is a secondary stain used to stain decolorised bacteria (Gram negative bacteria) *e.g.,* Safranine, neutral red, dilute carbol fuchsin; or to provide a colored background as in ZN staining *e.g.,* Methylene blue, Malachite green, picric acid.

Fixative. Fixes the smear (film) to the slide. Fixative can be physical (heating gently) or chemical (methanol).

SMEAR PREPARATION (OR) METHODS OF MAKING FILM

Before staining, the material concerned must be suitably prepared. This involves making slides of films, smears or sections.

Slides. The slides and coverslips used should be clean and grease-free; they should be boiled in a detergent solution for 5 to 10 minutes, scrubbed, rinsed well and stored in alcohol until required.

Films/Smears. Films are made either by spreading a loopful of liquid (*e.g.,* broth culture, sputum, pus, urine etc.) thinly on a slide, or, if the sample is a bacterial culture on agar, by emulsifying a very small portion of the colony in a drop of water or physiological saline (normal saline) on the slide. It is important that films should be thin. They may be allowed to dry in air, or drying may be accelerated by holding the slides, high above a bunsen flame. The film should then be fixed by passing the slide, slowly through the flame 2 to 3 times.

BACTERIOLOGICAL STAINING METHODS

(Examination of dead bacteria in stained condition)

Staining is usually effected by the application of an aqueous (watery) solution or an alcoholic solution of the dye.

The staining procedures are broadly divided into :

1. Simple staining
2. Differential staining
3. Negative staining or background staining
4. Fluorescent staining
5. Impregnation methods
6. Special stains.

Simple staining

A single stain is used in simple staining. Simple stains include basic aniline dyes such as methylene blue, gention violet, carbol fuchsin (basic fuchsin), safranine.

The bacterial suspension is smeared on the surface of the slide, fixed by gentle heating and flooded with a dye solution (*e.g.,* methylene blue) for about one minute. The dye is washed off with water and the slide blotted dry.

Simple stains shows the presence of microorganisms and the cells in exudates. But, different bacteria take up the same color, as a single dye is used for staining (Fig. 3.2).

Uses :

1. For the examination of cerebrospinal fluid (CSF) in the diagnosis of pyogenic meningitis *e.g., Hemophilus influenzae* meningitis.

2. To demonstrate *Yersinia pestis* (plague bacillus) in pus or aspirated fluid.

Advantages :

1. Simple to perform
2. Margins of bacteria are seen clearly in contrast to other stains.

***Disadvantages* :**

1. Morphology of different bacteria cannot be made out as same color is taken up by the bacteria.

2. Cannot differentiate between Gram positive and Gram negative bacteria and hence antibiotic sensitivity cannot be made out.

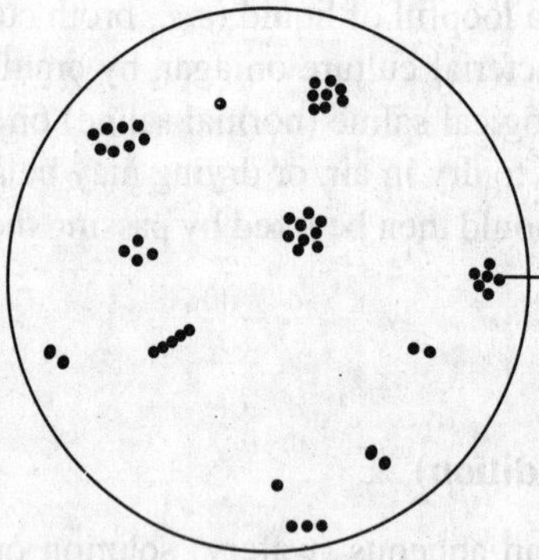

Fig. 3.2 Simple staining with methylene blue

Loeffler's methylene blue. Of the many preparations of methylene blue dye, Loeffler's methylene blue is most useful. It is made of methylene blue solution saturated in alcohol, dissolved in KOH (0.01 % in distilled water). It shows the characteristic morphology of pus cells, lymphocytes and other cells more clearly than Gram's or ZN stainings. Hence, it is widely used as a counterstain in Acid-fast (ZN) staining.

Polychrome methylene blue. This stain is prepared by allowing Loeffler's methylene blue to "ripen" for 12 months in half-filled bottles by shaking and aeration, during which time, the methylene blue slowly oxidizes to give a purple compound, that gives the stain its polychrome properties. It may be ripened quickly by the addition of 1% potassium carbonate. The stain is used to demonstrate McFadyean's reaction for the identification of anthrax bacilli in blood films.

Differential stains

Differential staining makes possible differentiating different types of bacteria or different parts of the same cell by differences in the staining pattern. Usually combinations of stains are used.

Differential stains are : Gram's staining, ZN staining.

Gram's staining. Gram's staining is the most widely used differential staining in microbiology, first developed by Hans Christian Gram (1884), a Danish physician. Gram's stain differentiates bacteria into two broad groups – Gram positive bacteria and Gram negative bacteria.

***Procedure* :**

Though, there are several variations of the Gram's staining, the basic principle is the same.

1. Primary staining of the smear with an aniline dye such as Gention violet or crystal violet for 1-2 minutes (Gention violet is a mixture of crystal violet and methyl violet dyes).

2. Pour off the excess stain, then wash off the rest with Gram's iodine.

Cover the smear with fresh Gram's iodine solution, and allow to act for 1 minute. Iodine acts as a mordant.

3. Pour off the iodine and hold the slide at a steep slope. Then pour decolorising agent, such as acetone or alcohol, slowly drop-wise from one end of the slide. The purple color starts running off. This decolorisation is carried on for a few seconds (2-3 seconds) only when acetone is used and for 30 secs when absolute alcohol is used.

4. Counterstaining with a dye of contrasting color such as saffranine, dilute carbol fuchsin or neutral red for 30 seconds.

Gram positive bacteria are those that take up and retain violet color and resist decolorisation, appearing violet/purple.

Gram negative bacteria are those that are decolorised completely and take up saffranine counter-stain, appearing red/pink.

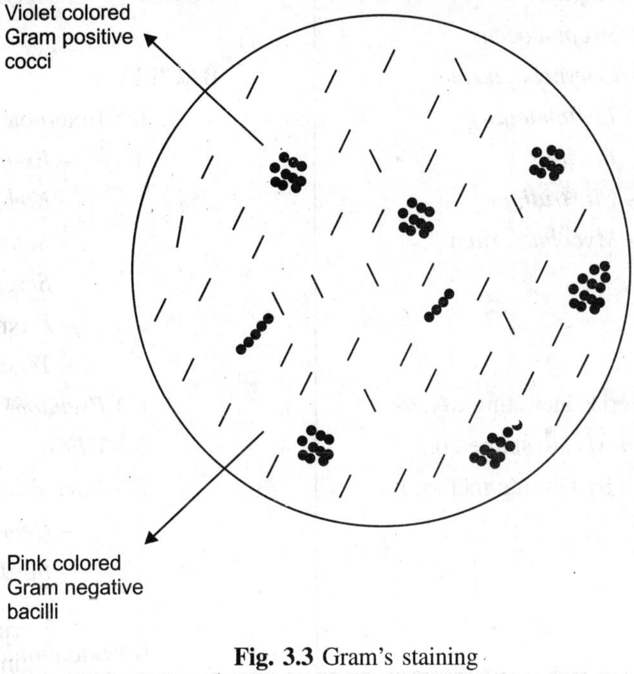

Fig. 3.3 Gram's staining

Mechanism of Gram's reaction. Many theories have been postulated to explain the mechanism of Gram's reaction. They are as follows:

1. Gram positive bacteria have a more acidic protoplasm (pH 2-3) and retain basic dye (crystal violet) more strongly than Gram negative bacteria (pH 4-5).

2. Gram's reaction may be related to the chemical composition of cell walls and permeability differences in the two groups of bacteria, towards dye-iodine complex.

In Gram positive bacteria, the cell walls are thicker, have numerous teichoic acid cross-linkages and less lipids. They get dehydrated causing decreased porosity in the cell walls, trapping dye-iodine complex, during treatment with acetone/alcohol; appearing violet (Gram positive).

Gram negative bacterial cell walls are thinner, have a smaller amount of peptidoglycan, less extensively cross-linked and contain a high percentage of lipids. They dissolve during treatment with acetone/ alcohol, forming larger pores in the cell wall, causing out-flow of dye-iodine complex and take up counter stain, thus appearing red/pink (Gram negative).

3. It has been found that Gram positivity depends on the integrity of cell wall and presence of specific Magnesium-ribonucleate-protein complex.

Thus, Gram positive bacteria may become Gram negative, if the cell is ageing, mechanically ruptured or by the action of ribonuclease.

Table 3.1 Gram Positive and Negative Bacteria

Gram positive bacteria	*Gram negative bacteria*
COCCI – *Staphylococcus* – *Streptococcus* BACILLI – *Corynebacterium* – *Lactobacillus* – *Bacillus* – *Clostridium* – *Mycobacterium* (Some, Mycobacteria, including *Mycobacterium tuberculosis* are stained only faintly or not at all by Gram's method)	COCCI – *Neisseria* BACILLI (*a*) Enterobacteria – *Escherichia coli* – *Klebsiella* – *Salmonella* – *Shigella* – *Proteus* – *Yersinia* (*b*) *Pseudomonas* (*c*) *Vibrio* (*d*) *Parvobacteria* – *Hemophilus* – *Bordetella* – *Brucella* (*e*) *Bacteroides*

Acid-fast staining/Ziehl-Neelsen's (ZN) staining

Acid-fast staining was first developed by Paul Ehrlich (1882) and later modified by Ziehl and Neelsen (1885).

Principle: Some bacteria, such as mycobacteria are resistant to aniline dyes and the dye cannot penetrate into bacilli, because their surface is coated with a unsaponifiable wax. However, by using a strong solution of carbol fuchsin, that contains phenol (acts as a mordant), and by application of heat, the dye can be made to penetrate the bacillus. Once stained, they cannot be decolorised even with strong mineral acids. Hence, they are called **Acid-fast Bacilli (AFB)**. Some of them are also not decolorised by alcohol. Therefore, they are called as **"Alcohol-fast"**.

Acid fastness is due to the presence of fatty acids, lipids and higher alcohols. A saponifiable wax, called mycolic acid (long chain fatty acid) is present in all Acid-fast bacilli. Acid-fastness is lost when the tubercle bacilli are exposed to Isoniazid (INH), but not by other drugs.

Procedure: 1. Flood the smear with strong carbol fuchsin solution and heat the slide from below, intermittently, gently, until steam rises for 3 to 5 minutes. Care should be taken to see that the stain neither boils nor evaporates; then wash well with water.

2. Decolorize with:

(*a*) 20% sulphuric acid for about 1 minute, wash the slide and pour on fresh acid. Repeat this procedure several times (5 to 6 times atleast), each time for 1 minute, till the red color is changed to yellowish brown. 20% H_2SO_4 is used, when it is desired to stain all AFB.

(*b*) 3% Hydrochloric acid in 95% ehtanol, if only tubercle bacilli is to be shown. Other mycobacteria are only acid-fast, whereas *Mycobacterium tuberculosis* is both acid and alcohol-fast.

(*c*) 5% sulphuric acid, to show the leprae bacilli (*Mycobacterium leprae*) in skin clippings or smears or sections.

3. Counterstain with Loeffler's methylene blue or malachite green or picric acid for 15 to 20 seconds.

Wash and blot dry, using blotting paper and examine under oil immersion lens of microscope (Fig. 3.4).

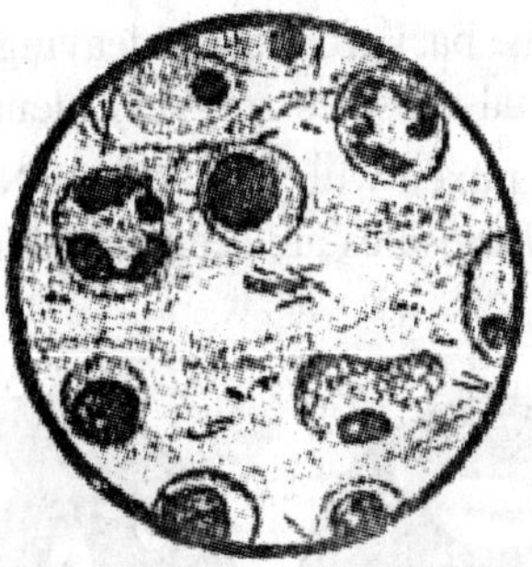

Pink coloured tubercle bacilli in sputum smear against a blue back ground

Fig. 3.4 Ziehl-Neelsen's Staining

Acid-fast bacilli appear bright pink, while other organisms, tissue cells and debris are stained blue (methylene blue) or green (malachite green) or yellow (picric acid) according to the counterstain used.

Acid-fast organisms :

1. All mycobacteria are acid-fast *e.g., Mycobacterium tuberculosis, Mycobacterium bovis, Mycobacterium leprae,* atypical mycobacteria.

2. *Nocardia asteroides, Nocardia braziliensis*.

3. *Cryptosporidium*-a protozoan coccidian parasite, which causes opportunistic infections in AIDS, is acid-fast.

4. Bacterial spores are weakly acid-fast.

Fluorochrome staining for tubercle bacilli. Auramine 'O' dye can be substituted for carbol fuchsin in the Ziehl-Neelsen method, so that tubercle bacilli fluoresce and become easier to detect. Heating is unnecessary.

1. Stain a thin heat-fixed sputum smear with the Auramine solution for 15 minutes at room temperature.

2. Wash off with tap water.

3. Cover the slide with acid-alcohol decolorizing solution for 5 minutes.

4. Wash off with tap water and rinse well.

5. Cover the slide with potassium permanganate solution for 30 seconds.

6. Wash well with tap water. Dry in air, do not use blotting paper.

7. Examine the slide by fluorescence microscope. Tubercle bacilli are seen as yellow luminous rods in a dark field.

Silver impregnation method

Impregnation is done by precipitating a solution of metallic salts, such as silver salts, on the surface of organisms.

Impregnation methods are used to demonstrate very slender bacteria such as spirochetes and bacterial flagellae that are too thin to be seen under ordinary microscope. These slender organisms and thin flagellae are made thicker by coating or impregnating silver salts on their surface, so that they become visible under ordinary microscope.

Negative staining/background staining

Negative stains act by coloring the background and leaving the bacteria as clear objects. Negative staining is used to demonstrate bacterial capsules and very slender bacteria such as spirochetes.

In negative staining, bacteria are mixed with India Ink or Nigrosin and spread on a glass slide and examined under microscope. Bacterial capsules are seen unstained, as bright halos against a uniformly blackstained background (Fig. 3.5).

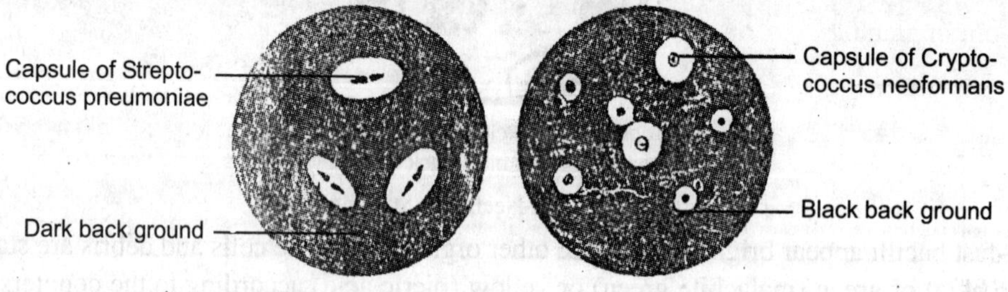

Fig. 3.5. Negative staining (Indian ink/Nigrosin preparation)

In negative staining, either wet films or dry films can be prepared. Dry film method is used for permanent preparations.

Special stains for Corynebacterium diphtheriae, (Stains to demonstrate metachromatic granules)

Certain bacilli possess volutin granules in the protoplasm which aid in the identification of diphtheria bacilli. Several special and differential stains are used to stain diphtheria bacilli and to demonstrate their metachromatic granules.

1. Albert's stain
2. Neisser's stain
3. Ponder's stain
4. Pugh's stain.

1. Albert's stain.

1. Prepare a thin smear of throat swab from a patient or culture, dry it.
2. Stain with Albert's stain (Albert's solution A) for 3 to 5 minutes.
3. Wash with a few drops of Albert's iodine.
4. Stain with Albert's iodine (Albert's solution B) for 1 to 2 minutes.

Wash with water and blot dry. Observe under the oil-immersion objective.

The metachromatic (volutin) granules of *Corynebacterium diphtheriae* stain bluish-black and the bacterial protoplasm green.

2. *Neisser's stain.*

1. Stain the smear with Neisser's methylene blue for 3 minutes.
2. Wash off with dilute iodine and leave some of this solution on the slide for 1 minute.
3. Wash in water.
4. Counterstain with neutral red solution for 3 minutes.

Wash in water and dry. Observe under oil immersion lens. By this method the bacilli exhibit deep blue granules and the bacterial protoplasm takes pink color.

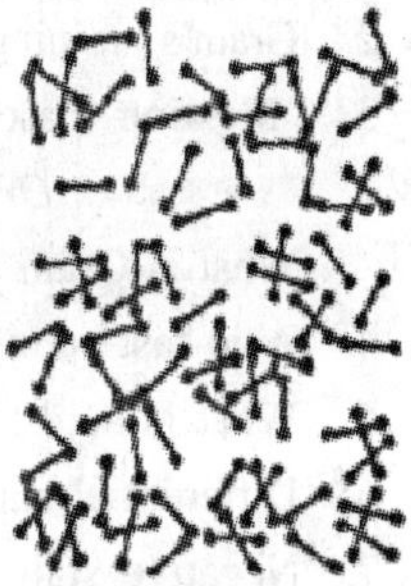

Fig. 3.6. Diphtheria bacilli under Albert's stain.

3. *Ponder's stain.*

1 Stain the smear with Ponder's stain for 1-2 minutes.
2. Wash with water and blot dry. Examine under oil immersion objective.

The volutin granules stain dark blue, whereas the bacillus pale blue.

4. *Pugh's stain.*

1. Stain the smear with Pugh's stain (toluidine blue) for 2 to 3 minutes.
2. Wash with water and blot dry. Examine under oil immersion objective. The volutin granules stain reddish purple and the remainder of the organism light blue.

Vital staining

Microorganisms may be stained in the living state. Many dyes are toxic and kill the cells on staining. Non-toxic staining, during which the cells retain their viability, is known as vital or intravital staining *e.g.,* Methylene blue dye test for *Toxoplasma.*

Supervital staining

The staining of living cells after their removal from the host has been referred to as supervital or supravital staining, where the cells remain viable during the staining process.

Excess stain, if any can be removed by blotting paper.

For permanent preparations, the edges of coverslips may be sealed with nail polish. Lactic acid is a preservative, phenol is a disinfectant and cotton blue provides blue color to fungal filaments.

QUESTIONS

Essay Type Questions

1. Describe in detail the Gram's staining.
2. Give an account of differential stains.

Short Notes

1. Simple staining.
2. Gram's staining.
3. Mention reasons behind Gram positivity of bacteria.

   Or

   What is Gram positivity due to ?
4. Acid-fast stain or Ziehl-Neelsen's stain.
5. What is acid-fastness due to ?
6. Differential stains.
7. Negative staining.
8. Impregnation methods.
9. Albert's stain.
10. Mention stains to demonstrate volutin granules of diphtheria bacilli.

4

Morphology of Bacteria

SIZE OF BACTERIA

Micron. The unit of measurement used in Bacteriology is the micron or micrometre. Most of the cocci have a diameter of 1 micron (μ) and bacilli measure 2-5 microns in length and 0.5-1 micron in width.

1 Micron (μ) or 1 micrometre (μm) = One thousandth of a millimetre

The unit micron is also used to measure the size of protozoan parasites, parasitic eggs and larvae.

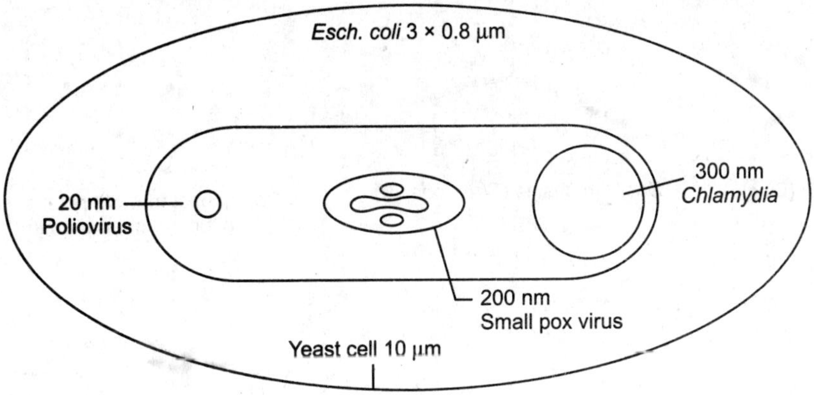

Fig. 4.1 Comparative sizes of certain microbes

Microsocpic measurements

Micrometer (μm) –	One millinth (10^{-6}) of a meter	or	one thousandth of a mm
Nanometer (nm) –	One billionth of a meter (10^{-9})	or	one millinth of a mm
Angstrom (Å) –	1/10 th of nm (one ten billionth of a meter (10^{-10})		

NANOMETER (nm) AND ANGSTROM UNIT (Å)

These units are used to measure the size of viruses and various cell organelles.

1 Millimicron (mμ)	–	one thousandth of a micron
or		or
1 Nanometer (nm)	–	one millionth of a millimetre
1 Angstrom unit (Å)	–	one tenth of a nanometre

MORPHOLOGY (SHAPES) OF BACTERIA

Bacteria can be classified into various groups, based on their shape.

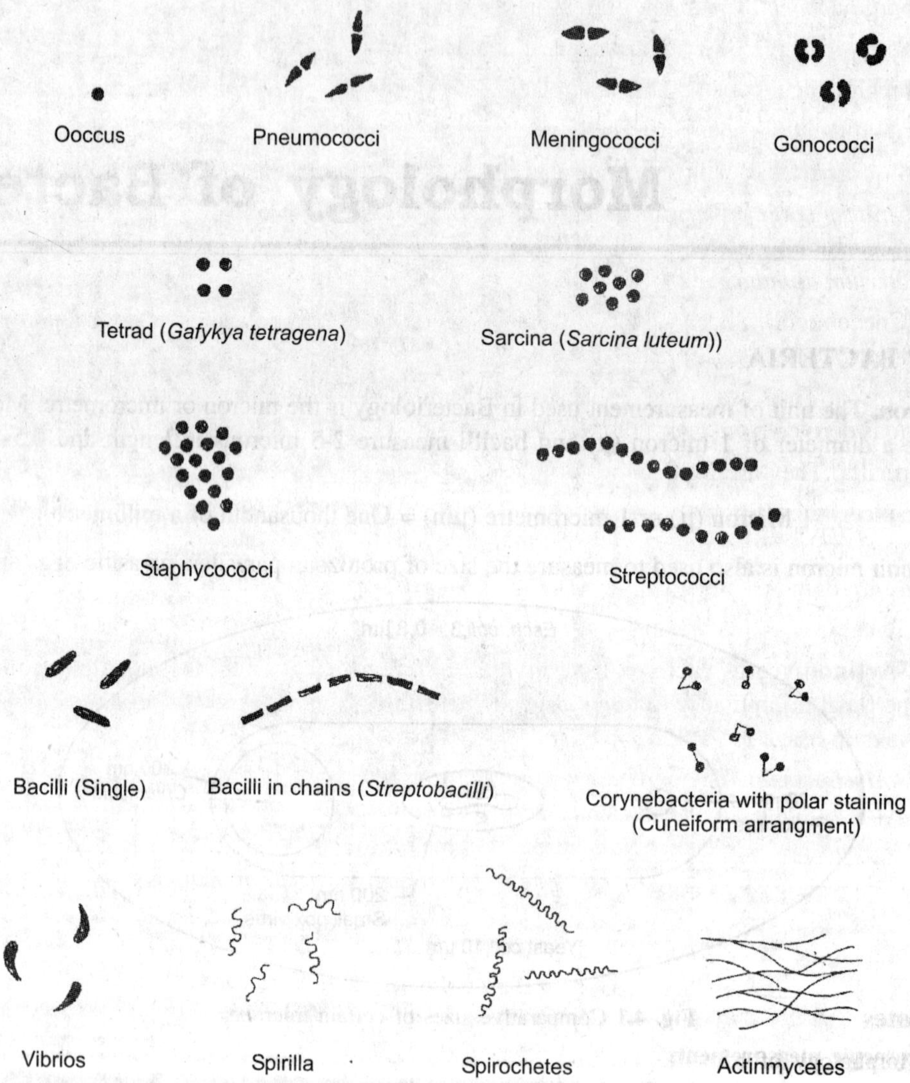

Fig. 4.2 Some morphological forms of bacteria

I. Cocci (Kokkos-berry). They are spherical or oval shaped cells. The cocci can be arranged in different ways and different names are given according to their arrangement.

1. ***Dipococci.*** Cocci may be present in pairs

e.g, Pneumococci – cells are lanceolate or flame shaped, Gram positive diplococci

Meningococci – cells are oval shaped, Gram negative diplococci.

Gonococci – cells are kidney or bean seed shaped, Gram negative diplococci.

2. ***Tetrads***. Cocci are present in groups of four *e.g., Gaffykya* tetragena.

3. ***Sarcina.*** Cocci are present in groups of eight *e.g., Sarcina luteum.*

4. ***Staphylococci.*** Cocci are present in grape like bunches.

5. ***Streptococci.*** Cocci are arranged in chains.

II. Bacilli (Baculus rod). They are rod shaped organisms. *e.g., E.coli, Clostridium, Mycobacterium*

Based on their arragnement, bacilli can be further named.

1. ***Streptobacilli.*** Bacilli are arranged in chains *e.g., Streptobacillus moniliformis, Bacillus anthracis.*

2. ***Chinese letter pattern or cuneiform arrangement.*** The bacilli are arranged at right angles to each other, resembling letters V or L, similar to chinese letter pattern or cuneiform arrangement *e.g., Corynebacterium diphtheriae.*

III. Coccobacilli. Short rod shaped organisms or small ovoid organisms are called coccobacilli *e.g., Brucella, Bordetella*

IV. Vibros. They are comma shaped organisms. They can be described as curved bacilli. The name vibrio is derived from their vibratory motility. *e.g., Vibrio cholerae, Campylobacter, Helicobacter.*

V. Spirilla. They are rigid spiral forms *e.g., Spirillum minus.*

VI. Spirochetes (Speira = spiral; chaite = hair like). They are flexuous spiral shaped organisms having several coils. These coils may be arranged in two ways :

1. Relaxed coils – *Borrelia, Leptospira.*
2. Tight coils – *Treponema.*

VII. Actinomycetes (actis = ray; mykes = fungus). The are branching filamentous forms, having superficial resemblance to fungi. They are called as actinomycetes, because they look like radiating sun rays in tissue lesions. *e.g., Actinomyces, Nocardia.*

VIII. *Mycoplasma.* They are cell wall deficient and hence do not possess a stable morphology. They occurs as spherical, oval, bacillary and filamentous forms. Bacteria lose their cell wall either spontaneously or in the presence of salts, penicillin like agents. Such cells are called L-forms, protoplasts or spheroplasts. *e.g., Mycoplasma pneumoniae, M.hominis, Ureaplasma urealyticum.*

QUESTIONS

Short Notes

1. Morphology of bacteria/shapes of bacteria.
2. Cocci
3. Morphological classification of bacteria.
4. Micron.
5. Nanometer.
6. Angstrom unit.
7. Size of bacteria.

5

Bacterial Anatomy/Ultrastructure of Bacterial cells

- *Introduction*
- *Cell envelope*
- *Cell wall*
  - *– Chemical composition*
  - *– Gram positive bacterial cell walls*
  - *– Gram negative bacterial cell walls*
  - *– Differences between Gram positive and Gram negative bacaterial cell walls*
  - *– Demonstration*
  - *– Functions*
- *Cytoplasmic membrane*
- *Mesosomes*
- *Cytoplasm*
- *Cytoplasmic inclusions*
  - *– Ribosomes*
  - *– Volutin/metachromatic granules*
  - *– Lipid granules*
  - *– Polysaccharide granules*
  - *– Vacuoles*
- *Bacterial nucleus (Nucleoid)*
- *Plasmids and episomes*
- *Glycocalyx, capsule, slime layer*
  - *– Chemical composition*
  - *– Demonstration*
  - *– negative staianing*
  - *– Quellung reaction*
  - *– Functions*
- *Flagellae*
  - *– Parts of flagellum*
  - *– Arrangement*
  - *– Demonstration*
  - *– Functions*
- *Fimbriae*
- *Bacterial spores (Endospores)*
  - *– Structure*
  - *– Shape and position*
  - *– Demonstration*
  - *– Uses*
- *Pleomorphism and Involution forms*
- *Protoplasts*
- *L-phase organisms*

INTRODUCTION

Bacteria are prokaryotic unicellular microorganisms, enclosed by a thin, elastic membrane known as plasma membrane. Outside, and closely covering this, there is cell wall; these two together are called "cell envelope". The cell envelope encloses protoplasm, that is differentiated into cytoplasm and nuclear material. The cytoplasm contains ribosomes, mesosomes, vacuoles and inclusion granules. Some bacteria may be enclosed by a viscous material known as capsule. Some bacteria carry filamentous appendages protruding from the cell membrane – the flagellae which are organelles of locomotion, and the pili or fimbriae which are organelles of adhesion (Fig. 5.1).

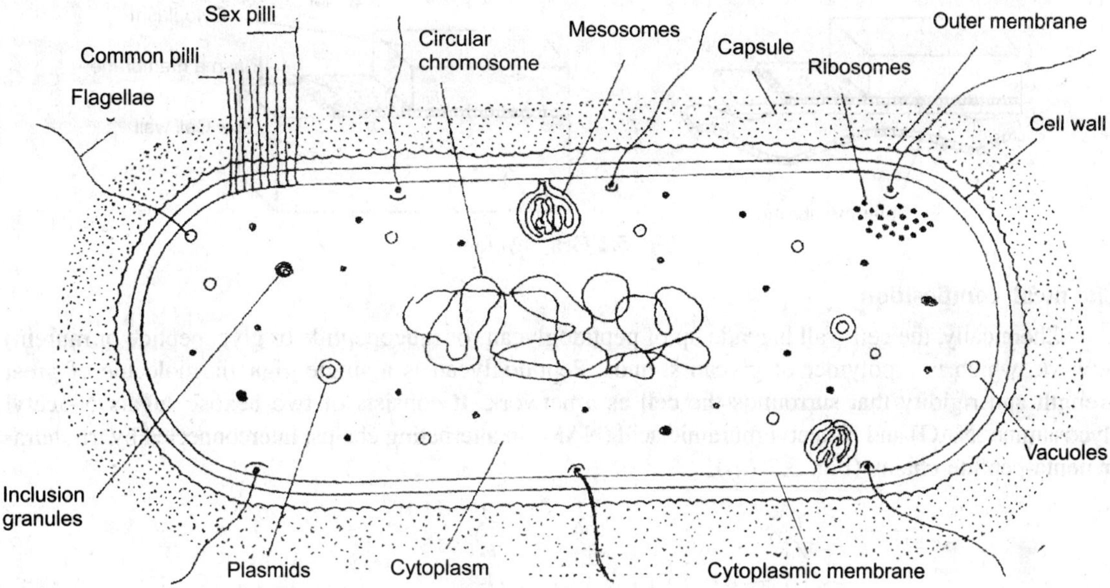

Fig. 5.1 The structure of bacterial cell

CELL ENVELOPE

Various layers that surround the bacterial cell are collectively referred to as "cell envelope". The structure and organization of cell envelope differ in Gram positive and Gram negative bacteria.

The cell envelope in Gram positive bacteria consists of plasma membrane and cell wall and in some bacteria an outer layer called the capsule.

The cell envelope in Gram negative bacteria contains plasma membrane, cell wall, outer membrane and in some capsule. The plasma membrane in Gram negative bacteria is sometimes called "inner membrane" and the space between inner membrane and outer membrance is called the "**periplasmic space**".

CELL WALL

Cell wall encloses the protoplast and lies immediately external to the cytoplasmic membrane. It accounts for about 20-30% dry weight of the cell. It measures 10-25 nm in thickness. The cell walls of Gram negative bacteria are thinner (10-15 nm) and those of Gram positive bacteria are thicker (20-25 nm) (Fig. 5.2).

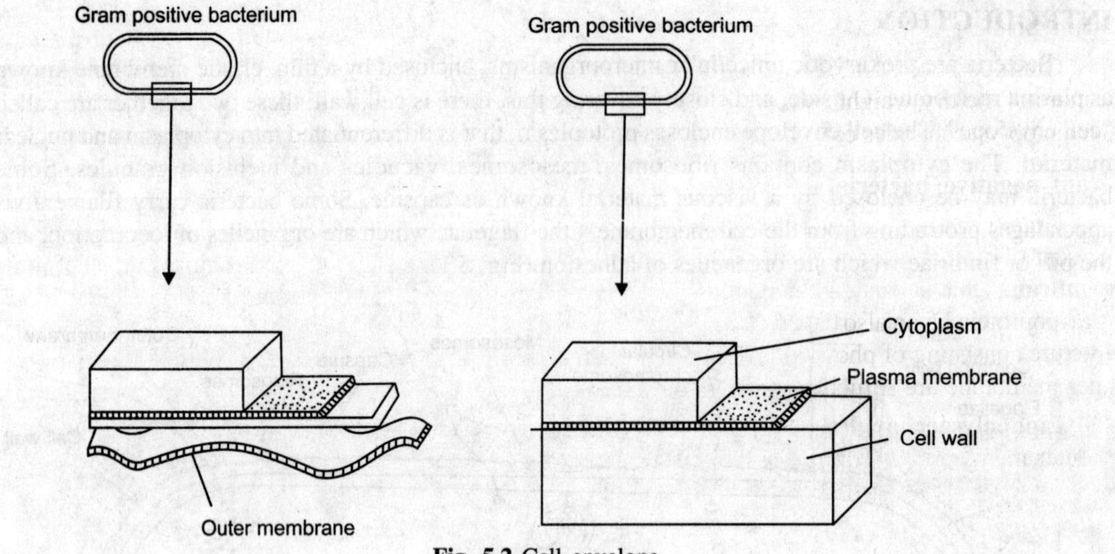

Fig. 5.2 Cell envelope

Chemical composition

Chemically, the cell wall is made up of peptidoglycan (or mucopeptide or glycopeptide or murein) network, which is a polymer of glycan strands. Peptidoglycan is a single gigantic molecule of great strength and rigidity that surrounds the cell as a network. It consists of two hexose sugars N-acetyl glycosamine (NAG) and N-acetyl muramic acid (NAM) in alternating chains, interconnected by tri-, tetra- or penta-peptide chains (Fig. 5.3 (*a*)).

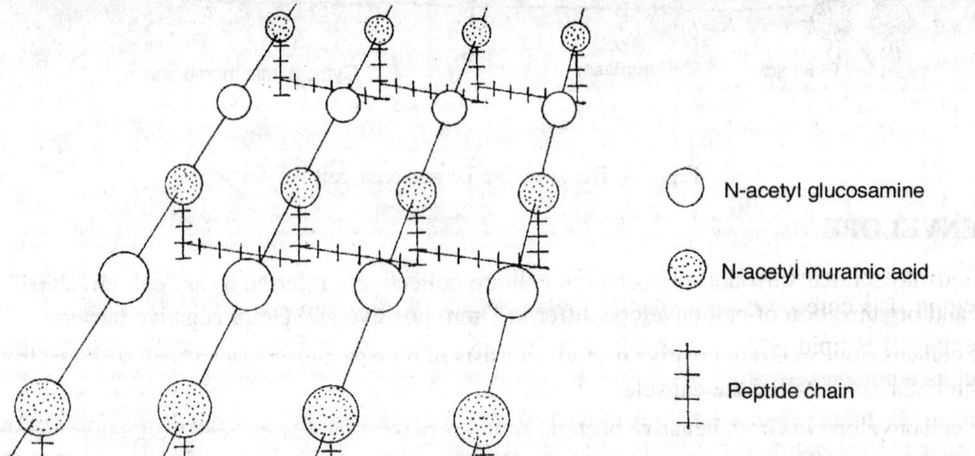

Fig. 5.3 (***a***) The structure of bacterial cellwall

Lysozyme, an enzyme normally present in tissue fluids, lyses susceptible bacteria, by splitting the cell wall mucopeptide linkages between NAG and NAM. It can completely destroy the cell wall of Gram positive bacterium, producing a "**protoplast**"; while the cell walls of Gram negative bacteria are more resistant to lysozyme and lose less of their cell wall producing a "**spheroplast**".

Gram positive bacterial cell walls

Gram positive bacterial cell walls contain large amount of peptidoglycan, account for 50 per cent or more of the dry weight of the cell wall and are thicker. Many Gram positve bacterial cell walls also contain polysaccharides called "**Teichoic acids**", which are polymers of glycerol and ribitol phosphates.

Gram negative bacterial cell walls

Gram negative bacterial cell walls contain less amount of peptidoglycan, account for only 5 to 10 per cent of the dry weight of the cell wall and are thinner. These cell walls have an additional "**outer membrane**" that surrounds the peptidoglycan layer. The outer membrane is anchored to peptidoglycan by a lipoprotein layer, also called Braun's lipoprotein. The outer layer of the outer membrane is a bilayered structure consisting of phospholipids, proteins and lipopolysaccharides (LPS). The phospholipids of the outer membrane are similar to those in the cytoplasmic membrane.

Lipopolysaccharides are characteristic to Gram negative bacteria and found on the outer surface of outer membrane. It comprises three parts, which are covalently linked (Fig. 5.3 (*b*)).

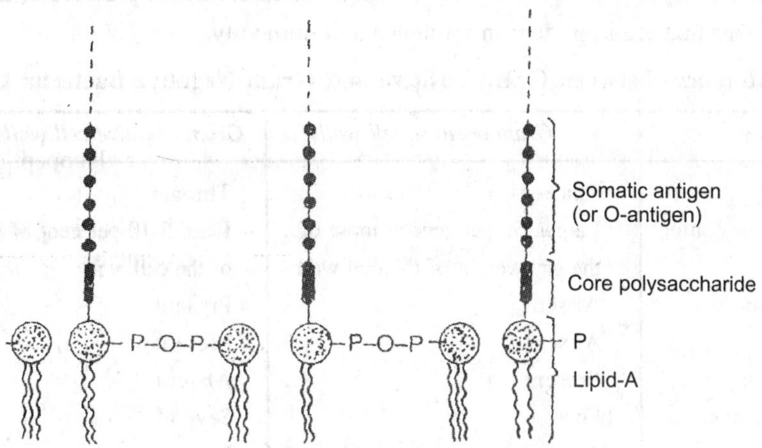

Fig. 5.3 (*b*) Lipopolysaccharide.

1. Region I is a polysaccharide. It extends like whiskers (hair like) from the membrane surface into the surrounding medium. It is also called somatic antigen or O-antigen. It was first extracted by Boivin, hence known as Boivin antigen.

2. Region II is core polysaccharide located at the membrane surface.

3. Region III is lipid A, firmly embedded in the outer membrance. It is also knwon as **endotoxin** and can act as a poison – causing fever, diarrhea, lysis of RBC, and fatal shock.

Outer membrane contains various proteins, known as **outer membrane proteins (OMP)**, which include porins and receptors.

Porins are special proteins that form diffusion channels; that are selectively permeable allow smaller molecules and act as a barrier for larger molecules. Various porins are specific for different kinds of small molecules, and some can allow passage of larger, essential molecules such as vitamin B_{12}. Porins allow secretion of extracellular enzymes. Porins facilitate signal transdusion. Some outer membrane proteins act as receptor sites for attachment of bacteriophages and bacteriocins. The region between outer membrane and plasma membrane is called **"periplasmic space".** It contains hydrolytic enzymes, binding proteins and oligosaccharides, that play an important role in osmotic regulation.

Demonstation of cell wall. Cell wall can be demonstrated by :

1. Microdissection.
2. Mechanical rupture of cell.
3. Electron microscope.
4. Differential staining procedures.
5. Plasmolysis–when bacterial cells are placed in hypertonic solution, cytoplasm loses water by osmosis and shrinks, while cell wall retains the original shape and size and appears like a bacterial ghost under the microscope.

Functions of cell wall:

1. accounts for the characteristic shape of the cell.
2. confers rigidity and ductility on the cell and gives mechanical support to the cell.
3. plays an important role in cell division by forming cross walls to separate the daughter cells.
4. supports weak cytoplasmic membrane against high internal osmotic pressure of the protoplasm.
5. carries antigens that are important in virulence and immunity.

Table 5.1 Differences between Gram Positive and Gram Negative Bacterial Cell Walls.

Character	*Gram positive cell walls*	*Gram negative cell walls*
1. Thickness	Thicker	Thinner
2. Peptidoglycan content	Larger, 50 per cent or more of the dry weight of the cell wall	Less, 5-10 per cent of the dry weight of the cell wall
3. Outer membrane	Absent	Present
4. LPS	Absent	Present
5. Teichoic acids	Present	Absent
6. Variety of aminoacids	Few	Several
7. Aromatic and sulphur containing aminacids	Absent	Present
8. Lipids	Absent, Mycolic acids present in mycobacteria	Present, possess endotoxic activity
9. Lipoproteins	Absent	Present.

CYTOPLASMIC MEMBRANE

Immediately beneath the cell wall is the cytoplasmic membrane; also called plasma membrane or cell membrane.It is thin, elastic and semipermeable, composed of phospholipids (20 to 30 per cent) and proteins (50 to 70 per cent). The phospholipids form a bilayer in which proteins are firmly held. It possesses unit membrane structure.

Functions :

1. Plasma membrane carries specific enzymes called permeases, that transport small molecules into the cell by active transport.

2. Cell membrane also contians various enzymes, some of which are involved in energy production and cell wall synthesis.

3. The plasma membrane is selectively semi-permeable for the penetration of water soluble molecules. It allows the entry and exit of small molecules such as nutrients and waste products by simple diffusion.

MESOSOMES

Mesosomes are sites of respiratory enzymes and are analogous to mitochondira. They are vesicular, convoluted or multilaminated membranous bodies, formed by invagination or infolding of plasma membrane into the cytoplasm. They consist of convoluted tubules and vesicles. They are especially prominent in Gram positive bacateria. Mesosomes are also known as "chondroids" (Fig. 5.4).

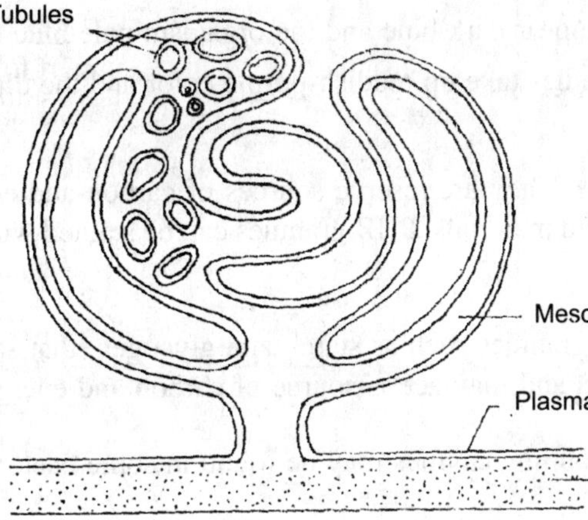

Fig. 5.4 Mesosome

CYTOPLASM

Cytoplasm is a colloidal system of viscous watery solution or soft gel, containing a variety of organic and inorganic solutes. It does not exhibit cytoplasmic streaming. Cell organelles such as ER, Golgi bodies, mitochondria, are absent.

The cytoplasm is largely consists a high percentage of water, alongwith nucleic acids, proteins, carbohydrates, lipids, inorganic ions and several low molecular weight compounds.

Cytoplasm stains uniformly in young cultures, but becomes granular with age and shows barred or beaded appearaance in old cells.

CYTOPLASMIC INCLUSIONS

Cytoplasm contains ribosomes, several inclusion storage granules, nucleoid and vacuoles.

Ribosomes. They are present in the cytoplasm freely and are centres of protein synthesis. They may be found together on mRNA strand to form polysomes. Ribosomes in bacteria consists of two subunits – the larger 50S subunit and the smaller 30S subunit, together they form the 70S bacterial ribosome (the 'S' refers to the "svedberg unit", a measure of rate of sedimentation when centrifuged at high speed. Since both shape and size determine the rate of sedimentation, the 'S' units do not add up arithmetically).

Volutin granules or Metachromatic granules or Babes-Ernst granules. They are characteristically present in diphtheria bacilli (*Corynebacterium diphtheriae*) as round, dark bipolar bodies. The name 'volutin' refers to the bacterium *Spirillum volutans* in which these granules were first found. They take up reddish purple color when stained with Loeffler's methylene blue (stain red with blue dye) and therefore called metachromatic granules.

They are composed of polymetaphosphate and considered to be reserve sources of energy. They can to demonstrated by special stains;

1. Albert's stain– Volutin granules appear bluish black and diphtheria bacilli light green.
2. Neisser's stain– The granules appear deep blue colored and the bacillie pink color.
3. Ponder's stain– The granules appear dark blue and the organism pale blue color.
4. Pugh's stain– The volutin granules take up reddish-purple color and the diphtheria bacilli light blue color.

Poly β-hydroxy butyrate (PHB). They are reserve sources of carbon and energy and are clear, round areas and chloroform-soluble lipid materials. PHB granules can be stained with lipid soluble dyes such as Nile blue or sudan black.

Polysaccharide. Polysaccharide granules such as starch and glycogen, that stain blue and brown with iodine respectively, may be found and may act as source of carbon and energy.

Vacuoles. Vacuoles are fluid containing cavities may be found in some bacterial cells.

BACTERIAL NUCLEUS (or) NUCLEOID

Bacteria possess a prokaryotic nucleus. They have no nuclear membrane or nucleolus and DNA is not associated with any protein. The DNA material is located or concentrated near the centre of the cell called the "nucleoid".

The nucleoid consists of a single circular chromosome, made up of a single molecule of double-stranded DNA, arranged in the form of a circle. It is haploid and replicates by simple fission. Mitosis is absent. It carries hereditary genetic information.

The nuclear material can be demonstrated by acid or ribonuclease hydrolysis and subsequent staining by fuelgen technique.

PLASMIDS AND EPISOMES

Plasmids are small circular, covalently closed, double-stranded DNA molecules found in cytoplasm. They are self-replicating extrachromosomal genetic elements that reproduce themselves and are thus conserved, apart from chromosome, through successive cell divisions and segregate into daughter cells.

Plasmids that may also become integrated into the chromosome are sometimes called episomes.

Plasmids may be transmitted from one bacterium to another bacterium either through conjugation or through the agency of bacteriophages by transduction. They are not essential for the life of the cell. They inhabit, but may confer on it certain properties like toxin production, drug resistance or resistance to heavy metals which may constitute a survival advantage.

Some plasmids, such as F factor endow the host celll with maleness or ability to conjugate with other cells. Following conjugation, the recipient acquires the plasmid, becoming male or donor cell in the process. The basis of maleness is the ability to form sex pili which are coded for by the plasmid (F factor).

Penicillinase plasmids which induces resistance in Staphylococci are transmitted from cell to cell through transduction.

R-plasmids confer drug resistance and readily transmitted from cell to cell by mechanisms of gene transfer. It is known as **transferable** or **infectious drug resistance**.

GLYCOCALYX, CAPSULE, SLIME LAYER

Many bacteria secrete a viscous, jelly-like, gelatinous material, that surrounds the cell wall is called "Glycocalyx". When glycocalyx is organized into a sharply defined structure and is attached firmly to the cell wall, it is a "capsule" *e.g., Streptococcus pneumoniae, Bacillius anthracis, Clostridium welchii, Klebsiella pneumoniae, Hemophilus influenzae, Neisseria meningitidis.*

When a capsule is too thin to be seen under light microscope, and detectable only by indirect, serological means or by electron microscope, it may be termed "Microcapsule". When glycocalyx is disorganized without any definite shape, and seen as a loose undemarcated secretion and surrounds bacterial cells, as "matrix", in which several bacterial cells may be embedded; then it is termed "Slime layer" *e.g., Leuconostoc.* Some bacteria may have both capsules and slime layer *e.g., Streptococcus salivarius.*

Capsular gel consists largely of water and has only a small content (2 per cent) of solids. Bacteria producing large amount of capsular material, produce mucoid growth on agar medium, with a stingy consistency when touched with the wire loop. Capsulated strains form smooth (S) colonies whereas noncapsulated strains form rough (R) colonies. Capsule may be lost either spontaneously or due to mutations and is associated with loss of virulence.

Capsular material is soluble in water and may diffuse into liquid culture medium or infective exudates and tissues, and therefore called "**Specific soluble substance (SSS)**".

Under electron microscope, capsules are seen as a mesh or network of fine strands. Capsule may be chemically composed of polysaccharide *e.g., Streptococcus pneumoniae*; or polypeptide *e.g., Bacillus anthracis*; or hyaluronic acid *e.g., Streptococcus pyogenes.*

Demonstration of Capsules. Capsule have no affinity for basic aniline dyes and cannot be stained by ordinary methods such as Gram's and Leishman stains.

Capsules can be demonstrated by 1. Negative staining, 2. capsule swelling reaciton (quellung reaction), 3. special staining methods such as Hiss stain, in which copper salts are used as mordants.

Negative Staining. When capsulated bacteria are mixed with Indian ink or nigrosin, and spread on a glass slide and examined under microscope; capsules can be seen as unstained bright halos against black dark background.

Capsule Swelling Reaction or Quellung Reaction. Capsular material is antigenic, and therefore may be demonstrated by serological methods. When a suspension of capsulated bacteria is mixed on a slide with a drop of type specific anticapsular serum and a loopful of methylene blue solution, and examined under the microscope, the capsule becomes swollen, refractile and prominent.

Quellung (= swelling) reaction was first described by Neufeld (1902). It was widely employed for typing of pneumococci when lobar pneumonia used to be treated with specific anticapsular serum, before sulphonamides were discovered.

Functions of capsules :

1. Capsules protect pathogenic bacteria from being engulfed by phagocytes *i.e.,* inhibit phagocytosis and confer or promote virulence or greater infective ability.
2. Capsule protect bacteria by preventing adsorption and lysis by bacteriophages and from lytic enzymes and drugs.
3. Capsular vaccines may be used for immunization against diseases caused by capsulated bacteria.

FLAGELLAE

All motile bacteria, except spirochetes possess one or more long, unbranched hair like or thread like filamentous appendages, called flagellae, which are organelles of locomotion. They originate in the cytoplasm, extend through cytoplasmic membrane and extruded out through the cell wall. Each flagellum is a long, thin filament, twisted spirally (helical shape) in an open, regular wave form, which effect cork-screw like propulsive movements. Flagellae are usually several times longer than the cell, measuring 15 to 20 μ in length.

Parts of flagellum. Each flagellum has three distinct parts – basal body, hook and filament or shaft.

Basal body. It is embedded in cell envelope and consists of a small central rod surrounded by a series of rings. Gram negative bacteria have two pairs of rings, with the outer rings anchored to the cell wall and the inner rings attached to the cytoplasmic membrane. These rings are called sequentially as follows:

M ring – attached to plasma membrane

S ring – located in the periplasmic space above the plasma membrane.

P ring – attached to the peptidoglycan

L ring – attached to lipopolysaccharide.

In Gram positive bacteria, only one pair of rings is present, the outer set of rings (P ring and L ring) are absent. One ring, called M ring is embedded in the plasma membrane and the other S ring is attached to the inside of the peptidoglycan (cell wall) layer (Fig. 5.5).

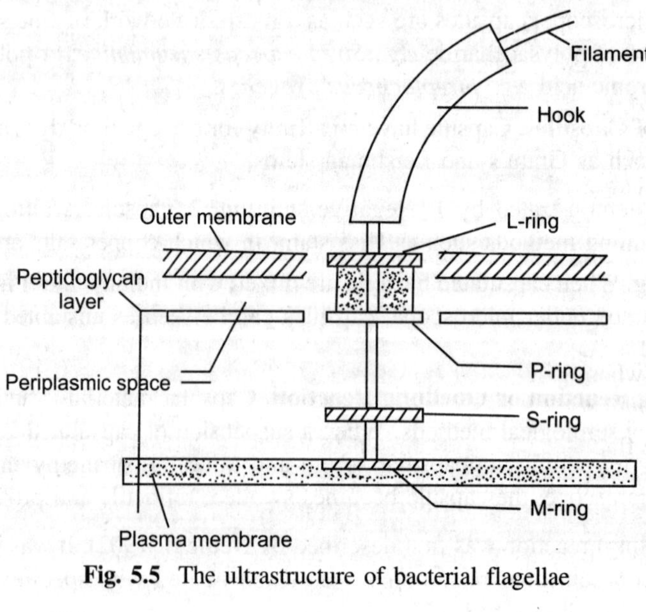

Fig. 5.5 The ultrastructure of bacterial flagellae

Hook. Hook connects the basal body with the filament. The hook of Gram positive bacterial flagellum is longer than that of the Gram negative bacterial flagellum. Hook arises from basal body and positions the filament along its long aixs during motility.

Filament or shaft. It is external to the cell surface twisted helically and connected to the hook at the cell surface. The filament is composed of protein molecules called "flagellin" similar to keratin or myosin. These flagellin molecules are made within the cell and then passed along the hollow core of the flagellum to be added to the distal end of the fialment. Thus, a flagellum grown at its tip rather than at its base.

Arrangement.

Based on number and arrangement of flagellae, bacteria can be classified into different groups. The bacteria which do not possess flagellae may be termed "Atrichous". When bacteria contian flagellae at one or both ends. They are termed "Polar" flagellae (Fig. 5.6).

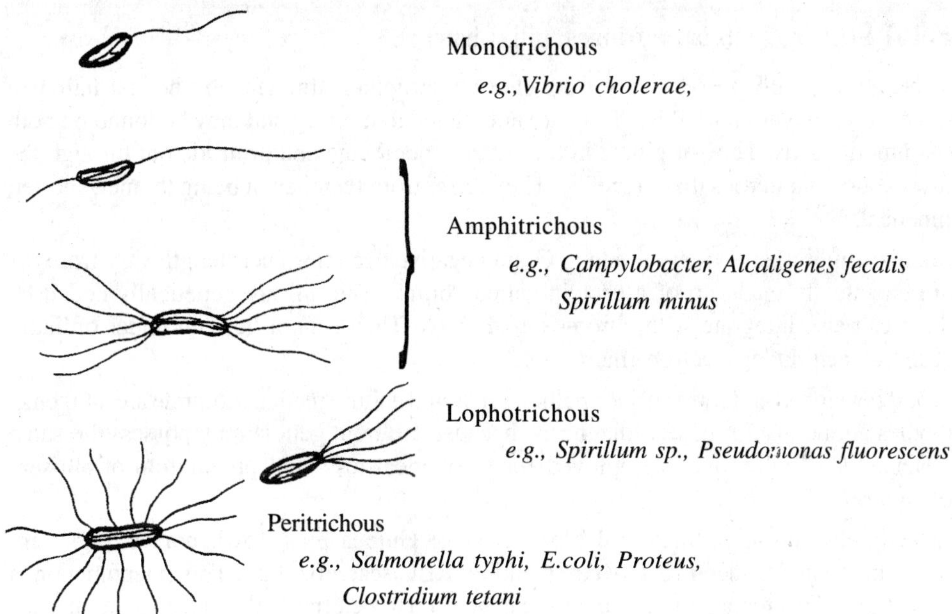

Fig. 5.6 Number and arrangement of flagellae

1. ***Monotrichous*** (Greak monos = single; trichos = hair) – consists of a single polar flagellum *e.g., Vibrio cholerae, Campylobacter sp.*

2. ***Amphitrichous*** – when bacteria has flagellae at both the ends. It could be a single flagellum at either end *e.g., Campylobacter sp., Alcaligenes fecalis*;

3. ***Lophotrichous*** – when a bacterial cell possesses a tuft of flagellae at one end, it is known as lophotrichous *e.g., Spirillum sp., Helicobacter pylori.*

4. ***Peritrichous*** – when flagellae are present all around the bacterial cell surface, it is called peritrichous. *e.g., E.coli, Salmonella typhi, Proteus sp., Clostridium tetani.*

Cocci rarely have flagellae. But some cocci such as *Rhodococcus* are flagellated. Spirochetes are actively motile but do not contain external filaments instead they possess special flagellae called "axial filaments or periplasmic flagellae or endoflagellae", that arise at cell poles and wind around the cell body beneath the outer membrane of cell wall in the periplasmic space. They are responsible for cork-screw like rotatory movement of spirochetes.

Demonstration of flagellae. Flagellae can be demonstrated by several methods :

1. in electron microscope.

2. by silver impregnation methods, where the flagellae are made thick by impregnating or depositng silver salts on their surface so that they become visible under the microscope.

3. by dark field microscopy.

4. by special staining methods such as Leifson's staining.

5. the presence of flagellae can be inferred by demonstrating motility. The motility can be demonstrated (*a*) by hanging drop experiment or (*b*) by noting spreading or swarming growth on a semisolid agar medium.

Functions : Flagellae are organelles of locomotion.

FIMBRIAE (or) PILI (Latin; fimbriae = fringes; pili = hair)

Many Gram negative bacilli possess very fine, shorter, straighter, thinner, non-helical hair like surface appendages called pili (singular pilus). Thay are not related to motility and may be found on both motile as well as nonmotile cells. They originate in the plasma membrane and protrude out through the cell envelope. They are more numerous than flagellae. They differ from flagellae in being thinner, shorter, straighter and nonhelical.

Fimbriae (singular fimbria) are widely found in Gram negative bacteria. Their length vary from 0.1 μ to 2 μ. They are chemically made up of a protein called "pilin". The pili are genetically coded by plasmid DNA which can also integrate with chromosomal DNA. They cannot be seen under ordinary microscope, but can be seen under electron microscope.

Fimbriae are best developed and form surface pellicles in liquid culture media. Fimbriae are antigenic. But fimbrial antibodies are not useful in sero-diagnosis, because different genera may possess the same fimbrial antigen. Hence bacterial antigens employed for serological tests and preparation of antisera must be devoid of fimbriae.

Many fimbriated cells can agglutinate red blood cells of Guinea pigs, fowl, horses, pigs very strongly, human RBC moderately, sheep RBC weakly and ox RBC scarcely at all. This phenomenon is called "Hemagglutination". This hemagglutination test can be used to determine the presence or absence of fimbriae. This hemagglutination is specifically inhibited by D-mannose or methyl-α-D-mannoside.

Fimbriae have been classified into the following major groups :

I. Based on function, pili are classified into 2 groups :

1. *Common pili or ordinary pili.* Help in adhesion to host cells or nutritionally favourable environments.

2. *Sex pili.* They are special type of fimbriae, which are longer and fewer in number than other fimbriae. They are found on male or donor or + strains and help in the attachment to female or recipient or – strains through hollow conjugation tubes and aid in gene transfer. The formation of sex pili or maleness is determined by F-plasmid or fertility factor.

II. Based on susceptibility to specific bacteriophages, pili are classified into different types *e.g.,* F, I.

III. Based on morphology, pili are classified into six morphological types or groups (Types 1 to 6).

BACTERIAL SPORES (or) ENDOSPORES

Bacterial spores are highly resistant resting dormant forms. They are commonly found in *Bacillus* and *Clostridium* species. Bacterial spores are formed inside the cell, hence called as endospores. Each bacterium forms one spore, which on germination forms a single vegetative cell. Sporulation in bacteria, therefore, is not a method of reproduction. The spores are highly resistant to heat, UV radiation, mechanical disruption, chemical disinfectants and desiccation and can remain viable for many centuries. The extremely high resistance of spores is due to

1. low content of water
2. absence of metabolism and enzyme activity
3. high content of calcium and dipicolinic acid
4. impermeability of spore layers (spore cortex and spore coat).

The spores can be killed by moist heat at 100-120°C for a period of 10 min or preferably by autoclaving.

Spore structure.

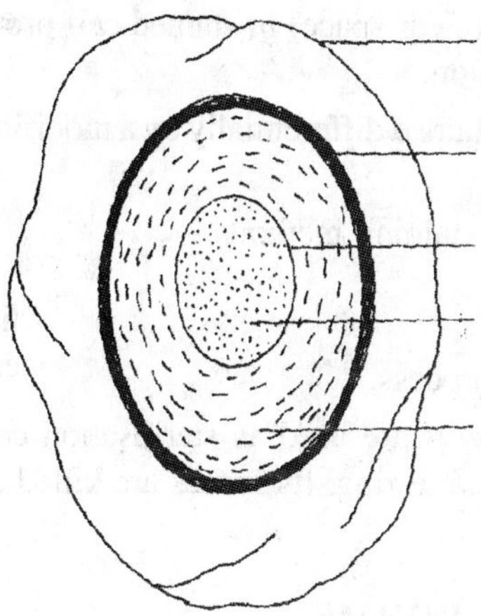

Fig. 5.7 Structure of a bacterial spore

The core of a fully developed spore has homogenous protoplasm, containing chromosome, enzymes of glycolysis and protein synthesis. The protoplast is surrounded by a membrane called "spore wall". It contains normal peptidoglycan, from which the cell wall of future vegetative bacterium develops. Outside the spore wall is a thick "spore cortex" consisting of dipicolinic acid, calcium and an unusual type of peptidoglycan. Spore cortex is surrounded by "spore coats", usually two or upto three may be present. Spore coat is highly impermeable and responsible for the resistance of spores. Outside the spore coats, there is a wrinkled outerlayer with ridges and folds, known as "exsoporium", contianing mainly lipoprotein and some carbohydrate.

Shapes and Position of Spores. The spores may be spherical, oval or elongated in shape. The spores may be narrower than the cell or broader causing bulging of parent cell. Spores may occupy terminal, subterminal or central (equatorial) position. In *Clostridium* species the spores are broader than bacillary body and gives a swollen appearance, resembling a spindle. Bacteria may be classified based on the shape and position of spores.

1. Spores are spherical in shape and terminal in position and broader than vegetative cell giving the bacillus a drum-stick appearacne, *e.g., Clostridium tetani.*

2. Spores are oval in shape and terminal in position and broader than parent cell, giving the bacillus a tennis racket appearance, *e.g., Clostridium tertium.*

3. Spores are oval and subterminal in position between the center and one of the poles of the bacillus and broader than parent cell casuing bulging, *e.g., Clostridium welchii (perfringens), Clostridium septicum, Clostridium sporogenes.*

4. Spores are spherical and equatorial in position; narrower than parent cell and do not bulge cell, *e.g., Bacillus anthracis.*

Demonstration of Spores. The spores can be demonstrated by several methods.

1. Spores are seen as refractile bodies within parent cell in unstained preparations, under phase-contrast microscope.

2. Spores can be seen as unstained haloes (clear space) in stained cell protoplasm in simple stains and Gram's staining, since spores resist coloration.

3. Spores are slightly acid-fast and may be stained differentially by a modificaiton of Ziehl-Neelsen's staining.

4. Spores can be demonstrated by special staining methods –

Uses of Spores :

1. Spores are used to define sterilisation process.

2. The spores of *Bacillus stearothermophilus* are used as sterilisation controls to determine the efficiency of moist heat sterilisation by biological testing. Its spores are killed at 121°C for 12 minutes by moist heat.

PLEOMORPHISM AND INVOLUTION FORMS

During the course of growth, bacteria of a single strain may exhibit variation in size and shape, a phenomenon known as pleomorphism. The cells may become swollen, spherical, pear-shaped, elongated filaments and filaments with localized swellings. These abnormal cells are called "involution forms". This phenomenon is commonly seen in *Streptobacillus moniliformis, Yersinia pestis, Neisseria gonorrhoeae* and *Corynebacterium diphtheriae.*

Pleomorphism occurs in ageing cultures on artificial media, particularly in the presence of antagonistic substances such as penicillin, sodium chloride. These involution forms are non-viable; some of them may grow and revert back to normal form when transferred to a suitable medium.

PROTOPLAST

A protoplast is a cell wall deficient microbial form, bounded by cytoplasmic membrane and do not contain any cell wall material.

Protoplasts are readily produced from Gram positive bacteria by treatment with lysozyme enzyme or egg-white which lyses mucopeptide linkages. Protoplasts are osmotically sensitive or fragile and undergo rapid lysis in hypotonic or isotonic solutions. Because of this protoplasts can be maintained in intact form only in hypertonic solutions. Protoplasts when maintained in osmotically protective medium, they remain viable, metabolize and grow. They do not divide or multiply. They cannot form cell wall and cannot revert back to their parent form.

SPHEROPLASTS

Spheroplast is a cell wall deficient microbial form differs from protoplast in that it contains outer membrane and some amount of cell wall material.

Spheroplasts are readily produced from Gram negative bacilli in the presence of penicillin and other antibiotics, which inhibit the synthesis of peptidoglycan; or by culturing on media lacking nutrients such as diaminopimelic acid, lysine or a hexosamine derivative, which are required for cell wall synthesis.

Spheroplasts are not as osmotically sensitive as protoplasts, since they contain residual cell wall material. Spheroplasts may reproduce and multiply and are capable of growing on ordinary agar medium. They can synthesize their cell wall and revert back to their original parent form when transferred to a medium lacking cell wall inhibitor.

L-FORMS (L-PHASE) OF BACTERIA

L-forms were discovered by Klieneberger-Nobel (1935, 1942) in *Streptobacillus moniliformis*, at Lister Institute, London; hence the name.

L-forms are cell wall deficient, capable of multiplication and develop either spontaneously, or in the presence of antibiotics which inhibit cell wall synthesis such as penicillin or chemical agents such as salt (NaCl). In other words, protoplasts and spheroplasts that are capable of multiplicaiton are called L-forms. L-forms are usually unstable, and their morphological abnormality is maintained only in the presence of inducing agents and may revert back to their normal parent form, when inducing agent is absent. Some times L-forms may be stable, and become permanent feature of the organism and cannot revert back to their parent form, even in the absence of inducing agent. For example, Mycoplasmas represent stable L-forms derived from an unknown parent form.

L-forms do not possess definite shape and size, because of the absence of cell wall. They vary in size from minute bodies of 0.1 μ to 10 – 20 μ in diameter. The smallest forms can pass through bacteria-stopping filters. Their shape varies, may occur as granules and filaments of various sizes. The granules may be coccoid, balloon, disc, ring or star shaped. The filaments are slender of varying lengths.

The colonies of L-phase organisms are typically biphasic and exhibit fried-egg appearance with a central, opaque, dark, thick centre extending deep into the medium surrounded by a lace like textured flat, translucent peripheral zone. Since the colonies are highly fragile, L-forms are best examined in situ in an agar block bearing the growth under microscope. L-forms can be maintained by culturing in a soft agar medium containing 20% horse serum.

QUESTIONS

Long Essay

1. Describe briefly the anatomy of bacterial cell.

Short Notes

1. Cell envelope.
2. Bacterial cell wall.
3. Periplasmic space.
4. Porins.
5. Lysozyme.
6. Draw a neat diagram of bacterial cell and label its parts.
7. Mesosomes.
8. Volutin granules or Metachromatic granules or Babes-Ernst granules.
9. Bacterial nucleus.
10. Capsule or bacterial capsule.
11. Negative staining.
12. Capsule swelling reaction or quellung reaction.
13. Plasmids or episomes.
14. Filamentous appendages of bacteria.
15. Bacterial flagellae.
16. Fimbriae or pili.
17. Sex pili.
18. Bacterial spores or endospores.
19. Pleomorphism and involution forms.
20. Protoplasts.
21. Spheroplasts.
22. What are the similarities and differences between protoplasts and spheroplasts ?
23. L-forms.

6

Bacterial Nutrition

- *Nutritional classification*
- *Autotrophs or Lithotrophs*
  - *– Photoautotrophs or Photolithotrophs*
  - *– Chemoautotrophs or Chemolithotrophs*
- *Heterotrophs or organotrophs*
  - *– Photoheterotrophs or Photoorganotrophs*
  - *– Chemoheterotrophs or chemoorganotrophs*
- *Nutritional requirements of bacteria*
  - *– Water*
  - *– Source of energy*
  - *– Source of carbon*
  - *– Source of nitrogen*
  - *– Hydrogen, oxygen, sulfur and phosphorous*
  - *– Macronutrients/Inorganic salts/minerals*
  - *– Micronutrients/Trace elements*
  - *– Growth factors/bacterial vitamins*
- *Physical (Environmental) growth requirements of bacteria*
  - *– Oxygen requirement*
  - *– Carbondioxide requirement-capnophiles*
  - *– O-R potential (Eh)*
  - *– pH*
  - *– Temperature*
  - *– Light*
  - *– Effect of moisture and desiccation*
  - *– Effect of osmotic pressure*
  - *– Effect of mechanical and sonic stress*

NUTRITIONAL CLASSIFICATION

Bacteria may be classified nutritionally into various nutritional forms.

I. Based on energy requirements, bacteria are classified into two types.

1. Phototrophs – derive energy from sunlight
2. Chemotrophs – derive energy from oxidation of chemical compounds.

II. Based on the ability to synthesize essential metabolites, bacteria are classified into two types.

1. Autotrophs (Lithotrophs) – can synthesize their own metabolites.

2. Heterotrophs (organotrophs) – cannot synthesize their own metabolites, hence, depend upon preformed readymade organic compounds.

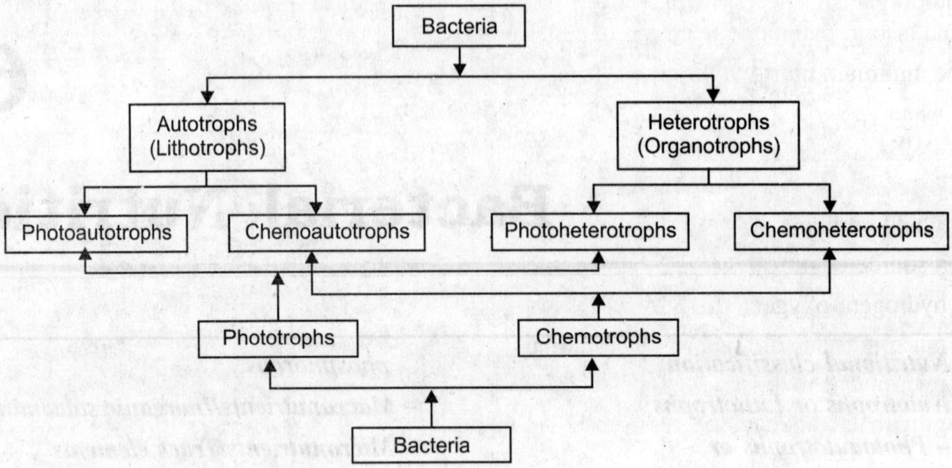

Fig. 6.1

AUTOTROPHS (OR) LITHOTROPHS

They can utilise atmospheric CO_2 and are capable of independent existence in soil and water. They are vitally important in agriculture and maintenance of soil fertility; they are of no medical importance.

Autotrophs can be further subdivided into two groups.

Photoautotrophs/photolithotrophs/photosynthetic autotrophs. They utilise sunlight as a primary source of energy and carry out photosynthesis to synthesize organic compounds from CO_2, *e.g., Chlorobium, Chromatium, Cyanobacteria.*

Chemoautotrophs/chemolithotrophs. They derive their energy by oxidation of inorganic compounds. Chemoautotrophs can be further subclassified into groups based on the type of inorganic compound used as a source of energy. *e.g.,* Nitrifying bacteria, sulphur bacteria, iron bacteria, hydrogen bacteria.

HETEROTROPHS (ORGANOTROPHS)

They cannot synthesize their own metabolites and depend upon preformed readymade organic compounds such as amino acids, nucleotides, lipids, carbohydrates and growth factors or coenzymes.

Heterotrophs are further subclassified into two groups.

Photoheterotrophs/photoorganotrophs. They utilise sunlight as a source of energy and organic compounds such as alcohols, fatty acids and amino acids as a source of carbon. *e.g., Rhodospirillum.*

Chemoheterotrophs/chemoorganotrophs. Majority of heterotrophs are chemoheterotrophs. They utilise organic compounds as a source of energy as well as directly as a source of carbon. They constitute medically important bacteria, that can be grouped into commensals and parasites. Parasitic bacteria may be pathogens or nonpathogens. *e.g., Salmonella typhi, Mycobacterium tuberculosis.*

NUTRITIONAL REQUIREMENTS OF BACTERIA

Microorganisms need a variety of chemical compounds as nutrients for their growth and multiplication and also to maintain the structure and organization of the cell.

The minimum nutritional requirements are

1. water
2. a source energy
3. a source of carbon (for the majority of bacteria, the same nutrient may serve both the purposes of energy and carbon).
4. a source of nitrogen
5. hydrogen, oxygen, sulphur and phosphorous
6. macronutrients/inorganic salts/minerals
7. micronutrients/trace elements
8. growth factors/bacterial vitamins.

Water

Water is the major constituent of bacterial cell and an integral part of the protoplasm. It is a prime nutritional requirement. Water participates in the metabolic reactions and acts as a medium for the entry of nutrients and for the excretion of waste products. Thus, water acts as a life supporting medium.

Source of Energy

Bacteria which derive their energy from sunlight are called phototrophs and those that obtain energy from chemical reactions are called chemotrophs. Usually carbohydrates are the sources of energy; amino acids and nucleotides may also serve as energy source. For the majority of bacteria the same nutrient may serve both the purposes of energy and carbon.

Source of Carbon

Carbon is one of the most important chemical required as building block for microbial growth. All microorganisms require carbon in some or other form.

The microorganisms that use organic compounds such as carbohydrates, lipids, aminoacids, nucleotides as their major carbon source are called heterotrophs; and those that use CO_2 as sole source of carbon are called autotrophs.

Source of Nitrogen

Nitrogen is the essential part of aminoacids, that together form proteins. Nitrogen serves mainly as a source of structural unit. Bacteria are particularly versatile in the utilization of nitrogen. Some bacteria use atmospheric gaseous nitrogen for cell synthesis through a process called nitrogen fixation, which is vital for the maintenance of soil fertility in agriculture. Others use inorganic nitrogen compounds such as nitrates, nitrites or ammonium salts, while some require organic nitrogen compounds such as amino acids or peptides.

Hydrogen, Oxygen, Sulfur and Phosphorous

Hydrogen and oxygen form part of many organic compounds. Water also serves as the source of hydrogen and oxygen. Hydrogen serves as the main electron donor and oxygen as the chief electron acceptor. Sulphur and phosphorous, the constituents of certain aminoacids and nucleotides are also required in smaller amounts. Phosphorous is essential for the synthesis of ATP and nucleic acids. ATP is a compound that is extremely important for energy storage and transfer. Sulphur is needed for the biosynthesis of the aminoacids cysteine, cystine and methionine.

Macronutrients/Inorganic Salts/Minerals

Bacteria require a supply of inorganic salts, particularly the anions phosphates, sulphates and the cations sodium, potassium, magnesium, iron, and calcium. These are normally present in the natural environments where bacteria live, but will have to be supplied in culture media.

Micronutrients/Trace Elements

Most microorganisms require manganese, zinc, copper, cobalt, molybdenum, selenium, boron and nickel in minute quantities. These trace elements are usually supplied in adequate amounts as impurities in major inorganic salts.

Growth Factors/Bacterial Vitamins

Some bacteria require certain organic compounds in minute quantities for growth. These are known as growth factors. In many cases, these growth factors are identical with the vitamins belonging to the B-complex group and hence known as "Bacterial vitamins".

e.g., Hemophilus influenzae requires X and V factors

Salmonella typhi requires tryptophan

Gonococci requires glutathione

Brucella abortus requires niacin

Growth factors may be of two types :

1. ***Essential growth factors.*** They are essential for the growth and the growth does not occur in their absence.

2. ***Accessory growth factors.*** They are not essential for the growth, but when present can enhance growth.

PHYSICAL/ENVIRONMENTAL GROWTH REQUIREMENTS

Bacteria require environmental factors for growth in optimum concentrations. They are as follows:

1. Oxygen
2. Carbondioxide
3. Oxidation-reduction potential (Eh)
4. pH
5. Temperature
6. Light
7. Moisture and drying
8. Osmotic effect
9. Mechanical and sonic stress.

Oxygen requirement

The proper oxygen tension is essential for balanced growth. The bacteria which require oxygen for growth are known as "**Aerobes**"and those that do not require oxygen are known as "**Anaerobes**".

Based on the influence of oxygen on growth and viability, bacteria may be classified into different groups.

1. ***Obligate aerobes.*** They grow only in the presence of oxygen. Oxygen is used as terminal electron acceptor. *e.g., Pseudomonas, Mycobacterium.*

2. ***Facultative anaerobes.*** They can grow in the presence or absence of oxygen. *e.g.,* Staphylococci, *Salmonella, E.coli.*

3. ***Microaerophiles.*** They are aerobes which grow best with less oxygen than found in air *e.g., Campylobacter.*

4. ***Obligate anaerobes.*** They can grow only in the absence of oxygen, presence of small amounts of oxygen may be toxic and kills the bacterium. They do not use oxygen as an electron acceptor. Anaerobic bacteria use nitrates and sulphates (inorganic compounds) as terminal electron acceptors. In the absence of oxygen, energy is produced by fermentation. *e.g., Clostridium, Bacteroides.*

5. ***Aerotolerant anaerobes.*** They are anaerobes which are not readily killed by oxygen. *e.g.,* most Streptococci, *and* Lactobacilli.

In the presence of oxygen, hydrogen peroxide, superoxide radicals and other toxic peroxides accumulate. The enzymes superoxide dismutase and catalase, which splits superoxide radicals and hydrogen peroxide is present only in aerobic bacteria but absent in anaerobes. Moreover, obligate anaerobes may possess enzymes that are active only in the reduced state.

Carbondioxide requirement

All bacteria require small amounts of carbondioxide for their growth. This is provided by the atmospheric air or endogenously by the metabolic reactions within the cell.

Capnophiles. Some bacteria grow best at a high CO_2 tension than those found in atmosphere. Several bacteria are stimulated by partial pressures that are greater than those normally found in air. These bacteria, which have high CO_2 requirement are called capnophilic bacteria. *e.g., Brucella,* gonococci, meningococci etc. require 3–10% CO_2 for their primary isolation from clinical specimens. Hence, these cultures are incubated in a CO_2 incubator (capnoeic incubator) or candle jar, that provides 3–10% CO_2.

Oxidation-Reduction Potential (Eh) Requirement

The growth of the aerobic and anaerobic bacteria is greatly dependent upon the oxidised or reduced state of the environment than the presence or absence of oxygen.

For most bacteria, the optimum Eh is about + 0.2 to + 0.4 millivolts at pH 7. Obligate anaerobes are unable to grow, unless the Eh is atleast as low as – 0.2 millivolts.

During the growth of both aerobic and anaerobic bacteria, there is a progressive decrease in the Eh of the environment.

pH requirement

Bacteria are very sensitive to variations in pH. Each microorganism has a "**pH range**" and the growth does not occur above the maximum or below the minimum of this range. Every microorganism has a well-defined pH optimum, at which it grows best. Majority of bacteria grow best at neutral or very slightly alkaline reaction *i.e.,* 7.2 to 7.6. These are called **neutrophiles**, since they grow at and around neutral pH. But some microorganisms grow best at acidic pH, known as "**acidophiles**". *e.g.,* Lactobacilli. Fungi and yeasts grow best at acidic pH. Some bacteria are very sensitive to acid, but tolerant of alkali and grow at alkaline pH. They are known as "**alkaliphiles** or **basophiles**". *e.g., Vibrio cholerae* grows at a pH of 8.5 to 9.

The pH of a culture medium is adjusted by adding NaOH (alkali) if the pH is acidic or HCl (acid) if the pH is alkaline.

Temperature requirement

Bacteria differ in their requirements of temperature for growth. For each species, there is a "**temperature range**", and growth does not occur above the maximum or below the minimum of the range. The temperature at which growth occurs best is known as the "**optimum temperature**". Most pathogenic bacteria grow best at an optimum temperature of 37°C. In the laboratory, bacteria are grown at this optimum temperature in a thermostatically controlled incubator.

Based on temperature requirement, microorganisms can be broadly classified into five groups :

1. Psychrophiles
2. Mesophiles
3. Thermophiles

Psychrophilic bacteria are those which grow best at temperatures below 20°C, usually quite well at 0°C and in some cases even at – 7°C. These microorganisms grow in refrigerated and frozen foods and cause spoilage.

Mesophilic bacteria are those which grow at a temperature range of 25 to 40°C. Some mesophiles have a wide growth temperature range *e.g.,* 5 to 43°C for *Pseudomonas aeruginosa*; whereas some others have a more restricted range of temperature *e.g.,* 30 to 39°C for gonococci. A few mesophiles can grow at temperatures below 5°C, as in a domestic refrigerator or at temperatures above 45°C.

Many saprophytes of soil and water are mesophilic. Parasites of humans and warm-blooded animals are also mesophilic.

Thermophilic bacteria are those which grow at high temperatures between 55 and 80°C. They are usually non-parasitic. They may cause spoilage of under processed canned foods. Some bacteria such as *Bacillus stearothermophilus* and *Clostridium botulinum* form spores that are extremely heat resistant.

Light requirement. Many bacteria, except phototrophic organisms require darkness for growth and viability. Sunlight, UV light and ionizing radiations can kill microorganisms. Hence, cultures are incubated in an incubator under dark to protect them from sunlight, clinical specimens containing meningococci. *e.g.,* CSF, should not be exposed to sunlight.

Effect of Moisture and Desiccation

There is a wide variation in the ability of bacteria to survive drying. Bacterial spores (*e.g.,* anthrax spores, tetanus spores) are extremely resistant to desiccation and can survive many years in a moisture free environment.

Vegetative bacteria are much less resistant to drying and require moisture. It is for this reason culture media should be fresh and contain water of condensation. Otherwise delicate organisms like Streptococci, gonococci and meningococci cannot grow well.

Treponema pallidum and gonococci cannot withstand drying and die quickly whereas *Staphylococcus aureus*, tubercle bacillus can withstand drying for weeks.

Delicate, nonsporing organisms can survive drying for many years, if they are desiccated rapidly, completely while frozen and maintained in vacuum in the dark. This is the basis of preservation of cultures by "**Freeze-drying** or **Lyophilisaiton**".

Effect of Osmotic Pressure

Bacteria are more tolerant to osmotic variation than most other cells due to the mechanical strength of their cell walls.

When bacteria are placed in hypertonic solution (*e.g.,* 20% NaCl), water (solvent) passes out, from the interior of the cell through semipermeable cell membranes, into the solution surrounding the cell (by osmosis), so that cells become dehydrated, resulting in shrinkage of cell. This phenomenon is called "**Plasmolysis**". Here, the cell wall retains the original shape and size, appearing as bacterial ghost. Plasmolysis occurs more readily in Gram negative than in Gram positive bacteria.

Some bacteria can grow and tolerate high salt concentrations. They are known as halophilic organisms, usually found in sea water. Some pathogenic bacteria such as *Staphylococcus aureus* can grow in the presence of 8–10% NaCl and *Enterococcus* at a concentration of 6.5% NaCl.

When bacteria are placed in hypotonic solution (*e.g.,* distilled water, 0.01% NaCl), the water enters the cell from the surroundings causing swelling and may even burst the cell. This phenomenon is called "**Plasmoptysis**" or "**Imbibition**".

Effect of mechanical and sonic stress. Though bacteria have tough cell walls, they may be ruptured by mechanical stresses, such as grinding or vigorous shaking with glass beads. They may also be disintegrated by exposure to ultrasonic vibrations.

QUESTIONS

Essay Type Questions:

1. What are the heterotrophic bacteria ? Discuss the nutritional and physical requirements for the growth of the bacteria.

Short Notes:

1. Heterotrophs.
2. Growth factors/bacterial vitamins.
3. Oxygen requirement of bacteria.
4. Capnophilies.
5. Psychrophiles.
6. Thermophiles.
7. Mesophiles.
8. Lyophilisation/freeze drying.
9. Plasmolysis.
10. Plasmoptysis.

7

Growth and Multiplication of Bacteria

- *Reproduction in bacteria*
- *Generation time/Population doubling time*
- *Batch cultures*
- *Bacterial counts*
  - *– Total count*
  - *– Viable count*
- *Bacterial growth curve*
- *Continuous cultures*

REPRODUCTION IN BACTERIA

Bacteria reproduce asexually by transverse binary fission. When a bacterium size increases and reaches its critical stage, it divides and produces two daughter cells. Bacterial cell division consists of following stages :

1. DNA replication. The two strands of DNA separate and each strand replicates to form a new complementary strand. Nucleus replicates by simple fission. Mitosis is absent.

2. The replicated double stranded DNA molecules are distributed into two daughter cells equally.

3. The cell divides into two by an inward growth of cytoplasmic membrane across the cell, known as transverse septum or cross wall. Mesosome (chondroid) attached to the cytoplasmic membrane plays an important role in the formation of transverse septum. This is followed by the formation of cell wall material, and finally the two daughter cells separate. Sometimes, the daughter cells may remain together, even after cell division.

GENERATION TIME/POPULATION DOUBLING TIME

The time required for a cell to divide to form two daughter cells or the interval of time between two cell divisions is known as generation time or population doubling time.

Bacteria multiply by binary fission, in which each cell produces two daughter cells. Thus, if we start with a single bacterium, the increase in population is by geometric progression :

$$1 \rightarrow 2 \rightarrow 2^2 \rightarrow 2^3 \rightarrow 2^4 \rightarrow 2^5 \dashrightarrow 2^n$$

Therefore, a single bacterial cell can theoretically give rise to 10^{21} progeny in 24 hours.

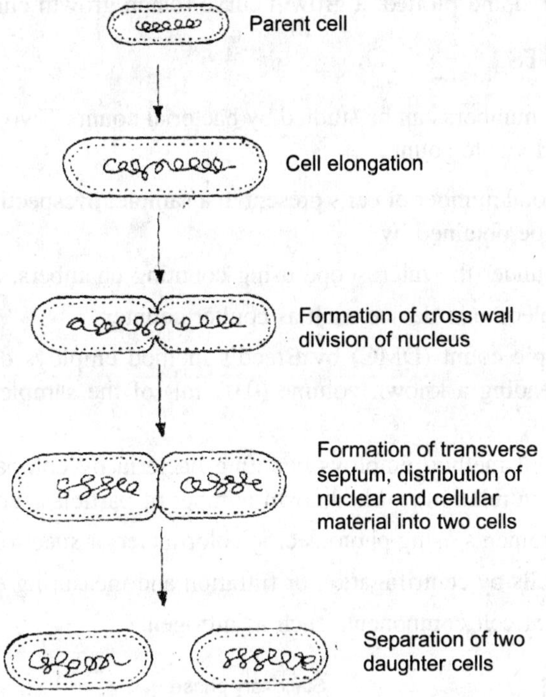

Fig. 7.1 Reproduction/multiplication of bacteria by transverse binary fission.

Table 7.1 Generation times of some bacteria

Microorganism	*Generation time*
Escherichia coli	20 minutes
Staphylococcus aureus	30 minutes
Mycobacterium tuberculosis	20–24 hours
Mycobacterium leprae	20–30 days

The generation time of most of the medically important bacteria is about 20 minutes. It varies with the species and environmental conditions. Generation times in nature are usually much longer than in culture media.

BATCH CULTURE

When microorganisms are cultivated in a liquid medium, in a closed system such as in a conical flask or a large fermentor vessel; that is when they are incubated and grown in a single batch of medium, the multiplication of bacteria, after some time, comes to a halt, due to depletion of nutrients and accumulation of toxic waste metabolites; because no fresh medium is provided during incubation. Such culture is known as "Batch culture" and grown each time by inculating into fresh medium, in batches. Such a closed system culture is very useful in studying the growth characters of microorganisms.

If the number of cells present at different time intervals after inoculation, in a limited volume of liquid medium is measured and plotted, a growth curve (batch growth curve) is obtained (Fig. 7.2).

BACTERIAL COUNTS

Bacterial growth in numbers can be studied by bacterial counts. Two types of bacterial counts can be made. Total count and viable count.

Total count is the total number of cells present in a sample, irrespective of whether they are living or not. Total counts can be obtained by

1. Direct counting under the microscope using counting chambers.
2. Counting in an electronic device such as coulter counter.
3. Direct microscopic count (DMC) by Breed's method employs direct counting using stained smears prepared by spreading a known volume (0.01 ml) of the sample over a measured area (one square cm) of a slide.
4. Proportional count method employs counting bacteria by comparing the number of cells in smears in proportion (or in relation) to the known number of particles such as tiny plastic beads.
5. Turbidity measurements using photoelectric colorimeter or spectrophotometer or nephalometer.
6. Separating the cells by centrifugation or filtration and measuring their wet or dry weight.
7. Chemical assay of cell components such as nitrogen.

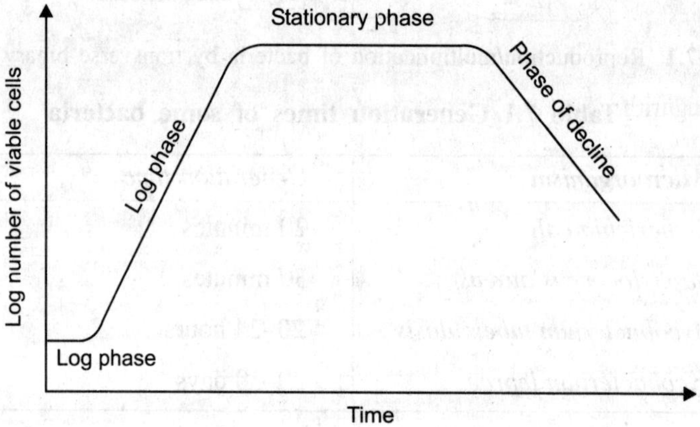

Fig. 7.2 (*a*) Growth curve for viable count.

Viable count measures only those cells capable of growing and producing a colony on a suitable nutrient medium. In other words, it measures the number of living cells, that is, cells capable of multiplication.

Viable counts are obtained by

1. Standard plate count (SPC) by pour plate method,
2. Membrane filter method, and
3. Mean probable number (MPN) or presumptive coliform count used in the bacteriological analysis of water.

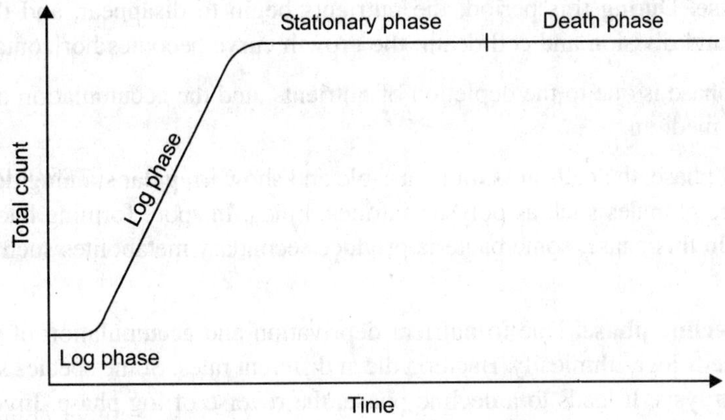

Fig. 7.2 (*b*) Growth curve for total count

BACTERIAL GROWTH CURVE

Growth curve is a graphic representation of rate of multiplication (or number) of cells plotted against time. For all organisms including microbes the growth curve is sigmoid.

When bacteria are cultivated in a liquid medium, in a closed system and bacterial counts are made at regular time intervals and plotted in relation to time; a growth curve is obtained. The growth curve shows four distinct phases Fig.7.2.

1. Lag phase.
2. Log phase/Logarithmic phase/Exponential phase.
3. Stationary phase
4. Death phase/phase of decline.

1. Lag phase. When a microorganism is inoculated into a fresh culture medium, usually no immediate increase in cell numbers or mass occurs because no cell division occurs. Therefore, this period is called the lag phase. It is the time taken by the organism to adjust physiologically to the given conditions and build up an internal supply of metabolites.

The duration of the lag phase varies with the species, amount of inoculum, nature of culture medium and environmental factors such as pH, temperature etc. The bacteria will have maximum size towards the end of lag phase.

Log phase/Logrithmic phase/Exponential phase. Following the lag phase, the cells grow at constant rate, start dividing by binary fission and their numbers increase exponentially or by geometric progression with time. There is a linear relationship (strength line on the graph) between the time and logarithm of the number of cells. That is why, sometimes infection overtakes body defences and gets out of control.

During log phase the cells are smaller in size, young, actively multiplying, the metabolic activity is at its peak, and the population is most uniform in terms of chemical and physiological properties, and stain uniformly. Therefore, log phase is most suitable for studying biochemical and physiological properties of cells.

Stationary phase. During this period, the nutrients begin to disappear, and there is a balance between cell growth and division and cell death; the growth curve becomes horizontal or plateau.

The stationary phase is due to the depletion of nutrients, and the accumulation of toxic metabolic wastes in the culture medium.

In the stationary phase, the cells are Gram variable and show irregular staining due to the presence of intracellular storage granules such as polysaccharides, lipids. In spore forming bacteria, sporulation occurs in this phase. In this phase, some bacteria produce secondary metabolites such as exotoxins and antibiotics.

Death phase/Decline phase. Due to nutrient deprivation and accumulation of toxic metabolites leads to the death of cells logarithmically. Bacteria die at different rates. Some species such as gonococci die rapidly due to autolysis. It leads to a decline phase, the reverse of log phase. Involution forms are common in phase of decline.

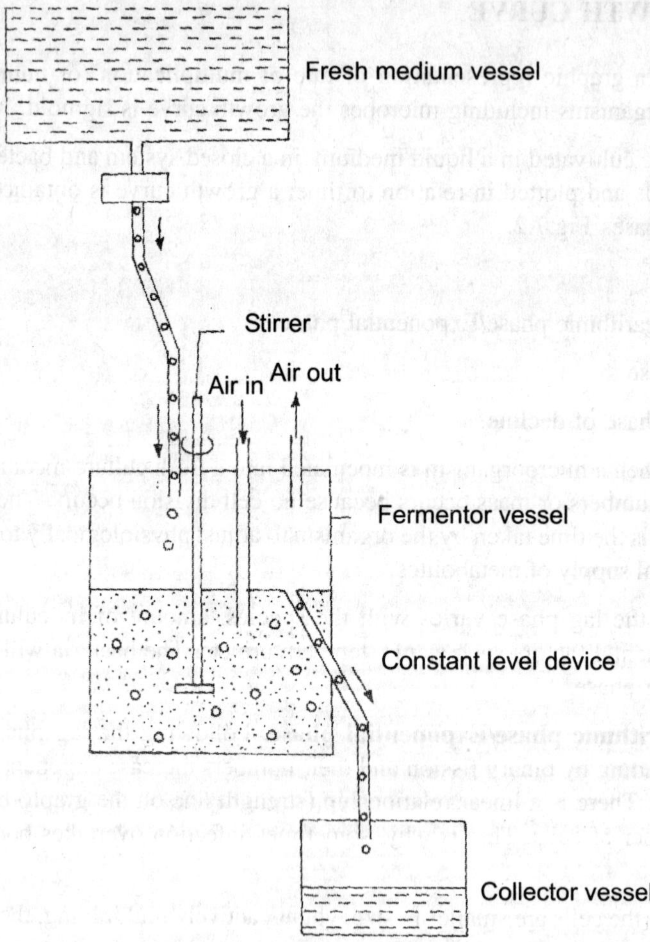

Fig. 7.3 Chemostat for continuous cultures

CONTINUOUS CULTURES

Batch culture is the usual method of growing bacteria. However, it is possible to grow microorganisms in an open system, through continuous provision of nutrients and removal of wastes, so that cells continuously multiply and remain in logarithmic phase and at a constant biomass concentration. This method is called continuous culture, may be similar to a situation occurring in human and animal disease.

Continuous cultures are useful, 1. for the production of industrially important fermentation products, 2. in selective isolation of certain rare microorganisms and, 3. for research studies, to obtain population at logarithmic phase, which can grow continuously in limiting concentrations of nutrients.

Chemostat. It is a continuous system cultivator in which the sterile nutrient medium is continuously fed into the culture vessel at the same rate as media containing waste products, old and dead cells of microorganisms is removed. The level of growth is controlled by maintaining in fixed, limiting concentration of an essential nutrient.

QUESTIONS

Short Notes

1. Reproduction in bacteria/binary fission.
2. Generation time/population doubling time.
3. Batch culture.
4. Bacterial counts.
5. Total count.
6. Viable count.
7. Bacterial growth curve/growth phases of bacteria.
8. Continuous cultures.
9. Chemostat.

8

Sterilization

- *Introduction*
- *Definition*
- *Sterilization methods*
- *Heat sterilization*
  - *Dry heat sterilization*
    - *Red heat*
    - *Flaming*
    - *Incineration or burning*
    - *Hot air oven*
    - *Sterilization controls*
  - *Moist heat sterilization*
    - *Mode of action of steam*
    - *Moist heat below 100°C*
    - *Inspissation*
  - *Moist heat at 100°C*
    - *Tyndallization*
  - *Moist heat at above 100°C*
    - *Autoclaving*
  - *Sterilization controls*
- *Ionizing radiation/Cold sterilization*
  - *Gamma rays*
- *Gaseous chemosterilizers*
  - *Ethylene oxide*
  - *Formaldehyde gas/fumigation*
  - *Beta propiolactone*
- *Liquid chemosterilizers*
  - *Formalin solution*
  - *Glutaraldehyde (cidex)*
  - *Iodine*
- *Filtration*
  - *Applications*
  - *Types of bacterial filters*
  - *Diatomaceous earthenware candle filters*
  - *Unglazed porcelain/ceramic filters*
  - *Asbestos disk (seitz) filters*
  - *Sintered glass filters*
  - *Membrane filters*
  - *Sterilization controls*

INTRODUCTION

The sterilization procedures are important particularly in the microbiological laboratories and in hospital practice. In microbiological work the sterilization of culture media, glass ware, containers and instruments is essential for the isolation and maintenance of pure cultures. In hospital practice, the sterilization of instruments, dressings, drugs and other supplies is important for the prevention of infection.

Sterilization procedures are also important and widely practiced in food, drug and pharmaceutical industries.

DEFINITION

Sterilization can be defined as a process by which any article, surface, culture medium, specimen or material is freed from all living microorganisms including vegetative cells and their spores.

METHODS OF STERILIZATION

Sterilization may be accomplished by physical, chemical and mechanical methods.

Physical Methods

I. Heat. A. *Dry heat* :

1. Red heat
2. Flaming
3. Incineration or burning
4. Hot air oven

B. *Moist heat* (*steaming*)

1. Steaming below 100°C or below atmospheric pressure
   – Inspissation
2. Steaming at 100°C or at atmospheric pressure
   – Tyndallization
3. Steaming under pressure, above 100°C or above atmospheric pressures
   – Autoclaving

II. Ionizing radiation (cold sterilization)

– Gamma rays
– Particulate high energy electrons.

Chemical methods/chemosterilants/chemical sporicidal agents

III. Gaseous chemosterilizers

1. Ethylene oxide gas
2. Formaldehyde gas
3. Betapropiolactone

IV. Liquid chemosterilizers

1. Formalin (formaldehyde solution)
2. Glutaraldehyde solution
3. Iodine

V. Filtration

1. Diatomaceous earthenware candle filters *e.g.*, Berkefeld filters, Mandler filters.
2. Unglazed, porcelain filters *e.g.*, Chamberland filters.

3. Asbestos disk filters *e.g.,* Seitz filters.
4. Sintered glass filters (fritted glass filters/Morton filters).
5. Membrane filters (ultra filters).

HEAT STERILIZATION

Heat is the simplest and reliable means of sterilization. Practical procedures by which heat is employed are divided into 2 categories – dry heat and moist heat.

A. Dry Heat Sterilization

The lethal effect of dry heat is due to :

– oxidative damage to cell constituents
– protein denaturation
– increased levels of electrolytes.

1. Red heat. Inoculation wires, wire loops, points of forceps and spatulas are held in Bunsen flame till they become red hot, to sterilize them.

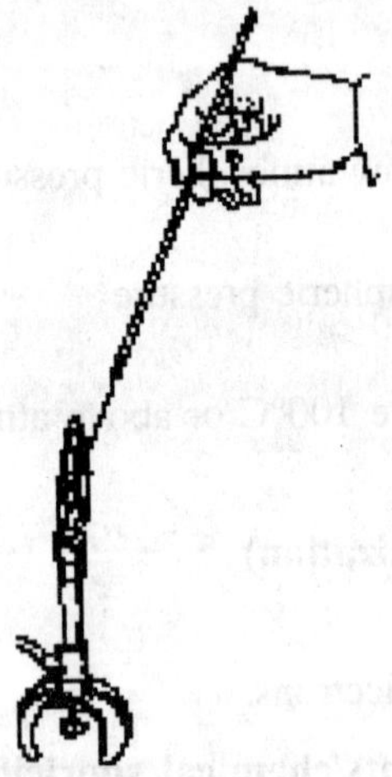

Fig. 8.1 Method of sterilization by read heat (dry heat). Inoculation loop heated to redness before and after inoculation. Aseptic technique to prevent contamination.

If inoculation loops contain infectious proteinaceous material, it should be washed in chemical disinfectant before heating to avoid the spread of infected particles by spattering.

2. Flaming. Scalpels, needles, necks of flasks, mouths of culture tubes, glass slides, coverslips etc. could be passed a few times through the bunsen flame without allowing them to become red hot.

Needles, scalpels, basins, inoculation loops are sometimes treated by immersing in methylated spirit and burning off the alcohol

3. Incineration or burning. It is an efficient method for the sterilization and disposal of hazardous infectious hospital waste. Soiled dressings, pathological materials, animal carcasses, infected linen/bedding, sharp needles and other clinical waste are literally burned to ashes at temperatures of 870°C to 980°C in incinerator by electricity.

Plastics such as disposable syringes, rubber catheters, culture plates, specimen containers made of polyvinyl chloride (PVC) and polyethylene may emit dense black smoke when incinerated. They can be autoclaved before disposal.

4. Hot air oven/Hot air sterilizer. It is the most important, widely used and the best method of sterilization by dry heat.

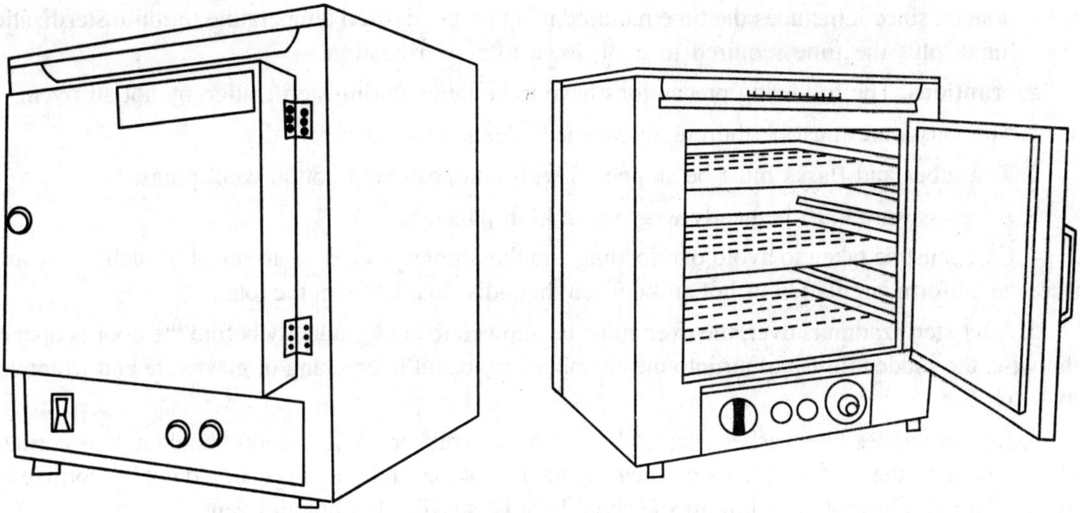

Fig. 8.2 Hot air oven.

Principle. Dry heat is transferred from source to load (article) by conduction or radiation. Since hot air is a bad conductor of heat with less penetrating power; high temperatures and long exposure times are required for dry heat sterilization than moist heat sterilization.

Uses. Hot air oven is used for the sterilization of following items :

1. Glass ware such as test tubes, conical flasks (or any other flasks), petri plates, pipettes, measuring cylinders, ampoules etc.

2. Glass syringes.

3. Surgical metal instruments like needles, fine cannulae, forceps, scissors, scalpels etc.

4. Materials such as oils, petroleum jelly, waxes, glycerol, fats, grease and liquid paraffin which are impervious to steam.

5. Sulphonamides.

6. Powders, talc, dusting powder that may form paste by steam can be sterilized by dry heat in hot air oven.

Cotton wool plugs, wrappings of kraft paper, aluminium tins, aluminium tubes, aluminium foils may be used to retain sterility after processing.

Structure of hot-air oven. Hot air oven consists of an insulated double walled cabinet made of aluminium or stainless steel and is constructed to withstand high temperatures. It is heated by electricity and has a thermostat, which regulates the temperature inside the chamber at a desired level, and a thermometer is fitted for recording the temperature. Large hot air ovens may have a motor and fan fitted either at the bottom or back of the oven to circulate hot air uniformly throughout the chamber. The shelves (partitions) within the oven are perforated to ensure proper air circulation.

Temperature and holding period used for sterilization. Sterilization in hot air oven is done by two methods :

(*i*) using a temperature of 160°C for one hour

(*ii*) using a temperature of 180°C for 30 minutes. Infact, the total heating cycle time is much longer, since it includes the time required to attain the desired temperature, prior to sterilization time, plus the time required to cool down after sterilization.

Precautions. The following precautions have to be taken during sterilization by hot air oven.

1. The glassware must be thoroughly washed, cleaned and perfectly dry.

2. Test tubes and flasks must be stoppered with non-absorbent cotton wool plugs.

3. All glass ware must be neatly wrapped in kraft paper.

4. Care must be taken to avoid overloading and the articles should be arranged in such a way as to ensure the uniform circulation of hot air between the individual items in the load.

5. After sterilization is over, the oven must be allowed to cool gradually before the door is opened. Otherwise, the sudden inrush of air into the chamber may result in cracking of glassware and wrappings may catch fire.

6. Rubber articles like washers, caps, gloves, plastics, rubber tubings, corks should not be sterilized by hot air oven as they get melted by dry heat. Similarly fabrics and dressings should not be sterilized as they get charred. Fluids and culture media should not be sterilized in hot air oven.

Sterility tests for dry heat sterilization or sterilization controls for hot air oven.

To determine the efficiency of dry heat sterilization, various sterilization controls are employed. They are as follows :

Physical methods. 1. By recording temperature with centigrade thermometers.

2. Thermocouple measurement.

A thermocouple is inserted inside any article in the hot air oven chamber and its wire leads are carried out to a potentiometer which indicates the temperature inside the chamber during sterilization.

3. **Chemical methods – Browne's tube.** Browne's tube contains a red color indicator solution which turns green when adequate temperature is maintained for a fixed time by dry heat sterilization and is a convenient method for routine use.

4. **Biological method/bacteriological test.** For determining efficiency of dry heat sterilization by microbiological testing, paper strips impregnated with 10^6 spores of a non-toxigenic strain of *Clostridium tetani* are placed in envelopes and inserted into hot air oven chamber. After sterilization is over, the strips are taken out and inoculated into RCM broth or thioglycollate broth and incubated for sterility test under strict anaerobic conditions at 37°C for 5 days.

MOIST HEAT STERILIZATION

Moist heat (steaming) under pressure is the only method of sterilization that is both reliable, widely applicable and efficient and always should be the method of choice, wherever applicable.

Moist heat kills bacteria by

– denaturation of enzymes and proteins

– coagulation of cytoplasm.

1. Moist heat below 100°C or steaming below atmospheric pressure.

Inspissation and serum inspissator. Inspissation is a process used to sterilize and solidify culture media containing substances like serum, egg and other coagulable proteins, which cannot withstand high temperatures, in an apparatus called inspissator.

Culture media such as Lowenstein-Jensen (LJ) media, Dorset's egg media and Loeffler's serum slope are rendered sterile and solid, simultaneously by inspissation.

Inspissator consists of a chamber made of copper plate with a water jacket around it and the chamber can be closed with a glass lid. The temperature is regulated automatically by a thermostat. There are small openings in the inner wall communicating with the top of the water chamber above the level of the water, so that water vapor (steam) can enter the interior of the inspissator, and the medium is exposed to moist heat.

The tubes or bottles containing media are kept in a slanting position inside the chamber and exposed to a temperature of 80–85°C for 30 minutes on three successive days, without disturbing their position. Hence, the sterilization takes place by the principle of tyndallization. The first day heating kills all vegetative bacteria; spores, if present, being in a favorable medium, will germinate and be killed on subsequent heatings.

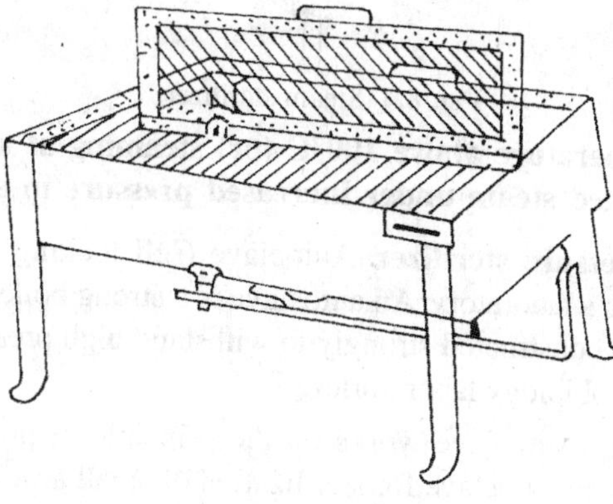

Fig. 8.3 Inspissator.

2. Moist heat at 100°C or steaming at atmospheric pressure –

Tyndallization/fractional sterilization/intermittent sterilization. This method was introduced by John Tyndall, hence known as Tyndallization.

This method is used to sterilize culture media which might damage at higher temperature, such as sugar media, media containing gelatin, milk etc., with a free-flowing steam at atmospheric pressure.

A Koch steamer or Arnold steamer is widely used for tyndallization. It is a vertical metal cylinder or rectangular vessel, with a removable conical lid, with an opening at the top for escaping of steam. At the bottom, there is a water reservoir, which can be heated either by using electricity or gas. A perforated tray situated above the water bears the articles to be sterilized.

The tubes and flasks plugged with cotton wool are arranged in wire baskets and covered with kraft paper to avoid damping of plugs with condensed steam.

The container and the medium are simultaneously sterilized. Tyndallization is done by heating to 100°C for 30 minutes (or 20 to 45 min.) on three successive days. The principle is that first exposure kills all vegetative bacteria, and between heatings, spores, if present, being in a favorable medium will germinate and be killed on second day and third day heatings. Since, sterilization is done by heating intermittently or in fractions, it is also called intermittent sterilization or fractional sterilization.

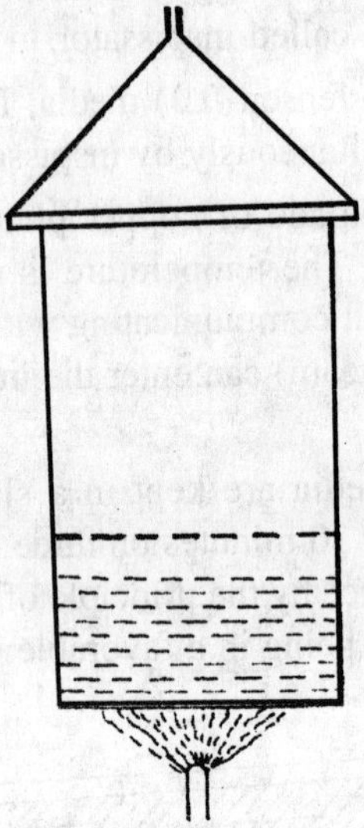

Fig. 8.4 Steam sterilizer.

3. Moist heat at a temperature above 100°C (or) steaming at a temperature above atmospheric pressure (or) saturated steam under increased pressure in an autoclave.

Autoclave (or) high pressure sterilizer. Autoclave (self-locking) was originally designed by Chamberland (1880) in Pasteur's laboratory. An autoclave is a strong boiler or cylinder with a lid which can be hermetically sealed and constructed strongly to withstand high pressures. Autoclave is an essential equipment required in microbiology laboratories.

Principle of autoclaving. Autoclave works on the principle of pressure cooker. Infact, a large pressure cooker can be used as an autoclave for sterilization of small articles in clinics and laboratories.

When the water is boiled within a closed vessel at increased pressures, the boiling point of water will rise above 100°C, depending on the pressure employed. Thus an increase in pressure yields an increase in effective temperature. This is the principle employed in the pressure cooker and autoclave.

Table 8.1 Temperatures attained at Different Pressures

Steam pressure	*Temperature attained*
0 lb/in^2 (atmospheric pressure)	100°C
5 lb/in^2	108°C
10 lb/in^2	115.5°C
15 lb/in^2	121°C
20 lb/in^2	127°C
25 lb/in^2	135.5°C
30 lb/in^2	133.5°C

The sterilization by steam under pressure depends upon four properties of dry, saturated steam :

– high temperature

– ability to form water by condensation

– liberation of latent heat when steam condenses on a cooler surface

– instantaneous contraction in volume that sucks more steam during condensation.

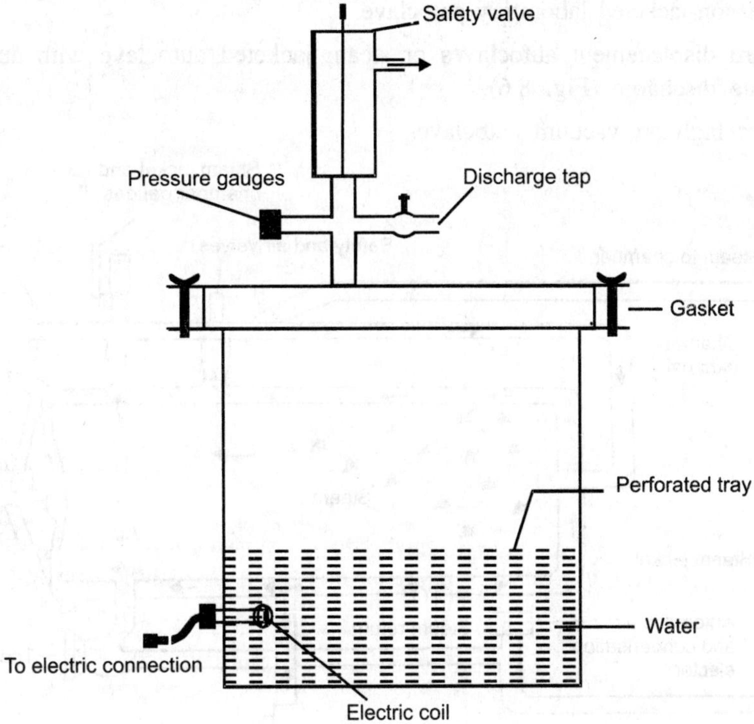

Fig. 8.5 A simple non-jacketed autoclave

Holding period. In autoclave, sterilization is done by steaming under 15 lb/in^2 (1.05 kg/cm^2) pressure for 15 min, where the temperature is attained to 121°C. Some laboratories employ a holding period of 20–30 min.

Articles to be sterilized in an autoclave : Autoclave is generally used for the sterilization of following articles :

– surgical dressings

– surgical instruments

– culture media

– liquids which can withstand high temperatures

– dilution blanks (measured quantities of normal saline or distilled water in test tubes or bottles)

– rubber articles like tubing, washers, caps etc.

– rubber gloves

– discarded media with growth.

Substances that are immiscible in water, such as greases, waxes, fats and oils cannot be sterilized by autoclaving, as steam cannot penetrate into them.

Types of autoclaves : Several types of autoclaves are available.

1. A simple non-jacketed laboratory autoclave.
2. Downward displacement autoclaves or steam jacketed autoclave with automatic air and condensate discharge (Fig. 8.6).
3. Automatic high pre-vacuum autoclaves.

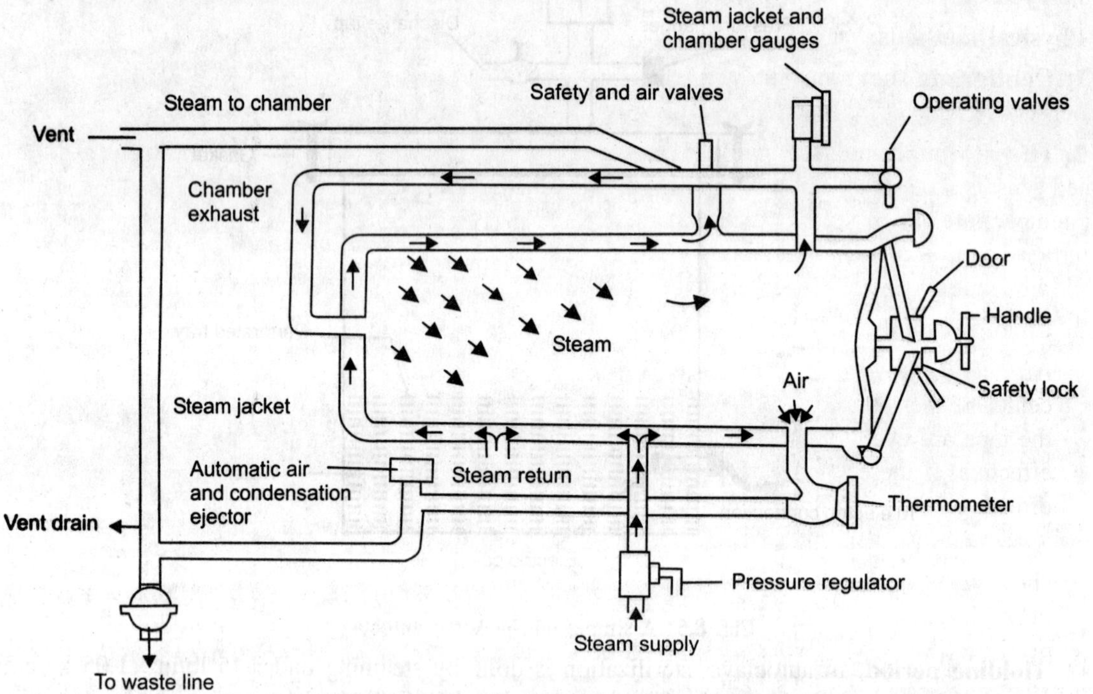

Fig. 8.6 Steam-jacketed autoclave with automatic gravity discharge of air condensate and system for drying by vacuum and intake of filtered air

Simple laboratory autoclave. It consists of a vertical or horizontal cylinder made up of strong gun metal or stainless steel. It may be single chambered or double chambered. The articles/items to be sterilized are placed in a perforated vessel or tray above the water level. The lid is fastened by screw clamps, rendered air-tight by an asbestos gasket/washer. On the lid, there is a pressure gauge (indicates the steam pressure built up inside), a discharge tap (for discharge of air and steam mixture) and a safety valve (that can be set to release steam at the chosen pressure). The cylinder contains water upto a certain level and is heated by electric heater.

Autoclaving. Sufficient water is poured into the cylinder and the articles to be sterilized are placed on a perforated tray above the water level. The discharge tap is opened and the lid is tightened with screw clamps. The water in the chamber is heated by electricity. When water begins to boil the air-steam mixture escapes through discharge tap and it is closed when the chamber is filled with steam. When the steam pressure rises to 15 lb/in^2 inside the chamber, a temperature of 121°C is attained and should be maintained for 15–20 minutes. It is the temperature that kills the organisms and spores.

Then the heater is switched off and autoclave is allowed to cool down slowly so that the pressure comes down to atmospheric pressure. The discharge tap is opened and air allowed to enter the chamber and the lid can be opened. Autoclave should not be opened under positive pressure as it may cause explosion, scalding and the liquids may boil and spill over.

Sterilization controls for moist-heat sterilization or sterility tests for autoclaving

To determine the efficiency of moist heat sterilization or autoclaving various sterilization controls are employed.

Physical methods:

1. Centigrade thermometers in the outlet drain records temperature inside the autoclave chamber, which is displayed on dial.

2. Thermocouple measurement. Thermocouples are temperature-sensitive and electronically operated sensors (fine probes consisting of two different metals *e.g.,* copper and constantan) for measuring temperature and are more accurate than routine thermometers. A thermocouple is inserted inside a test article in the autoclave chamber and its wire leads are carried out through valves in the autoclave wall and linked to a galvanometer, the dial of which gives a reading of the temperature.

3. Chemical methods:

(*i*) **Autoclave tapes – Bowie-Dick test.** The test consists of placing autoclave tapes into the center of the load and examining the tape after the sterilizing cycle. If the diagonal lines in the tape are evenly changed and become dark colored, it indicates that the sterilization was effective. If there is no dark color in the diagonal lines, it indicates the sterilization was not effective.

(*ii*) **Adhesive indicator tapes (steritapes).** These are impregnated with a dye that show a color change from colorless (or white) to various shades-brown to grey to black on completion of sterilization.

4. Biological or bacteriological test. To determine the efficiency of moist heat sterilization, *Bacillus stearothermophilus* is used as indicator for microbiological testing. *Bacillus stearothermophilus* is a thermophile, grows optimally at 55-60°C. Its spores are killed at 121°C in about 12 min. Paper strips impregnated with 10^6 spores of *Bacillus stearothermophilus* are placed in envelopes and inserted into different parts of load in the autoclave chamber; and after sterilization, the strips are inoculated into a suitable medium and incubated for sterility test at 55°C for 5 days.

An autoclaved spore strip is cultured as a positive control and an uninoculated medium as negative control.

IONIZING RADIATION (COLD STERILIZATION)

Two sources of ionizing radiations are used :

1. Gamma rays
2. Particulate high energy electrons

Gamma Radiations

The application of ionizing radiation, particularly gamma radiation to sterilize biological materials and heat sensitive materials is called **"cold sterilisation"**, because ionizing radiations produce no heat in the material being irradiated. Thus, cold sterilization finds application in food and pharmaceutical industries and in medical field to sterilize heat-sensitive materials.

Gamma rays are high energy radiations emitted from certain radioactive isotopes such as cobalt-60 and cesium-137. Gamma rays are similar to X-rays but are of shorter wavelength. They have very high penetrative power and lethal to all life including microorganisms by causing damage to DNA and other vital cell constituents. Because of this, they can be used for sterilization of materials of considerable thickness or volume *e.g.,* packaged items.

The items can be packed before sterilization in sealed aluminium foil or plastic packs contained in outer carton ready for despatch; can be sterilized by gamma rays, avoiding any handling and recontamination after sterilization.

Gamma rays are used for sterilizing disposable items such as plastic syringes, needles, suture materials, scalpel, blades, rubber gloves, catherters, swabs, culture plates, animal feeds, cardboard, oils, greases, fabrics and metal foils.

Chemical sterilants may be gases or liquids.

GASEOUS CHEMOSTERILIZERS

1. Ethylene Oxide Gas. Ethylene oxide is a highly reactive colorless liquid with a boiling point of 10.8°C; above this temperature it is a gas and it is used in this gaseous state for sterilization of heat-sensitive materials. It is highly flammable and carries the risk of explosion even in low concentrations. This problem can be overcome by mixing ethylene oxide with inert diluents like CO_2, Freon and nitrogen. These mixtures are non-flammable and retain the microbicidal and sporicidal activity.

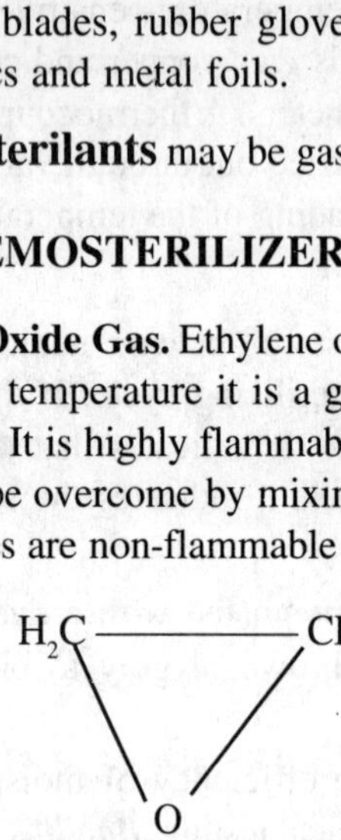

Molecular structure of ethylene oxide

The action of ethylene oxide depends upon temperature, concentration, time and presence of water vapor (humidity). Usually 10% ethylene oxide mixture (CO_2 or freon or nitrogen) and 30% humidity are used.

The gas can be used at low temperature, does not corrode or damage materials and used for sterilizing materials which would be ruined by both heat and ionizing radiation. It is used to sterilize plastic syringes, needles, transfusion sets, polythene tubing, respirators, heart-lung machines, cardiac catheters and pacers, sutures, surgical equipment, dental equipment, hospital bedding, blankets, books, ophthalmic and anesthetic equipment, endoscopes, electronic and medical equipment, biological materials, crude drugs, powders and culture media. Items such as syringes can be packed first and sterilized.

Ethylene oxide gas has been used for sterilization of space craft components.

Ethylene oxide acts by inactivating enzymes and other proteins by alkylating the amino, carboxyl, hydroxyl and sulphydryl groups.

2. Formaldehyde Gas or Fumigation. Formaldehyde gas is used for the sterilization of instruments, heat-sensitive catheters, clothing, bedding, woolen blankets, furniture, foot wear etc. It is mainly used for the sterilization of enclosed areas such as operation theaters, wards, sick rooms, babies' incubators, respiratory ventilators and laboratories by fumigation. The temperature and humidity affects the action of formaldehyde. The temperature must be 22°C and the humidity between 60 and 80%.

Fumigation can be achieved by several ways

- formaldehyde gas can be sprayed
- formalin solution can be heated so that it liberates fumes
- paraformaldehyde solid can be heated so that it liberates gaseous vapors, as it is highly volatile
- formalin solution can be added to potassium permanganate to generate gas. Usually 150 gms of $KMnO_4$ to 280 ml formalin for every 1000 cu.ft (28.3 cu.mt) of room volume. The reaction produces considerable heat and so heat resistant vessels should be used.

After starting generation of formaldehyde vapor the doors, windows and other outlets should be sealed and left unopened for atleast 48 hrs.

The gas is irritant and toxic when inhaled and carcinogenic. Its irritant action can be neutralized by exposure to ammonia vapor.

3. Beta Propiolactone (BPL). It is a colorless liquid at room temperature, with a high boiling point of 155°C. It is more active for sterilization and more efficient for fumigation than formaldehyde. But it is not widely used due to its carcinogenicity and lack of penetrating power. Liquid BPL is used in the preparation of veterinary vaccines.

LIQUID CHEMOSTERILIZERS

4. Formalin (Formaldehyde) Solution. It is marketed in aqueous solution as formalin, which contains 37 to 40% (w/v) formaldehyde. Methanol is added to (10 to 15%) to prevent polymerization of formaldehyde.

Formalin solution has several uses :

- for sterilization of clean instruments, furniture, fibres, leather etc.
- to preserve anatomical specimens
- 10% formalin solution is used for killing bacterial cultures and suspensions
- to destroy anthrax spores in hair, wool and hair brushes
- as a fixative for fixation of tissue specimens
- as a microbicidal agent in the preparation of killed vaccines
- to prepare toxoids from toxins

5. Glutaraldehyde. It is usually employed as a 2% buffered solution "cidex". It has a broad spectrum of action against viruses, fungi, fungal spores, bacteria, bacterial spores and tubercle bacilli. Its antimicrobial action is due to cross-linking and precipitation of proteins.

It is used to sterilize urological instruments, instruments with lenses, rubber anaesthetic tubes, face maskes, plastic endotracheal tubes, bronchoscopes, metal instruments, polythene tubing, fibre-optic endoscopes, cystoscopes. It does not corrode lenses, metal or rubber. It is less toxic and less irritant to the eyes and the skin than formaldehyde.

Glutaraldehyde is stable in acidic pH. But is most active in alkaline solution. It is unstable under alkaline pH due to gradual polymerization. Hence, the alkali has to be added to the glutaraldehyde, shortly before use. For example, cidex 25%, an aqueous solution of glutaraldehyde is diluted to 2% with an alkali (0.3 % Na_2CO_3) and can be used for sterilization of articles.

6. Iodine. It is sporicidal, bactericidal, fungicidal, virucidal and amoebicidal. Iodine kills microorganisms by denaturation of enzymes by oxidizing sulfhydryl groups and by binding to tyrosine.

FILTRATION

Filtration is used to sterilize heat labile liquids such as antibiotic solutions, sera, carbohydrate solutions, pharmaceutical fluids and certain laboratory media.

Several types of filters are available. They render liquids bacteria-free but not virus-free or *Mycoplasma*-free.

Filtration is usually carried out under carefully controlled negative pressure, the fluid being sucked through the filter into receiving flask, which is connected to an exhaust pump.

Uses or Applications of Filtration

1. Used for sterilization of heat-labile liquids such as carbohydrate solutions, sera, antibiotic solutions, blood products and other parenteral and ophthalmic fluids.
2. Used to obtain bacteria-free filtrates of toxins, enzymes and bacteriophages.
3. To separate microorganisms which are scanty in fluids.
4. For clarification of water.
5. For microbiological analysis of water. The organisms from water or infected fluids may be recovered on the surface of the filter discs and placed on suitable culture media to obtain the viable count.
6. For sterilization of certain culture media.

Types of Filters

Several types of filters are used for filtration.

1. Diatomaceous earthenware candle filters, *e.g.,* Berkefeld filters, Mandler filters.
2. Unglazed porcelain filters, *e.g.,* Chamberland filters.
3. Asbestos disk filters, *e.g.,* Seitz filters.
4. Sintered glass filters (fritted glass filters/Morton filters).
5. Membrane filters (ultra filters).

Diatomaceous Earthenware Candle Filters

These filters are usually made in the form of hollow candles open at one end. A metal nozzle is inserted and cemented in the open end.

Berkefeld German filters are made from kieselguhr (infusorial earth), a fossilised diatomaceous earth.

Mandler American filters are made from kieselguhr (60-80%), asbestos (10-30%) and plaster of paris (10-15%).

These filters are manufactured in different grades of porosity, They are mainly used for the clarification of water. They can be cleaned with sodium hypochlorite, but without scrubbing.

Unglazed Ceramic Filters or Porcelain Filters.

Filters of this type are hollow cylinders and unglazed except for a short distance at the open end. They are made up of hydrous aluminium silicate (kaolin) and sand. They are manufactured in different grades of porosity and used for large-scale clarification of water. They can be cleaned with sodium hypochlorite and by scrubbing.

e.g., **Chamberland** (French)–designed for the filtration of small quantities of liquid.

For use, the candle is mounted in a silicone rubber bung, which fits over the glazed portion and filtration is effected from within outwards.

Asbestos Disk Filters

These filters are made up of compressed filter sheet of asbestos fibres. They have high adsorbing capacities and tend to alkalinate solutions being filtered. Asbestos filters include – seitz filters.

Sietz filters are made from chrysotile type of asbestos, chemically composed of magnesium silicate. They are available in different grades of porosity. Seitz filters have a pore size of between 0.5 μm and 0.75 μm.

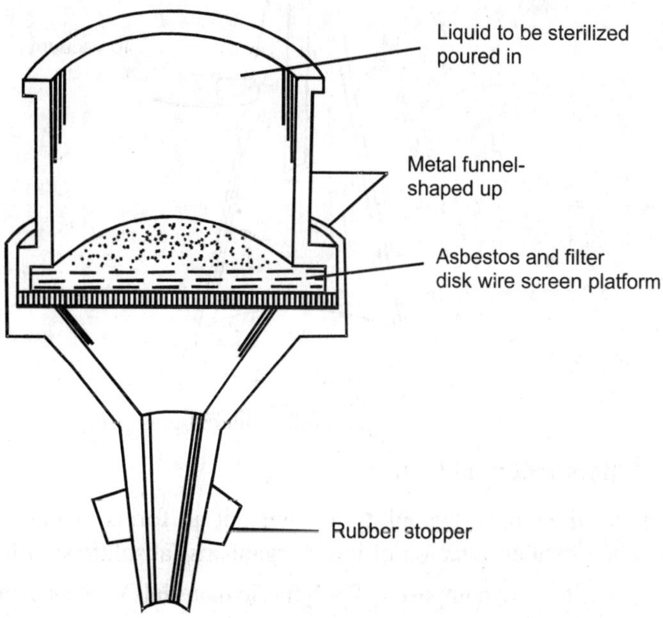

Fig. 8.7 Sietz filter

They are particularly useful in the laboratory for removing bacteria from serum and fluid culture media. Seitz filters are also used to sterilize hydatid fluid.

The filter disc is fitted to a funnel like structure supported on a metal mount and is inserted rough side up ensuring that the metal support grid is in position. The filter is attached to a vacuum flask through a silicone rubber bung. The whole assembly can be sterilized by autoclaving. After use, the filter is discarded.

Sintered Glass Filters/Fritted Glass Filters

They are prepared by molding finely pulverized glass in disk from. Glass for such a filter is ground into fine mesh powder of uniform size and then fused (fritted) in a furnace by heating sufficiently to leave small pores. This is then sealed into the body of the funnel and thoroughly cleaned by treating with H_2SO_4 containing sodium nitrate. The acid treatment quickly oxidizes and dissolves organic matter, if any. The acid is removed later by repeated washing with distilled water.

The funnel fitted with sintered glass filter disc is then attached to a collecting flask either by a rubber stopper or through a ground glass joint.

Fritted glass filters are available in various pore sizes – EC (extracoarse), C (coarse), M (medium), F (fine) and UF (ultrafine).

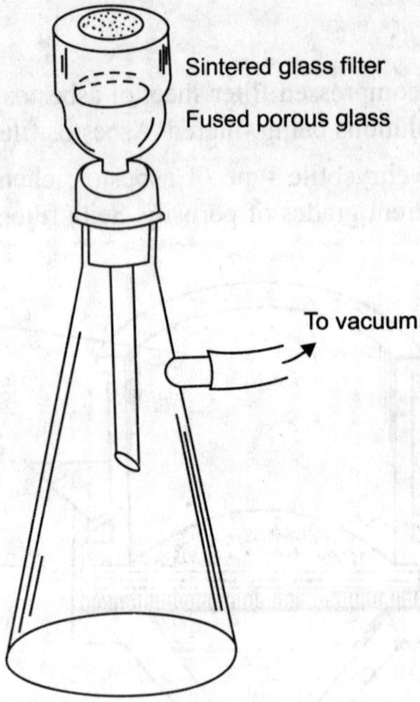

Fig. 8.8 Sintered glass filter.

Membrane Filters (Ultra Filters)

Membrane filters have the ability to filter out all forms of microorganisms and are the best and most useful when total elimination of microorganisms (absolute sterility) is required.

Membrane filters are composed of polymeric materials such as cellulose nitrate, cellulose diacetate, polycarbonate and polyester.

The older type membrane filters are composed of cellulose nitrate and are called Gradocol membrane filters, whereas the modern filters are made of cellulose acetate and are known as millipore filters (as they were originally manufactured by Millipore Corporation, USA). They are available in a range of pore sizes from 12 μm down to 0.015 μm.

The membrane filters have a highly uniform pore size and the pores occupy 80-85% of total filter volume and the cellulose matrix occupying only 15 to 20%, which facilitates high flow rate of liquids. Moreover, membrane filters are resistant to dilute acids, alkalies etc.; free of biological inhibitors, remain stable at high temperatures and high pressures and thus are superior to other filters. The membranes allow large volumes of liquid to pass through rapidly under suction.

QUESTIONS

Essay Types Questions

1. Define sterilization. Classify the methods of sterilization. Describe various methods of sterilization.
2. Define sterilization. Classify the methods of sterilization. Write briefly all about autoclave.
3. Define and classify the methods of sterilization. Describe moist heat sterilization.
4. Define sterilization. Classify the methods of sterilization be heat. Write in detail about dry heat sterilization.
5. Define and classify sterilization. Describe the various types of filters and their applications.

Short Notes

1. Define sterilization and mention two important uses of autoclave.
2. Explain how autoclave function. Specify the commonly used temperature, pressure and quality control measures.
3. Incineration.
4. Hot air oven.
5. Sterilization controls for dry heat sterilization/hot air oven.
6. Inspissation or serum inspissator.
7. Tyndallization or intermittent sterilization or fractional sterilization.
8. Articles sterilized in an autoclave.
9. Autoclave.
10. Sterilization controls for autoclave.
11. Cold sterilization.
12. Use of ionizing radiation in sterilization of lab. material.
13. Sterilization by radiation and its practical applications.
14. Filtration.
15. Bacterial filters.
16. Asbestos disc filters.
17. Seitz filters.
18. Membrane filters.
19. Gaseous sterilization.
20. Fumigation.
21. Chemical sporicidal agents.
22. Applications (uses) of filtration.
23. Sintered glass filters (fritted glass filters).
24. Gamma radiation.

9

Disinfection

- *Definition*
- *Mode of action*
- *Methods of disinfection*
  - *– Disinfection by moist heat*
  - *– Pasteurisation*
  - *– Boiling*
- *Nonionizing radiation*
  - *– UV radiation*
- *Chemical disinfectants*
  - *– Aldehydes*
  - *– Alcohols*
  - *– Phenolics*
  - *– Diguanides*
  - *– Halogens*
  - *– Surface active agents*
  - *– Salts of heavy metals*
  - *– Oxidising agents*
  - *– Dyes*
- *Testing of antimicrobial potency of disinfectants and antiseptics*
  - *– Tube dilution technique*
  - *– Agar plate technique*
  - *– Phenol coefficient technique*
  - *– Rideal walker test*
  - *– Chick Martin test*
  - *– Kelsey-Sykes capacity tests*
  - *– In-use tests*

DEFINITION

Disinfection is defined as the destruction of many microorganisms, but not usually spores. The term "Disinfection" is usually applied to the treatment of inanimate objects.

Disinfectants are chemical substances that are used for disinfection. Chemical disinfectants are strongly microbicidal and are generally used to eradicate microorganisms from inanimate materials. Disinfectants kill vegetative bacteria, fungi viruses but not usually spores.

Antisepsis refers to prevention of infection, usually by inhibiting the growth of bacteria.

Antiseptics are chemical disinfectants that can be safely applied to skin and mucus membrane surfaces.

Any given chemical can be used as disinfectant at a high concentration, and as an antiseptic at very low concentrations.

MODE OF ACTION

Chemical disinfectants and antiseptics kill microorganisms by various mechanisms

1. Coagulation of proteins
2. Disruption or damage to cell membrane which results in alteration of cell permeability
3. Removal of free sulfhydryl groups from the active sites of enzymes, so that enzyme activity is destroyed, so that cell dies
4. Substrate competition – A chemical compound resembling the essential substrate misleads the enzyme by competing for substrate, so that metabolism is prevented causing cell death

METHODS OF DISINFECTION

Disinfection by moist heat

1. Pasteurization
2. Boiling

Non-ionizing radiation

1. UV radiation

Chemical disinfectants

1. Aldehydes – formaldehyde, Glutaraldehyde
2. Alcohols – Ethyl alcohol, Isopropyl alcohol
3. Phenolics – Phenols, Cresols, Hexyl resorcinol, Lysols, Hexachlorophene, Chloroxylenol (Dettol)
4. Diguanides – Chlorohexidine (Hibitane)
5. Halogens – Iodine compounds, chlorine compounds.
6. Surface active agents
   – anionic detergents–soap
   – cationic detergents (Quaternary ammonium compounds) – cetrimide, benzalkonium chloride
7. Salts of heavy metals – Mercury compounds, silver nitrate, copper sulphate, Zinc compounds
8. Oxidizing agents- hydrogen peroxide, potassium permanganate
9. Dyes – Aniline dyes, Acridine dyes
10. Acids
11. Alkalies

These methods of disinfection should always be preceded by a thorough cleaning with a detergent and hot water, of the item to be disinfected, which will remove the majority of microorganisms present.

Disinfection by Moist Heat

1. Pasteurization. It was devised by Louis Pasteur to prevent spoilage of wine and beer. It is now widely used it kill majority of microorganisms in milk, cream, alcoholic beverages (winr and beer) and food industries.

There are three methods of pasteurization

(*i*) Holder method (or) low temperature holding method (LTH) – milk is heated at 62.8°C (145°F) for 30 minutes, followed by cooling to 13°C.

(*ii*) Flash method (or) High temperature short time method (HTST) – Milk is heated to a temperature of 71.7°C (161°F) for 15 seconds, followed by sudden cooling to 13°C.

(*iii*) Ultra high temperature (UHT) method –The milk is heated to a very high temperature of 130°C for 1 or 2 seconds and then rapidly cooled.

Coxiella burnetti, the causative agent of Q fever may survive holder method but can be killed in other methods.

Pasteurization is not a method of sterilization, and it only reduces the microbial count.

2. Boiling. Total immersion of contaminated materials, objects and instruments in boiling water at 100°C for 5 min. can bring about disinfection. This required 5 min. time is measured from the time when the water actually boils again after the last instruments have been immersed. Sterile forceps may be used to remove instruments from boiler after processing.

Non-ionizing Radiation

UV RAYS: UV radiation can be produced artificially by mercury vapor lamps. UV rays are effective against both Gram positive and Gram negative bacteria and Viruses. It has low penetrating power and its main application is to reduce the bacteria in air, water and on contaminated surfaces.

UV radiation is mainly used

– to disinfect drinking water and to obtain a Pyrogen-free water

–for air disinfection in hospital wards, operation rooms, laboratories, ventilated safety cabinets and enclosed areas such as entry ways and corridors.

UV radiation is absorbed by the proteins and nucleic acids and kills microorganisms by the chemical reactions it sets up in the bacterial cell.

Prolonged exposure to sunlight and fresh air is the most pleasant and perhaps an oldest anti-infection method.

The disadvantages of UV radiation :

– Causes damage to eyes, hence dark glasses must be worn or light source must be screened

– Excessive exposure to skin produces burns

Chemical Disinfectants

1. Aldehydes

Formaldehyde can be used in liquid form or gaseous form.

Formaldehyde gas is used for fumigation of operation theatres, sick rooms, wards, laboratories, post-mortem rooms, terminal room disinfection of premises occupied by TB, anthrax cases, safety cabinets, respiratory ventilators and babies incubators.

Formaldehyde gas can be liberated by spraying or by heating formalin solution or by heating solid paraformaldehyde. The atmosphere must have a humidity of over 60% (Preferably 80-90%) at a temperature of 18°C.

Formaldehyde is highly toxic and irritating. This effect can be neutralized by exposure to ammonia.

Small articles, instruments, blankets, surfaces of mattresses, shoes, hair brushes are disinfected in a cabinet, by exposure to formaldehyde gas for atleast three hours, by boiling formalin.

Glutaraldehyde is an effective disinfectant against both Gram positive and Gram negative bacteria, including tubercle bacilli and sporicidal. It is used to treat heat sensitive articles such as respirators, fibre-optic endoscopes, corrugated rubber anaesthetic tubes, plastic endotracheal tubes, metal instruments, polythene tubing and lensed instruments such as bronchoscopes and cystoscopes. It has no deleterious effect on cements or lenses of these instruments and is an advantage over formaldehyde.

Glutaraldehyde is less corrosive than hypochlorites and therefore can be used to disinfect centrifuges and automated equipment.

2. Alcohols. Isopropyl alcohol, ethyl alcohol and methylated spirit (denatured alcohol) are bactericidal in aqueous solutions at a concentration of 70-75%. They are effective against Gram positive bacteria, Gram negative bacteria, Acid fast bacilli and viruses. They can kill vegetative cells, but are non-sporicidal and non-fungicidal. Since, alcohols are volatile they are used as rapidly drying antiseptics for skin, and disinfectants for inanimate surfaces.

Alcohols are used as skin antiseptics before and after venepuncture, cutaneous injections and hypodermic injections, for hand disinfection and applied as hand rubs on dry skin. 70% alcohols in combination with chlorhexidine (0.5%), Iodine (1 to 2%), laurolinium acetate (5%) are superior to alcohol alone .

The presence of organic matter delays the action of alcohols. Hence, they are used as disinfectants on physically clean surface; such as thermometers, instruments and equipment such as trolley tops, clean glass slides, mouths of culture bottles.

There is a gradual increase in the bactericidal action of alcohols, as their molecular weight increases. Thus, the bactericidal activity of isopropanol is greater than ethanol and being less volatile, widely used for the sterilization of thermometers. Whereas, alcohols with a molecular weight higher than that of propyl alcohol are not miscible in water, and are not used as disinfectants.

Methyl alcohol is less bactericidal than ethanol and it is highly poisonous. The fumes may produce permanent damage to eyes and not generally used.

3. Phenolics. Phenols were the first antiseptics used in surgery by Joseph Lister (1865)

Phenols are widely used as disinfectants and antiseptics and used for decontamination of infective discharges, spillages, bathrooms, bed pans, environmental surfaces, walls, floors, furniture, instruments bedding and as aerial disinfectants.

Phenols is also used as a preservative in sera and vaccines at a conc. of 0.5%.

Phenols are bactericidal to both Gram positive and Gram negative bacteria whereas spores are resistant. Phenols are active at acidic pH and their activity is reduced at alkaline pH. Presence of organic matter delays or inactivates the action of phenols. They may be bactericidal or bacteriostatic depending on the concentration used.

Phenol (carbolic acid) – at 2 to 5% aqueous solution used to disinfect materials such as sputum, urine, feces and contaminated instruments and utensils. Because phenol is toxic and has an unpleasant odor, it is replaced by several chemically related compounds.

Due to early recognition in the field of disinfection, phenol is used as the standard disinfectant against which the efficiency and activity of others is measured.

Cresols – ortho, meta and para cresols are more bactericidal than phenol and employed as a mixture of tricresol. Their emulsions in liquid soaps and alkalies are used for practical applications.

Hexylresorcinol is used in a solution of glycerin and water. It is a strong surface-tension reductant, which accounts for its bactericidal action and used as general antiseptic.

Lysols are made of a soap solution containing phenolic compounds (o-phenyl phenol, o-benzyl-p-chlorophenol, xylenols) used to disinfect inanimate objects such as floors, walls, table surfaces, contaminated hospital items such as rectal thermometers, excreta and secretions from infected patients.

Hexachlorophene is a chlorinated phenolic bacteriostatic agent active against Gram positive bacteria such as *Staphylococci* and not active against Gram negative bacteria. It is used to reduce staphylococcal sepsis in maternity and neonatal units. In combination with soap it is used for hand washing and skin cleaning in operation theatres and clinical areas

Chloroxylenol (Dettol) is popularly used as disinfectant and antiseptic and active against both Gram positive and Gram negative bacteria.

Clear soluble phenolics-such as hycolin, clearsol, stericol and sudol are more efficient than phenol and more resistant to inactivation by organic matter.

Mode of action of phenols. 1. Alter the semipermeability of cell membrane causing leakage of vital intracellular constituents.

2. Causing denaturation and inactivation of proteins such as enzymes.

4. Diguanides or Biguanides

Chlorhexidine (Hibitane; 1, 6-di-4´-chloro phenyl guanido hexane) – It is the most widely used nontoxic, non-irritating skin antiseptic in medical dental and veterinary practice. It is very active against Gram positive bacteria (*e.g.*, Staphylococci) and moderately active against Gram negative bacteria, but less active against *Pseudomonas* and *Proteus* sp. It has no action against spores, tubercle bacilli fungi and viruses. Its action is inactivated by organic matter, pus, serum, soaps, hard water, anionic compounds and some plastics. It is available as a dihydrochloride, diacetate and gluconate. The most widely used one is chlorhexidine gluconate in 0.5%, 2%, 4% concentrations.

Uses – a general antiseptic for skin and mucus membrane surface

– used before operation, lumbar puncture or bone marrow aspiration

– 4% solution in a compatible detergent (Hibiscrub) is used as antiseptic for hand washing of hospital staff and preoperative scrub for surgeons.

– 0.5 to 1% solution in isopropyl alcohol (Hibisol) is used for rapid hand antisepsis in hospitals. The alcohol present results in a rapid antibacterial effect together with drying of the hands.

– chlorhexidine-cetrimide mixture (Savlon) is a useful antiseptic for wounds.

– Skin disinfection in urology and gynaecology.

5. Halogens – Halogens are strong oxidizing agents. Iodine (skin antiseptic) and chlorine (water disinfectant) are frequently used.

Iodine – It is one of the oldest and most effective disinfectant. It is sporicidal, bactericidal, fungicidal, virucidal and amoebicidal. Iodine kills microorganisms by denaturation of protein enzymes by oxidizing sulphydryl groups and by binding to tyrosine.

Iodine is used as skin antiseptic, to disinfect small quantities of water and food utensils. Iodine vapor is sometimes used to disinfect air. It is traditionally used as antiseptic in the form of "tincture of Iodine". The term "tincture" refers to an alcoholic solution of a medicinal substance. Several preparations of Iodine are used.

Aqueous solution of Iodine consists of 5% Iodine, 10% potassium Iodide in distilled water.

Alcoholic solution of Iodine consists of 7% Iodine, 5% potassium Iodide in 83% alcohol.

Tincture of Iodine consists of 2% Iodine, 2% sodium iodide diluted in 70% alcohol.

Iodophores are compounds of iodine with detergents have the advantages of non-staining and non-irritating to the skin. Povidone Iodine is used for hand washing, surgical scrubbing, preparation of the skin prior to invasive procedures such as injection, aspiration and surgery and for prophylaxis against post-operative infections.

Chlorine. It is most widely used either in the form of gas or in certain chemical combinations.

Compressed and liquefied chlorine gas is the choice for disinfection of drinking water or municipal water supplies, swimming pools and for the treatment of effluents and used at a concentration of 0.5 to 1.0 PPM (mg/Lit). Many compounds of chlorine are more convenient to use than chlorine gas. *e.g.*, Inorganic chlorine compounds such as hypochlorites – *e.g.*, calcium hypochlorite ($Ca(OC1)_2$) and sodium hypochlorite (NaOC1). Calcium hypochlorite is used for sanitizing utensils in restaurants and equipment in food and dairy plants.

A solution of 1% sodium hypochlorite is used for personal hygiene and to disinfect baby-bottles. High concentrations, such as 5-12% are used as household bleaches, disinfectants and as sanitizers in dairy and food processing plants and for kitchen hygiene. Sodium hypochlorite kills spores, bacteria, fungi, protozoa and viruses. It is particularly useful because of its activity against HIV and Hepatitis B virus .The disadvantages being corrosion of metals and its action can inactivated by the presence of organic matter.

Organic chloramines are used as antiseptics and for dressing wounds.

Dakin's solution (surgical chlorinated soda solution) and electrolytic sodium hypochlorite are used for wound irrigation and dressings.

Mode of action of chlorine. When added to water, hypochlorites and chloramines undergo hydrolysis giving rise to hypochlorous acid which changes to nascent oxygen, which is a powerful oxidizing agent that can severely damage vital cell constituents.

6. *Surface active agents/surfactants/surface tension depressants/wetting agents/synthetic detergents.* Compounds that have the property of concentrating at interfaces and alter the energy relationships at interfaces producing a reduction of surface tension of interfacial tension causing disruption of cell membrane are called as surface active agents.

They possess wetting and cleansing properties and disinfectant activity. They are used in laundry, disk washing powders, shampoos, other washing preparations and for hand washing.

They are of 4 types – anionic, cationic, non-ionic and amphoteric (Tego) compounds. Among these anionic and cationic detergents are very useful for disinfection and cleaning purposes.

Anionic surface active agents – Detergents in which a long-chain hydrocarbon has a negative charge are called anionic e.g. soaps, fatty acids and bile salts. They dissociate in aqueous solution to form a large, complex anion, which is responsible for lowering surface tension.

They are mainly effective against Gram positive bacteria, Acid fast bacilli and some viruses.

Soft soaps derived by combination of unsaturated fatty acids (*e.g.*, oleic acid) with NaOH or KOH are more efficient than hard soaps formed by combination of saturated fatty acids (*e.g.*, coconut oil) with NaOH or KOH.

Cationic surface active agents/quaternary ammonium compounds. Possess both bactericidal and detergent properties. They are active against Gram positive bacteria but less active against Gram negative bacteria. *Pseudomonas aeruginosa*, *Proteus* and tubercle bacilli are particularly resistant. Selective media for the cultivation of *Pseudomonas aeruginosa* contains cetrimide, and is known as **cetrimide agar**. They are sporistatic and funsistatic and are active against enveloped viruses but not against non-enveloped viruses.

They are most active at alkaline pH. Acid, organic matter, blood inactivates them. Their action is neutralized by anionic surface active agents, soaps, hard water and various chemicals.

Examples for Quaternary ammonium compounds are:

1. Cetyl trimethyl ammonium bromide (cetrimide or cetavlon)
2. Benzalkonium chloride (zephiran)
3. Cetyl pyridinium chloride
4. Laurolinium acetate (laurodin)

They possess a peculiar adsorptive property which is of practical importance. When applied to skin they form an antibacterial surface film. They are readily adsorbed to glass ware and to fabrics. They are, therefore, widely used for the disinfection of food utensils in hotels and restaurants, milk containers in dairy industry, blankets in hospitals.

They are widely used for preoperative skin preparation of the skin and mucus membrane surfaces, as surgical scrub and as antiseptic for abrasions and wounds. They are also used for disinfection of bench-tops, floors and other surfaces in laboratories.

7. Salts of heavy metals. The term "heavy metals" refers to metals such as mercury, silver, copper, zinc and lead. They are protein coagulants and combine with free sulphydryl (–SH) groups of enzymes and thus kills the bacteria.

Mercuric chloride ($HgCl_2$) was widely used as a general disinfectant. Organic mercury compounds such as Merbromin (mercurochrome), thiomersal (merthiolate), nitromersol (metaphen) were used for treatment of minor cuts, wounds and infections. Merthiolate (1 in 10,000) is used for inactivation of vaccines and preservation of sera and antitoxins.

1% silver nitrate ($AgNO_3$) was widely used to disinfect the eyes of infants at birth to prevent ophthalmia neonatorum, a gonococcal infection. Currently, it is sometimes replaced either by antibiotics such as penicillin or erythromycin or by antiseptics such as chlorhexidine. Sponges or layers of gauze impregnated with 0.5% silver nitrate has been used to prevent infections of burns.

Copper sulphate is an effective algicide in open bodies of water such as tanks, reservoirs and pools.

8. Oxidizing agents. Hydrogen peroxide, potassium permanganate, ozone, chlorine dioxide, peracetic acid are some oxidizing agents find application in disinfection and antisepsis.

Hydrogen peroxide is active against both Gram positive and Gram negative bacteria and sporicidal at high concentrations. It is used as antiseptic for cleansing wounds, abscesses, for the removal of adhering dressings and for irrigation. It liberates oxygen when in contact with organic material. The effervescence helps mechanically to loosen slough and pus in a wound.

Potassium permanganate is used as mouth wash, gargle and for wound cleaning. It is also used to purify well water. Ozone (O_3) is bactericidal, sporicidal and virucidal and used to disinfect vegetables and fruits.

9. Dyes. Two groups of dyes, the aniline dyes and the acridines can be used as skin and wound antiseptics. Both are bacteriostatic at high dilution but are of low bactericidal activity.

Aniline dyes (Triphenyl methane dyes). Crystal violet, brilliant green, malachite green are included in this group. They are more active against Gram positive bacteria than Gram negative bacteria. Hence, selective media prepared by incorporating these dyes are used to grow coliform bacilli (Gram negative bacilli such as *E.coli*) in bacteriological analysis of water.

These dyes have no action on tubercle bacilli. Hence, malachite green is used as a selective agent in **Lowenstein-Jensen (LJ) medium** for the cultivation of tubercle bacilli.

Acridine dyes. Proflavine, acriflavine, euflavine and aminacrine are included in this group. Though they are more active against Gram positive bacteria than Gram negative bacteria, they are not as selective as the aniline dye. Their action is usually not affected by the presence of organic matter. Presently, they have less application and are used to some extent for the treatment of burns, wounds, ophthalmic application and for bladder irrigation.

TESTING OF ANTIMICROBIAL POTENCY OF DISINFECTANTS AND ANTISEPTICS

There are several procedures available to evaluate antimicrobial potency of chemical agents

1. Tube dilution technique
2. Agar plate technique
3. Phenol, coefficient technique
   (*a*) Rideal-walker test
   (*b*) Chick-Martin test
4. Kelsey-Sykes capacity tests
5. In-use tests

Tube Dilution Technique

The disinfectant is made into several dilutions and an equal amount (*e.g.*, 5 ml) of each dilution is taken into sterile test tubes. Then a specific amount (*e.g.*, 0.1 ml) of the test organism is added to each tube and incubated. At regular intervals of time subcultures are made and incubated and examined for growth.

"No growth" indicates the dilution at which the chemical agent has killed the test organism when exposed to a particular period of time.

Agar-Plate Technique

The test organism is inoculated on to nutrient agar and the chemical is placed in the center of the placed. If the chemical agent is in liquid form, an absorbent paper disk impregnated with the solution can be placed on the agar medium or a small volume of solution can be held in a hollow cylinder set upon the agar surface. After incubation, the plate is observed for a zone of inhibition.

Alternatively, the chemical can be incorporated into the nutrient agar and then poured into the plates. The medium is inoculated with the test organism, incubated and examined for microbial growth.

Phenol Coefficient Technique/Rideal-Walker Test

It is used extensively to test disinfectants. The Rideal-walker test compares the action of the antiseptic or disinfectant with that of phenol on *Salmonella typhi* in distilled water. It is expressed in terms of phenol coefficient.

$$\text{Phenol coefficient} = \frac{\text{Dilution of the disinfectant which kills the test organism in the given time}}{\text{Dilution of the phenol which kills the test organism in the same time}}$$

The disinfectant is made into several dilutions in one set and similarly phenol is taken in several dilutions in another set. To each of these tubes, the test organism (*Salmonella typhi*) is added and allowed to react over a definite time interval – 2.½, 5, 7 and 10 minutes at 37°C for two days and observe for growth (turbidity).

The Rideal-Walker test is performed in distilled water, which does not give any similarity of the disinfecting action under a practical condition, where much organic material is present.

If the phenol coefficient is 1 or less than 1, the chemical agent is said to be a good disinfectant or antiseptic.

Chick-Martin test. It is same as Rideal-Walker test, but done in the presence of organic matter such as feces or yeast.

Kelsey-Sykes Capacity Tests. Capacity tests measure the capacity of a disinfectant to retain its activity when repeatedly used microbiologically .These tests simulate practical disinfecting situations.

In Kelsey-sykes test, the test organism such as *Staphylococcus aureus*, *E.coli*, *Pseudomonas aeruginosa*, *Proteus vulgaris* is added to disinfectant in three successive lots at 0, 10 and 20 minutes. The organism is in contact with the disinfectant for 8 minutes, so that samples are transferred at 8, 18 and 28 minutes respectively to a nutrient medium. The disinfectant is assessed based on its ability to kill bacteria as judged by growth on nutrient medium. The test is carried out under both clean and dirty (in the presence of organic matter such as yeast or feces) conditions.

In-use Tests. These tests are used to monitor not only the performance of a disinfectant but also how it is being used.

In-use tests are realistic as they test a disinfectant's action in use in the hospital at the time of tests.

Samples of the disinfectant dilutions in use in the hospital are taken (usually 1 ml) and added to nutrient broth (usually 9 ml). This 1 in 10 dilution of disinfectant in nutrient broth is inoculated on to two agar plates using 10 drops of diluted disinfectant per plate, using a sterile Pasteur pipette. One plate is incubated at 37°C for 2-3 days and the other plate is incubated at room temperature.

If a few colonies appear, it does not imply the failure of in-use test, since disinfection is partial removal of organisms. However, if more than 5 colonies appear on the plate, it suggests that the disinfectant action is not effective.

Regular in-use tests are valuable for helping supervise the correct use of disinfectants in the hospital.

QUESTIONS

Essay Type Questions

1. Define disinfection. Name various disinfectants and describe in detail.
2. Give an account of testing antimicrobial potency of disinfectants and antiseptics.

Short Notes

1. Define disinfection.
2. Describe mode of action of disinfectants.
3. Pasteurization.
4. Name two uses of UV radiation.
5. Uses of aldehydes.
6. Uses of alcohols.
7. Phenols.
8. Chlorhexidine or Diguanides.
9. Halogens.
10. Quaternary ammonium compounds.
11. Oxidizing agents.
12. Testing of disinfectants.
13. Phenol coefficient (or) Rideal-walker test.
14. Chick-Martin test.
15. Kelsey-Sykes test.
16. In-use dilution test.

10

Culture Media

- *Definition*
- *Ingredients/constituents of culture media*
- *Classification of culture media*
- *Defined/synthetic media*
- *Semidefined media*
- *Simple media/Basal media*
- *Enriched media*
- *Enrichment media*
- *Selective media*
- *Differential media*
- *Indicator media*
- *Transport media*
- *Anaerobic media*
- *Sugar media/sugar fermentation test*

DEFINITION

Culture medium can be defined as an artificial food provided in the petriplates, test tubes, bottles to grow/cultivate, to isolate, to identify and to study growth, biochemical, antigenic and other characteristics of bacteria in the laboratory.

An ideal culture medium must give a rapid and good growth from a small inoculum and ideally from a single cell. It should make possible for all the characteristics of the isolate to be demonstrated.

INGREDIENTS/CONSTITUENTS OF CULTURE MEDIA

Many ingredients are incorporated to prepare culture media.

Water. Water is very essential for life as an hydrogen or electron donor in metabolism, and as a medium in which enzymatic activities takes place. Usually demineralized water or glass-distilled water is used in the preparation of culture media.

Electrolytes. NaCl or other electrolytes may be incorporated in the culture medium in optimum concentrations, as per the requirements of microorganisms.

Meat extract/lab lemco/beef extract. Meat extract is an essential ingredient in many culture media. It is prepared by boiling finely grinded meat or beef from which a soluble extract is obtained, which is concentrated by evaporation to a dark paste or powder. Commercially prepared meat extract is known as lab-lemco. It contains many water-soluble compounds and protein degradation products such as albumoses, gelatin, peptones, proteoses and amino acids; and other nitrogen compounds, creatine, purines etc. It also contains inorganic salts, growth factors and some carbohydrates.

Peptone. Peptone is a common ingredient of culture media. It provides nitrogen requirement of pathogenic bacteria. It is obtained by digestion of protein material with proteolytic enzymes such as pepsin, trypsin or papain. Peptone is a complex mixture of proteoses, polypeptides, amino acids, inorganic salts such as phosphates, potassium and magnesium and certain growth factors such as riboflavin and nicotinic acid.

Peptone is supplied as golden granular powder with a low moisture content. It is water soluble, does not coagulate on heating and can be incorporated in culture media. Commercially available digest broths can be used instead of peptone.

Different brands of peptone will have differences in composition and growth promoting properties. Also, there may be variations between different batches of the same brand. Special brands of peptone such as neopeptone, proteose peptone and mycological peptone are available for special uses.

Yeast extract. It is prepared from washed cells of baker's yeast or brewer's yeast. Yeast cells are allowed to undergo autolysis by mild heating at 55°C or hydrolysed with HCl on proteolytic enzymes. The extract is concentrated to thick paste or powder form by evaporation. Yeast extract contains a wide range of nutrients such as amino acids, inorganic salts, carbohydrates, vitamins and growth factors.

Blood. Blood is used to enrich culture media, to cultivate microorganisms with fastidious growth requirements. Usually 5–10% defibrinated sheep blood is used. Horse blood or Rabbit blood can be used. But human blood should not be used as it may contain antibodies, bactericidal and other inhibitory agents to human pathogens.

Gelatin. Gelatin is a protein of animal source. Initially gelatin was tried as a solidifying agent in culture media, but at incubation temperature at 37°C, it melts into liquid, hence its use was abandoned. Certain bacteria utilize and liquefy gelatin by producing gelatinase.

Agar-Agar. Agar powder is used as a solidifying agent to prepare solid culture media. It melts at 98°C and solidifies at 42°C and provides a smooth surface on solid medium. It is not used up as a nutrient by the bacteria. Hence, agar is most satisfactory and preferred solidifying agent.

It is prepared from sea weeds (Red Algae belonging to Rhodophyceae) such as *Gelidium*, *Pterocladia* and *Eucheuma* species. The main constituent of agar is a long-chain polysaccharide; in addition, it may contain inorganic salts and protein like materials. Agar is manufactured either in long shreds or in powder form. It varies in its composition from batch to batch. Special brands of agar such as NewZcaland agar and Japanese agar are available for special purpose.

Routinely in culture media, agar is used at a concentration of 2% to prepare a good solid medium When agar concentration is decreased to 0.2 to 0.5%, semisolid agar or sloppy agar is obtained, which enables motile organisms to spread. The agar concentration may be further decreased to 0.05 to 0.1% to prevent convection currents of air in thioglycollate media. The agar concentration can be increased to 6% to prevent swarming growth of *Proteus* and *Clostridium tetani*.

In gel diffusion 0.1 to 0.2% agar gel or agarose gel is used.

Table 10.1 Agar Concentrations in Different Media.

Culture media	*Conc. of agar*	*Use*
Solid media	2%	solidifying agent
	6%	to prevent swarming of bacteria
Semi-solid media/ sloppy agar	0.2 to 0.5%	to enable motile organisms spread; to separate motile organisms from a mixture of motile and nonmotile organisms
Thiglycollate media (anaerobic medium)	0.02 to 0.01%	to prevent convection currents in the medium

CLASSIFICATION OF CULTURE MEDIA

Based on the functions, culture media are classified into several types.

– simple media or ordinary media or basal media

– complex media

– synthetic or defined media

– semidefined media

– special media – they are further classified into

– enriched media

– enrichment media

– selective media

– differential media

– indicator media

– transport media

– sugar media (carbohydrate media)

– anaerobic media.

DEFINED MEDIA/SYNTHETIC MEDIA

These media are used to study metabolic requirements of the bacteria. These media are prepared from pure chemical compounds; hence, known as synthetic media. The exact chemical composition of the medium is known, hence called defined media.

SEMI–DEFINED MEDIA

When the chemical composition of the medium is approximately known it is called semidefined or semisynthetic media *e.g.,* peptone water medium.

Peptone water. It is a simple, basal medium since it's chemical composition is approximately known, it is also called semisynthetic media. It contins peptone 1%; NaCl 0.5% and distilled water, with a pH adjusted to 7.4.

Uses. 1. It acts as a simple medium for the growth of many organisms, particularly Gram negative bacilli.

2. It is used to test indole production.

3. It is used to prepare sugar media.

4. Peptone water at an alkaline pH of 8.6; known as **alkaline peptone water**, used for enrichment of *Vibrio cholerae* from feces samples.

SIMPLE MEDIA/BASAL MEDIA

Simple media are those which contain only basic nutrients required for the growth of ordinary organisms, and used as a general purpose media. *e.g.,* peptone water, nutrient broth and nutrient agar. These simple media can be used as a base to prepare enriched media; hence known as basal media.

Nutrient broth. It is a simple basal liquid medium, supports growth of many organisms. It contains 1% peptone, 1% meat extract (lab lemco), 0.5% NaCl and distilled water, with a pH adjusted to 7.4

Nutrient broth is used as a base to prepare many other culture media. It is also used to study growth curve.

There are three types of nutrient broth –

1. Meat infusion broth – It is an aqueous extract of lean meat to which peptone is added.
2. Meat extract broth – It is a mixture of meat extract and peptone.
3. Digest broth – It is an aqueous extract of lean meat, that has been digested with a proteolytic enzyme so that additional peptone need not be added.

Nutrient agar. Nutrient agar is the simplest and commonest medium used routinely in microbiology laboratories, to grow non-fastidious bacteria. It is prepared by adding agar at a concentration of 2% to the nutrient broth. Nutrient agar is commonly referred to as "agar medium".

Composition :

Peptone –	1%
Meat extract (lablemco) –	1%
NaCl –	0.5%,
Agar –	2%
Distilled water –	100 ml

pH 7.4.

Nutrient agar is used in the form of slopes, butts in test tubes or plates in petridishes.

Uses. Nutrient agar is used

1. to study colony characteristics
2. to detect pigment formation
3. to maintain stock cultures
4. for antibiotic sensitivity testing
5. pure growth of the bacterium on nutrient agar medium is used for slide agglutination and other tests.

Semi-solid agar. When agar concentration in agar medium is decreased to 0.2 to 0.5% a semisolid agar or sloppy agar is formed, which enables motile organisms to spread (by using craigie's tube). When agar concentration is further decreased to 0.05% to 0.1%, agar prevents convection currents and prevents the diffusion of air in thioglycollate media, used for the growth of anaerobic and microaerophilic organisms.

Firm agar. When agar concentration is increased to 6%; it prevents the swarming growth of *Proteus* species and *Clostridium tetani* and enable them to form discrete colonies.

ENRICHED MEDIA

They are prepared by adding blood, serum, egg, milk, glucose etc. to a basal medium. In other words, a simple basal medium is enriched by adding highly nutritious substances such as blood, serum, egg, milk glucose etc.

Enriched media are used for the cultivation of bacteria that possess fastidious growth requirements (complex growth requirements) or that are exacting in their growth requirements. *e.g.*,

1. Blood agar – It is used for the cultivation of Streptococci, pneumococci, *Hemophilus*.
2. Chocolate agar – It is used for the cultivation of *Hemophilus*, meningococci and gonococci.
3. Loeffler's serum slope – It is used for the cultivation of *Corynebacterium diphtheriae*.
4. Dorset's egg medium – It is used for the cultivation of *Mycobacterium tuberculosis* and *Corynebacterium diphtheriae*.
5. Milk agar – It is used to cultivate Staphylococci, to promote their pigment production.
6. Lowenstein-Jensen (LJ) medium used for the cultivation of *Mycobacterium tuberculosis*. Since LJ medium contains egg, it can be grouped under enriched media. But it also contains malachite green, a selective agent; hence widely referred to as selective media.

Blood agar. It is a solid enriched medium, widely used in medical bacateriology, to isolate fastidious bacteria. It is prepared by adding 8–10% sheep blood or horse blood to sterile melted nutrient agar at 50–55°C. Defibrinated blood is preferred to citrated blood to prepare blood agar medium. It is used for the cultivation of bacteria such as Streptococci, pneumococci, gonococci and *Hemophilus* species. Blood agar can be used as an indicator medium to indicate hemolysis property of Streptococci and Staphylococci. It is also used as differential medium to differentiate alpha (α) hemolytic Streptococci, beta (β) hemolytic Streptococci and gamma (γ) hemolytic streptococci.

Chocolate agar/heated blood agar. It is an enriched solid medium, suitable for the cultivation of *Hemophilus influenzae*, pneumococci, meningococci and goncocci.

It is prepared by adding 8–10% defibrinated blood to sterile, melted nutrient agar at 50–55°C; in a boiling water bath at 75°C; by gentle agitation of blood and agar until the medium becomes chocolate-brown in colour. It can also be prepared by heating blood agar plates at 70–80° C for 10 minutes.

Chocolate agar is essentially the same as blood agar, except during preparation RBC are lysed releasing intracellular nutrients such as hemoglobin, hemin ("X" factor), and the co-enzyme NAD ("V" factor). Lysis of RBC gives the medium a chocolate-brown colour from which this medium gets its name. Chocolate agar is the most suitable medium for the cultivation of *Hemophilus influenzae*, because it requires "X" and "V" growth factors for its growth.

Loeffler's serum slope. It is an enriched solid medium preferred for the primary culture of *Corynebacterium diphtheriae*. In this medium, diphtheria bacilli grow very rapidly within 6 to 8 hours of inculbation and luxuriant growth occurs within 12 to 18 hours. Further, smears from growth stained by Albert's or Ponder's or Neisser's method shows typical morphology with well formed metachromatic granules.

On Loeffler's serum slope, diphtheria bacilli form colonies which are small, circular white opaque discs at first, but enlarge on continued incubation and acquire a distinct yellow tint.

Loeffler's serum slope is also used for subculture diphtheria bacilli from potassium tellurite blood agar medium. It is used for growing pure cultures for toxigenicity testing.

Loeffler's serum slope is made up of sheep or horse serum, nutrient broth and glucose. It is sterilised and solidified simultaneously by inspissation.

Dorset's egg media. It is a solid enriched medium prepared by mixing egg and nutrient broth sterilised and solidified by inspissation.

Uses. 1. It is used for the cultivation of *Corynebacterium diphtheriae*.

2. Dorset's egg medium with glycerine is used as a selective medium for the cultivation of *Mycobacterium tuberculosis*.

3. It is used for the preservation of cultures, particularly to prevent S→R (smooth to rough) variation (*e.g., Salmonella typhi*).

Milk agar. It is an enriched solid medium prepared by adding 8–10% milk to nutrient agar. It enhances the pigment production by Staphylococci. The pigments of Staphylococci does not diffuse into the medium. Hence pigmented (colored) colonies are particularly marked against the opaque milky white background. *e.g.,*

1. *Staphylococcus aureus* produces golden-yellow colonies.
2. *Staphylococcus albus* (*epidermidis*) produces white colonies.
3. *Staphylococcus citreus* produces lemon-yellow colonies.

Pigment production can also be enhanced by the addition of 1% glycerol monoacetate into nutrient agar.

ENRICHMENT MEDIA

Enrichment media are essentially liquid media, containing specific nutrients required to enhance the growth of a particular bacterial pathogen, that may be inhibitory to nonpathogenic commensals. In other words, some chemical substances are incorporated into liquid media, which cause enrichment of the required pathogenic bacterium and inhibits the growth of unwanted bacteria from a mixture of organisms such as feces, throat swab etc. *e.g.,*

1. Selenite F broth (F for feces) for enrichment of typhoid and paratyphoid bacilli from fecal samples.

2. Tetrathionate broth for enrichment of *Salmenella* species from feces.

3. Alkaline peptone water (pH 8.6) for enrichment of *Vibrio cholerae* from feces.

4. Monsur's taurocholate tellurite peptone water (pH 9.2) can also be used for enrichment of *Vibrio cholerae* from feces.

5. Bile broth used for isolation of *Salmonella* from blood.

6. Salt broth containing 8–10% NaCl is used for enrichment of *Staphylococcus aureus*.

Selenite F broth. It is an excellent and widely used liquid enrichment medium, used for the isolation of *Salmonellae* from *feces*, sewage, food stuffs and other materials containing mixed bacterial flora. It is prepared from peptone, lactose, sodium acid selenite and phosphate buffer with pH adjusted to 7.1.

Feces sample is added to selenite-F broth (F for fecal) broth and incubated at 37°C for 6–8 hrs. and subcultured on to solid media. Sodium selenite can be utilised by Salmonellae, but toxic to *E.coli* and other enterobacteriaceae members. Selenite is reduced by Salmonellae and produce alkali, that increases the pH decreasing toxicity. Hence, phosphate buffer is added to prevent this.

Selenite F broth is a brick red or orange colored liquid. a slight amount of red precipitate may form but this does not interfere with the enrichment.

Tetrathionate broth. It is a liquid enrichment medium used for the enrichment of Salmonellae from fecel samples. The medium contains nutrient broth, calcium carbonate, sodium thiosulphate and iodine. Phenol red is the indicator. These substances ibhibit the growth of coliform bacilli, while permitting typhoid and paratyphoid bacilli to grow freely. Tetrathionate broth is not as efficient as selenite F broth for enrichment of *Salmonellae*, because it may permit the growth of *Proteus* species. Feces is inoculated into tetrathionate broth and incubated for 6–18 hours and a subculture is made on Mac Conkey agar or DCA medium.

SELECTIVE MEDIA

Selective media are solid media, in which chemical substances are incorporated, which promotes the selective growth of required bacterial pathogens and suppress the growth of unwanted, commensal, non-pathogenic bacteria.

Selective media and enrichment media are essentially similar; the only difference is that selective media are solid, while enrichment media are liquid. *e.g.,*

1. Thayer-Martin medium for the isolation of gonococci and meningococci.
2. LJ medium for the isolation of tubercle bacilli.
3. Potassium tellurite chocolate agar for the isolation of diphtheria bacilli.
4. Wilson Blair's brilliant green bismuth sulphite agar medium – for the isolation of typhoid and paratyphoid bacilli.
5. Deoxycholate citrate (DCA) agar for the isolation of *Shigellae.*
6. TCBS (Thiosulphate, citrate, bilesalts, sucrose) agar for the isolation of *Vibrio cholerae.*

Potassium tellurite blood agar/McLeod's medium. It is a selective medium used for the cultivation of *Corynebacterium diphtheriae*. This special medium is devised by McLeod with heated Rabbit's blood and potassium tellurite (0.04%) and called it chocolate tellurite agar.

Potassium tellurite acts as a selective agent inhibiting the growth of other organisms, particularly commensals of throat. Diphtheria bacilli reduce tellurite to metallic tellurium, which gets incorporated in the colonies giving them a black or grey color. The growth may be slow and colonies appear on two days of incubation.

Based on colony morphology on potassium tellurite chocolate agar medium, McLeod classified diphtheria bacilli into three biotypes:

1. Gravis – Daisy head colonies
2. Intermedius – Frog's egg colony
3. Mitis – Poached egg colony.

Wilson and Blair's bismuth sulphite agar. It is a selective medium for the isolation of typhoid and paratyphoid pacilli from feces samples. It is prepared by adding bismuth sulphite-phosphate-glucose mixture and iron- citrate-brilliant green mixture to nutrient agar. Brilliant green and bismuth sulphite act as selective agents and inhibit the growth of coliforms including *Shigellae* and *Proteus* species.

Salmonella typhi and *Salmonella paratyphi* 'B' reduce sulphite to sulphide in the presence of glucose and hence produce black colonies with a metallic sheen due to the formation of iron-sulphide (H_2S positive). *Salmonella paratyphi* 'A' and *Salmonella cholera-suis* which does not forms H_2S, produce green colored colonies.

Fecal culture on Wilson and Blair's medium is particularly valuable in patients of enteric fever on anti-biotics, as the drug does not eliminate the bacilli from the gut as rapidly as it does from the blood. Also, to trace carriers, swabs left in the sewage drainers (sewer-swab technique) or membrane filters through which sewage is filtered; can be cultured on this medium.

TCBS agar. Thiosulphate citrate bile sucrose (TCBS) agar is the most widely used selective plating medium for the isolation of *Vibrio cholerae* from feces. It gives good growth of *Vibrio cholerae* and *Vibrio parahemolyticus* and other vibrios, inhibits the growth of enterobacteria, and Gram positive bacteria.

The pH of the medium is alkaline 8.6. Bromothymol blue is the indicator. It appears dark green colored, transparent on which *Vibrio cholerae* produces large yellow convex colonies due to sucrose fermentation. *Vibrio parahemolyticus* does not ferment sucrose hence produce green colored colonies.

Lowenstein-Jensen (LJ) medium. It is a selective medium for the cultivation and differentiation of human and bovine types of tubercle bacilli and atypical mycobacteria.

It contains mineral salts, starch, glycerol, asparagine, malachite green and egg. Mycobacteria obtain their nitrogen from asparagine and the carbon from glycerol. Malachite green acts as a selective agent and inhibits contaminants. The medium is sterilised and solidified simultaneously by inspissation in inspissator. No agar is present in the medium. Coagulation of egg gives the solid surface. Clinical specimens are decontaminated and also concentrated for bacilli by Petroff's technique and then inoculated into the medium. Growth occurs in 4–6 weeks.

Mycobacterium tuberculosis grows luxuriantly and produces large, dry, rough, heaped up colonies with a wrinkled surface. It is called "Eugonic" growth. Colonies are creamy white initially, becoming yellowish or buff coloured later. In comparison, *Mycobacterium bovis* growus sparsely and produces small, flat, smooth, moist and small discrete colorless colonies known as "dysgonic" growth.

The most widely employed medium for routine culture is LJ medium, without starch, as recommended by International union against tuberculosis (IUAT).

Deoxycholate citrate agar. DCA is a selective medium suitable for the isolation of Shigellae and Salmonellae. It is prepared by adding sodium citrate, sodium thiosulphate, ferric citrate, lactose and a bile salt (sodium deoxycholate) to nutrient agar. Neutral red is the indicator. Bile salts inhibit the growth of Gram positive organisms and to a certain extent the coliforms. Some coliforms may grow and produce pink colonies due to lactose fermentation, whereas non-lactose fermenters (NLF) produce palc, colorless colonies. Medium contains ferric citrate and H_2S producing bacteria form iron sulphide and the colony shows a central black dot.

DIFFERENTIAL MEDIA

Differential media are those in which chemical substances are incorporated which enable it bring out different characteristics of different bacteria; so that colonies of one particular species can be differentiated visually from those of another. *e.g.*, MacConkey agar, Eosin-Methylene blue (EMB) agar.

MacConkey's agar/Bile salt lactose neutral red agar. It is a differential medium widely used in the primary isolation, identification and differentiation of Gram negative bacilli, belonging to family enterobacteriacease.

It contains peptone, meat extracat, NaCl, bile salt, lactose and neutral red indicator. Bile salt inhibits the growth of Gram positive bacteria. Some bacteria ferment lactose and produce acid which decreases medium pH and causes the neutral red indicator to give a pink or red color to colonies. They are known as Lactose fermenters (LF). Non-lactose fermenters (NLF) form colorless, pale colonies. Some organisms ferment lactose late, and called as Late-Lactose fermenters (LLF).

LF-*e.g., Esch.coli*, *Klebsiellae* sp.

Colonies of *Esch.coli* are pink, moist, large, partially translucent or opaque discs.

Colonies of *Klebsiellae* are pink, large, dome shaped, mucoid with varying degrees of stickyness.

NLF – *e.g., Salmonella, Shigella.*

LLF – *e.g., Shigella sonnei.*

INDICATOR MEDIA

Indicator media are those which indicate a property of the bacterium. These media contain an indicator which changes color when a bacterium grows in it. *e.g.,*

1. MacConkey agar indicates lactose fermenting property. LF produce pink colonies and NLF produce colorless colonies due to neutral red indicator.
2. Wilson and Blair's bismuth sulphite agar medium indicates H_2S production due to the reduction of sulphite to sulphide in the presence of glucose. *S.typhi*, *S.paratyphi* B and *S.paratyphi* C produce black colonies with metallic sheen due to H_2S production whereas *S.paratyphi* A and *S.cholera-suis* form green colonies, as they do not produce H_2S.
3. Potassium tellurite chocolate agar indicates reduction of tellurite by forming tellurium metal, which accumulates in the colonies of diphtheria bacilli forming black colonies.

TRANSPORT MEDIA

When the patient is not close to the laboratory, there is a risk that the pathogen in a specimen may not survive or may be overgrown by non-pathogens during the time it takes to transport the specimen to the laboratory. For this purpose, special media have been devised termed as "transport media". Enrichment media can be used to transportation of specimens. Transport media can also be used for preservation of bacteria in clinical specimens. *e.g.,*

1. Stuart's transport medium for gonococci.
2. Sach's buffered glycerol saline for enteric bacilli in feces.
3. Pike's medium for *Streptococcus pyogenes*, pneumococci and *Hemophilus influenzae* in nose and throat swabs.
4. Cary-Blair medium for *Vibrio cholerae* and *Campylobacter.*
5. V-R fluid (pH 9.2) for *Vibrio cholerae*.
6. Alkaline peptone water (pH 8.6) for *Vibrio cholerae.*

ANAEROBIC MEDIA

They are used for the cultivation of anaerobic bacteria. These media contain a reducing substance which absorbs all the oxygen and creates an anaerobic condition, which favours the growth of anaerobes. *e.g.,*

1. Robertson's cooked (chopped) meat (RCM) broth.
2. Thioglycollate medium.

RCM broth. (Robertson's cooked meat broth) – It is used for the cultivation of anaerobic bacteria; also used for the preservation of aerobic bacteria.

The medium contains meat infusion or nutrient broth, minced, cooked ox heart tissue. Broth is layered over by liquid paraffin to prevent the entry of air. Chopped meat contains unsaturated fatty acids which act as reducing agent and absorb oxygen; hematin catalyses this reducing action; and sulphydryl groups create a low redox potential; all these factors favor the growth of anaerobic bacteria. Particularly *Clostridium* species. The specimen is inoculated deep in the medium in contact with the meat.

RCM broth detects proteolytic and saccharolytic activities of anaerobic bacteria. Proteolytic Clostridia blacken the meat with the formation of foul smelling sulphur compounds *e.g., Clostridium histolyticum.* Saccharolytic *Clostridia* turn meat red slightly with sour smell. *e.g., Clostridium welchii (perfringens).*

Clostridium tetani does not have saccharolytic property and shows only mild proteolytic activity and hence no change in the meat appearance. Only prolonged incubation give slight blackening.

Thioglycollate medium/broth. It is an anaerobic medium. The medium contains reducing agents such as sodium thioglycollate, glucose, vitamin-C (ascorbic acid), cysteine and agar at a concentration of 0.05%, with methylene blue.

Thioglycollate acts as a reducing agent and creates an anaerobic environment deeper in the tube, allows anaerobic bacteria to grow. Glucose and thioglycollate maintain the anaerobic condition. Agar (0.05%) prevents convection currents of air. Methylene blue act as an oxidation-reduction potential indicator. Methylene blue remains colorless throughout the medium except at the surface where oxygen may be present.

SUGAR MEDIA/SUGAR FERMENTATION TEST

Bacteria differ widely in their ability to metabolise/ferment carbohydrates, and produce either only acid or both acid and gas. Hence, carbohydrate fermentation is used for characterisation and identification of bacteria, particularly important in the study of Gram negative bacilli. Sugar media are used to test fermentation.

Carbohydrate media consists of peptone water, 1% sugar and Andrade's indicator. The sugars may be glucose, lactose, sucrose, maltose, xylose, mannitol etc. Andrade's indicator consists of acid fuchsin and NaOH. The medium is distributed in the test tubes and a small inverted tube called "Durham's tube" completely filled with liquid and containing no air bubbles is placed isnide, and sterilised. The color of the medium is light yellow.

The test bacterium is inoculated and incubated. Acid production is indicated by the development of pink color. Gas accumulates in the inner Durham's tube.

Phenol red indicator can also be used. Then the original color of the medium is red and turns yellow on acid production.

Bromocresol purple indicator can also be used. Then the original color of the medium is purple and turns yellow on acid production.

To test sugar fermentation of bacteria with fastidious growth requirements, such as Streptococci, pneumococci, gonococci, meningococci and diphtheria bacilli, **Hiss's serum water** is used. It is a sugar medium enriched with serum.

QUESTIONS

Short Notes

1. Meal extract/lablemco.
2. Peptone.
3. Agar/Agar-agar.
4. Defined media/synthetic media.
5. Semidefined media.
6. Peptone water medium.
7. Simple media/ordinary media/Basal media.
8. Nutrient broth.
9. Nutrient agar.
10. Enriched media.
11. Blood agar-constituents, preparation and uses.
12. Chocolate agar.
13. Loeffler's serum slope.
14. Dorset's egg media.
15. Milk agar.
16. Name four commonly used enriched media and their uses.
17. Enrichment media.
18. Selenite F broth.
19. Tetrathionate broth.
20. Name any two enrichment media and their uses.
21. Selective media.
22. Name four commonly used selective media and their uses.
23. wilson and Blair's medium.
24. Potassium tellurite blood agar.
25. TCBS agar.
26. Lowenstein - Jensen (LJ) medium.
27. Deoxycholate citrate agar (DCA).
28. Differential media.
29. Macconkey agar.
30. Indicator media.
31. Transport media.
32. Name four transport media and their uses.
33. Anaerobic media.
34. Name two anaerobic media and their uses.
35. RCM broth.
36. Thioglycollate medium/thioglycollate broth.
37. Sugar media/carbohydrate media/carbohydrate (sugar) fermentaion.

11

Isolation of Bacteria, Cultivation Methods for Bacteria, Inoculation of Culture Media, Culturing Microorganisms

- *Inoculation*
- *Primary culture*
- *Isolate*
- *Subculture*
- *Axenic culture*
- *Inoculation wire loop*
- *Straight wire*
- *Spud/L-shaped wire*
- *Spreader*
- *Pasteur pipette*
- *Methods of cultivation*
  - *Streak culture/ surface plating*
  - *Stroke culture*
  - *Stab culture*
  - *Lawn/Carpet culture*
  - *Pour plate culture*
  - *Liquid culture*
  - *Sweep plate method*
  - *Cough plate method*
- *Anaerobic methods of cultivation*
  - *Glove boxes (anaerobic chambers)*
  - *Anaerobic bags/pouches*
  - *Reduction of oxygen in the media*
  - *Mc Intosh Field's anaerobic jar*
  - *Absorption of oxygen*
  - *Candle jar method*

INOCULATION

The process of seeding bacteria (or) a specimen containing bacteria in to culture media is called "inoculation".

PRIMARY CULTURE

When an organism is isolated for the first time directly from a sample is called "Primary culture" or "Primary isolation".

ISOLATE

Each primary culture isolated/cultivated in pure culture from a natural source is called an isolate.

SUBCULTURE

The periodic transfer of cultures to fresh media under sterile, aseptic conditions and its subsequent growth is termed "Subcultures" or Secondary cultures", Where bacteria are transferred or cultured from one medium to another medium.

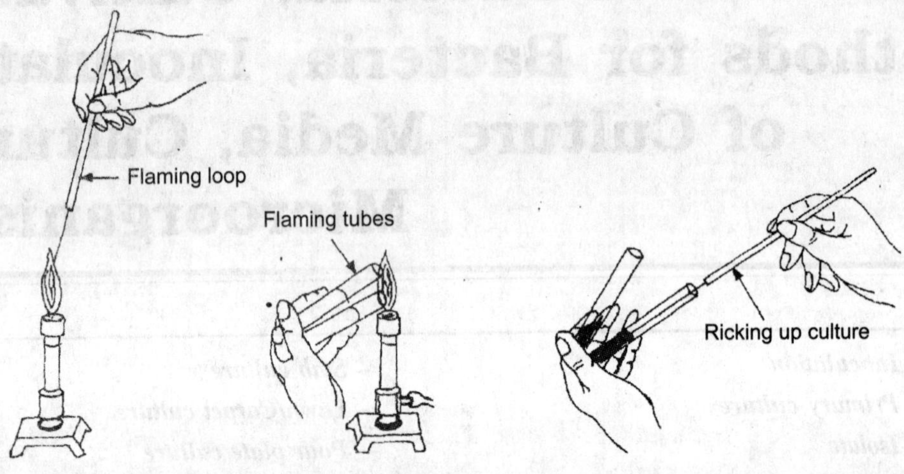

Fig. 11.1 The process of picking up inoculum from a culture tube for transfer to another slant (subculturing).

Subcultures are usually done

1. to obtain a pure growth of the bacterium
2. to study the characteristics/properties of the isolated organism
3. to maintain/preserve stock cultures

AXENIC CULTURE

It is a pure culture of an organism of a single species (*e.g.*, bacterium, fungus, protozoan etc.) growing in a medium free of other living organisms.

For inoculation of a specimen in to culture medium, the following instruments are used.

INOCULATION WIRE LOOP

It consists of a nichrome wire of thickness 23 SWG and of 3 inches length, mounted in a glass or metal holder. The other end of wire is drawn in to a flat, circular, completely closed loop of 2–4 mm internal diameter. Instead of nichrome wire, platinum or Eureka may be used.

The wire loop is sterilized by holding it vertically in a Bunsen flame so that the whole length becomes red hot at the same time. The advantages of nichrome, platinum and eureka wires are that they get heated quickly and cooled quickly. It is allowed to cool down before touching any specimen or culture.

It is used for inoculation of clinical specimens on to the culture media or transfer of the material on to the slide to prepare smears etc. A standard wire loop for urine culture should deliver 0.01 ml of urine for quantitative estimation of bacteria in urine.

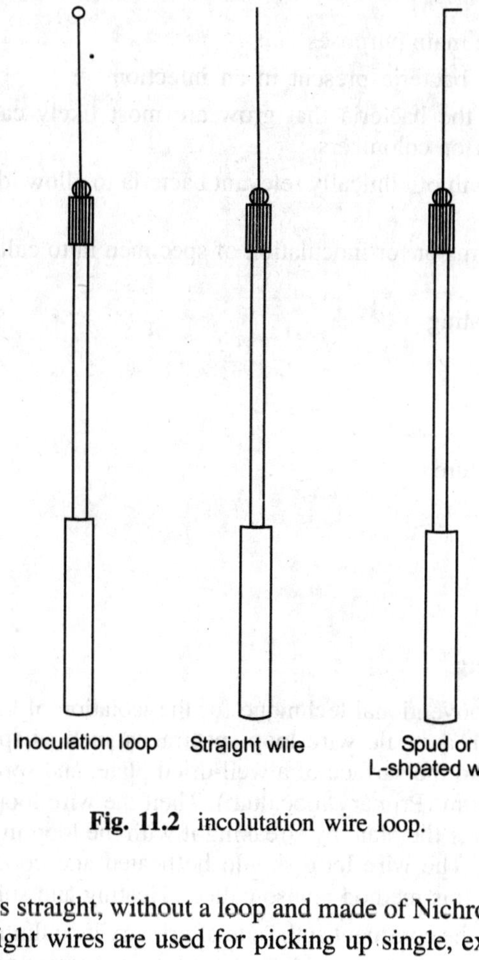

Fig. 11.2 incolutation wire loop.

STRAIGHT WIRE

This inoculation wire is straight, without a loop and made of Nichrome or platinum or Eureka with a length of 4.5 inches. Straight wires are used for picking up single, exact colonies and for deep stab inoculation.

SPUD/L-SHAPED WIRE

It is a straight wire bent at right angles into L-shaped and tip is flattened. It is used to handle tenacious growths such as fungal colonies, to pick up sticky colonies of Actinomycetes and for scraping the medium.

SPREADER

It is a capillary tube bent at right angle. This is used for spreading or carpetting the liquid culture on the solid medium employed for antibiotic sensitivity testing and phage typing.

PASTEUR PIPETTE

It is single glass tube drawn into a long tapering end, as a capillary pipette. It is sterilised in hot air oven at 160°C for 1 hour. It is used with a rubber teat.

It is used for transferring liquid cultures, liquid media, antigen and antisera etc. It is used for inoculation of media for biochemical tests and for serological tests.

METHODS OF CULTIVATION

Bacterial cultivation serves three main purposes

1. to grow and isolate all bacteria present in an infection
2. to determine which of the bacteria that grow are most likely causing infection and which are likely contaminants or colonizers
3. to obtain sufficient growth of clinically relevant bacteria to allow identification and characterization.

For culturing microorganisms or for inoculation of specimen in to culture media various methods are employed.

1. Steak culture/surface plating
2. Stroke culture
3. Stab culture
4. Shake culture
5. Lawn culture/carpet culture
6. Pour plate culture
7. Liquid culture
8. Sweep plate method
9. Cough plate method

Streak Culture/Surface Plating

It is routinely employed conventional technique for the isolation of bacteria in pure culture from various clinical specimens. With a sterile wire loop specimens such as sputum, pus, feces, CSF and aspirated fluid is transferred on to the surface of a well-dried plate, and spread over a small area at the periphery. It is known as inoculum (Primary inoculum). Then the wire loop is sterilized again and the inoculum is distributed thinly over the plate by streaking it with the loop in a series of parallel lines, in different segments of the plate. The wire loop should be heated and cooled (sterilized) between the different sets of streaks. Hence, this method is also called "Heating and subsequent streaking".

On incubation, growth may be confluent at the site of primary inoculum, but becomes progressively thinner, and well separated, discrete colonies appear over the final series of streaks.

Surface plating can also be done by successive or consecutive rubbing, and grid plate method.

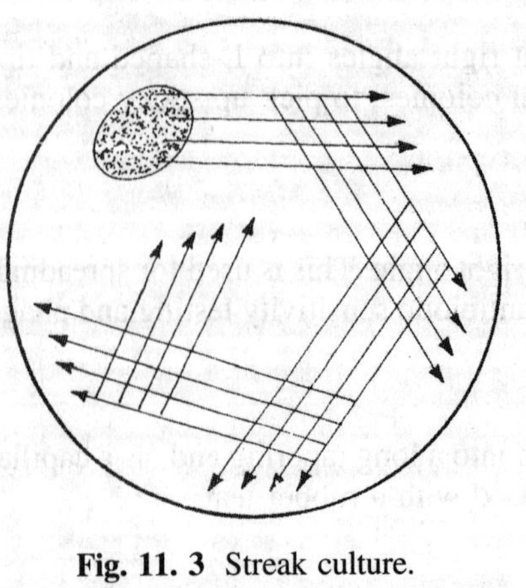

Fig. 11. 3 Streak culture.

Stroke Culture. Stroke cultures are made in test tubes or bottles containing agar slope or slant. The agar medium is allowed to set in tubes in a slanting position at 45° angle. The specimen or a colony is taken with a sterile wire loop and inoculated on to a slope by strokes, by holding the tube horizontally. If there is a butt, inoculation in to butt is done by stabbing with a straight wire.

Stroke cultures are employed 1. for obtaining pure growth of the bacterium, 2. for slide agglutination tests, 3. for biochemical tests and other diagnostic tests.

e.g., Inoculation of Nutrient agar slant, Loeffler's serum slope, TSI agar and Sabouraud's agar medium etc.

Stab Culture. The agar medium for stab culture is allowed to set in upright position in test tubes providing a flat surface at the top of the medium.

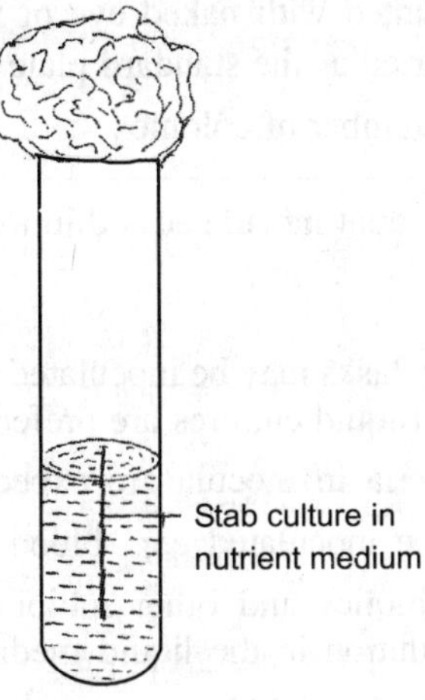

Fig. 11.4 Stab culture.

A straight wire of 4.5 inches length is sterilized and the colony is picked up and inoculated by puncturing or stabbing deep in to the medium (such as nutrient gelatin or glucose agar).
Stab cultures are used

1. to test gelatin liquefaction or production of gelatinase, which liquefies gelatin.

2. to study the oxygen requirement of the bacterium to differentiate aerobic and anaerobic bacteria. Aerobic bacteria grow on the surface, where oxygen is available .Anaerobic bacteria grow deep in the medium, where oxygen is not available, whereas facultative anaerobes grow along the stab on the surface as well as deep in the medium.

3. for maintenance or preservation of stock cultures

4. to study the motility of bacteria in "semi-solid agar".

Lawn Culture/Carpet Culture

Lawn cultures are prepared by flooding/spreading the surface of the agar plate with a liquid culture or bacterial suspension. The excess fluid can be pipetted out. Alternatively, a sterile swab soaked in bacterial culture can be rubbed over the entire surface of the medium.

The lawn culture provides a confluent, uniform surface growth of the bacterium and is useful for– 1. Antibiotic sensitivity testing by disc diffusion method, 2. Phage typing, 3. Obtaining a large amount of growth as in the preparation of large amount of bacterial suspensions to produce antigens or vaccines.

Pour Plate Culture

Pour plate cultures are used to estimate colony count or viable count or standard Plate count (SPC) of bacteria and fungi in water, milk and soil samples. Pour plate method is also useful for quantitative urine cultures.

The sample is diluted several times (serial dilutions) and a small volume (usually 1 ml) of the diluted sample is mixed with 10-15 ml agar medium in a test tube, that is molten and cooled to 45°C; and the mixtures are shaken or rolled between the palms (as in shake cultures) and poured immediately in to sterile petriplates. Most bacteria and fungi are not killed by a brief exposure to the warm agar. After the agar is hardened, each cell is fixed in its place and forms an individual colony upon incubation. The total number of colonies equals the viable microorganisms in the diluted sample. The colonies can be seen trapped deep inside the medium.

The visible colonies can be counted with naked eye or in a colony counter and the number of colonies per ml of the sample is reported as the standard plate count (SPC) per ml.

$$\text{Number of cells per ml} = \frac{\text{Number of colonies}}{\text{Amount inoculated} \times \text{dilution}}$$

Liquid Cultures

Liquid media in tubes, bottles or flasks may be inoculated with a sterile wire loop or by adding the inoculum with pipettes and syringes. Liquid cultures are preferred

1. When concentration of bacteria in inocula are expected to be small *e.g.*, sterility tests.
2. When large inocula are to be inoculated *e.g.*, blood culture.
3. For inocula containing antibiotics and other inhibitory substances, as these are rendered diluted and ineffective by dilution in the liquid media *e.g.*, blood culture.
4. When large yields are desired, the yield being enhanced by agitation, aeration *e.g.*, production of alcohols and antibiotics.
5. For biochemical tests *e.g.*, sugar fermentation and IMViC reactions.
6. For enrichment media *e.g.*, selenite F broth.
7. For presumptive coliform test in bacteriological analysis of water.

The major disadvantage of liquid culture is that it does not provide a pure culture from mixed inocula.

Sweep Plate Method

The edges of the petriplate with culture medium is rubbed over the cloth with the medium facing it. The dust particles alongwith microorganisms stirred up from the fabric and get settled on the culture medium. Colonies develop on incubation, which can be counted and viable counts made.

Cough Plate Method

Cough plate method is used to collect specimens directly from patients at bed side suffering from whooping cough (pertussis) caused by *Bordetella pertussis*.

Bordet-Gengou glycerine-potato-blood agar plate is held about 10-15 cm infront of the patient's mouth, during a spontaneous or induced paroxysm of coughing, so that respiratory exudates impinge directly on the medium. The plate is incubated for 48-72 hours. *Bordetella pertussis* produces colonies resembling mercury drops or bisected pearls when growth is confluent, silvery or aluminium paint like appearance is seen.

The colonies should be first examined by Gram's staining and then confirmed by slide agglutination test with specific antiserum.

ANAEROBIC METHODS OF CULTIVATION

Anaerobic bacteria do not require oxygen for their growth. In the presence of oxygen, hydrogen peroxide which is toxic to growth accumulates. The enzyme catalase which splits hydrogen peroxide is absent in anaerobes. Hence, special methods have been devised to process specimens and cultivate anaerobic bacteria in oxygen-free atmosphere.

Various anaerobic methods of cultivation are listed here below :

I. Gloves boxes (Anaerobic chambers).

II. Anaerobic bags/Anaerobic Pouches.

III. Anaerobic media/Reduction of oxygen in the media

(*i*) RCM broth.

(*ii*) Thioglycollate medium.

IV. Mc Intosh-Filds's anaerobic Jar

V. Absorption of oxygen

1. Chemical method
2. Biological method.

Glove Boxes/Anaerobic Chambers/Anaerobic Cabinets

Glove boxes are used for processing of specimens, incubation of cultures, periodic examination of culture plates, subcultures, and to make prereduction of media for anaerobic organisms in an oxygen-free atmosphere.

Anaerobic Bags/Anaerobic Pouches

They are useful for laboratories processing small number of specimens. They can be used to transport specimens, and also to incubate one or two agar plates.

Reduction of Oxygen in the Media/Anaerobic Media

These media contain a reducing agent which absorbs all the oxygen and creates an anaerobic condition, which favours the growth of anaerobes.

(i) RCM broth. It contains meat infusion or Nutrient broth and minced, cooked beef heart tissue. Liquid paraffin is layered over the broth to prevent the entry of air. Chopped meat contains unsaturated fatty acids which act as reducing agent and absorb oxygen, hematin catalyses this reducing action, and sulphydryl groups create a low redox potential ; All these factors favour the growth of anaerobic bacteria, particularly *Clostridium* species.

(ii) Thioglycollate medium. It contains reducing agents sodium thioglycollate, glucose, Vitamin-C, cysteine and agar at a concentration of 0.05%, with methylene blue as indicator.

Thioglycollate acts as a reducing agent and creates an anaerobic environment. Glucose and thiogly-collate maintain the anaerobic condition. Agar (0.05%) prevents convection currents, which prevents diffusion of air in to the medium.

Mc-Intosh-Filde's Anaerobic Jar

To grow anaerobes on the surface of solid media it is necessary to provide an atmosphere free of oxygen. This is achieved by the use of anaerobic jars, such as Mc Intosh-filde's and Baird and Tatlock anaerobic jar.

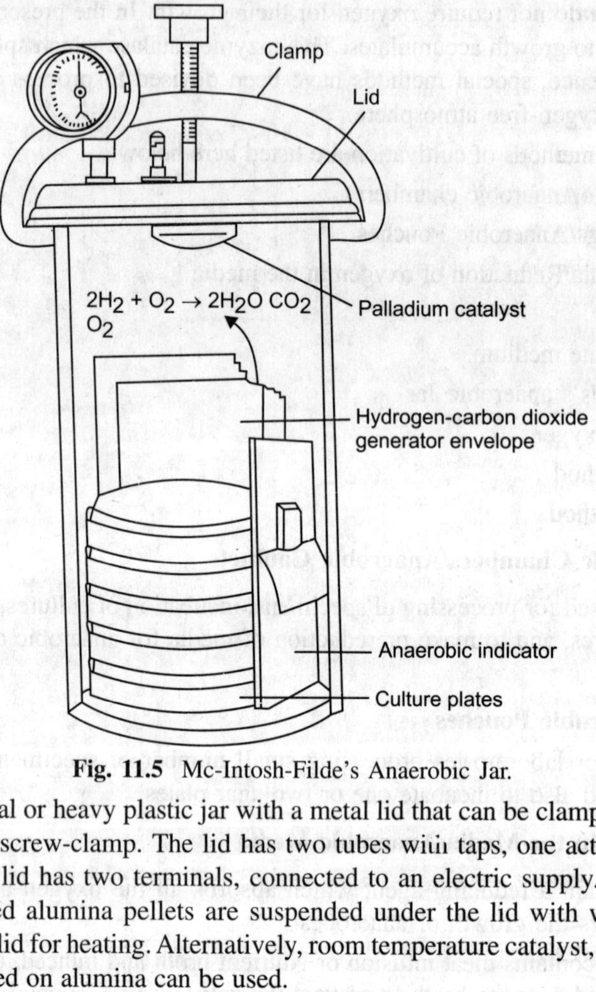

Fig. 11.5 Mc-Intosh-Filde's Anaerobic Jar.

It consists of a metal or heavy plastic jar with a metal lid that can be clamped down on a gasket to make it air-tight with a screw-clamp. The lid has two tubes witu taps, one acting as the inlet and the other as the outlet. The lid has two terminals, connected to an electric supply. One or more capsules containing palladiumized alumina pellets are suspended under the lid with wires and connected to electric terminals on the lid for heating. Alternatively, room temperature catalyst, called Deoxo pellets, in which palladium is coated on alumina can be used.

Inoculated culture plates are placed inside the jar with medium upside and lid downwords, as soon as they are seeded, and the lid is clamped air-tight. Following procedures are adopted to provide anaerobiosis in anaerobic jars, with an increased CO_2 concentration, as CO_2 enhances the growth of many anaerobes.

(i) Displacement of oxygen or evacuation-replacement method. The outlet valve is connected to a vacuum pump and the air is removed from the sealed jar by drawing a vacuum of 25 inches of mercury (62.5 cm or 625 mm of Hg). This process is repeated two times, filling the jar with an oxygen-free gas such as nitrogen, between evacuations. Finally, the jar is filled with a gas mixture containing 80% nitrogen, 10% hydrogen and 10% CO_2 (or 90% hydrogen and 10% CO_2). The inlet valve is then closed and the jar is incubated at 37°C when room temperature catalyst is used, there is no need of heating.

(ii) Displacement and combustion of oxygen. The electric terminals are connected to a current supply so that palladiumized asbestos is heated. This acts as a catalyst for the combination of hydrogen with residual oxygen present in the jar. This method of displacement of oxygen combined with combustion ensures complete anaerobiosis, but rarely carries the risk of explosion.

(iii) Gas pak system. The Gas pak is at present the method of choice for producing anaerobiosis in anaerobic jars.

It is a disposable aluminium foil packet, commercially available, containing pellets of sodium borohydride and cobalt chloride and of citric acid and sodium bicarbonate. They generate hydrogen and CO_2 on addition of water, hence known as "hydrogen and CO_2 generator envelope"

The Gas pak envelope is kept in the jar, with water added along with inoculated plates and the lid is tightened. The Gas pak chemicals generate H_2 and CO_2 and the presence of a catalyst enables the combination of H_2 and oxygen to produce anaerobic environment. Production of heat within a few minutes and subsequent development of moisture on the walls of the jar are indications that the catalyst and Gas pak envelope are functioning properly.

However Methylene blue or resazurin indicators can be used to verify anaerobiosis. Methylene blue becomes colorless in the absence of oxygen; whereas it becomes blue colored when exposed to oxygen.

Absorption of oxygen

Anaerobiosis can be produced by absorption of oxygen from closed systems either by chemical method or biological method.

Chemical Methods

(i) Alkaline pyrogallol. It absorbs oxygen. It is used in various modifications.

(a) Spray anaerobic dish. It is a glass dish with its bottom partitioned in to two halves, and the top accommodating one half of a Petri dish carrying the medium. Pyrogallic acid and NaOH are placed in the separate halves at the bottom of the dish. The inoculated culture plate is inverted on the top of the dish and sealed air-tight. The dish may be tilted slightly to mix the chemicals.

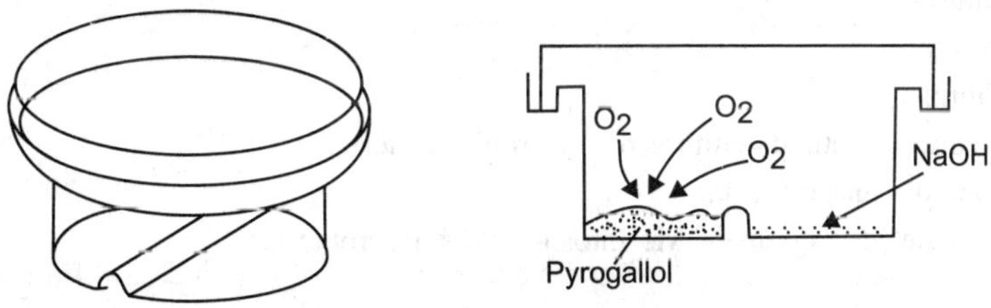

Fig. 11.6 The spray plate.

(b) Alkaline pyrogallol in an ordinary petri plate. This method employs a disc of filter paper having the same diameter as a Petri dish. It is placed on top of one half of the dish, and pyrogallol and sodium carbonate in dry powder form is spread on it. The inoculated plate is inverted over the filter paper and sealed tight with molten wax. The dry pyrogallol and sodium carbonate is activated by the moisture within the closed system, and complete anaerobiosis develops within about two hours.

(ii) Rosenthal method. Anaerobiosis within jars can be produced with a mixture of chromium and sulphuric acid. Oxygen is reduced to water.

(iii) Phosphorous stick method. Inoculated plates are kept in a closed air-tight jar. Yellow phosphorous sticks are burnt in the jar to absorb oxygen. The phosphorous continues to burn till all the oxygen gets exhausted and ultimately only the inert gases and partial vacuum remain. A small container of water should be kept to absorb phosphorous pentoxide formed due to phosphorous burning.

Biological Method

Absorption of oxygen from jars is attempted by incubating cultures with germinating seeds, chopped vegetables (Potatoes), and aerobic organisms such as *Pseudomonas aeruginosa* and *Serratia marcescens*. Anaerobiosis produced by biological methods is slow and ineffective.

QUESTIONS

Essay Type Questions

1. Give an account of various methods of anaerobic culture of bacteria.
2. Enumerate the growth requirements of bacteria. Describe in detail the anaerobic methods of cultivation.

Short Notes

1. Inoculation wire loop.
2. Spud.
3. Pasteur pipette.
4. Surface plating/streak cultures.
5. Stroke culture.
6. Stab culture.
7. Lawn culture/carpet culture.
8. Pour plate method.
9. Liquid cultures.
10. Cough plate method.
11. Primary cultures.
12. Subculture.
13. Axenic culture.
14. Anaerobic culture methods/culture of anaerobic bacteria.
15. Mc Intosh-Field's anaerobic jar.
16. Draw a neat labeled diagram of Mc Intosh-Field's anaerobic jar.
17. Gas pak.
18. Alkaline pyrogallol method.
19. Candle jar.
20. RCM broth.
21. Thioglycollate medium.

12

Biochemical Tests for the Identification of Bacteria

• ***IMViC Reactions***	• ***Catalase test***
– Indole test	• ***Oxidase test***
– Methyl red test	• ***Phynyl alanine deaminase test***
– Voges-Proskauer test	• ***TSI agar***
– Citrate utilization test	• ***Oxidation-Fermentation test/Hugh & Leifson's test***
• ***Urease test***	

IMViC REACTIONS

IMViC is a sigla, refers to Indole test, Methyl Red test, Voges-Proskauer test and Citrate utilization tests. '*i*' is added for the easiness of pronounciation. IMViC reactions are widely used for the identification and differentiation of intestinal Gram negative bacilli.

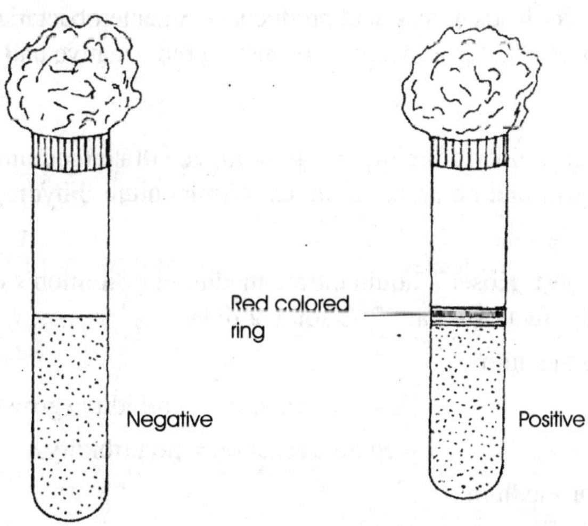

Fig. 12.1 Indole test.

Indole Test

Some bacteria decompose the amino acid tryptophan to form indole, which is tested for by a colorimetric reaction with Kovac's (or Ehrlich's) reagent.

The test bacterium is inoculated into peptone water medium and incubated at 37°C for 1-2 days. To this culture add few drops of Kovac's reagent or Ehrlich reagent and shake gently. A red color ring in the top alcohol layer indicates a positive reaction.

Kovac's reagent is composed of p-dimethyl amino benzadehyde, Amyl or isoamyl alcohol, conc. HCl.

E.coli and *Vibrio cholerae* are indole positive, whereas *Klebsiella* and *Salmonella* are indole negative.

Methyl Red Test

The test is employed to detect the production of acid during the fermentation of glucose and maintenance of a pH below 4.5 in an old culture, tested by Methyl Red reagent.

The test bacterium is inoculated into glucose phosphate peptone water medium and incubated at 37°C for 1-2 days. Add a few drops of methyl red reagent, mix and read. Positive tests are bright red and negative are yellow. If the results are equivocal, the test can be repeated with cultures incubated for 5 days. For some organisms, incubation at 30°C for 5 days may be preferable.

Voges-Proskauer Test/Acetoin Production

Some bacteria ferment carbohydrates with the production of acetyl methyl carbinol (acetoin) or its reduction product 2, 3 butylene glycol, which is oxidized to diacetyl. It is tested by a colorimetric reaction with a guanidine group under alkaline conditions.

The test bacterium is inoculated in to Glucose phosphate peptone water medium and incubate at 37°C or 30°C for 1-2 days only.

Add 1 ml of 40% Potassium hydroxide and 3 ml of a 5% solution of α-naphthol in absolute alcohol (Barrit's reagent). A positive reaction is indicated by the development of a pink color in 2-5 minutes, becoming crimson in 30 minutes.

This test is usually done in conjunction with methyl red test, since the production of acetyl methyl carbinol or 2:3 butylene glycol leads to less acid production. An enterobacterial organism is usually either methyl red positive and voges-Proskaver negative or methyl red negative and Voges-Proskauer positive.

Citrate Utilization Test

The test is based on the ability of an organism to utilize citrate (sodium citrate) as the sole carbon and energy source for growth and an ammonium salt (Ammonium dihydrogen phosphate) as the sole source of nitrogen.

For citrate utilization test, Koser's liquid citrate medium or Simmon's citrate agar may be used to inoculate test bacterium and incubated at 37°C for 1-2 days.

Koser's liquid citrate medium –

Positive reaction = turbidity (growth)
Negative reaction = no turbidity

Simmon's citrate agar medium –

Positive reaction = blue color and streak of growth. Utilization of citrate changes the pH of the medium to alkaline (formation of NaOH) which is indicated by color change from green to blue (bromothymol blue indicator).

Negative reaction = Original green color and no growth.

UREASE TEST/CHRISTENSEN'S AGAR MEDIUM

Some bacteria are able to decompose urea to form Ammonia and Carbon dioxide by means of the enzyme urease.

The test is done in Christensen's agar medium. It is composed of peptone, sodium chloride, dipotassium hydrogen phosphate, Phenol Red indicator, Urea, glucose and agar by dissolving in distilled water with a pH of 7.0. The medium can be used as liquid by omitting the agar.

The test bacterium is inoculated on to slope and incubated at 37°C. Examine after overnight incubation, No test is reported negative until after 4 days incubation.

Breakdown of urea with production of ammonia is indicated by the change in color of the medium from yellow to pink, due to phenol red indicator.

Proteus, *Klebsiella* and *Ureaplasma* are urease positive. *Helicobacter pylori* produces abundant urease, which is utilized as a rapid diagnostic test.

CATALASE TEST

Some bacteria produce catalase enzyme, which catalyzes the release of oxygen from hydrogen peroxide (H_2O_2).

$$H_2O_2 \xrightarrow{\text{Catalase}} H_2O_2 + \frac{1}{2} O_2$$

A small amount of culture to be tested is taken with a sterile wire loop or thin glass rod and is inserted into hydrogen peroxide solution, held in a small tube. Production of gas bubbles indicates catalase production. Alternatively a loop full of hydrogen peroxide may be added to colonies on nutrient agar. Prompt effervescence indicates catalase production. *Staphylococcus aureus* and Enterobacteriaceae members are catalasc positive.

Since blood contains catalase, cultures from media containing blood are not suitable for catalase test.

Nichrome wire loop should never be used to pick up colonies because iron component of nichrome wire loop will give false positive reaction.

OXIDASE TEST

Oxidase test depends on the presence of oxidases in bacteria that will catalyze the transport of electrons between electron donors in the bacteria and a redox dye (tetramethyl-p-phenylene diamine). The dye is reduced to a deep purple color.

The test can be done in two ways.

1. Plate method. A freshly prepared 1% solution of tetra methyl-p-phenylene diamine dihydrochloride is poured over the colonies on agar plates. The oxidase positive colonies rapidly develop a purple color.
2. Filter paper method or Kovac's method-strips of whatman's No. 1 filter paper are soaked in a freshly prepared 1% solution of tetramethyl-p-phenylene diamine dihydrochloride, and laid in a

Petri dish. The colony to be tested is smeared over it. A positive reaction is indicated by a deep purple color, within 5-10 seconds and a negative reaction by absence of coloration.

Neisseria, Alcaligenes, Aeromonas, Vibrio, Campylobacter, Pseudomonas and *Hemophilus* are oxidase positive, whereas enterobacteriaceae species give negative reactions.

PHENYL ALANINE DEAMINASE TEST

This test indicates the ability of bacteria like *Proteus* to deaminate phenyl alanine with production of phenyl pyruvic acid which will react with ferric salts to give a green color.

Test bacterium is inoculated in to Nutrient agar or Yeast extract agar containing DL-phenyl alanine and incubated at 37°C for 4-24 hrs. Add a few drops of 10% ferric chloride solution to run down on to the slope. If the test is positive, a green color will develop in the fluid and in the slope.

TRIPLE SUGAR IRON AGAR (TSI AGAR)

It is used for differentiation and preliminary identification of Gram negative bacilli, originally designed as a multi test medium, now mainly used as a standard test for H_2S. It is a composite medium consisting glucose, lactose, sucrose with phenol red indicator to detect gas production and ferric ammonium citrate to demonstrate hydrogen sulphide (H_2S) production. The medium is distributed in tubes with a butt and slant.

After inoculation of test bacterium and overnight incubation

1. If the slant remains red (alkaline) and butt becomes yellow glucose is fermented, but sucrose and lactose are not fermented.
2. If both slant and butt become yellow (acid) all sugars are fermented.
3. If both slant and butt remain red (alkaline) all sugars are not fermented.
4. Air bubbles in the butt indicates gas production.
5. Blackening of the medium indicates H_2S production.

OXIDATION-FERMENTATION (O.F) TEST/HUGH AND LEIFSON'S TEST

This test is done to detect whether a bacterium utilizes glucose oxidatively or fermentatively in Hugh and Leffson's (O.F) semisolid medium containing carbohydrate (usually glucose) and pH indicator, bromothymol blue.

The test bacterium is stab-inoculated into duplicate tubes of medium; the medium in one tube is covered with sterile liquid paraffin; both the tubes are incubated. If acid is produced only at the surface of the medium, where conditions are aerobic, the metabolism of glucose is oxidative. If acid is found throughout the tube; including the lower layers where conditions are anaerobic, the metabolism is fermentative.

Fermentative organisms such as Enterobacteriaceae, *Aeromonas, Vibrio* produce acid reaction throughout the medium in the covered (anaerobic) as well as the open (aerobic) tube.

Oxidizing organisms such as *Pseudomonas* produce an acid reaction only in the open tube.

Organisms such as *Alcaligenes fecalis* that cannot break down the carbohydrates aerobically or anaerobically produce an alkaline reaction in the open tube and no change in the covered tube.

QUESTIONS

Short Notes

1. IMViC reactions.
2. Indole test.
3. Meth;yl red test.
4. Citrate utilisation test.
5. Urease test.
6. TSI agar.
7. O-F test.

13

Classification of Microorganisms/ Microbial Taxonomy

- *Taxonomy*
- *Nomenclature*
- *Species concept and intraspecies classification*
- *Taxonomy ranks*
- *Kingdoms of organisms*
- *Differences between prokaryotes and eukaryotes*
- *Methods of classification*
  - *– Phylogenetic*
  - *– Based on staining reaction*
  - *– Based on chemical composition*
  - *– Biochemical classification*
  - *– Nutritional*
  - *– Morphological*
  - *– Serological*
  - *– Adansonian*
  - *– Genetic analysis*
  - *– Molecular*
- *Bergey's manual classification*

TAXONOMY

Taxonomy is concerned with the systematic arrangement of organisms into groups or categories called "Taxa" or "Divisions". The science of taxonomy can be divided into three parts.

1. Classification – The orderly arrangement of units into groups of larger units.
2. Nomenclature – The naming of units, characterised by classification.
3. Identification – Microorganisms are identified by comparing the characteristics of an "unknown" to the "known" units.

The major characteristics of microorganisms that have to be observed or determined to classify microorganisms include morphological, cultural, physiological, metabolic, antigenic, genetic and chemical composition.

NOMENCLATURE

Two kinds of names are given to bacteria.

1. Common name or casual name may vary from place to place and useful for communication at the local level.
2. Scientific name or international name is given by using the bionomial system of Linneaus according to International code of nomenclature of bacteria, prepared by the International committee on systematic bacteriology. The first part of the name begins with capital letter, indicates 'Genus' name, which is usually Larin or Greek noun. Genera may be masculine (ending in – us), feminine (ending in – lla, ada) or neuter (ending in – um). Second part is "species" name, which is a specific epithet and uncapitalized.

Table 13.1 Common and Scientific Names of some Bacteria

Common name	*Scientific name*
Gonococcus	*Neisseria gonorrhoeae*
Tubercle bacilli	*Mycobacterium tuberculosis*
Diphtheria bacilli	*Corynebacterium diphtheriae*
Typhoid bacilli	*Salmonella typhi*
Tetanus bacilli	*Clostridium tetani*

A satisfactory binomial system of nomenclature has not been evolved for viruses even today.

SPECIES CONCEPT IN MICROBIOLOGY/INTRA-SPECIES CLASSIFICATION

The basic taxonomic group in biology is the "Species". **Species** is defined as a group of individuals that are similar in characters, adopted to a particular ecological habitat and a way of life, and are capable of interbreeding freely and producing fertile offspring.

The above definition of species is most suitable for plants and animals which reproduce sexually. But it cannot satisfy the condition in prokaryotes and some lower eukaryotes, which are haploid and reproduce by asexual methods. Therefore, in microbiology the term "species" is defined as a collection of "strains" that share many stable properties in common and differ significantly from one another in many ways. However, a species may be divided into two or more "subspecies" based on minor but consistent phenotypic variations within the species.

A **"STRAIN"** is a population of organisms that descends from a single organism or pure culture isolate or from a particular source, such as patient.

Strains within a species may differ slightly from one another in many ways. They are named according to the differences they exhibit *e.g.,*

Table 13.2 Classification of Species

Biotypes	– strains with biochemical or physiological differences.
Serotypes	– possess distinctive antigenic characters.
Phagotypes	– differ in susceptibility to bacteriophages.
Morphotypes	– differ morphologically.
Pathotypes	– differ in pathogenicity to certain hosts.
Colicin types	– differ in their ability to produce bacteriocins.

One strain of a species is designated as the **"Type strain"**. It is usually one of the first strains studied and is often more fully characterized than other strains. Only those strains very similar to the type strain are together form a species. Type strains are generally deposited in "Type culture collection centre" as a reference and maintained in International reference laboratories.

TAXONOMIC RANKS

Microorganisms are grouped into various "taxa", based on resemblances and relatedness. Kingdoms are divided successively into divisions, classes, orders, families, tribes, genera and species.

"GENUS" is a collection of similar species, one of them being the type species, which serves as a permanent example of the genus. A group of similar genera form a "Family", a group of similar families an "order", a group of similar orders a "class", a group of similar classes a "division" and a group of similar divisions a "kingdom", and thus goes the taxonomic hierarchy.

Table 13.3 Taxonomy of some Bacteria

Taxonomic rank	*Examples*		
Kingdom	Prokaryotae	Prokaryotae	Prokaryotae
Division	Gracilicutes	Gracilicutes	Tenericutes
Class	Scotobacteria	Scotobacteria	Mollicutes
Order	Eubacteriales	Spirochaetales	Mycoplasmatales
Family	Enterobacteriaceae	Leptospiraceae	Mycoplasmataceae
Genus	*Escherichia*	*Leptospira*	*Mycoplasma*
Species	*Escherichia coli*	*Leptospira icterohaemorrhagiae*	*Mycoplasma pneumoniae*

KINGDOMS OF ORGANISMS

Linnaeus (1735) divided all organisms into two kingdoms – plant and animal. Linnaeus put protozoa in the animal kingdom, and the other microorganisms with the plants. But this classification was impractical for microorganisms, some of which are plant-like, others animal-like, and others with characteristics of both.

Ernst Haeckel (1865) established a third kingdom, called protista, to include microorganisms having characteristics of both plants and animals.

Microorganisms are divided into two categories, based on the nuclear structure.

1. Prokaryotes (pro=first, primitive; karyon = nucleus) *e.g.*, Bacteria, blue green algae (cyanobacteria)
2. Eukaryotes (Eu=advanced, well developed) *e.g.*, Algae, fungi, protozoa.

Table 13.4 Differences between Prokaryotes and Eukaryotes

Feature	*Prokaryotes*	*Eukaryotes*
Group of organisms	Bacteria, Blue green algae	Algae, Fungi Protozoa
NUCLEUS		
– Nuclear membrane	Absent, genetic material free	Present
– Nucleolus	Absent	Present
– Chromosomes	Single, circular	More than one, linear
– Nuclear division	By simple fission, mitosis and meiosis absent	Mitosis and meiosis present
– Deoxyribonucleoprotein	Absent (histones)	Present
CYTOPLASM		
– Cytoplasmic streaming	Absent	Present
– Pinocytosis	Absent	Present
– Lysosomes	Absent	Present
– Golgi bodies	Absent	Present
– Endoplasmic reticulum	Absent	Present
– Mitochondria	Absent	Present
– Mesosomes	Present	Absent
CHEMICAL COMPOSITION		
– Sterols	Absent	Present
– Muramic acid	Present	Absent
– Diaminopimelic acid	Present in some	Absent

METHODS OF CLASSIFICATION/CLASSIFICATION SCHEMES/ CLASSIFICATION SYSTEMS

There are several approaches to bacterial classification and various schemes have been devised.

Phylogenetic (Evolutionary) Classification

During Post Darwinian period organisms are classified according to their evolutionary relationships. Haeckel placed all the microorganisms under protista kingdom, by separating them from plant and animal kingdoms. R.H. Whittaker developed a phylogenetic five kingdom classification of living forms – Monera, protista, fungi, plantae and animalia. Microorganisms are included in the first three kingdoms, while all prokaryotes are included under monera.

Classification Based on Staining Reaction

Based on Gram's staining, bacteria are divided into Gram positive and Gram negative bacteria. This is an important medical classification that depends on the cell wall composition.

Similarly, based on acid-fast staining, bacteria can be divided into acid fast bacilli and non-acid fast bacilli.

Classification Based on Chemical Classification

Based on chemical composition microorganisms can be classified. For example, the prokaryotic cell wall contains N-acetyl muramic acid, which is absent in eukaryotic cell wall. Similarly, sterols are present in eukaryotic cell membrane, while they are absent in prokaryotic cell membrane.

Biochemical Classification

Microorganisms can be classified based on various biochemical properties. *e.g.,*

1. Based on lactose fermentation, enterobacteriaceae members can be classified into lactose fermenters (LF), non-lactose fermenters (NLF) and late lactose fermenters (LLF).

Nutritional Classification

Based on energy requirements, bacteria are classified into two types – phototrophs and chemotrophs.

Similarly, based on the ability to synthesize essential metabolites, bacteria are classified as Autotrophs and heterotrophs.

Morphological Classification

Based on morphology bacteria are divided into various groups, as follows :

I. Filamentous bacteria or higher bacteria *e.g.,* Actinomycetes, Mycobacteria

II. True bacteria or lower bacteria – *e.g.,*

1. Gram positive bacilli : Aerobes – *Corynebacterium, Bacillus, Listeria.*
   Anaerobes – *Clostridium, Lactobacillus, Eubacterium.*
2. Gram positive cocci : Staphylococci, Streptococci, Enterococci, pneumococci
3. Gram negative cocci : Aerobes – *Neisseria* (gonococci and meningococci)
   Anaerobes – *Veillonella.*
4. Gram negative bacilli :
   Aerobes – Enterobacteria – *Escherichia, Klebsiella, Proteus, Salmonella, Shigella, Yersinia*
   Pseudomonads – *Pseudomonas, Alcaligenes*
   Parvobacteria – *Hemophilus, Bordetella, Brucella, Pasteurella,*
   Anaerobes – *Bacteroides, Fusobacterium*
5. Gram negative vibrios : *Vibrio, Spirillum, Campylobacter, Helicobacter*

III. Spirochetes – *Borrelia, Treponema, Leptospira.*

IV. Mycoplasmas – *Mycoplasma, Ureaplasma.*

V. Rickettsiae – *Rickettsia, Coxiella, Bartonella.*

VI. Chlamydiae – *Chalmydia.*

Serological/Antigenic Classification

Microorganisms possess many different kinds of antigens. Microorganism or some part of the organism is injected into an animal and subsequently the blood serum of the animal is tested for the presence of antibodies.

Adansonian Classification/Numerical Taxonomy/Phenetic System of Classification/Taxometrics

It was first suggested by Michael Adanson, the 18th century botanist, hence called Adansonian taxonomy. It proved to be a powerful tool in microbial taxonomy as it is more useful for classification of strains within a larger group that shares major characteristics. The use of computers extended the scope of numerical taxonomy.

This system determines the degree of relationship between strains by a statistical coefficient by scoring a large number of phenotypic characters such as morphological, cultural, biochemical, physiological, serological and ecological etc., all of which are given equal weight. Hence, it is called "phenetic system".

"Similarity coefficient" is obtained when shared positive characters are considered. It does not take into account negative characters. Whereas a "Matching coefficient" is obtained when both positive and negative shared characters (matches) are taken into account. These matches can be expressed as a per centage as S_M (simple matching coefficient) which can be expressed as follows :

$$S_M = \frac{N_S}{N_S + N_D} \times 100$$

S_M = Simple matching coefficient
N_S = Number of shared (similar) characters
N_d = Number of different characters.

The similarities are analysed by computers to indicate degrees of similarity for a group of different microorganisms to yield "groups or clusters" and the strains are arranged into "phenons (phenetic groups)". These similarity values between measured characters yield a check board of entries, a square table of similarities known as "Similarity matrix (S-matrix) or **dendrogram** or phenogram". Thus dendrogram shows heirarchial relationships between organisms.

Genetic Analysis as a Basis of Classification

The study of chromosomal gene exchange through transformation, transduction and conjugation in prokaryotes is sometimes useful in their classification. Based on susceptibility to bacteriophages, bacterial species can be divided into several phage types.

Plasmids are also important in taxonomy because they are present in most bacteria and carry genes coding for phenotypic traits.

Macromolecular Classification/Molecular Classification

Comparison of macromolecules such as proteins, enzymes and nucleic acids indicate relatedness between organisms and is useful in taxonomy.

1. *Comparison of proteins*. The amino acid sequences of proteins reflect mRNA sequences and therefore closely related to the structures of the genes coding for their synthesis. Hence, comparisons of proteins from different microorganisms are very useful taxonomically.

2. *Nucleic acid (DNA) base composition*. In double-stranded DNA, three hydrogen bonds join guanine and cytosine ($G \equiv C$) base pairs, and two bonds connect adenine and thymine (A=T) base pairs. As a result, DNA with a greater G + C content will have more hydrogen bonds, and its strands will separate only at higher temperature, that is, it will have a higher melting point. DNA melting can be followed spectrophotometrically because the absorbance at 260 nm UV light by DNA increases during strand separation.

$$\text{Mol \% G + C} = \frac{G + C}{G + C + A + T} \times 100$$

G+C content is determined by acid hydrolysis method, thermal denaturation (melting tempe-rature) method and Buoyant density method. By measuring the G + C content of bacteria, it can be shown that there is a wide range in the G + C component of DNA varying from about 25 to 80 moles % in different genera. However, for any one species, the G + C content is relatively fixed, which provides a basis for classification.

3. *Nucleic acid hybridization/DNA homology*. DNA homology experiments are used for detecting similarities between closely related organisms, whereas RNA homology experiments are used to detect more distantly related organisms. They indicate taxonomic and phylogenetic relationships.

If a mixture of single-stranded DNA formed by heating dsDNA is cooled (annealing), strands with complementary base sequences will reassociate to form stable dsDNA. Single strands of DNA from two bacterial species can be compared by hybridization *in vitro*.

4. *Ribosomal RNA (rRNA) sequencing.* The structure of ribosomal RNA (rRNA) appears to have been highly conserved during the course of evolution and close similarities in nucleotide sequences reflect phylogenetic relationships. Investigation of similarities in oligonucleotides derived from rRNA are increasingly used in taxonomic studies.

BERGEY'S MANUAL OF SYSTEMATIC BACTERIOLOGY

It is well known as "Bible of Microbiology". Chester (1899-1901) published a manual of determinative bacteriology, which embodies classification of bacteria. This was modified by David Bergey into what is popularly now called "Bergey's manual of determinative bacteriology". The first edition was published in 1923. This has been updated and eigth edition was released in 1974.

Bergey's manual has been updated again in 1984 into "Bergey's Manual of Systematic Bacteriology" published in four volumes by R.G.E. Murray et al. In this edition, prokaryotes are classified into four divisions as, shown below :

Division I – Gracilicutes

Division II – Firmicutes

Division III – Tenericutes

Division IV – Mendosicutes

All the bacteria are divided in these divisions into 33 sections. Volume I has 11, Volume II has 6, Volume III has 8 and Volume IV has 8 sections.

QUESTIONS

Essay Type Questions

1. Explain different methods of classification of bacteria.

Short Notes

1. Species concept in microbiology.
2. Strain.
3. Role of taxonomy in infectious diseases.
4. Prokaryote.
5. Differences between prokaryotes and eukaryotes.
6. Morphological classification of bacteria.
7. Adansonian classification/numerical taxonomy/phenetic system of classification.
8. Dendrogram/similarity matrix.
9. G + C content/G + C ratio.
10. Nucleic acid hybridization.
11. Bergey's manual classification.

14

Antibiotic Sensitivity Tests

- *Definitions*
  - *Antimicrobial agent*
  - *Chemotherapeutic agent*
  - *Chemotherapy*
- *Chemotherapeutic Index*
- *Antibiotics*
- *Spectrum of activity of antimicrobial agents*
  - *Narrow spectrum antibiotics*
  - *Broad spectrum antibiotics*
- *Mode/mechanism of action of antimicrobial agents*
- *Antibiotic sensitivity tests*
  - *Dilution methods*
  - *Diffusion tests–Disc-diffusion (Kirby-Bauer) test*
- *Antibiogram*
- *Assay of antibiotics*
- *Bacteriocins*

DEFINITIONS

Antimicrobial Agent

Any chemical substance which inhibits the growth or causes death of a microorganism is known as antimicrobial agent.

Chemotherapeutic Agent

Synthetic chemicals that are used to kill or inhibit the growth of microorganisms in the body tissues are called chemotherapeutic agents.

Chemotherapy

The term chemotherapy is introduced by Ehrlich, to denote the treatment of a microbial disease by the administration of the drug which kills or inhibits the growth of pathogen, without any toxic action on the tissues, in therapeutic concentrations.

CHEMOTHERAPEUTIC INDEX

Chemotherapeutic agent must possess selective toxicity against the pathogen and should act at a concentration that can be tolerated by the host tissues. This selective toxicity is expressed in terms of "chemotherapeutic index", which compares the maximum dose that can be tolerated by the host without causing death, known as "maximum tolerated dose", with the minimum dose that cures the particular infection, known as" minimum curative dose".

$$\text{Chemotherapeutic index} = \frac{\text{Maximum tolerated dose}}{\text{Minimum curative dose}}$$

The chemotherapeutic index provides a rough guide to the degree of selective toxicity, and therapeutic value of a chemical. A high value of chemotherapeutic index indicates that the chemotherapeutic agent is highly efficient against the pathogen and less toxic to the host.

ANTIBIOTICS

Antibiotics are defined as natural antimicrobial agents produced by microorganisms, that is capable in small concentractions to kill or inhibit the growth of other microorganisms.

The ability to produce antibiotics is particularly common among soil microorganisms and therefore, antibiotics are widely distributed in nature; where they play an important role in regulating the microbial population of soil, water, sewage and compost. Of many antibiotics that have been purified, only a few have been nontoxic to be of use in medical practice. Those that are currently of greatest use have been derived from a small group of microorganisms belonging to genera *Penicillium*, *Streptomyces*, *Cephalosporium*, *Micromonospora* and *Bacillus*.

SPECTRUM OF ACTIVITY OF ANTIMICROBIAL AGENTS

Based on the spectrum of activity, antibiotics are classified into two types.

1. Narrow Spectrum Antibiotics are those which can kill or inhibit the growth of only a few species of microorganisms. *e.g.*, Penicillin—mainly active against Gram positive bacteria. Aminoglycosides, such as gentamycin and streptomycin are mainly active against Gram negative bacteria. Metronidazole-mainly active against anaerobic bacteria and some protozoans.

2. Broad spectrum antibiotics are those which can kill or inhibit the growth of many different species of microorganisms, including both Gram positive and Gram negative bacteria. *e.g.*, Tetracyclines, ampicillin, cephalosporins, and quinolones. They are often used for the "blind" treatment of infections. Unfortunately there is much abuse of broad spectrum antibiotics in clinical practice.

MODE/MECHANISM OF ACTION OF ANTIMICROBIAL AGENTS

Antimicrobial agents kill or inhibit microorganisms by several mechanisms –

1. Inhibition of cell wall synthesis.

   e.g., Penicillins, bacitracin, cephalosporins, cycloserine, vancomycin and ristocetin

2. Inhibition or alteration of cell membrane permeability.

   e.g., Amphotericin B, colistin, imidazoles, nystatin, polymyxins.

3. Inhibition of protein synthesis.

e.g., Chloramphenicol, erythromycins, lincomycins, tetracyclines, Aminoglycosides – Amikacin, Gentamycin, Kanamycin, neomycin, netilmycin, streptomycin, Tobramycin etc.

4. Inhibition of transcription and nucleic acid synthesis.

e.g., Nalidixic acid, novobiocin, pyrimethamine, rifampin, sulfonamides, trimethoprim.

5. Antimetabolite action (antagonistic to metabolites).

e.g., Sulfonamides, sulfones, trimethoprim and PAS (paraamino salicylic acid)

ANTIBIOTIC SENSITIVITY TESTS

Strains of microorganisms differ in their degree of susceptibility to antibiotics and chemotherapeutic agents. The susceptibility of an organism may change with time. It is therefore important for the physician to know the identity of the microbe causing the infection, as well as its susceptibility to antibiotics, so that the specific, correct antibiotic can be selected for treating the infection.

The susceptibility of the pathogen to various antibiotics and chemotherapeutic agents is determined by two methods.

1. Dilution tests
2. Diffusion tests.

1. Dilution Method. It is of two types: 1. Tube dilution or broth dilution method, and, 2. Agar dilution method. Dilution tests are generally used-when therapeutic dose is to be regulated as in the treatment of endocarditis, for tests on slow growing bacteria such as tubercle bacilli, and when small degrees of resistance are to be demonstrated.

1. *Tube Dilution Method or Broth Dilution Technique.* It is used to determine the minimum inhibitory concentration (MIC) and the minimum bactericidal concentration (MBC) of an antibiotic for a pathogen.

The tube dilution method uses a series of test tubes containing sterile culture medium, usually Mueller-Hinton broth and various concentrations of each of a variety of antibiotics. All tubes are inoculated with the microorganism to be tested and then incubated. Control consists of drug-free broth. Then the tubes are examined to see which antibiotics have inhibited the growth of the organism. For each antibiotic MIC is determined.

Minimum inhibitory concentration (MIC) is defined as the lowest concentration (or highest dilution) of the drug/antibiotic that inhibits the growth, as determined usually by the lack of turbidity. The antibiotics having the lowest MIC values would have the highest antimicrobial activity.

Minimum bactericidal concentration (MBC) is defined as minimum concentration of an antibiotic required to kill a defined per cent (usually 99.9%) of bacteria when a mixture of bacteria and antibiotic are incubated together.

The MBC is determined by inoculating a drug-free medium from each test tube that showed no growth in MIC determination. The MBC is determined by the growth pattern seen after incubation. The MBC may be equal to or greater than the MIC.

Determination of MBC is not routinely performed but is indicated in the treatment of endocarditis by Streptococci and other organisms, to adjust the dose and combination of antibiotics.

Broth dilutions can be performed in a microtitre plate. The technique has been highly automated.

2. Agar Dilution Technique. It is more convenient when several strains are to be tested at the same time. In this method serial dilutions of the drug are prepared in Mueller-hinton agar, melted to 45°C and then poured into plates. Several strains can be inoculated on each plate containing antibiotic. Following incubation, the MIC, lowest concentration of the drug that inhibits colony formation is determined.

Diffusion Tests. In diffusion tests, the drug is allowed to diffuse through a solid medium so that a concentration gradient is established, the concentration being higher near the site of the drug and gradually decreases with distance. The test strain is inoculated on the medium and on incubation, its sensitivity to the drug is determined from the inhibition of its growth.

The most commonly employed method is use of discs of antibiotic impregnated filter paper known as disc-diffusion test. The concentration of drug in discs may be as per Kirby-Bauer or I.C.S. recommendations.

Disc-Diffusion Test/Kirby-Bauer Disc Diffusion Method

It is a qualitative method to determine susceptibility of bacteria to drugs, employing discs made of filter paper (Whatman No. 2 filter paper) about 6 mm in diameter, impregnated with appropriate concentrations of the drug, as per Kirby-Bauer or I.C.S. methods. The discs are stored dry with a desiccant, in the cold (Refrigerator). The potency of the discs is periodically tested, using control standard strains of known sensitivity, such as *Staphylococcus aureus*, oxford strain NCTC 6571.

Preparation of Inoculum. The colonies of test strain may be inoculated into peptone water or nutrient broth and incubated at 37°C for 4 – 8 hours, till light to moderate turbidity develops. The inoculum may be adjusted to give a uniform, dense but not confluent growth.

Antibiotic sensitivity medium. To determine susceptibility to antibiotics, usually Mueller-Hinton agar medium is used as a standard sensitivity medium. Nutrient agar is also routinely used, but it should not be preferred as it contains inhibitors of sulphonamides, trimethoprim and other sulphur containing drugs. These inhibitors may be neutralized by the addition of lysed horse blood. For fastidious pathogens such as Streptococci and pneumococci, blood agar plates may be used.

Inoculation. Inoculation on to Mueller-Hinton agar may be done by two methods-

1. The broth culture of inoculum may be poured on to the surface of solid medium and the plate is tilted for uniform spreading; and then excess fluid may be pipetted off.

2. A sterile cotton swab is soaked in inoculum, and pressed against the upper inside wall of the tube to remove excess fluid and rub it over the surface of solid medium three times, turning the plate 60° angle between each swabbing.

Application of discs. Antibiotic-impregnated filter paper discs are applied gently under sterile conditions with a sterile forceps. Discs are placed flat on the surface and firmly applied to ensure adhesion. The discs should preferably be deposited with centres at least 25 mm to 30 mm apart.

Mechanical devices of disc dispensers are available, which deliver all discs simultaneously on to the surface of solid medium.

Incubation. For most organisms incubation at 35°C to 37°C for 18 hrs or overnight is sufficient. In case of fastidious pathogens the incubation may be done in the presence of increased CO_2 concentration.

Reading results. After incubation, the plates are examined for zones of inhibition of growth, around the discs. Growth will be inhibited around discs containing antibiotics to which the bacterium is susceptible, but not around those to which it is resistant. The diameter of the zone of inhibition may be measured with a ruler or Vernier calipers in millimeters (mm).

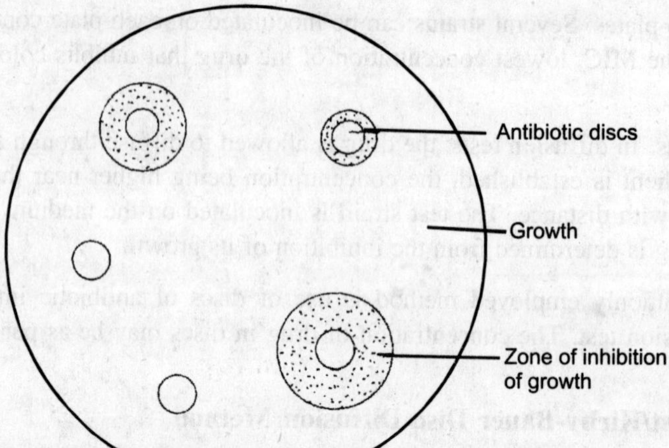

Fig. 14.1 Disc diffusion test

Interpretation of results. The results are interpreted and reported as "sensitive," "moderately sensitive" and "resistant" by referring the diameter of zone inhibition with standard interpretation tables.

Sensitive – zone size equal to, wider than or not more than 3 mm smaller than the control.

Intermediate (Moderately sensitive) – zone size greater than 3 mm, but smaller than the control by more than 3 mm.

Resistant – zone size 3 mm or less.

Factors affecting disc diffusion test. The accuracy of disc diffusion test depends on

– disc concentration,

– diffusibility of the drug,

– nature, composition and depth of the medium,

– pH of the medium,

– size of inoculum,

– incubation temperature,

– incubation period or length of incubation,

In a rotary plating method, the control organism is inoculated in the centre and the test organism at the periphery of the plate leaving a gap of 2-3 mm between test and control inocula, where antibiotic discs are applied.

ANTIBIOGRAM

The sensitivity pattern of a microorganism to a series of antibiotics is called antibiogram. This antibiogram is useful –

– as a guide for antibiotic therapy

– as a marker in the identification of an organism, usually in epidemiological studies.

Most infections are treated on an empirical basis; chemotherapy may be guided by predictable sensitivities or fixed antibiograms for commonly occurring bacterial pathogens. It saves time, allow treatment to begin, and reduce the amount of unnecessary work carried out in the laboratory.

Fixed antibiograms for some common bacterial pathogens are as follows :

Streptococci – Penicillin, erythromycin, vancomycin

Staphylococci – Flucloxacillin, clindamycin, fusidic acid, Gentamycin, vancomycin.

Anaerobiccocci – Penicillin, erythromycin, metronidazole

Enterococci – Ampicillin, vancomycin

E. coli and *Proteus* – Gentamycin, trimethoprim, ciprofloxacin, co-trimoxazole.

Pseudomonas – Gentamycin, ceftazidime, azlocillin, ciprofloxacin.

Hemophilus – Amoxycillin, co-trimoxazole, tetracycline chloramphenicol, erythromycin

Bacteroides – Metronidazole, co-trimoxazole,

Salmonella typhi,
S. paratyphi B – Chloramphenicol Ampicillin, co-trimoxazole, Amoxycillin.

ASSAY OF ANTIBIOTICS

Determination of the antibiotic content of a microbial culture, a patient's blood sample or other body fluids, an antibiotic tablet or similar specimens can be done by two methods.

1. Chemical assay. 2. Biological assay.

Chemical Assay

If an antibiotic occurs as part of a solid specimen, such as a powder or tablet, its concentration can be determined by a chemical assay method and expressed in micrograms of the antibiotic per milligram of the specimen.

Chemical assay methods are generally more accurate and require less time than biological methods, but they are less sensitive. Moreover, they may not always be reliable, since antibiotics may degrade into biologically inactive forms that the chemical assay cannot distinguish from the active form.

Microbiological Assay

In biological assay, living microorganisms are used to measure the amount of antimicrobial activity present in an antibiotic-containing specimen. It is based upon comparing the antimicrobial activity of the specimen with that of a standard preparation of the antibiotic under standard conditions.

The biological assay of antibiotics is performed by using either the tube dilution or disc plate technique. In tube dilution technique, two series of tubes are prepared: a standard set using tubes of media containing known (measured) amounts of the antibiotic, and a test sample set using tubes of media containing unknown amounts of the same antibiotic. The tubes are inoculated with a test bacterium, incubated and then observed for growth. By comparing the end points of growth of the known and the unknown, the antibiotic content of the sample can be determined.

BACTERIOCINS

Many gram negative bacteria produce antibiotic-like bactericidal substances active against some other strains of the same or closely related specie. They are called bacteriocins.

The bacteriocins produced by coliform bacilli such as *E. coli* are called colicins, Pseudomonads produce pyocines (aeruginocines) *Bacillus megaterium* produce megacins, *Corynebacterium diphtheriae* produce diphthericins, *Yersinia pestis* produces pesticins and so on.

Bacteriocins are proteins, and when seen under electron microscope, appear like tail structures of phages. They also resemble phages in their ability to adsorb on specific receptor sites on susceptible bacterial cells; some of the receptor sites may be same for both phages and bacteriocins.

The production of bacteriocins is determined by the presence in bacteria of plasmids (colicinogenic factors or col factors), known as bacteriocinogen, that are transmitted from cell to cell by conjugation, transduction. Certain physical (UV rays) and chemical agents (nitrogen mustard) may induce bacteriocin production by the bacteria possessing plasmids.

Bacteriocin typing may be used as a tool for epidemiological studies. Bacteriocin typing is based on the ability of bacteriocins produced by the test strain to kill standard indicator strains of bacteria.

QUESTIONS

Essay Type Questions

1. Define antibiotic. Write in brief the mode of action of antibiotics. List the various methods of antibiotic susceptibility testing

Short Notes

1. Chemotherapeutic index.
2. MIC.
3. Disc diffusion test.
4. Kirby-Bauer method.
5. Explain the different methods of antibiotic sensitivity testing.
6. Bacteriocins.
7. Tube dilution method of antibiotic susceptibility testing.
8. Assay of antibiotics.
9. Antibiogram.

15

Microbial Genetics

- *Introduction*
- *Structure of DNA*
- *Structure of RNA*
- *Central dogma of molecular biology*
- *Regulation (control) of gene expression*
- *Variability in microorganisms*
  - *Genotypic*
  - *Phenotypic*
- *Mutations*
  - *Definitions*
  - *Spontaneous mutations*
  - *Induced mutations*
  - *Mutagens*
  - *Biochemical mutations*
  - *Conditional mutations*
  - *Point mutations*
  - *Frame-shift mutations*
  - *Base-pair mutations*
  - *Reversion mutations*
  - *Inversion*
  - *Detection of mutations (selection of mutants)*
- *Mechanisms of gene transfer (genetic recombination)*
  - *Transformation*
  - *Conjugation*
  - *Sexduction*
  - *Transduction*
  - *Lysogeny*
- *Genetic engineering/Gene cloning/DNA recombinant technology*
- *Restriction endonucleases*
- *DNA fingerprinting*
- *Restriction fragment length polymorphism (RFLP)*
- *Polymerase chain reaction (PCR)*
- *Transposable elements (Jumping genes)*
- *Blotting techniques*
  - *Southern blotting*
  - *Northern blotting*
  - *Western blotting*
- *Plasmids or episomes*
- *DNA probes*

INTRODUCTION

Genetics is the study of heredity and variation, seeking to understand the similarities and differences between parents and their daughter cells.

In all living organisms, the hereditary information resides or is encoded in nucleic acids – DNA and RNA. Nucleic acids are called "life molecules", because they are store house of genetic information. The genetic information in bacteria, as in all cells, is contained in the specific sequence of nucleotides in the cell's Deoxyribonucleic acid (DNA). Thus, DNA is the store house of genetic information required for protein synthesis.

BACTERIAL NUCLEUS

Bacteria possess a prokaryotic nucleus, consisting of a single circular chromosome, made up of a single molecule of double-stranded DNA, of abut 1000 to 1300 μ length. Some viruses may possess RNA genome.

STRUCTURE OF DNA

DNA possesses a double-helix structure (Watson and Crick - 1953). The DNA molecule consists of two helically twisted strands, connected together in the form of a double helix. Each strand consists a back bone of deoxyribose (a pentose sugar) and phosphate groups, linked covalently by phosphodiester bonds. The purine and pyrimidine nitrogenous bases are covalently connected to deoxyribose sugar molecules. Purine bases are adenine (A) and guanine (G) and the pyrimidines thymine (T) and cytosine (C).

The double stranded nature of the molecule is stabilised by hydrogen bonding between the bases on the opposite strands in such a manner that adenine base of one strand always binds, via two hydrogen bonds, to the thymine base of the other strand, or vice versa, (A = T). Likewise, the guanine base of one strand always binds by three hydrogen bonds to the cytosine base of the other strand, or vice versa (G ≡ C). Thus, adenine and thymine form a complementary base pair, and guanine and cytosine form another. A molecule of DNA will, therefore contain as many units of adenine as thymine, and of guanine as cytosine, but the ratio of each pair of bases $\frac{(A+T)}{(G+C)}=1$, though constant for each species, varies widely from one bacterial species to another.

Each strand has a 5′ and a 3′ hydroxyl terminus. Both the strands of DNA run antiparallel, with the 5′ terminus of one strand opposed to the 3′ terminus of the other.

The DNA molecule is a polynucleotide, a polymer consisting of several nucleotides. Each **"nucleotide"** consists of pentose sugar deoxyribose, a phosphate group and a nitrogenous base (purine or pyrimidine).

Deoxyribose sugar and a nitrogenous base together called as **"nucleoside"**.

A nucleoside and phosphate together called as **nucleotide.**

The strand completes a turn each 34Å; each nucleotide occupies 3.4Å; thus, there are ten nucleotides per turn.

The order of nitrogenous bases along a DNA or RNA strand is known as the "**base sequence**". Genetic information is stored in the DNA as a **"code or codon",** consisting of a sequence of 3 bases, *i.e.*, the code is **"triplet".** Each codon specifies for a single amino acid, but more than one codon may exist for the same amino acid. *e.g.*, the codons (triplets) AGA, AGG, CGC, CGU, CGA and CGG code for the same amino acid arginine.

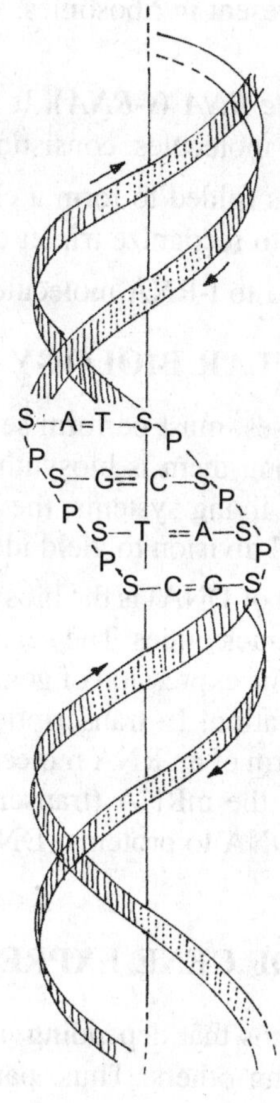

Fig. 15.1 DNA double hellix

Three codons UAA, UAG, and UGA do not code for any amino acid and are called **"non-sense codons".** They act as punctuation marks (stop codons), terminating the message for the synthesis of a polypeptide. A segment of DNA carrying codons specifying for a particular polypeptide is called a **"gene"** or **"cistron".** A DNA molecule consists of large number of genes, each of which contains thousands of nucleotides.

STRUCTURE OF RNA

RNA is a polymer of ribonucleotides, frequently occurs in single stranded form. It is found in cytoplasm and ribosomes.

RNA is structurally similar to DNA, except for two major differences. It contains the sugar ribose (instead of deoxyribose in DNA) and the base uracil (instead of thymine in DNA). Thymine is absent in RNA.

On the basis of structure and function, three distinct types of RNA can be distinguished.

1. *Messenger RNA* (*m-RNA*). DNA acts as a template for the synthesis of m-RNA, and therefore, the bases will be complementary to each other. The m-RNA is formed on DNA template by transcription and carries message-specific sequence of nucleotides in triplet codons, passes from nucleus to cytoplasm to convey message to ribosomes for the synthesis of protein molecule.

2. *Ribosomal RNA (r-RNA).* It is present in ribosomes, where messages of m-RNA are translated into amino acid structure of proteins.

3. *Transfer RNA (t-RNA)* or *soluble RNA (s-RNA).* It is present mainly in cytoplasm. They are relatively small, single stranded, globular molecules, consisting about 75 – 100 nucleotides.

Each single stranded t-RNA remains folded to form a clover-leaf structure, containing four main arms or loops. The anticodon loop helps to recognize triplet codon on mRNA.

Amino acids in cytoplasm are linked to t-RNA molecules, which carry them to the ribosomes.

CENTRAL DOGMA OF MOLECULAR BIOLOGY

Living organisms from man to viruses, must perform several actions in order to carry out normal life processes. The important action among them is biosynthesis of nucleic acid and protein. Nucleic acid (DNA) is the genetic material in all living systems, the duplication of which is necessary for the passage of genetic information during cell division to yield identical daughter cells.

The duplication of DNA (replication of DNA) is the biosynthesis of an exact copy of parental DNA molecules from the monomeric deoxyribonucleotides. The genetic information is preserved by duplicating the nucleotide sequence of parent DNA. The expression of genetic information of genes in DNA involves the processes of transcription and translation. In transcription, the genetic information stored in the base sequence of DNA is copied in the form of an RNA molecule (mRNA). In the process of translation, the genetic information, now present in the mRNA (transcript) is utilized to direct the synthesis of proteins. The flow of information from DNA to proteins (DNA → RNA → Polypeptides) is called the "central dogma of molecular biology".

REGULATION (OR) CONTROL OF GENE EXPRESSION

Every cell has regulatory mechanisms that depending upon the current environment, allow some genes to be transcribed, while preventing others. Thus, particular genes act at particular time in a organism. Based on the nature of gene expression, two types of genes are known.

1. *Constitutive genes.* An enzyme or protein is always produced by the cell, whether or not the substrate present. This means that the gene for that enzyme or protein is always transcribed. They are known as constitutive genes *e.g.*, glycolysis enzymes. They are not regulated and they are not under the control of inducers or repressors.

2. *Inducible genes* or *regulated genes*. An enzyme or protein is produced by the cell only when needed and only in the presence of a particular substrate. The substance that initiates enzyme induction iss called "inducer", the substance that represses enzyme production is called a "co-reprocessor". *e.g.*, β-galactosidase, which splits lactose is produced by *E.coli*, only when the substrate lactose is present. If lactose is absent, the enzyme is not synthesized. This phenomenon is called "enzyme induction" and "enzyme repression". This strategy avoids waste and overproduction of products that are already present.

In bacteria, the genes that code for the enzymes of a metabolic pathway are usually arranged in a consecutive manner to form a functional unit called an "operon". In bacteria the process of gene expression is mainly regulated at transcriptional level.

Enzyme induction. *Esch.coli* can utilize lactose as a source of energy. The enzyme β-galactosidase is produced only in the presence of lactose and its production is switched off when not required. Lactose (substrate) is called "inducer" and β-galactosidase is called "inducible enzyme".

Operon. The genes associated with fermentation of lactose in *E.coli* are present in "**lac operon**", which contains following structural genes, involved in a common regulatory system.

lac Y gene – codes for a permease required for active transport of lactose into cells.

lac Z gene – codes for the synthesis of β-galactosidase which splits lactose into glucose and galactose.

lac A gene – codes for a transacetylase enzyme that reduces the toxicity of some galactosides by transferring acetyl groups.

lac I gene – codes for the repressor, a regulatory protein.

When the substrate (inducer) is absent, the lac operon can be switched off by the attachment of a repressor molecule to a specific region of the DNA, known as the "operator", which lies between the promotor and the lac Z gene. When the inducer is present, the repressor is released from the operator, and transcription takes place.

The repressor is an allosteric molecule with two active sites. One recognizes operator of the lac operon and binds to it to prevent transcription. The other recognizes inducer (lactose) and binds to it and gets released from operator, so that transcription can resume.

VARIABILITY IN MICROORGANISMS

Genetic information is transmitted from parents to progeny with great accuracy, carrying specific traits from generation to generation. However, genetic variability is also necessary for a biological species. Living organisms maintain a proper balance between these two properties *i.e.,* variability and constancy. Variability is associated with two properties of an organism, its genotype and phenotype.

Genotype

The sum total of genes that make up the genetic apparatus or genetic constitution of a cell is known as its genotype. It is stable, permanent and hereditary, that is transmitted to its progeny.

The genotype includes inheritable complete genetic potential of the cell, all of which may or may not be expressed at a time, in a given environmental situation. In a bacterial cell, genotype includes the chromosomal DNA plus any plasmid DNA that may be present; In an eukaryotic cell, it includes the chromosomal DNA plus the DNA of the mitochondrion.

Phenotype

The phenotype is the physical expression of a genotype in a given set of environmental conditions. A cell may exhibit different phenotypic appearances in different situations. *e.g.,*

1. ability of microbes to utilize specific chemicals as energy sources

2. presence or absence of bacterial flagellae

Genotypic variations. Genotypic changes are due to alterations in genome or genotype.

Genotypic variations are stable, permanent, heritable and not influenced by the environment. They may occur by, 1. mutations, 2. one of the methods of genetic exchange or gene transfer or genetic recombination. They are :

(*i*) Transformation (*ii*) Conjugation

(*iii*) Sexduction (*iv*) Transduction

(*v*) Lysogency (*vi*) Transposition

Phenotypic variations. Both the genotype and environment influence the phenotype of an organism.

Phenotypic variations are temporary, not heritable, limited in range by the genotype, influenced by the environment. Phenotypic changes caused by changes in the environment, will return back to original phenotype, if the original environmental conditions are restored. *e.g.*,

1. *Salmonella typhi* is normally flagellated but when grown in phenol agar, the flagellae are not synthesized. When it is subcultured on to medium without phenol, the flagellae are resynthesized.

2. *E.coli* produces β-galactosidase enzyme for lactose fermentation, only when lactose is present whereas the enzyme is not produced when lactose is not available.

MUTATIONS

Mutation is defined as a random, undirected, heritable variation caused by an alteration in the nucleotide sequence at some point of the DNA of the cell.

Any gene can undergo mutation. Mutated gene will have an altered nucleotide sequence, and the protein coded by it may have an altered amino acid sequence.

The importance of mutations lies in the field of drug resistance and the development of live attenuated vaccines.

Mutant strain. A cell of an organism carrying a mutated gene (with altered nucleotide sequence) is called a mutant.

Wild strain. The organism or cell with a normal, nonmutated gene is called wild type.

Mutagenesis. The process of mutation is called mutagenesis.

Mutagen. Any agent physical or chemical, which increases the frequency of mutations is called mutagen.

Mutations can be classified into various types as described herebelow :

Spontaneous Mutations

Mutations which occur under natural conditions are called "spontaneous mutations".

Mutation is a natural event, taking place all the time at its particular frequency in all dividing forms of life. Each gene undergoes mutation with a fixed frequency. Mutation rates of individual genes in bacteria range from 10^{-2} to 10^{-10} per bacterium per division.

Spontaneous mutations usually arise due to errors in DNA replication or tautomerism or damage to DNA. Spontaneous mutations are usually rare and may be dominant or recessive. Recessive mutations are more frequent.

Induced Mutations

Though mutations occur spontaneously, its frequency can be increased by several physical and chemical agents, called **mutagens**; and mutations induced by mutagens are called induced mutations.

Physical mutagens. Physical mutagens include radiations such as

Non-ionizing – UV rays or over exposure to sunlight.

Ionizing – X-rays, gamma rays, beta rays, alpha rays.

Chemical mutagens. They can be classified according to the way in which they bring about mutations.

(*i*) ***Base analogues.*** Chemical substances resembling bases are called base analogues. A base analogue may be incorporated into newly synthesized DNA, instead of a normal base *e.g.,* 5-Bromouracil, 2-amino purine, 2, 6 diaminopurine, 5-bromodeoxyuridine and nitrogen mustard.

(*ii*) ***Agents that modify purines and pyrimidines.***

e.g., Deaminating agents – nitrous oxide, hydroxyl amine

Alkylating agents – dimethyl sulphate, ethyl methane sulphonate, ethyl ethane sulphonate, nitrosoguanidine.

(*iii*) ***Intercalating substances.*** They produce distortion in DNA. *e.g.,* fluorescent acridine dyes such as proflavine, acridine orange.

(*iv*) ***Chemicals in cigarette smoke.*** Polycyclic aromatic hydrocarbons such as benzopyrene in smoke induce cancer.

Biological mutagens. **Transposons**–small, mobile pieces of DNA, contain genetic information and insert themselves into chromosomes at numerous locations, randomly. They cause mutations by interrupting the nucleotide sequence of the genes into which they are inserted.

Biochemical Mutations

In some mutations, the organism loses the ability to synthesize an essential metabolite, and unable to grow in a medium that does not contain this essential metabolite and therefore require this nutrients. These mutants are called "**auxotrophs**". Thus, an auxotroph is a microbial cell that, through mutation has lost the ability to synthesize an essential metabolite, and gained a growth requirement for this metabolite, which must be supplied in the medium for its growth; whereas the wild type strains capable of growing on minimal media are known as "**prototrophs**".

Conditional Mutations

They are expressed only under certain environmental conditions. For example, temperature sensitive (ts) mutant of *E.coli,* which behaves normally below 34°C and as a mutant above 39°C. It is known "conditional mutant". Temperature sensitive mutation creates a gene product that is functional at low temperature but inactive at high temperature. The reverse relationship is called cold-sensitive.

Point Mutatons

They are produced when a single base is substituted for another in a gene. They are of several types.

(*i*) ***Silent mutations or neutral mutations.*** The altered nucleotide sequence continues to code for the same amino acid as before, hence there will be no change in phenotypic expression.

(*ii*) ***Non-sense mutation.*** The nucleotide substitution produces a nonsense condons such as UAA, UAG and UGA, resulting in premature polypeptide chain termination.

(*iii*) ***Missense mutations.*** One base of a codon may be substituted by another base. The changed codon may code for another amino acid. As a result, there is a simple change of one amino acid in polypeptide chain.

Frame Shift Mutations

A mutation in which there is deletion or addition of one or a few nucleotides is called a frame shift mutation. The name is derived from the fact that there is a shift in the reading frame either backwards or forwards by one or two nucleotides. This usually leads to the formation of a nonfunctional protein.

(*i*) ***Addition or insertion mutations.*** Addition of one or few bases to a nucleotide chain.

(*ii*) ***Deletion nucleotides.*** Removal of one or a few bases from a nucleotides chain.

Base Pair Substitutions

They occur due to incorporation of wrong bases during replication of DNA due to tautomerism. Base pair substitutions are categorised into two major types.

(*i*) ***Transitions.*** They are the most common type of substitutions where a purine base is replaced by another purine base and a pyrimidine by another pyrimidine.

(*ii*) ***Transversion.*** They are substitutions where a purine base is substituted by a pyrimidine base or vice versa. This type of substitution is very rare.

Reversion Mutations

The effect of a mutation on the phenotype can be reversed, so that the original phenotype is brought back. This reversal may be due to true reversion or suppression.

(*i*) ***True reversion or back mutations.*** True reversion is restoration at the site of mutation. In true reversion, there is a reversal of original genetic exchange. Such a mutation is called "back mutation".

(*ii*) ***Suppression.*** A change at a site different from the mutation, causes suppression of mutation resulting in phenotypic restoration of gene function.

Suppressor mutations are of two types :

(*a*) ***Intragenic suppression.*** A mutation in a gene is suppressed by another mutation in the same gene.

(*b*) ***Extragenic or intergenic suppression.*** A mutation in a gene is overcome by a mutation in another gene.

Inversion

If a segment of DNA is removed and reinserted in a reverse direction, it results in an inversion mutation.

Detection of Mutations or Selection of Mutants

There are several experiments to detect mutants. The most important are :

1. Replica plating technique.
2. Penicillin enrichment technique.
3. Fluctuation tests.
4. Ames test.

1. *Replica plating technique.* Nutritional mutants (auxotrophs) can be detected by the technique of replica plating. A nutritional mutant that has developed a requirement for a growth factor is called an "auxotroph" and the wild type parent from which the auxotroph was derived is called a "prototroph".

The technique involves imprinting of colonies from a master plate on to an agar plate lacking the nutrient, using a sterile velvet cloth covered on a cylinder, called velvet disk replicator. Here the colonies of the parental type will grow normally, whereas those of the mutant will not. Thus, the inability of a colony to grow on the replica plate will be a signal that it is a mutant. The colony on the master plate corresponding to the vacant spot on the replica plate can then be picked, purified and characterized.

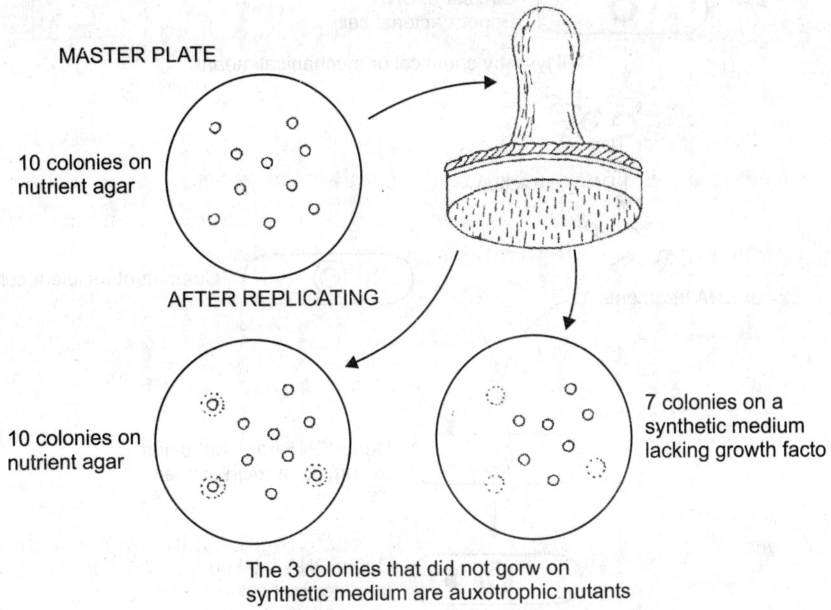

Fig. 15.2 Replica plating to detect auxotrophic mutants

MECHANISMS OF GENE TRANSFER (OR) GENETIC EXCHANGE (OR) GENETIC RECOMBINATION IN BACTERIA

In bacteria, gene transfer that can lead to genetic recombination, may occur by any one of following methods.

1. Transformation or Griffith phenomenon.
2. Conjugation.
3. Sexduction.
4. Transduction.
5. Lysogeny.
6. Transposition.

Transformation or Griffith Phenomenon

Some bacteria can take up or acquire DNA fragments or genes from surroundings, that is released into the environment due to bacterial death or lysis.

It is first discovered by Griffith (1928) hence known as Griffith phenomenon. Griffith found that mice died when injected with a mixture of live noncapsulated (Rough or R) pneumococci and heat killed capsulated (Smooth or S) pneumococci, neither of which proved fatal when injected separately. From blood cultures of dead mice, the live capsulated (S) pneumococci was isolated, which shows that some factor from heat-killed capsulated pneumococci (S) had transferred the genetic information for capsule synthesis to the live noncapsulated (R) pneumococci.

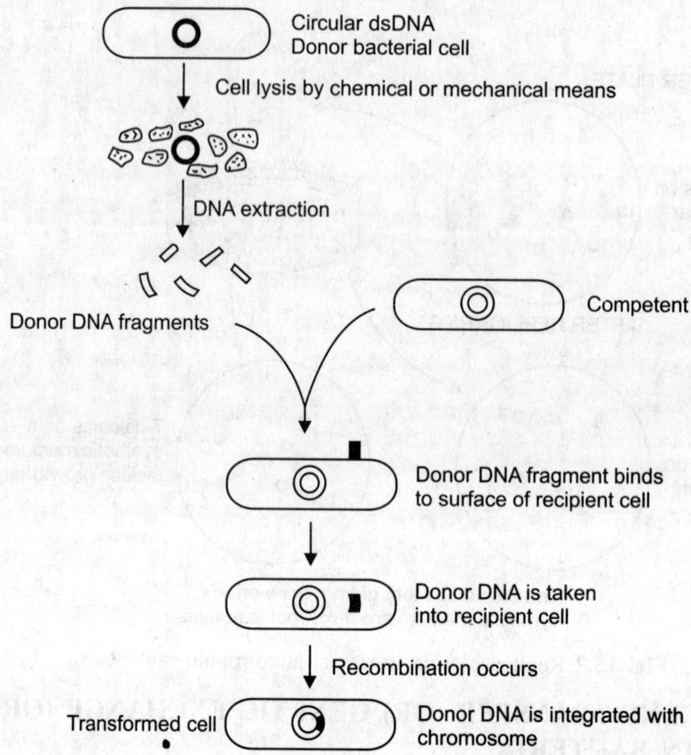

Fig. 15.3 Transformation

It is found in both Gram positive and Gram negative bacteria. Transformation has been studied mainly in pneumococci, *Bacillus* species and *Hemophilus influenzae*. Any character may be transferred by transformation. The fragments of DNA involved in transformation may carry about 10 to 50 genes.

Transformation can be used as a genetic tool for gene mapping and the quantitative determination of gene dosages.

Conjugation

It was first discovered by Lederberg and Tatum (1946) in *E.coli* K12 strain, for which they were awarded Noble prize, since it opened up the era of molecular genetics.

Conjugation is a process whereby DNA is transferred by cell to cell physical contact, from one bacterium to another. This may be regarded as a primitive means of sexual reproduction. Conjugation takes place between a "male cell" or "donor cell" or "+ strain" and a "female cell" or "recipient cell" or "– strain". The donor status or maleness of a cell is determined by the presence in it of a plasmid which codes for special fimbriae, called "sex pili". This plasmid is called fertility factor (F factor) or sex factor or transfer factor. It contains genetic information necessary for the synthesis of sex pilus or F pilus. Cells carrying F factor are called F^+ cells and cells without F factor are called F^- cells.

When F^+ and F^- cells are mixed together ($F^+ \times F^-$ cross), the end of the F^+ sex pilus binds to a nearby F^- cell and then retracts, pulling the F^- and F^+ cells into close contact. A conjugation tube is formed between two cells by sex pilus. The plasmid DNA (F factor) replicates and a copy of it passes from the F^+ cell into F^- cell, through conjugation tube. As a result, the recipient acquires donor status and can in turn conjugate with other female (– strain) cells. In this way, the conjugation process can continue until all the F^- cells in the culture are converted. In an $F^+ \times F^-$ cross, it is usually only the donor's F plasmid that moves to the F^- cell, and do not transfer any chromosomal genes.

Genetic mapping by interrupted mating is one of the most powerful genetic tools of conjugation. It is the most common mode of spread of drug resistance among Gram negative bacilli.

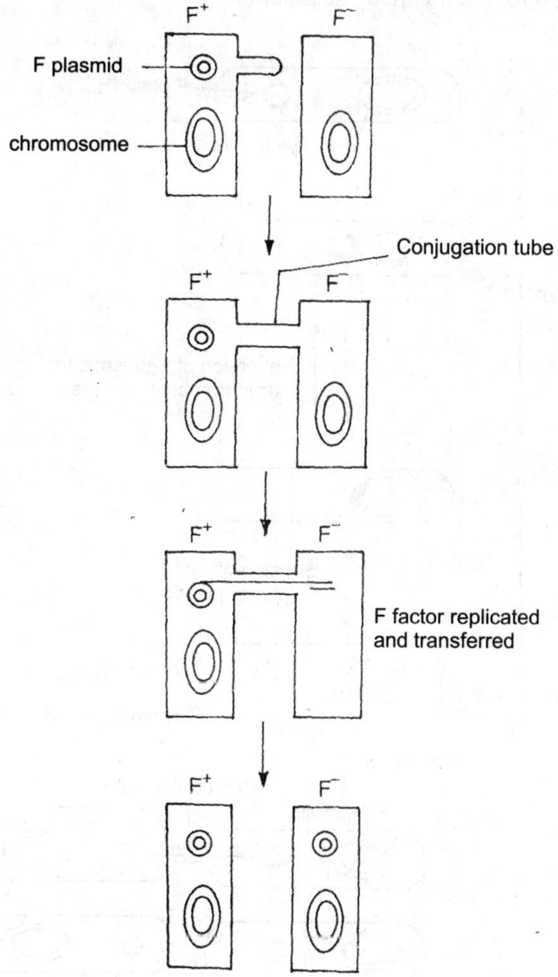

Fig. 15.4 Bacterial conjugation

Sexduction

In conjugation F^+ cells can transmit only F factor to F^- cells and do not transmit any chromosomal genes. However, there are exceptions. Certain F^+ cells can transfer chromosomal genes to F^- cells at rates atleast 1000 times greater than normal F^+ cells. These special donor cells are called "High-frequency recombination (Hfr) cells". They are F^+ cells in which the F plasmid has become integrated into the bacterial chromosome and replicates synchronously with it.

The conversion of F^+ cell into Hfr state is reversible. When the F plasmid reverts from the integrated to the free state, it may sometimes carry with it some chromosomal genes from the bacterial chromosome. Such F factor possessing some chromosomal genes is called "F prime factor" of "F′ factor" and the cells are "F prime cells" or "F′ cell".

When F′ cell mates with a recipient, it transfers, alongwith the F plasmid, the host chromosomal genes incorporated with it. This process of transfer of host genes through the F factor, resembles transduction, and has, therefore, been called "sexduction".

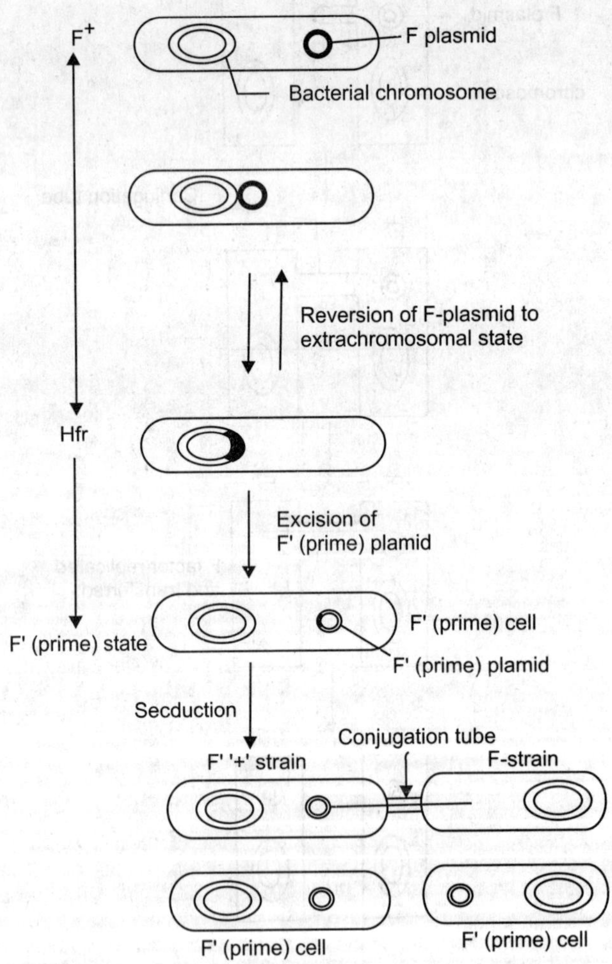

Fig. 15.5 F^+ to Hfr interconversion and sexduction

Transduction

Transduction is a process where DNA is transferred from cell to cell through the agency of bacteriophages. In other words, it is a method of gene transfer in which a virus (phage) acts as a vehicle for carrying DNA from a donor bacterium to recipient bacterium.

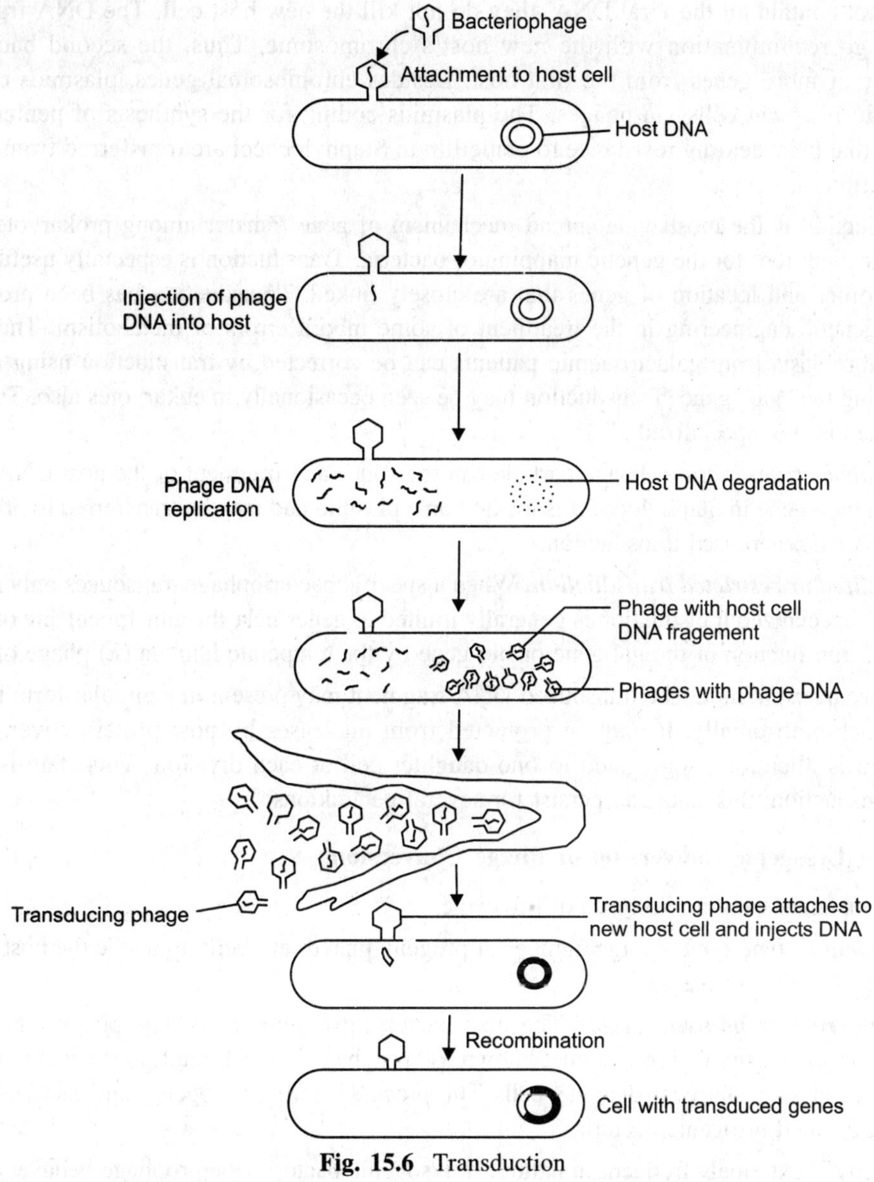

Fig. 15.6 Transduction

Viruses that attach (infect) bacteria are called bacteriophages or simply phages. A phage consists of a nucleic acid, usually DNA, surrounded by a protein coat to form a head and a tail that helps the phage to attach to the surface of a susceptible host bacterium. After the phage injects its DNA into the host cell, the phage DNA is replicated rapidly, which then directs the synthesis of new phage proteins. The DNA and proteins, then assemble to form daughter phages, which are released due to the lysis of host bacterium.

During the assembly of phage progeny inside the bacterial cell, "packaging errors" may occur; a fragment of bacterial DNA may be incorporated into daughter phage head instead of the phage DNA. Any phage carrying such bacterial DNA is called "transducing phage", because, if it infects another bacterium, it injects the bacterial DNA fragment into the new host. Because the transducing phages do not contain all the viral DNA, they do not kill the new host cell. The DNA fragment can then under go recombination with the new host's chromosome. Thus, the second bacterial host acquires one or more genes from the first host. Besides chromosomal genes, plasmids can also be transferred to recipient cells via phages. The plasmids coding for the synthesis of penicillinase (β-lactamase), that provide drug resistance to penicillin in Staphylococci are transferred from cell to cell by transduction.

Transduction is the most wide spread mechanism of gene transfer among prokaryotes and provides an excellent tool for the genetic mapping of bacteria. Transduction is especially useful for determining the order and location of genes that are closely linked. Transduction has been proposed as a method of genetic engineering in the treatment of some inborn errors of metabolism. The metabolic defects in fibroblasts from galactosaemic patients can be corrected by transduction using the lambda phage carrying the "gal" gene. Transduction may be seen occasionally in eukaryotes also. Transduction may be generalised or specialized.

Generalised transduction. Phage particle can transduce any fragment of the host DNA randomly. *e.g.,* penicillinase gene in Staphylococci is located on a plasmid and may be transferred to other Staphylococcal cells by generalised transduction.

Specialized or restricted transduction. When a specific bacteriophage transduces only a particular genetic trait. Specialized transduction is generally limited to genes near the attachment site of temperate phages. *e.g.,* transduction of the gal gene or bio gene by the temperate lambda (λ) phage of *E.coli.*

Abortive transduction. The transduced DNA fragment may present in a circular form in the cytoplasm, extrachromosomally. It may be protected from nucleases by host protein cover. It can not replicate and is, therefore, segregated to one daughter cell at each division. This state is known as abortive transduction; this state can persist for several generations.

Lysogeny or Lysogenic Conversion or Phage Conversion

Bacteriophages exhibit two types of life cycle.

1. ***Virulent or lytic cycle*** – large number of progeny phages are built up inside the host bacterium, which ruptures to release them.

2. ***Temperate or nonlytic cycle*** –The host bacterium is unharmed. The phage DNA becomes integrated with the bacterial chromosome, known as "prophage", which multiplies synchronously with the host DNA and is transferred to daughter cells. This process is called "lysogeny" and bacteria harbouring prophages are called lysogenic bacteria.

Lysogeny is extremely frequent in nature. In lysogenic bacteria, the prophage behaves as an additional fragment of the bacterial chromosome, coding for new characters. This process by which the prophage confers genetic information to a bacterium is called "lysogenic conversion" or "phage conversion". *e.g.,* diphtheria bacilli acquire toxigenicity on lysogenic conversion with beta phage. Elimination of the phage, renders it nontoxigenic.

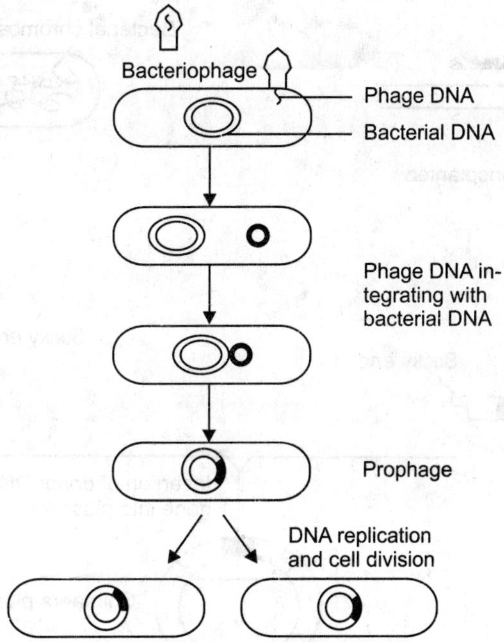

Fig. 15.7 Lysogeny

GENETIC ENGINEERING (OR) GENE CLONING (OR) RECOMBINANT DNA TECHNOLOGY

The basic steps in producing a genetically engineered bacterium are as follows :

1. Isolation of genes from donor DNA by

(*a*) Shotgun method – by using restriction endonucleases

(*b*) Obtaining from m-RNA by hybridization method or reverse transcriptase method.

2. Plasmid DNA is isolated to serve as the "carrier" or "vector" for the particular gene. Bacteriophages (*e.g.,* Lambda phage) can also be used as vectors.

3. Plasmid DNA is subjected to the action of same restriction enzymes. Since both donor DNA and plasmid DNA are treated with the same enzyme, a "restriction endonuclease", that cleaves or cuts the DNA in such a way as to form complementary single-stranded ends ("sticky ends"). These ends are capable of joining to other fragments of DNA having the same complementary single-stranded ends.

4. Foreign DNA or isolated genes from donor are mixed with plasmid DNA (vector) fragments. The sticky ends of the donor DNA joins with sticky ends of plasmid DNA by hydrogen bonding, thus forming a modified plasmid which now carries the donor DNA fragment, known as "chimaera plasmids" or "recombinant DNA".

Another enzyme called "DNA ligase" Together with ATP forms covalent bonds between sugar-phosphaste linkage.

5. The recombinant chimaera plasmids are placed or inserted into recipient bacteria, usually by transformation. *E.coli* is the most important bacterium used as cloning organism in genetic engineering. Yeasts are safer than *E.coli* for recombinant DNA studies, because they do not live in humans and are not pathogenic to man.

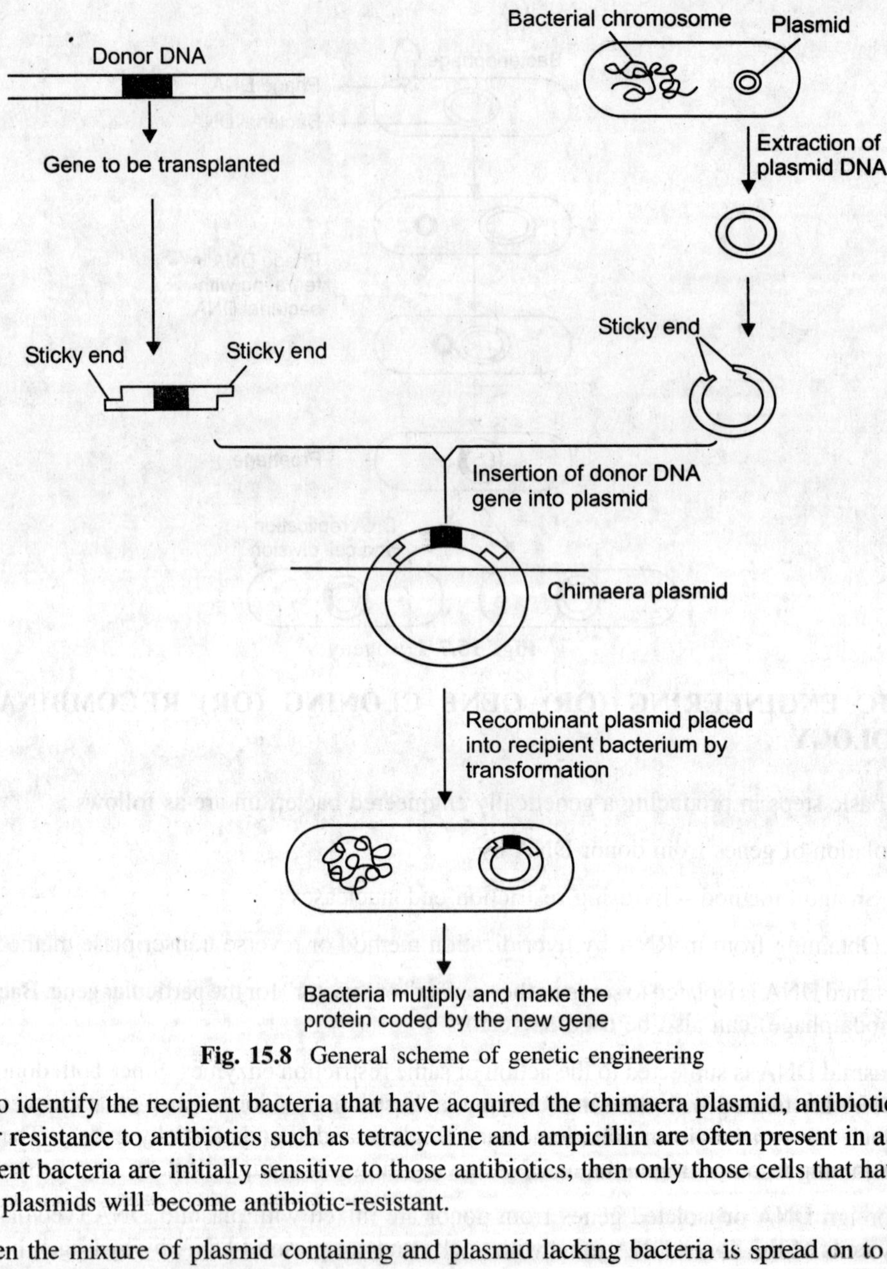

Fig. 15.8 General scheme of genetic engineering

6. To identify the recipient bacteria that have acquired the chimaera plasmid, antibiotics are used. Genes for resistance to antibiotics such as tetracycline and ampicillin are often present in a plasmid. If the recipient bacteria are initially sensitive to those antibiotics, then only those cells that have acquired chimaera plasmids will become antibiotic-resistant.

When the mixture of plasmid containing and plasmid lacking bacteria is spread on to agar media containing the antibiotics, only the bacteria that contain the chimaera plasmid will be able to form colonies.

7. Once colonies of plasmid containing bacteria that either have the gene or can make the product of the transplanted gene are identified; cells are inoculated on agar medium and upon incubation form colonies, which contain large population of identical cells, called a "clone", in which the new gene is present in every cell. Thus, the new gene is inherited, called a "cloned gene". Since, a plasmid is the vehicle, by which the new gene is placed into recipient bacterial cell, the plasmid is called a "cloning vector". Some times bacteriophages are used as "cloning vectors", when yeast cells are used as recipients.

Recombinant DNA technology is useful in the production of

1. Hormones – *e.g.,* Human insulin, growth hormone, thymosin alpha–1 (effective against brain and lung cancer) and beta endorphin (pain killer produced by the brain).
2. Vaccines – *e.g.,* Hepatitis B vaccine, rabies vaccine, foot and mouth disease vaccine.
3. Enzymes – *e.g.,* Streptokinase or urokinase (used to dissolve blood clots).
4. Monoclonal antibodies by the production of hybridomas.
5. Biologically active substances such as interferon, interleukin-II, tumor necrosis factor, clotting factor VIII, erythropoietin.
6. **Gene therapy** – It aims at inserting one or few genes into target tissues such as bone marrow or chromosomes by using plasmids or Retroviruses as vectors. Many genetic disorders like hemophilia, phenyl ketonuria, sickle cell anemia, thalassemia, alkaptoneuria, galactosemi etc., which are due to defective genes can be cured by replacing with correct genes.

RESTRICTION ENDONUCLEASES (Molecular scissors)

Restriction endonucleases are enzymes produced by bacteria, that identify and destroy foreign DNA, that might enter a cell, particularly bacteriophages.

Restriction enzymes are broadly of three types. The type I and type III enzymes recognize and bind to specific base sequences and cut the DNA at a site away from the point of attachment.

Type II enzymes are most useful in genetic engineering experiments. They recognize certain sites of DNA, consisting short, specific nucleotide sequences of 4 to 6 base pairs with palindromic sequences *i.e.,* a sequence of nucleotide bases that can be read same in both the 3′ to 5′ and 5′ to 3′ direction; and makes a cut in deoxyribose-phosphate back bones of both DNA strands, like a pair of scissors cutting a piece of tape.

Restriction endonucleases recognize and cleave at specific sites on DNA. This cleavage positions may be "even" or "staggered".

In "even cleavage" the cuts on the two strands at the same position, exactly opposite each other, resulting in DNA fragments with blunt ends or non-sticky ends.

DNA FINGERPRINTING

This technique is now widely used in research and a variety of legal situations to help identity individuals

1. to identity criminals in forensic science.
2. to determine paternity.
3. to study genetic variations among populations.
4. to diagnose various hereditary and infectious diseases.

DNA fingerprinting can be done with minute quantities of DNA; for example, from a single strand of hair, a drop of semen, a spot of blood, saliva residue on cigarette butts; from these specimens, DNA can be amplified by PCR and used in DNA fingerprinting.

In each person, certain DNA segments contain base sequences that are repeated several times. Both the number of repeat copies in one region and the number of regions subject to repeat are different from one person to another. Except for identical twins, the chance that two people would have the same DNA fingerprint is about 1 in 10 billion.

In DNA finger printing a technique called "Restriction Fragment Length Polymorphism (RFLP)" is used. The technology includes following steps :

1. Extraction of DNA (from blood, amniotic fluid, hair, semen etc.).

2. The DNA is cut into fragments by using restriction endonucleases.

3. The DNA fragments are then separated by gel electrophoresis.

4. Then specific base sequences in DNA fragments are identified by using radioactive isotope labelled DNA probes of known base sequence.

5. DNA probes pair with complementary base sequences. These are then subjected to autoradiography to set band like pattern called DNA fingerprints.

6. Such DNA fingerprints are compared to identify criminals or to solve disputed paternity etc.

RESTRICTION FRAGMENT LENGTH POLYMORPHISM (RFLP)

Refers to inherited differences in sites for restriction enzymes (for example, caused by base changes in the target site) that result in differences in the lengths of the fragments produced by cleavage with the relevant restriction enzyme. RFLPs are used for genetic mapping to link the genome directly to a conventional genetic marker. It is widely used in DNA finger printing to solve paternity dispute.

POLYMERASE CHAIN REACTION (PCR)

PCR is an *in vitro* DNA amplification method for producing large amounts of DNA (unlimited number of copies of DNA) from very tiny initial quantities of DNA, impossible to detect by routine methods. The PCR technique involves a repeated cycling process composed of 3 stages.

1. Denaturation – Double-stranded DNA is heated at 90 – 95°C for 60 seconds to form two single stranded DNAs.

2. Annealing – Specific oligonucleotide primers (15 – 22 bases) are added by reducing temperature to 40 – 50°C. They are allowed to react for 60 to 120 seconds so that they bind (hybridize) to their complementary bases on single stranded DNA.

3. Extension of annealed primers at 72°C for 60 to 180 seconds by sequential addition of nucleotides at 3′ end by DNA polymerase. Usually Taq polymerase, a heat stable DNA polymerase is used. It is produced by a thermophilic bacterium, *Thermus aquaticus* found in hot springs that produce enzymes resistant to high temperature.

These three steps constitute one cycle and generally 25 to 50 cycles are performed, using an automated thermal device which is usually completed within 3 to 4 hours. The product of first cycle becomes template for next cycle. By the third cycle double stranded DNA molecules, whose ends are defined by the two oligonucleotides, begin to appear and accumulate exponentially. By the twenty-fifth cycle, millions of copies are formed.

Large amounts of DNA can be produced from minute amounts present in water, food, blood, hair, semen, saliva and clinical samples taken from patients.

PCR has several applications in basic research, forensic (legal) medicine, clinical diagnosis, immunology and in molecular biology and human genetics

1. to study the structure of genome and DNA sequencing

2. in the early diagnosis of infectious diseases to detect and identify viral and bacterial pathogens, genetic disorders and cancer.

3. to obtain large amounts of DNA for subsequent analysis, as in forensic science.

4. to obtain genetic mapping of genes.

5. in immunology widely used to characterize HLA, T-cell receptors, antibody diversity and quantification of lymphokines.

6. used in epidemiological, phylogenetic and developmental studies.

7. to detect mutations, polymorphisms, gene defects, tumor cell markers.

TRANSPOSABLE ELEMENTS (OR) JUMPING GENES (OR) GENES WITH MOBILITY

Transposable elements are pieces (specific sequences) of DNA that move from one genetic element to another, from one plasmid to other or within the chromosome or plasmid to chromosome or vice versa. They do not exist as separate entities within the bacterial cell because do not contain information for self replication and depend on chromosomal or plasmid DNA. Thus they must either be incorporated into a plasmid or the chromosome. Transposable elements were first discovered by Barbara McClintock (1930) in Maize. They are found widely in bacteria.

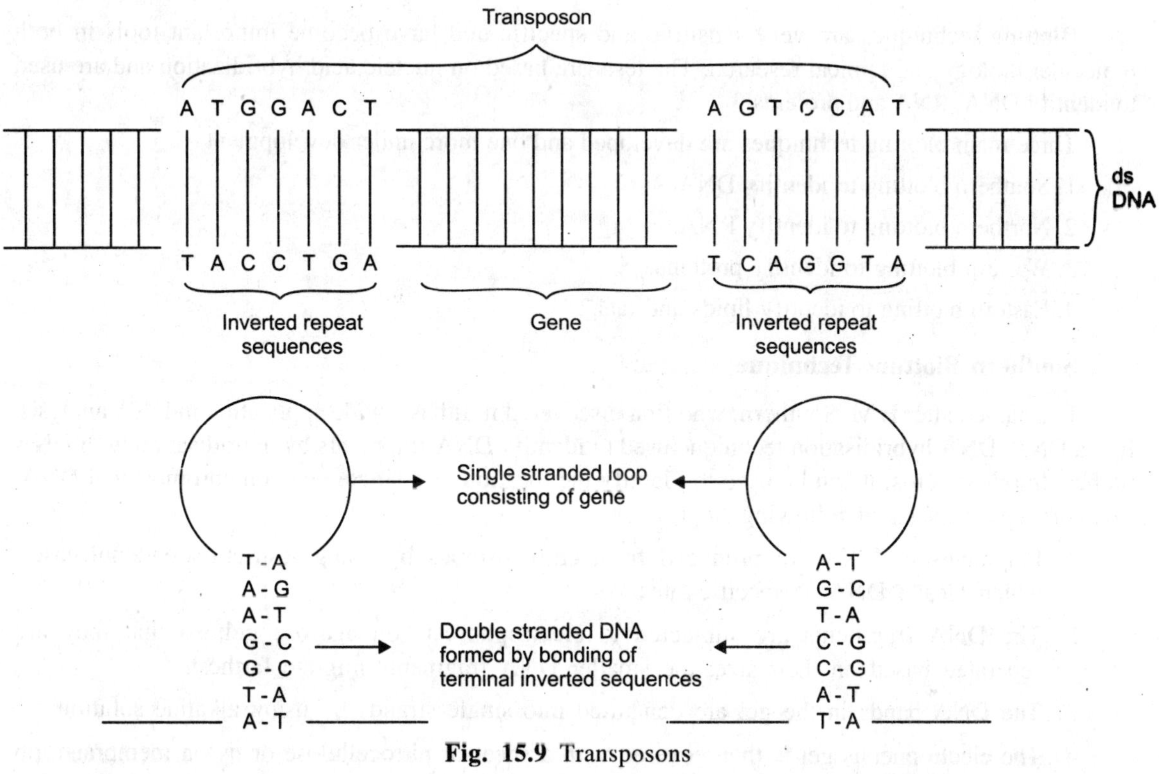

Fig. 15.9 Transposons

Transposable elements are of two types : 1. Insertion sequences (IS), 2. Transposons. They differ in size and gene content.

Insertion sequences. They are small (1–2 Kb) consisting a central coding sequence and flanking short, inverted repeat sequences at either end. They contain genes that encode for information required for movement among plasmids and chromosomes and for replicative recombination. Usually they do not alter phenotype of the cell.

Transposon. They are larger (4 – 25 Kb) composite elements contain genes for movement as well as genes that encode for various functions such as drug resistance and toxin production. They can alter the phenotype of the cell. Transposons contain one or more genes in the centre, and the two ends carrying very long "inverted repeat" sequences of nucleotides, *i.e.,* nucleotide sequences complementary to each other but in the reverse order. Because of this, transposons can form a single stranded loop carrying the gene, and a double-stranded stem formed by hydrogen bonds between the terminal inverted repeat sequences.

Bacteriophage mu is a large transposable element and inserts in many sites on *E.coli* chromosome. Because of the ability of transposable elements to insert into a large number of sites both on the chromosome and on plasmids, they are popularly called "**jumping genes**", and this phenomenon is known as **"transposition".**

Transposition requires an enzyme "transposase" which is coded by is and transposons by may also be coded by the chromosome, plasmid or phage to which transposable element is inserted.

BLOTTING TECHNIQUES

Blotting techniques are very sensitive and specific and have become important tools in both molecular biology and clinical research. The tests are based on nucleic acid hybridization and are used to identify DNA, RNA and proteins.

Three main blotting techniques are developed and one more under development

1. Southern blotting to identify DNA.
2. Northern blotting to identify RNA.
3. Western blotting to identify proteins.
4. Eastern blotting to identify lipids and fats.

Southern Blotting Technique

It is named after E.M. Southern, who first discovered it. It has a wide application in DNA analysis. It is a DNA–DNA hybridisation technique used to identify DNA fragments by hybridisation with DNA probes. In other words, it can be used to identify the location of a single gene on chromosomal DNA. The technique consists of following steps.

1. Fragments of DNA are produced from chromosomes by using restriction endonulceases, which cleave DNA at specific sites.
2. The DNA fragments are subjected to electrophoresis on agarose gel, so that they are separated based on their size; the smaller DNA fragments migrate farthest.
3. The DNA bands in the gel are denatured into single strands by using alkaline solution.
4. The electrophersis gel is then covered with a sheet of nitrocellulose or nylon membrane, on to which DNA fragments are transferred and immobilised or blotted.
5. This nitrocellulose membrane with adsorbed DNA fragments is treated and incubated with radioactive isotope labelled single stranded DNA probe. These will hybridise with homologous DNA to form radioactive double-stranded DNA probes, which can be detected by autoradiography.

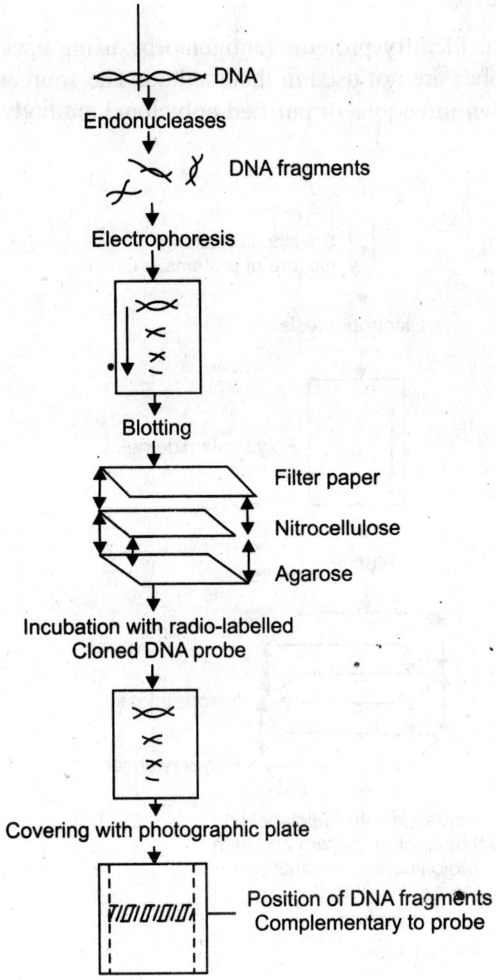

Fig. 15.10 Southern blotting

Northern Blotting Technique

It is used to identify RNA (messenger RNA) by hybridisation with labelled DNA or RNA probes. With this method the transcripts of specific genes can be studied and measured.

Since, it is an analogous procedure for the analysis of RNA, and patterned after southern blot it has been called "northern blotting" as opposite to southern blotting.

Here the RNA (mRNA) mixture is separated, according to size by gel electrophoresis and then transferred and immobilized or blotted on nitrocellulose membrane or on a chemically reactive paper prepared by diazotization with aminobenzyloxymethyl paper. RNA fragments that bind to this membrane or paper can be hybridized with radiolabelled DNA, which can be detected by autoradiography.

Western Blotting Technique

This technique is used to identify proteins (antigens) by using specific antibodies as analytical probes. Thus, nucleic acid probes are not used in this method. The sources of antibody probes may be serum from patients with known infections or purified polyclonal antibody preparations or monoclonal antibodies.

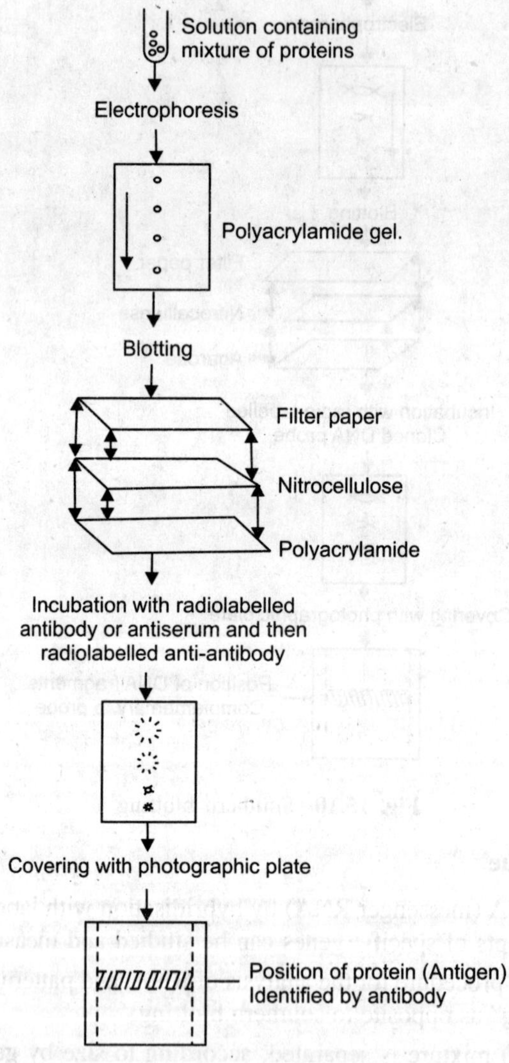

Fig. 15.11 Western blotting

Since this test is used for the identification of protein antigens, it is known as "immunoblotting" or "western blotting" in conformity with other blotting techniques.

Protein antigen mixture is first separated into its components by polyacrylamide gel electrophoresis, and then blotted on to nitrocellulose membrane. It is then incubated with specific antibody. This primary antibody binds to its target protein antigen and is immobilised on the nitrocellulose blotting support.

This antigen-antibody complex can then be identified with radioactive or enzyme labelled antibodies (anti-antibody) to primary antibodies, and can then be visualised by autoradiography. If required the labelled anti-antibody can be removed and the protein antigens can be studied further.

Western blot test is very popular as a confirmatory test for AIDS.

PLASMIDS OR EPISOMES OR EXTRA CHROMOSOMAL GENETIC ELEMENTS

Plasmids are small, circular, covalently closed, double-stranded DNA molecules found in cytoplasm. They are self-replicating.

They are not essential for the normal life of the bacteria, but confer on it certain survival advantages such as toxigenicity, drug resistance etc.

Plasmids containing information for self-transfer to another cell by conjugation are called conjugative or transmissible plasmids.

e.g., F-factor, R-factor, Col-factor. They are commonly found in Gram negative bacilli such as *E.coli, Klebsiella, Shigella, Salmonella, Proteus* etc.

F-factor or Sex factor or Transfer factor or F-plasmid

F-factor is a transfer factor that contains the basic genetic information for extrachromosomal existence, self-transfer by conjugation and for the synthesis of sex pilus (F-pilus).

Cells that contain F-factor are called F^+ cells. F-factor codes for the synthesis of sex pilus, which mates with F^- cell by forming a conjugation tube and promotes transfer of plasmid DNA from one bacterium to another, quickly converting F^- population into F^+.

R-factors or R-plasmids or Resistance factors or Resistance transfer factor (RTF)

R-plasmids carry genes (determinants) for resistance to various antibiotics They are numerous among intestinal Gram negative bacilli and responsible for the spread of multiple drug resistance among them.

Indiscriminate use of antibiotics can increase the incidence of antibiotic-resistant bacteria. Transfer of multiple drug resistance was demonstrated between *E.coli* and *Shigella* strains both *in vitro* and *in vivo*. This resistance is plasmid mediated and is transferred by conjugation. This mechanism of drug resistance is known as "**infectious** or **transferable** or **episomal drug resistance**". Bacteria carrying R-factors can be transmitted from animals to man. Hence, indiscriminate use of antibiotics in veterinary practice or in animal feeds can also lead to an increase of multiple drug resistance in the community.

R-plasmid consists of two components – 1. the resistance transfer factor (RTF), which is responsible for conjugational transfer, and 2. the resistance determinant (r-det) for each of several drugs. Both of them together (RTF + r-det) constitute the whole R-plasmid. R-factor can have several r-determinants, and resistance to as many as eight or more drugs can be transferred simultaneously. Some times, the RTF may dissociate from the r-determinants, and the two components can exist as separate plasmids. The RTF can have determinants other than drug resistance, coding for the synthesis of enterotoxin, hemolysins in some enteropathogenic *E.coli* (EPEC).

Col-Factor or Colicinogenic Factors or Bacteriocinogenic Plasmids

Col-factors contain a gene that directs the host bacterium to synthesize a bacteriocin-antibiotic like substance which specifically and selectively lethal to other bacteria.

Col-factor contains genes that promote self-transfer by conjugation, self-replication and capable of transferring chromosomal segments.

DNA PROBES

Each species will have a unique DNA base sequence, that differentiates it from every other species. If this sequence can be identified and isolated, a chemical label (such as radioactive isotopes) can be attached to it so that this labelled DNA sequence can be used as a probe to detect. Complementary DNA sequences present in a given sample by hybridization reactions.

Hybridization is a process in which two single strands of nucleic acid with complementary base sequences bind together to form a stable double-stranded molecules.

Labelled DNA probes that are specific for particular pathogens can be used to detect and identify pathogen specific DNA present in clinical samples, directly; even without any isolation of pathogen.

DNA probes have already been used to identify a wide variety of pathogens such as viruses, bacteria and parasites. Commercial kits using DNA kits for diagnostic use are available. DNA probes have also been developed to detect and identify specific antibiotic resistance genes, so that antimicrobial sensitivity of an organism can be determined directly from clinical sample, without primary isolation and growth.

QUESTIONS

Essay Type Questions

1. Describe the mechanisms of genetic exchange or gene transfer among bacteria.
2. Describe mutations and their importance in clinical microbiology.

Short Notes

1. Central dogma of molecular biology.
2. Regulation or control of gene expression.
3. Operon or lac operon.
4. Genotype.
5. Phenotype and phenotypic variations.
6. Mutations.
7. Mutagens.
8. Replica plate technique.
9. Transformation or Griffith phenomenon.
10. Bacterial conjugation.
11. Transduction.
12. Specialized transduction.
13. Lysogenic conversion.
14. Describe the principles of genetic engineering or gene cloning or recombinant DNA technology.

15. Applications of genetic engineering.
16. Restriction endonucleases.
17. DNA finger printing.
18. RFLP.
19. Auxotroph.
20. PCR.
21. Transposons or transposable elements or jumping genes or insertion sequences or transposition.
22. Blotting techniques.
23. Southern blotting.
24. Northern blotting.
25. Western blotting.
26. Plasmids or episomes or extrachromosomal genetic elements.
27. R-plasmids.
28. RTF.
29. F-factor.
30. Hfr.
31. Sexduction.
32. F′ cell.
33. DNA probes.
34. Col-factor.

16

Drug Resistance

- *Introduction*
- *Biochemical mechanisms of drug resistance*
- *Chromosome mediated/mutational drug resistance*
- *Extrachromosomal or plasmid mediated or infectious or transmissible drug resistance*
- *Drug dependence*
- *Prevention of drug resistance*

INTRODUCTION

Strains of microorganisms differ in their degree of susceptibility to antibiotics and chemotherapeutic agents. The susceptibility of an organism to any particular drug may change with time. An organism that had once been highly susceptible to a drug may develop resistance, over time. There are different mechanisms by which microorganisms exhibit resistance to drugs.

BIOCHEMICAL MECHANISMS OF DRUG RESISTANCE

1. Microorganisms may produce enzymes that destroy the active drug. *e.g.,* Staphylococci resistant to penicillin G produce penicillinase (β-lactamase) that destroys the active drug. similarly, Gram negative bacilli resistant to chloramphenicol produce chloramphenicol acetyl transferase enzyme.
2. Microorganisms may change their permeability to the drugs. Microbes may cease active uptake of certain drugs *e.g.,* resistance to tetracyclines and polymyxins.
3. Microorganisms develop an altered metabolic pathway that bypasses the reaction inhibited by the drug. *e.g.,* some bacteria have developed resistance to sulphonamides by acquiring the ability to synthesize PABA by utilizing preformed folic acid.

GENETIC MECHANISMS OF DRUG RESISTANCE

Microorganisms may develop drug resistance due to genetic changes mediated by either chromosome or extrachromosomal genetic elements.

(a) Chromosome Mediated Drug Resistance or Mutational Drug Resistance

Mutations confer resistance to only one drug at a time. Mutational drug resistance can be overcome by high dosage of drug as the degree of resistance is usually low. It can be prevented by treatment with a combination of drugs as in tuberculosis. Resistant mutants may be metabolically defective and their virulence may be low (live attenuated vaccines).

For many antibiotics, a particular mutation produces only a slight increase in resistance; but a series of consecutive mutations can produce a step-wise increase in resistance, usually seen with penicillin. Mutation can result in the loss of penicillin-binding proteins (PBPs) making such mutants resistant to β-lactam drugs.

Resistance to streptomycin arises quite readily be a "single large-step mutation" in many bacteria, posing a serious problem in clinical practice, as in the treatment of tuberculosis, the mutants may vary widely in the degree of resistance, some exhibiting low resistance, while others may be highly resistant, and some mutants may become streptomycin-dependent for growth.

(b) Extrachromosomal Resistance or Infectious Drug Resistance or Transmissible Drug Resistance

R-plasmids carry genes (determinants) for resistance to various antibiotics. They are numerous among intestinal Gram negative bacilli and responsible for the spread of multiple drug resistance among them.

R-plasmids can confer simultaneous resistance to several antibiotics used to treat infections successfully. Transfer of multiple drug resistance was demonstrated between different genera of bacteria. For example, between *Shigella* and *E.coli*. This mechanism of drug resistance is known as "infectious drug resistance" or "transferable drug resistance". The degree of resistance is usually high and cannot be prevented by a combination of drugs.

Bacteria carrying R-factors can be transmitted from animals to man. Hence, indiscriminate use of antibiotics in veterinary practice or in animal feeds can also lead to an increase of multiple drug resistance in the community.

R-plasmid consists of two components – 1. the resistance transfer factor (RTF), and 2. the resistance determinant (r-det) for each of several drugs. Both of them together (RTF + r-det) constitute the whole R-plasmid. R factor can have several r-determinants, and resistance to as many as eight or more drugs can be transferred simultaneously. Sometimes, the RTF may dissociate from the r-determinants, and the two components can exist as separate plasmids. In such cases, though the host bacterium remains drug resistant, the resistance is not transferable.

Transferable drug resistance can be transferred between different bacteria by the transfer of plasmids and genetic material through following mechanisms :

1. Conjugation
2. Sexduction
3. Transduction
4. Lysogeny
5. Transformation
6. Transposition.

Table 16.1 Differences between Mutational and Transferable Drug Resistance.

Mutational drug resistance	*Infectious (transferable) drug resistance*
1. Mutations confer resistance usually to one drug at a time	Mediated by plasmids, may confer resistance to multiple drugs or all drugs used in treatment, simulta neously
2. Degree of drug resistance is low	Degree of drug resistance is usually high
3. It can be overcome by administering high dose of drug	It cannot be overcome by high drug dosages
4. It can be prevented by treatment with a combination of drugs (multidrug therapy)	It cannot be prevented by a combination of drugs
5. Mutational drug resistance does not spread from cell to cell	Transferable drug resistance spreads to other cell of same or different species by various methods of gene transfer such as conjugation, transduction, transformation, transposition etc.
6. Resistant mutants are usually metabolically defective	Drug resistant strains are metabolically normal
7. The virulence of resistant mutants may be decreased	Virulence is not decreased

DRUG DEPENDENCE

Certain organisms not only develop resistance to a drug but require it and depend on it for growth. This has been best demonstrated with streptomycin, When streptomycin is used for treatment of tuberculosis, the tubercle bacilli develop resistance by mutations, with varying degrees some of which may become drug dependent.

PREVENTION OF DRUG RESISTANCE

The emergence of drug resistance can be prevented by following ways.

1. Indiscriminate use of antibiotics must be avoided.
2. It is essential to use the correct dosage and schedule (complete course) of the antibiotic to overcome the infection early.
3. Maintain sufficiently high levels of the drug in the tissues to inhibit both the original population and first step mutants.
4. Use a mixture of drugs that have different modes of action so that the organism cannot quickly undergo adaptation. Multi-drug therapy may prevent the emergence of mutants *e.g.,* rifampin and isoniazid in the treatment of tuberculosis.
5. Antibiotics used in vetefinary practice can lead to emergence of drug resistant strains, that may be transferred to humans.
6. Incorporation of antibiotics in animal feeds may cause animals to grow more rapidly, but associated with increase of drug resistant strains in farm workers. Hence, use of antibiotics in animal feeds must be controlled.

7. The drug of choice has to be replaced at the first sign of resistance by the organism.

8. Antibiotics should only be used in situations where a bacterial infection is either proven or strongly suspected.

9. The drug chosen should be targeted for the specific organism to be eradicated rather than opting for a more broad-spectrum drug.

QUESTIONS

Essay Type Questions

1. Describe the genetic mechanisms of drug resistance with examples.
2. Describe various mechanisms of drug resistance in bacteria.

Short Notes

1. Drug resistance.
2. Transferable drug resistance or infectious drug resistance.
3. Mutational drug resistance.
4. Control of drug resistance.

17

Infection and Host-Parasite Interactions

- *Definitions*
- *Infection and Infestation*
- *Types of infections*
- *Sources of infections*
  - *Human patients*
  - *Human carriers*
  - *Animals*
  - *Insects*
  - *Mechanical vectors*
  - *Biological vectors*
  - *Water*
  - *Food*
  - *Soil*
- *Portals of entry (Mode of transmission)*
  - *Direct contact*
  - *Indirect contact*
  - *Inhalation/Air-borne transmission*
  - *Ingestion/food and water borne transmission*
  - *Venereal transmission*
  - *Vertical transmission*
  - *Congenital infections*
  - *Perinatal infections*
  - *Inoculation/percutaneous transmission*
  - *Zoonotic transmission*
  - *Insects*
  - *Iatrogenic transmission*
  - *Laboratory infections*

DEFINITIONS

Saprophyte. (Sapros = decayed ; phyton = plant) – Any microorganism (or plant) living on dead or decaying organic matter is known as saprophyte. They are free living in soil and water and carry out biodegradation of organic matter in nature. They cannot invade living tissues, and only on very rare occasions enter into parasitic relationship with man.

Parasite. Parasite is an organism living in or on another living organism (host) for food and shelter, benefitting at the expense of the host.

By convention, when the word "parasite" is used, it refers specifically to a protozoan or helminthic organism.

Ectoparasite is an organism, which lives on the surface of its host *e.g.,* lice, ticks, mites and leeches.

Endoparasite is an organism, which lives inside the body of the host; in the tissues, blood, body cavity, digestive tract and other organs.

Commensal. (Com = with ; Mensa = table ; living together) Commensals live in complete symbiosis (friendship) with the host, without causing any damage or lesion or invasion. They constitute the normal flora of the body *e.g., Staphylococcus epidermidis* (*albus*). They are normally non-pathogenic, hence known as "non-pathogens". But some commensals are capable of causing infections, when transferred to an abnormal site for example, *Escherichia coli* is normally a harmless commensal in the gut, but causes infection in a wound or urinary tract. *Streptococcus viridans*, a normal mouth commensal, can cause subacute bacterial endocarditis, when it enters blood stream, after a tooth extraction. *Clostridium welchii*, a normal intestinal commensal can cause gangrene in locally damaged tissues.

Pathogen. (Patho = disease ; gen = to produce) – A microorganism capable of causing a disease is called a pathogen.

Host. Host is a person or animal including birds and arthropods that provide lodgement and nourishment to an infectious agent under natural conditions.

INFECTIONS

The entry, lodgement and multiplication of an infectious agent in the body of man and animals is called infection. An infection may or may not lead to a disease state.

Infectious disease. A clinically manifested disease of man or animals resulting from an infection.

Contagious disease. An infectious disease that is transmitted by direct contact. *e.g.,* sexually transmitted diseases.

Communicable disease. It is a disease due to an infectious agent or its toxic products capable of being transmitted directly or indirectly from man to man, animal to animal or from the environment to man.

INFESTATION

It is defined as the lodgement, development and reproduction of parasites (particularly helminthes) in the host.

It is also defined as the lodgement, development, and reproduction of arthropods (insects such as lice, ticks and mites) on the skin of the body or in the clothing of humans.

TYPES OF INFECTIONS

Primary infection. It is an initial (or first) infection caused by a microorganism.

Reinfection. When the same (or a single) microorganism cause infections repeatedly, subsequent infections are termed reinfections.

Secondary infections. When a new microorganism sets up an infection in a host whose resistance is lowered by a pre-existing disease, it is termed secondary infection.

Opportunistic infections. When the host resistance is impaired, as in immunocompromised patients, a non-pathogenic organism may set up infection, which is known as opportunistic infection. For example, opportunistic infections are very common in AIDS due to immunodeficiency.

Vertical infection. Infections transmitted from one generation to another either congenitally (transplacentally) or perinatally (just before or during birth) are known an vertical infections. *e.g.*, syphilis, AIDS, rubella, CMV, toxoplasmosis.

Mixed infection. When more than one microorganism infects a host simultaneously it is called a mixed infection.

Focal infection. It refers to localised or circumscribed chronic infection or sepsis in the body; in areas like gums of teeth, tonsils, nasal sinuses, appendix etc.

Cross infection. When a patient is suffering from a disease, a new infection is set up from another host or exogenous source, termed as cross infection.

Nosocomial/hospital-acquired infection. Cross infections in hospitals are called hospital-acquired infections; developing in hospitalized patients, which were not present or in incubation at the time of their admission; originating from patient (endogenous) himself or external source (exogenous).

Iatrogenic infection. It is a physician induced infection resulting from diagnostic, preventive (immunization) or therapeutic (drug therapy) procedures.

Subclinical/inapparent infection. It is an infection, where clinical effects are not apparent.

Atypical infection. Atypical infection is one in which the typical or characteristic clinical manifestations of the particular infectious disease are not present.

Exogenous infection. It is an infection caused by the entry of organism from an external source such as food, water, air, fomites or other persons.

Endogenous infection. It is an infection caused by a microorganism, derived from the host's body itself; and is often due to lowering of resistance of the host. It is often an opportunistic infection caused by commensals. *e.g., E .coli* derived from bowel may cause urinary tract infection.

Latent infection. It is an infection in which infecting organism is quiescent, but may reactivate. Some microorganisms following infection, may remain in the tissues for long periods, without producing any symptoms, in a latent or hidden form proliferating and producing clinical disease, when the host resistance is lowered. This is termed latent infection.

e.g., Herpes simplex virus (HSV) infections, Brill-Zinsser disease, slow virus infections.

Bacteremia. Presence or circulation of viable bacteria in the blood stream is called bacteremia. Transient bacteremia occurs in healthy persons during chewing, brushing of teeth and while straining during excretion of feces.

Septicemia (Sepsis). A systemic disease or blood poisoning in which microorganisms multiply in the blood stream, form toxic products, producing clinical signs and symptoms such as fever.

Sepsis may occur as a complication of intravenous catheterisation or child birth (puerperal).

Pyemia. Pyemia is a condition where pyogenic bacteria produce septicemia with multiple abscesses in the internal organs of the body.

Epidemic (epi = upon ; demos = population). It refers to increased occurrence of disease and a larger number of diseased or infecting individuals in a particular location; spreads rapidly involving many persons at the same time in an area. *e.g.*, influenza.

Epizootic. An epidemic that occurs in animals is called epizootic. *e.g.*, plague in rats.

Endemic. A disease constantly or persistently present at some rate of occurrence in a defined population or geographical area. *e.g.*, typhoid fever.

Enzootic. An endemic occurring in animals is called enzootic. *e.g.*, plague in rats, brucellosis in cattle.

Pandemic. An epidemic that spans the world is called pandemic disease; spreading through many areas of the world involving very large numbers of people within a short period.

e.g., influenza, cholera, plague, enteroviral conjunctivitis.

SOURCES OF INFECTION

The term "source of infection" refers to the location (*e.g.*, man, animals, fomites etc.) from which the pathogen is disseminated to the host.

Human Patients

Infections due to some microorganisms are acquired mainly or exclusively from patients with active infection. *e.g.*, pulmonary tuberculosis, leprosy, whooping cough, syphilis, gonorrhoea, measles, small pox, mumps and influenza.

Human Carriers

Carrier is defined as an infected person, who harbours the pathogen, without any clinical disease (asymptomatic infection), and acts as a potential source of infection for others.

Carriers play an important role in the epidemiology of the disease. *e.g.*, Marry Mallon ("Typhoid Mary"), a New York cook, who over a period of 15 years, caused atleast seven outbreaks affecting over 200 persons. Carriers are of several types :

Healthy carrier is an individual who harbours the pathogen but is not ill.

Incubatory carrier is an individual who is incubating the pathogen in large numbers, during the incubation period of an illness, but is not yet ill.

Convalescent carrier is an individual who has recovered from the infectious disease, but continues to harbour large numbers of the pathogen.

Temporary carriers harbour the pathogen for less than 6 months.

Chronic carriers harbour the pathogen for long periods – months, years or life.

Contact carrier is one who acquires the pathogen from a patient.

Paradoxical carrier is one who acquires the pathogen from another carrier.

Animals

Some pathogens that are primarily parasites of different animals, may spread from the infected animal to man and called "zoonoses". Many animals serve to maintain the parasite in nature by acting as

"Reservoir hosts" or "Amplifying hosts". Some diseases are endemic among animals, known as "enzootic", whereas epidemics that occur in animals are known as "epozootic". e.g., bacterial zoonoses – Anthrax, plague, Brucellosis, bovine tuberculosis, Leptospirosis, Viral zoonoses – rabies, cowpox, lymphocytic choriomeningitis. Parasitic zoonoses – hydatid disease, leishmaniasis, fish tape worm, beef tape worm.

Insects

Insects such as mosquitoes, flies, lice, ticks, mites and fleas that transmit infections are called vectors. Vectors are classified into two types based on mode of transmission.

(*i*) ***Mechanical vectors.*** They transmit the pathogen mechanically, through soiling of its legs or probascis. There is no development or multiplication of the pathogen on or within the vector *e.g.*, transmission of dysentery bacilli or typhoid bacilli by domestic fly.

(*ii*) ***Biological vector.*** The pathogen undergoes development or multiplication or both in vector and requires an incubation period before transmission. *e.g.*,

Female anopheles mosquito – malaria

Aedes aegypti mosquito	– yellow fever
Culex mosquito	– filariasis, Japanese B encephalitis
Rat flea	– plague
Louse	– epidemic typhus
Tick	– spotted fevers, relapsing fever
Mite	– scrub typhus
Tsetsefly	– African sleeping sickness (Trypanosomiasis)
Sandfly	– Leishmaniasis

Water

Water acts as a source of infection due to contamination with pathogens from humans or animals (usually excreta). Water-borne diseases may be due to the presence of a pathogen or an aquatic host in it.

Water borne diseases

I. Due to the presence of pathogens

1. Bacteria	*Vibrio cholerae, Salmonella* sp, *Shigella, Esch.coli, Vibrio Parahemolyticus, Yersinia enterocolitica, Campylobaer, Leptospira.*
2. Viruses	Hepatitis 'A' virus, Poliovirus (enteroviruses), Rotavirus.
3. Protozoa	*Entamoeba histolytica, Giardia lamblia, Cryptosporidium, Acanthamoeba, Naegleria fowleri.*
4. Helminthes	Round worm, whip worm, pin worm

II. Due to the presence of an aquatic host

1. Cyclops	Guinea worm, fish tape worm
2. Snail	*Schistosoma*

Food

Many diseases are transmitted by foods contaminated with pathogens or their toxins. Foods may be contaminated by flies mechanically or by carriers due to handling or eating utensils infected by handling or washing in contaminated water.

e.g., Staphylococcus aureus, Clostridium botulinum, Clostridium welchii (Type A), *Bacillus cereus, Salmonella* species, *Campylobacter jejuni, E.coli, Shigella, Yersinia enterocolitica, Vibrio parachemolyticus, Listeria monocytogenes* etc. may be transmitted by contaminated food. Tape worm infestations may be transmitted by undercooked pork or beef.

Soil

Some infectious diseases of man are caused by saprophytes derived from the soil, vegetation etc. The soil derived infections are not infectious from one man to another.

e.g., Tetanus, gas gangrene, maduramycosis, sporotrichosis, histoplasmosis, coccidioidomycosis; hook worm and round worm.

METHODS/MODES/ROUTES OF TRANSMISSION/PORTALS OF ENTRY

Humans may acquire microorganisms by various routes referred to as the 'modes of transmission".

1. Direct contact
2. Indirect contact
3. Inhalation/Air-borne transmission
4. Ingestion/food and water-borne transmission
5. Venereal transmission
6. Vertical transmission
7. Inoculation/percutaneous transmission
8. Zoonotic transmission
9. Insects
10. Iatrogenic transmission
11. Laboratory infections.

Direct Contact

Direct contact implies an actual physical interaction with the infectious source. This route is frequently called person-to-person contact, which occurs primarily –

(*i*) by touching of bodies as in handshaking,

(*ii*) by kissing

(*iii*) by contact of clothing, *e.g.,* HSV-I, boils, Staphylococcal infections.

(*iv*) by sexual contact

Indirect Contact

Indirect contact refers to the transmission of the pathogen from the source to the host via an inanimate objects, known as "Fomites". *Pseudomonas* bacteria are easily transmitted by this route. Pens and pencils shared by school children may act as fomites in the transmission of diphtheria and face towels in trachoma.

Fomites : Surgical instruments, thermometers, eating utensils, spoons, drinking cups, bedding, clothing, pillows, towels, handkerchiefs, doctor's coats, nurses uniform, pens, pencils, toys, pockets, books, door handles, taps, etc.

Inhalation/Air-Borne Transmission

Microorganisms that cause respiratory infections occur in nasal and oral secretions of individuals. During coughing, sneezing, singing or talking, aerosols may be expelled. These droplet nuclei remain suspended in air for hours or days and may be carried long distances. *e.g.,* common cold, influenza, chicken pox, measles, mumps, pneumonia, diphtheria, tuberculosis, meningitis and pertussis.

Some pathogens that inhabit soil may be raised as dust and transmitted through inhalation. *e.g.,* histoplasmosis, coccidioidomycosis.

Ingestion/Food and Water-Borne Transmission

In alimentary tract infections, pathogens are discharged in the feces of infected persons, and are transmitted by fecal-oral routes.

Intestinal infections may be transmitted by following ways :

1. Contamination of water supplies with excreta – water-borne infection.
2. Through contaminated or uncleaned fingers – hand to mouth infection. Nurses may infect their hands in attending patients and in touching bed-pans.
3. Contamination of food – due to a carrier handling the food or mechanically by insects – food-borne infection.
4. Contamination of vegetables and fruits grown fertilised with feces (sewage).
5. Through fomites such as door handles, water taps, lavatory seats contaminated by patients or carriers.

e.g. Cholera, enteric fever (salmonellosis), dysentery, intestinal tuberculosis, Type A hepatitis, enteroviral infections (poliomyelitis), intestinal parasitic infestations.

Venereal Transmission

The diseases that are transmitted by sexual contact are called venereal diseases or sexually transmitted diseases (STD).

e.g. Syphilis, gonorrhoea, chancroid, granuloma inguinale, lymphogranuloma venereum (LGV), AIDS, HSV-2.

Vertical transmission/congenital infections/teratogenic infections/transplacental transmission

The infections that are transmitted from one generation to another, either transplacentally (congenital) or perinatally are known as vertical infections. These infections usually lead to the deformity or malformations in the developing embryo. Hence, they are also called teratogenic infections.

Congenital infections are those diseases, that are acquired by the fetus in utero, through the transplacental route.

e.g. Congenital syphilis, AIDS, congenital toxoplasmosis, congenital rubella syndrome, congenital cytomegalovirus infections.

Congenital infections during first three months of pregnancy may lead to abortion, still birth, miscarriage, premature delivery and a wide range of congenital defects or malformations (teratogenic) such as cardiac defects, blindness, deafness, mental retardation etc.

Perinatal infections are those diseases, that are acquired either during birth or just before birth leading to neonatal complications. *e.g,,* neonatal herpes with HSV-2 and ophthalmia neonatorum by gonococci.

Inoculation/Percutaneous Transmission

Infections may be transmitted by inoculation through the skin or mucus membranes to deeper tissues. *e.g.,* surgery, trauma, injections, dressing of surgical wounds, insect bites etc.

Diseases such as syphilis, AIDS and Type B hepatitis may be introduced by injection of serum, plasma or blood, particularly among intravenous drug addicts. Infection by inoculation may be iatrogenic when it is due to unsterile syringes, surgical instruments and catheters.

In some occasions, the pathogens may be directly implanted or inoculated into the tissues. Inoculation of rabies virus by dog bite, implantation of gas gangrene and tetanus spores in the depth of wounds, and injection of Arboviruses by mosquitoes are examples.

Zoonotic Transmission

See sources of infection.

Insects

See sources of infection.

Iatrogenic Transmission

Infections caused as a result of health care are called iatrogenic or physician induced infections. It refers to adverse consequences resulting due to physician's professional health care activities such as diagnostic, preventive (immunization) and therapeutic procedures. Modern methods of treatment such as exchange transfusion, dialysis and heart and transplant surgery have increased the possibilities for iatrogenic infections.

e.g. Administration of injections, lumbar puncture, aplastic anemia following the use of chloramphenicol, purpura following administration of sedormid, childhood leukemia due to prenatal X-rays, AIDS, hepatitis B following blood transfusion.

Laboratory infections

Technicians, nurses and other paramedical laboratory workers occasionally become infected from cultures or from infectious materials collected from patients or experimental animals. When working with dangerous pathogens such as sputum samples for AFB and blood samples for screening AIDS and Type B hepatitis, special care should be taken to prevent laboratory infections.

QUESTIONS

Essay Type Questions

1. What is an infection ? Describe various types of infections.

2. Describe in detail the sources of infections to humans beings.
3. Describe the portals of entry or routes of transmission or methods of transmission of infections.

Short Notes

1. Define and differentiate primary, secondary, opportunistic and reinfections.
2. Cross infections.
3. Iatrogenic infections.
4. Define epidemic, endemic, pandemic and sporadic.
5. Define bacteremia, septicemia and pyemia.
6. Define exogenous and endogenous infections.
7. Carrier.
8. Zoonoses.
9. Define and mention two zoonotic infections.
10. Name two zoonotic bacterial diseases.
11. Name four parasitic zoonotic diseases.
12. Name four viral zoonotic diseases.
13. Name two fungal zoonotic diseases.
14. Vectors/biological vector/mechanical vector.
15. Name any four water-borne diseases.
16. Fomites.
17. Droplet nuclei/name any four air-borne diseases.
18. Vertical infections/teratogenic infections/congenital infections.
19. Define and differentiate secondary infection and opportunistic infections.

18

Microbial Pathogenicity

- *Pathogenicity*
- *Virulence*
- *Exaltation*
- *Attenuation*
- *Factors determining virulence/pathogenicity*
  - *Communicability of transmissibility*
  - *Adhesion or colonization*
  - *Invasiveness/Aggressiveness*
  - *Toxigenicity/Bacterial toxins*
  - *Exotoxins*
  - *Endotoxins*
  - *Extracellular enzymes*
  - *Resistance to phagocytosis*
  - *Survival within phagocytes*
  - *Infective dose*
  - *Routes of infection*
  - *Plasmids*
  - *Bacteriophages*

PATHOGENICITY

Pathogenicity is defined as the capacity of a microbial species to produce disease. *e.g., Mycobacterium tuberculosis*, *Salmonella typhi* are referred to as pathogenic.

VIRULENCE

Virulence is defined as the degree or intensity of pathogenicity in a strain or clone of microorganism. *e.g.,* The species *Mycobacterium tuberculosis* may contain several strains with varying degrees of virulence.

EXALTATION

Enhancement of virulence is known as **"exaltation"**, which can be achieved by serial passage in favourable and susceptible hosts.

ATTENUATION

Reduction in virulence is known as **"attenuation"**, which can be achieved by following means

(*i*) by serial passage through unfavourable host (other than natural host) (*ii*) by repeated subcultures

(*iii*) by growth under high temperature

(*iv*) by growth in the presence of weak antiseptics

(*v*) by prolonged storage in cultures

(*vi*) by desiccation

(*vii*) by mutations.

e.g., Sabin's oral polio vaccine (OPV) is a live attenuated strain (a mutant); BCG (Bacillus Calmette-Guerin) is a live attenuated vaccine, attenuated by 239 serial subcultures over a period of 13 years in a glycerine-bile-potato medium.

FACTORS DETERMINING VIRULENCE/PATHOGENICITY

In order to cause infectious disease, a pathogen must be able to

1. infect the host
2. adhere to, colonize or invade the host
3. grow and multiply in the host tissues
4. resist host defence mechanisms
5. damage the host.

There are several factors, which contribute to or determine virulence, known as virulence determinants or aggressins.

Communicability or Transmissibility

The ability of a parasite to spread from one host to another is known as communicability, which determines the survival and distribution of a parasite in a community.

The infections in which the pathogen is shed in oral or nasal secretions as in respiratory infections and in feces as in intestinal infections, are highly communicable.

Adhesion and Colonization

After being transmitted to host, the pathogen must be able to adhere to and colonize host cells and tissues. Microorganisms adhere with a high degree of specificity to particular tissues, with various kinds of adhensins. *e.g.,* Fimbriae or pili, glycocalyx or capsue, slime or biofilms, hemagglutinin, adherence proteins such as ligands, colonisation factors, IgA protease, fibronectin.

Invasiveness/Aggressiveness

It refers to the ability of a pathogen to spread or invade and multiply in healthy tissues, usually by producing lytic substances or passively through disrupted skin and mucosal surfaces.

Highly invasive pathogens produce generalised or spreading type of lesions *e.g.,* streptococcal septicemia following wound infections; whereas less invasive pathogens cause more localised lesions *e.g.,* staphylococcal abscess. Some pathogens are non-invasive but can cause fatal diseases *e.g.,* tetanus by *Clostridium tetani.*

Toxigenicity/Bacterial Toxins

Some microorganisms produce poisonous substances known as "Toxins". They are of two types.

I. Exotoxins – excreted into the surrounding medium.

II. Endotoxins – retained within the cell as an integral part of cell wall.

Exotoxins

1. Proteins (polypeptides) with a mol. wt. 10,000 – 900,000.
2. Heat labile, can be inactivated by heating at 60–80°C.
3. Soluble.
4. Excreted (secreted) from the microbial cells into the surroundings (into the culture medium or into the circulatory system and tissues of a host).
5. Do not require cell lysis or bacterial death for their release. Toxins can be separated from cultures by physical methods such as filtration.
6. Possess enzymatic action.
7. Associated with specific diseases.
8. Possess specific pharmacological effects.
9. Possess specific tissue affinities.
10. Most lethal substances known; highly potent.
11. Active in very minute doses and pssesses very high toxicity. Active in micrograms or less for laboratory animals.
12. It can be inactivated by formaldehyde, phenol, acids, betapropiolactone, iodine, heat into antigenic **"toxoids"**, which can be used for immunisation *e.g.,* tetanus toxoid, diphtheria toxoid.
13. Strongly antigenic (immunogenic), both toxins and toxoids stimulate the formation of antibodies, known as "antitoxins".
14. Antitoxins can neutralise toxins specifically, *e.g.,* Tetanus antitoxin (ATS), diphtheria antitoxin.
15. Cannot produce fever in the host (not pyrogenic).
16. Cannot produce shock.
17. Often given the name of the disease they produce. *e.g.,* cholera toxin, diphtheria toxin, tetanus toxin.
18. Produced mainly by Gram positive bacteria and by some Gram negative bacteria.

Endotoxins

1. Lipopolysaccharides (LPS).
2. Relatively heat stable, can withstand heat over 60°C for many hours.
3. They form an integral part of the outer membranes of cell wall, as a component of somatic antigen (O-antigen).
4. They are released upon cell lysis or cell death only.
5. Do not possess enzymatic action.
6. Do not possess specific pharmacological effects.
7. Do not possess specific tissue affinities.
8. Action is common to all endotoxins; non-specific.
9. Less potent than exotoxins; active in very large doses only.
10. Weakly antigenic.
11. Cannot stimulate the formation of antitoxins; can stimulate the formation of antibodies to polysac-

charide moiety (somatic or O-antigen).

12. Cannot be rendered nontoxic when combined with homologous antibody.
13. Cannot be converted to toxoids.
14. Pyrogenic; often produce fever in host.
15. Can produce shock, known as endotoxic shock.
16. Present in Gram negative bacteria *e.g., Salmonella, Shigella, Escherichia, Neisseria* etc.
17. Biological activity or toxicity of endotoxins, is largely due to lipid A.
21. ***Biological effects of endotoxins or endotoxic shock*** are as follows :

Pyrogenicity, lethal action, hypotension, activation of complement, leucopenia, clotting of limulus lysate, polyclonal activation of B-lymphocytes, local Shwartzmann reaction, macrophage migration inhibition, stimulates natural killer (NK) cells, stimulates macrophages to produce cytokines such as inter leukin-1, tumour necrosis factor (TNF), and colony stimulating factor (CSF), disseminated intravascular coagulation, induction of prostaglandins and leucotrienes, stimulates non-specific resistance to infections.

Table 18.1 Differences between Exotoxins and Endotoxins

Exotoxins	*Endotoxins*
1. Proteins (polypeptides) with a molecular weight of 10,000-900,000	Lipopolysaccharides
2. Heat labile; can be inactivated by heating at 60–80°C	Relatively heat stable; can withstand heat over 60°C for many hours
3. Excreted (secreted) from the microbial cells into the surroundings (into the culture medium or into the circulatory system and tissues of a host)	They form an integral part of the outer membranes of cell wall as a component of somatic antigen (O-antigen)
4. Do not require cell lysis or bacterial death for their release; toxins can be separated from cultures by physical methods such as filtration	They are released upon cell lysis or cell death only
5. Possess enzymatic action	Do not possess enzymatic action
6. Possess specific pharmacological effects	Do not possess specific pharmacological effects
7. Possess specific tissue affinities	Do not possess specific tissue affinities
8. Highly potent; active in very minute doses only	Less potent than exotoxins; active in very large doses only
9. Strongly antigenic	Weakly antigenic
10. Can be converted to antigenic toxoids by inactivation with formaldehyde, betapropiolactene, iodine, phenol, acids and heat; which can be used for immunisation	Cannot be converted to toxoids
11. Both toxins and toxoids stimulate the formation of antibodies known an "antitoxins".	Cannot stimulate the formation of antitoxins; can stimulate the formation of antibodies to polysaccha-

	ride moie ty (somatic antigen or O-antigen)
12. Antitoxins can neutralise toxins specifically	Cannot be rendered non-toxic when combined with homologous Antibody.
13. Cannot produce fever in the host (not pyrogenic)	Pyrogenic; often produce fever in the host
14. Cannot produce shock	Can produce shock, known as endotoxic shock
15. Produced mainly by Gram positive bacteria and by some Gram negative bacteria	Present in Gram negative bacteria only
e.g., Clostridium tetani, Clostridium botulinum, Corynebacterium diphtheriae, Vibrio cholerae	*e.g., Salmonella, Shigella, Escherichia, Neisseria* etc.

Extracellular enzymes

Some bacterial products enhance virulence by promoting invasiveness into the tissue and by inhibiting host's resistance.

Hyaluronidase hydrolyzes hyaluronic acid, an intercellular cement substance and helps the pathogen to penetrate the tissues. Hence, it is called "Spreading factor". *Staphylococcus aureus, Streptococcus pyogenes* and *Clostridium welchii* etc. produce hyaluronidase.

Lecithinase destroys membrane lipids and collagenase collagen, a tissue fiber found in muscles; produced by *Clostridium welchii* and responsible for its virulence.

Fibrinolysin (streptokinase) produced by *Streptococcus pyogenes* breaks down fibrin barrier and promote spreading of streptococcal lesions.

Depolymerizing enzymes such as mucinase, lipases, proteases, nucleases, neuraminidase etc. may contribute to virulence.

Staphylococcus aureus produces coagulase enzyme which converts fibrinogen into fibrin; which is deposited around the lesion, and protects bacteria from host phagocytes.

Hemolysins are substances that lyse RBC, releasing their hemoglobin known as **hemolysis.**

Resistance to Phagocytosis

Capsules inhibit phagocytosis thereby promote virulence. Capsulated bacteria such as Pneumococci, *Klebsiella pneumoniae, Hemophilus influenzae* are highly virulent. When they lose capsules (by mutations), they become avirulent.

Survival Within Phagocytes

Intracellular patahogens use different strategies to resist intracellular killing mechanisms of macrophages and other phagocytes and may multiply intracellularly. *e.g., Mycobacterium tuberculosis* and *Salmonella typhi.*

Infective dose

Virulence is estimated in terms of the number or weight of microorganisms or micrograms of toxin required to kill a particular species of animal. This is called Minimum lethal dose (MLD). Minimum Infecting Dose (MID) is the minimum number of bacteria required to produce clinical disease or death, in a susceptible animal under standard conditions. As different animals exhibit differences in susceptibility to various microorganisms, these doses are more accurately expressed as LD 50 and ID 50, which is defined as the dose requried to infect or kill 50 per cent of the animals tested under standard conditions.

Routes of Infection

Bacteria can survive and multiply only when introduced by optimal routes and related to the modes by which different bacteria are able to initiate tissue damage and establish themselves. For example, cholera vibrios are infective orally but cannot cause infection when introduced subcutaneously.

Plasmids

Plasmid mediated factors are associated with virulence. In *E.coli* both enterotoxin genes and colonisation factor genes are coded for by plasmids. R factors increase the severity of clinical disease by conferring multiple drug resistance on bacteria.

Bacteriophages

Phage directed virulence is characteristically seen in *Corynebacterium diphtheriae* and *Clostridium botulinum*. The diphtheria bacilli are harmless by themselves; but when it is infected with β-phage (corynephage), the phage DNA (prophage) codes for the synthesis of diphtheria toxin, which is responsible for the clinical manifestations of diphtheria disease. Similarly *Costridium botulinum* (types C and D) produces toxin, coded by Tox^+ bacteriophages.

QUESTIONS

Essay Type Questions

1. Describe the factors determining microbial pathogenicity and virulence.

   Or

   Describe bacterial virulence factors.

   Or

   Write a note on virulence factors in bacteria .
2. Describe bacterial toxins.

Short Notes

1. Differentiate pathogenicity from virulence.
2. Virulence.
3. Attenuation.
4. Virulence factors.
5. Bacterial toxins.
6. Exotoxins.
7. Endotoxins.
8. Toxoids.
9. Endotoxic shock.
10. Name any four extracellular enzymes produced by bacteria.
11. What is the difference between attenuation and exaltation ?
12. Name any two bacterial appendages that offer resistance to phagocytosis.
13. Define MLD and MID.
14. Define LD 50 and ID 50.
15. Name two phages which code for the synthesis of bacterial toxins. What diseases they cause ?
16. Hemolysins.
17. Name any four bacteria that produce toxins and the diseases caused by them.

PART-II

IMMUNOLOGY

19

History of Immunology

The discipline of immunology grew out of the observation that individuals who had recovered from certain infectious diseases were thereafter protected from the disease. The latin term *immunis*, meaning "exempt", is the source of the English word **"immunity"**. In general, it means the state of protection from infectious disease.

It has been noticed from very early days that persons surviving an attack of small pox did not develop the disease, when exposed to the infection subsequently. This observation had been applied for the prevention of the disease by producing a mild form of small pox intentionally (variolation). This practice, prevalent in India, China and other ancient civilisations from time immemorial, was introduced in England by Lady Mary Wortley Montague (1718) who had observed the custom in Turkey. Variolation was effective but hazardous.

Edward Jenner (1749–1823) observed the immunity to small pox in milk maids who were exposed to occupational cowpox infection. Jenner introduced the technique of vaccination against small pox by injecting cowpox material from disease pustules into man (in 1796). Jenner published his findings in 1798 in a pamphlet "*An inquiry into the cause and effect of variole vaccine*"

An accidental observation by Louis Pasteur (1822–1895), that chicken cholera bacillus cultures left on the bench for several weeks lost their pathogenic property but retained their ability to protect the birds against subsequent infections by them led to the discovery of the process of **attenuation** and the development of live vaccines. He attenuated cultures of anthrax bacillus by incubation at high temperature (42–43°C) and proved that inoculation of such cultures into animals induced specific protection against anthrax, which was demonstrated by a public experiment (1881). Pasteur coined the term **"vaccine"** (vacca = cow) for such prophylactic preparations, the commemorate the first of such preparations, namely cowpox, employed by Jenner for protection against small pox.

Pasteur developed a vaccine against Rabies (hydrophobia), which made a great impact in medicine. In a series of studies, Pasteur established that the rabies virus was present in the brain of infected animals. By serial intracerebral passage in rabbits, he obtained the fixed virus and demonstrated that dogs could be rendered immune by a series of injections of fixed virus of graded doses. This vaccine was prepared by drying pieces of spinal cord from rabbits infected with the fixed virus for various periods of time. In July 1885, Joseph Meister, a nine year old boy, severely btitten by a rabid dog and in grave risk of developing rabies, was given a course of 13 inoculations of the infected cord vaccine by Pasteur. This dramatic event was acclaimed as a milestone in the development of medicine.

The Pasteur Institute, Pairs was built by public contributions and similar institutions were established soon in many other countries for the preparation of vaccines and for investigation of infectious diseases.

Elie Metchnikoff (1833), a Russian-French biololgist, discovered the phenomenon of phagocytosis, the cellular concept of immunity. In Italy where he has gone on research visit, he studied the transparent larvae of star fish and noticed some of their cells could engulf and digest foreign protein particles. These cell eaters are called **phagocytes**. He continued his work on phagocytic action at Pasteur Institute, Paris and found that in human blood a large proportion of the leucocytes are phagocytic and attack invading bacteria. This, in turn, results in increased numbers of leucocytes in the infected areas followed by the inflamed area becoming hot, red, swollen and painful due to dead phagocytes forming pus. He spent his last two decades on the study of human ageing, since he believed that phagocytes eventually begin to digest the host cells aided by the effects of intestinal bacteria and that effectively combating them would increase the life span of human being.

A specific humoral factor or **antibody** was described by Von Behring and Kitasato (1090) in the serum of animals which had received sublethal doses of tetanus toxin. Pfeiffer (1893) demonstrated bactericidal effect in *vivo* by injecting live cholera vibrios intraperitoneally in guinea pigs previously injected with killed cholera vibrios. The vibrios where shown to undergo lysis. The humoral nature of such lytic activity was proved by Bordet (1895), who defined the two components participating in the reaction, the first being heat stable antibody and the second being heat labile component. Wright (1903) discovered opsonisation, in which antibodies and phagocytic cells act in conjunction.

Robert Koch (1890) had noticed that when the tubercle bacillus or its protein was injected into a guinea pig already infected with the bacillus, an exaggerated response took place-a hypersensitivity reaction, known as **Koch's phenomenon**. Portier and Richet (1902), studying the effect of the toxic extracts of sea anemones in dogs made the same observation that dogs which had prior contact with the toxin were abnormally sensitive to even minute quantities of it subsequently. This phenomenon was termed **anaphylaxis**. Theobald Smith (1902) had noticed a similar phenomenon (theobald smith phenomenon) in guinea pigs following widely spaced injections of toxin-antitoxin mixtures. Later, many similar reactions were observed, both experimentally and in nature, of injury, disease or even death resulting from repeated contacts with antigens. The importance of this phenomenon, in the pathogenesis of many human diseases, led to the development of discipline of allergy.

Sir Frank MacFarlane Burnet proposed **clonal selection theory** (1957) to explain antibody synthesis. Burnet (1967) developed the concept of **immunological surveillance**, according to which the primary function of the immune system is to preserve the integrity of the body, seeking and destroying all "foreign" antigens, whether autogenous or external in origin.

Understanding of the immunological basis of transplantation, Medawar and Burnet made successful transplants possible by immunosuppression and proper selection of donors based on histocompatibility.

Blood transfusion became scientifically feasible only after the discovery of blood groups by Landsteiner. Landsteiner (1900) cross tested serum form himself and five of his colleagues against their blood cells. There distinct patterns of agglutination were observed. Cells which failed to agglutinate with any of the serum samples were designated group 'O' while cells agglutinating in the two different patterns were called groups A and B, respectively. The fourth group AB was described later by his pupils Von Decastallo and Sturli (1902). In 1930, Landsteiner was awarded the Nobel prize for his discovery of human blood groups. Using rabbit antisera to different samples of human red cells, Landsteiner and Levine (1926) discovered the MN and P antigens. Landsteiner and Weiner

(1940) raised rabbit and guinea pig antisera against Rhesus monkey erythrocytes and tested them against human red cells. This led to the discovery of the rhesus (Rh)) factor.

The earliest example of autoimmunity was the observation by Metalnikoff (1900) what guinea pigs injected with their own spermatozoa produced sperm immobilising antibodies. Dameshek and Schwartz (1938) established the autoimmune basis of the hemolytic anemia.

Some of the outstanding contributions to the development of Immunology are listed herebelow.

India and China (ancient times) – practice of "variolation" in which protection against small pox was obtained by inoculating live organisms from disease pustules.

Edward Jenner (1798) – protective effect of vaccination with nonvirulent cowpox against small pox infection.

Louis Pasteur (1879) – Fowl cholera vaccine using old cultures of cholera bacilli.

Louis Pasteur (1881) – Vaccine for anthrax using attenuated organisms.

Metchnikoff (1883) – role of phagocytes in immunity.

Louis Pasteur (1885) – Rabies vaccine prepared by using spinal cord extracts saved the life of Joseph Meister.

Von Behring (1890) – recognized antibodies in serum to diphtheria toxin.

Kitasato and Von Behring (1890) – discovered tetanus antitoxin.

Roux and Martin (1894) – produced antitoxin by immunizing horses.

Denys and Leclef (1895) – phagocytosis greatly enhanced by immunization.

Paul Ehrlich (1896) – introduced methods of standardizing toxins and antitoxins.

Gruber and Durham (1896) – described the phenomenon of agglutination.

Paul Ehrlich (1898) – side chain theory of antibody formation

Bordet (1899) – lysis of cells by antibody requires cooperation of serum factors now collectively termed complement.

Landsteiner (1900) – human ABO groups and natural isohemagglutinins.

Richet and Portier (1902) – anaphylaxis (opposite of prophylaxis).

Wright (1903) – relation of opsonic activity to phagocytosis.

Wasermann (1906) – applied complement fixation test to the diagnosis of syphilis.

Leonor Michaelis (1907) – described the phenomenon of precipitation.

Calmette and Guerin (1921) – developed BCG vaccine against tuberculosis by attenuation of a strain of *Mycobacterium bovis*.

Zinsser (1925) – contrast between immediate and delayed hypersensitivity.

Heiderberger and Kendall (1930–35) – quantitative precipitin studies on antigen-antibody interactions.

Landsteiner and Wiener (1940) – discovered Rh factor.

Mac Farlane Burnet (1960) – Clonal selection theory of antibody formation.

Peter B. Medawar (1960) – proved immunological basis for allograft rejection, contributed to elucidation of induced immunological tolerance.

Rodney Porter and Gerald Edelman (1972) – structure and chemical nature of Immunoglobulins.

Kohler and Milstein (1975) – production of monoclonal antibodies by hybridoma technology.

Rosalyn Yalow (1977) – developed and defined Radioimmunoassay (RIA).

George Snell, Jean Dusset and Baruj Bencerraf (1980) – MHC and genetic control of Immune response; described analogies; between mouse and human histocompatibility system, identified immune response genes.

Neils K. Jerne (1984) – described biological selection theory of antibody formation and also accounted for immunological tolerance.

Susumu Tonegaeva (1987) – generation of antibody diversity.

J. Murray (1990) – first successful transplant of living donor kidney to host.

E.D. Thomas (1990) – pioneered procedures for chemical management of Graft versus host reaction in tissue or organ transplantation.

Sabin (1990) – introduced oral poliovaccine by using attenuated mutant poliovirus.

Peter C. Doherty, Rolf M. Zinker Magel (1996) – cell mediated immune defenses.

20

Immunity

- *Definition*
- *Classification*
- *Innate immunity (Nonspecific immunity)*
  - *Species immunity*
  - *Racial immunity*
  - *Individual immunity*
- *Mechanisms of Innate (Nonspecific) immunity*
  - *Skin and Mucus Membranes*
  - *Antimicrobial Substances or Chemical Mediators*
  - *Cells involved in innate immunity*
  - *Inflammation*
  - *Fever*
  - *Microbial antagonism*
- *Factors influencing the level of innate immunity*
- *Acquired immunity*
  - *Actively acquired immunity*
    - *Active natural immunity*
    - *Active artificial immunity*
  - *Passively acquired immunity*
    - *Passive natural immunity*
    - *Passive artificial immunity*
- *Local immunity*
- *Herd immunity*
- *Infection immunity (premunition)*
- *Adoptive immunity*

DEFINITION

Immunity is the ability to resist damage from foreign substances such as microorganisms and harmful chemicals such as toxins released by microorganisms.

The ability to ward off disease through our defenses is called resistance.

CLASSIFICATION

INNATE IMMUNITY/NATIVE IMMUNITY/NON-SPECIFIC IMMUNITY

It is the resistance which an individual possesses by virtue of his/her genetic and body constitution. Thus, it is inborn.

In Innate immunity, the body is born with the ability to recognize and destroy certain foreign substances, but the ability to destroy them does not improve each time the body is exposed to them due to lack of immunological memory.

Innate Immunity can act against many microorganisms in general due to the absence of specificity, hence also called as Non-specific immunity.

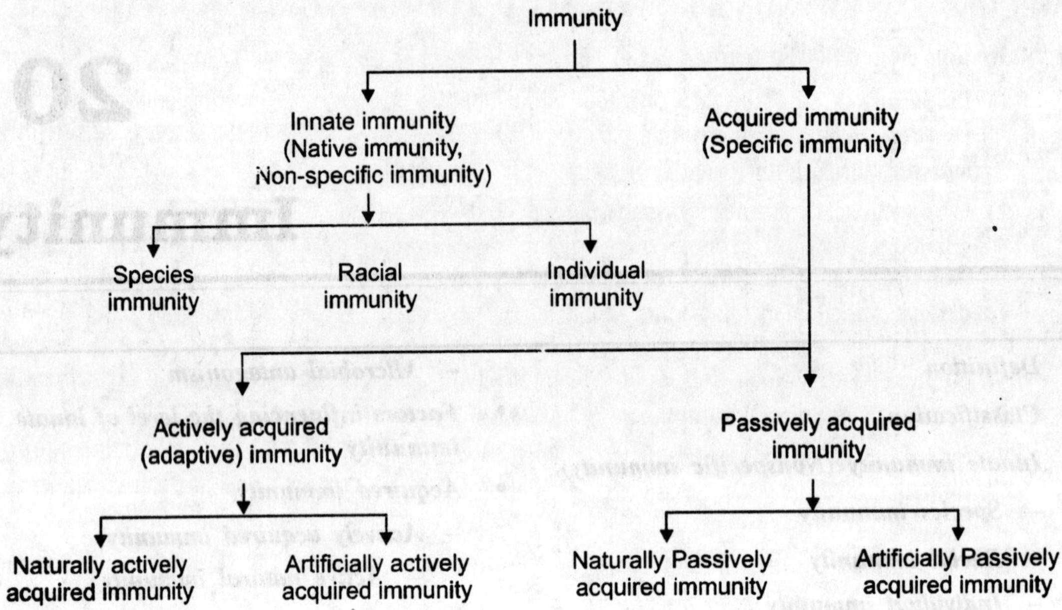

Species Immunity

Resistance to infection varies with the species. Species immunity is the resistance exhibited by all members of a species towards a pathogen. e.g.,

1. Humans are resistant to plant pathogens.
2. Ground squirrels are resistant to *Yersinia pestis*, whereas humans are susceptible.
3. Humans are susceptible to measles infection, whereas dogs are resistant.
4. Dogs can contract dog distemper, whereas humans are resistant to it.

Basic anatomical, physiological and biochemical characteristics of a species can determine whether a microorganism can be pathogenic for that species.

Racial Immunity

Within a species, different races may exhibit differences in their resistance, due to genetic factors. e.g.,

1. Africans are resistant to malarial infection due to the absence of a specific component on RBC membrane to which malarial parasite binds in order to invade and multiply.
2. Algerian sheep are resistant to anthrax.
3. Negroes are more susceptible to TB than Caucasians.

Individual Immunity

Different individuals in a race exhibit differences in innate immunity and is known as individual immunity. It is probably due to a combination of nonspecific and specific resistance factors inherited from their parents. Thus, some people have many more colds during the winter than do others.

Homozygous twins may exhibit similar degrees of resistance or susceptibility to some infections such as TB and leprosy.

MECHANISMS OF NONSPECIFIC IMMUNITY (INNATE IMMUNITY)

I. Skin and Mucus Membrane

(1) Epidermis of skin forms a physical barrier to the entrance of microorganisms. Healthy skin possesses bactericidal activity because of low moisture, acidic pH, presence of salt in sweat and unsaturated fatty acids of sebum.

(2) Hair in nose filters microorganisms and dust. The mucus traps microorganisms and cilia of ciliated epithelium propels microorganisms and dust from upper respiratory tract back to pharynx where they tend to be swallowed or coughed out. Cough reflex is an important defense mechanism. Particles that manage to reach alveoli are phagocytosed by alveolar macrophages. The nasal and respiratory secretions contain mucopolysaccharides which can combine with viruses and inactivate them. This entire defense system can be suppressed by alcohol, narcotics, cigarette smoke, hypoxia, acidosis.

(3) Saliva washes microorganisms from surfaces of teeth and mucus membranes of mouth. The intestinal wall is covered by mucus which traps microorganisms and forms small masses that are propelled by peristalsis.

(4) Lachrymal secretions (tears) in eyes dilute and wash away irritating substances and microorganisms.

(5) The flushing action of urine flushes and washes microorganisms from urethra.

II. Antimicrobial Substances (or) Chemical Mediators of Non-specific Resistance

(1) Lysozyme present in tears, saliva, nasal secretions, tissue fluids and perspiration can kill or inhibit the growth of microorganisms.

(2) The acidic pH of the gastric juice destroys microorganisms swallowed into the stomach.

(3) The acidic pH of adult vagina makes it inhospitable of many pathogens.

(4) Complement causes cytolysis of microorganisms, promotes phagocytosis and contributes to inflammation.

(5) Interferons protect uninfected cells from viral infections.

(6) Kidneys contain sperminc, an antibacterial substance.

(7) Beta lysins, basic polypeplides such as leukins from leucocytes, plakins from platelets, kinins from plasma proteins; lactoferrin in milk-all are antibacterial.

(8) Pyrogens released by neutrophils, monocytes and other cells stimulate fever production.

(9) Several plasma proteins, collectively known as "**acute phase proteins**" show an increase in concentration following infections or tissue injury e.g., C-Reactive protein (CRP), mannose-binding protein, alpha-1 acid glycoprotein, serum amyloid P component.

Acute phase proteins enhance host resistance, minimize tissue injury and promote resolution and repair of inflammatory lesions.

CRP and some other acute phase proteins activate alternate complement pathway.

(10) Histamine, prostaglandins, leukotriences increase vascular permeability and cause vasodilatation.

III. Cells Involved in Innate Immunity (or) Cells of Nonspecific Resistance

(1) Phagocytic cells ingest invading microorganisms and other foreign particulate matter and in most cases, kill and digest them.

There are two types of phagocytic cells – macrophages or monocytes and polymorpho nuclear neutrophils (PMN) which form a large circulating pool of phagocytic cells.

Circulating monocytes leave the blood and enter into tissues to become macrophages.

When macrophages leave the blood and migrate through tissue to infected areas, they are called tissue macrophages. They also migrate to the lungs, spleen and other sites where microorganisms are likely to occur.

Some fixed macrophages, called histiocytes enter certain tissues and organs and remain there. They are found in the liver (Kupffer cells), lungs (alveolar macrophages), nervous system (microglial cells), lymph nodes (dendritic macrophages), bronchial tissue, spleen, peritoneal cavity and bone marrow.

(2) Natural killer (NK) cells are large granular lymphocytes and kill virus-infected cells and tumor cells. They may also provide nonspecific resistance against intracellular protozoan and fungal parasites. Interferons enhance the natural killing activity of NK cells.

(3) Basophils and mast cells release chemicals that promote inflammation.

(4) Eosinophils release chemicals that inhibit inflammation.

IV. Inflammation

It is an important non-specific defense mechanism which destroys and removes microorganisms or its products and repairs tissues.

The process of inflammation may be divided into the following stages.

1. Initiation–damaged or invaded tissue.
2. Tissue response–chemical factors released–histamines, kinins, and prostaglandins cause vasodilatation and increased permeability of blood vessels.
3. Leucocyte response-phagocytes engulf microorganisms and damaged tissue cells. Blood clotting, pus and abscess formation occurs.
4. Resolution–tissue repair.
5. Cure-healthy tissue.

V. Fever

Fever is an abnormally high body temperature. Fever following infections is believed to be beneficial to the host. It increases the phagocytic activity and the rate of induction of inflammation and immune response. The high temperature reached during fever inhibits or kills infecting microorganisms. *Treponema pallidum* (syphilis) and Gonococci (gonorrhoeae) are actually killed by fever temperature.

Fever stimulates the production of interferons and promotes their action and aids in recovery from viral infections. Metabolic and physiological processes are speeded up that aid repair.

VI. Microbial Antagonism

The normal resident flora of skin, gastrointestinal tract prevents colorization by pathogens. The importance of normal bacterial flora in native immunity is exemplified by the extreme susceptibility of germ free animals to infections.

FACTORS INFLUENCING THE LEVEL OF INNATE IMMUNITY

Several factors influence the level of innate immunity.

1. Age

Persons in young and old age are highly susceptible to infectious diseases than adults. In fetus and newborn babies, the immune system is immature whereas in old people, it is due to warning of their immune responses.

2. Malnutrition

In malnutrition both humoral and cell mediated immune responses are reduced and may be the cause of immunodeficiency.

3. Hormonal Influences

The susceptibility to infectious disease increases in diabetes mellitus, hypothyroidism and adrenal dysfunction. Corticosteroids depress immune response by their anti-inflammatory and antiphagocytic effects. The increased steroid level during pregnancy may be related to the increased susceptibility of pregnant women to infections.

ACQUIRED IMMUNITY

The resistance that an individual acquires during life is known as acquired immunity. It is of two types – Actively acquired and Passively acquired.

Table 20.1 Differences between Active and Passive Immunity

Actively acquired immunity	*Passively acquired immunity*
1. Produced by active functioning of the immune system.	Received passively, no involvement of immune system.
2. Stimulated by infections, antigens (vaccines, allergens).	Acquired by administration of antibodies or sensitized T-cells.
3. Provides effective and long-lasting immunity.	Immunity is less effective and transient.
4. There is a lag phase (latent period) required for the formation of antibodies.	Offers immediate protection.
5. Immunological memory is present. Subsequent contact with antigen will have a booster effect.	No memory. Subsequent administration of antibodies is less effective due to immune elimination.
6. Negative phase may occur due to the combination of antigen with preexisting antibody.	No negative phase.
7. Not applicable in immunodeficient hosts.	Applicable in immunodeficient hosts.
8. Active immunization is mainly employed for prophylaxis.	Passive immunization has therapeutic and prophylactic uses.

Actively acquired immunity may be natural or artificial. Similarly passively acquired immunity may be natural or artificial. Thus, there are four ways to acquire acquired immunity.

1. Actively naturally acquired.
2. Actively artificially acquired.
3. Passively naturally acquired.
4. Passively artificially acquired.

ACTIVELY ACQUIRED IMMUNITY

When an individual is naturally or artificially exposed to infections or antigens, results in stimulation and active functioning of the immune system leading to humoral immunity or cell mediated immunity. This is called actively acquired immunity.

It affords durable and long lasting immunity. It may persist for few weeks (common cold) to life long (chicken pox).

It sets in after a latent period/lag phase, required for the synthesis of antibodies.

There may be a negative phase during the development of active immunity due to the combination of antigen with pre–existing antibody and the immunity may be lower than it was before antigenic stimulus.

Immunological memory is present. Subsequent contact with the same specific antigen will have a booster effect on immune response.

Active Natural Immunity is due to natural exposure to antigen from infections (disease or subclinical infections). *e.g.*, – Many people, if exposed to polio virus repeatedly during childhood will develop natural active immunity.

Persons who recover from viral diseases such as small pox, chicken pox, and measles will develop life long natural active immunity.

Active Artificial Immunity – when an antigen is deliberately introduced into an individual to stimulate his/her immune system, the immunity developed is known as Active artificial immunity. This process is "**vaccination**" and the introduced antigen is a "**vaccine**". Injection of the vaccine is the usual mode of administration, although ingestion (Sabin's OPV) is sometimes used.

The vaccine usually consists of a dead or live microorganism, altered microorganism, part of the microorganism or a product of the microorganism. The antigen has been changed so that it stimulates the immune system, without producing disease.

Active artificial immunity is the preferred method of acquiring immunity because it produces long lasting immunity without any disease.

The first injection of the antigen stimulates a primary response, and the booster doses causes immunological memory, which produces high levels of antibody, memory cells and long-lasting protection.

Examples of vaccines are as follows :

Bacterial Vaccines

Live – BCG for TB.

Killed – TAB for enteric fever

– cholera Vaccine for cholera.

Bacterial products – Tetanus toxoid, Diphtheria toxoid.

Subunit – Vi antigen for typhoid.

Viral Vaccines

Live – Sabin's OPV for poliomyelitis

– 17 D Vaccine for yellow fever

MMR for measles, mumps, Rubella.

Killed – Salk's vaccine for poliomyelitis

– Rabies (semple) vaccine

– Japanese B encephalitis vaccine

Subunit – Hepatitis B vaccine

PASSIVELY ACQUIRED IMMUNITY

Passive immunity occurs when another person or animal develops antibodies and the antibodies are transferred to a non-immune individual, who did not produce antibodies and there is no involvement of immune system.

It is received passively by the recipient by injection of readymade preformed antibodies.

There is no lag phase, protection being effective immediately following passive immunization but protection is transient and less effective than active immunity.

There is no negative phase. Subsequent administration of antibodies is less effective due to **"immune elimination"**.

Passive immunity is preferred in some situations when immediate protection is required.

Passive Natural Immunity results when antibodies are transferred from mother to child. During her life the mother has been exposed to many antigens, either naturally or artificially and she therefore has antibodies against many of these antigens. These antibodies protect the mother and the developing fetus against disease.

The antibody IgG can cross the placenta from mother to fetus and provides **natural passive immunity** to the fetus.

If the mother nurses her child, IgA in the mother's milk, particularly in colostrum provides natural passive immunity to the child.

Passive Artificial Immunity – It is achieved by administration of specific antibodies or sensitized T-lymphocytes e.g., Tetanus antitoxin (antitetanus serum, ATS), Diphtheria antitoxin, pooled human gamma globulin against Hepatitis B, convalescent sera and antirabic serum.

Passive immunization may also be used to suppress active immunity in Rh negative women with Rh positive baby by the administration of anti-Rh antibody (IgG).

Achieving passive artificial immunity usually begins with vaccinating an animal such as horse. After the animal's immune system responds to the antigen, antibodies (sometimes T-cells) are removed from the animal and injected into the individual requiring immunity. In some cases a human who has developed immunity is used as a source.

Passive artificial immunity provides immediate protection for the individual recieiving the antibodies and is therefore preferred when there might not be time for the individual to develop his own immunity. But it involves the risk of hypersensitivity (**serum sickness**).

However, this technique provides only temporary immunity because the antibodies are metabolized and eliminated (**Immune elimination**).

When passive artificial immunity is achieved by injecting sensitized T-lymphocytes or an extract of lymphocytes, called transfer factor; it is known as "**Adoptive immunity**".

LOCAL IMMUNITY

Besredka (1927) introduced the concept of local immunity, which provides defense against infections at mucosal, surfaces or at the site of entry of pathogen. IgA constitutes the major component of local immunity. e.g.,

(1) In prophylaxis of poliomyelitis, injection of Salk's killed polio vaccine induces humoral immune response, and neutralizes the poliovirus when it enters the blood circulation, thus offering protection to the individual. But, it will not prevent the multiplication of virus at the site of entry, *i.e.*, intestinal mucosa and its excretion in feces. This is achieved by the administration of Sabin's live attenuated oral polio vaccine (OPV) which induces local intestinal immunity and offers protection to both individual as well as community.

(2) In Influenza, active immunization with killed vaccine induces systemic immunity, but the level of antibodies may not be high enough in respiratory tract to prevent infection. Whereas the administration of live attenuated virus vaccine intranasally provides local immunity.

IgA, particularly secretory IgA, produced locally by plasma cells present in secretory glands or mucosal surfaces, is present in saliva, tears, colostrum, mucus secretions of respiratory tract and intestine and provides local defense against microorganisms.

HERD IMMUNITY

It refers to overall level of immunity in a community.

When large number of persons in a herd are resistant to a pathogen, the herd immunity to that pathogen is said to be good. When herd immunity is low, epidemics may occur due to the presence of a large number of susceptible individuals.

The development of herd immunity is relevant in the control of epidemics.

INFECTION IMMUNITY or PREMUNITION

The presence of active infection in the patient offers protection against reinfections. The protection to reinfections lasts only as long the original infection remains active. Once the disease is cured, the patient becomes susceptible to reinfections. This is known as infection immunity or premunition, and is seen in syphilis and malaria.

ADOPTIVE IMMUNITY

It is an artificial passive immunization method where immune competent cells or sensitized T-cells are injected into the patient. This is known as adoptive immunity. Instead of whole lymphocytes, an extract of lymphocytes called "**Transfer factor**" may be used.

Adoptive immunity finds application in tumour immunotherapy where cells that have antitumor activity are injected into the blood of a cancer patient.

QUESTIONS

Essay Questions

1. Define and classify immunity. Describe the mechanisms of native immunity.

(or)

Define and classify immunity. Describe in detail non-specific immune mechanisms of the body.

2. What is Innate immunity ? Discuss its mechanism. Briefly describe the cells involved in Innate Immunity.
3. Define and classify immunity. Describe acquired immunity with examples.
4. Classify immunity. Describe Active immunity with examples.

Short Notes

1. Define and classify immunity.
2. Innate immunity (or) Native immunity (or) nonspecific immunity.
3. Species immunity.
4. Mechanisms of nonspecific immunity/Innate immunity.
5. Chemical mediators of nonspecific immunity.
6. Cells involved in Innate immunity (or) cells of nonspecific resistance.
7. Active immunity.
8. Passive immunity.
9. Artificial active immunity.
10. Passive artificial immunity.
11. Differences between active and passive immunity.
12. Local immunity.
13. Herd immunity.
14. Infection immunity (or) premunition.
15. Adoptive immunity.
16. Factors influencing Innate immunity.

21

Antigens/Immunogens (Vaccines, allergens, precipitinogens, agglutinogens)

- ***Definition***
- ***Complete antigen***
- ***Haptens***
- ***Antigenic determinant or Epitope***
- ***Paratope***
- ***Cross-reactions***
- ***Factors determining antigenicity***
  - ***Foreignness***
  - ***Size***
  - ***Chemical nature***
  - ***Susceptibility to tissue enzymes***
- ***Types of antigens***
  - ***Species specific antigens***
  - ***Isoantigens***
  - ***Organ specific antigens***
  - ***Autospecific antigens***
  - ***Heterophile antigens***
- ***Super Antigens***
- ***T-cell dependent (TD) and T-cell independent (TI) antigens***

DEFINITION

An antigen has been defined as any substance living or nonliving, which when introduced parenterally into humans or animal body, stimulates the formation of opposite substances called antibodies (humoral immunity), with which it reacts specifically and in an observable manner.

Some antigens may also sensitize specific T-lymphocytes leading to cell mediated immunity or may cause immunological tolerance.

Thus, as per the definition, an antigen can perform two important functions.

1. Inducing an immune response, known as immunogenicity.

2. Specific reaction with antibodies or sensitized T-cells, known as immunological reactivity.

COMPLETE ANTIGEN

Any antigen which can carry out the above two functions is known as "complete antigen".

HAPTENS

Haptens are substances, which cannot induce the formation of antibodies (not immunogenic) by themselves, but can react with specific antibodies, e.g., Capsular polysaccharide of Pneumococci, cardiolipin, Forssmann antigen, Polysaccharide 'C' of β-hemolytic Streptococci.

Penicillin is an hapten. It can breakdown and bind to serum proteins to form a combined molecule that can produce allergic reaction such as rash and fever, rarely death.

Haptens may be converted to complete antigens by combining with a large inert carrier molecule.

ANTIGENIC DETERMINANT (or) EPITOPE

The smallest unit of antigenicity is known as antigenic determinant or epitope. It is a small area on the antigen, usually consisting four or five monosaccharide or aminoacid residues possessing a specific chemical structure, spatial (steric) configuration and electric charge, capable of sensitizing lymphocytes and of reacting with its complementary site on the specific antibody or T-cell receptor.

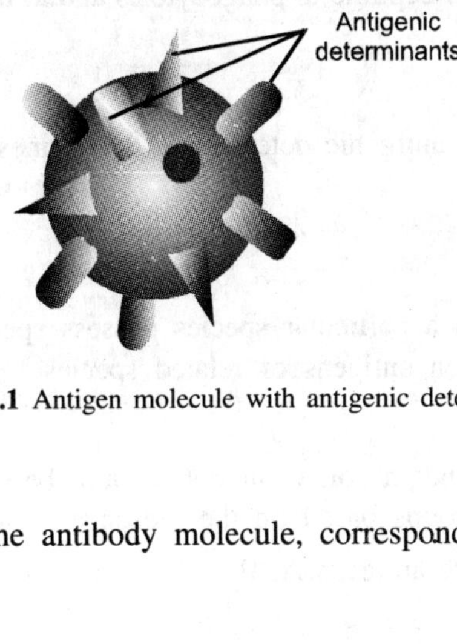

Fig. 21.1 Antigen molecule with antigenic determinant.

PARATOPE

The combining area on the antibody molecule, corresponding to the epitope is called the paratope.

CROSS-REACTION

The reaction of antibody with an antigen or hapten other than one that induced its formation is called a cross-reaction.

The presence of the same or similar epitopes (antigenic determinants) on different antigens is responsible for cross-reactions. Examples for cross-reacting antigens.

(1) Epstein-Barr virus and sheep RBC

(2) Rickettsiae and *Proteus vulgaris* OX19, OX2 strains and *Proteus mirabilis* OX K.

FACTORS DETERMINING ANTIGENICITY

Several factors determine antigenicity.

Foreignness

Only antigens which are foreign to the individual can induce immune response.

Size

Antigenicity is directly related to the size of antigen molecules. Large molecules are strongly antigenic, whereas low molecular weight substances are weakly antigenic or nonantigenic.

Low molecular weight substances can be rendered antigenic by adsorbing them on large inert particles such as latex, bentonite or Kaolin.

Chemical Nature

Most of the natural antigens are proteins and polysaccharides. Lipids and nucleic acids are weakly antigenic and their antigenicity can be increased by combining with proteins.

Proteins are better antigens than polysaccharides. However, not all proteins are antigenic e.g., gelatin, histones, protamines.

The presence of tyrosine, an aromatic aminoacid is essential for the antigenicity of proteins.

Susceptibility to Tissue Enzymes

Only substances which are susceptible to phagocytosis and to the action of intracellular enzymes can act as antigens.

Antigenic Specificity

The spatial configuration of antigenic determinant determines the antigenic specificity.

TYPES OF ANTIGENS

Species Specific Antigens

Tissues of all individuals in a particular species possess species specific antigens. However, cross reactions may occur between antigens of related species.

Isospecific Antigens

Isoantigens are antigens found in some but not all members of a species. A species my be further classified into different groups based on the presence or absence of isoantigens.

e.g.,
- Human erythrocyte antigens A, B
- Rh antigen
- Histocompatibility antigens.

Organ Specific Antigens

Some organs such as brain, kidney, lens protein share the same antigen in different species, which are known as organ specific antigens.

Autospecific Antigens

Self antigens or autologous antigens are usually non-antigenic. But, **sequestrated antigens** or **hidden antigens** such as lens protein of the eye, which is enclosed in a capsule and antigens such as spermatozoa that are absent during embryonic life and develop later are not recognized as self antigens and may induce immune response.

Heterophile Antigens (Heterogenetic antigens)

The same or closely related antigens may sometimes occur in different biological species, classes and kingdoms. These are known as heterogenetic or heterophile antigens.

e.g., Forssmann antigen, which is a lipid-carbohydrate complex, is found in animals, birds, plants and bacteria. It is absent in Rabbits, so anti-Forssmann antibody is prepared in these animals.

Heterophile antigens are responsible for some diagnostic serological reactions (heterophile reactions) in which antigens unrelated to causative agents are employed.

e.g., Weil-Felix reaction in typhus fever caused by Rickettsiae employs *Proteus vulgaris* OX2, OX19 and *Proteus mirabilis* OX K antigens.

Paul-Bunnel test in infectious mononucleosis caused by Epstein–Barr virus employs sheep RBC as antigen.

Cold agglutination test for primary atypical pneumonia caused by *Mycoplasma* employs human 'O' group RBC at 4°C.

Streptococcus MG agglutination test for primary atypical pneumonia cause by *Mycoplasma* employs *Streptococcus* MG antigen.

SUPER ANTIGENS

Super antigens are proteins that stimulate the immune system much more extensively than do normal antigens e.g., Staphylococcal enterotoxin-A, TSST-1 (Staphylococcal toxic shock syndrome type-1), Staphylococcal exfoliative toxin and streptococcal pyrogenic exotoxin A.

Super antigens stimulate the proliferation of many different T cell clones. They can bind directly to the outer surface of the MHC molecule without being processed by the antigen-presenting cell. They stimulate T cells bearing a particular β chain of TCR. Thus, super antigens can activate many more T-helper cells than a normal antigen does. This exaggerated T-cell activation leads to massive secretion of cytokines, causing multisystem dysfunctions, as seen in staphylococcal toxic shock syndrome.

T-CELL DEPENDENT (TD) AND T-CELL INDEPENDENT (TI) ANTIGENS

Based on the ability to induce antibody formation by B lymphocytes, antigens are classified as T-cell dependent (TD) and T-cell independent (TI) antigens.

TD antigens require the participation of T-lymphocytes, whereas TI antigens do not require the cooperation of T-lymphocytes for antibody formation.

Table 21.1 Differences between TD and TI Antigens

T-cell dependent (TD) antigens	*T-cell independent (TI) antigens*
1. Structurally complex.	Structurally similar, contain limited number of epitopes.
2. Antigenic over a wide dose range.	Antigenicity is critically dose dependent.
3. Do not cause immunological tolerance.	Too much dose may result in immunological tolerance, whereas too little is nonantigenic.

4. They induce full gamut of Ig types – IgM, IgG, IgA and IgE.	Antibody response is limited to IgM and IgG.
5. Produce immunological memory.	Do not produce immunological memory.
6. Require preliminary processing.	Do not require preliminary processing.
7. Rapidly metabolized in the body. e.g., RBC, Plasma proteins, several protein-hapten complexes.	Metabolized very slowly. e.g., Pneumococcal capsular polysaccharide, bacterial lipopolysaccharide, flagellar protein (flagellin).

QUESTIONS

Essay Question

1. Define antigen. Describe the properties of antigens. Add a note on factors that determine antigenicity.

Short Notes

1. Define antigen or Immunogen.
2. Complete antigen.
3. Haptens (or) Definition and example of hapten.
4. Antigenic determinant (or) epitope.
5. Epitope and paratope.
6. What is cross-reaction ?
7. Mention the properties of antigen (or)
   What are the main attributes that make a substance a good antigen ? (or)
   What are the factors that determine antigenicity ?
8. Types of antigens.
9. Heterophile antigens (or) Heterophile reactions.
10. Differences between T-cell dependent and T-cell independent antigens.
11. TD antigens.
12. TI antigens.
13. Super antigens.

22

Immunoglobulins (Gamma globulins, antisera, immune sera, antibodies)

- *Introduction*
- *Definition*
- *Structure*
- *Ig determinants*
- *Physical and chemical properties*
- *Classes of Immunoglobulins*
  - *IgG*
  - *IgM*
  - *IgA*
  - *IgD*
  - *IgE*
- *Abnormal Immunoglobulins*

INTRODUCTION

Following introduction of an antigen into humans or animals, opposite substances called antibodies appear in the serum, which react with the antigen specifically and in an observable manner. Sera having high antibody levels following infection or immunization are called "**immune sera**" or "**antisera**".

Tiselius (1937) separated plasma proteins into albumin, globulins (alpha, beta and gamma globulins). Albumin is the protein present in highest concentration, which contributes to the colloidal osmotic pressure of plasma and also acts as a nonspecific transport protein. Globulins include specific transport proteins (e.g., transferrin for iron), clotting factors, the complement system and inactive precursors of certain hormones (e.g., angiotensinogen). Gamma globulins act as circulating antibodies important in specific immune process, also known as Immunoglobulins (Fig. 22.1).

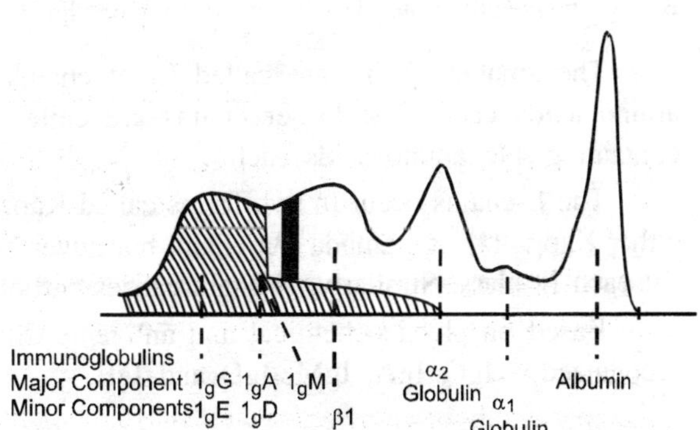

Fig. 22.1 Electrophoretic pattern of plasma proteins.

Antibodies are produced from B lymphocytes, following antigenic stimulation.

DEFINITION

WHO (1964) introduced the term "Immunoglobulin (Ig, γ)" and defined as **"proteins of animal origin possessing antibody activity and for certain other proteins related to them by chemical structure"**. As per this definition, besides antibody globulins, the abnormal proteins found in myeloma, macroglobulinemia, cryoglobulinemia and L and H chains (subunits of immunoglobulins) are also considered as Immunoglobulins.

The term **"Immunoglobululin"** indicates a structural and chemical concept, while the term "antibody" is a biological and functional concept. All antibodies are immunoglobulins, but all immunoglobulins may not be antibodies.

STRUCTURE

Immunoglobulins constitute 20–25% of the total serum proteins. Immunoglobulins are glycoproteins, composed of four polypeptide chains, held together by disulfide bonds and are arranged in the form of a flexible 'Y', with a hinge region. (Fig. 22.2)

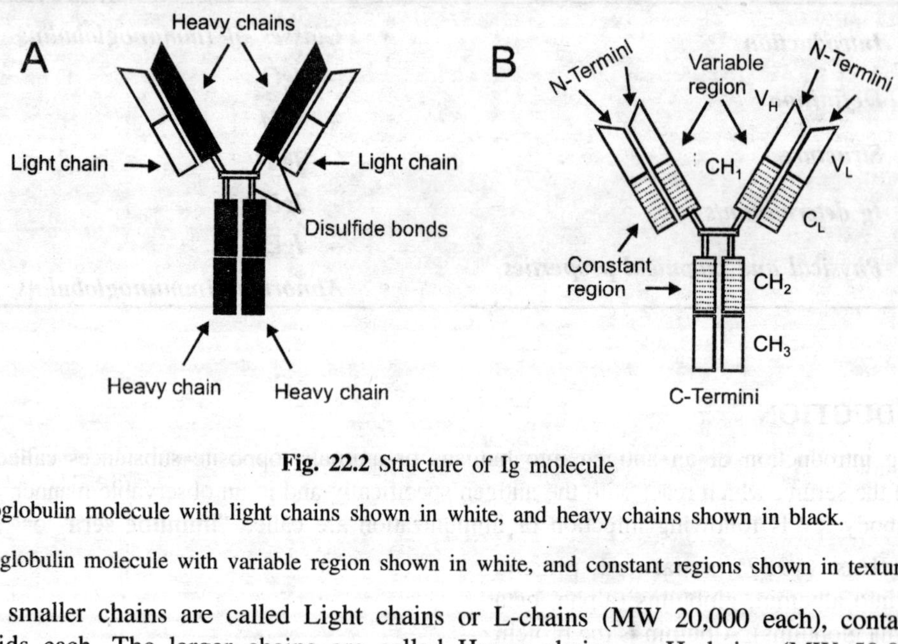

Fig. 22.2 Structure of Ig molecule

A. Immunoglobulin molecule with light chains shown in white, and heavy chains shown in black.

B. Immunoglobulin molecule with variable region shown in white, and constant regions shown in textured gray.

The smaller chains are called Light chains or L-chains (MW 20,000 each), containing 214 amino acids each. The larger chains are called Heavy chains or H-chains (MW 50,000 each), containing 446 amino acids each.

The L-chains occur in two forms called Kappa (*k*) and Lambda (λ). A molecule of Ig may have either Kappa (*k*) or Lambda (λ) chain, but never both together. The H-chains are structurally distinct for each Ig class. Similarly, H-chain carries carbohydrate moiety which is distinct for each Ig class.

Based on physicochemical and antigenic differences 5 classes of immunoglobulins have been recognized – IgG, IgA, IgM, IgD and IgE.

Fig. 22.1 Different Immunoglobulins and their H Chains

Ig class	*H-chain*
IgG	gamma (γ)
IgA	alpha (α)
IgM	mu (μ)
IgD	delta (δ)
IgE	epsilon (ε)

Both L and H chains contain two different regions :

(1) Constant regions (C_L and C_H) have amino acid sequences that do not vary between antibodies of the same subclass.

(2) Variable regions (V_L and V_H) have amino acid sequences that are different for all antibodies.

The stalk of the 'Y' is termed the "**crystallizable fragment** (F_C)". It is composed of only H-hains with carboxy terminal end. It contains the site at which the antibody molecule can bind to cell. It determines the biological properties of Ig molecules such as complement fixation, placental ransfer, skin fixation and catabolic rate.

The top of the 'Y' consists of both L and H chains with aminoterminus and constitute two antigen–binding fragments ($F(ab)_2$)" or "paratopes", that can bind to antigenic determinant sites epitopes).

The F_C fragments are composed of only constant regions, whereas $F(ab)_2$ fragments have both onstant and variable regions. The portion of H-chain, present in $F(ab)_2$ fragment is called F_d piece.

Each Ig chain has internal disulphide links or intrachain disulphide bonds (in addition to interchain isulphide bonds) forming loops, within each chain, known as "domain". These domains can be alled as VL_1, VL_2 etc. and VH_1, VH_2 etc., for those present in variable regions of L and H chains espectively; Similarly CL_1, CL_2 etc. and CH_1, CH_2 etc., for those present in constant regions.

The region between CH_1 and CH_2 domains is called hinge region. It is highly fragile. When xposed to enzymes such as papain, Ig molecule will be cleaved at hinge region to produce two Fab agments and one F_C fragment. (Fig. 22.3)

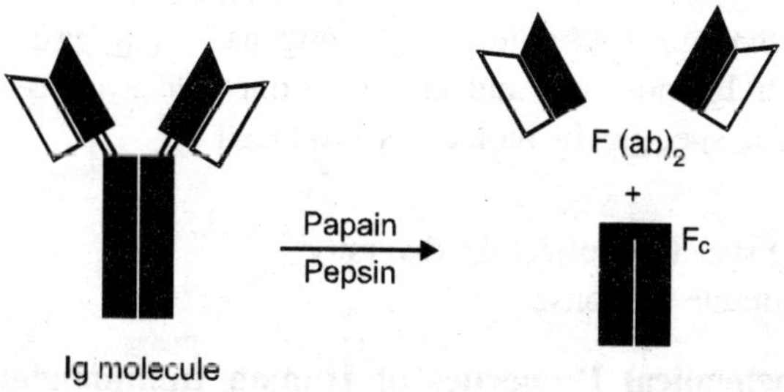

Fig. 22.3. Cleavage of Ig molecule at hinge region by proteolytic enzymes.

The amino acid sequences of variable regions of L and H chains are not uniformly variable ong their length, but consist of relatively invariable and some highly variable regions, known as ıypervariable regions" or hot spots and are involved in the formation of antigen-binding sites. They e **complementarity determining regions** (CDRs), which can make contact with specific epitope.

Within two of the major Ig classes, there are subclasses. For example, IgG can be grouped into 4 subclasses (IgG_1, IgG_2, IgG_3 and IgG_4) and IgA into two subclasses (IgA_1 and IgA_2).

Ig DETERMINANTS

Each Ig subclass has differences in the amino acid sequences, which determine the antigen specificity.

1. Isotypes (iso=same)

These determinants are common to or shared by all members of a species. These isotypic markers distinguish H chain classes (IgG–γ, IgA–α, IgM–μ, IgD–δ, and IgE–ε) and subclasses (IgG_1–γ_1, IgG_2–γ_2, IgG_3–γ_3, IgG_4–γ_4, IgA_1–α_1, and IgA_2–α_2) as well as k and λ L chains. They are located in the constant domains of Ig chains in all individuals. Each isotype is encoded by a gene that is characteristic for a particular species and is present in all the members of that species. Antibodies to these determinants may be raised by injecting Immunoglobulins from one species to another species.

2. Allotypes

Allotypic markers occur for Ig molecules, with the same isotype but with amino acid sequences that differ from one person to another. Everyone ("allo") of them cannot have the same IgG or IgM. Allotypes are variations that exist between individuals of same species. They are distinct aminoacid residues located primarily in γ and α H chains and k (kappa) L chains. Allotypic determinants reflect genetic polymorphism of Immunoglobulins within one species. Allotype markers are useful in testing paternity and population genetics.

3. Idiotypes

These are located in the hypervariable regions (V regions) of L and H chains and are analogous to epitopes of antigens. Idiotypes are specific for each Ig molecule and are sometimes useful in identifying marker for specific Ig molecules produced by a single clone of cells.

The many variations of Ig structure reflect the diversity of antibodies generated by immune response.

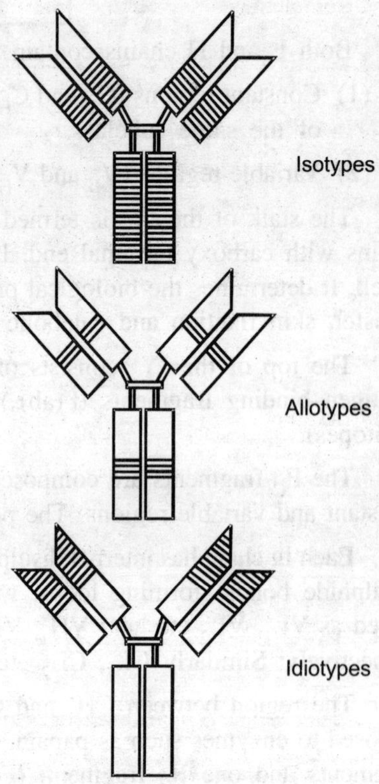

Fig. 22.4 Isotypic, allotypic and Idiotypic determinants Ig molecules.

Table 22.2 Physicochemical Properties of Human Immunoglobulin Classes

Property	*Immunoglobulin classes*				
	IgG[a]	IgM	IgA[b]	IgD	IgE
Heavy chain	γ_1	μ	α_1	δ	ε
Mean serum concentration (mg/ml)	9	1.5	3.0	0.03	0.00005

Percent of total antibody	80–85	5–10	5–15	<1	0.002–0.05
Valency	2	5(10)	(2–4)	2	2
Mass of heavy chain (kDa)	51	65	56	70	72
Mass of entire molecule (kDa)	146	970	160[C]	184	188
Placental transfer	+	–	–	–	–
Half-life in serum (days)[d]	23	5	6	3	2
Complement activation					
Classical pathway	++	+++	–	–	–
Alternative pathway	–	–	+	–	–
Induces mast cell degranulation	–	–	–	–	+
Major characteristics	Most abundant Ig in body fluids; neutralizes toxins, opsonizes bacteria, activates complement, maternal antibody	First to appear after antigen stimulation; very effective agglutinator; expressed as membrane-bound antibody on B Cells	Secretory antibody; protects external sufaces	Present on B-cell surface; B-cell recognition of antigen	Anaphylactic-mediating antibody: resistance to helminths
% carbohydrate	3	7–10	7	12	11

[a]Properties of IgG subclass 1.

[b]Properpties of IgA subclass 1.

[c]sIgA = 360 – 400 kDa

[d]Time required for half of the antibodies to disappear.

IMMUNOGLOBULIN CLASSES

There are 5 different classes of Immnoglobulins – IgG, IgA, IgM, IgD and IgE.

IgG

It is the major Ig in human serum, accounts for about 80% of the total Ig pool in serum. It is present in blood plasma and tissue fluids. It has a molecular weight 150,000(7S). Normal serum concentration is 8–16 mg/ml. There are 4 subclasses, namely IgG_1, IgG_2, IgG_3 and IgG_4. The production of IgG occurs later in an immune response. Its presence in serum indicates remote or chronic infection. It has a half life of approximately 23 days.

The major functions of IgG are as follows :

1. IgG is the major humoral line of defense.
2. Neutralizes toxins and viruses.
3. Fix complement well and cause the lysis of bacteria, enveloped viruses and infected or aged cells.

4. **Act against bacteria and viruses by opsonization to promote phagocytosis.**
5. **It is the only maternal Ig that is transported across the placenta and provides natural passive immunity to the child.**
6. **Anti-Rh (anti-D) antibodies are IgG type. When IgG is administered passively, it suppresses the homologous antibody synthesis by a feed back process. This property is utilized in the isoimmunization of women by the administration of anti-Rh (anti-D) IgG during delivery.**

IgM

It accounts for about 10% of the Ig pool, with a serum concentration of 0.5–2 mg/ml. It has a half life of about 5 days. It is a polymer (pentamer) of five molecules, held together by a special **joining (J) chain**. It is a large molecule (MW 10,00,000) and therefore called as millionnaire molecule (Fig. 22.5). It is the first class of antibody produced in immune response, about 4 days after immunization (antigenic stimulus) and reaches peak concentrations by about first week and then rapidly falls because of its short life span. Hence, their demonstration in serum indicates recent or acute infection.

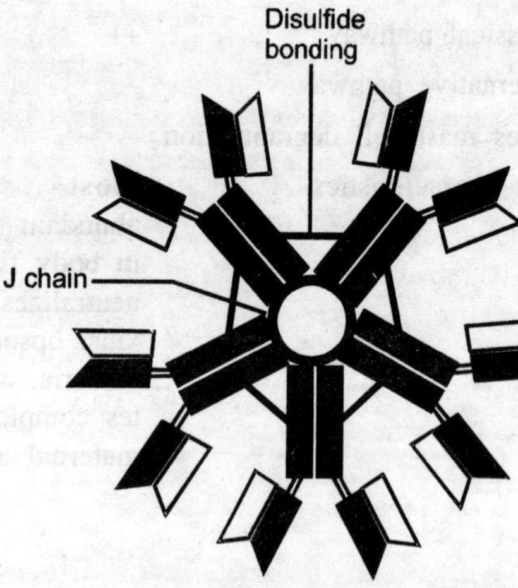

Fig. 22.5 IgM Molecule.

This class contains special antibodies such as blood group antibodies (anti–A and anti–B) and heterophile antibodies. It is largely confined to intravascular space, and responsible for protection against blood invasion by microorganisms. Treatment of serum with the mercaptoethanol selectively destroys IgM without affecting IgG antibodies.

As IgM is not transported across the placenta, its presence in the fetus or newborn indicates congenital infection.

IgM can fix complement extremely well (30 times better than IgG), and therefore can effectively cause the lysis of bacteria, enveloped viruses and infected or aged cells.

Monomeric IgM is found in the membranes of B-lymphocytes and acts as a specific receptor for antigen. IgM also enhances phagocytosis.

IgA

It accounts for about 15% of the Ig pool. In serum, IgA is present primarily as a monomer, but in mucus secretions as a dimer, held together by a J-chain (Fig. 22.6). Normal serum concentration is 0.6–4.2 mg/ml. It has a half life of 6–8 days.

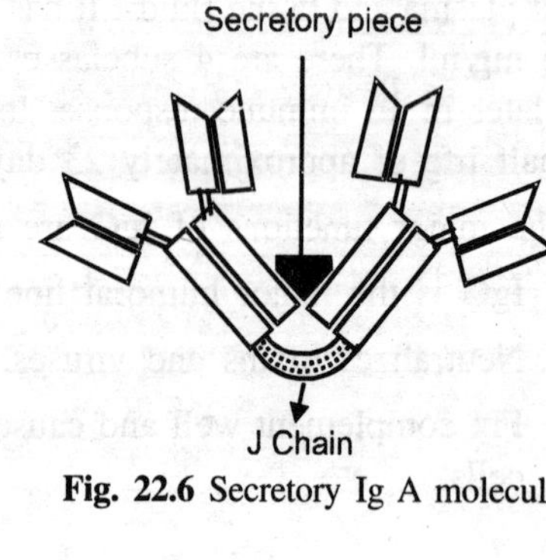

Fig. 22.6 Secretory Ig A molecule.

It provides humoral immunity (Local immunity) in mucus secretions such as tears, saliva, intestinal mucus, semen and colostrum (first breast milk). During the transport of IgA from the Mucosa Associated Lymphoid Tissues (MALT) to mucosal surfaces, it acquires a protein called "**Secretory (S)**

piece", hence, it is known as "**Secretory IgA** (sIgA). It is the primary Ig of secretory immune system. It plays a major role in protecting surface tissues in respiratory tract, intestine and urogenital system against infectious microorganisms. IgA is resistant to proteases and neutralizes toxins, allergens, bacteria and viruses before they can enter the body through the mucus membranes.

sIgA present in breast milk provides **natural passive immunity** against enteric pathogens to the intestine of the new born.

In the intestine, sIgA attaches to viruses, bacteria and protozoan parasites such as *Entamoeba histolytica* and prevents their adhesion and entry through mucus membrane surfaces.

IgA, also activates alternate complement pathway and promotes phagocytosis.

IgA has two subclasses – IgA_1, and IgA_2. Serum IgA is a monomeric 7S molecule (MW about 160,000). Secretory IgA is a much larger molecule than serum IgA (MW about 400,000).

IgD

It is found in trace amounts in the blood serum 3 mg per 100 ml, without a well-known function. It is mostly intravascular. They are found on the surface of B lymphocytes, alongwith IgM and may act as a receptor or recognition molecule for antigens to stimulate antibody production. It has a half life of 3 days.

IgE

It is the antibody that is responsible for hypersensitivity to several antigens – from mosquito bites to pollens. It is an 8S molecule (MW about 190,000) with a half life of two days.

IgE is also known as **reaginic antibody** and found only in trace amounts in serum, but it is found attached to the surface of basophils and mast cells. When two IgE molecules on the surface of these cells are cross-linked by binding to the same antigen, the cells are activated to release granules, which contain pharmacologically active substances such as histamine, which cause allergic conditions such as asthma, anaphylaxis, eczema etc. It also stimulates eosinophilia and gut motility that help in the elimination of helminthic parasites. IgE also causes skin sensitization.

IgE differs from other immunoglobulins in several aspects.

(1) IgE can be detected by Radio allergosorbent test (RAST), ELISA and passive agglutination tests but cannot be detected by conventional serological tests.

(2) IgE is species specific (homocytotropic) only human IgE can fix to the surface of human cells.

(3) IgE is heat sensitive (unlike other antibodies) and is inactivated at 56°C in one hour.

(4) It can fix complement and does not pass through placenta.

(5) It can be destroyed by mercaptoethanol.

IgE is mainly produced in the linings of respiratory and intestinal tracts. IgE levels will be increased in **Type–I hypersensitivity** (Anaphylaxis, Atopy) and in children with a high load of intestinal parasitic infections.

ABNORMAL IMMUNOGLOBULINS

(1) **Bence-Jones proteins** are so called because of their discovery by Henry Bence Jones (1847) and are typically found in multiple myeloma. These are light chains (k or λ) of

immunoglobulins that are synthesized in excess. In about 20% of the patients of multiple myeloma, they are excreted in urine and damages the renal tubules.

Bence Jones proteins can be identified in urine by its characteristic property of coagulation when heated to 50°C, but redissolving at 70°C.

(2) Heavy chain disease is a lymphoid neoplasia, characterized by the overproduction of the F_C portions of Ig heavy chains.

(3) Cryoglobulinemia is a condition in which there is a formation of gel or precipitation on cooling the serum, which redissolves on warming. It may be found in myelomas, macrogloblinemias and autoimmune diseases such as systemic lupus erythematosus. The cryoglobulins are either IgG, IgM or their mixed precipitates.

(4) Waldenstrom's macroglobulinemia is a condition in which there is an excess production of myeloma proteins (M proteins) and of their light chains (Bence Jones proteins).

QUESTIONS

Essay Questions

1. Describe the structure, classes and functions of Immunoglobulins.
2. What are Immunoglobulins ? Outline the role they play in host defence.

Short Notes

1. Immunoglobulins.
2. IgG.
3. Draw a neat labelled diagram of IgG.
4. IgA (or) Structure of IgA.
5. IgM.
6. IgE (or) reagin antibodies.
7. Abnormal Immunoglobulins.
8. Bence-Jones proteins.

23

Monoclonal Antibodies

- *Definition*
- *Production*
- *Uses*
- *Polyclonal antibodies*

INTRODUCTION

Antibodies produced by a single clone (a single antibody forming cell or a single Blymphocyte/ plasma cell) and directed against a single antigenic determinant are called "**Monoclonal antibodies**".

However, antibodies produced by infection or immunization are polyclonal because natural antigens possess several epitopes.

PRODUCTION

Monoclonal antibodies against any desired antigen can be produced on a large scale by **hybridoma technology**, developed by Kohler and Milstein (1975), for which they were awarded Nobel prize (1984).

Hybridomas are somatic cell hybrids produced by fusing antibody forming spleen cells with myeloma cells. The resultant hybrid retains the antibody producing capacity of the spleen cell and the ability of the myeloma cells to multiply indefinitely.

Animals (mice) are immunised with the desired antigen. Once the animal starts producing antibodies, their spleen is removed and the spleen cells are separated from each other and fused with myeloma cells (**Myeloma** is a cancer or continuous proliferation of antibody forming cell) by the addition of polyethylene glycol, which promotes membrane fusion. These fused cells derived from spleen cells and myeloma cells are called "**hybridomas**".

The mutant myeloma cells are grown in culture which do not form immunoglobulins and are deficient in the enzyme "**hypoxanthine phosphoribosyl transferase (HPRT)**".

The fused cells are transferred to a culture medium containing hypoxanthine, Aminopterin and thymidine (**HAT medium**). Aminopterin is a poison that blocks a specific metabolic pathway in cells. Myeloma cells lack HPRT enzyme that allows their growth in the presence of aminopterin. However, the pathway is by-passed in spleen cells provided with the intermediate metabolites hypoxanthine and thymidine. As a result, the hybridomas grow in the HAT medium, but the myeloma cells die due to deficiency of HPRT enzyme and metabolic defect and cannot employ the bypass or salvage pathway.

When the culture is initially established using the HAT medium, it contains lymphocytes, myeloma cells and hybridomas. The unfused splenic lymphoid cells die naturally in culture within a week or two as they cannot replicate indefinitely, and the myeloma cells die in the HAT as just described. In contrast, the fused cells survive because they have the immortality of the myeloma and the metabolic bypass of the splenic lymphoid cells.

Hybridomas are then separated into individual wells of plastic dishes and allowed to grow into clones. Each hybridoma clone may produce monoclonal antibody; the antibodies in each well are screened to see which hybridoma is producing the particular antibody required.

Once the particular hybridoma is identified, it may be recloned by cell culture or it may be maintained *in vivo* by injection into the peritoneal (abdominal) cavity of living animals. Cell culture yields about 100 μg of monoclonal antibody; *in vivo* culture yields about 1000 μg or more of monoclonal antibody per ml of ascitic fluid from peritoneal cavity.

Hybridomas may be frozen for prolonged storage.

USES

Monoclonal antibodies are important because they are homogenous, highly specific and produced readily in large quantities.

They bind to one and only one antigen, and are therefore monospecific. Monoclonal antibodies against several antigens are now available commercially. They have several diagnostic, therapeutic and research applications. They are useful

(1) in tissue typing
(2) in blood grouping
(3) in the identification and epidemiological study of infectious microorganisms.
(4) in the identification of tumor antigens and other surface antigens.
(5) in the classification of leukemias.
(6) in the identification of functional populations of different types of T-cells.

Anticipated future uses include.

(1) passive immunization against infectious agents and toxic drugs.
(2) tissue and organ graft protection.
(3) Stimulation of tumor rejection and elimination.
(4) Manipulation of immune response.
(5) preparation of more specific and sensitive diagnostic procedures.
(6) to deliver antitumor agents such as lethal doses of radiation and anticancer drugs to tumor cells to destroy them.

POLYCLONAL ANTIBODIES

Polyclonal antibodies are effective immunosuppressants and are generally prepared by immunizing animals with human lymphocytes e.g., **antilymphocyte serum (ALS)** or antilymphocyte globulin. Their primary effect is to inhibit cell mediated immune responses.

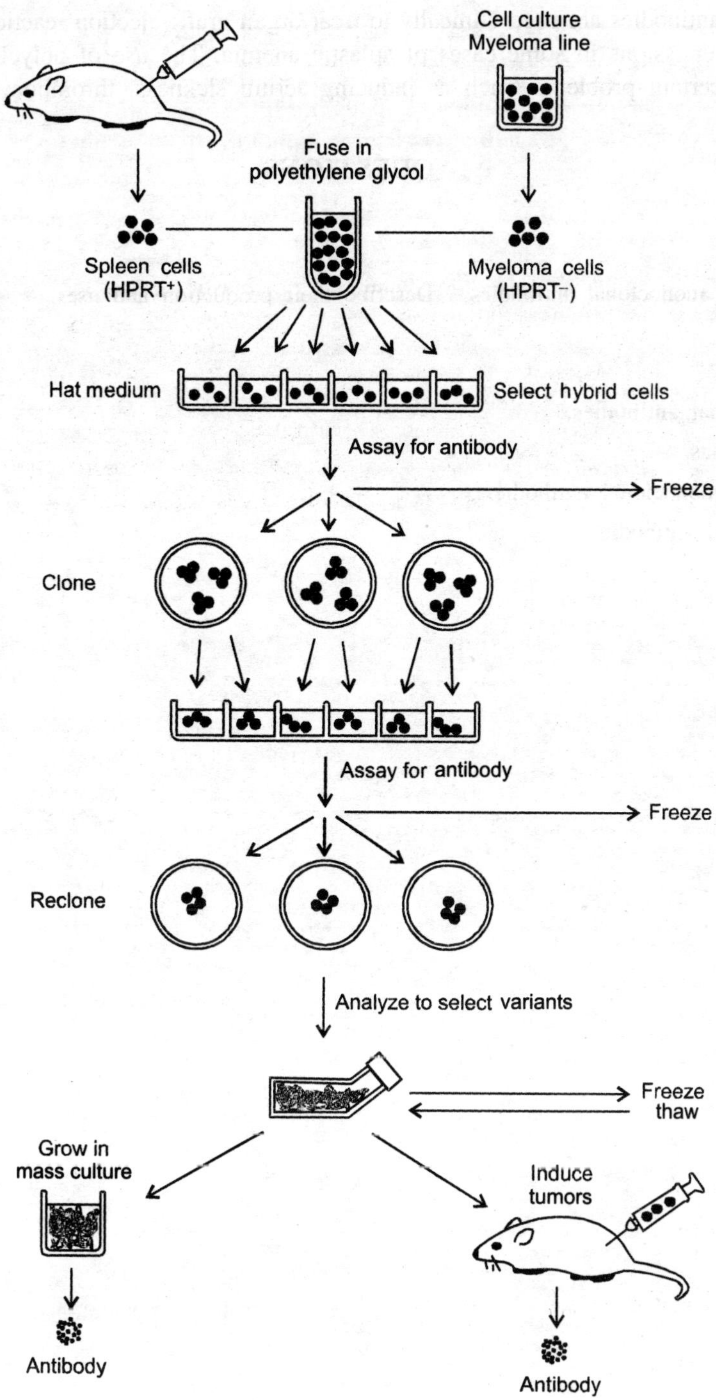

Fig. 23.1 Production of monoclonal antibodies.

Polyclonal antibodies are used clinically to treat organ graft rejection reactions, GVH reactions and to promote remissions in some cases of aplastic anemia. The use of polyclonal antibodies are associated with certain problems, such as inducing serum sickness, thrombocytopenic purpura.

QUESTIONS

Essay Question

1. What are monoclonal antibodies ? Describe their production and uses.

Short Notes

1. Monoclonal antibodies.
2. Hybridomas.
3. Uses of monoclonal antibodies.
4. Polyclonal antibodies.

24

Antigen-Antibody Reactions

- ***Introduction***
- ***Affinity and Avidity***
- ***Sensitivity and Specificity***
- ***Titre***
- ***Mechanism of Ag-Ab reaction***
- ***Zone phenomenon***
- ***List of antigen-antibody reactions***
- ***Precipitation reactions***
  - ***Definition***
  - ***Applications***
    - ***Ring test***
    - ***Slide test***
    - ***Tube test***
    - ***Immunodiffusion***
    - ***Immunoelectrophoresis***
    - ***Electroimmunodiffusion***
- ***Agglutination reactions***
  - ***Definition***
  - ***Applications***
  - ***Slide agglulination test***
  - ***Tube agglutination test***
  - ***Passive agglutination test***
  - ***Reverse passive agglutination***
  - ***Coagglutination***
  - ***Coombs test (Antiglobulin test)***
  - ***Viral hemagglutination***
  - ***Hemagglutination inhibition test***
- ***Complement–Fixation test***
- ***Immunofluorescence***
- ***ELISA***
- ***Radioimmunoassay***
- ***Immunoelectroblot tests***
- ***Immunochromatographic tests***
- ***Immunoelectron microscopic tests***
  - ***Immunoelectron microscopy***
  - ***Immunoferritin test***
  - ***Immunoenzyme test***
- ***Neutralisation tests***
- ***Opsonization***

INTRODUCTION

The reactions between antigens and antibodies *in vivo* form the basis of antibody mediated immunity in infectious diseases or of tissue injury in some types of hypersensitivity and autoimmune diseases.

In the laboratory (*in vitro*) antigen-antibody reactions are useful in the diagnosis of infectious diseases, in the identification of infectious organisms and antigens such as enzymes and in epidemiological surveys.

AFFINITY AND AVIDITY

Affinity (intrinsic affinity) is the intensity of attraction between antigen and antibody molecules.

Avidity (functional affinity) is the binding strength between antigen and antibody molecules.

SENSITIVITY AND SPECIFICITY

Sensitivity refers to the ability of a serological test to detect even very minute quantities of antigen or antibody. When a serological test is highly sensitive, false negative results will be absent or minimum.

Specificity refers to the ability of a serological test to detect reactions between homologous antigens and antibodies only, and not with other. When a serological test is highly specific, false positive reactions will be absent or minimum.

TITRE

Titre is a unit used for the measurement of antibodies.

Titre can be defined as the highest dilution (or lowest quantity) of the serum which gives a visible reaction with the antigen in a particular test.

MECHANISM OF ANTIGEN-ANTIBODY REACTIONS (MARRACK'S HYPOTHESIS)

The mechanism of Antigen-Antibody reaction can be explained according to Marrack's lattice hypothesis.

The multivalent antigens react with bivalent antibodies in varying quantities. But agglutination or precipitation occurs only when a large lattice of antigen-antibody complex is formed, which occurs when antigen and antibody are found in equal concentrations (zone of equivalence). (Fig. 24.1)

ZONE PHENOMENON

Prozone is of importance in clinical serology, as sometimes sera rich in antibody may give a false negative result, unless several dilutions are tested.

If to the same amount of antibody in a series of tubes, increasing quantities of antigens are added, precipitation or agglutination occurs best in one of the middle tubes where antigen and antibody are found in equal concentrations. It is called "Zone of equivalence".

In the initial tubes, where antibody is in excess, the precipitation or agglutination will be absent. It is called "**prozone**".

In the later tubes, where the antigen is in excess, the precipitation or agglutination will be absent. It is called "**postzone**".

If the amounts of antigen-antibody complexes in different tubes are plotted on a graph, the resulting curve will have three phases.

(1) an ascending zone, prozone or zone of antibody excess.

(2) a peak, zone of equivalence.

(3) a descending zone, postzone or zone of antigen excess.

This phenomenon is called zone phenomenon. To avoid prozone phenomenon in clinical serology, several serum dilutions should be tested.

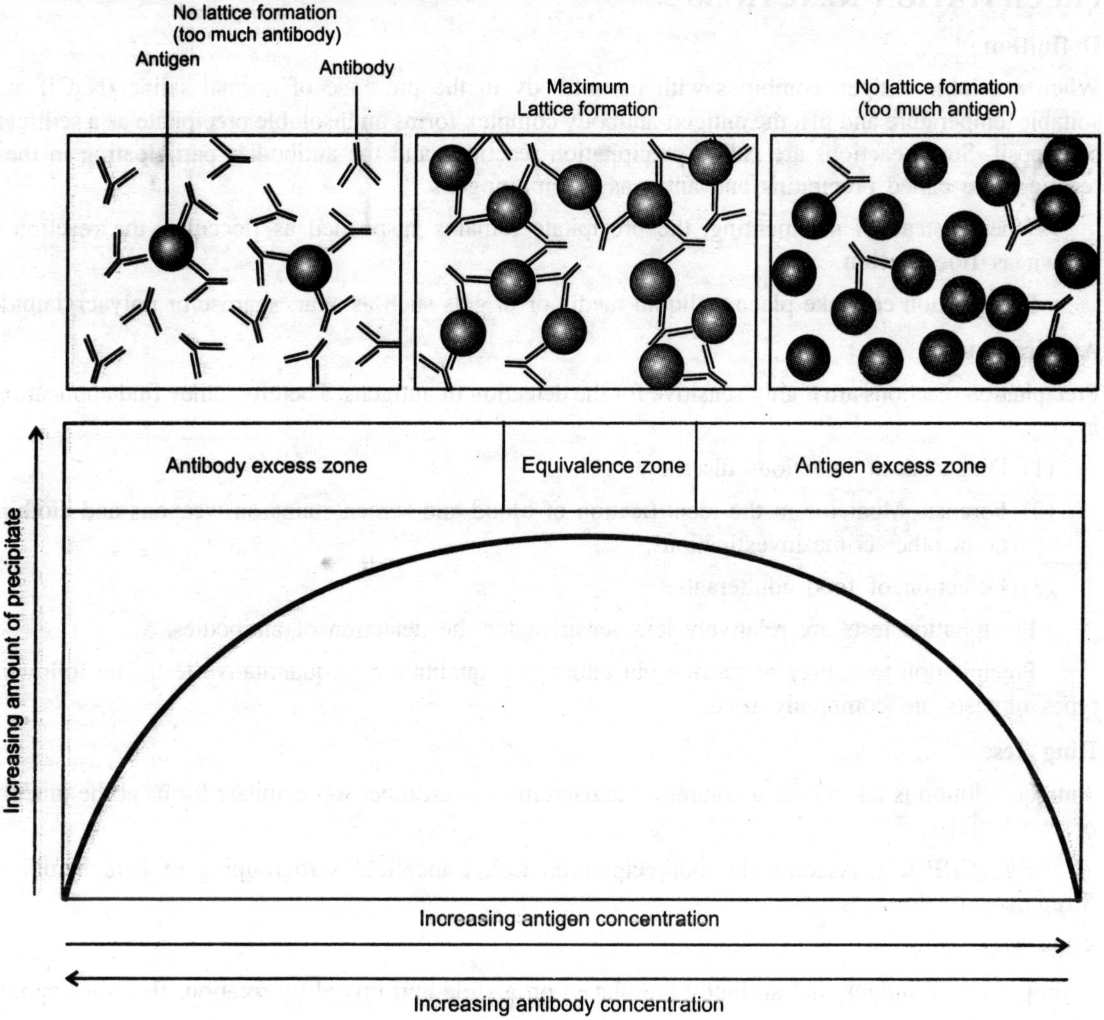

Fig. 24.1 Mechanism of antigen-antibody reaction and zone phenomenon

LIST OF ANTIGEN-ANTIBODY REACTIONS

1. Precipitation (flocculation) reactions
2. Agglutination reactions
3. Complement fixation tests
4. Neutralisation tests
5. Opsonisation
6. Immunofluorescence (IF)
7. Radioimmunoassay (RIA)
8. Enzyme linked immunosorbent assay (ELISA)
9. Immuno-electroblot techniques.

10. Immunochromatographic tests

11. Immunoferritin tests

PRECIPITATION REACTIONS

Definition

When a soluble antigen combines with its antibody in the presence of normal saline (NaCl) at a suitable temperature and pH, the antigen-antibody complex forms an insoluble precipitate as a sediment or deposit. Such reactions are called precipitation reactions and the antibodies participating in these reactions are called precipitins and antigens precipitinogens.

When instead of sedimenting, the precipitate remains suspended as floccules, the reaction is known as **flocculation**.

Precipitation can take place in liquid media or in gels such as agar, agarose or polyacrylamide.

Applications

Precipitation reactions are highly sensitive for the detection of antigens. Therefore, they find applications in

(1) Diagnosis of infectious diseases.

(2) Forensic Medicine in the identification of blood and semen stains on weapons and clothing or in other crime investigations.

(3) Detection of food adulterants.

Precipitation tests are relatively less sensitive for the detection of antibodies.

Precipitation tests may be carried out either as a qualitative or quantitative test. The following types of tests are commonly used.

Ring Test

Antigen solution is taken over a column of antiserum in a test tube. A precipitate forms at the junction of two liquids.

e.g., CRP test, Ascoli's thermoprecipitation test, Lancefield serogrouping of beta hemolytic Streptococci.

Slide Test

A drop each of antigen and antibody are placed on a slide and mixed by rotation, floccules appear.

e.g., VDRL test for syphilis is a slide flocculation test.

Tube Test

The antigen solution and antiserum (Patient's serum) are taken in a test tube mixed, incubated and then observed for precipitation. Usually several tubes with different dilutions of antigen are set up since precipitation may be inhibited in the postzone region.

e.g., Kahn test is a tube flocculation test used for the diagnosis of syphilis.

Immunodiffusion (or) Precipitation In Gel (or) Gel Precipitation

When precipitation is allowed to occur in a gel, the reaction is visible as a distinct band, which is stable and can be stained for preservation. As each antigen-antibody reaction gives rise to a line of precipitation, the number of different antigens in the sample can be made out. Immunodiffusion also indicates identity, cross-reaction and non-identity between different antigens.

Gel precipitation can be done by several ways

(*i*) **Single diffusion in one dimension (oudin method)** – Soluble antigen is directly layered over the antibody-containing gel. The antigen diffuses into the gel and forms a line of precipitation (Fig. 24.2).

(*ii*) **Double diffusion in one dimension (Oakley-Fullthorpe method)** – This method separates antigen and antibody solutions with a layer of clear agar. This results in the diffusion of both soluble antigen and antibody into the agar and the formation of a precipitation ring (Fig. 24.3).

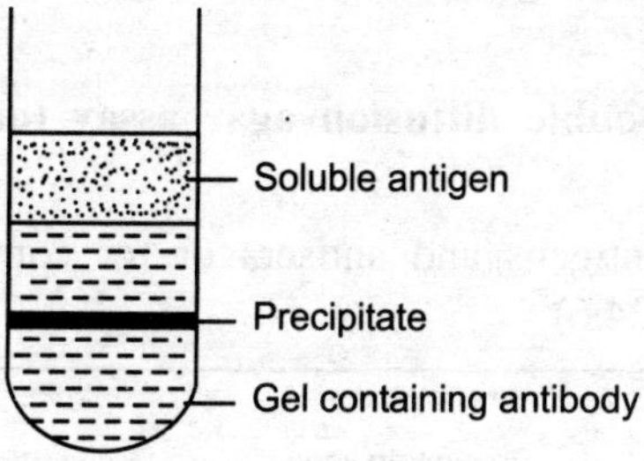

Fig. 24.2 Single diffusion in one dimension (Oudin method)

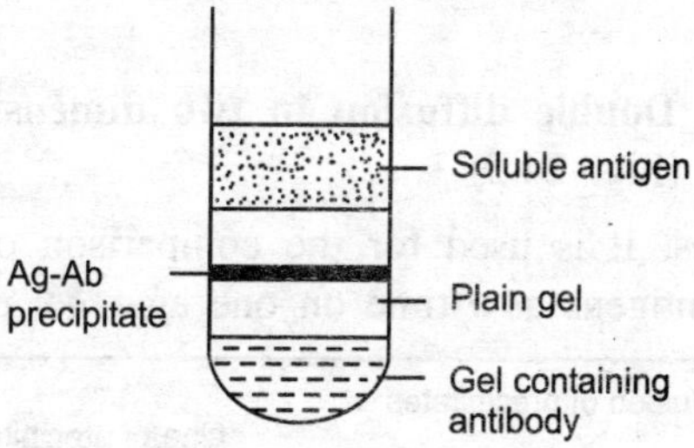

Fig. 24.3 Double diffusion in one dimension (Oakley method)

(*iii*) **Single diffusion in two dimensions (or) Single Radial immunodiffusion (Mancini method)** – It is a quantitative immunodiffusion test used to quantitate serum proteins, immunoglobulins, complement factors and other substances (Fig. 24.4).

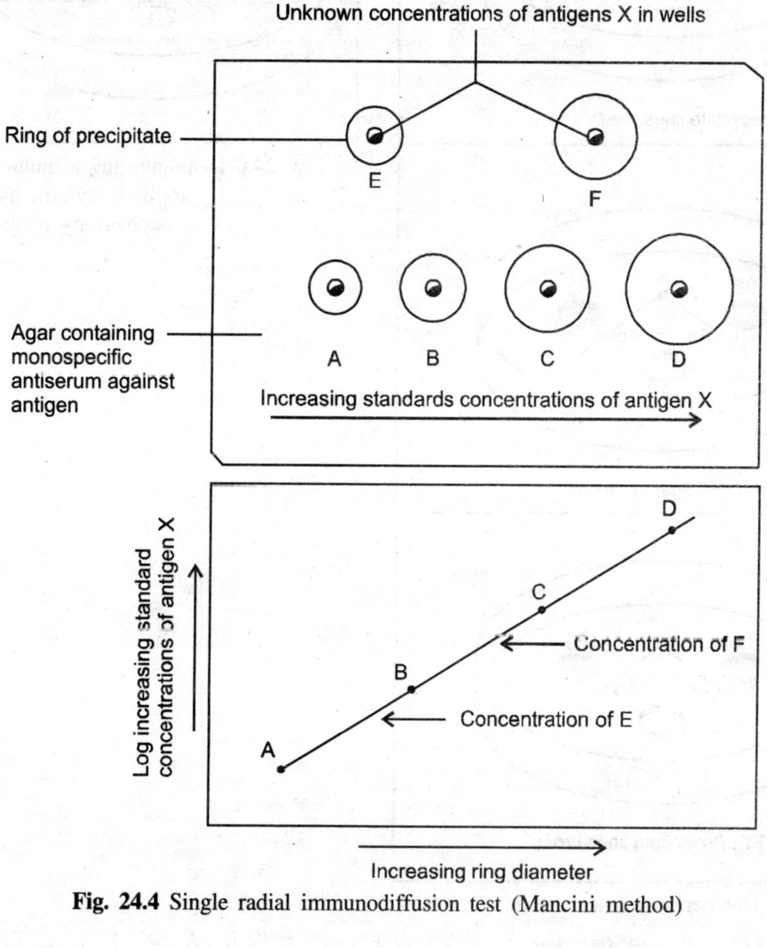

Fig. 24.4 Single radial immunodiffusion test (Mancini method)

Monospecific antibody is added to molten agar and poured on slides or petridishes and allowed to set. Wells are cut and filled with known amounts of various dilutions of reference standard antigen solutions. The unknown test antigen is added to a separate well, and allowed to diffuse. A ring of precipitate forms around each well, and the diameter of the ring is proportional to the antigen concentration in the well. The wider the ring, the greater the antigen concentration. The diameters of the rings formed by the standard antigen concentrations are measured and plotted as a function of antigen concentration. Concentration values for the test antigens are then read from the plotted graph.

(*iv*) **Double diffusion in two dimensions (or) Double diffusion agar assay (ouchterlony method)** (Fig. 24.5)

Uses. It is used for the comparison of various antigens and antisera or for comparison of several antigens at a time on one agar gel plate. (Fig. 24.6)

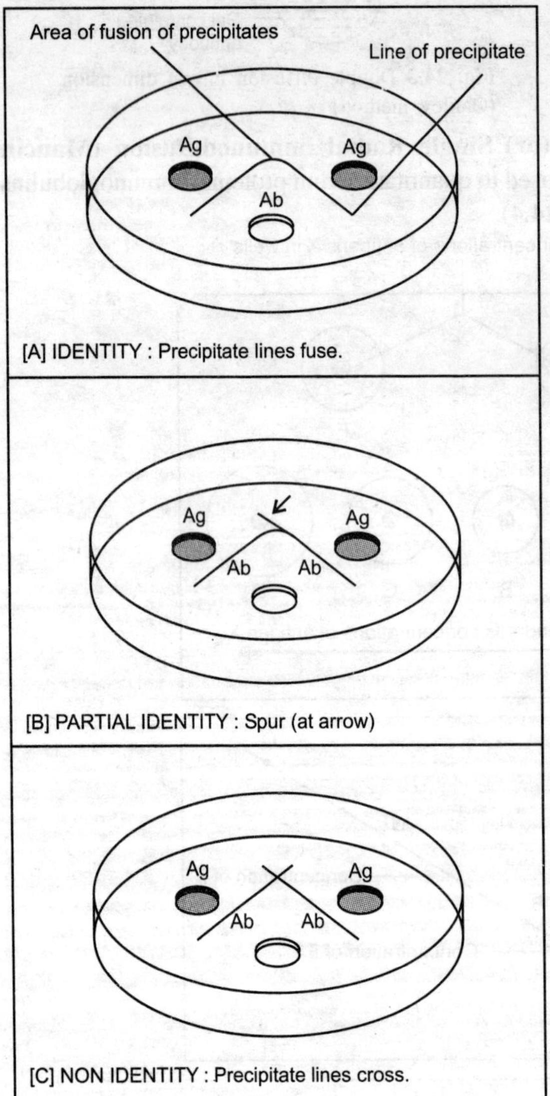

Fig. 24.5 Ouchterlomy test.

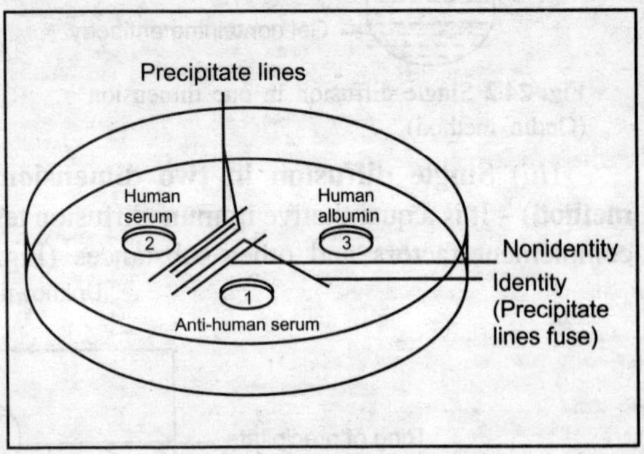

Fig. 24.6 Distinguishing a multicomponent antigen-antibody system by the ouchterlony method.

– It is also used to detect enterotoxin in cases of suspected food poisoning.

– To detect antibodies against specific pathogens in the diagnosis of infectious diseases. It was widely used for the diagnosis of small pox.

– Elek test for toxigenicity of diphtheria bacilli is a special variety of double diffusion in two dimensions.

The test is performed by pouring molten agar on to glass slids or petridishes and allowing it to settle. Test solutions of antigen and antibody are added to separate opposing wells punched in agar. The antigen and antibody diffuse from the wells to form a precipitate at the equivalence zone.

If the two adjacent precipitation lines fuse (V-shaped), it indicates reaction of identity or similarity between two antigens.

If the two adjacent precipitation lines fuse and form a spur or projection (Y-shaped, the stem of Y called spur), it indicates reaction of partial identity (cross-reactivity) of the antigens.

If the two adjacent precipitation lines cross each other (X-shaped), it indicates reaction of non-identity.

Immunoelectrophoresis

It was devised by Grabar and Williams. It combines the techniques of immunodiffusion and electrophoresis. It has the advantage of greater resolution by its ability to separate components of complex antigen mixtures. It can resolve as many as 39 individual antigens in a mixture.

This technique is used to analyze serum proteins and immunoglobulins (Fig. 24.7).

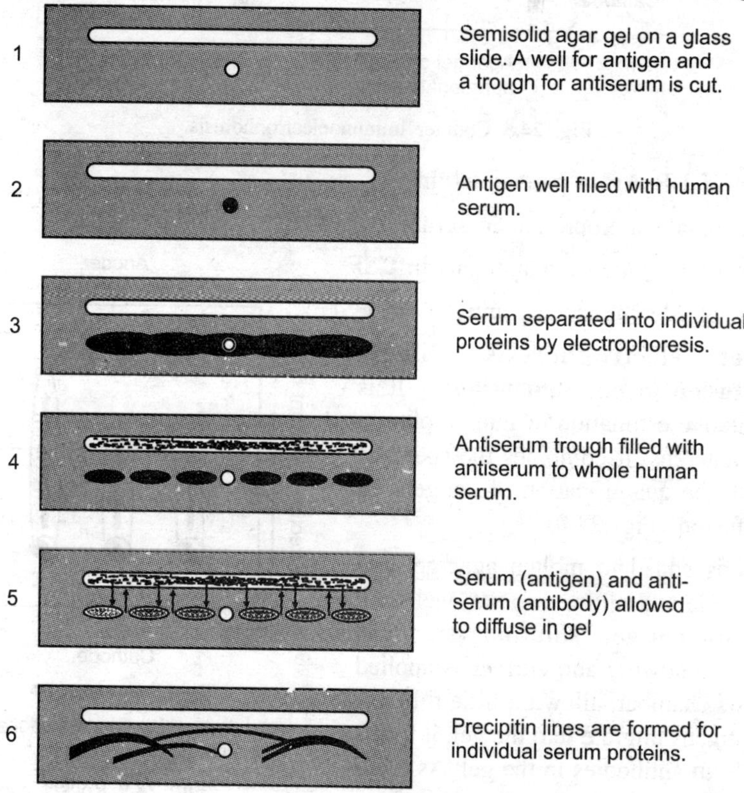

Fig. 24.7 Immunoelectrophoresis.

The test is performed in two stages.

I. Agar gel is taken on a slide and a well is cut and filled with an antigen mixture such as human serum. Electric current is applied in an electrophoresis chamber. As a result, antigens are separated and distributed as separate spots based on their electrical charge. Positively charged proteins move to the negative electrode and negatively charged proteins move towards the positive electrode.

II. A rectangular trough is then cut parallel to the electrophoretic separation and filled with appropriate antibody, and incubated. The antigens and antibodies diffuse into the gel and form a complex pattern of arc shaped precipitation bands that can be better visualized by staining.

Electroimmunodiffusion (Electroimmunoassay)

There are several methods of doing these tests.

(*i*) **Counter current immunoelectrophoresis (CIEP) (or) Double electroimmunodiffusion in one dimension.** It is used for detecting antigens and antibodies, which have opposite charges and move towards each other in an electric field, by forming a line of precipitation where specific antigen and antibody meet in equivalent amounts (Fig. 24.8).

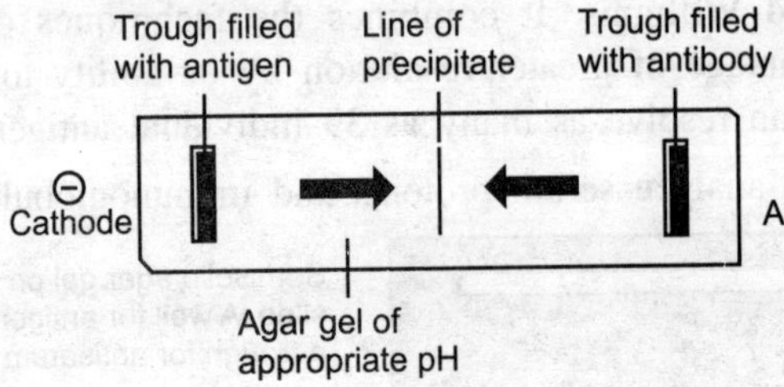

Fig. 24.8 Counter immunoelectrophoresis

Uses. (1) detection of HBsAg in patient serum

(2) detection of alphafetoprotein in serum

(3) detection of *Cryptococcus* antigens in CSF

(4) detection of Meningococcal antigens in CSF.

(*ii*) **Rocket electrophoresis (Single electroimmunodiffusion in one dimension)** – It is used for the quantitative estimation of human plasma antigens and viral antigens. It combines the speed of electrophoresis with the quantification of antigens of Radial immunodiffusion (Fig. 24.9).

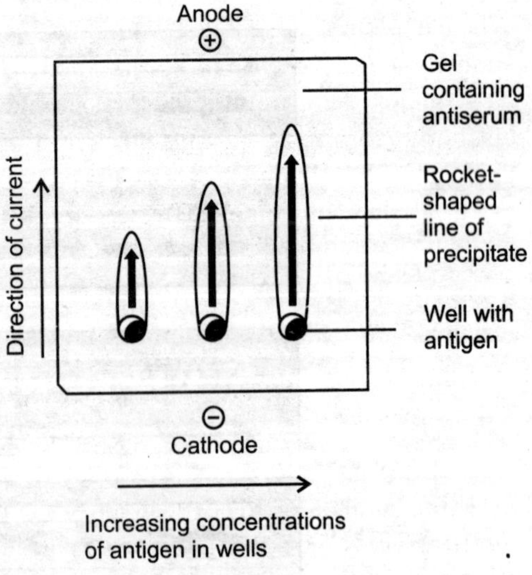

Fig. 24.9 Rocket electrophoresis

The antibody is added to molten agar gel and poured on a glass slide and allowed to set; wells are cut and filled with antigen solution (standard concentrations and unknowns) and current is applied in an electrophoresis chamber, allowing little time for diffusion. When antigens migrate into the gel, it forms precipitation lines with antibodies in the gel. As more antigen arrives, the precipitate at the advancing front dissolves, while the precipitate at the sides remains; this gives a rocket like configuration. Hence, the procedure is commonly called rocket immunoelectrophoresis.

The area of each rocket, or its height is directly proportional to the initial concentrations of antigen.

(*iii*) **Laurell's electroimmunodiffusion in two dimensions.** It is used to quantify each of several components in an antigen mixture. In this method the antigen mixture is first electrophoretically separated into different components, followed by immunodiffusion in gel containing antibody, so that rocket like precipitation lines are produced. Thus, this technique is similar to Immunoelectrophoresis. (Fig. 24.10)

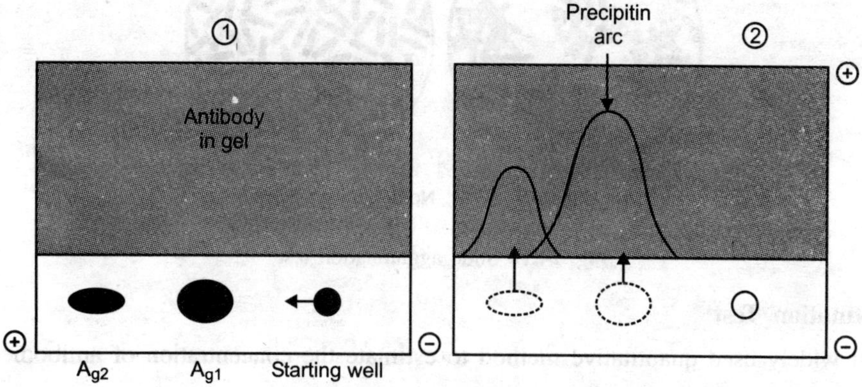

Fig. 24.10 Laurell's two dimensional rocket electrophoresis

(1) Antigens are separated by their electrophoretic mobility on first run.

(2) The second run at right angles to the first drives the antigens into the antigserum containing gel to form precipitation rockets.

AGGLUTINATION REACTIONS

Definition

When a particulate antigen combines with its antibody in the presence of normal saline (NaCl) at a suitable temperature and pH, the antigen-antibody complexes form large clumps or aggregates or agglutinates, that are visible and can be seen with unaided eye. Such reactions are called Agglutination reactions (Fig. 24.11).

The antibodies participating in these reactions are called "agglutinins" and antigens are "agglutinogens".

Applications

Agglutination tests are more sensitive for detecting antibodies. They can be used either qualitatively or for quantitative assay of antibodies.

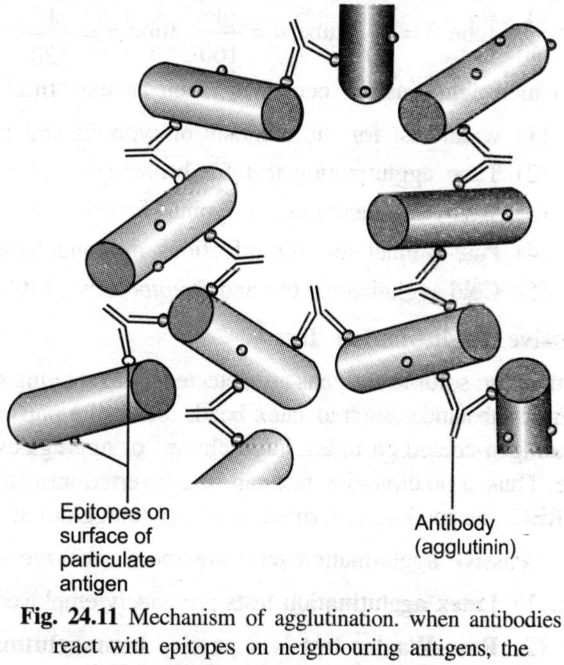

Fig. 24.11 Mechanism of agglutination. when antibodies react with epitopes on neighbouring antigens, the particulate antigens clump into visible aggregates

Slide Agglutination Test

It is mainly used for the identification of bacterial isolates from clinical specimens and for blood grouping (to type RBC) and **cross-matching.**

When a drop of specific antiserum is added to a smooth, saline suspension of a particulate antigen and mixed on a slide, agglutination occurs by formation of clumps and clearing of the drop, which is usually visible to the naked eye (Fig. 24.12).

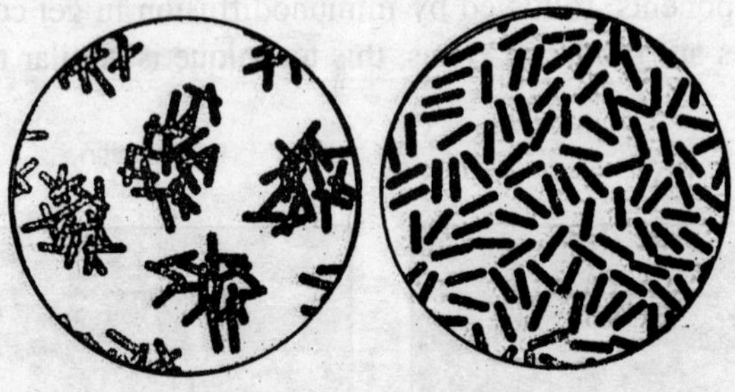

Fig. 24.12 Slide agglutination test

Tube Agglutination Test

It is the most widely used quantitative method to estimate the concentration of antibodies in serum specimens.

The test is performed by adding a fixed amount of particulate antigen to a series of tubes containing doubling dilutions of the antiserum (patient's serum); for example, tube 1 = $\frac{1}{20}$, tube 2 = $\frac{1}{40}$, tube 3 = $\frac{1}{80}$, tube 4 = $\frac{1}{160}$, tube 5 = $\frac{1}{320}$ and so on. The reciprocal of the highest dilution in which agglutination occurs is taken as the "titre" of the antiserum. (Fig. 24.13)

e.g.,(1) widal test for the dianosis of typhoid and paratyphoid fevers.

(2) Tube agglutination test for brucellosis.

(3) Weil-Felix reaction for typhus fevers.

(4) Paul-Bunnel test for infectious mononucleosis.

(5) Cold agglutination test and *Streptococcus*. MG agglutination test for primary atypical pneumonia.

Passive Agglutination Test

In this test, soluble antigens are detected by first being made to adhere to the surfaces of inert particulate carrier substances such as latex beads, bentonite particles and RBC. When specific antiserum is added to antigen-coated particles, large clumps or aggregates are formed, that are easily visible to the naked eye. Thus, a precipitation test can be converted into an agglutination test (Fig. 24.14). When the carrier is RBC, the method is termed passive hemagglutination.

Passive agglutination tests are more sensitive for detecting antibodies.

e.g.,(1) **Latex agglutination tests** are widely employed for the detection of ASLO, CRP, RA factor etc.

(2) **Rose-Waaler test** is a **passive hemagglutination test** (sensitized sheep RBC agglutination test) used to detect RA factor.

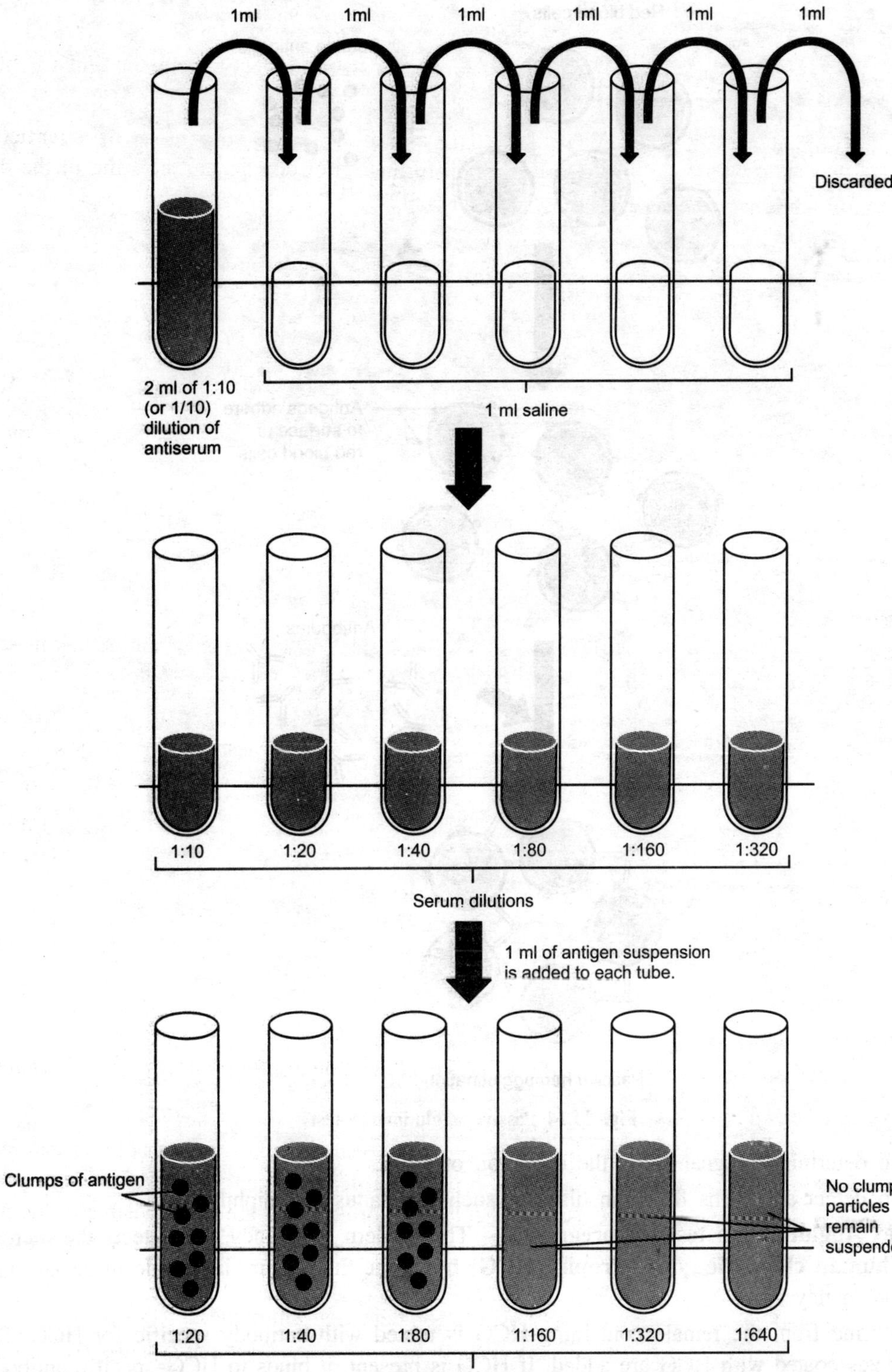

Fig. 24.13 Procedure for making doubling dilution for tube agglutination test

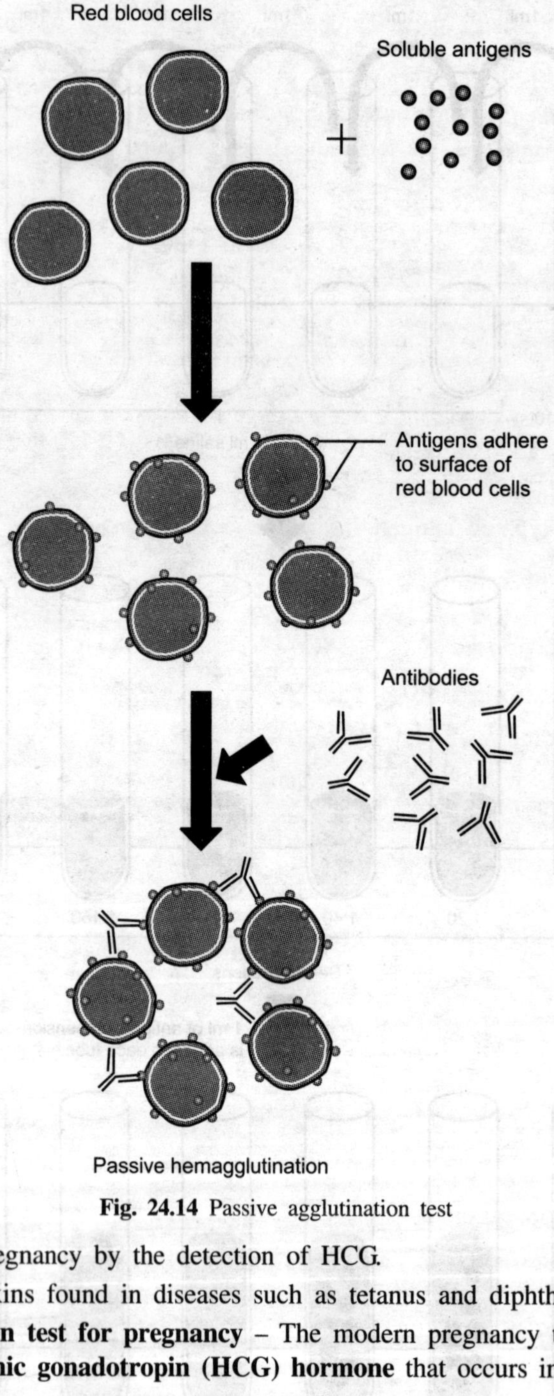

Fig. 24.14 Passive agglutination test

(3) To determine pregnancy by the detection of HCG.

(4) To detect antitoxins found in diseases such as tetanus and diphtheria.

Latex Agglutination test for pregnancy – The modern pregnancy test detects the increased levels of **human chorionic gonadotropin (HCG) hormone** that occurs in female urine and blood early in pregnancy.

The urine from the female containing HCG is mixed with antibody specific for HCG. Then, latex particles coated with HCG are added. If HCG is present, it binds to HCG–specific antibodies, thereby preventing them from agglutinating the latex particles coated with HCG. Therefore, in a positive test there will be no agglutination.

In a negative test, the latex particles coated with HCG are agglutinated by antibody to HCG.

Reverse Passive Agglutination Test

When instead of the antigen, the antibody is attached to carrier particles such as latex or bentonite in tests for estimation of antigens, the technique is known as reverse passive agglutination test. e.g., detection of HBsAg in patient's serum.

Coagglutination

In this method *Staphylococcus aureus* (cowan I strain) cells are used as carriers of antibodies, because protein–A on their cell wall can react with F_C region of immunoglobulin molecules, while leaving the Fab region free to combine with a specific antigen.

Thus *Staphylococcus aureus* (cowan I strain) cells with attached IgG antibodies on their protein-A of cell wall against a specific antigen will agglutinate bacteria that have that specific antigen. This is called co-agglutination. (Fig. 24.15)

It has several important diagnostic applications such as streptococcal grouping, Gonococcal typing and detection of typhoid antigen from enteric fever cases etc.

Coombs Test (Antiglobulin Test)

It is used to detect incomplete antibodies (nonagglutinating or antierythrocyte antibodies). The major applications of coombs test are –

(1) evaluating hemolytic disease of the new born.

(2) diagnosis of autoimmune hemolytic anemia.

(3) erythrocyte (RBC) typing in blood banks.

The test may be direct or indirect (Fig. 24.16)

Principle. Anti-Rh antibodies when react with RBC (coated on RBC) fail to produce agglutination. The addition of an antiglobulin antiserum (coombs serum) produced in heterologous species (e.g., Rabbit antihuman γ-globulin), produces marked agglutination.

Direct coombs test. Detects antibodies that are adherent to RBC taken directly from a sensitized individual.

When RBC from infants suffering from hemolytic anemia is mixed with coombs serum agglutination results.

Indirect coombs test. It is a two-stage reaction for detection of incomplete antibodies in patient's serum.

The patient's serum is first incubated with test RBC (Rh +ve), so that antibody coats RBC.

In the second step coombs antiglobulin serum is added so that antibody-coated RBC are agglutinated.

Hemagglutination. Different types of hemagglutination with examples are as follows.

(1) Viral hemagglutination e.g., Influenza virus agglutinates RBC.

(2) Passive hemagglutination e.g., **Rose-waaler test** is a sensitized sheep RBC agglutination test, used to detect RA factor.

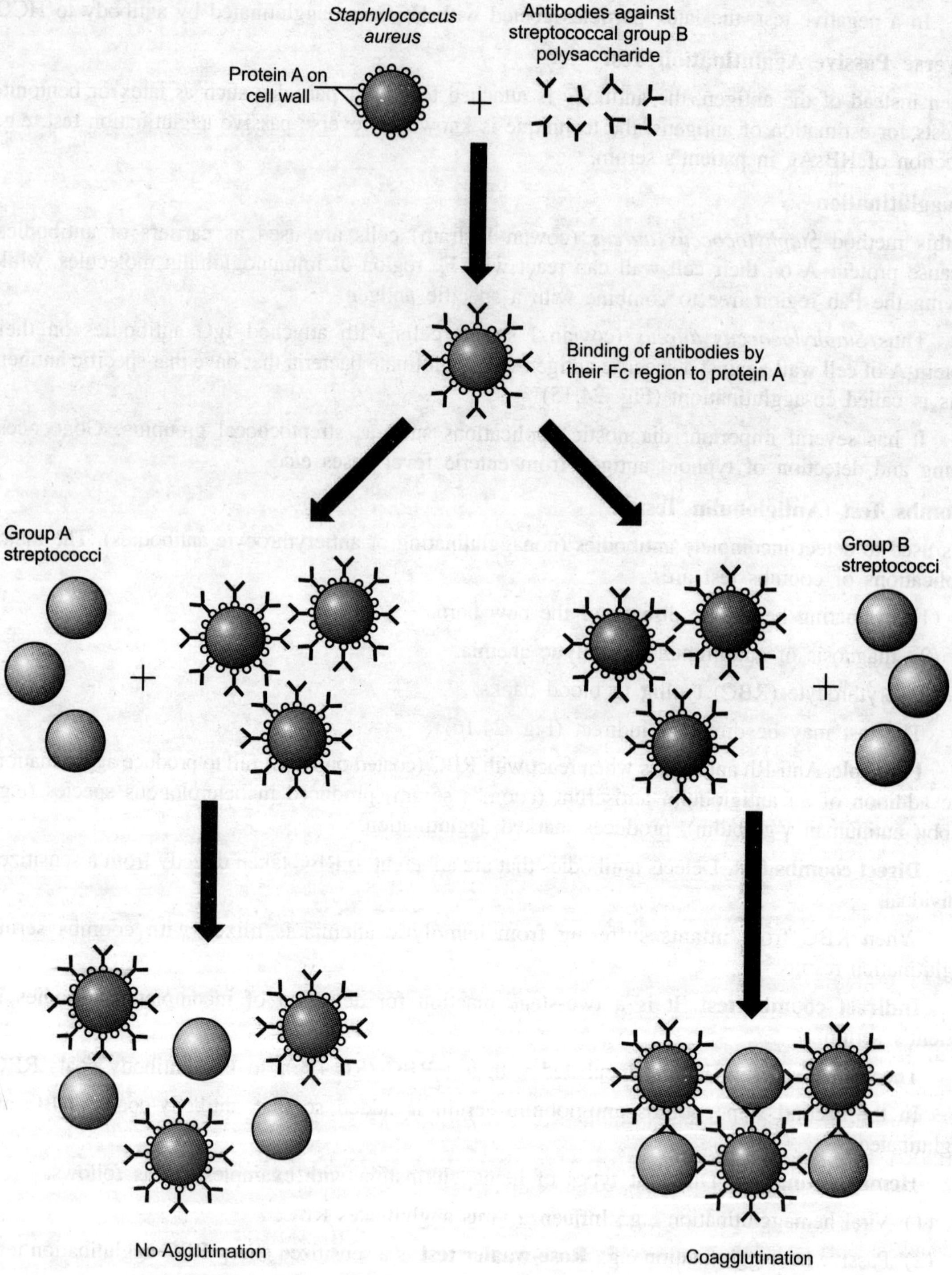

Fig. 24.15 Bacterial coagglutination test for determining the serological groups of streptococci. Antibodies are bound by their Fc region to protein A on the *Staphylococcus aureus* cell wall. The *S. aureus* cells become carriers of antibodies (to group B streptococci in the case shown). No agglutination occurs with group A streptococci (bottom left). Coagglutination occurs in the presence of group B streptococci (bottom right)

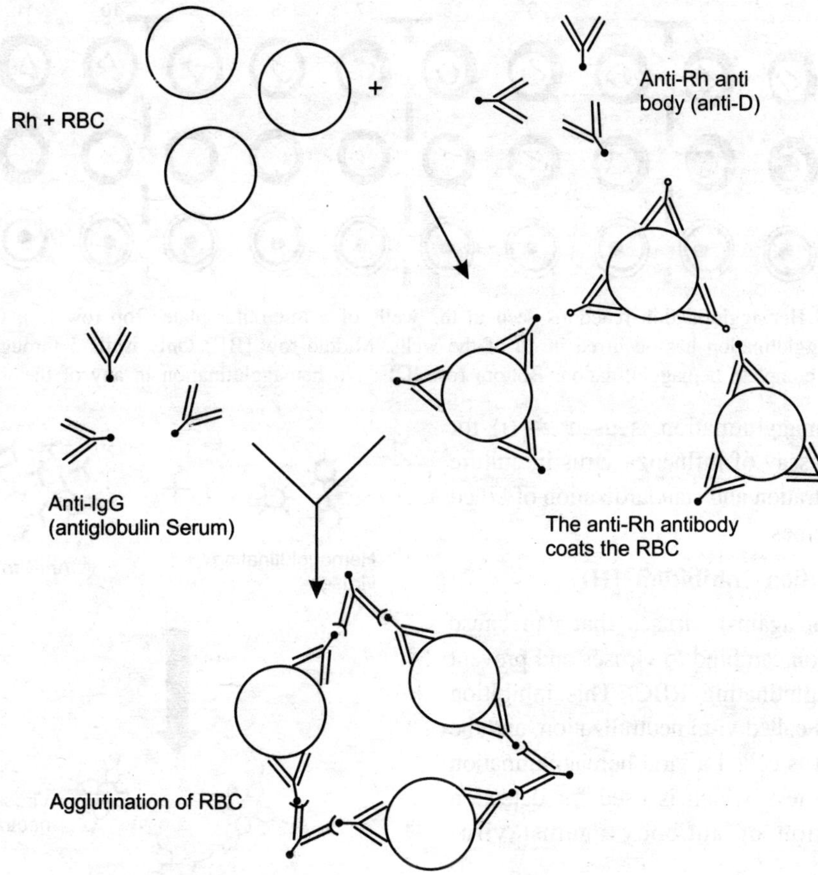

Fig. 24.16 Coombs test (antiglobulin test)

(3) Indirect hemagglutination (IHA) test used in the serodiagnosis of several parasitic, bacterial diseases e.g., IHA for malaria, TPHA for syphilis.

(4) Fimbrial hemagglutination is used to detect the presence of fimbriae.

Viral Hemagglutination

Certain viruses have the ability to agglutinate RBC from chicken, Guinea pig and humans and is known as viral hemagglutination (Fig. 24.17).

When RBC are added to serial dilutions of the viral suspension (or of serum from a virus-infected patient) in tubes or plastic trays, RBC which are not agglutinated settle at the bottom in the form of a button, while the agglutinated cells spread as an even coating in a shield like pattern (Fig. 24.18).

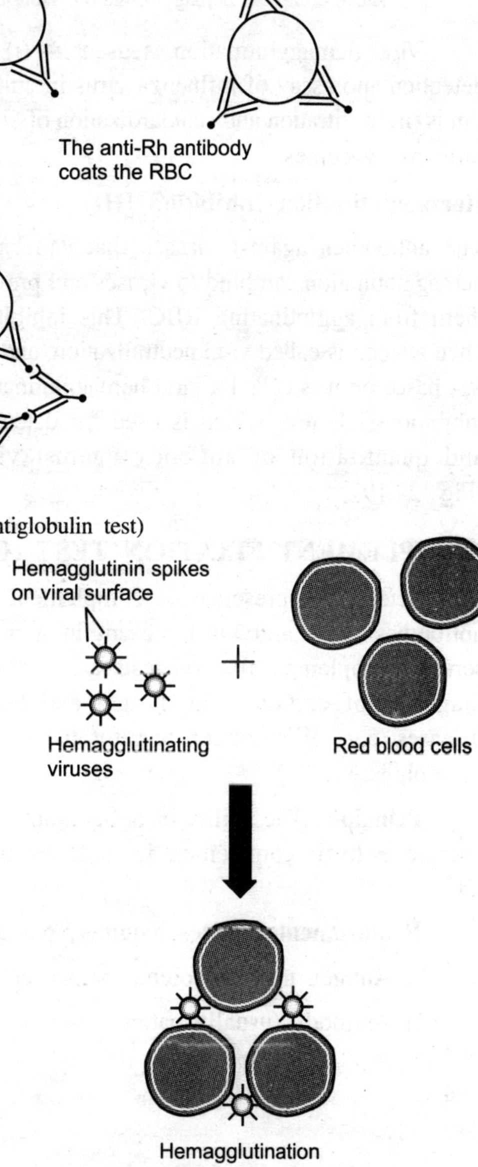

Fig. 24.17 Viral hemagglutination

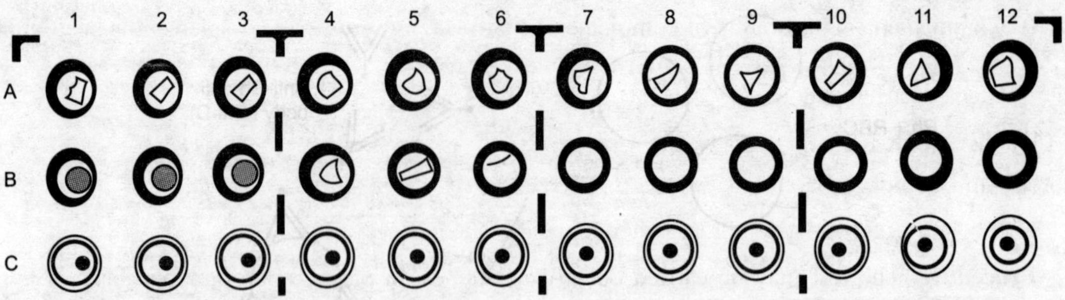

Fig. 24.18 Hemagglutination reactions seen in the wells of a microtiter plate. Top row [A]: Complete hemagglutination has occurred in all of the wells. Middle row [B] : Only wells 3 through 6 show complete hemagglutination. Bottom row [C] : No hemagglutination in any of the wells.

Viral hemagglutination is used — (i) for detection and assay of influenza virus in culture fluids (ii) for titration and standardization of killed influenza vaccines.

Hemagglutination Inhibition (HI)

The antibodies against viruses that can cause hemagglutination can bind to viruses and prevent them from agglutinating RBC. This inhibition phenomenon is called viral neutralization, and the test based on it is called a viral hemagglutination inhibition (HI) test, which is used for detection and quantitation of antibody against virus (Fig. 24.19).

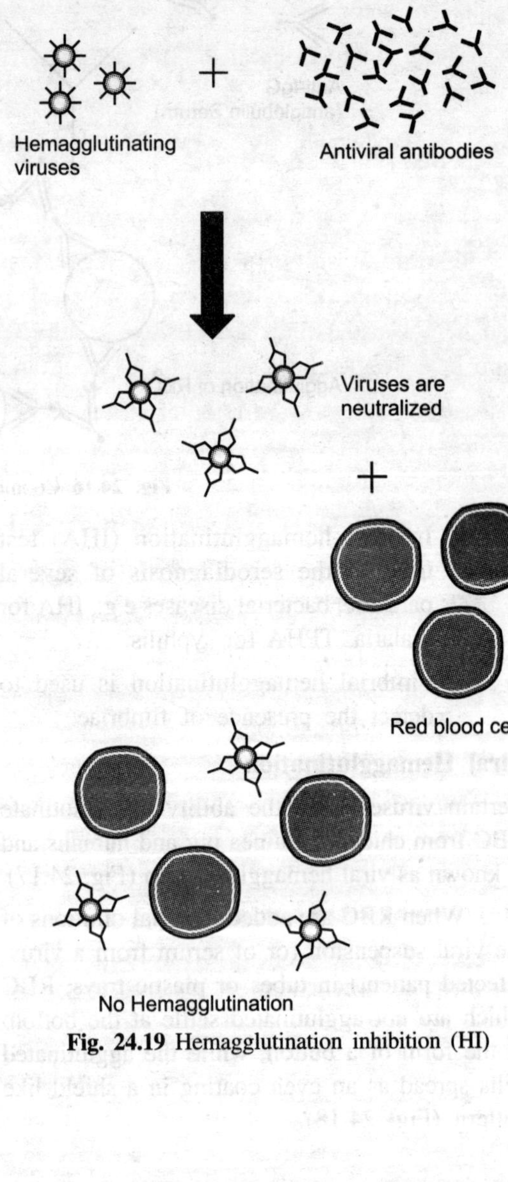

Fig. 24.19 Hemagglutination inhibition (HI)

COMPLEMENT FIXATION TEST (CFT)

CFT detects the presence of complement fixing antibodies (IgM and IgG) present in a patient's serum. Complement-fixation tests are used in the diagnosis of certain viral, fungal and bacterial diseases. e.g., Wassermann test for the diagnosis of syphilis.

Principle. The ability of antigen-antibody complexes to fix complement is made use of in CFT.

Requirements. The test requires 5 reagents.

(1) Antigen may be soluble or particulate.

(2) Antibody (usually patient's serum).

(3) Complement – The source of complement is Guinea pig serum. As complement is heat-labile, the serum should be freshly drawn or preserved either in lyophilized or frozen state or by Richardson's method.

(4) Sheep RBC.

(5) Amboceptor, an antibody to sheep RBC raised in rabbits.

Sheep RBC and amboceptor together known as hemolytic system.

Procedure. The test may be carried out in small tubes, in plastic microtitration plates or even in automated system. (Fig. 24.20)

The test is performed in the two stages.

The test serum from the patient must first be inactivated at 56°C for 30 min. to destroy its complement activity.

I stage – known antigen + test serum + complement mixture is incubated at 37°C for 30 min or longer.

The antigen–antibody reaction cannot be seen at the end of this stage, since all components are soluble.

II stage – Sheep RBC + Amboceptor are added.

Reading Results. In the first stage, if complement has been fixed because of an antigen–antibody reaction, it is no longer available for the lysis of sheep RBC in stage II. Therefore, if there is no hemolysis; it indicates positive result, because the complement fixing antibodies in the test serum have reacted with antigen in I stage and utilized (fixed) the complement.

If there is hemolysis, it indicates negative result, because complement is available for hemolysing the sheep RBC in II stage, therefore, no antibodies specific for the known antigen were present in the patient's serum.

Immunolabelled Tests and Conjugates Used In Them

There are several serological tests in which either antigen or antibody is labelled.

1. Immunofluorescent tests – conjugates used are fluorescein isothiocyanate, Lissamine Rhodamine conjugated with antigen or antibody.
2. Radioimmunoassay (RIA) – Radioactive isotopes ^{125}I and ^{32}P are conjugated/labelled with antigen or antibody.
3. ELISA – horse radish peroxidase, Alkaline phosphatase are labelled with either antigen or antibody.
4. Immunoferritin labelled tests – Ferritin labelled antibody is the conjugate.

IMMUNOFLUORESCENCE

Fluorescence is the property of absorbing light rays of one particular wavelength and emitting rays with different wavelengths.

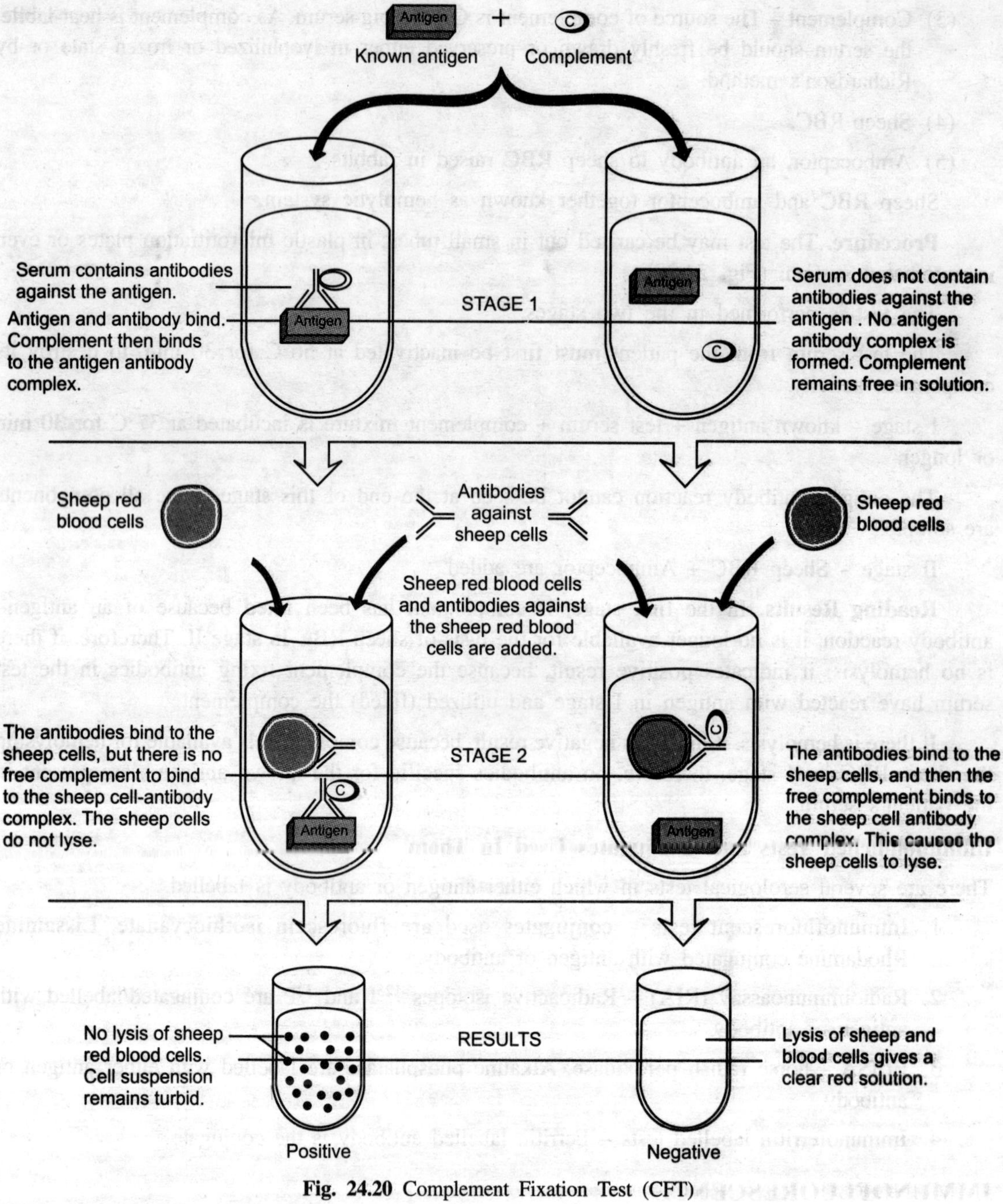

Fig. 24.20 Complement Fixation Test (CFT)

Fluorescent dyes show up brightly under UV light as they convert UV light (invisible light) into visible light. Such fluorescent dyes can be conjugated to antibodies and such **labelled antibodies** can be used to detect and identify antigens in tissues.

The technique is of 2 types.

1. Direct Immunofluorescence. The specimen (cells or microorganisms) containing the antigen are fixed on to a slide. Then specific Fluorescein labelled antibodies are added to the slide and incubated. The slide is washed to remove any unbound antibody and examined with the **Fluorescence** Microscope for a yellow-green fluorescence, which reveals the antigen location (Fig. 24.21).

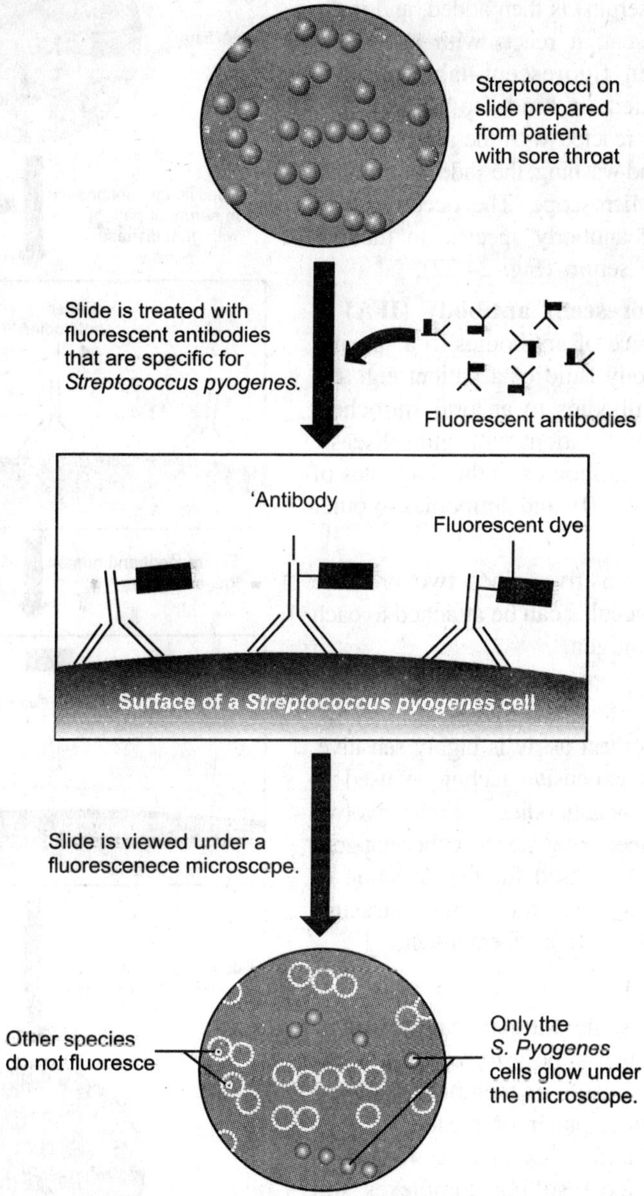

Fig. 24.21 Direct fluorescent antibody (DFA)

Direct fluorescent antibody (DFA) technique is usually used to identify a **particular kind of** microorganism in a clinical specimen e.g., *Streptococcus pyogenes* in a throat swab **from a patient.**

Direct immunofluorescence is used to identify antigens found on surface of Group A **streptococci** and to diagnose EPEC, *Neisseria meningitidis*, *Salmonella typhi*, *Shigella sonnei, Listeria monocytogenes,* *Hemophilus influenzae* and the Rabies virus.

2. Indirect Immunofluorescence. In this technique, a known antigen is fixed on to a slide. The test antiserum (patient's serum) is then added, and if the specific antibody is present, it reacts with antigen to form a complex. When fluorescent–labelled anti-immunoglobulin is added, it binds to the specific antibody that has already reacted with the antigen in the smear. After incubation and washing, the slide is examined with the Fluorescence Microscope. The occurrence of fluorescence shows that antibody specific to the test antigen is present in the serum (Fig. 24.22).

The **indirect fluorescent antibody (IFA)** is used to detect the presence of antibodies to a specific microorganism in the body fluid of a patient e.g., (1) the presence of IgG antibodies to an oral spirochete in the serum or saliva of a patient with gum disease. (2) *Treponema pallidum* antibodies in the diagnosis of syphilis (FTA-ABS, FTA-200), and antibodies to other microorganisms.

The IFA is more sensitive, since two or more labelled antiglobulin molecules can be attached to each antibody bound to its antigen.

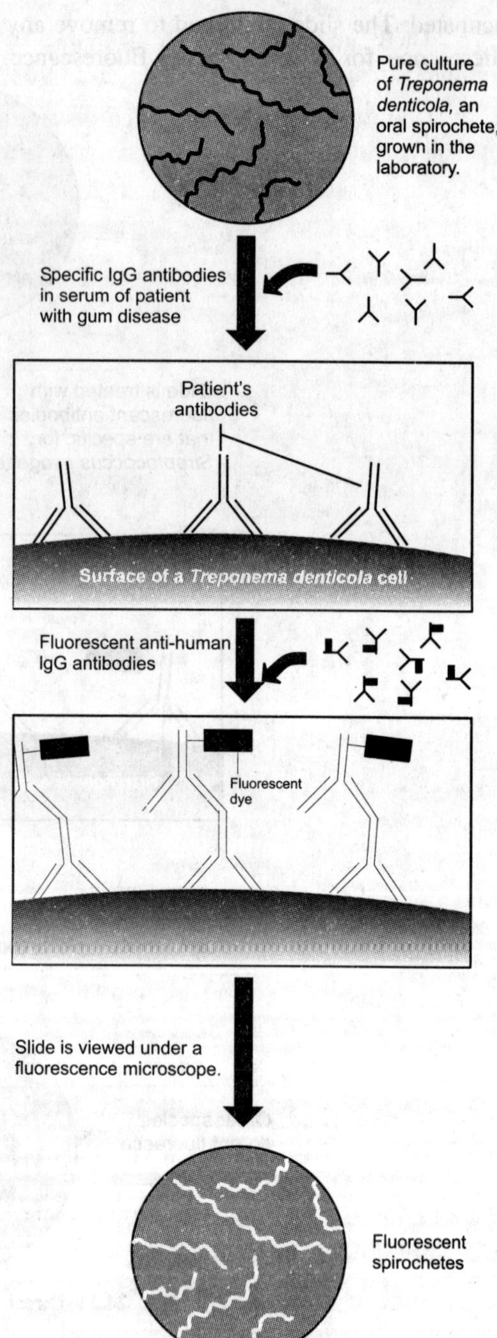

Fig. 24.22 Indirect fluorescent antibody (IFA) technique

ELISA

Enzyme-linked immunosorbent assay is highly sensitive, highly specific and less expensive technique used in serology to detect antigens or antibodies. This test involves the linking of various "label" enzymes to either antigens or antibodies. The ELISA is used for the detection of many infectious viruses, bacteria, fungi, parasites (protozoa) and drugs, toxins, food allergens etc.

ELISA is based on two principles —

(1) Antibodies and some antigens can adsorb to a solid support such as polystryrene, polyvinyl or polycarbonate wells or membranes (discs) of polyacrylamide, paper or plastic.

(2) Antigens and antibodies can be linked to enzymes, with the resulting complexes still fully functional, both immunologically and enzymatically.

Enzyme activity is used to measure the quantity of antigen or antibody present in the test sample Enzymes used in ELISA include β-galactosidase, glucose oxidase, peroxidase, and alkaline phosphatase. The test is usually done using microtiter plates (96-well) suitable for automation.

There are 2 basic ELISA techniques – The double-antibody-sandwich technique and the **indirect** immunosorbent technique.

Double Antibody Sandwich Assay. It is used for the detection of **antigens (e.g., HBsAg in** patient's serum). (Fig. 24.23)

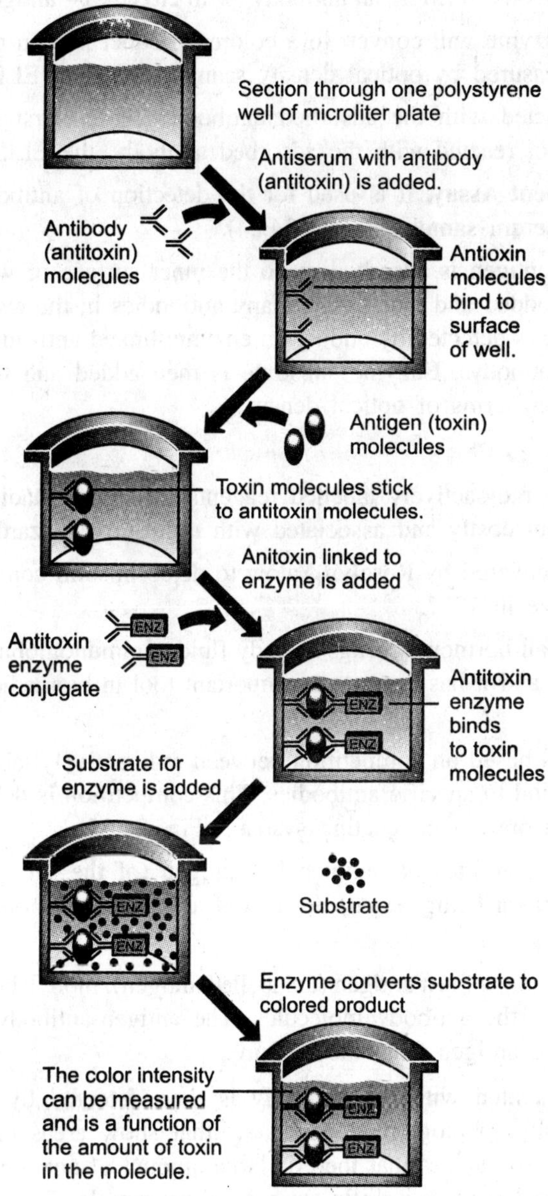

Fig. 24.23 Double-antibody-sandwich ELISA technique for the detection and measurement **of antigen. The** detection of staphylococcal enterotoxin in a food extract is illustrated. The presence **of as little as 0.4 ng of** toxin per mililiter of food extract can be detected by the ELISA technique. (Note that the necessary washing after each step is not shown)

In this technique, specific antibody is placed in wells of a microtiter plate (or it may be attached to a membrane) and the antibody adheres to the inner surface of each well. The test antigen is added to each well. If the antigen reacts with the antibody, the antigen is retained when the well is washed to remove unbound antigen.

An antibody-enzyme conjugate specific for the antigen is then added; it will bind to the antigen already fixed by the first antibody, forming an antibody (with enzyme) – antigen-antibody "sandwich".

A substrate that the enzyme will convert to a colored product is then added, and any resulting product is quantitatively measured by optical density scanning with an ELISA Reader.

If the antigen has reacted with the adsorbed antibodies in the first step, the ELISA test is positive. If the antigen is not reacted with the adsorbed antibody, the ELISA test is negative.

Indirect Immunosorbent Assay. It is used for the detection of antibodies (e.g., antibodies to HIV and Rubella virus in serum samples). (Fig. 24.24).

In this technique, the antigen is adsorbed on to the inner surface of well wall. Test antiserum (usually patient's serum) is added and incubated. If any antibodies in the test antiserum have bound to the antigen, their presence is detected by adding an enzyme-linked anti-immunoglobulin (anti-anti-body or antibody against antibody). Enzyme substrate is then added and the color change can be detected by ELISA Reader in terms of optical density.

Radioimmunoassay (RIA)

Immunological assays using radioactively labelled reagents are called Radioimmunoassays (RIAs). RIAs are highly sensitive but costly and associated with radioactive hazard.

The technique was discovered by Rosalyn Yalow to detect insulin concentration in plasma, for which she won a noble prize in 1977.

RIAs are available for all hormones, drugs in body fluids, immunoglobulins, tumor antigens and viral antigens (e.g., HBsAg) and it has become an important tool in biomedical research and clinical practice.

Principle. The assay is based on competition between radioactively labeled antigens (e.g., ^{125}I) and unlabelled antigens to bind to specific antibodies. This competition is determined by the level of the unlabelled (test) antigen present in reacting system. (Fig. 24.25)

Procedure. Measured quantities of radiolabeled antigen (of the same kind being tested) and antibody (specific to the antigen being tested) are mixed and incubated, one mixture with and one without added test sample.

At increasing concentrations of test antigen (unlabelled antigen), more labelled antigen is displaced or prevented from binding to the antibody molecules. The antigen-antibody complex is washed to remove unbound radiolabeled antigen from the mixture.

The radioactivity associated with the antibody is then detected by means of radioisotope analyzers and autoradiography (photographic emulsions that show areas of radioactivity). A little amount of bound radioactivity indicates that there is large amount of antigen; and a large amount of bound radioactivity indicates that there is little antigen in the sample.

A standard calibration curve is plotted on graph by taking the ratio of bound radiolabeled antigen to free radiolabeled antigen against varying known amounts of unlabelled antigen and the antigen concentration of the test sample can be read from this curve.

IMMUNOELECTROBLOT TECHNIQUES

In **Immunblot** techniques, antibodies detect individual proteins (antigens) in complex mixtures. The technique combines the sensitivity of enzyme immuno-assay with much greater specificity. e.g., Western blot.

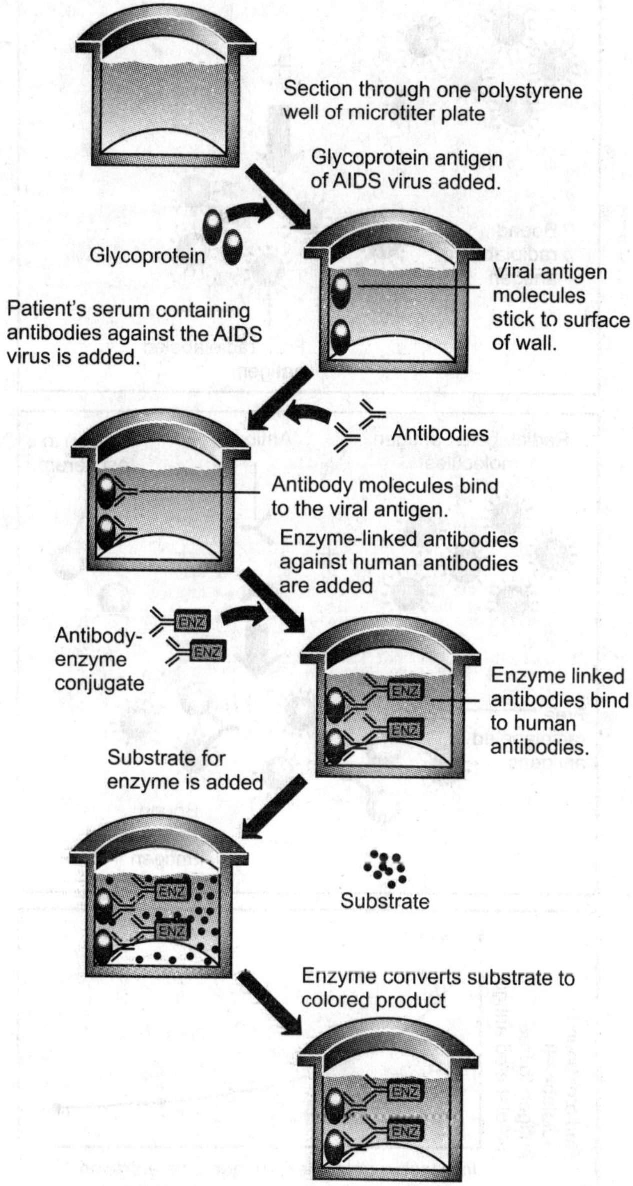

Fig. 24.24 Indirect immunosorbent ELISA technique for the detection and measurement of antibody. The example illustrated here is the detection of antibodies against the AIDS virus (human immunodeficiency virus) in a patient's serum. (Note that the necessary washing after each step is not shown.)

Western Blotting. It is used as a **confirmatory test** for the serodiagnosis of **HIV infection**.

This technique is used to identify proteins (antigens) by using specific antibodies as analytical

probes. The sources of antibody probes may be serum from patients with known infections or purified polyclonal antibody preparations or monoclonal antibodies.

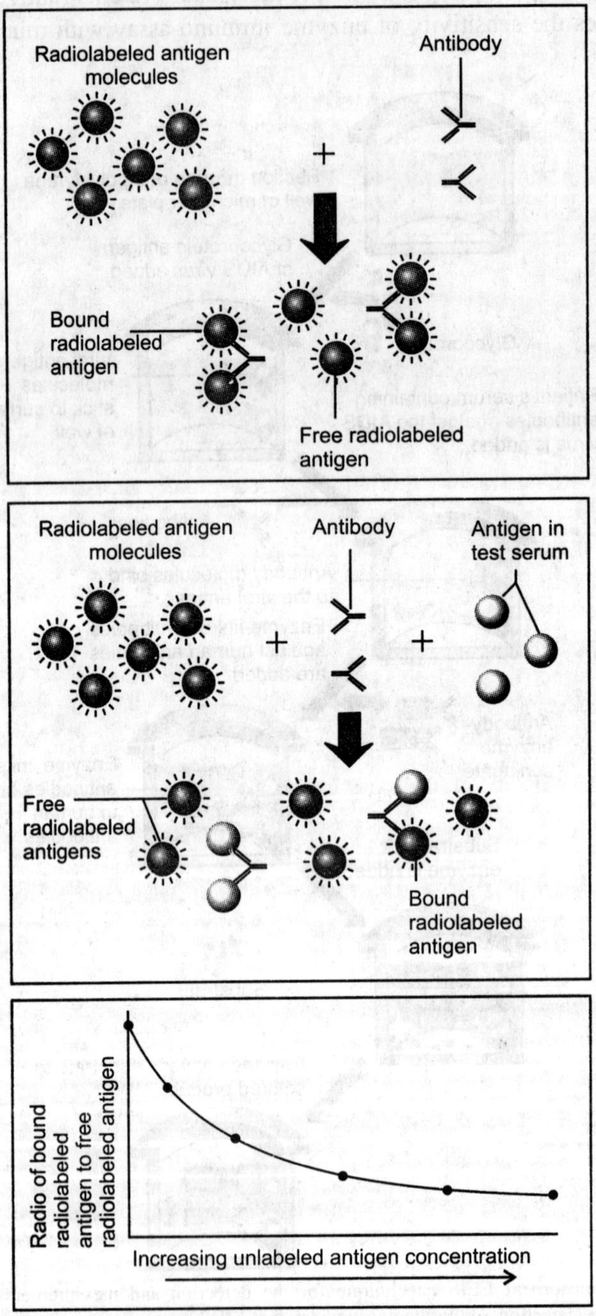

Fig. 24.25 Radioimmunoassay. [A] Radiolabeled antigens bind to specific antibodies. [B] Unlabeled antigen (variable amount in test sample) competes with labeled antigen (fixed amount) for antibody-combining sites (fixed amount of antibodies). [C] As the amount of unlabeled antigen increases, the ratio of antibody-bound labeled antigen to unbound labeled antigen decreases, as shown in the radioimmunoassay calibration curve

Protein antigen mixture is first separated into its components by polyacrylamide gel electrophoresis and then blotted on to nitrocellulose membrane. It is then incubated with specific antibody (Patient's serum). This primary antibody binds to its target protein antigen and is immobilised on the nitrocellulose blotting support. This antigen-antibody complex can then be identified with radioactive or enzyme labelled antibodies (anti-antibodies or antihuman gamma globulin) to primary antibodies, and can then be visualised by autoradiography. If required the labelled anti-antibody can be removed and the protein antigens can be studied further.

When enzyme tagged antihuman gamma globulin is added to detect primary antibody, Enzyme substrate is added subsequently. The substrate changes color in the presence of enzyme and permanently stains the nitrocellulose paper.

IMMUNOCHROMATOGRAPHIC TESTS

Immunochromatographic technique has wide application in serodiagnosis due to its simplicity, economy and reliability.

A one-step qualitative immunochromatographic test for HBsAg will be as follows:

The test system is a small cassette containing a membrane impregnated with anti-HBsAg antibody-colloidal gold dye conjugate. The membrane is exposed at three windows on the cassette. The test serum is dropped into the first window. As the serum travels upstream by capillary action, a colored band appears at the second window (test site) if the serum contains HBsAg indicating a positive reaction. Absence of a colored band at the test site indicates a negative reaction. Simultaneously a colored band should appear in every case at the third window, which forms an inbuilt control, in the absence of which the test is invalid.

IMMUNOELECTRON MICROSCOPIC TESTS

Immunoelectron Microscopy

Antigen-Antibody reactions can be visualised by electron microscope. When viral particles are mixed with specific antisera and observed under the electron microscope, they are seen to be clumped. e.g., detection of Hepatitis A virus and Rotavirus from fecal samples.

Immunoferritin Test

Antigen-Antibody reactions can be visualised by electron microscope with the help of appropriate markers. Ferritin, an electron dense substance from horse spleen can be conjugated with antibody, and such labelled antibody reacting with an antigen can be visualised under the electron microscope.

Immunoenzyme Test

Antigen-Antibody reactions can be visualised by electron microscope with the help of appropriate markers such as enzymes e.g., peroxidases, glucose oxidase, phosphatases, tyrosinase etc.

Some stable enzymes, such as peroxidases, can be conjugated with antibodies. Tissue sections carrying the corresponding antigens are treated with peroxidases, labelled antisera. The peroxidase bound to the antigen can be visualised under the electron microscope, by treatment with enzyme substrate.

NEUTRALIZATION TESTS

Neutralization tests are antigen-antibody reactions that determine whether the activity of a toxin or virus has been neutralized by antibody. Laboratory animals or tissue culture cells are used as

"indicator systems" in these tests. The toxin or virus to be assayed has known effects on the **indicator system**. The effect in the animal might be death, paralysis or skin lesions.

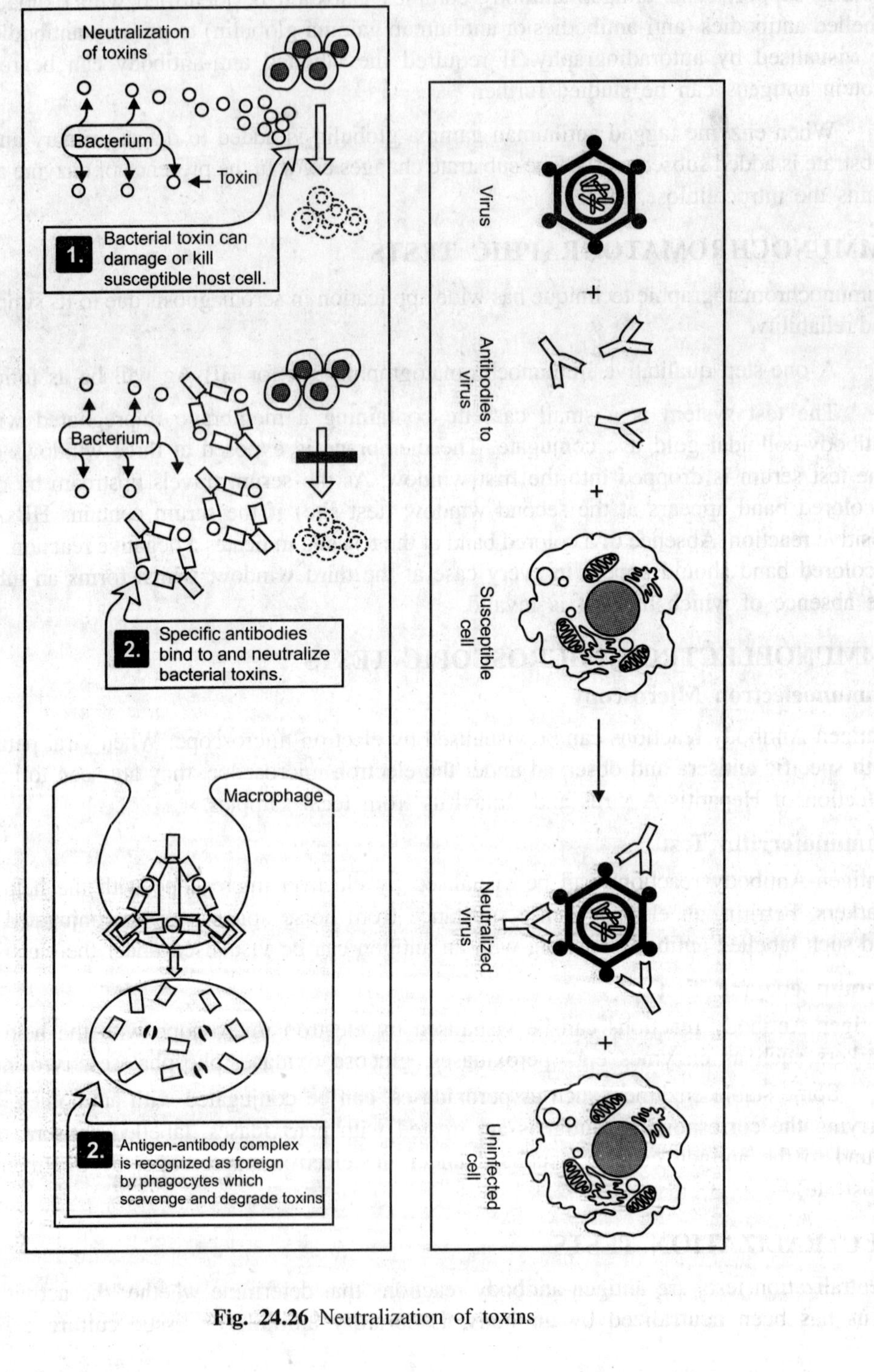

Fig. 24.26 Neutralization of toxins

For example, when the exotoxin of *Clostridum botulinum* is suspected of causing food poisoning in a person, a sample of either suspect food or the serum, stools or vomitus of the patient is collected. Two groups of indicator mice are used. The control group receives the botulinum antitoxin and the experimental group does not. Filtrates of the samples are injected into both groups of mice. If toxin is present, all mice except those receiving the antitoxin will die, and the test is positive for botulism.

Viral neutralization are frequently used to detect viral infections. Suspected blood serum containing viral antibodies can be introduced into tissue culture cells or embroynated eggs. If antibodies are present against the virus, viral neutralization will occur and prevent the virus from infecting the culture cells. No cytopathic effect is seen.

The mechanism of neutralisation of toxins is illustrated in Fig. 24.26.

OPSONIZATION

Opsonization (Greek; Opson = prepare victims for) is a process in which microorganisms or other particles are coated by antibody and/or complement, thereby being prepared for "recognition" and ingestion by phagocytic cells.

Opsonins are substances that make an antigen more susceptible to phagocytosis. Antibodies (IgG) act as opsonins by connecting to the antigen at $F(ab)_2$ site and to the macrophages by F_C receptor. This binding forms a bridge between the phagocyte and the antigen. The macrophage then phagocytoses the antigen and antibody (Fig. 24.27)

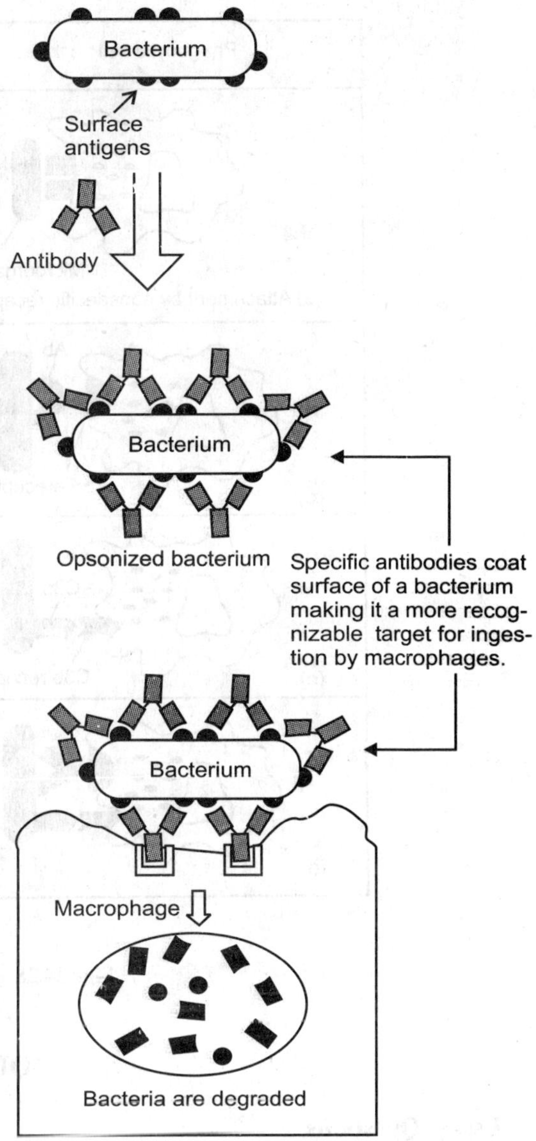

Fig. 24.27. Opsonization of bacteria.

When antigen-antibody complexes activate complement pathway, C3b fragment assembles on the surface of microorganisms. Both neutrophils and macrophages possess surface receptors for C3b. A bridge is formed between microorganisms and phagocytic cells via complement that aids in phagocytosis. (Fig. 24.28)

If both antibody and C3b opsonize, binding is greatly enhanced. (Fig. 24.29)

The **opsonic index** is defined as the ratio of the phagocytic activity of patient's blood for a given bacterium, to the phagocytic activity of blood from a normal individual. It is measured by incubating fresh citrated blood with the bacterial suspension at 37°C for 15 minutes and estimating the average number of phagocytosed bacteria per neutrophils (phagocytic index) from stained blood films.

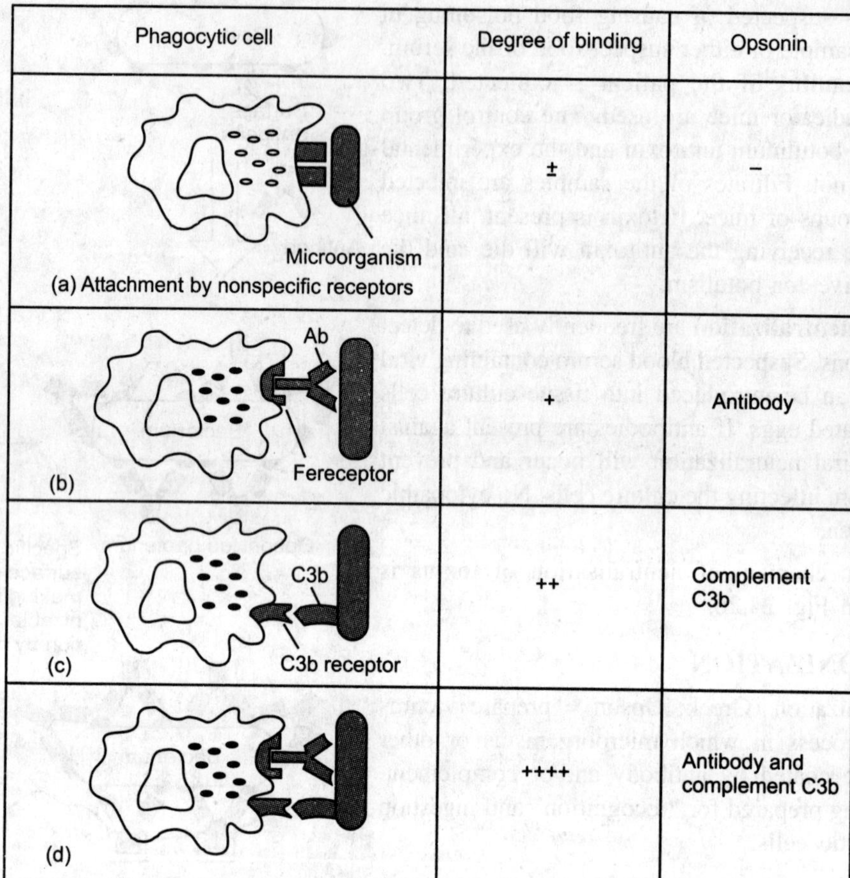

Fig. 24.28. Degree of opsonization

QUESTIONS

Essay Questions

1. Name the various antigen-antibody reactions. Describe the precipitation reactions.
2. Define agglutination. Explain the different methods of agglutination with an example for each (or) Describe the mechanism and applications of agglutination reactions.

Short Notes

1. Mechanism of Ag-Ab reactions/precipitation/Agglutination (or) Marrack's hypothesis.
2. Zone phenomenon (or) prozone.
3. Avidity and affinity.
4. Sensitivity and specificity of a serological test.

5. Titre.
6. Precipitation tests in diagnostic microbiology.

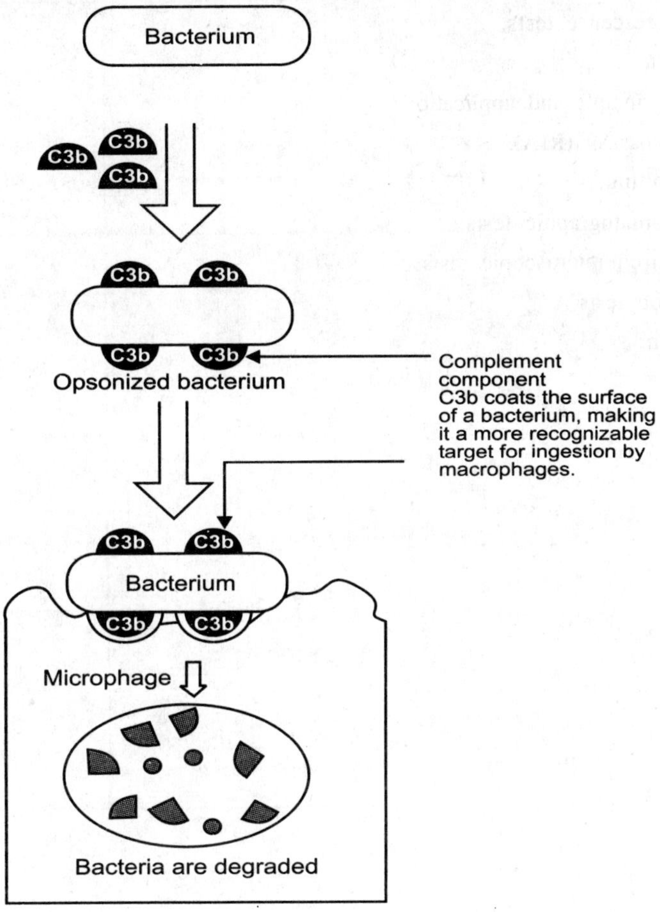

Fig. 24.29 Opsonization of bacteria

7. Ring test.
8. Immunodiffusion (or) gel diffusion.
9. Radial immunodiffusion.
10. Ouchterlony procedure (or) Double diffusion in two dimensions.
11. Electroimmunodiffusion.
12. CIEP.
13. Rocket electrophoresis.
14. Agglutination reactions.
15. Coombs test (or) Antiglobulin test.
16. Passive agglutination test.
17. Co-agglutination.

18. Reverse passive agglutination.
19. Complement fixation test (or) CFT.
20. Neutralization tests.
21. Immunofluorescence tests.
22. Opsonization.
23. ELISA–its principle and application.
24. Radioimmunoassay (RIA).
25. Western blotting.
26. Immunochromatographic tests.
27. Immunoelectron microscopic tests.
28. Neutralisation tests.
29. Opsonization.

25

The Complement System

- *Definition*
- *Pfeiffer's phenomenon*
- *Inactivation of serum*
- *Components of C*
- *C cascade*
- *Classical pathway*
- *Alternative pathway (properdin pathway)*
- *Properdin*
- *Biological effects of C*
- *C 1 inhibitor*
- *Biosynthesis of C components*
- *Deficiency diseases of C system*
- *Conglutinin or conglutination*

DEFINITION

Complement (C) is defined as a group of proteins present in normal serum, that are activated characteristically by antigen-antibody interaction, and subsequently mediate a number of biologically significant consequences such as cell lysis, immobilisation etc.

PFEIFFER'S PHENOMENON

Pfeiffer (1894) demonstrated that cholera vibrios were lysed when injected intraperitoneally into specifically immunized Guinea-pigs. This "**bacteriolysis *in vivo***" is known as Pfeiffer's phenomenon and is due to the activation of complement by antigen-antibody complexes.

INACTIVATION OF SERUM

C as a whole is heat labile. Its activity undergoes spontaneous denaturation slowly at room temperature and being destroyed in 30 min. at 56°C.

A serum, when heated at 56°C for 30 min in a water bath, will be deprived of its complement activity, is then said to be "inactivated" and the process is known as "Inactivation of serum".

COMPONENTS OF C

The complement system contains as group of about 20 chemically and immunologically distinct serum proteins comprising C components, the properdin system and the control proteins.

The complement (C) is a complex of a nine different protein fractions called C1 and to C9. C1 is made up of three protein subunits called C1q, C1r, and C1s. Thus C is made up of a total of 11 different proteins.

C components once activated react in a sequence as a cascade. C proteins are named C1 to C9 in the sequence of cascading reaction, except that C4 comes after C1, before C2. (Fig. 25.1).

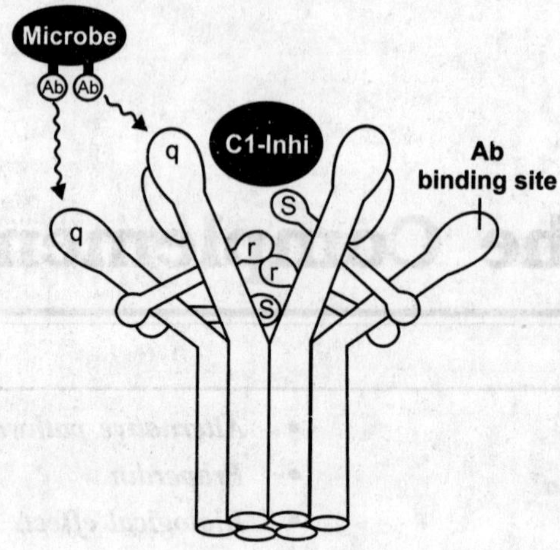

Fig. 25.1. C1 complex.

C CASCADE

The model commonly used to explain C activity in immune cytolysis is the lysis of erythrocyte (E) sensitised by its antibody (A). The erythrocyte (E) antibody (A) complex is called EA, and when C components are attached to EA, the product is called EAC, followed by the components that have reacted (e.g., EAC 14235).

When a C component acquires enzymatic activity it is indicated by a bar over the component number. For example, the enzymatically activated C1 is shown as $\overline{C\,1}$.

Fragments cleaved from C components during the cascade reaction are indicated by small letters (e.g., C3a, C3b).

Inactivated forms of C components are indicated by the suffix "i" (C4i).

Once activated, C components react sequentially in a cascade fashion or like a row of falling dominoes. Some complement proteins act as protease enzymes, cleaving and activating the next protein in the sequence. The larger fragments usually join the cascade. The smaller fragments possess inflammatory effects.

Based on C3 activation, there are two pathways—classical and alternative pathways.

Table 25.1: Proteins of the Complement Cascade in Serum

Protein	*Fragment*	*Function*
Recognition Unit		
C1	q	Binds to the Fc portion of antigen-antibody complexes
	r	Subunit of C1; activates Cls
	s	Cleaves C4 and C2 due to its enzymatic activity

Activation Unit		
C2		Causes viral neutralization
C3	a	Anaphylatoxin, immunoregulatory
	b	Key component of the alternative pathway and major opsonin in serum Induces leukocytosis
C4	a	Anaphylatoxin
	b	Causes viral neutralization; opsonin
Membrane Attack Unit		
C5	a	Anaphylatoxin; principal chemotactic factor in serum; induces neutrophil attachment to blood vessel walls
	b	Initiates membrane attack
C6, C7, C8, C9		Participate with C5b in formation of the membrane attack complex that lyses targeted cells
Alternative Pathway		
Factor B		Causes macrophage spreading on surfaces; precursor of C3 convertase
Factor $\overline{D}$		Cleaves Factor B to form active C3Bb in alterantive pathway
Properdin		Stabilizes alternative pathway C3 convertase
Regulatory Proteins		
Factor H		Promotes C3b breakdown and regulates alternative pathway
Factor I		Degrades C3b and regulates alternative pathway
C4b binding protein		Inhibits assembly and accelerates decay of C4bC2a
C1 INH complex		Binds to and dissociates Clr and Cls from Cl
S protein		Binds fluid-phase C5b67; prevents membrane attachment

CLASSICAL PATHWAY

It refers to a chain of cascade reactions in which C components react in a specific sequence following activation of C1 and typically causing immune cytolysis is known as the classical pathway. It consists of following steps.

(1) C1 binds to the antigen-antibody (EA) complex. The recognition unit of C1 is C1q, which reacts with F_C piece of bound IgM or IgG (IgG3, 1, and 2). C1q binding in the presence of calcium ions leads to sequential activation of C1r and C1s.

(2) Activated $\overline{C1s}$ is an esterase (C1s esterase) which cleaves C4 into C4a (an anaphylatoxin) and C4b which binds to cell membrane alongwith C1.

(3) $\overline{C14b}$, in the presence of magnesium ions cleaves C2 into C2a, which binds to cell membrane alongwith C14b and C2b (kinins released into fluid phase). $\overline{C1\,4b\,2a}$, has enzymatic activity and is referred to as the classical pathway C3 convertase.

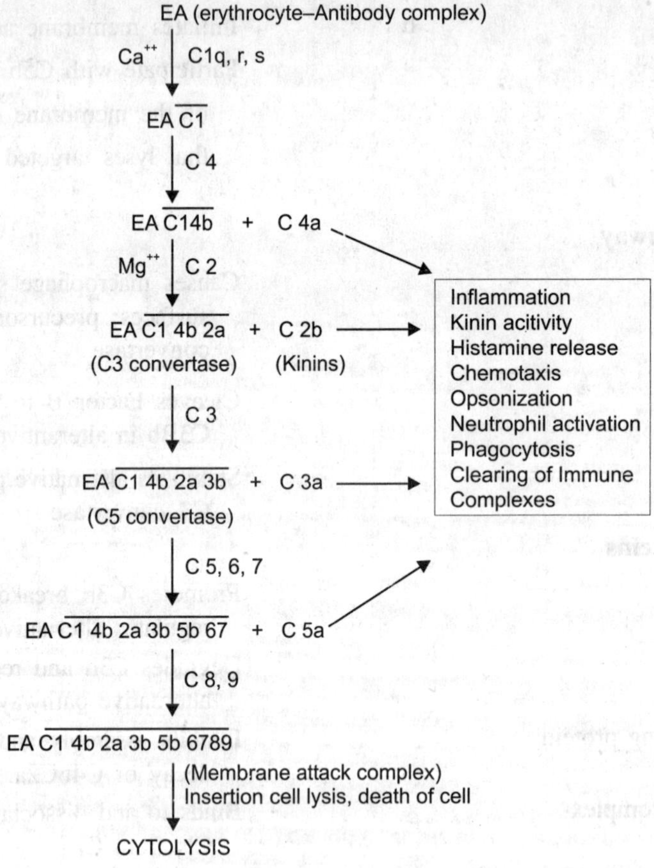

Fig. 25.2 Classical pathway.

(4) C3 convertase splits C3 into two fragments C3a (an anaphylatoxin) and C3b which remains cell bound alongwith C14b2a to form $\overline{C1\,4b\,2a\,3b}$, which has enzymatic activity and is called C5 convertase (C3a interacts with tissue leucocytes called mast cells which release mediators of the inflammatory response).

(5) C5 convertase cleaves C5 into C5a (an anaphylatoxin) and C5b which continues with the cascade C6 and C7 then join together forming $\overline{C5\,b\,67}$, which binds to the cell membrane and prepares it for lysis by C8 and C9 which join the reaction subsequently, known as "membrane attack complex ($\overline{C5\,b\,6789}$) that creates pores by forming a channel across the plasma membrane of the target cell. This channel allows potassium ions to leave the cell and water and sodium to ente:; the cell swells and lyses. (Fig. 25.3) (C5a is a chemotactic factor that attracts phagocytes).

The classical pathway is generally activated by antigen-antibody complexes. Besides antigen-antibody complexes; DNA, CRP, trypsin like enzymes or some retroviruses can also activate complement.

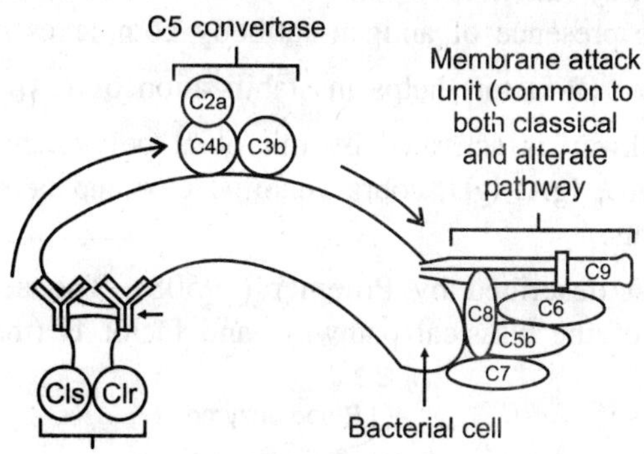

Fig. 25.3. Complement mediated cell lysis

ALTERNATIVE C PATHWAY (PROPERDIN PATHWAY)

The central process in the complement cascade is the activation of C3. In the classical pathway, C3 is activated by $\overline{C142}$, known as classical C3 convertase. The activation of C3 without prior participation of C142 is known as the "alternative pathway".

It plays an important role in the innate, nonspecific immune defense against intravascular invasion by bacteria and some fungi that occur before the development of specific antibodies.

The alternative pathway is activated by microbial polysaccharides (zymosan from yeast cell wall), endotoxins of Gram negative bacilli, protozoa, IgA, IgD, cobra venom factor and the nephritic factor present in serum of glomerulonephritis patients. The alternative pathway can occur in body fluids rather than on a cell surface and does not require the presence of antigen-antigbody complexes or the C1 recognition unit.

The alternative pathway begins with the cleavage of C3 into C3a and C3b by an enzyme present in the blood. These fragments are produced at a slow rate and do not carry out the next step, the cleavage of C5, because free C3b is rapidly cleaved into inactive fragments by serum protein factors H and I.

However, when C3b binds to lipopolysaccharides, endotoxins, aggregates of IgA or IgE, Zymosan etc., it becomes stable. A protein in blood termed Factor B adsorbs to bound C3b and is cleaved into two fragments by factor D, leading to the formation of active enzyme $\overline{C3bBb}$. This complex is sometimes called the C3 convertase, because it cleaves more C3 to C3a and C3b. $\overline{C3bBb}$ is extremely labile and is stabilized by properdin (factor P), another serum protein, to form C3B b b P complex. When a second C3b molecule is added to the C3b B b P complex, a conformational change occurs that makes it into an enzyme, C5 convertase ($\overline{C3bBb3b}$).

This C5 convertase then cleaves C5 to C5a and C5b, leading to further steps in the cascade, similar to classical pathway.

PROPERDIN

Properdin system is a group of serum proteins, which play an important role in the innate nonspecific immune defense against intravascular invasion by bacteria and some fungi that occur before the development of specific antibodies.

The properdin pathway (alternative pathway) occurs in body fluids rather than on a cell surface and does not require the presence of antigen-antibody complexes or C1 recognition unit.

The properdin factor (P-factor) helps in stabilization of $\overline{C3bBb}$ in alternative pathway.

The alternative pathway is activated by microbial polysaccharides (zymosan from yeast cell wall), endotoxins, protozoa, IgA, IgD, cobra venom factor and nephritic factor present in serum of glomerulonephritis patients.

Properdin was first described by Pillemer (1950S). The action of the properdin pathway requires Mg^{++} (like C4 of the classical pathway) and factor B (that resembled C2).

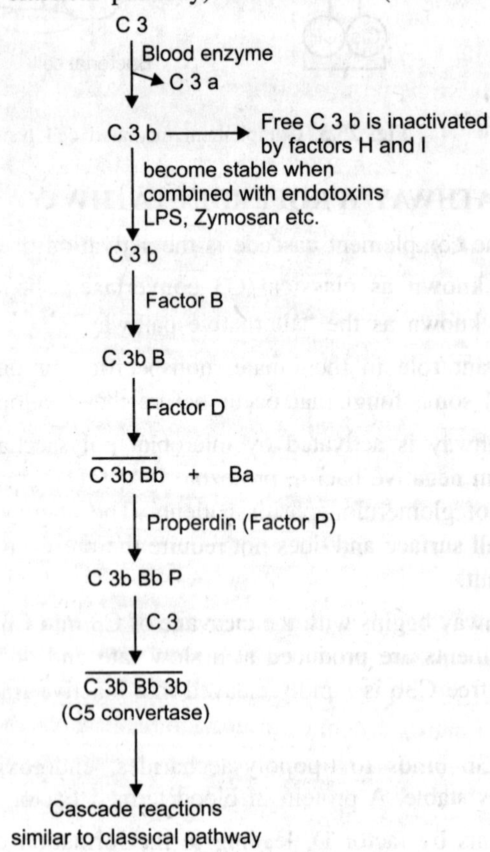

Fig. 25.4 Alternative Complement pathway.

Properdin factor in serum when combined with zymosan, a yeast cell wall polysaccharide, selectively consumes C3, without requiring C1, C4 and C2. This is known as alternative pathway (properdin pathway) of complement activation.

BIOLOGICAL EFFECTS OF C

Complement system is protective by three general ways; (1) early steps of cascade stimulate the inflammatory response (2) Intermediate steps of cascade release substances that attract phagocytic cells and render them highly active (3) Once activated, the C system results in the assembly of lytic complexes that cause lysis of invading microorganisms.

Complement mediates several important biological functions.

(1) The classical and alterantive pathways results in **bacteriolysis** and **cytolysis**. Gram negative bacteria are sensitive to lysis. Gram positive bacteria are killed without lysis.

(2) C facilitates **opsonization** by promoting the uptake and destruction of pathogens by phagocytes. Several C receptors are present on the surface of macrophages, monocytes and neutrophils, which stimulate phagocytosis and removal of immune complexes.

(3) C bound to antigen-antibody complexes adheres to RBC. This reaction is called "**immune adherence**", contributes to defense against pathogens by promoting phagocytosis.

(4) C exhibits antiviral activity. The neutralization of viruses requires the participation of C.

(5) C also effects **immobilization** of motile organisms.

(6) C fragments released during cascade reaction help in amplifying the **inflammatory response**. C2 kinins are vasoactive amines and increase capillary permeability and smooth muscle contraction. C4a, C3a and C5a are anaphylotoxic (release histamine) and chemotactic.

(7) It also interacts with the coagulation, fibrinolytic and kininogenic systems of blood.

C also participates in the pathogenesis of several diseases.

(8) The C receptor (CR 2) on B lymphocytes acts as a receptor for Epstein-Barr (EB) virus and contributes to the pathogenesis of infectious mononucleosis.

(9) C participates in the Type II (cytolytic and cytotoxic) hypersensitivity reactions e.g., The lysis of RBC following incompatible blood transfusion; thrombocytopenia in sedormid purpura.

(10) C also participates in the pathogenesis of Type III (immune complex) hypersensitivity reactions e.g., nephrotoxic nephritis, serum sickness, Arthus phenomenon.

(11) C plays a major role in the pathogenesis of autoimmune hemolytic anemia, paroxysmal nocturnal hemoglobinuria and hereditary angioneurotic edema. C components level in blood decreases in several autoimmune diseases such as SLE and Rheumatoid arthritis.

(12) In endotoxic shock, there is a massive C3 fixation and platelet adherence. The lysis of platelets and the release of platelet factor leads to the disseminated intravascular coagulation and thrombocytopenia.

C1 INHIBITOR

Normal serum contains an inhibitor of C1 esterase (C1s INH) known as C1 inhibitor. It does not prevent the normal progress of the C cascade but checks its autocatalytic prolongation. It is an alpha neuraminoglycoprotein and heat labile. It also inhibits many other esterases found in blood such as plasmin, kininogen and Hageman factor.

BIOSYNTHESIS OF C COMPONENTS

C components are synthesized in various organs of the body.

C component	*Site of synthesis*
C1	intestinal epithelium
C2, C4	Macrophages
C5, C8	Spleen
C3, C6, C9	Liver
C7	Unknown

DEFICIENCY DISEASES OF C SYSTEM

Deficiency	*Disease*
C1 inhibitor	Hereditary angioneurotic edema
C1, C2, C4 (early components of classical pathway)	SLE and other collagen diseases
C5 to C8	Bacteremia (mainly with Gram negative diplococci), Toxoplasmosis

C deficiencies result in host with an inability to eliminate microbial antigens or immune complexes. Recurrent bacterial and fungal infections and collagen diseases also occur.

CONGLUTININ AND CONGLUTINATION

Bovine blood contains an abnormal protein called conglutinin (K) which causes clumping of particles or cells coated with C, a process known as conglutination. Conglutinin reacts only with bound C3.

Conglutinin requires Ca^{2+} for its activity and acts as an antibody to C, but it is not an Ig. Antibodies with conglutinin-like activity can be produced by immunization with C-coated materials.

It may also occur in humans and other mammals as autoantibodies to fixed C. Their titres increase in infections and autoimmune diseases associated with increased fixation of C *in vivo.*

QUESTIONS

Essay Question

1. Define complement. Describe the C cascade reactions. Add a note on biological functions of complement.

Short Notes

1. Complement or components of C.
2. Classical pathway.
3. Alternative pathway.
4. C3.
5. Activation of alternative pathway.
6. Pfeiffer's phenomenon.
7. Properdin.
8. Conglutinin or Conglutination.
9. Inactivation of serum.
10. C1 inhibitor.
11. Biosynthesis of C.
12. Deficiency diseases of C system.

26

Major Histocompatibility Complex

- *Introduction*
- *MHC Complex or HLA Complex of genes*
- *HLA molecules*
  - *HLA class I antigens*
  - *HLA class II molecules*
  - *HLA class III molecules*
- *MHC Restriction*
- *Costimulation*
- *HLA typing*

INTRODUCTION

Almost all human tissue cells contain surface antigens on their plasma membranes, known as "histocompatibility antigens".

They bind to antigens and present them to T-cells and are responsible for antigen recognition by the T-cell receptor. They are also responsible for rejection of allografts. They are helpful in maximizing protection against microbial infections.

"Major histocompatibility complex (MHC)" is a general term and refers to any histocompatibility antigen complex involved in antigen presentation to T-cells.

The major antigens determining histocompatibility in humans are alloantigens, characteristically found on the surface of leucocytes. Human MHC antigens are therefore called "Human leucocyte antigen (HLA) complex" and MHC complex of genes with HLA complex.

HLA COMPLEX OF GENES/MHC COMPLEX OF GENES

MHC complex possesses a cluster of genes on the short arm of one chromosome pair 6. It consists of 3 separate classes of genes coding for 3 different classes of proteins. (Fig. 26.1)

(1) Class I genes comprising A, B and C loci, coding for class I antigens that determine histocompatibility and the acceptance or rejection of allografts.

(2) Class II genes or the D region comprising DR, DQ and DP loci, coding for class II antigens that regulate the immune response.

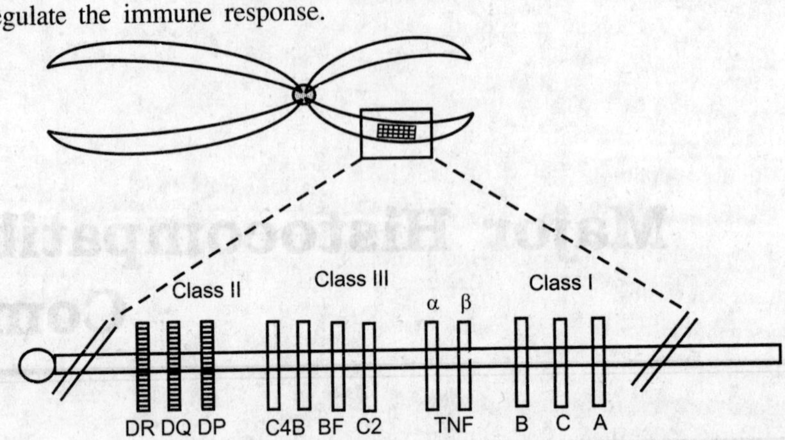

Fig. 26.1 MHC complex LOCI on chromosome 6

3. Class III genes or the complement region containing genes for complement components C2 and C4 of the classical pathway, as well as properdin factor B of the alternative pathway, Tumor necrosis factor (TNF) alpha and beta and heat-shock proteins.

Each individual has 2 sets of these genes, one from each parent; a person can have any combination of 8 different MHC or HLA molecules. Only one gene of each pair can code for an antigen in a given individual, and these antigens are different from one individual to another. The closer two individuals are related, the more similar are their histocompatibility antigens.

The Immune response (Ir) genes which control immunological responses to specific antigens are believed to be situated in the Class I region, associated with DR locus.

HLA MOLECULES

HLA antigens are two-chain glycoprotein molecules anchored on the surface membrane of cells.

HLA Class I Antigens

They are found virtually on all nucleated cells. They are the main antigens involved in graft rejection and cell mediated cytolysis. Class I molecules may also function as components of hormone receptors.

Class I molecules consists of a heavy peptide chain, called alpha chain, which is linked non-covalently to a smaller peptide called β_2 microglobulin (beta chain). (Fig. 26.2)

The beta chain has a constant amino acid sequence and is coded for by a gene on chromosome 15. The alpha chain consists of three globular domains (alpha 1, alpha 2 and alpha 3) which protrude from the plasma membrane and a short hydrophilic sequence carries the C-terminus into the cytoplasm.

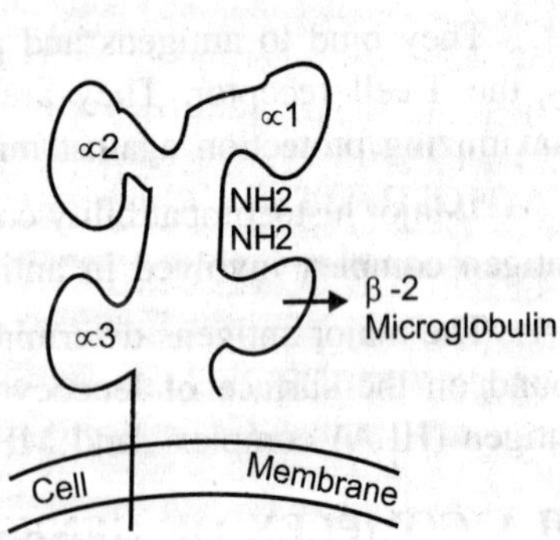

Fig. 26.2 HLA Class I molecule

The distal domains (alpha 1 and alpha 2) have highly variable amino acid sequences and are folded to form a cavity or groove between them.

Protein antigens processed by macrophages or dendritic cells to form small peptides are bound to this groove for presentation to CD8 T-cells. The T-cell will recognize the antigen only when presented as a complex with the MHC Class I molecule and not otherwise. This phenomenon is called "MHC Restriction". When so presented, the CD8 cytotoxic Killer cell destroys the target cell such as a virus infected cell.

Class I antigens serve to identify all cells of the body as "self". They also stimulate antibody production when introduced into a host with different Class I antigens. This is the basis for HLA typing when a patient is being prepared for an organ transplant.

HLA Class II Molecules

They are more restricted in distribution, being found only on cells of the immune system such as macrophages, dendritic cells, Langerhans cells, activated T-cells and particularly on B-cell. (Fig. 26.3)

Class II antigens are heterodimers, consisting of an alpha and beta chain; noncovalently associated transmembrane glycoproteins. Each chain has two domains, the proximal domain being the constant region and the distal domain variable. The two distal domains (alpha 1, beta 1) constitute the antigen-binding site, for recognition by CD4 lymphocytes, in a fashion similar to the recognition of the class I antigen peptide complex by CD8 T-cells. HLA Class II molecules are primarily responsible for graft versus host (GVH) reaction and mixed leucocyte reaction (MLR).

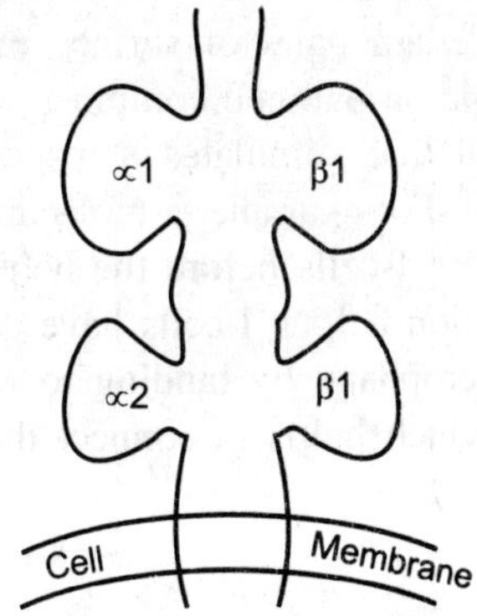

Fig. 26.3 HLA Class II molecule.

Class II antigens do not stimulate antibody production but are required for T-cell communication with macrophages and B lymphocytes.

Part of the T-cell receptor must recognize a class II antigen on the adjacent cell before the T-cell can secrete lymphokines necessary for the immune response.

HLA Class III Molecules

They are heterogenous. They include complement components C2 and C4 of the classical pathway, as well as properdin factor B of the alternative pathway, Tumour necrosis factor (TNF) alpha and beta and heat shock proteins.

MHC RESTRICTION

B-cells respond to antigens that are either in solution or on a cell surface, but a T-cell characteristically responds to processed antigens on the macrophages or dendritic cells only when they are presented along with the self-MHC antigen. This phenomenon is known as MHC restriction. Both Class I and Class II antigens operate in this phenomenon.

CD8 cytotoxic killer cells can recognize and destroy the target cells (such as virus infected cell) when it is presented by Class I MHC molecules.

CD4 lymphocytes (helper T-cells) can recognize and accept antigen processed by macrophages only when the macrophages bear the same Class II MHC molecules on the surface. For T-cells participating in delayed hypersensitivity, the antigen has to be presented along with Class II MHC determinants.

The major biological function of MHC restriction is to exercise a genetic control on the entire specific immune system through an action on T_H cell generation.

COSTIMULATION

The combination of a MHC-II with an antigen is usually only the first signal necessary to produce a response from a B or T-cell. In many cases costimulation by a second signal is required. Costimulation is usually achieved by cytokines.

Certain pairs of surface molecules can also be involved in costimulation. When the surface molecule on one cell combines with the surface molecule on another cell, the combination can act as a signal that stimulates a response from one of the cells, or the combination can hold the cells together. For example, a molecule called B7 on macrophages must bind with a molecule called CD28 on helper T-cells before the helper T-cells can respond to the antigen presented by the macrophage. In addition helper T-cells have a glycoprotein, called CD4, which helps to connect helper T-cells to the macrophage by binding to MHC Class-II antigen. Cytotoxic T-cells have a glycoprotein called CD8, which helps to connect them to body cells displaying MHC Class-I antigens. (Fig. 26.4 and Fig. 26.5)

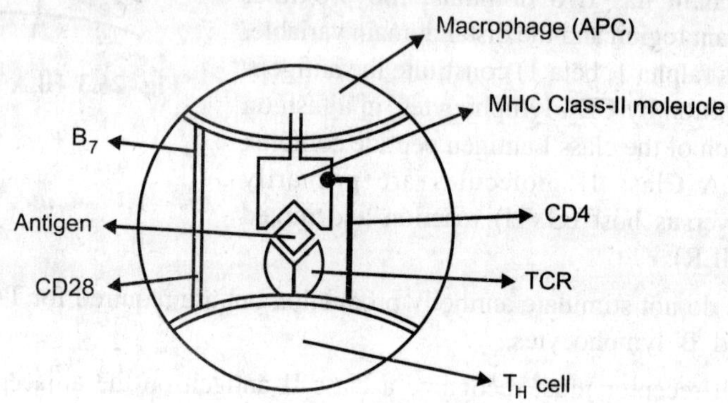

Fig. 26.4 CD4 binds to MHC-II molecules.

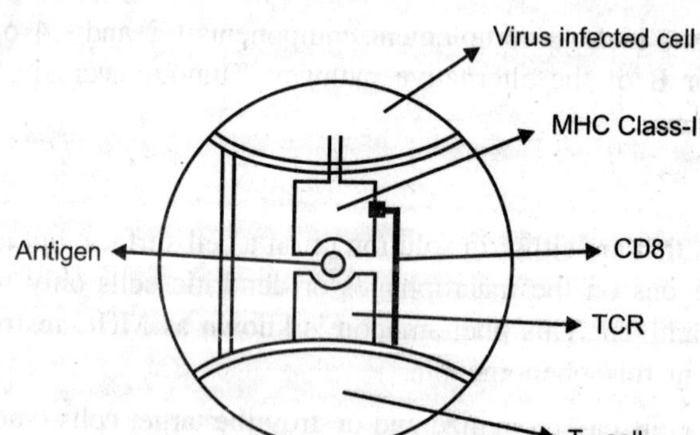

Fig. 26.5 CD8 binds to MHC-I molecules

HLA TYPING/TISSUE TYPING

HLA typing is used

1. for testing compatibility between recipients and potential donors before tissue transplantation
2. in disputed paternity
3. in anthropological studies
4. for establishing disease associations.

Histocompatibility is tested by HLA typing and tissue matching. The standard serological typing method is **Microcytotoxicity test,** which tests for complement mediated lysis of peripheral blood lymphocytes with a standard set of typing sera. Lymphocyte suspensions are added to microwells of tissue typing trays predispensed with a panel of HLA typing sera, each containing antibodies to a specific HLA antigen, and incubated with complement. Cells carrying antigens corresponding to the HLA antiserum are killed by complement mediated cell lysis. This can be detected by adding trypan blue or eosin which stains only dead cells. The lymphocytes are presumed to have HLA antigens corresponding to the specificities of the antisera that caused cell death, as indicated by the staining.

Antisera for HLA typing were originally obtained from multiparous women, placental fluid and from multiple blood transfusion recipients, who have antibodies to paternal or donor HLA antigens. At present monoclonal antibodies are widely used.

RFLP, southern blotting, PCR methods can also be used for tissue typing.

Among a set of HLA donors, the best donors can be chosen by tissue matching. This is done by **mixed lymphocyte reaction** (MLR) or mixed lymphocyte culture (MLC) and primed lymphocyte typing.

In MLR, the T-lymphocytes in culture, when exposed to HLA incompatible antigens, will undergo blast transformation, the intensity of the reaction being a measure of the antigenic disparity between the donor and recipient lymphocytes. The test is a one-way test in which the donor lymphocytes are killed only the recipient lymphocytes are permitted to be transformed in response to the incompatible antigens on the donor cells.

QUESTIONS

Essay Question

Give an account of MHC (or) Describe HLA system of antigens.

Short Notes

1. MHC
2. HLA (or) HLA antigens
3. HLA Class I antigens
4. Describe HLA antigens. Add a note on their role in immunity.
5. HLA typing
6. Microcytotoxicity test
7. MHC Restriction
8. MHC Complex or MHC Genes.

27

Organs, Tissues and Cells of The Immune System/Structure and Functions of The Immune System

- *Introduction*
- *Lymphoid cells*
- *Immune response*
- *Organs and tissues of the immune system (lymphoid organs)*
- *Primary (central) lymphoid organs*
  - *Thymus*
  - *Bursa of fabricius*
  - *Bone marrow*
- *Secondary (peripheral) lymphoid organs*
  - *Spleen*
  - *Lymph nodes*
  - *MALT*
- *Lymphocytes*
- *Differential characteristics of T cells and B cells*
- *Development of T cells*
- *T lymphocytes*
- *Development and maturation of B lymphocytes*
- *B lymphocytes*
- *Plasma cells*
- *Null cells/Large granular lymphocytes (LGL)*
  - *Natural killer (NK) cells*
  - *Killer (K) cells/ADCC cells*
  - *Lymphokine activated killer (LAK) cells*
- *Phagocytes/Macrophages*
- *Phagocytosis*
- *Antigen presenting cells (APCs)*
  - *Macrophages*
  - *B-lymphocytes*
  - *Dendritic cells*
  - *Langerhans' cells*
- *Neutrophils*
- *Eosinophils*
- *Basophils and Mast cells*
- *Mitogens*

INTRODUCTION

The immune system is an organization of organs, tissues, cells and molecules with specialized roles in defending against microorganisms, viruses, cancer cells and nonself proteins (*e.g.,* organ transplants). The cells of the immune system are present throughout the host's body. Some become residents within tissues, where they respond to local trauma and alarm; others circulate in body fluids and are recruited to the sites of infection. The cells responsible for both nonspecific and specific immunity are the white blood cells called leukocytes. In defending the host against pathogenic microorganisms, leukocytes cooperate with each other first to recognize the pathogen and then to destroy it.

LYMPHOID CELLS

Lymphocytes (Latin; lympha = water, cyte = cell) are the major cells of the specific immune system. Lymphocytes can be divided into three populations – T cells, B cells, and Nuli cells. B lymphocytes reach maturity within the bone marrow, circulate in the blood, and also settle in various lymphoid organs. T lymphocytes mature in the thymus gland; they can remain in the thymus, circulate in the blood, or reside in lymphoid organs such as the lymph nodes and spleen. (Fig. 27.1)

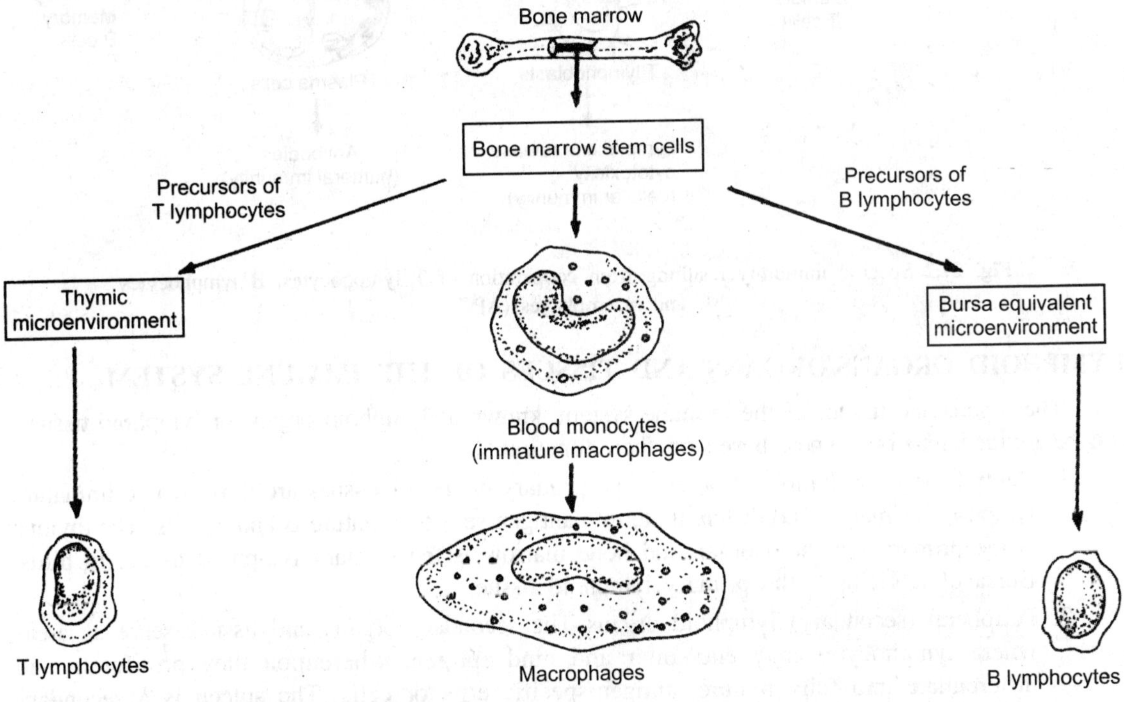

Fig. 27.1 Pathways of development of cells in the dual immune system

IMMUNE RESPONSE

The specific reactivity induced in a host by an antigenic stimulus is known as "Immune response". (Fig. 27.2)

Immune response to an antigen is of two types –

1. Humoral Immune response or Antibody mediated immunity – mediated by antibodies produced by plasma cells, that are transformed B lymphocytes.

2. Cellular Immune response or cell mediated immunity–mediated directly by sensitized T lymphocytes.

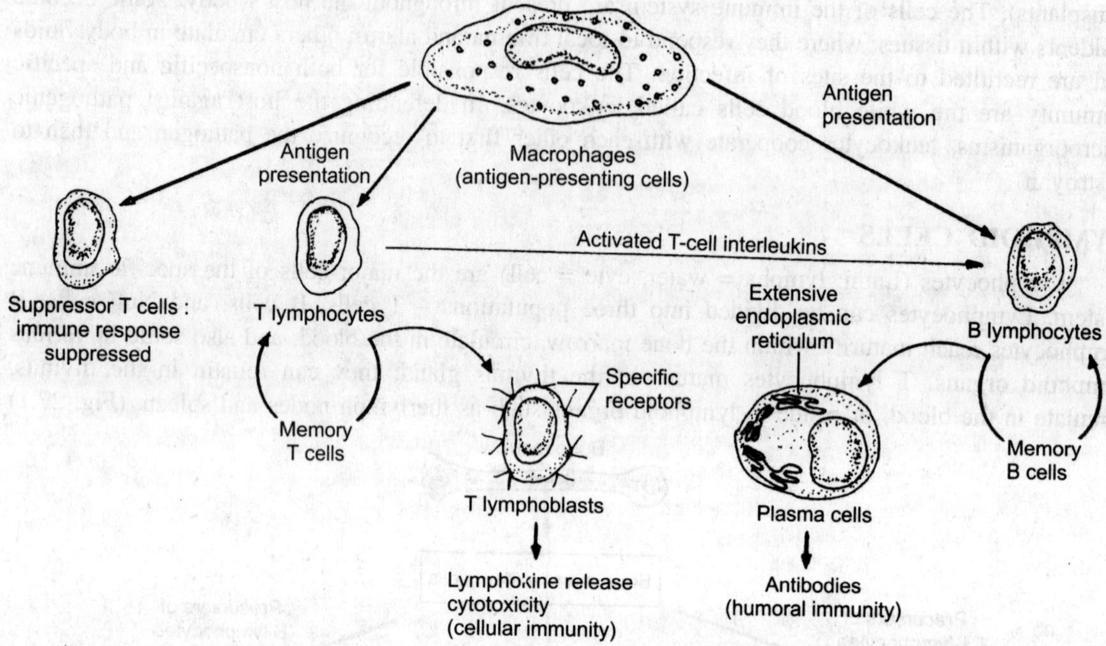

Fig. 27.2 Specific immunity resulting from cooperation of T lymphocytes, B lymphocytes and macrophages (APC)

LYMPHOID ORGANS/ORGANS AND TISSUES OF THE IMMUNE SYSTEM

The organs and tissues of the immune system, known as lymphoid organs or lymphoid tissues, can be divided into two types, based on their function.

1. Central (primary) lymphoid organs–The primary organs or tissues are those where immature lymphocytes mature and differentiate into antigen-sensitive mature B and T cells. The thymus is the primary lymphoid organ and bone marrow is the primary lymphoid tissue. In birds, Bursa of fabricius is the primary lymphoid tissue.
2. Peripheral (secondary) lymphoid organs–The secondary organs and tissues serve as areas where lymphocytes may encounter and bind antigen, whereupon they proliferate and differentiate into fully mature, antigen-specific effector cells. The spleen is a secondary lymphoid organ and the lymph nodes and Mucosal-associated lymphoid tissues (MALT) are the secondary lymphoid tissues.

PRIMARY (CENTRAL) LYMPHOID ORGANS

Immature undifferentiated lymphocytes are generated in the bone marrow, and mature and become committed to a particular antigenic specificity within the primary lymphoid organs/tissues. The two most important of these in mammals are the thymus and bone marrow.

Thymus

It is a lymphoid organ located above the heart, behind the upper part of the sternum, extending into the neck on the front and sides of trachea. It develops from the epithelium of third and fourth pharyngeal pouches, at about sixth week of embryonic life.

The embryonic thymus consists of epithelial cells surrounded by a thin capsule. In embryonic life, mesenchymal stem cells (precursors of lymphocytes) from the yolk sac, fetal liver and bone marrow reach the thymus and differentiate into the thymic lymphoid cells (thymocytes) by about eighth week. (Fig. 27.3)

The thymus has two lobes surrounded by a fibrous capsule. Septa arising from the capsule divide the gland into lobules, each containing an outer cortex and inner medulla.

Prothymocytes, from the bone marrow, migrate through blood stream, enter the cortex and divide. Thus, cortex is crowded with actively proliferating small lymphocytes. The medulla consists mainly of epithelial cells and mature lymphocytes, in the middle of which are the Hassall's corpuscles. (Fig. 27.4)

The primary function of the thymus is the production of thymic lymphocytes or T lymphocytes, responsible for cell mediated immunity and also humoral immunity by T_H cells.

Thymus is the major site for lymphocyte proliferation in the body. However, most cells die in the process. Of the lymphocytes produced only 5% leave the thymus in viable state. It is believed that this destruction in thymus may eliminate lymphocyte clones that react against self. The lymphocyte proliferation in thymus is not dependent on antigenic stimulation (unlike in peripheral lymphoid organs).

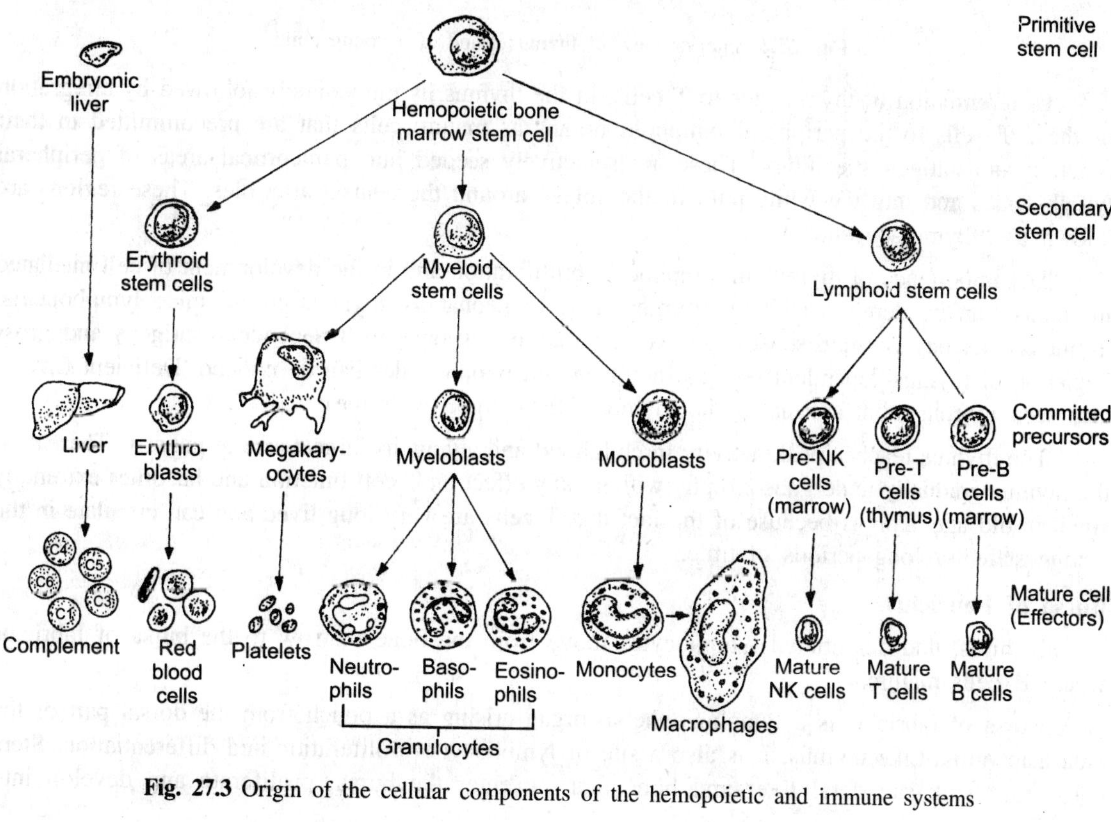

Fig. 27.3 Origin of the cellular components of the hemopoietic and immune systems

In thymus, the lymphocytes acquire new surface antigens (Thy antigens). Thymus confers immunological competence on the lymphocytes during their stay in the organ. In other words, the lymphocytes are educated to acquire immunocompetence, so that they become capable of mounting immune response against appropriate antigens. This is effected under thymic microenvironment and several hormones like thymosin, thymopoietin and thymulin produced by thymic epithelium.

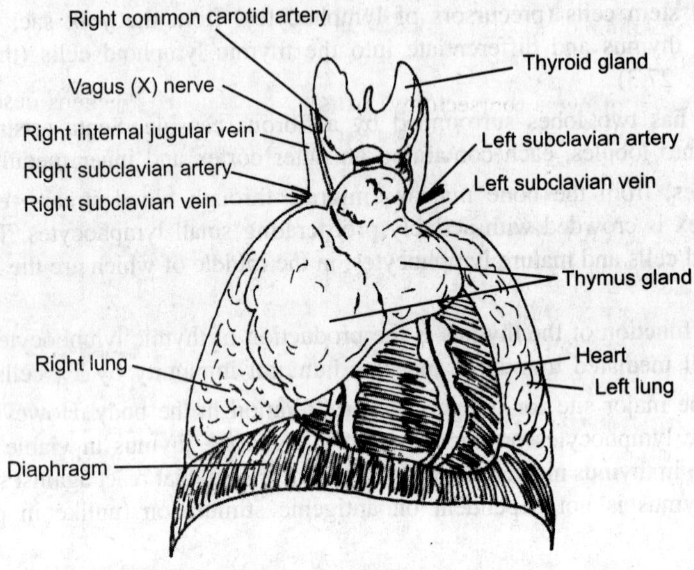

Fig. 27.4 Anterior view of thymus gland of a young child.

Differentiation of thymocytes to T cells, in the thymus, is immediately followed by emigration of these T cells to the peripheral lymphoid organs as mature cells that are precommitted to their function and antigen specificity. These are selectively seeded into paracortical areas of peripheral lymph nodes and into the white pulp of the spleen around the central arterioles. These regions are known as "thymus-dependent".

The importance of thymus in lymphocyte proliferation and in the development of cell mediated immunity can be demonstrated by **thymectomy**. In neonatally thymectomised mice lymphopenia, immunodeficiency (**runt disease**), decreased antibody response to T-dependent antigens and gross depletion of thymus-dependent regions in spleen and lymph nodes can be noticed. Deficient CMI is also seen in congenital aplasia of the thymus (Di George Syndrome).

The thymus reaches peak activity in childhood and attains its largest size at puberty. Thereafter, the thymus gradually undergoes atrophy without any effect on T cell function and becomes extremely small in old age. This is because of the fact that T cells are very long-lived and can circulate in the resting state for long periods of time.

Bursa of Fabricius

In birds, undifferentiated lymphocytes move from the bone marrow to the bursa of fabricius where B cells mature.

Bursa of fabricius is a lymphoepithelial organ arising as a pouch from the dorsal part of the cloaca in birds. Like thymus, it is also a site of lymphocytic proliferation and differentiation. Stem cells from yolk sac, fetal liver and bone marrow enter the bursa, proliferate and develop into immunocompetent bursal lymphocytes or B lymphocytes or B cells (B for bursa or bone marrow). These B cells migrate and seed selective areas in the peripheral lymphoid organs–the mantle, germinal follicles and perifollicular regions of the spleen, and the far cortical areas and medullary cords of lymph nodes. These are known as "bursa dependent" or "thymus independent areas". Following appropriate antigenic stimulation, B lymphocytes transform into plasma cells and secrete antibodies.

It becomes a lymphoid organ by about the 15th day of embryonation, develops full functional ability near hatching and atrophies at puberty.

Surgical removal of bursa (bursectomy) from newly hatched chickens destroys their subsequent ability to produce antibodies without affecting their ability to mount cell mediated immune response.

Bone Marrow

In mammals, the bone marrow is the site of B-cell maturation and is equivalent of the bursa of fabricius. Thus, mammalian bone marrow is the site of hemopoiesis and differentiation of stem cells to B cells.

Like thymic selection during T-cell maturation, a selection process within the bone marrow eliminates B cells with self-reactive antibody receptors (the acquisition of tolerance).

SECONDARY (PERIPHERAL) LYMPHOID ORGANS

Lymphocytes differentiate and mature in the primary lymphoid organs and proceed via circulation to the secondary lymphoid organs. Here, they bind to antigen and undergo further antigen-dependent differentiation. From secondary lymphoid organs, these lymphocytes move from one lymphoid organ to another through the blood and lymphatics, a process known as lymphocyte recirculation.

The spleen is the most highly organized secondary lymphoid organ and the lymph nodes the most highly organized secondary lymphoid tissue.

Spleen

Spleen is a large, encapsulated secondary lymphoid organ located in the abdominal cavity. There are two types of tissues in the spleen —

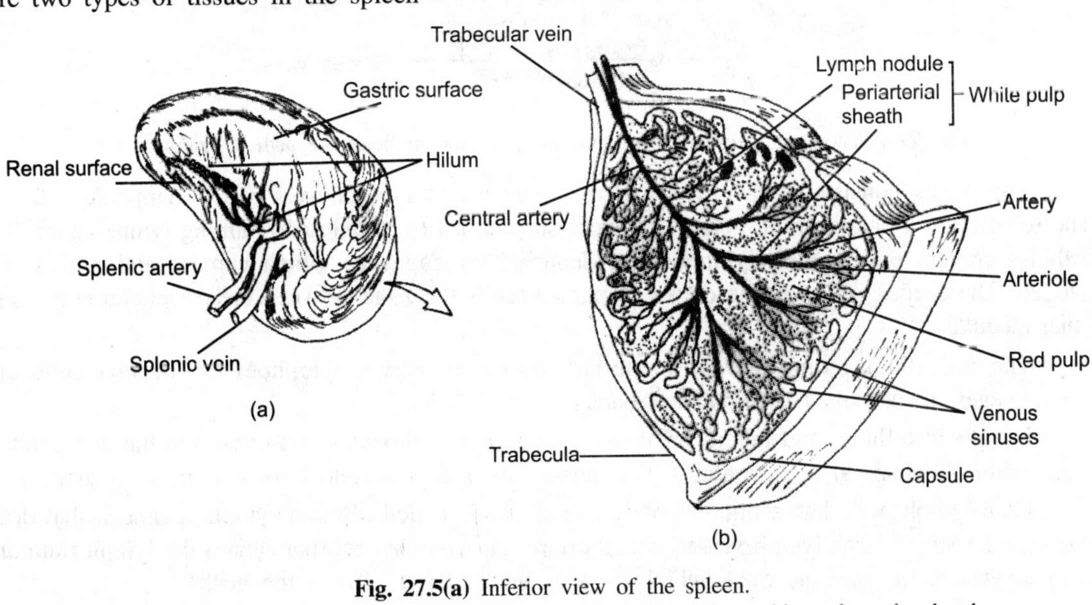

Fig. 27.5(a) Inferior view of the spleen.
(b) Section of spleen showing the arrangement of arteries, veins, white pulp and red pulp.

1. The lymphoid or white pulp of the cortex consisting primarily of lymphocytes and macrophages, and
2. The erythroid or red pulp of the medulla consisting of erythrocyte-rich blood. (Fig. 27.5)

Arteries entering the spleen are surrounded by a sheath of T cells and macrophages, known as periarteriolar sheath. Within this sheath are present lymphoid follicles known as primary follicles of B cells.

The spleen specializes in filtering the blood and trapping blood-borne microorganisms and antigens. Once trapped by macrophages and dendritic cells, the pathogen is phagocytosed and antigens are presented to B and T cells, which become activated to carry out their immune functions.

Presentation of antigens to the splenic lymphocytes results in the formation of secondary follicles containing germinal centres of dividing and differentiating B cells.

Lymph Nodes

Lymph nodes are small bean shaped organs lie at the junctions of lymphatic vessels, distributed throughout the body forming a part of lymphatic network. They are surrounded by connective tissue capsules from which trabeculae penetrate into the nodes. They consist of an outer cortex and inner medulla. (Fig. 27.6)

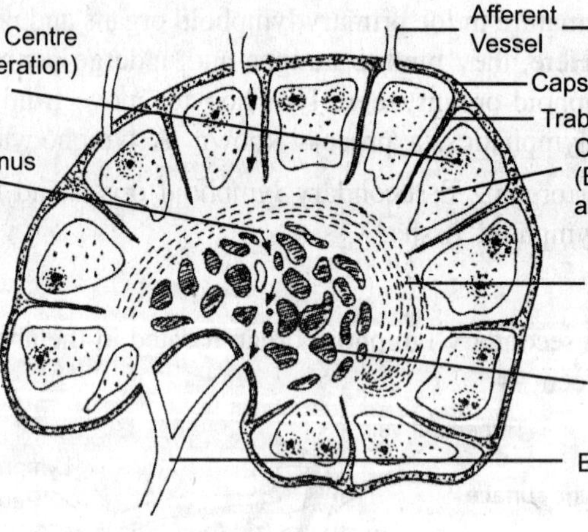

Fig. 27.6 Schematic diagram of a lymph node. Arrows indicate the path of lymph flow.

The cortex consists of several rounded aggregates of lymphocytes called lymphoid follicles. The follicle has a pale-staining germinal centre, surrounded by small dark-staining lymphocytes. The follicles contain proliferating lymphocytes, dendritic marcophages which capture and process the antigen. The deeper region of the cortex or paracortex is the zone between the peripheral cortex and inner medulla.

The medulla is composed of medullary cords, in which lymphocytes, plasma cells and macrophages are arranged as elongated bands.

Lymphoid follicles and medullary cords contain B lymphocytes and constitute bursa-dependent areas while paracortical area contains T lymphocytes and constitute bursa-independent areas.

Each lymph node has a number of lymph channels called afferent lymph channels, that drain into it and a single large lymph vessel, called efferent lymph channel that carries the lymph fluid and lymphocytes to the thoracic duct, which empties into a large vein in the neck.

Lymph nodes filter out harmful microorganisms and antigens from the lymph. Pathogens and antigens are trapped by phagocytic and dendritic cells. Fixed macrophages then phagocytose the foreign material. It is within the lymph nodes that B cells proliferate into antibody-secreting plasma cells. Dendritic cells serve as antigen presenting cells and T helper cells promote the B-cell immune response.

MALT

All lymphoid tissues found in submucosal regions of the body can be viewed as a single functional unit, called the **"Mucosa Associated Lymphoid Tissues (MALT)"**. They are present in the mucosa lining the alimentary, respiratory, genitourinary, skin and other surfaces. They are the sites of secondary development of lymphocytes, which is antigen-specific.

The lymphoid tissues in the gut (*e.g.*, tonsils, adenoids, Peyer's patches, lymphoid follicles) are called **"Gut Associated Lymphoid Tissues (GALT)"**, those in the respiratory tract are called **"Bronchus Associated Lymphoid Tissues (BALT)"** and those in the skin are called **"Skin Associated Lymphoid Tissues (SALT)"**.

MALT contains phagocytic cells and lymphoid cells (both T and B cells). The predominant Ig produced in the mucosa is secretory IgA (sIgA); other Immunoglobulins IgG, IgM and IgE are also formed.

GALT contains a full range of lymphoreticular cells, T and B cells and macrophages. In Peyer's patches, microfold cells sample foreign antigens from the gut lumen, and macrophages process the antigens for presentation to CD^+4 (T_4) lymphocytes. These CD^+4 cells produce cytokines IL-2, IL-4 and IFN-γ that stimulate follicle B lymphocytes to become IgA producing cells, IgA is released into the intestinal lumen as sIgA after being connected to secretory component by epithelial cells. GALT provide a major defense against food-borne pathogens (*e.g., Staph aureus, Bacillus cereus, E. coli, Cryptosporidium*, Rota virus, Norwalk virus etc.).

LYMPHOCYTES

The cells capable of responding to antigens are the lymphocytes, which are one of the classes of white blood cells. They are found in peripheral blood, lymph, lymph nodes and lymphoid organs.

Based on size, lymphocytes are classified into small (5-8 mm), medium sized (8-12 mm) and large (12-15 mm) lymphocytes. Small lymphocytes are most abundant. They consist of a spherical nucleus with prominent nuclear chromatin and a thin rim of cytoplasm, containing scattered ribosomes but ER and other organelles are absent. They are capable of slow motility and during movement assume a "hand-mirror" form, with the nucleus in front and the cytoplasm as a tail behind.

Based on life span, lymphocytes are classified into short lived and long lived lymphocytes. Short lived lymphocytes have a life span of about two weeks and serve as effector cells in the immune response. Long lived cells have a life span of about three years or more, or even for life, and act as store houses of immunological memory; therefore known as memory cells.

Lymphocyte production, differentiation and maturation takes place in the central lymphoid organs and then enter into blood circulation, peripheral lymphoid organs and tissues and mix together in a process known as "lymphocyte recirculation".

Mature lymphocytes, also called naive cells, will be educated or acquire immunocompetence in central lymphoid organs and become Immunocompetent cells (ICC).

Lymphocytes serve the following functions:

1. Recognition of antigen. Lymphocytes have antigen recognition mechanisms on their surface, enabling each cell to recognise only one antigen.
2. Induction of immune response or tolerance to specific antigen.
3. Storage of immunological memory.

A number of surface antigens or markers have been identified on lymphocytes and other leucocytes by means of monoclonal antibodies. These markers reflect the stage of differentiation and functional properties of the cells. "International workshops for Leucocyte Differentiation Antigens" introduced a **CD (cluster of differentiation)** number, by comparing the specificities of leucocytes with different antisera. When a cluster of monoclonal antibodies react with a particular antigen, it was defined as a separate marker and given a CD number. Thus, the term "CD" refers to cluster of differentiation designation assigned to leucocyte cell surface glycoprotein molecules which are identified by their reaction by a given group of monoclonal antibodies. Over 200 CD markers have been identified so far.

The involvement of lymphocytes with the immune response and various diseases can be assessed by enumeration of specific cells bearing particular membrane proteins called "Cluster of differentiation (CD) molecules". CDs are functional cell surface proteins or receptors that can be measured *in situ* and from peripheral blood, biopsy samples or other body fluids.

CDs have both biological and diagnostic significance. In normal persons, the concentration of these molecules in serum is very low. When one's immune system is activated in response to disease, the concentration of these molecules usually rises and fluctuates. Monitoring CD levels may help in the management of the disease. For example, circulating levels of CD54 are directly related to the progress and prognosis of the skin cancer metastatic melanoma. CD23 is a B cell growth factor, and increased levels are associated with chronic lymphocytic leukemia. CD35 is a potent agent for the suppression of complement-dependent tissue injury in autoimmune disease. Elevated levels of CD8 have been found in childhood lymphoid malignancies and AIDS cases. CD4 molecule is a cell surface receptor for HIV.

Table 27.1 Some Functional Examples of Cluster of Differentiation Molecules (CDs)

CD Molecule	*Function*
CD2	The CD2 molecule is a glycoprotein present on T cells, thymocytes and NK cells. It functions as an intercellular adhesion molecule and binds to the human leukocyte function-associated antigen-3 or LFA-3 (CD58). CD2 may be involved in the attachment of T_H cells to antigen-presenting cells and cytotoxic T cells to target cells, and in other cellular interactions. It also is a signal-transducing molecule and may help stimulate T cells to proliferate and secrete cytokines.
CD4	The CD4 molecule is a glycoprotein found primarily on T cells associated with helper/inducer regulatory functions and to a lesser degree on monocytes and macrophages. It is a cell adhesion molecule with great affinity for class II MHC.
CD8	The CD8 molecule is a polypeptide found on the surface of cytotoxic T cells, It is a molecule that participates in the interaction of class I MHC found on target cells.
CD23	CD23 is a protein found on the surface of IgM-bearing B cells, eosinophils, macrophages, and platelets. Soluble CD23 is a B-cell growth factor and upregulates IgE synthesis in conjunction with interleukin-4 released from T cells.

CD35	CD35 is a glycoprotein present on erythrocytes, PMNs, monocytes, all B and some T cells, mast cells, and in soluble form in the plasma. It is the receptor for complement C3b/C4b. The functions of CD35 vary according to the cell type possessing the receptor. For example, CD35 on erythrocytes binds immune complexes bearing C3b or C4b and promotes their clearance from the circulation. On B cells, CD35 augments the maturation of these cells into antibody-secreting cells. It also aids leukocytes in binding and phagocytosing C3b-or C4b-coated objects.
CD54	CD54, also known as intercellular adhesion molecule-1 (ICAM-1), is a protein that is an important early marker of immune activation and response. It is a ligand for the lymphocyte function-associated antigen-1 (LFA-1) found on lymphocytes, monocytes, and neutrophils. The CD54/LFA-1 interaction is important in T-cell-antigen-specific responses and lymphocyte emigration into inflammatory sites. CD54 also is found on mucosal epithelial cells and erythrocytes. Recent evidence suggests CD54 is the cellular receptor for the human rhinovirus and *Plasmodium falciparum*-infected erythrocytes.

Lymphocytes are divided into three main groups—

1. T lymphocytes or thymus derived lymphocytes.
2. B lymphocytes or Bone marrow derived lymphocytes (In birds, bursal lymphocytes).
3. Null cells.

T and B lymphocytes can be differentiated by their surface markers (distinct membrane glycoproteins), whereas null cells do not possess surface markers.

Table 27.2 Differential Characteristics of T Cells and B Cells

T Lymphocytes	*B Lymphocytes*
1. Maturation and differentiation takes place in thymus.	1. Maturation and differentiation takes place in lymphoid tissue or bone marrow.
2. Mobility is great.	2. Mobility is very little.
3. Complement receptors are absent.	3. Complement receptors are present.
4. Surface Immunoglobulins are absent. Instead they have T cell receptor (TCR).	4. Surface Immunoglobulins IgM, IgD are present. TCR is absent.
5. CD3 receptors (surface markers) are present.	5. CD3 receptors are absent.
6. Thymus specific antigens are present.	6. Thymus specific antigens are absent.
7. Cytoplasmic surface projections (microvilli) are absent.	7. Possess an extensively filamentous surface with numerous microvilli.
8. Receptors for F_C piece of IgG are absent.	8. Possess receptors for F_C piece of IgG.
9. T cells bind to sheep RBC by CD2 antigen forming rosettes (SRBC rosette or E rosette).	9. B cells bind to sheep RBC coated with antibody and complement, forming EAC (Erythrocyte antibody complement) rosettes, due to the presence of a C3 receptor (CR2) on the B cell surface. This CR2 receptor also acts as a receptor for EB virus. T cells do not possess this.

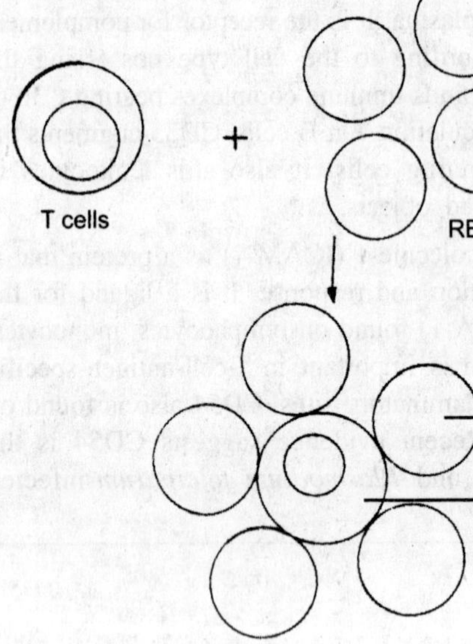

Fig. 27.7 T cell resette (E-rosette).

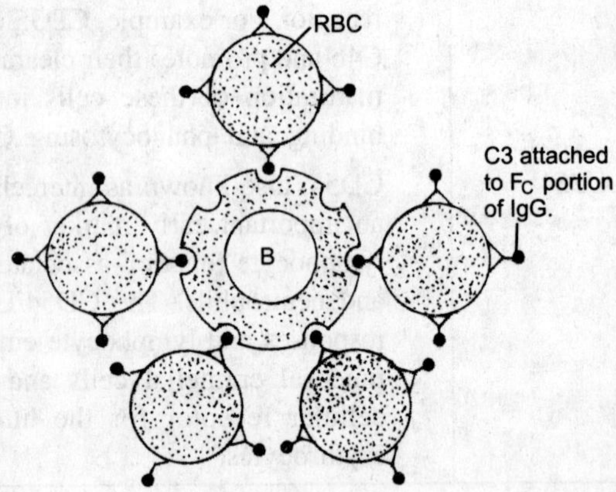

Fig. 27.8 B cell rosettes (EAC rosettes)-rosette formed with IgG coated RBC binding to the receptor for F_C cluster of C3 receptor around B lymphocyte.

10. Undergo blast transformation on treatment with mitogens such as phytohemagglutinin (PHA), concanavalin A and anti-CD3.	10. Undergo blast transformation on treatment with bacterial endotoxins, *Staphylococcus aureus* (cowan I strain), Epstein-Barr (EB) virus.
11. Distribution is high in blood, lymph and lymphoid tissues.	11. Distribution is high in spleen, lymph nodes, bone marrow and other lymphoid tissues; low in blood.
12. Mediate cell mediated immunity and humoral immunity.	12. Mediates humoral immunity.
13. Secrete lymphokines upon activation undergo clonal proliferation and secrete lymphokines.	13. Upon antigenic stimulation undergo clonal proliferation and differentiate into plasma cells and memory cells. Plasma cells secrete antibodies.

DEVELOPMENT OF T CELLS

The precursors of the T cell (pro-T cell) is derived from the hematopoietic stem cell in the fetal yolk sac, liver and post natal bone marrow. Subsequent development takes place in the thymus.

Pro-T cells entering the thymus bear CD34 surface marker. On entering thymus, in the thymic cortex they express a few more lineage specific markers such as surface CD7, CD2 and cytoplasmic CD3 (CCD3), and become pre-T cells. These cells are now called CD7+, CD2+, CCD3+.

Within these cells T cell receptor (TCR) synthesis takes place by TCR gene rearrangement that leads to a functional TCR gene that recognizes only one specific antigen. (Fig. 27.9)

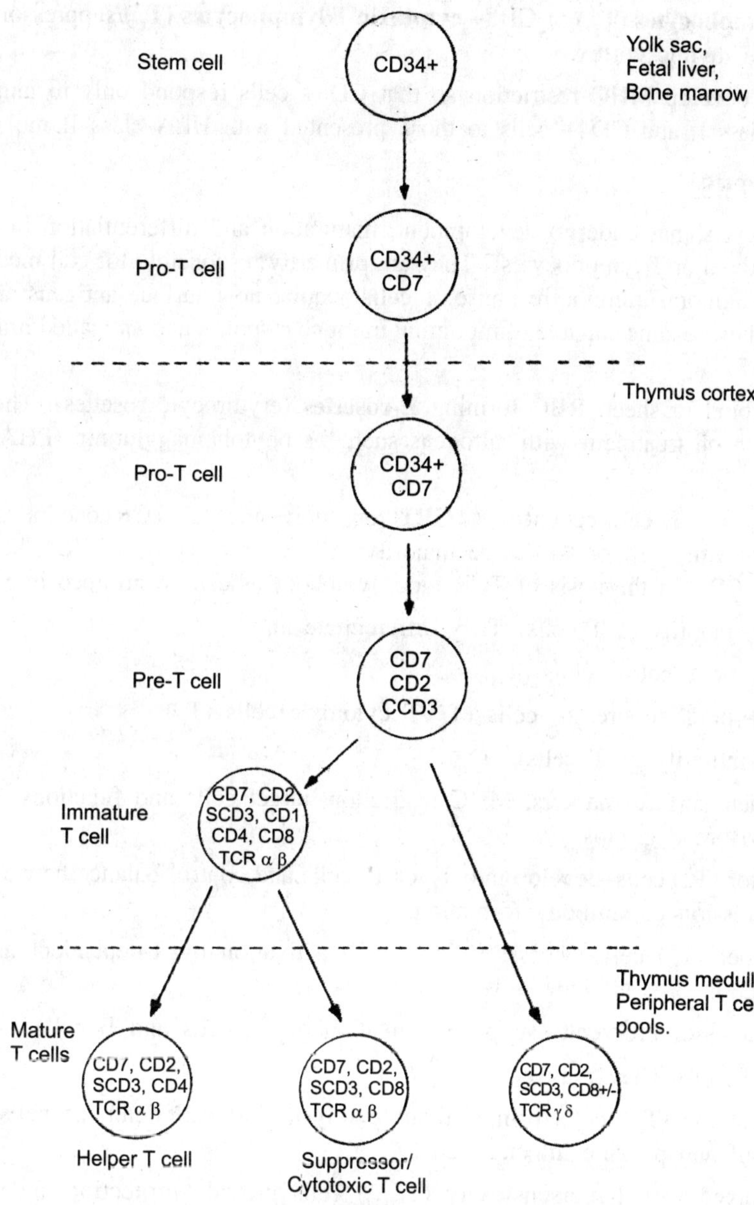

Fig. 27.9 Development of T lymphocytes

TCR occurs as two pairs of glycoprotein chains-either αβ or γδ. Pre-T cells differentiate into two lineages, expressing either αβ (alpha, beta) or γδ (gamma, delta) TCR chains. Large majority of T cells carry αβ TCR whereas a minority of cells carry γδ TCR. The CD3 in the cytoplasm complexes with TCR and is, subsequently co-expressed on the surface.

Contact with self antigens within the thymus leads to the destruction of immature T cells, carrying the corresponding TCR, so that self tolerance is established within the thymus.

TCR-γδ cells expresses CD8 molecule on the surface and leave the thymic cortex. On the other hand, TCR-αβ cells express both CD4 and CD8 molecules on the surface, which become either

CD4+ helper T lymphocytes (T_H) or **CD8+ cytotoxic T lymphocytes (T_C)**/suppressor T lymphocytes (T_S) and leave the thymic cortex.

T cells also develop MHC restriction so that CD8+ cells respond only to antigens presented alongwith HLA class I, and CD4+ cells to those presented with HLA class II molecules.

T LYMPHOCYTES

The lymphocytes that undergo development, maturation and differentiation in the thymus are called "thymus derived or T lymphocytes". They are primarily responsible for cell mediated immunity and can also help humoral immune response. T cells acquire new surface antigens and are educated in thymus so that they become capable of mounting immune response and are called immunocompetent cells.

T cells can bind to sheep RBC forming **E-rosettes** (erythrocyte rosettes). They can undergo blast transformation on treatment with mitogens such as phytohemagglutinin (PHA), concanavalin A (con A).

T cells possess **"T cell receptor (TCR)"** on their surface. TCR occurs as two pairs of glycoprotein chains-either αβ or γδ. Large majority of T cells carry αβ TCR, whereas a minority of cells carry γδ TCR. On the basis of TCR type, lymphocytes can be grouped into different types.

1. TCR–αβ (majority of T cells)–They differentiate into
   (*a*) CD4+ or T helper cells (T_H)
   (*b*) CD8+ or T suppressor cells (T_S)/T cytotoxic cells (T_C)
2. TCR–γδ (minority of T cells).

Based on their surface markers, MHC restriction, target cells and functions, T cells may be classified into two broad groups:

1. T-Regulator (T_R) cells–develop into T_H or T_S cells and control balance between enhancement and suppression of antibody formation.
   (*a*) T-helper (T_H) cells–necessary for B cell activation by T-dependent antigens and for activation of T-effector cells.
   (*b*) T-suppressor (T_S) cells–suppress activation of T_H cells and B cells.
2. Effector T cells–They may be
   (*a*) T-cytotoxic (T_C) cells–brings about cytolysis and cell death of cells recognized as nonself and parasite infected cells.
   (*b*) T-delayed type hypersensitivity (T_{DTH}) cells provide protection against intracellular infectious agents, mediates inflammation and activates macrophages in delayed type IV hypersensitivity.
   (*c*) T cells, which undergo mixed lymphocyte reaction (MLR).

T cells are classified into different antigenic subsets based on surface glycoproteins and designated with a CD number. The term "CD" refers to cluster of differentiation designation assigned to leucocyte cell surface glycoprotein molecules which are identified by their reaction by a given group of monoclonal antibodies.

CD3–All T cells have CD3 proteins on their surface in association with T cell receptors. The CD3 is a complex of five transmembrane proteins involved with transmitting the information or signal from outside of the cell (T cell receptor) to the inside. One of the CD3 transmembrane proteins, the zeta chain, is linked to a tyrosine kinase, called "fyn", which is involved with signal transduction.

CD4—CD4+ cells possess a surface glycoprotein, termed CD4, usually on helper T lymphocytes, that recognizes MHC class II molecules on antigen-presenting cells. CD4 is a single transmembrane glycoprotein.

CD4 cells make up about 65% of peripheral T cells and predominate in the blood, thymic medulla and tonsils. CD4 lymphocytes perform the following helper functions:

1. They help B cells develop into antibody producing plasma cells and thus in antibody formation.
2. They help CD8 T cells to become activated cytotoxic T cells.
3. They help macrophages to effect delayed hypersensitivity (cell mediated immunity).

These functions are performed by two subpopulations of CD4 cells. The CD4+ T_H cells responding to the antigen differentiate either into T_{H1} or T_{H2} subtypes that guide the immune response predominantly to the cell mediated or humoral response, respectively. (Fig. 27.10)

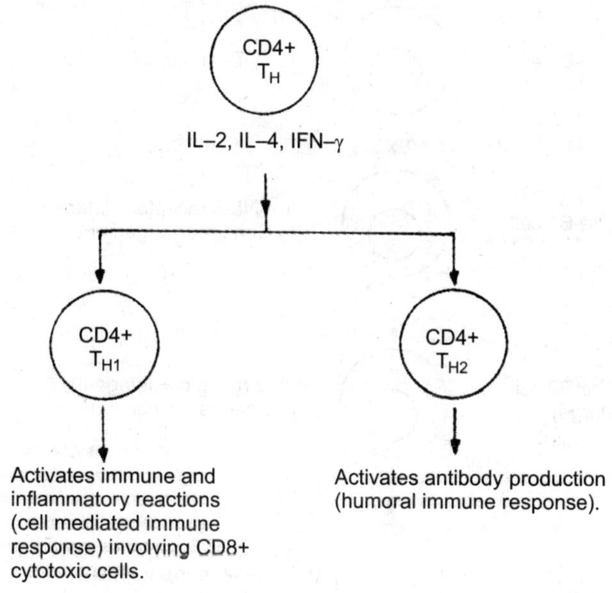

Fig. 27.10 Functions of T lymphocytes

T_{H1} cells help the cell mediated immune response by producing primarily IL-2 and γ-IFN, whereas T_{H2} cells perform the B cell helper function by producing primarily IL-4 and IL-5.

Macrophages produce IL-12, which increases the number of T_{H1} cells, thereby enhancing cell mediated immune responses. Gamma interferon inhibits the production of T_{H2} cells. Thus IL-12 and γ-IFN act as a regulator of the balance between T_{H1} and T_{H2} cells.

CD8–T lymphocytes are subdivided into 2 major groups on the basis of whether they have CD4 or CD8 proteins on their surface. Mature T cells have either CD4 or CD8 proteins but not both.

CD8+ lymphocytes possess a surface glycoprotein, termed CD8, usually on suppressor T cells/ cytotoxic T cells, that recognizes MHC class I molecules on target cells. CD8 consists of two transmembrane polypeptides.

CD8 lymphocytes perform cytotoxic functions. They kill tumor cells, virus-infected cells, allograft cells either by the release of the perforins, which destroy cell membranes or the induction of **programmed cell death (apoptosis)**. CD8 cells predominate in bone marrow, gut lymphoid tissue and constitute about 35% of peripheral T cells.

DEVELOPMENT AND MATURATION OF B LYMPHOCYTES (Fig. 27.11)

I. Antigen independent or **primary development** of B cells takes place in the bone marrow in the early fetal life and continues at low level throughout life. They arise from hemopoietic stem cell in the bone marrow. The primary development of B-cells is under genetic control. Mature B cells develop through several successive stages.

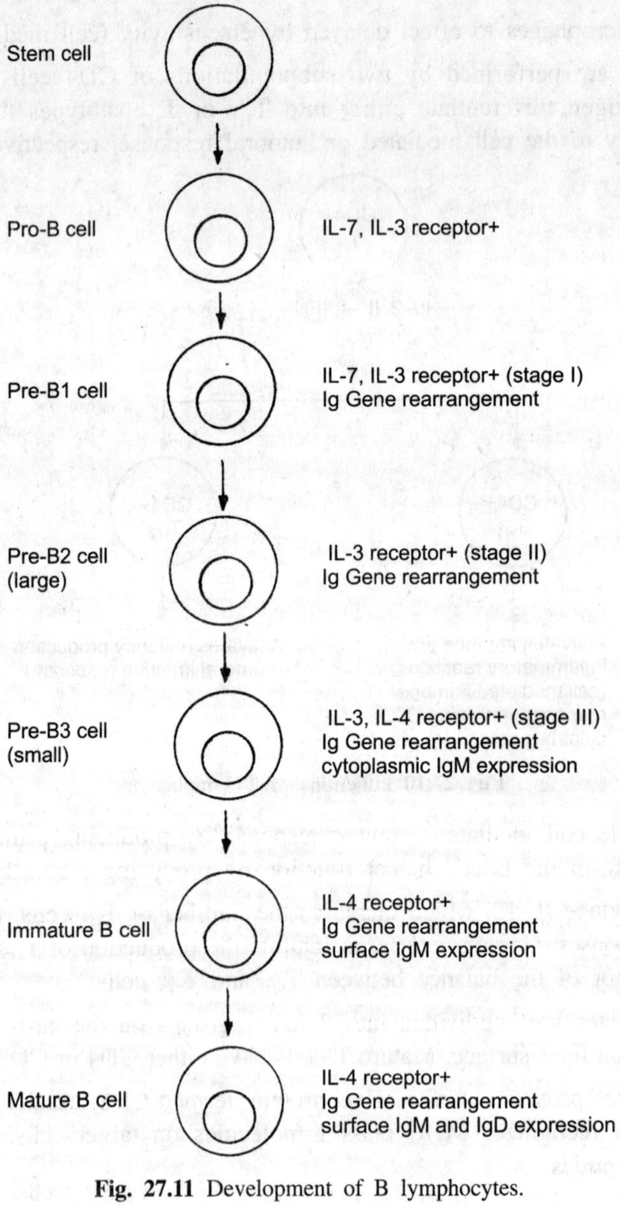

Fig. 27.11 Development of B lymphocytes.

In the bone marrow B cells express surface IgM and IgD and become mature B cells, which leave the bone marrow and settle down in the peripheral lymphoid organs.

The expression of specific surface markers, and rearrangement of the Immunoglobulin genes generates B cells with a diverse antigen specificity. Immature B cell clones that react with self antigens are eliminated so that immunological tolerance is established.

II. Antigen dependent or Secondary development of B cells takes place in the germinal center of the peripheral lymphoid organs, leading to the formation of plasma cells, which produce antibodies specific to the stimulating antigen. This secondary development is dependent on the active cooperation and the help signal from helper T cells (T_H).

On contact with appropriate antigen, the mature B cell undergoes clonal proliferation. Majority of activated B cells are transformed into plasma cells and some activated B cells become long-lived memory cells.

In secondary development, the plasma cells produce antibodies of IgM class initially and switch on IgG production later, and also associated with affinity maturation.

B LYMPHOCYTES

The lymphocytes derived from bone marrow are called bone marrow derived lymphocytes or B cells. In birds, B cells are developed from Bursa of fabricius (a lymphoid organ present on the dorsal part of cloaca). The distribution of B cells is high in spleen, lymph nodes, bone marrow and other lymphoid tissues but low in blood.

Mature B cells possess surface immunoglobulins IgM and IgD. They possess surface receptors for F_C portion of IgG. Immature cells do not possess these Ig receptors. B cells have an extensive filamentous surface with numerous microvilli.

Receptors for C3 component of complement are found on most B cells. These are known as complement receptors (CRs). These receptors are believed to play a role in the regulation of the B cell response to antigen. B cells bind to sheep RBC coated with antibody and complement, forming EAC-rosettes (Erythrocyte Antibody Complement rosettes), due to the presence of C3 receptor (CR2) on B cell surface. This CR2 receptor also acts as a receptor for Epstein-Barr (EB) virus. B cells undergo blast transformation on treatment with bacterial endotoxins, *Staphylococcus aureus* (cowan I strain), EB virus.

The **primary development (antigen independent)** of B cells is under genetic control and takes place in the bone marrow throughout life at low level.

The **secondary development (antigen dependent)** of B cells requires the active cooperation and help signal from helper T cells (T_H) and takes place in the germinal center of the peripheral lymphoid organs, leading to the formation of plasma cells, which produce antibodies specific to the stimulating antigen. Some activated B cells become long lived memory cells.

B lymphocytes primarily mediated humoral immune response or antibody mediated immunity and their main function is to produce specific antibodies against the antigen. Surface IgM of the mature B cells serve as an antigen recognition receptor. B cells also serve as an efficient antigen presenting cell (APC), particularly during the secondary immune response to derive help signals from T_H cells necessary for antibody class switching, affinity maturation and memory cell production.

PLASMA CELLS

Upon antigenic stimulation, B cells undergo rapid clonal proliferation and blast transformation. Majority of activated B cells transform into plasma cells and some become long lived memory cells.

A mature plasma cell is structurally designed to be an Ig or antibody secreting cell. It is a large, oval cell (about twice the size of a small lymphocyte) with an eccentrically placed oval nucleus containing large blocks of chromatin located peripherally, presenting a cart wheel appearance. The cytoplasm is large and contains abundant Endoplasmic reticulum (ER) and well developed Golgi apparatus.

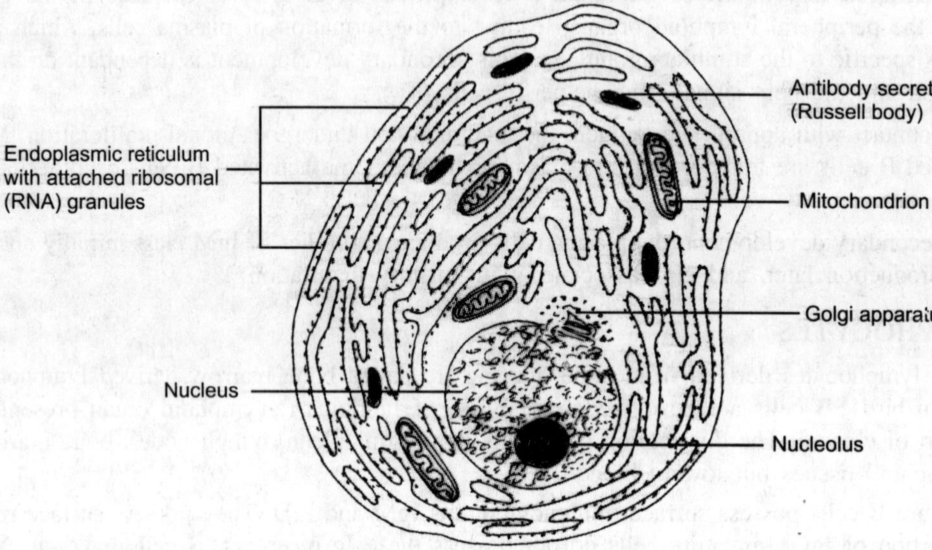

Fig. 27.12 Plasma cell

Plasma cells are end cells and have a life span of 5 to 7 days. A plasma cell manufactures an antibody of a single specificity, of a single Ig class and allotype, and of a single light chain type only. An exception is seen in primary antibody response, when a plasma cell is producing IgM initially, may later be switched to IgG production.

Thus, plasma cells are literally protein factories that produce about 2,000 antibodies per second in their brief 5 to 7 day life span.

NULL CELLS/LARGE GRANULAR LYMPHOCYTES (LGL)

Null cells are a small proportion (5%) of lymphocytes which lack the surface markers and other characteristics of T and B cells and arise in the bone marrow and thymus. They are nonphagocytic but can kill malignant, virus infected and transplanted cells by a direct cytotoxic action.

Null cells are large with abundant cytoplasm containing azurophilic granules, hence known as large granular lymphocytes (LGL); a characteristic feature which helps in distinguishing them from T and B cells.

Null cells are of 3 types–

1. Natural killer (NK) cells
2. Killer (K) cells, and
3. Lymphokine activated killer (LAK) cells

Natural Killer (NK) Cells

They mediate direct cytotoxicity and kills mainly malignant cells and virus infected cells. Their cytotoxicity is neither antibody dependent nor MHC restricted. NK cell activity is natural and non-immune and form a part of innate immunity. NK cells are active in severe combined immunodeficiency diseases, where both T and B cells are absent. NK cells are activated by interferons. IL-2 acts as a growth factor for NK cells.

NK cells have CD16 and CD56 on their surface. They can bind to glycoprotein receptors on the surface of target cells and release many cytolytic factors (*e.g.*, perforin resembling C9) which produce transmembrane pores, through which cytotoxic factors (*e.g.*, TNF-β) enter the cell and destroy it. This phenomenon is called **apoptosis** or programmed cell death.

NK cells are, thus, important in immune surveillance and natural defence against virus infected and malignant cells. (Fig. 27.13)

Killer (K) Cells/Antibody Dependent Cellular Cytotoxic (ADCC) Cells

These large granular lymphocytes or null cells possess surface receptors for F_C portion of IgG. They are capable of killing or lysing target cells sensitised with IgG antibody. This is known as "**antibody dependent cellular cytotoxicity** (ADCC)" and is different from the action of cytotoxic T cell which is independent of antibody.

Lymphokine Activated Killer (LAK) Cells

These null cells are NK cells treated with interleukin-2 (IL-2). They are cytotoxic to a wide range of tumor cells. LAK cells can be used in the treatment of some tumors such as renal cell carcinoma.

PHAGOCYTES/MACROPHAGES

Phagocytic cells ingest invading microorganisms and other foreign particulate matter and in most cases, kill and digest them. There are two types of phagocytic cells :

1. Monocytes in blood; when monocytes enter into tissues they become macrophages.
2. Polymorphonuclear neutrophils (PMN)–They form a large circulating pool of phagocytic cells.

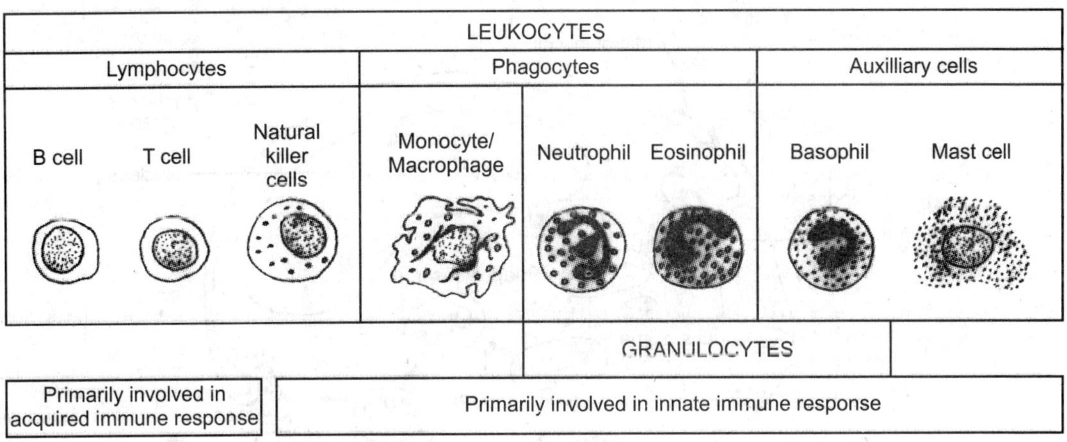

Fig. 27.13 Major cell types involved in the immune response

Macrophages are found in the lymph nodes (dendritic macrophages), spleen, perivascular connective tissues, connective tissues of the skin, lungs (alveolar macrophages), serous cavities, liver (kupffer cells), bone marrow (osteoclasts), nervous system (microglial cells) and synovium (type A lining cells).

Phagocytes carryout several important functions:

1. The primary function is **phagocytosis**. Antibody coated (opsonized) microorganisms are phagocytosed more readily. They accumulate in areas of inflammation and tissue damage and carry out phagocytosis.
2. They function as **antigen-presenting cells (APC)**. They trap the antigen and process the phagocytosed particles and provide it in optimum concentration to T_H cells in association with MHC class II molecules.
3. Macrophages can be activated by lymphokines, C components or interferon. Activated macrophages are not antigen specific and cause antigen-nonspecific lysis of bacteria.
4. They remove immune complexes and other immunologically active substances from blood.
5. They become giant cells in response to lymphokines secreted by T_{H1} cells. Giant cells coalesce to become epitheloid cells (found in granulomatous disease) which are effective in containing intracellular pathogens.
6. Activated macrophages produce IL-1, IL-6 and TNF α/β that are vital to antigen specific activation of CD4+ T_H cells. IL-1 induce the synthesis of IL-2 by the activation of T cells.
7. They produce several other biologically active substances such as hydrolytic enzymes, binding proteins (fibronectin, transferrin) and some complement components.

PHAGOCYTOSIS

Monocytes, macrophages and neutrophils ingest and digest bacteria and other foreign particles by phagocytosis. Phagocytosis is more efficient when bacteria are opsonized *i.e.*, coated with antibody or complement activation products, such as C3b, known as opsonins. Phagocytosis is carried out in 3 stages: (Fig. 27.14)

(*i*) Recognition and binding

(*ii*) Ingestion

(*iii*) Digestion

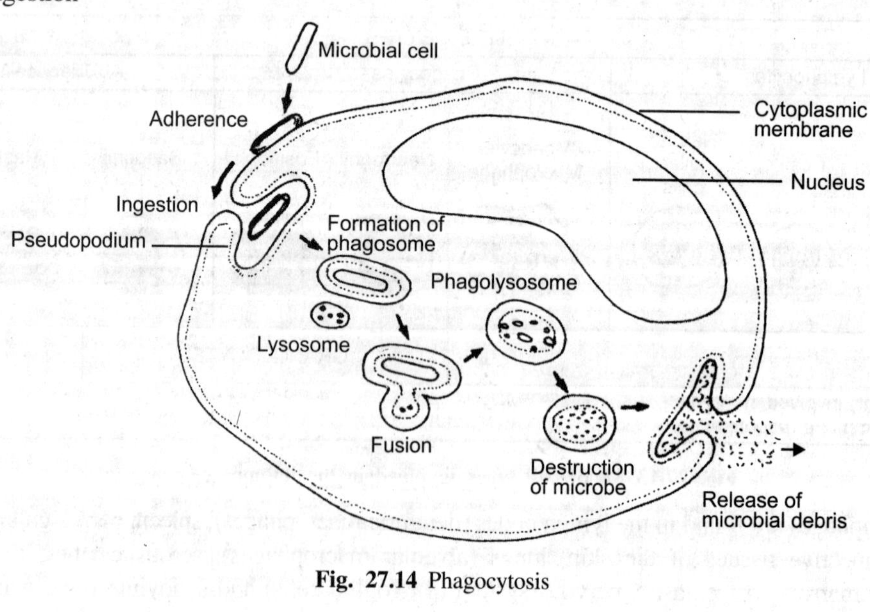

Fig. 27.14 Phagocytosis

Phagocytes recognize and bind to invading microorganisms with the receptors on their surface to the microbial surface structures or opsonins. After the phagocyte attach a microbe to its surface, it sends out projections called pseudopodia that surround the microbe. These pseudopodia fuse and form a phagocytic vacuole called "phagosome or endosome" containing the microbe. The phagosome then pinches off from the membrane and enters the cytoplasm.

The lysosome fuse with the phagosome and form a digestive vacuole called "phagolysosome". The lysosomes contain digestive enzymes and toxic microbicidal substances and initiate intracellular killing and digestion of the microorganism. Digestion is carried out in two phases-oxygen dependent phase and oxygen independent phase.

In **oxygen dependent phase**, the activated phagocytic cell increases its oxygen consumption and ATP generation needed for phagocytosis, known as "**Respiratory burst**", This generates highly toxic oxygen metabolites such as superoxide, singlet oxygen, hydrogen peroxide, hydroxyl radicals, hypochlorites, and in the case of neutrophils, hypohalite ions (chloride, iodide, bromide). These products alongwith myeloperoxidase constitutes a highly toxic microbicidal system and destroy/kill invading microorganisms. Children with **chronic granulomatous disease** have defects in the oxygen dependent phase of killing. Therefore, they are susceptible to a wide range of pyogenic bacterial infections.

In **oxygen independent phase** lysosomal hydrolases such as lysozyme, phospholipase, ribonuclease, deoxyribonuclease, proteases and acidic pH-collectivity destroy the trapped microbe. Oxygen independent killing follows the fusion of the lysosome and the phagosome; whereas this fusion is not necessary for oxygen dependent killing or respiratory burst.

Microbes vary in their response to phagocytic activity. Gram positive bacteria are rapidly destroyed. Gram negative bacteria are relatively resistant to digestion.

Intracellular pathogens such as *Mycobacterium tuberculosis*, *Mycobacterium leprae*, *Listeria monocytogenes*, *Legionella pneumophila*, *Toxoplasma gondii*, *Trypanosoma cruzi* and some fungi and some other microbes are resistant to phagocytic action and may multiply within the phagocytes.

ANTIGEN PRESENTING CELLS (APC)

The term "Antigen-presenting cell (APC)" refers to cells that constitutively express class II MHC molecules and so can present antigen to helper T cells. APCs can also perform nonspecific immunological functions such as phagocytosis and cytotoxicity. Induction of humoral or cell mediated immunity cannot occur efficiently in the absence of APCs.

The major classes of cells that function as APC are–

1. **Macrophages** include monocytes (blood macrophages) and histiocytes (tissue macrophages). They trap the antigen and process the phagocytosed particles and provide it in optimum concentration to T_H cells in association with MHC class II molecules.
2. **B-Lymphocytes** serve as an efficient antigen presenting cell, particularly during the secondary immune response to derive help signals from T_H cells necessary for antibody class switching, affinity maturation and memory cell production.
3. **Dendritic cells** are derived from bone marrow and are usually found in blood and peripheral lymphoid organs. The dendritic cells, when present in skin (dermis) are known as "Langerhans cells". The dendritic cells that are found throughout T-cell zones of lymphoid organs are called "interdigitating cells". Dendritic cells are highly pleomorphic, with a small central body and many long needle-like processes.

They possess MHC class II antigens, and are highly efficient in capturing and presenting antigens to T cells, particularly during immune response. They do not possess surface immunoglobulins and receptors for F_C portion of IgG and sheep RBC.

4. **Langerhans' cells**–The dendritic cells present in skin (dermis) and submucosa are known as Langerhans' cells. They possess features of macrophages and dendritic cells. They process and present antigens that reach dermis. The processing and presentation of antigen by macrophages to T cells require that both the cells possess surface determinants coded by the same MHC genes. T cells can accept the processed antigen only if it is presented by macrophages carrying on its surface the self-MHC determinant known as "Immune associated (Ia) antigen". When the macrophage bears a different Ia antigen, it cannot cooperate with T cell. This is known as MHC restriction.

NEUTROPHILS (Fig. 27.13)

They constitute 60% of the leucocytes in blood circulation. Their primary function is phagocytosis of foreign or dead cells and pinocytosis of pathological immune complexes. They can also exhibit antibody-dependent-cell mediated cytotoxicity (ADCC). The phagocytic property of neutrophils is nonspecific, except for its augmentation by opsonins, They are capable of rapid activation and mobilization in response to chemotactic stimuli such as bacterial products or activated components of complement (C5a). They constitute predominant cell type in acute inflammation. A variety of receptors for F_C portion, CR1 and CR2 are displayed following activation.

EOSINOPHILS (Fig. 27.13)

They account for 3-5% of the white blood cells. They are found in large numbers in allergic inflammation, parasitic infections and around antigen-antibody complexes. They primarily inhabit tissues rather than blood stream. These are granulocytes containing prominent acidophilic granules-small, round, homogenous ones and the large ovoid ones. The granules contain a variety of hydrolytic enzymes which bring about extracellular killing of large parasites. They can engulf and remove immune complexes by phagocytosis/pinocytosis. They possess receptors for F_C portion of immunoglobulins and can mediate ADCC. They can bind to worm larvae such as schistosomulae coated with IgG, degranulate and release toxic proteins which are damaging to the parasites.

BASOPHILS AND MAST CELLS (Fig. 27.13)

Basophils constitute less than 1% of white blood cells. Basophils are found in blood circulation and when they are found in tissues are called mast cells. Their cytoplasm has large numbers of prominent basophilic granules containing pharmacological mediators-histamine, heparin, serotonin and other hydrolytic enzymes that mediate Type I hypersensitivity (Anaphylaxis and Atopy). IgE antibodies get attached F_C receptors on the surface of mast cells and basophils. When stimulated with allergen, granules release their contents. Basophils also possess surface receptors for F_C portion of IgG and complement receptors (CRs) for C3a, C3b and C5a.

MITOGENS

Mitogens are substances that induce blast transformation and cell division of lymphocytes and other cells *e.g.*,

1. Plant lectins such as phytohemagglutinin and concanavalin A (con A) can activate T lymphocytes.

2. Antilymphocyte globulin (heterologous antisera) activate both T and B cells.
3. Anti-CD3 monoclonal antibody activates only those T cells that bear TCR complex.
4. *Staphylococcus aureus* (cowan I strain) protein A specifically stimulates B cells (T independent).
5. Pokeweed mitogen activates B cells (T independent).

QUESTIONS

Essay Questions

1. Describe the development of T and B lymphocytes.
2. Mention the distinguishing characters of T cells and B cells and describe the development of T cells.
3. Give an account of lymphocytes.
4. Describe T lymphocytes (or) Describe the role of T lymphocytes in immunity.

Short Notes

1. Role of thymus in immunity
2. Bursa of fabricius
3. MALT
4. GALT
5. Lymphocytes
6. CD
7. Differences between T and B cells
8. Development of T cells
9. TCR
10. T lymphocytes
11. CD3
12. CD4
13. CD8
14. Functions of T lymphocytes
15. Development of B lymphocytes
16. B lymphocytes
17. Plasma cells
18. Null cells (or) Large granular lymphocytes (LGL)
19. Natural killer cells or NK cells
20. Killer cells or K cells or ADCC cells
21. LAK cells
22. Phagocytes (or) Macrophages
23. Phagocytosis
24. Antigen presenting cells or APC
25. Dendritic cells
26. Langerhans' cells
27. Mast cells
28. Mitogens.

28

Immune Response

- *Definition*
- *Types of immune responses*
- *Generation of immune response*
- *Interactions of immune cells and cytokines during immune response*
- *Immunological memory*
- *Immunological tolerance*
- *Immunological paralysis*
- *Sulzberger-Chase phenomenon*
- *Comparision and contrast of CMI and AMI*

DEFINITION

The specific reactivity induced in a host by an antigenic stimulus is known as "Immune response".

The immune response includes reactions against any antigen, living or nonliving. It may lead to consequences that are beneficial, indifferent or injurious to the host. It also includes the state of specific nonreactivity (Immunological tolerance) induced by certain types of antigenic stimuli.

TYPES OF IMMUNE RESPONSE

The immune response to an antigen is of two types.

1. Humoral immune response or antibody mediated immunity (AMI).
2. Cell mediated immune response (CMI).

The two types of immune responses are usually developed together, though at times one or the other may be predominant or exclusive. They usually act in conjunction but may sometimes act in opposition.

Humoral Immune Response (AMI)

It is mediated by antibodies produced by plasma cells, that are transformed B lymphocytes.

AMI is primarily directed against

(*i*) Extracellular bacterial infections.

(*ii*) Respiratory and intestinal viral infections

(*iii*) Recurrence of viral infections.

(*iv*) Toxin-induced diseases.

(*v*) Infections in which virulence is related to polysaccharide capsules (*e.g.*, Pneumococci, Meningococci, *Haemophilus influenzae*).

AMI also leads to the development of immediate (Types I, II, III) hypersensitivity reactions and certain autoimmune diseases.

Cell Mediated Immune Response (CMI)

It is mediated directly by sensitized T lymphocytes and macrophages, without involving antibodies and B lymphocytes.

CMI serves the following immunological functions :

(*i*) Immunity against obligate and facultative intracellular bacterial diseases *e.g.*, Tuberculosis, Leprosy, Brucellosis, Listeriosis etc.

(*ii*) Immunity against viral, fungal (*e.g.*, histoplasmosis, coccidioidomycosis, blastomycosis) and parasitic (e.g., Leishmaniasis, Malaria, Toxoplasmosis, Trypanosomiasis etc.) diseases.

(*iii*) Immunity against tumor cells (cancer) and Immunological surveillance.

(*iv*) Transplantation immunity–participates in graft rejection and Graft-versus-host (GVH) reaction.

(*v*) Delayed (Type IV) hypersensitivity (DH).

(*vi*) Pathogenesis of certain autoimmune diseases *e.g.*, thyroiditis, encephalomyelitis.

GENERATION OF IMMUNE RESPONSE

Immune response against an invading pathogen is specific and comprehensive, and is mediated by a number of developmentally independent but functionally interacting families of lymphocytes. The functions of the each type of lymphocytes are closely integrated with the function of the other cell types of the immune system.

For example, macrophages and APC trap and present the antigen to the CD4+ T_H lymphocytes. While the T-lymphocytes produce cytokines that activate macrophages to become more efficient. Likewise, the antibody makes a generalized response of phagocytes specific by opsonisation, and that of complement system specific by activating the complement by the classical pathway. A successful immune response depends on a close functional collaboration among all the components.

Moreover, macrophages and other APCs also help in growth and multiplication of T_H cells by producing specific cytokines. These cytokines determine to a large extent the nature of the subsequent specific response *i.e.*, whether the response will predominantly be cell mediated or humoral immune response.

T_{H1} cells help the cell mediated immune response by producing primarily IL-2 and gamma interferon, whereas T_{H2} cells perform the B cell helper function by producing primarily IL-4 and IL-5.

Macrophages produce IL-12, which increases the number of T_{H1} cells, thereby enhancing cell mediated immune responses. Gamma interferon inhibits the production of T_{H2} cells. Thus IL-12 and IFN-γ act as a regulator of the balance between T_{H1} and T_{H2} cells (Fig. 28.1).

IMMUNOLOGICAL MEMORY

Immunological memory is a characteristic feature of acquired immune response of lymphocytes. The primary antibody response prime or sensitize the immune system so that it possesses specific immunologic memory. A second encounter with a given antigen produces a secondary immune response faster, greater and long lasting than the primary immune response.

Clonally differentiated T and B cells produced during a primary immune response, which are "primed" or "sensitized" to mediate a secondary immune response to the original antigen are known as "memory cells".

Only T cell dependent antigens can induce this immunologic memory. Though the serum will contain antibodies as a result of the primary immune response, they will be gradually metabolised and eliminated. Usually the B cells undergo chronic low-level reactivation as a result of immune responses to other related antigens. Therefore, low levels of antibodies to many antigens exist in the serum at any time. Such antibodies are called "Natural antibodies". Their presence reflects the cumulative immunologic memory of the host.

The major result of immunologic memory is the "anamnestic response", which may confer life long immunity on the host.

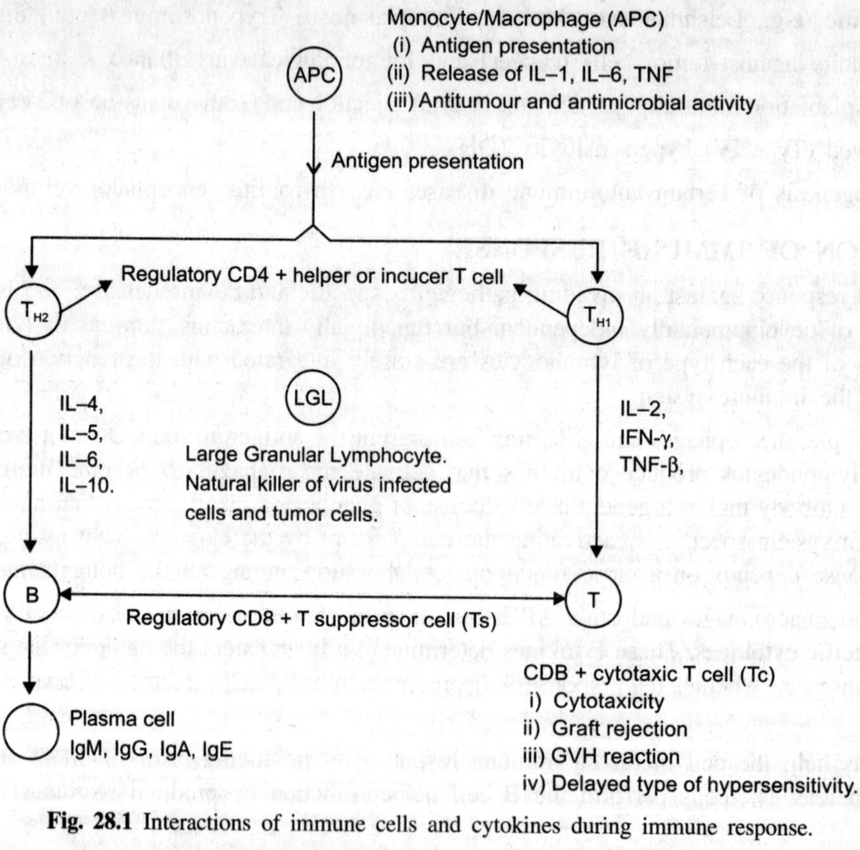

Fig. 28.1 Interactions of immune cells and cytokines during immune response.

IMMUNOLOGICAL TOLERANCE

Immunological tolerance or immunological unresponsiveness is the condition in which contact with an antigen specifically abolishes the capacity to mount an immune response against that particular antigen on subsequent contacts. This nonreactivity is specific to the particular antigen, immune response to other antigens being unaffected.

Any antigen that comes in contact with the immunological system during embryonic life would be recognised as a self antigen and would not induce any immune response. Tolerance could be induced against foreign antigens if they were administered during embryonic life. Twins exhibit immunological tolerance due to the sharing of same placental blood supply during intrauterine life.

The immune system is constantly exposed to self antigens without stimulating lymphocytes, a phenomenon called "self-tolerance". Self-tolerance is not inherited but somatically acquired. It is antigen specific. Self-tolerance is achieved through clonal deletion of self-reactive lymphocytes.

The central mechanism in tolerance induction may be elimination of T_H cells, thereby preventing B cell activation. In some cases, the access of antigen to immunocompetent cells is interfered or the antibody synthesized is neutralised or destroyed. Induction of tolerance is very difficult in adults already immunised against the antigen.

Usually high doses of antigen induce B cell tolerance and repeated minute doses of antigen induce T cell tolerance. Tolerance to humoral and cellular types of immunity is usually induced simultaneously.

Tolerance can be overcome spontaneously or by injection of cross-reacting antigens. For example, tolerance to bovine serum albumin in Rabbits can be abolished by immunization with cross-reacting human serum albumin. In general, tolerance to living agents is long lasting than that to nonliving substances.

IMMUNOLOGICAL PARALYSIS (FELTON'S PHENOMENON)

When an antigen is given in large doses, it may completely paralyse the immune system without any antibody response. This phenomenon was called immunological paralysis by Felton.

SULZBERGER-CHASE PHENOMENON

Sulzberger and Chase demonstrated that if certain antigens are given orally before parenteral administration into Guinea pigs, the animals developed specific tolerance to the given antigen. This is known as Sulzberger-Chase phenomenon.

COMPARISON AND CONTRAST OF CMI AND AMI

(1) CMI provides immunity against obligate and facultative intracellular bacterial, viral, fungal and parasitic diseases; immunity against tumor cells (cancer) and provides immunological surveillance.

Humoral immunity is directed primarily against extracellular bacterial infections, respiratory and intestinal viral infections, toxin-induced diseases and infections in which virulence is related to polysaccharide capsules (*e.g.,* Pneumococci, Meningococci, *Haemophilus influenzae*).

(2) CMI participates in graft rejection and GVH. Transplantation immunity is predominantly cell mediated. The first set response is brought about exclusively by T lymphocytes.

Antibodies are formed more rapidly and abundantly during second set response than during first set response, and participate in second set response alongwith cell mediated immunity.

(3) CMI is responsible for delayed (Type IV) hypersensitivity. Humoral immunity leads to the development of immediate (Type I, II and III) hypersensitivity.

(4) Both CMI and humoral immunity can produce certain autoimmune diseases.

(5) CMI is brought about by T lymphocytes whereas humoral immunity is produced by B lymphocytes.

(6) In CMI, activated T cells produce certain low molecular weight, biologically active substances called cytokines (interleukins) which effect the manifestations of CMI.

In humoral immunity, stimulated B cells are transformed to plasma cells, which produce antibodies.

(7) The terms primary and secondary response are primarily associated with antibody formation but the T cell also follows the same pattern.

(8) Humoral immunity can be passively transferred by serum transfer. Whereas CMI cannot be transferred with serum. CMI can be passively transferred with sensitized T cells or their extract (transfer factor).

(9) In both types of immunity, the antigen is trapped and presented by macrophages, dendritic cells, langerhans cells in association with MHC class II molecules to the CD4+T_H cells bearing specific TCR.

(10) The CD4+T_H cells responding to the antigen differentiate either into T_{H1} or T_{H2} subtypes that guide the immune response predominantly to the cell mediated or humoral response, respectively.

(11) In CMI, T_{H1} cells respond to intercellular pathogens and recognize the antigen by its TCR. The stimulated T cells undergo blast transformation and clonal proliferation and produce biologically active mediators, known as cytokines or Interleukins, which activate macrophages, enabling them to kill intracellular pathogens. The T_{H1} cells also recruit CD8+ cytotoxic T cells, which recognize the target, in association with MHC class I molecules, secrete cytokines to destroy them. They specifically kill the target cells such as tumor cells, virus-infected cells and graft cells.

In humoral immunity, T_{H2} cells stimulate the specific clone of B cells. The activated B cells multiply and mature into plasma cells that secrete specific antibodies of IgM type and some cells convert to memory cells in primary immune response. During secondary response, the memory cells mount a rapid and more effective antibody response which is IgG (class switch) with an increasing affinity (affinity maturation).

With nonprotein antigens such as bacterial capsular polysaccharides, the humoral response does not require the cooperation of T_H cells.

QUESTIONS

Essay Question

1. Compare and contrast the cell mediated immunity and humoral immunity with respect to their activity.

Short Notes

1. Define immune response.
2. Generation of immune response.
3. Immunological memory.
4. Describe interactions of immune cells and cytokines during immune response.
5. Immunological tolerance.
6. Immunological paralysis or Felton's phenomenon.

29

Cell Mediated Immune Response

- ***Definition***
- ***Induction of CMI***
- ***Cytokines***
  - ***Interleukins (IL)***
  - ***Colony stimulating factors (CSFs)***
  - ***Tumor necrosis factor (TNF)***
  - ***Interferons***
  - ***Chemokines***
  - ***Other cytokines***
  - ***Migration inhibition factor (MIF)***
- ***Transfer factor (TF)***
- ***Immunomodulators***
- ***Detection of CMI***
  - ***Intradermal tests***
  - ***Macrophage migration inhibition test***
  - ***Lymphocyte blast transformation test (or) MLR***
  - ***Cell mediated cytotoxicity or target cell lysis***
  - ***Enumeration of T cells and subpopulations***

DEFINITION

Cell mediated immunity (CMI) refers to specific acquired immunity, accomplished by effector T cells and macrophages, without involving antibodies and B lymphocytes.

CMI serves the following immunological functions :

(1) Immunity against obligate and facultative intracellular bacterial diseases *e.g.*, Tuberculosis, Leprosy, Brucellosis, Listeriosis etc.

(2) Immunity against viral, fungal (*e.g.*, histoplasmosis, coccidioidomycosis, blastomycosis) and parasitic (*e.g.*, Leishmaniasis, Malaria, Toxoplasmosis, Trypanosomiasis etc.) diseases.

(3) Immunity against tumor cells (cancer) and Immunological surveillance.

(4) Transplantation immunity-participates in graft rejection and Graft-versus-host (GVH) reaction.

(5) Delayed (Type IV) hypersensitivity (DH).

(6) Pathogenesis of certain autoimmune diseases e.g., thyroiditis, encephalomyelitis.

INDUCTION OF CMI

CMI is best developed following infections with intracellular parasites. Only T cell dependent antigens can induce CMI. Killed vaccines and other nonliving antigens do not induce CMI, unless administered with the Freund type of adjuvants. The application of certain chemicals on the skin induces delayed hypersensitivity. (Fig. 29.1).

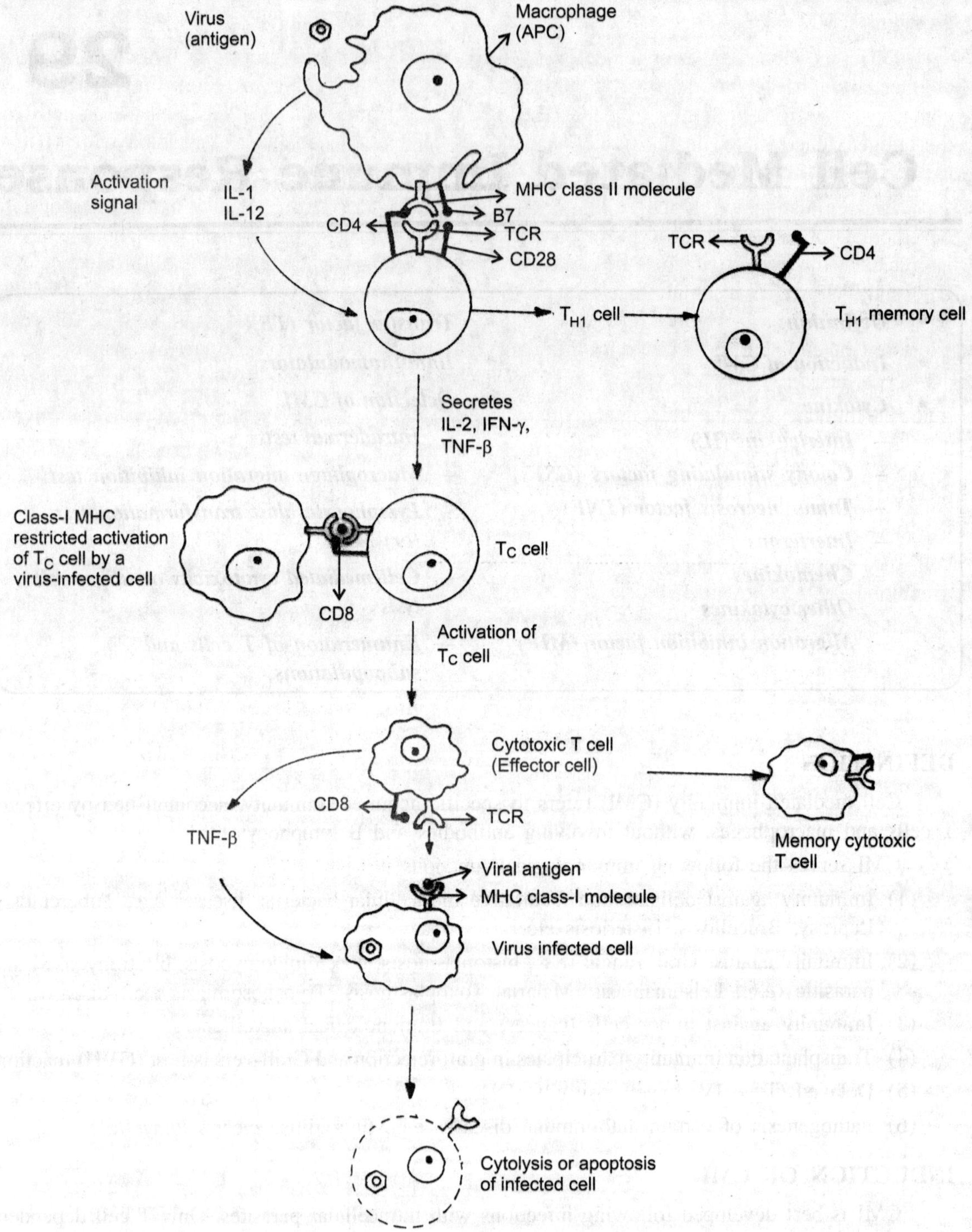

Fig. 29.1 Cell mediated immune response

Each T cell bears on its surface a specific receptor, called TCR for one epitope and combines only with antigens carrying that epitope. On contact with the appropriate antigen, T cells undergo blast transformation, clonal proliferation and differentiation into memory cells and effector cells providing CMI.

Different clones of lymphocytes constantly traffic from one secondary lymphoid organ to another through the blood and lymphatics. Lymphocyte trafficking increases the probability of contact with antigen presented by APC. The APCs such as macrophages and Langerhans cells trap the antigens encountered in the tissues, and process and present them in association with MHC–II to the CD4+T_H cells bearing a specific TCR.

Antigen recognition by the T_H cell is the most crucial stage in the acquired immune response for development of subsequent CMI and/or humoral immunity against a specific pathogen. The role of APC is crucial in this regard which is more than a mere presentation of the antigen. APCs produce IL-1, IL-6 and TNF-α. IL-1 stimulates the responding clone of T_H cell to produce IL-2, and to express receptor for IL–2 on the surface at the same time. IL-2, in turn, acts on T_H cells through IL–2 receptor expressed on the surface to cause its differentiation and proliferation *i.e.,* clonal expansion.

The CD4+T_H cells responding to the antigen differentiate either into T_{H1} or T_{H2} subtypes that guide the immune response predominantly to the cell mediated or humoral immune response, respectively.

T_{H1} type response is the usual response in case of intracellular pathogen. The T_{H1} cells recruit CD8+cytotoxic T lymphocytes bearing specific TCR and activate them to specifically kill the infected cells. Cytotoxic T cells target the infected cell by recognizing the antigen fragment presented in association with the MHC-I on its surface secrete lymphokines and destroy the cells (Fig. 29.2). T_{H1} cells also recruit macrophages and activate them to become giant cells that finally coalesce to form granuloma, as seen in tuberculosis.

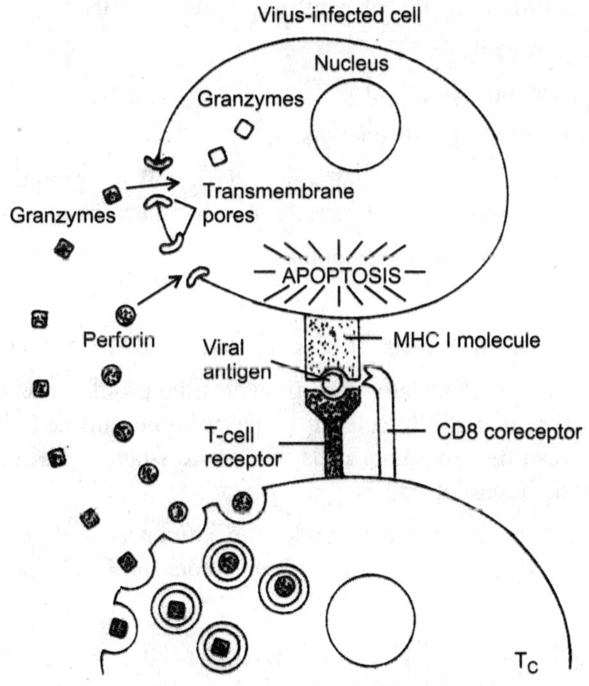

Fig. 29.2 Destruction of a virus infected target cell by an Effector Cytotoxic T cell (T_C). When a T_C cell contacts target cell, the T_C cell secretes perforins that forms transmembrane pores in the target cell's plasma membrane, allowing the contents to leak out

CYTOKINES

Cytokines are low molecular weight proteins produced by cells that stimulate or inhibit the differentiation, proliferation or function of other cells. Similar substances produced by activated T cells are called "Lymphokines" and those produced by macrophages or monocytes are called "monokines". The term "Interleukin (IL)" is given to those cytokines that act on or signal between cells of the immune system.

Cytokine production is regulated by exogenous stimuli such as antigens and mitogens, as well as by endogenous factors such as neuroendocrine hormonal peptides (corticosteroids, endorphins) and products of lipoxygenase and cyclooxygenase pathways. They also regulate each other by positive and negative feed backs.

Cloning of cytokines and the availability of monoclonal antibodies against them have helped to characterise them better. A number of cytokines possess therapeutic application and can be used in the management of inflammatory, infectious, autoimmune and neoplastic conditions.

Thus cytokines include interleukins, colony stimulating factors, tumour necrosis factors, interferons, chemokines and others.

I. Interleukins

(a) Interleukin–1 (IL-1)

It is produced mainly by all nucleated cell types such as macrophages, monocytes and fibroblasts. IL-1 mediates a wide range of physiological, metabolic, inflammatory and hematological effects by acting on bone marrow, epithelial and synovial cells, fibroblasts, osteoclasts, hepatocytes, vascular endothelium etc. It occurs in two forms – IL-1 alpha and IL-1 beta. Its major functions are :

(*i*) Proliferation and differentiation of activated T and B cells.

(*ii*) Induces fever (pyrogenic).

(*iii*) Induce acute phase proteins.

(*iv*) Induces bone resorption by osteoclasts.

(*v*) Induce the production of prostaglandins (PGE_2), IL-6, granulocyte-macrophage colony stimulating factor (GM-CSF) and chemokines by macrophages and monocytes.

(*vi*) Activate neutrophils to produce cytokines.

(b) Interleukin–2 (IL-2)

It is produced by activated T cells. It was formerly known as T cell growth factor (TCGF).

IL-2 is a powerful immunomodulator and stimulates the proliferation of activated T and B cells and activates cytotoxic T cells and NK cells. It converts some null cells into lymphokine activated killer (LAK) cells which can destroy tumor cells that are resistant to NK cells. This property is used in the treatment of certain types of cancer.

IL-2 is released by T-helper (T_H) cells under the influence of IL-1. IL-2 is a potent activator of T cells and causes the expression of more IL-2 receptors on T cells so that they respond greatly to IL-2.

(c) Interleukin–3 (IL-3)

It is produced by T cells and mast cells. It stimulates the growth and differentiation of hematopoietic precursor stem cells. It is also known as multi-colony stimulating factor (multi-CSF).

(d) Interleukin–4 (IL-4)

It is produced by CD4+ T_H cells, mast cells, bone marrow stromal cells. It activates B cells and causes its proliferation and differentiation. Therefore, it was formerly known as B cell growth factor-I (BCGF-I). It also acts as a growth factor for T cells, mast cells and hematopoietic precursors. It enhances the action of cytotoxic T cells. It enhances IgG_1 and IgE production.

(e) Interleukin–5 (IL-5)

It is produced by CD4+T_H cells and mast cells. It was formerly known as B cell growth factor–II (BCGF–II). It causes proliferation of activated B cells, production of IgM and IgA, proliferation and maturation of eosinophils.

(f) Interleukin–6 (IL-6)

It is produced by CD4+T_H cells, macrophages, mast cells and fibroblasts. IL-6 has multiple biological activities on a variety of cells.

(*i*) Enhancing B cell replication, differentiation and Ig production.

(*ii*) Expression of IL-2 receptors on T cells so that T cells are stimulated to proliferate and differentiate. IL-6 synergises with IL-1 and TNF to costimulate T cells.

(*iii*) Induces the formation of acute phase proteins in liver cells.

(*iv*) Promotes hematopoiesis and thrombopoiesis.

(*v*) Supports the growth of transformed hepatocyte and myeloma cell lines in tissue culture.

(g) Interleukin–7 (IL-7)

It is produced from bone marrow stromal cells. It acts as B and T cell growth factor and causes proliferation of pre-B lymphocytes, T_H cells and activated mature T cells.

(h) Interleukin–8 (IL-8)

Produced by monocytes, causes activation and chemotaxis of neutrophils (neutrophil chemotactic factor).

(i) Interleukin–9 (IL-9)

Produced by T cells, causes growth and proliferation of T cells.

(j) Interleukin–10 (IL-10)

Produced by CD4+T_H cells, B cells and macrophages. It inhibits IFN-α secretion and inhibits mononuclear cell inflammation.

(k) Interleukin–11 (IL-11)

Formed by bone marrow stromal cells; induce acute phase proteins.

(l) Interleukin–12 (IL-12)

Produced by monocytes and macrophages. It causes proliferation of T_{H1} cells and activates NK cells. It was formerly called cytotoxic lymphocyte maturation factor (CLMF) or NK cell stimulatory factor (NKSF).

(m) Interleukin–13 (IL-13)

Formed by T cells. It inhibits mononuclear phagocyte inflammation and causes proliferation and differentiation of B cells.

II. Colony Stimulating Factors (CSFs)

They are cytokines that stimulate individual pluripotent stem cells in the bone marrow to produce large number of RBC, platelets, neutrophils, monocytes, eosinophils and basophils. They are named according to the stimulation of production of stem cell cultures *in vitro.*

The CSFs stimulate host defenses against infectious pathogens by increasing the number of phagocytes, modulate secretory function, chemotaxis and phagocyte killing by adjusting the rate of production of blood cells according to the requirements.

CSFs have clinical application in the treatment of hemopoietic disorders in diseases and malignancies.

(i) GM–CSF

Granulocyte-monocyte colony stimulating factor stimulates the growth of neutrophils and monocytes. It is produced by T cells, macrophages, fibroblasts, mast cells and endothelium.

(ii) G–CSF

Granulocyte CSF is produced by fibroblasts and endothelium; stimulates the growth of neutrophils.

(iii) M–CSF

Monocyte CSF is formed by fibroblasts, endothelium, epithelium and stimulates the growth of macrophages.

(iv) Multi–CSF

It is also known as IL-3. It is produced by T cells and mast cells. It stimulates the growth and differentiation of hematopoietic precursor stem cells.

(v) Steel factor

Produced by bone marrow stromal cells causes stem cell division.

III. Tumor Necrosis Factors (TNFs)

A serum factor found to induce hemorrhagic necrosis in certain tumors was named as tumor necrosis factor (TNF). The same substance was named as cachectin, since it causes wasting syndrome (cachexia) during chronic infections.

TNF occurs in two types– alpha (TNF-α) and beta (TNF-β).

TNF-α is produced by macrophages and monocytes. It exerts immunomodulatory influences on other cytokines. It resembles IL-1 in possessing a wide range of biological activities such as participation in the manifestations of endotoxic shock.

TNF-β (formerly known as lymphotoxin) is produced mainly by T_H cells.

TNFs exhibit a wide range of biological activities such as

(*i*) Tumor cytotoxicity

(*ii*) Cachexia (wasting syndrome)

(*iii*) Induction of acute phase proteins

(*iv*) Antiviral activity

(*v*) Antiparasitic activity

(*vi*) Induction of endotoxic shock

(*vii*) Induction of IFN-α, IL-1 (TNFα), GM-CSF and IL-6

(*viii*) Induction of phagocytic cells.

IV. Interferons (IFNs)

Interferons were originally identified as antiviral agents; now classified as cytokines. There are 3 types of IFNs.

(*i*) IFN-α (alpha Interferon) produced by leucocytes

(*ii*) IFN-β (beta Interferon) produced by fibroblasts.

(*iii*) IFN-γ (gamma Interferon) produced by T cells activated by antigens, mitogens or exposure to IL-2.

IFNs possess several biological effects :

(*i*) IFN-α and IFN-β are antiviral and associated in the expression of MHC class I molecules.

(*ii*) IFN-α is antiviral, activates macrophages and other cells, differentiation of cytotoxic T cells, synthesis of IgG_2 by activated B cells.

(*iii*) IFN-γ causes macrophage activation, promotes neutrophil and monocyte functions and antitumor activity.

V. Chemokines

They are produced by macrophages and T cells and are chemotactic for neutrophils and T cells and function as chemoattractants.

VI. Other Cytokines

TGF-β (Transforming growth factor beta) is produced by T and B cells and transforms fibroblasts by acting as a growth factor and promotes wound repair, inhibits T and B cell proliferation and hematopoeisis.

LIF (Leukemia inhibitory factor) is produced by T cells, causes proliferation of embryonic stem cells and chemotaxis and activation of eosinophils.

MSF (Macrophage stimulating factor) produced by T cells, stimulates macrophage migration to the site of action.

MAF (Macrophage activating factor) produced by T cells activates phagocytic function.

VII. Migration Inhibition factor *(MIF)* is produced by activated T_{DTH} (Delayed type hypersensitivity T cells). It inhibits the migration of macrophages away from the site of infection. This principle is employed in detection of CMI by macrophage migration inhibition test.

Specific T cells are activated at the site of delayed hypersensitivity reaction (*e.g.*, a positive intradermal tuberculin test), which amplify the reaction by releasing MIF. The released MIF causes the accumulation of macrophages at the site of reaction by inhibiting their migration.

CF (chemotactic factor) produced by T cells, stimulates chemotaxis of macrophages.

TRANSFER FACTOR (TF)

An extract of sensitised T lymphocytes is known as "transfer factor", that can be used for passive transfer of CMI, instead of sensitized T cells.

It is a low molecular weight polypeptide-poly nucleotide. TF transfers CMI to all the antigens to which the donor was sensitive. Humoral immunity is not transmitted by TF. Following the injection of TF, delayed hypersensitivity and other *in vitro* parameters of CMI can be demonstrated in the recipient.

TF may act by specific gene depression inducing antigenically uncommited lymphocytes to produce antigen-specific receptors.

TF has many clinical applications:

(*i*) To restore immunity in patients with T cell deficiencies (Wiskott–Aldrich syndrome).

(*ii*) To treat disseminated infections such as TB, leprosy, mucocutaneous candidiasis where CMI may be deficient.

(*iii*) To treat cancers such as malignant melanoma.

(*iv*) Can be used to treat certain autoimmune diseases (RA and SLE).

IMMUNOMODULATORS

Immunomodulators are biologic response-modifying compounds that affect the immune response either in a positive or negative fashion

e.g.,
- Gamma globulins
- Immunosuppressive drugs
- Cytokines
  - Interleukins – IL-2, IL-4, IL-10, IL-12
  - Interferons – IFN α, β and γ.
  - GM-CSF
  - TGF-β
- Complete Freund's adjuvant
- Anti-TNF antibodies
- Cytokine antagonists – IL-1 RA (Interleukin-1 receptor antagonist)
- Biochemical agents *e.g.*, levamisole
- Thymic hormones–thymosin, thymulin, thymopoietin.

DETECTION OF CMI

CMI can be detected by various tests :

In Vivo tests – Intradermal test to demonstrate delayed type hypersensitivity (DTH).

In Vitro tests –(i) Macrophage migration inhibition test.

(*ii*) Lymphocyte blast transformation test (or) Mixed lymphocyte reaction (MLR)

(*iii*) Cell mediated cytotoxicity (or) target cell lysis.

(*iv*) Enumeration of T cells and subpopulations.

Intradermal Test To Detect DTH

The antigen is injected intradermally in increasing doses. A hard, pale swelling with peripheral redness, measuring more than 5 mm in diameter, appearing in one to two days indicates a positive reaction, which is a type IV hypersensitivity reaction. A positive response indicates that the patient has active T cells that are specifically reacting with the antigen.

Macrophage Migration Inhibition Test

The test demonstrates the production of macrophage migration inhibitory factor (MIF) by sensitised T cells and its effect *i.e.*, inhibition of migration of macrophages from the site of antigen. The test is as follows :

(*i*) Capillary tubes are packed with a peritoneal exudate (consists of macrophages and lymphocytes) of guinea pig sensitized to a specific antigen by prior injection.

(*ii*) The tubes are placed in small tissue culture chambers containing culture media with and without the sensitizing antigen. The sensitised lymphocytes release MIF on contact with the specific antigen.

(*iii*) In the culture medium with the specific antigen, the motile macrophages are inhibited from migrating out of the end of the capillary tube by the MIF.

In the absence of sensitizing antigen, the macrophages migrate out from the end of the capillary tube in a fan-like pattern. (Fig. 29.3)

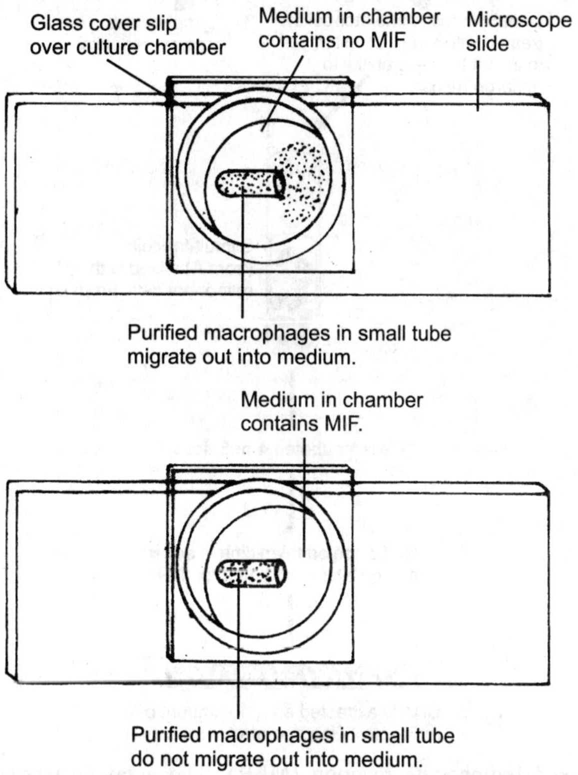

Fig. 29.3 Migration inhibition factor (MIF) test for cell-mediated immunity. Migration of motile macrophages is inhibited by lymphokine MIF. Macrophages migrate out of the open end of the capillary tube in a fanlike pattern unless inhibited by the presence of MIF

Mixed Lymphocyte Reaction (MLR) or Lymphocyte Blast Transformation Test

It measures the amount of cell proliferation stimulated by the presence of specific antigen.

The lymphocyte from two individuals are mixed together in a test tube. Each set of cells reacts against foreign histocompatibility antigens of other cells and become lymphoblasts, which begin to synthesize DNA and to multiply by mitosis. The cells are allowed to interact for 4 or 5 days. Then tritiated thymidine (Radiolabeled DNA precursor) is added and exposed to it for about 18 hours. The tritium (radio active isotype) will be incorporated into the newly synthesized DNA. The DNA is extracted and the radioactivity is determined, which gives a measure of the degree of cell proliferation.

The assay is most useful when only one set of cells is allowed to respond. The other set of cells are either irradiated or treated with mitomycin C (an antibiotic) to prevent proliferation or mitosis. This reaction is called "one way" MLR. (Fig. 29.4)

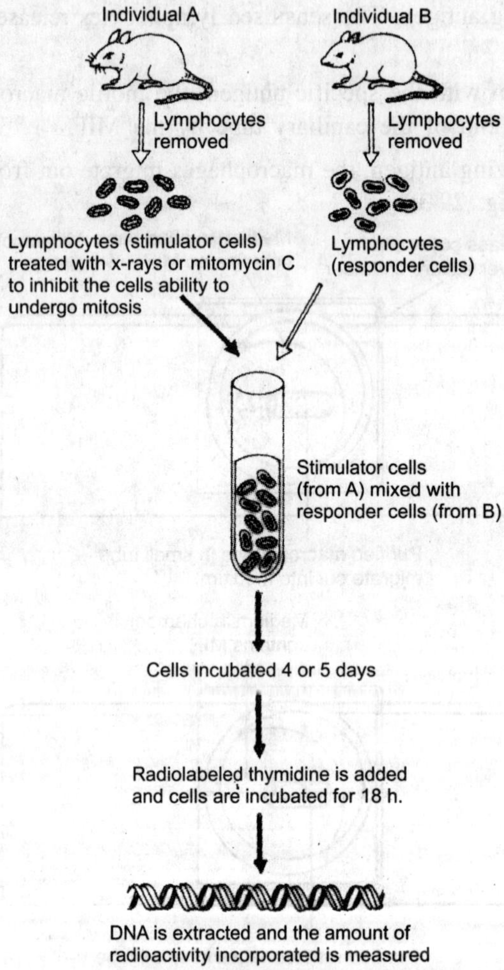

Fig. 29.4 The one-way mixed lymphocyte reaction (MLR). The assay is termed "one-way" because the stimulator cells from individual A have been irradiated or treated with mitomycin C (an antibiotic) to prevent them from synthesizing DNA, thereby preventing mitotic division. However, they continue to stimulate the responder cells from individual B, which continue to proliferate, i.e., incorporate radioactive thymidine

Cell Mediated Cytotoxicity (or) Target Cell Lysis

When lymphocytes from two individuals are allowed to react in a mixed lymphocyte culture, a subset of first individual's responder T cells are activated and lyse the second individual's stimulating cells and are called cytotoxic T lymphocytes (T_C). This lysis is specific for only target cells bearing the same epitopes as the stimulating cells. This phenomenon is called "target cell lysis" or "cell mediated cytotoxicity".

For the test, a population of viable lymphocytes are incubated with lymphocytes that are either irradiated or treated with mitomycin C. After 4–5 days, the cells are removed from the culture vessel, washed and suspended in various degrees of density. These cell suspensions are then mixed with a constant number of target cells whose cytoplasm has been labelled with radioactive chromium. After incubation for 4 hours the amount of target cell lysis is determined by the amount of radioactive chromium released into the medium.

Enumeration of T cells and Subpopulations

The cells are labeled with a monoclonal antibody tagged with a fluorescent dye (rhodamine or fluorescein). Single cells are passed through a laser light beam, and the number of cells that fluoresce are registered (counted) in a machine called Fluorescence-activated cell sorter (FACS).

QUESTIONS

Essay Questions

1. Give an account of cell mediated immunity.
2. Describe the various tests used for detection of CMI.

Short Notes

1. Cell mediated immune response.
2. Cytokines.
3. Interleukines.
4. IL-1.
5. Interleukin-2.
6. Interleukin-6.
7. Colony stimulating factor (CSF).
8. Tumor necrosis factor (TNF).
9. Types and uses of interferons.
10. Lymphokines.
11. MIF (or) Migration inhibition factor.
12. Transfer factor.
13. Immunomodulators.
14. Tests to detect CMI.
15. Macrophage migration Inhibition test.
16. Mixed lymphocyte reaction (MLR) or Lymphocyte blast transformation.

30

Humoral Immune Response (Antibody Mediated Immunity)

- ***Definition***
- ***Induction of AMI***
- ***Mechanism of antibody production***
- ***Primary and secondary immune responses***
- ***Ig class switching***
- ***Affinity maturation***
- ***Factors influencing antibody production***
  - ***Genetic factors***
  - ***Age***
  - ***Nutritional status***
  - ***Route of administration***
  - ***Size of antigen dose***
  - ***Number of antigen doses***
  - ***Multiple antigens***
  - ***Adjuvants***
  - ***Immunosuppressive agents***
- ***Theories of antibody production***
  - ***Instructive theories***
  - ***Direct template theory***
  - ***Indirect template theory***
  - ***Selective theories***
  - ***Side chain theory***
  - ***Natural selection theory***
  - ***Clonal selection theory***

DEFINITION

Humoral immune response (AMI) is mediated by antibodies produced by plasma cells, that are transformed B lymphocytes due to antigenic stimulation.

AMI is primarily directed against:

1. extracellular bacterial infections
2. Respiratory and intestinal viral infections
3. recurrence of viral infections
4. Toxin-induced diseases.
5. infections in which virulence is related to polysaccharide capsules (*e.g.,* Pneumococci, Meningococci, *Haemophilus influenzae*).

AMI also leads to the development of immediate (Types I, II, III) hypersensitivity reactions and certain autoimmune diseases.

INDUCTION OF AMI

The humoral immune response can be broadly divided into three stages:

1. The entry, distribution of antigen in tissues and its contact with an immunocompetent cell.
2. The processing and presentation of antigen to B cells and the control of antibody forming process.
3. The secretion of antibody and its distribution in blood and body fluids and the manifestation of its effects.

Antigens introduced intravenously are rapidly localised in the spleen, liver, bone marrow, kidneys and lungs. In contrast, antigens introduced subcutaneously are mainly localised in the draining lymph nodes, only small amounts being found in the spleen.

Different clones of lymphocytes constantly traffic from one secondary lymphoid organ to another through the blood and lymphatics, and come in contact with the antigen. The humoral response takes place in the germinal center of the secondary lymphoid tissues.

The macrophages, dendritic cells, langerhans cells trap the antigens, process them and present them in association with MHC class II molecules to the CD4+T_H cells bearing a specific TCR.

Antigen presenting cells produce IL-1, IL-6 and TNF-α. IL-1 stimulates the responding clone of T_H cells to produce IL-2 and to express receptor for IL-2 on the surface at the same time. IL-2, in turn, acts on T_H cells through the IL-2 receptor expressed on the surface to cause its differentiation and clonal proliferation.

The CD4+T_H cells responding to the antigen differentiate either into T_{H1} or T_{H2} subtypes that guide the immune response predominantly to the cell mediated or humoral response, respectively.

The T_{H2} cells stimulate the specific clone of B cells. The activated B cells recognize the same antigen (but a different epitope) which in the first place triggered the T_{H2} cells. Only with the help from T_{H2} cells, B cells multiply and mature into plasma cells that secrete specific antibodies of IgM type. This occurs during primary response or initial antigenic stimulus. Some B cells during the primary response convert to memory cells (Fig. 30.1).

On subsequent contact with the antigen, the memory cells mount a rapid and more effective response (known as secondary response), for they are already sensitized and recognize the antigen at once. When triggered by the antigen, memory cells convert to plasma cells, which produce IgG (class switch) with the same specificity, but with an increasing affinity (affinity maturation) to the antigen with the passage of time. Direct interaction between the T_{H2} cell and B cell is absolutely necessary for B cell response particularly in secondary response.

With non-protein antigens such as bacterial capsular polysaccharides, the humoral response does not require the cooperation of T_H cells (T-independent) and B cells respond directly. But this response is inefficient, short-lived and no memory cells are produced. Even on repeated subsequent contacts with the same antigen, class switching and affinity maturation do not occur. Thus, T-independent response can be converted to a T-dependent response by conjugating the polysaccharide antigen to a protein carrier.

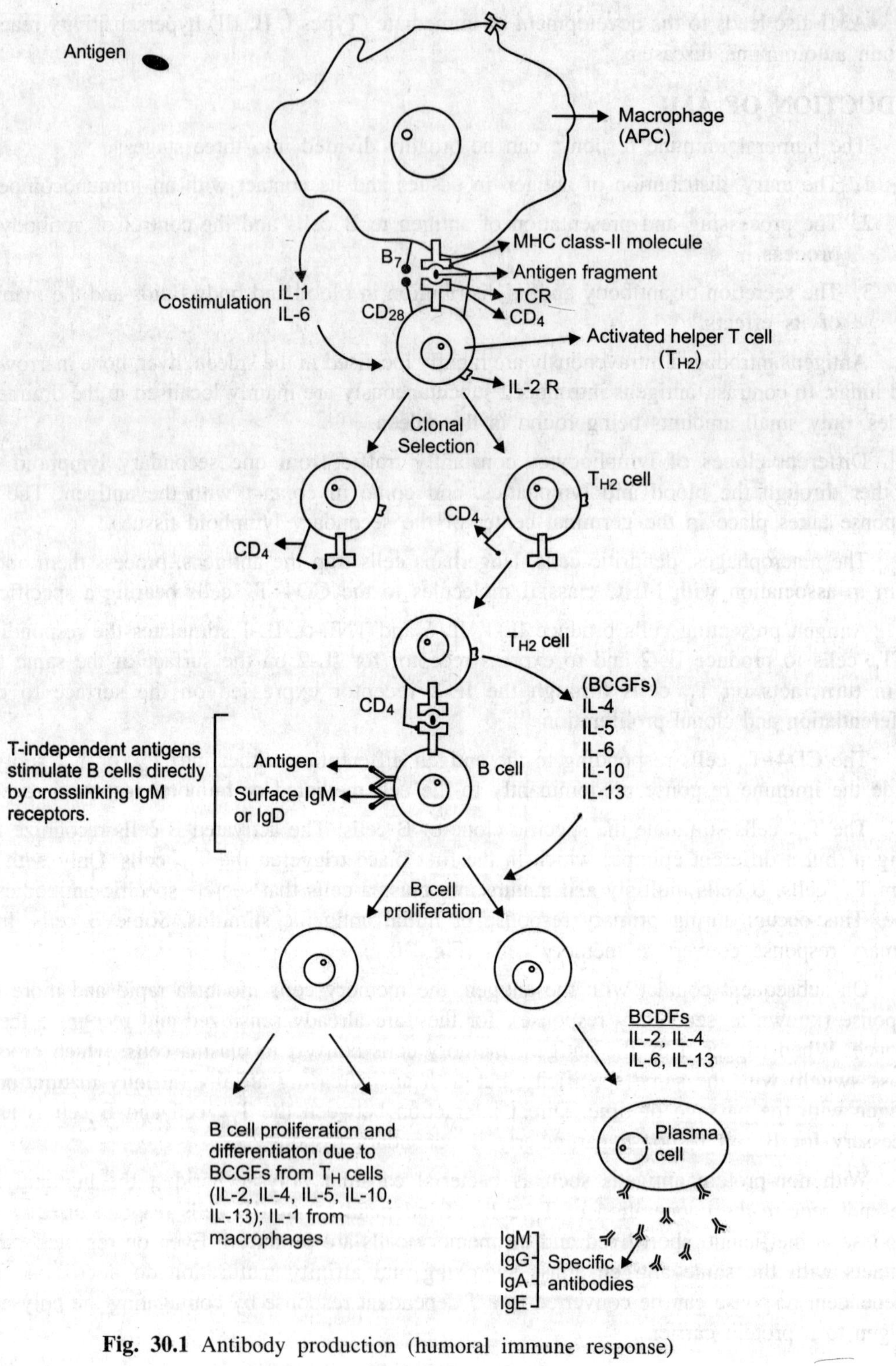

Fig. 30.1 Antibody production (humoral immune response)

MECHANISM OF ANTIBODY PRODUCTION

Immune response to an antigen is brought about by Antigen processing/presenting cells (APC- Macrophages and dendritic cells), T lymphocytes and B lymphocytes.

The antigens (such as bacteria and viruses) are captured and processed by APCs such as macrophages in their cytoplasm and present on their cell surface, epitopes complexed with MHC-class II molecules and are presented to T lymphocytes. This is essential for T cell dependent antigens, whereas T cell independent antigens do not require T cell cooperation for antibody production.

When the processed antigen is presented by antigen-presenting cell, in association with MHC class II molecules to the T lymphocytes (CD4+ T helper cells (or) T_H cells); only the T-helper cells carrying T cell receptor (TCR) to the epitope can recognize it.

B lymphocytes, which possess surface Ig and MHC class II molecules can also present antigens to T cells, particularly during the secondary response.

T_H cell is activated—(1) by combination of TCR with MHC class II and epitope complex on APC (2) by IL-1 produced by the APCs. Some T_H cells remain as memory cells (Fig. 30.1).

The activated T_H cell produces IL-2 and other cytokines such as B cell growth factor (BCGF) and the B cell differentiation factor (BCDF), which act on B cells carrying surface Ig for the epitope, to activate B cells causing cell growth, clonal proliferation and differentiation into plasma cells secreting antibody against the antigen. Some activated B cells become memory cells.

Cytotoxic T lymphocytes (CD8 cells or T_C cells) are activated on contact with the epitope complexed with MHC class-I molecules on APC. T_C cells are also stimulated by IL-2 produced by T_H cells. The stimulated cytotoxic cells release cytotoxins that destroys the target, which may be virus infected cell or tumor cell. Some T_C cells also become memory cells.

Conversely, in some cases suppressor T cells are activated, which suppress antibody formation either by restricting the supply of essential growth factor or by producing molecules that inhibit lymphocyte activation. This suppression gives rise to a state of immune tolerance in which the individual fails to respond to the activating antigen.

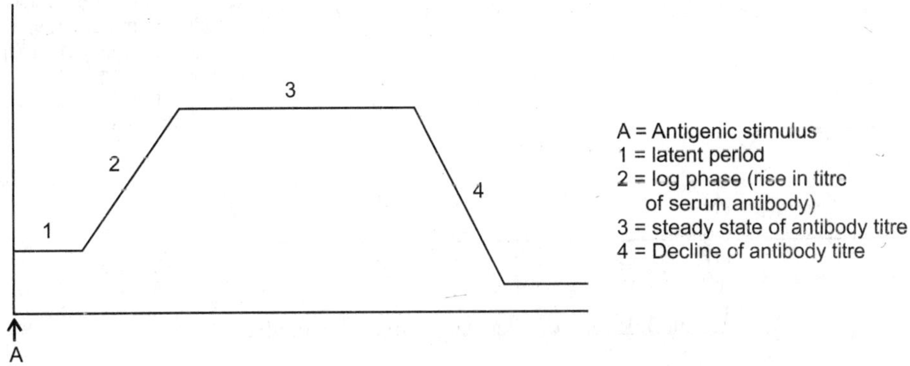

Fig. 30.2 Primary immune response

Antibody production follows a characteristic pattern consisting of (Fig. 30.2).

1. A lag phase, the immediate stage following antigenic stimulus during which no antibody is detectable in circulation.

2. A log phase in which there is steady rise in the titre of antibodies.
3. A plateau or steady state when there is an equilibrium between antibody synthesis and catabolism.
4. The phase of decline during which the catabolism exceeds the production and the titre falls.

PRIMARY AND SECONDARY HUMORAL IMMUNE RESPONSES

The antibody response to an initial antigenic stimulus differs qualitatively and quantitatively from the response to subsequent stimuli with the same antigen. The former is called primary response and the later secondary response.

The primary response is slow, sluggish, short-lived with a long lag phase and low titre of antibodies, usually of IgM type, that does not persist for long. In contrast, the secondary response is prompt, powerful and prolonged, with a short or negligible lag phase and a much higher level of antibodies (Fig. 30.3), usually of IgG type, that persists for long periods. The early antibody is more specific but less avid than the late antibody. The duration of the lag phase and the persistence of the antibody vary with the nature of the antigen. With some antigens such as diphtheria toxoid, the lag phase in the primary response may be as long as 2-3 weeks, while with pneumococcal polysaccharide, antibodies may appear within a few hours.

A single injection of an antigen helps more in sensitising or priming the immunocompetent cells producing the particular antibody than in the actual elaboration of high levels of antibody. Effective levels of antibody are usually induced only by subsequent injections of the antigen. It is for this reason that nonliving vaccines are given in multiple doses for active immunisation. The first injection is known as the "**priming dose**" or "**sensitising dose**" and subsequent injections as "**booster**" doses. With live vaccines, a single dose is sufficient as multiplication of the organism in the body provides a continuing antigenic stimulus that acts as both the priming and booster doses.

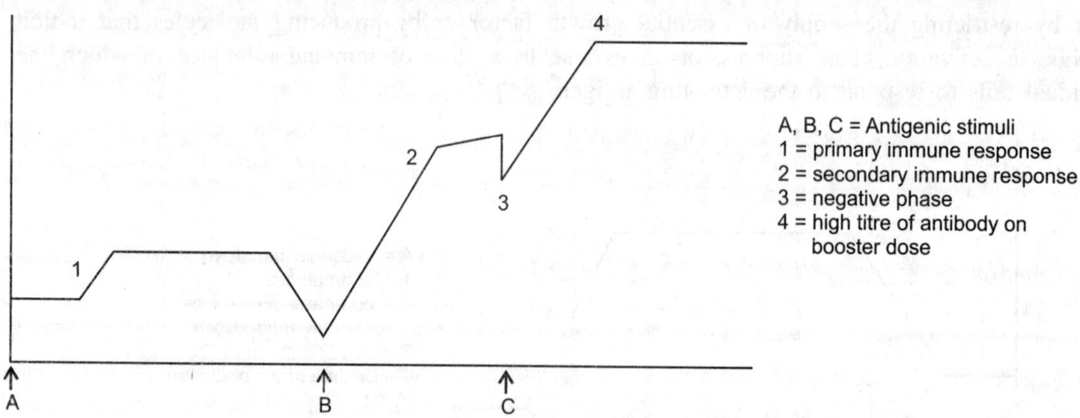

Fig. 30.3 Effect of repeated antigenic stimulus

Ig CLASS SWITCHING

When an antigen is encountered for the first time *i.e.,* during primary immune response, IgM class of antibodies are produced. If the same antigen is encountered subsequently *i.e.,* during secondary immune response, the same set of plasma cells or memory cells produce antibodies with the same specificity but of IgG class, which is known as class switch. Class switching occurs only with H-chains, whereas L-chains do not undergo class switching.

This process takes place in the germinal center and is irreversible. Help from the T_H cell is essential for class switching. On the long arm of the chromosome 14 from 3' to 5' end, a functional variable region (V_H) gene is followed by the C_H genes of different classes— μ, δ, γ–3, γ–1, α –1, γ –2, γ –4, ε and α–1 arranged in a sequential order. The class switch is achieved by splicing promoter of the μ gene infront of another downstream class-gene to be expressed next and deleting the intervening genes on the DNA.

AFFINITY MATURATION

Antibodies produced by a clone of plasma cells during the secondary response always bind the antigen with an increasing affinity with time. This process is called "affinity maturation". Help from the T_H cell and constant presentation of the antigen by Follicular dendritic cells (FDC) in the germinal center to the corresponding clone of B cells are essential for the process.

In the, germinal center, the clone of B cells responding to a specific antigen continuously undergoes random somatic hypermutation in the variable region genes of both the light and heavy chains of the antibody, which give rise to mutant B cells producing antibodies with slightly different specificity. The B cells producing the most avidly binding antibodies is selected in the germinal center to grow and proliferate. This is an ongoing process which leads to production of higher affinity antibodies with the passage of time.

ANAMNESTIC RESPONSE

The primary antibody response prime the immune system so that it possesses specific immunologic memory against a specific antigen. These memory cells may be activated in secondary response against a related antigenic stimulus (not the same specific antigen) and produce antibodies.

e.g., A person who suffered and recovered from typhoid fever or who had been immunized against typhoid fever may develop antityphoid antibodies in response to febrile viral infections. This phenomenon is called anamnestic response and is due to immunologic memory. Anamnestic response shows only a transient rise in titre of antibodies.

FACTORS INFLUENCING ANTIBODY PRODUCTION

Several factors influence AMI. They are as follows:

1. Genetic Factors

Immune response is under genetic control. Immune response genes (Ir genes) control immune response. Persons capable of responding to a particular antigen are called "responder" and those who cannot respond are called "non-responder".

2. Age

The embryo is immunologically immature. The fetus acquires capability to produce antibodies and induce CMI during last trimester (6-7 months). However, congenital infections may hasten the induction of immune response.

3. Nutritional Status

Protein calorie malnutrition and deficiency of essential amino acids (tryptophan, phenyl alanine, glycines, methionine, isoleucin) and vitamins (vitamin A, B-complex vitamins-riboflavine, pyridoxine, pantothenic acid, folic acid) suppress CMI and humoral immune response and decrease antibody synthesis.

4. Route of Administration

The humoral immune response is better following parenteral administration of antigen than through oral or nasal routes. However, oral or nasal route is most suitable for IgA production, and inhalation of pollen antigens induce IgE production.

The route of administration determines the type of antibody produced and also determines whether tolerance or antibody response results. Injection of protein antigens into the mesenteric veins or intrathymically usually induces tolerance. Application of simple chemicals to the skin usually leads to cellular immune response (delayed hypersensitivity) rather than antibody formation.

5. Size of Antigen Dose

Humoral immune response, to an extent, dose dependent. An antigen is effective only above a minimum critical dose. Further increase in dose enhances the intensity of the antibody response. But beyond a certain level, increase in the dose of antigen does not improve the antibody response but may even inhibit it and induce tolerance. The massive antigenic stimulus may paralyse the antibody producing system, a phenomenon known as "Immunological paralysis" by Felton.

6. Number of Antigen Doses

When antigens are administered repeatedly, the antibody response increases progressively; but after a critical stage, no further increase occurs.

7. Multiple Antigens

When a combination of two or more antigens are administered, the antibody response may be enhanced or decreased or remains unaffected *e.g.*,

(*i*) When toxoids are given along with bacterial vaccines (*e.g.*, DPT vaccine) the antibody response to the toxoids is increased.

(*ii*) When diphtheria and tetanus toxoids are given together, with one in high dose, the antibody response to the other is inhibited.

(*iii*) When two bacterial vaccines (*e.g.*, typhoid and cholera bacilli) are given together, the antibody response to each is not affected.

8. Adjuvants

The term adjuvant refers to any substance that enhances the antigenicity of an antigen. They delay the release of antigen from the site of injection and prolong the antigenic stimulus. They may confer antigenicity on nonantigenic substances, increase the concentration and persistence of the circulating antibody, induce or enhance the degree of CMI. Several substances can be used as adjuvants.

(*i*) **Aluminium hydroxide** or **aluminium phosphate** on to which the antigen is adsorbed, increase the stability and particle size and also promote the release of certain cytokines, such as IL-1. But they induce only humoral immunity. They cannot be frozen or freeze dried.

(*ii*) **Freund's incomplete adjuvant**-where the protein antigens are incorporated in the water phase of water-in-oil emulsion.

(*iii*) **Freund's complete adjuvant** is Freund's incomplete adjuvant along with a suspension of killed tubercle bacilli. It induces both humoral and CMI but produces local granuloma.

(*iv*) Muramyl dipeptides (MDP) from Mycobacterial cell walls, usually emulsified with oils, phospholipids or other surfactants can be used to induce humoral immune response without granuloma.

(*v*) LPS of Gram negative bacilli may act as adjuvants *e.g., Bordetella pertussis* acts as an adjuvant for diphtheria and tetanus toxoids in triple vaccine.

(*vi*) Silica particles, beryllium and endotoxins can be used as adjuvants. They activate macrophages.

(*vii*) Immunomodulators can be introduced into vaccines as adjuvants. IL-12 can promote helper T cell development and induces cell mediated immunity.

Adjuvants function in several ways

(*i*) by prolonging the retention of antigen and sustained release of antigen from depot.

(*ii*) by increasing the size of the antigen so that phagocytosis and presentation by macrophages is enhanced.

(*iii*) by stimulating the influx of macrophages or other immune cells such as T and B cells to the site of injection.

(*iv*) by promoting cytokine production.

(*v*) by stimulating CMI, promotes antitumor effect.

Adjuvants also produce "adjuvant diseases" such as allergic disseminated encephalomyelitis.

9. Immunosuppressive Agents

They inhibit/suppress the immune response. Immunosuppression may be necessary to prevent graft rejection in transplantation. Several agents can be used for immunosuppression.

(*i*) **X-irradiation–**Sublethal whole body irradiation suppresses antibody response. X-irradiation is more cytotoxic to replicating cells and has been used to prolong transplant survival and to control certain autoimmune conditions.

(*ii*) **Radiomimetic drugs (Alkylating agents)** *e.g.,* cyclophosphamide, nitrogen mustard, when administered 2-3 days after injection of antigen, completely suppresses the antibody formation. Cyclophosphamide is used in bone marrow recipients, selectively prevents B cell replication.

(*iii*) **Corticosteroids–**They are antiinflammatory drugs that suppress both T and B cell response. The act by inhibiting cytokine (*e.g.,* IL-1, IL-2 and TNF) production by macrophages and by lysing certain types of T cells and causes depletion of lymphocytes from blood and lymphoid organs.

(*iv*) **Antimetabolites–**They interfere with the synthesis of DNA, RNA or both and thus inhibit cell division and differentiation necessary for humoral and cellular immune responses. Many antimetabolites find clinical application in the prevention of graft rejection.

e.g.,	Folic acid antagonists	–	methotrexate
	Purine analogues	–	6-mercaptopurine, azothioprene
	Cytosine analogues	–	cytosine arabinoside
	Uracil analogues	–	5-fluorouracil

Azathioprene, used in renal transplants, inhibits T cells, but not B cell responses.

(*v*) **Drugs–**Cyclosporine, rapamycin, tacrolimus (FK 506). These drugs prevent the activation of T lymphocytes by inhibiting signal transduction within T cells by inhibiting calcineurin, a protein involved in the activation of the genes for IL-2 and the IL-2 receptor. Cyclosporine is widely used for preventing the rejection of transplants and is well-tolerated. Cyclosporine is a cyclic polypeptide derived from *Tolypocladium inflatum*, a soil fungus.

(*vi*) **Antilymphocyte serum (ALS)**–It is an heterologous antiserum raised against lymphocytes, by immunizing animals. Antiserum against thymus cells is called antithymocyte serum and the corresponding antibody globulin is called antilymphocyte globulin (ALG) and antithymocyte globulin.

ALS is used to prevent graft rejection. It acts against T lymphocytes and suppresses CMI specifically. ALS acts only on cells in circulation and not cells in lymphoid organs. ALS does not produce any side effects, whereas all other immunosuppressives have side effects.

(*vii*) **OKT3** is a murine monoclonal antibody against CD3, can block T cell function as well as lyse T cells.

THEORIES OF ANTIBODY PRODUCTION

Theories of immune response fall into two categories.

1. Instructive Theories

These theories postulate that an immunocompetent cell is capable of synthesizing antibodies of any specificity. The antigen encounters an immunocompetent cell and instructs it to produce the complimentary antibody *e.g.*, Direct template theory, Indirect template theory.

Direct template theory

These theories were proposed by Breinl and Haurowitz (1930), Alexander (1931) and Mudd (1932). According to these, antigen or the antigenic determinant enters antibody forming cells and serves as a "template" against which antibody molecules are synthesized so that they have combining sites complementary to the antigenic determinant. Pauling (1940) suggested that specificity was determined by the folding of the antibody polypeptide chains to form a tertiary structure fitting the antigenic determinant.

Indirect template theory

This theory was proposed by Burnet and Fenner (1949). According to this theory, antigenic determinant enters into the antibody producing cell and gets incorporated in its genome and transmitted to the progeny cells (indirect template). This theory, therefore, explained the specificity and the secondary response.

2. Selective Theories

These theories shift the emphasis from the antigen to the immunocompetent cell. They postulate that immunocompetent cells have only a restricted immunological range. The antigen exerts only a selective influence by stimulating the appropriate immunocompetent cell to synthesize an antibody. *e.g.*, Side chain theory, Natural selection theory, Clonal selection theory.

Side chain theory

This theory was proposed by Ehrlich (1900). According to this theory, immunocompetent cells have surface receptors, capable of reacting with antigens having complementary "side chains". Nutrients anchor to these receptors before assimilation. When foreign antigens are introduced into the body, they combine with those cell receptors which have a complementary fit. This inactivates the receptors and interferes with absorption of nutrients. As a compensatory mechanism, there is an overproduction of the same type of receptors, which spill over into the blood and circulate as antibodies. It explains the specificity of antibody response.

However, when Landsteiner demonstrated that antibodies could be formed not only against natural antigens but also against various synthetic chemicals, this theory was abandoned.

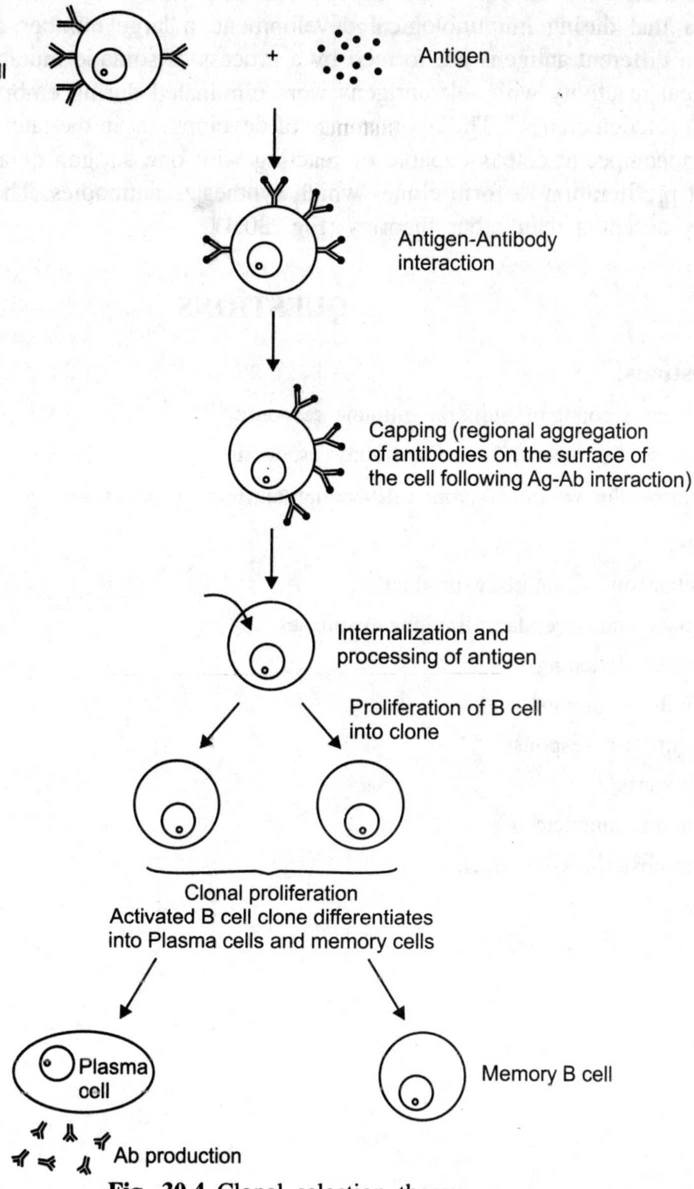

Fig. 30.4 Clonal selection theory

Natural selection theory

This theory was introduced by Jerne (1955). This theory postulates that about one million globulin (antibody) molecules were formed in embryonic life, which covers full range of antigenic specificities. These globulins are "natural antibodies". When an antigen is introduced, it combines selectively with the globulin molecule that has the nearest complementary fit. The globulin, with the combined antigen enters into the antibody forming cell and stimulated them to synthesize the same kind of antibody.

Clonal selection theory

This is a selective theory of antibody formation, proposed by Mac Farlane Burnet (1957). This theory states that during immunological development, a large number of lymphocytes capable of reacting with different antigens are formed by a process of somatic mutation. Clones of cells having immunological reactivity with self antigens were eliminated during embryonic life. Such clones are known as "forbidden clones". Their persistence of development in the later life leads to autoimmunity. Each immunocompetent cell is capable of reacting with one antigen or a small number of antigens leads to cell proliferation to form clones which synthesize antibodies. The clonal selection theory is more widely accepted than other theories (Fig. 30.4).

QUESTIONS

Essay Questions:

1. Give an account of humoral immune response.
2. Describe the mechanism of antibody production.
3. Describe the various factors influencing antibody production.

Short Notes:

1. Mechanism of antibody production.
2. Primary and secondary immune responses
3. Ig class switching.
4. Affinity maturation.
5. Anamnestic response
6. Adjuvants
7. Freund's complete adjuvant
8. Immunosuppressive agents
9. ALS
10. Clonal selection theory.

31

Immunization

INTRODUCTION

"Prevention is better than cure", and immunization is one of the most cost-effective ways of preventing infectious diseases.

VACCINATION AND IMMUNIZATION

The terms "immunization" and "vaccination" are often used interchangeably, but their meanings are different. Vaccination is the act of administering a vaccine. Immunization is a process by which immunity to a pathogen is elicited/induced by vaccination (active immunity) or transfered passively by administration of immune components (passive immunity).

VACCINE

The term vaccine refers to an antigenic preparation consisting of either cell suspension of live, attenuated strain (live vaccine) or inactivated strain (killed vaccine) of an organism or its antigenic constituents (subunit vaccine) or a product excreted/secreted by the cell such as an exotoxin, which is modified (toxoid) so that it is no longer toxic, but retains its antigenic properties.

TYPES OF IMMUNIZATION

Immunization is of three types:

– Active immunization

– Passive immunization

– Combined immunization

ACTIVE IMMUNIZATION

The immune system of the body can be stimulated to produce protective immunity against the infectious agent by injection of a vaccine or toxoid.

Development of active immunity by vaccination requires a period of time, and often, booster doses. The immunity induced is of long term. Immunological memory is present. Vaccines provide immunity by stimulating cell mediated immunity and/or production of antibodies.

Vaccines are made with either (1) killed microorganisms (2) live attenuated microorganisms (3) microbial extracts (4) vaccine conjugates or (5) inactivated toxins (toxoids).

1. Killed Vaccines

Bacterial vaccines are prepared from cultures grown on agar or broth media. Growth on agar is suspended in normal saline (0.85% NaCl). Bacterial cells in broth are washed by centrifugation with normal saline to remove extraneous materials. They are finally suspended in saline at a standard concentration or density. The bacteria are killed by heating at 60-65°C for 30-60 min and preserved or detoxified with 0.5% phenol or 0.2% merthiolate.

e.g., TAB vaccine against typhoid and paratyphoid fever
Cholera vaccine against cholera
Pertussis vaccine against whooping cough
Plague vaccine

Viral vaccines are prepared by cultivating viruses either in cell lines or embryonated eggs or animals. Vaccines prepared from these materials contain substances derived from the animal or tissue, which may occasionally cause hypersensitivity or other undesirable side reactions. These side effects are reduced by harvesting only portions of the infected tissue (*e.g.*, certain organs of inoculated animal, allantoic fluid of chick embryo etc.). The viruses are killed or inactivated with formaline, phenol or other substances.

e.g., Salk's polio vaccine against poliomyelitis
Influenza vaccine against influenza
Animal brain Rabies vaccine
Cell culture Rabies vaccine
Japanese encephalitis vaccine, Hepatitis A vaccine

2. Live Attenuated Vaccines

Some vaccines are prepared by live organisms, but their virulence is greatly diminished or attenuated. They produce Natural active immunity. Live vaccines initiate an infection without causing any injury or disease.

Attenuation or reduction of virulence can be achieved

1. by repeated subcultures.

2. by serial passage through unfavourable host.
3. by selection of mutants with low virulence.
4. by growth under high temperature or in the presence of weak antiseptics, desiccation.
5. by prolonged storage in cultures.

e.g., – Anthrax vaccine by cultivating at high temperature (40–43°C)

– BCG (Bacillus Calmette-Guerin) by repeated subcultures (239 times) of *Mycobacterium bovis* on glycerine-bile-potato medium over a period of 13 yrs.

– The live oral vaccine (typhoral) a mutant of *S. typhi* strain T_Y2 1a (Gal E mutant) against typhoid fever.

– Sabin's oral polio vaccine (OPV), a mutant strain

– Yellow fever vaccine (17D vaccine) by passaging into chick embryos

– Small pox vaccine

– MMR (Measles, Mumps, Rubella) vaccine

– Varicella vaccine against chicken pox

Some vaccines such as polio and typhoid vaccines are available both in live or killed versions.

3. Microbial Extracts

Instead of using whole organisms, vaccines can be composed of antigenic molecules extracted from the pathogen, from an acellular (noninfectious) filtrate of the culture medium in which the organism was grown or produced by recombinant DNA techniques.

e.g., Acellular pertussis (*Bordetella pertussis* antigen)
Anthrax (noninfectious filtrate from culture)
Hepatitis B vaccine
vi antigen for typhoid
Glycoprotein subunit vaccine for Rabies

4. Vaccine Conjugates

Covalent binding (conjugation) of an antigenic polysaccharide to a protein enhances the immune response, particularly in children below two years of age. Several conjugated polysaccharide vaccines are available.

e.g., – *Haemophilus influenzae* type B polysaccharide covalently conjugated to a protein antigen, such as diphtheria toxoid.

– Pneumococcal Polysaccharide vaccine

– Meningococcal Polysaccharide vaccines

5. Toxoids

Exotoxins are strongly antigenic. They are unstable. They lose toxicity on aging and are gradually converted into toxoids. The transformation of a toxin into toxoid can be achieved by

(*i*) prolonged incubation at 37°C
(*ii*) by treatment with 0.2 to 0.4% formalin
(*iii*) by acidic pH.

Toxoids retain the antigenic power of the original toxins but lack toxicity. Toxoids, therefore can be used to produce immunity against corresponding toxins.

For the production of toxins, specific strains of the bacterium that yield high quantities of toxin are selected. Incubation temperature, pH and composition of the culture medium are selected at optimum to obtain the greatest possible yield of the toxin. The diphtheria bacilli are grown aerobically to produce toxin, whereas the tetanus, gas gangrene and botulism bacilli require anaerobic conditions. After sufficient growth, the culture is passed through very fine-pored filters which remove the organisms. The filtrate contains the exotoxin liberated by the cells during their growth.

Toxin is converted into toxoid by treatment with 0.4 to 0.5% formalin and incubated at 37°C for a month or until animal tests show that no toxicity remains. Toxoid is partially purified by precipitation with ammonium sulphate. This toxoid protein is redissolved in buffered saline, is known as fluid toxoid or plain toxoid. When plain toxoid is injected, the soluble material is eliminated within a few hours and the antigenic stimulus is transitory. To prolong the antigenic stimulus and to potentiate the immune response, adjuvants are used *e.g.,* Alum-precipitated toxoids. When alum-precipitated toxoids are injected, the alum precipitate remains undissolved releasing its adsorbed toxoid slowly. This gives a prolonged and continuous antigenic stimulus which is highly effective.

e.g., Tetanus toxoid, Diphtheria toxoid.

ADJUVANTS

Substances that enhance the effectiveness of the antigens are called adjuvants. Adjuvants potentiate or augment the immune response to some vaccines.

Adjuvants act by

1. rendering soluble antigen into a particulate form and slowing down release of the antigen (depot effect), thus prolonging stimulation
2. mobilizing the antigen presenting cells (macrophages) into the site of injection.

Alum, a complex mixture of aluminium compounds including aluminium phosphate and aluminium hydroxide is used as adjuvant in adsorbed DPT and adsorbed DT vaccine.

IMMUNE RESPONSE TO VACCINES

Vaccines containing killed pathogens (*e.g.,* Salk's polio vaccine, hepatitis A vaccine) or antigenic components of pathogens (*e.g.,* hepatitis B vaccine) do not enter host cells, and therefore they give rise to a primary B-cell mediated humoral response. These antibodies are ineffective in attacking intracellular organisms. By contrast, live attenuated vaccines (usually viruses) do penetrate into cells. This results in the production of intracellular antigens that are displayed on the surface of the infected cell, prompting a cytotoxic T cell response, which is effective in eliminating intracellular pathogens.

TIMING OF VACCINATION

The infant's antibody-producing capacity develops slowly during the first year of life. Although the immune system is not fully developed, it is desirable to begin immunization at 2 months of age because diseases are common in this age group, and can be particularly severe (*e.g.,* whooping cough, *Haemophilus influenzae* meningitis).

Table 31.1 National Immunization Schedule

Age	*Vaccine*
*At birth	BCG, OPV-O dose
6 weeks	BCG (if not given at birth)
	DPT-1, OPV-1
10 weeks	DPT-2, OPV-2
14 weeks	DPT-3, OPV-3
9 months	Measles
16–24 months	DPT and OPV
5–6 years	DT**
10 years	TT***
16 years	TT
For pregnant women****	
Early in pregnancy TT-1 or booster	
One month after TT-1 TT-2	

* For institutional births only. OPV-O is additional, and not to be counted for the primary course of 3 doses starting at 6 weeks.

** A second dose of DT should be given at an interval of one month if there is no clear history or documented evidence of previous immunization with DPT.

*** The second dose of TT should be given at an interval of one month if there is no clear history or documented evidence of previous immunization with DPT, DT or TT.

**** For prevention of tetanus in the neonate primarily, but also in the mother.

WHO EPI IMMUNIZATION SCHEDULE

WHO (May, 1974) launched a global immunization programme known as "Expanded Programme of Immunization (EPI)" to protect all children of the world against six vaccine-preventible diseases-diphtheria, whooping cough, tetanus, poliomyelitis, tuberculosis and measles by the year 2000.

Table 31.2 WHO EPI immunization schedule

Age	*Vaccine*
Birth	BCG, OPV
6 weeks	DPT, OPV
10 weeks	DPT, OPV
14 weeks	DPT, OPV
9 months	Measles

This programme is now called Universal Child Immunization (UCI) (1990).

In addition, hepatitis B vaccine may be given at birth, 1 month and 6 months of age and booster dose at the age of 10 years. Children of the age of 15 months may be given MMR vaccine, followed by a booster at the age of 4-6 years.

RECOMBINANT DNA VACCINES

Genetically engineered (recombinant) strains of microorganisms produced by addition of the gene for expression of an appropriate protective antigen and by selective deletion of the virulence genes are emerging as potential vaccines.

e.g., Rabies vaccine, Hepatitis B vaccine.

DNA VACCINES

DNA vaccine is a nucleotide sequence encoding one or more microbial antigens, which is introduced into the host cell by means of a recombinant vector such as bacterial plasmid. Using the host cell's protein synthesis machinery, the plasmid DNA (recombinant) directs the synthesis of the antigenic microbial protein it encodes. This antigenic protein may leave the cells, which may be processed and presented to the immune system.

PASSIVE IMMUNIZATION

Passive immunization is achieved by injecting a recipient with preformed immunoglobulins or immunocompetent cells obtained from human serum (or occasionally equine serum *e.g.,* tetanus antitoxin, diphtheria antitoxin).

Passive immunization is used to provide immediate protection to individuals who have been exposed to an infectious organism and lack active immunity to that pathogen. Since passive immunization does not activate the immune system, immunological memory is absent. The immunity is short-lived for a few weeks to months, as the immunoglobulins are cleared from the recipient's serum.

Artificially, passive immunity is provided by injection of three types of immunoglobulin preparations.

1. Pooled Normal Immunoglobulin

Derived from pooled plasma of donors containing antibodies to the infectious agents currently prevalent in the population. It is used for prevention of an illness for which there is no specific immunoglobulin preparation. It is effective when given immediately before or after exposure to an infectious disease such as hepatitis A and Measles.

2. Specific Immunoglobulin (Hyperimmune sera)

This type of Immunoglobulin contains high concentrations of antibodies directed against a specific pathogen or toxin. It is prepared by active immunization of equine animals or obtained from the pooled blood of patients recovering from an infection.

e.g., Human Tetanus Immunoglobulin (HTIG)
Hepatitis B Immunoglobulin (HBIG)
Human Rabies Immunoglobulin (HRIG)
Varicella-Zoster Immunoglobulin (ZIG)

3. Monoclonal antibodies

Monoclonal antibody preparations are being developed against various infectious agents.

COMBINED IMMUNIZATION

(Combined passive and active immunization)–In some diseases (*e.g.,* tetanus, diphtheria, rabies) passive immunization is often undertaken in conjunction with inactivated vaccine products, to provide both immediate (but temporary) passive immunity and slowly developing active immunity. Both injections should be given at separate sites.

PRODUCTION OF ANTISERA

The term "antiserum" is applied to antibodies prepared in animals. The antisera for tetanus and diphtheria toxins is produced by active immunization of horses.

The antisera for agglutination tests in laboratories can be prepared by active immunization of Rabbits.

Large, healthy Rabbits are injected intravenously at intervals of 5 to 7 days with a saline suspension of 24 hr. culture, killed by exposure to one hour at 60°C. The following series of doses 1/20, 1/10, 1/5, 1/3 and 1/2 culture may be given. These doses are measured by emulsifying a slope culture in a given volume of saline. In the case of organisms of high toxicity; immunization can be started with even lower doses (1/100 of a culture).

With certain organisms, higher titres may be obtained if living organisms are injected. Small amounts (such as 0.01ml) of a young living broth culture should be injected intravenously. As the animal becomes immune, larger doses may be given.

When separate O and H agglutinating antisera are required for motile bacteria, immunization is best carried out with selected strains. For the production of O-antisera, a culture boiled for 2½ hr. or nonmotile variant can be used as a pure O antigen.

Seven to ten days after the last injection, a specimen of blood is withdrawn from an ear vein and the serum is tested for its agglutinating power towards the strain used for immunization. A series of dilutions is tested and if agglutination occurs in a 1 in 1600 or higher dilution, the animal is bled from the neck vessels or by cardiac puncture. The blood is allowed to clot in a sterile tube/bottle, placed overnight in the refrigerator, and the serum is then separated. 0.5% phenol is added to serum to prevent bacterial contamination. Glycerol may also be used as a preservative. The antisera may be preserved in sterile ampoules or glass tubes with ends sealed over the flame.

QUESTIONS

Essay Question

1. Give an account of various types of immunization.

Short Notes

1. Define vaccine
2. Active immunization
3. Killed vaccines
4. Live attenuated vaccines
5. Toxoids
6. National immunization schedule
7. Passive immunization
8. Production of antisera.

32

Hypersensitivity/Allergy

- *Definition*
- *Sensitising and shocking dose*
- *Classification*
- *Differences between immediate and delayed hypersensitivity*
- *Type–I hypersensitivity*
  - *Anaphylaxis*
  - *Atopy*
- *Type–II hypersensitivity*
- *Type–III hypersensitivity (Immune complex diseases)*
  - *Arthus phenomenon*
  - *Serum sickness*
- *Type–IV hypersensitivity (Delayed hypersensitivity)*
  - *Infection (Tuberculin type)*
  - *Contact dermatitis*
- *Type–V hypersensitivity (Stimulatory type)*
- *Jones–Mote reaction (or) cutaneous basophil hypersensitivity*
- *Shwartzmann reaction (Sanarelli-Shwartzmann reaction)*

DEFINITION

Hypersensitivity is a condition of increased immune sensitivity in which the body reacts to an antigen with an exaggarated immune response that usually harms the individual. It is also termed "Allergy".

In other words, hypersensitivity is an exaggarated immune response that results in tissue damage in a sensitised individual and is manifested on second or subsequent contact with specific antigen.

Antigens which can cause allergic symptoms are referred to as **allergens**.

An allergy is the unfortunate side effect of a correctly working immune system.

SENSITISING AND SHOCKING DOSE

The first (initial) contact with an antigen (allergen) sensitises the immune system, leading to the priming of specific T or B-lymphocytes. This is known as "**sensitising**" or "**priming dose**".

The second or subsequent contact with the same specific allergen produces the manifestations of hypersensitivity. This is known as "**shocking dose**".

CLASSIFICATION

(I) Based on the time required for the appearance of clinical reactions, on subsequent contact with the allergen; the hypersensitivity reactions may be classified into two types.

1. Immediate hypersensitivity (Antibody mediated)
   - Anaphylaxis
   - Atopy
   - Antibody mediated cell damage
   - Arthus phenomenon
   - Serum sickness
2. Delayed hypersensitivity (T-cell mediated)
   - Infection (tuberculin) type
   - Contact dermatitis type

(II) Robert Coombs and Peter Gell (1963) classified hypersensitivity reactions into four types based on the mechanisms of pathogenesis. Type V hypersensitivity is added to it recently.

1. Type I (Anaphylactic, IgE or reagin dependent) – Allergen reacts with IgE antibody fixed on basophils and mast cells causing release of histamine and other vasoactive amines *e.g.,* Anaphylaxis, Atopy.
2. Type II (cytolytic and cytotoxic) – Antibody (usually IgG, rarely IgM) reacts with cell associated antigens in the presence of complement. *e.g.*, hemolytic anemia (Rh incompatibility) and thrombocytopenic purpura.
3. Type III (Immune complex diseases) – Antigen-Antibody complexes are deposited on walls of blood capillaries causing activation of complement *e.g.*, Arthus reaction, serum sickness, glomerulonephritis.
4. Type IV (Delayed or cell mediated hyper-sensitivity) – Reactions between antigen and sensitized T-lymphocytes cause release of lymphokines leading to delayed hypersensitivity *e.g.,* Mycobacterial infections and contact dermatitis.
5. Type V (Stimulatory type) – Non-complement fixing antibodies directed against certain cell surface components may actually stimulate rather than destroy the cells.

Table 32.1 Differences Between Immediate and Delayed Hypersensitivity Reactions

	Immediate hypersensitivity	*Delayed hypersensitivity*
Onset of reaction	Appears within few minutes (immediately) and disappears rapidly.	Appears within 1–3 days (delayed) and lasts longer.
Sensitizing antigen	Induced by antigens or haptens by any route	Induced by living cells; antigens or haptens intradermally; antigens with adjuvants; or by skin contact

Mediators of hyper-sensitivity	Antibody mediated	T-cell mediated
Passive transfer	By transferring serum	By transferring sensitized T-cells or transfer factor
Basic lesion	Increased capillary permeability, exudation, contraction of smooth muscles.	Induration due to aggregation of cell infiltrates; no contraction of smooth muscles.
Skin test	Wheal and flare	Induration
Desensitization	Easy but short-lived	Difficult but long lasting.
Antihistamines	Beneficial	Not beneficial

TYPE I : HYPERSENSITIVITY

Anaphylaxis

It is a systemic form of Type I hypersensitivity. The allergens that can produce systemic Anaphylaxis include-antibiotics (penicillin); passively administered antisera (antitoxins) or heterologous serum therapy; insect venom from the stings or bites of wasps, hornets or bees.

Mechanism

On first contact with an allergen, B-lymphocytes are stimulated to differentiate into plasma cells and produce specific **IgE (reagin antibodies)**, and bind to the F_C receptors of **mast-cells or basophils** and sensitizes these cells, making the individual allergic to the allergen (Fig. 32.1).

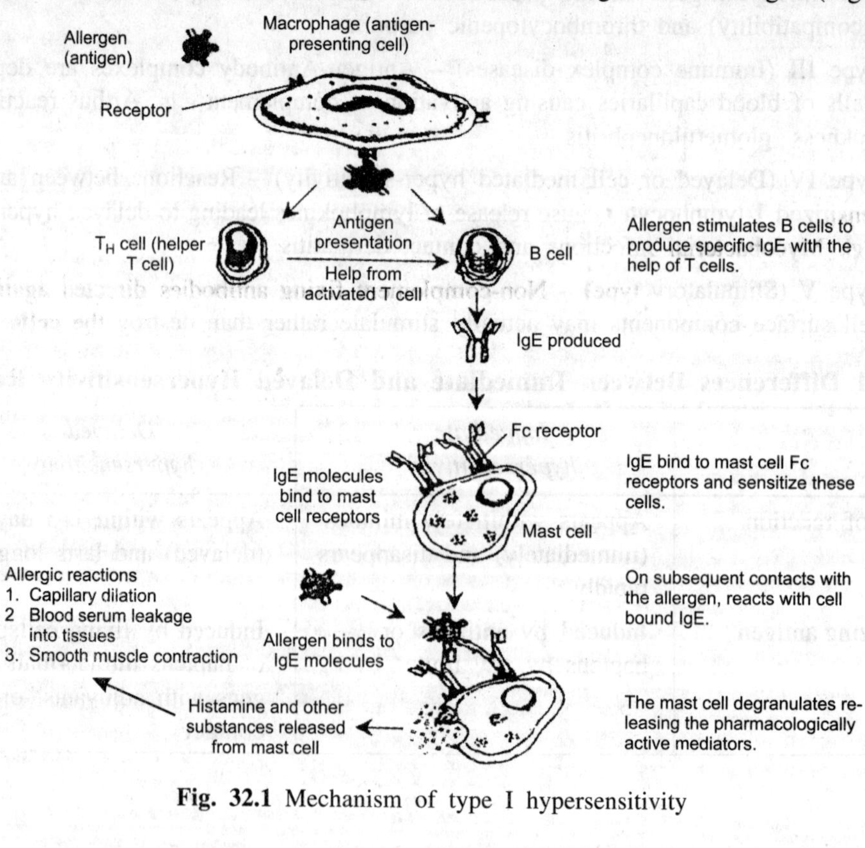

Fig. 32.1 Mechanism of type I hypersensitivity

When second or subsequent exposure to the same specific allergen occurs, the allergen attaches to the surface-bound IgE on the sensitized mast cells. Usually, the allergen reacts with adjacent IgE molecules, so that the gap between them is closed, so that mast cells are activated and their permeability to calcium ions is increased, causing degranulation (release the contents of basophilic granules). These granules contain biologically active or **pharmacologically active substances**, which are responsible for the manifestations of anaphylaxis.

Primary mediators (constitutive, preformed in granules) from mast cells triggered by cross-linking of IgE by antigen (allergen) or anaphylatoxins (C3a or C5a) :

- Histamine
- Serotonin
- Heparin
- Eosinophil chemotactic factor (ECF)
- Neutrophil chemotactic factor (NCF)
- Tryptase.

Secondary mediators, newly formed upon stimulation by mast cells, basophils and other leucocytes from arachidonic acid metabolic pathway :

- Slow reacting substance of anaphylaxis (SRS-A), also called leukotrienes (LT)-LTB4, LTC4, LT D4, LTE 4.
- Platelet activating factor
- Prostaglandins
- Thrombaxanes.

These pharmacologically active mediators trigger the following effects :

- Smooth muscle contraction
- Vasodilation (capillary dilation) – leads to reddening of the affected area
- Increased vascular permeability
- Blood serum leakage into tissues–edema formation
- Mucus secretion.

The area is typically infiltrated with neutrophils and eosinophils.

Cutaneous anaphylaxis

When a small dose of specific antigen is injected intradermally into a sensitized host, there will be a local wheal and flare reaction, which develops within few minutes and is known as cutaneous anaphylaxis, which is used in testing for Type–I Allergy.

Schultz-Dale phenomenon (Anaphylaxis *in vitro*)

Smooth muscle bits from intestine or uterus from sensitised animals kept in ringer's solution will contract vigorously, when specific antigen is added to it.

Anaphylactoid reaction

When certain substances such as peptone, trypsin are intravenously injected, produce a clinical reaction resembling anaphylactic shock. This is known as anaphylactoid reaction.

It is a nonspecific mechanism involving the activation of complement and the release of anaphylatoxins and has no immunological basis.

Passive cutaneous anaphylaxis (PCA) test is an *in vivo* method for detection of antibodies. A small dose of antibody is injected intradermally into a normal animal. After a gap of 4–24 hrs, the antigen alongwith Evan's blue dye is injected intravenously. There will be an immediate blueing at the site of intradermal injection due to vasodilation and increased capillary permeability *i.e.*, wheal and flare reaction. PCA test can be used to detect human IgG antibody which is heterocytotropic, capable of fixing to cells of other species, but not IgE, which is homocytotropic.

Atopy

It is a localized form of Type I hypersensitivity. Coca (1923) introduced the term "Atopy" to refer to naturally occuring familial hypersensitivity, characterized by allergic rhinitis (hay fever) and asthma.

The allergens (atopens) commonly involved are :

(1) Inhalants (air-borne allergens) – pollen, fungal spores, animal dander, house dust mites.

(2) Ingestants (food-borne allergens) – eggs, milk, fruits, fish.

Sensitization to these allergens is induced by natural contact. Atopy is hereditary and has genetical predisposition linked to MHC genotype. Atopic allergy is due to the production of IgE antibodies in large quantities. This is sometimes associated with a deficiency of IgA.

Mechanism

Same as anaphylaxis.

Clinical Symptoms

(1) **Hay fever (Allergic rhinitis)** – congested nasal passages, coughing, sneezing, itchy and tearing eyes (conjunctivitis). It involves upper respiratory tract.

(2) **Asthma** – It is an atopic allergy involving lower respiratory tract. The alveoli (air sacs) become overdistended and fill with fluid and mucus; the smooth muscles contract and narrows the lumen of the bronchi, which produces wheezing or whistling sound during exhalation.

(3) **Atopic dermatitis** – eruptions of skin (Hives) are a diagnostic sign of food allergy.

P-K Reaction

IgE is homocytotropic, that is only human IgE can fix to the human cells (species specific), which forms the basis of Prausnitz-Kustner (PK) reaction. It was originally used for detecting IgE antibody.

The serum from Kustner, who had atopic allergy to certain species of cooked fish is injected into prausnitz (who had no allergy) intradermally. After a gap of 24 hours, a small dose of cooked fish antigen is injected intradermally into the same site. Then, wheal and flare reaction developed immediately within few minutes.

This test also demonstrates the affinity of IgE for skin cells; and passive transfer of Type I allergy.

TYPE II : HYPERSENSITIVITY (COMPLEMENT MEDIATED CYTOLYTIC AND CYTOTOXIC REACTIONS)

Type II hypersensitivity is generally called a cytolytic and cytotoxic reaction, because it results in the destruction of host cells, either by lysis or toxic mediators.

In Type II hypersensitivity, IgG or IgM antibodies are directed against cell surface or tissue antigens; requires complement and occurs over several hours or days. (Fig. 32.2).

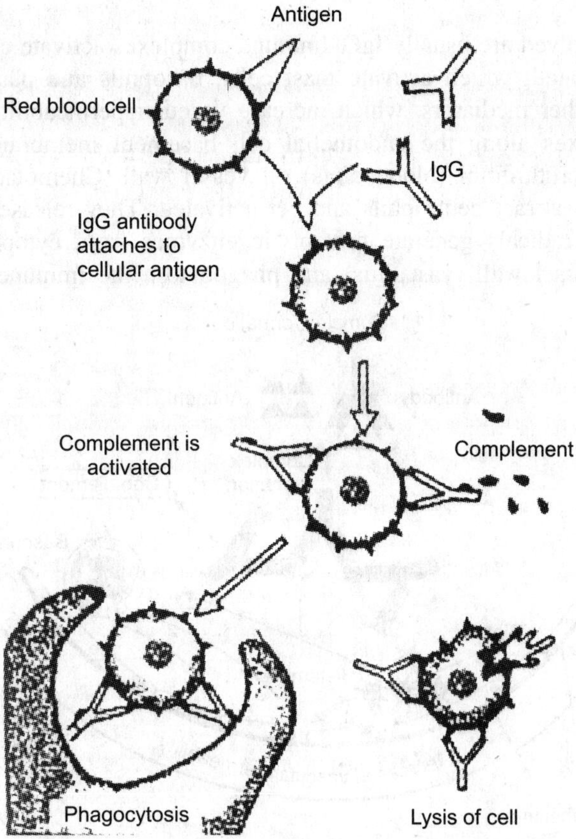

Fig. 32.2 Type II hypersensitivity. The action of antibody occurs through effector cells or the membrane attack complex, which damages target cell plasma membrane, causing cell destruction.

The antibodies interact with complement (C1q) and the effector cells through their F_C regions. Antibodies usually stimulate the complement pathway and a variety of effector cells (macrophages, neutrophils, NK cells, eosinophils and platelets) and cause the lysis of cells.

e.g., (1) When a person receives blood transfusion from a donor with a different blood group.

(2) Hemolytic anemia of newborn due to Rh incompatibility.

(3) Antierythrocyte antibodies in atuoimmune anemias.

(4) Thrombocytopenic purpura.

TYPE III : HYPERSENSITIVITY (IMMUNE COMPLEX DISEASES)

Immune complex allergic diseases are cutaneous Arthus reaction and systemic serum sickness. (Fig. 32.3)

Arthus Phenomenon

Arthus (1903) showed that the intradermal injection of a protein antigen into a hyperimmunized rabbit produces local inflammation which progressed to a hemorrhagic necroting ulcerating skin lesion. It is known as "Arthus phenomenon" and is a localized cutaneous inflammatory response to the deposition of immune complexes in dermal blood vessels.

Mechanism

The antibodies involved are usually IgG. Immune complexes activate complement and C3a, C5a anaphylatoxins are liberated, which activate mast cells, basophils and platelets to degranulate and release histamine and other mediators, which increase vascular permeability, permitting localization of the immune complexes along the endothelial cell basement membrane. This induces platelet aggregation to form microthrombi (blood clots) on vessel wall. Chemotactic factors from various complement components attract neutrophils and get activated. They release toxic chemicals such as oxygen containing free radicals generate proteolytic enzymes from cytoplasmic granules, causing damage to the blood vessel wall (vasculitis) and phagocytose the immune complexes.

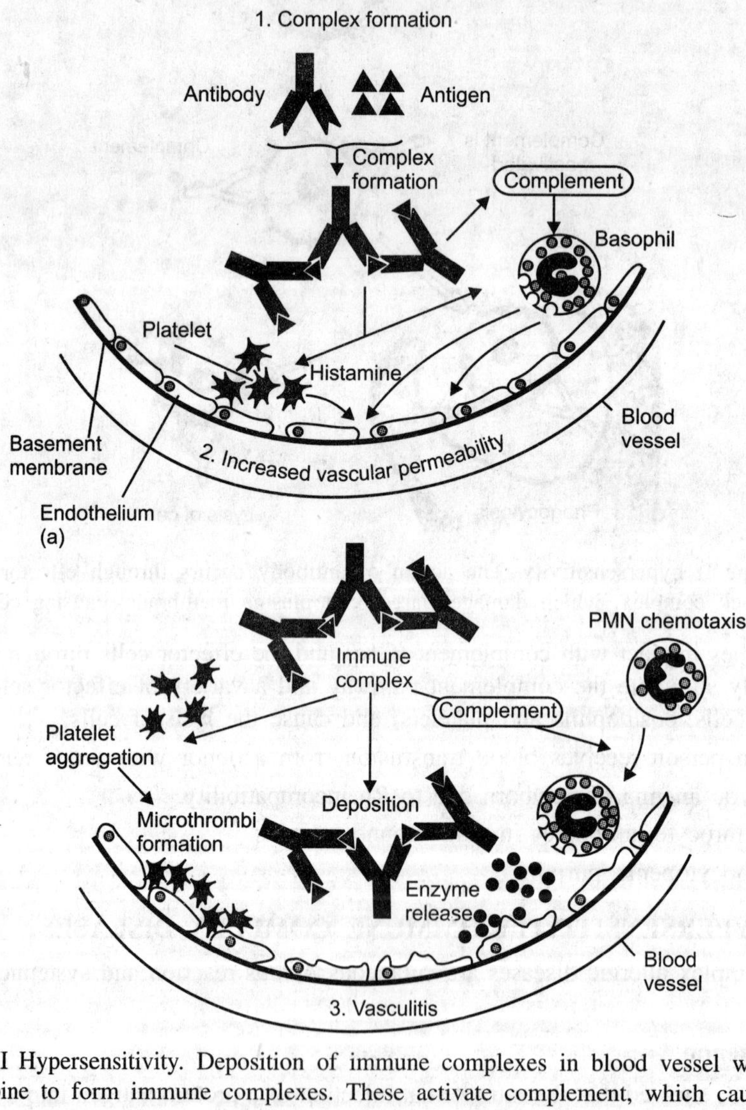

Fig. 32.3 Type III Hypersensitivity. Deposition of immune complexes in blood vessel walls. (a) Antibody and antigen combine to form immune complexes. These activate complement, which causes basophils and platelets to degranulate and release histamine and other mediators. These mediators increase vascular permeability. (b) The increased permeability allows the immune complexes to be deposited in the blood vessel wall. This induces platelet aggregation to form microthrombi (blood clots) on the vessel wall. PMNs, stimulated by complement, degranulate causing enzymatic damage to the blood vessel wall

e.g. (1) In **Farmer's lung disease**, the individual has circulating IgG antibodies to fungi, actinomycetes after being exposed repeatedly to moldy hay. When the allergens enter the alveoli of the lungs, local immune complexes are formed leading to inflammation.

(2) In **allergic pneumonitis**, immune complexes are formed in lungs, following repeated inhalation of allergens from molds, plants or animals.

Serum Sickness

It is an acute, self-limited systemic allergic disease caused by immune complex-activated complement-generated inflammation, after injection of a protein or haptenic drug, characterized by fever, dermatitis, lymphadenopathy and joint pains.

The disease occurs following heterologous serum therapy or gamma globulin for passive immunization, antilymphocyte serum (ALS) or antilymphocyte globulin for immuno suppressive therapy, vaccines, protein drugs and bee stings. A mild reaction may be caused by nonprotein drugs such as sulfonamides, penicillins and cephalosporins.

The severity of the disease is antigen dose-dependent. Serum sickness differs from other types of hypersensitivity reaction in that a single large dose of antigen can serve both as the sensitising dose and the shocking dose.

Mechanism

Same as Arthus reaction.

e.g.,(1) A persistent bacterial, viral or protozoan infection together with a weak antibody response, leads to chronic immune complex formation and their deposition in host tissues.

(2) The continuous production of autoantibody to self antigen during an autoimmune disease, such as systemic lupus erythematosus, can lead to prolonged immune complex formation and their deposition in tissues, overloading the Reticuloendothelial system.

(3) In post-streptococcal **glomerulonephritis**, the complexes of antibody and streptococcal antigen are deposited within the kidney glomeruli and produce Type III hypersensitivity reaction.

(4) Immune complex diseases may also occur in disseminated malignancies, Hepatitis type B and malaria.

TYPE IV : HYPERSENSITIVITY (DELAYED TYPE HYPERSENSITIVITY – DTH)

Type IV allergic diseases are mediated by specifically sensitized effector T-lymphocytes (T_{DTH} cells) and not by antibodies. The immunologic mechanism is often called "delayed hypersensitivity", and is also involved in cell mediated immunity, induced by intracellular microbial infections or haptens like simple chemicals applied on the skin, evolve slowly and consists of a mixed cellular reaction involving lymphocytes and macrophages.

The sensitised T lymphocytes (T_{DTH}, T_{H1}, T_{H2}, T_C) on contact with the specific antigen, release lymphokines which attract lymphocytes, macrophages and basophils to the affected tissue and results in extensive tissue damage. (Fig. 32.4)

Delayed hypersensitivity can be passively transferred by transferring sensitised T-cells or their extract, known as "transfer factor", but cannot be passively transferred by serum.

Delayed hypersensitivity reactions are of two types–Infection type (tuberculin hypersensitivity) and allergic contact dermatitis.

Some autoimmune diseases, graft rejection and killing of cancer cells also involves delayed hypersensitivity reactions.

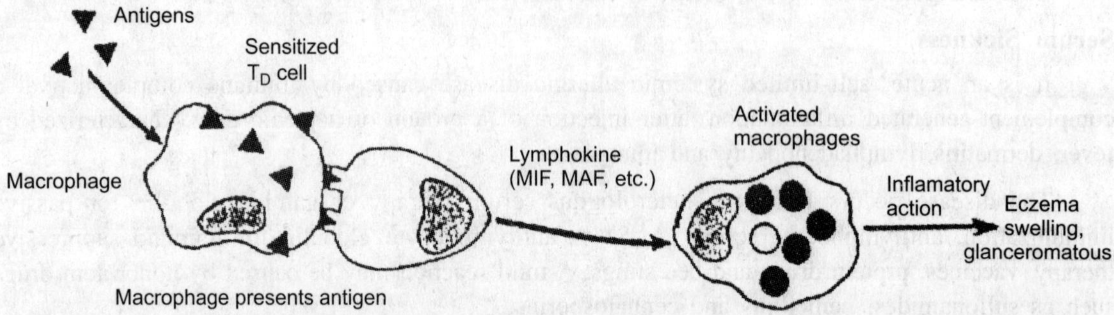

Fig. 32.4 Type IV hypersensitivity (cell mediated). The activation of T cells leads to the release of lymphokines and the activation of macrophages and cytotoxic T cells

Infection (Tuberculin) Type

When a small dose of tuberculin (partially purified protein obtained from the bacillus that causes tuberculosis) is injected intradermally into the skin of the forearm, the reaction begins in about 8 hours, and a reddened area surrounding the injection site becomes indurated with in 12 to 24 hours, reaching a peak in 48 hours and then subsides in a tuberculin-positive individual. The size of the induration is directly related to the amount of antigen that was introduced and to the degree of hypersensitivity of the tested individual.

The tuberculin test is negative and induces no response in unsensitised individual, who had no prior infection.

Tuberculin type hypersensitivity develops in many infections with bacteria, fungi, viruses and parasites especially in intracellular and chronic infections. Other microbial products used in Type IV skin testing are :

Histoplasmin for histoplasmosis

Coccidioidin for coccidioidomycosis

Lepromin for leprosy

Brucellin for brucellosis.

Contact Dermatitis

Allergic contact dermatitis is an eczematous skin disease caused by cell mediated hypersensitivity to environmental allergens. Both sensitization and elicitation of the reaction involve contact of the allergen with the skin.

Contact dermatitis is caused by haptens that combine with proteins in the skin to form the allergen that elicits the immune response. The haptens are the antigenic determinants, and the skin proteins are the carrier molecules for the haptens. Examples of these haptens include :

- Chemicals like dinitrochlorobenzene, picryl chloride
- Dyes

- Metals such as nickel and chromium
- Drugs such as penicillin and antibiotic ointments
- Cosmetics
- Plant materials (catechol molecules).

The haptens, alongwith carrier skin proteins are captured by Langerhans cells of skin, which migrate to the draining lymph nodes where they present the processed antigen along with MHC molecules to T cells. The sensitised T cells travel to the skin site, where on contact with allergen, get activated and release various lymphokines, which cause an influx of eosinophils and tissue damage. Activated cytotoxic T cells (T_C) mediate killing of target cells.

Contact with the allergen in a sensitised individual leads to "contact dermatitis", the lesions vary from macules and papules to vesicles that breakdown, leaving behind raw weeping areas typical of acute eczematous dermatitis.

The diagnosis is confirmed by "**Patch testing**". The allergen is applied to the skin under an adherent dressing. Sensitivity is indicated by itching appearing in 4–5 hours, and local reaction which may vary from erythema to vesicle or blister formation, after 24-48 hours.

TYPE V : HYPERSENSITIVITY (STIMULATORY TYPE)

This is an antibody-mediated hypersensitivity. Here antibody reacts with a key surface component such as hormone receptor and switches on or stimulates the cell. *e.g.,* thyroid hyperactivity in Grave's disease due to thyroid stimulating autoantibody.

Normally thyroid stimulating hormone (TSH) from pituitary gland binds to thyroid cell receptors. This activates adenyl cyclase in the membrane which converts ATP to AMP. The latter stimulates activity of thyroid cells to secrete thyroxin. The thyroid stimulating antibody present in the sera of thyrotoxic patients is an autoantibody directed against receptors for TSH. This antibody, therefore, binds to these receptors and brings about the same effect as that of TSH. (Fig. 32.5)

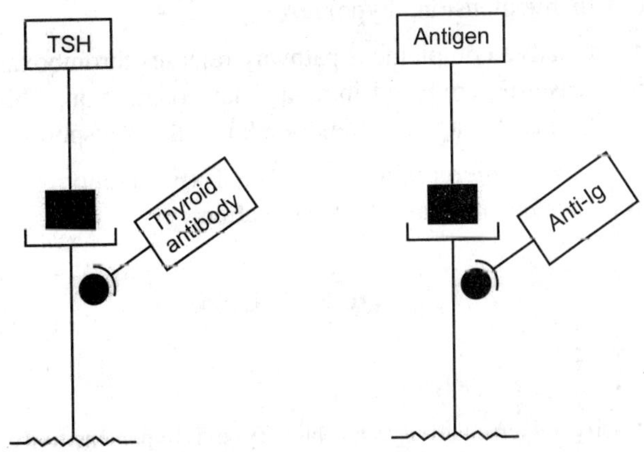

Fig. 32.5 Type V hypersensitivity. Stimulation of thyroid cell by antibody which causes membrane changes leading to cell activation

The situation is analogous to lymphocyte stimulation; the small lymphocytes with immunoglobulin surface receptors can be stimulated by changes induced through the receptor molecules either by binding of specific antigen or by an antibody to the immunoglobulin.

JONES-MOTE REACTION (OR) CUTANEOUS BASOPHIL HYPERSENSITIVITY

When some protein antigens are injected intradermally, a local reaction occurs, characterized by basophil infiltration. The reaction resembles tuberculin response, but it is not delayed hypersensitivity reaction, because it can be passively transferred by serum. This is known as Jones-Mote reaction or cutaneous basophil hypersensitivity.

SHWARTZMAN REACTION (OR) SANARELLI-SHWARTZMAN REACTION

Shwartzman (1928) showed that when a culture filtrate of *Salmonella typhi* is injected intradermally in a Rabbit, followed 24 hours later by the intravenous injection of the same material; a hemorrhagic necrotic lesion develops at the site of intradermal injection, pathogenesis is due to immune inflammation but not of immune origin.

The initial, preparatory dose is an endotoxin, which causes accumulation of leucocytes that condition the site by releasing lysosomal enzymes damaging capillary walls.

The later intravenous, provocative dose can be a variety of substances such as endotoxins, antigen-antibody complexes, starch, serum, kaolin etc., and causes intravascular clotting (thrombi), leading to necrosis of vessel walls and hemorrhage.

This reaction has no immunological basis–due to the absence of specificity and short interval between initial and provocative doses. If both the injections are given intravenously, the animal dies 12–24 hours after the second dose.

Sanarelli (1924) demonstrated a similar phenomenon in experimental cholera. Therefore, the reaction is also called "Sanarelli-Shwartzman reaction" or "generalized Shwartzman reaction".

Several diseases are associated with Shwartzman reaction –

(1) Purpuric rashes of meningococcal septicemia and acute hemorrhagic adrenal necrosis.

(2) Gram negative septicaemias may be accompanied by respiratory distress syndrome due to septic shock with hypotension, hypoxia.

(3) Activation of alternative complement pathway releases thromboxane and prostaglandins from platelets which cause disseminated intravascular coagulation. This is due to release of TNF and IL-1 and 6 by macrophages and endothelial cells in response to contact with endotoxins.

(4) *Staphylococcus aureus* enterotoxin can induce TNF secretion by macrophages and platelets, leading to disseminated intravascular coagulation.

QUESTIONS

Essay Questions

1. Define and classify hypersensitivity. Explain Type I hypersensitivity.
2. Define and classify hypersensitivity reactions. Describe anaphylaxis.
3. Describe various types of hypersensitivity reactions.

Short Notes

1. Define hypersensitivity.
2. Type–I hypersensitivity.

3. Anaphylaxis.
4. Pharmacological mediators of anaphylaxis.
5. Atopy.
6. P-K reaction.
7. Classification of hypersensitivity.
8. Coombs-Gell classification of hypersensitivity.
9. Type III hypersensitivity (or) Immune complex diseases.
10. Arthus phenomenon.
11. Serum sickness.
12. Type IV hypersensitivity (or) Delayed hypersensitivity (DTH).
13. Tuberculin test.
14. Contact dermatitis.
15. Cutaneous anaphylaxis.
16. Anaphylactoid reaction.
17. Passive cutaneous anaphylaxis (PCA).
18. Schultz–Dale phenomenon (or) Anaphylaxis *in vitro*.
19. Differences between Immediate and Delayed hypersensitivity.
20. Type–V hypersensitivity (or) Stimulatory type hypersensitivity.
21. Jones-Mote reaction (or) Cutaneous basophil hypersensitivity.
22. Shwartzman reaction (or) Sanarelli-Shwartzman reaction.

33

Autoimmunity

- *Definition*
- *Mechanisms of autoimmunity*
- *Autoimmune diseases*
- *Differences and similarities between organ-specific and non-organ-specific autoimmune diseases*
- *Diagnosis*
- *Treatment*

DEFINITION

Autoimmunity is a condition in which structural and functional damage is produced by the action of antibodies or immunocompetent cells against normal components (self antigens) of the body.

Autoimmunity literally means "protection against self" but it actually implies "injury to self" and therefore it has been criticised as a contradiction in terms. "Autoallergy" has been suggested as an acceptable alternative, but the term "autoimmunity" has the sanction of wide usage.

MECHANISMS OF AUTOIMMUNITY

(1) Certain self antigens are present in closed systems and are not accessible to immune system. They are called **hidden antigens** or **sequestrated antigens**.

e.g., (*a*) Lens protein of the eye is enclosed in its capsule and immunological tolerance against this antigen is not established during fetal life. Following cataract surgery or penetrating injury, when it leaks out into blood circulation, it may induce an immune response causing damage to the lens of the other eye.

(*b*) As spermatozoa develop only with puberty, the tolerance is not established during fetal life. When sperms are leaked into blood circulation (*e.g.,* orchitis following mumps) initiates immune response that leads to sterility.

(2) Cells or tissues may undergo antigenic alteration as a result of physical (irradiation, photosensitivity, cold allergy), chemical (drugs), or biological (viral infections, bacterial enzymes) influences. Such altered antigens are called "Neoantigens", which may induce an immune response.

(3) Autoimmunity may result due to cross-reacting organ-specific foreign antigens *e.g.*, neurological complications following antirabic immunization in humans with neural vaccine prepared from infected sheep brain, inactivated by phenol. When it is injected, antibodies are produced against sheep brain antigens that may damage nervous tissue of humans.

(4) Antigenic mimicry between infecting microorganisms and self antigens may cause autoimmunity.

e.g.,
- Arthritogenic *Shigella flexneri* and HLA–B27.
- *Mycobacterium tuberculosis* and joint membranes
- Coxsackie B virus and myocardium.
- *Streptococcus pyogenes* and myocardium and glomeruli (Rheumatic fever and glomerulonephritis).

(5) Polyclonal B-cell activation by chemicals (2-mercaptoethanol), bacterial products (lipopolysaccharide, purified protein derivative), enzymes (trypsin), antibiotics (nystatin) and infections with bacteria (*Mycoplasma*), viruses (EB virus) and parasites (*Plasmodium*) may result in autoimmunity.

(6) Breakdown of immunological homeostasis may lead to cessation of tolerance and the emergence of forbidden clones of immunocompetent cells capable of mounting immune response against self antigens.

(7) Increased helper T-cell activity and decreased suppressor T-cell activity may lead to autoimmunity.

AUTOIMMUNE DISEASES

Based on the site of involvement and nature of lesions, autoimmune diseases may be classified as

1. Hemocytolytic autoimmune diseases.
2. Localized or organ specific autoimmune diseases.
3. Systemic autoimmune diseases.
4. Transitory autoimmune diseases.

1. Hemocytolytic Autoimmune Diseases

(a) Autoimmune hemolytic anemia

Autoantibodies against RBC are produced.

(b) Autoimmune thrombocytopenia

Autoantibodies are produced against platelets *e.g.*, Thrombocytopenic purpura, Sedormid purpura.

(c) Autoimmune leucopenia

Autoantibodies are produced against leucocytes in patients with systemic lupus erythematosus and rheumatoid arthritis.

2. Localized or Organ-specific Autoimmune Diseases

(a) Autoimmune thyroiditis

(*i*) **Hashimoto's disease** (lymphadenoid goitre). Autoantibodies are produced against microsomal antigens and thyroglobulin. Thyroid gland enlarges with symptoms of hypothyroidism or myxedema.

(*ii*) **Thyrotoxicosis** (Grave's disease). Patients possess "long acting thyroid stimulator" which is an IgG antibody to thyroid membrane antigen and their combination stimulates excessive hormone secretion.

(b) Addison's disease

Antibodies are produced against adrenal gland cells.

(c) Autoimmune orchitis

It may occur as a complication of mumps.

(d) Myasthenia gravis

An antibody against acetyl choline receptor on neuromuscular junctions of striated muscles is present in these patients. This prevents acetyl choline from combining with its receptor, and impairs muscular contraction.

(e) Autoimmune diseases of the eye

Sometimes following cataract surgery or penetrating injuries into the eye, lens protein may leak into blood circulation and induce an immune response.

(f) Pernicious anemia

Autoantibodies produced against parietal cells of gastric mucosa may cause achlorhydria and atrophic gastritis. Similarly antibodies produced against intrinsic factor prevents absorption of vitamin B_{12}.

(g) Autoimmune diseases of the nervous system

e.g., neuroparalytic complications following antirabic immunization, Idiopathic polyneuritis (Guillain-Barre syndrome); Allergic encephalomyelitis.

(h) Autoimmune diseases of the skin

Pemphigus vulgaris is caused by an antibody to the intercellular cement substance. In bullous pemphigoid, antibodies are formed against dermal epithelial junction.

3. Systemic Autoimmune Diseases

(a) Systemic lupus erythematosus (SLE)

Patients have a variety of antibodies against cell nuclei, intracytoplasmic constituents immunoglobulins, thyroid, RBC, platelets, lymphocytes, clotting factors and neuronal cells.

LE cell phenomenon is noticed in SLE. LE cell is a neutrophil containing a large, pale, homogeneous body (LE body) almost filling the cytoplasm. The LE body is an immunologically damaged nucleus of a leucocyte. Sometimes, instead of being intracellular, the LE body can be seen freely surrounded by a rosette of neutrophils. The LE cell formation is due to an autoantibody, which can be demonstrated by incubating normal blood with serum from SLE patient. Immunofluorescence tests for antinuclear antibodies, RIA or ELISA for anti-DNA antibodies can be used for the diagnosis of SLE, but not specific as they may be positive in other autoimmune conditions.

(b) Rheumatoid arthritis

In rheumatoid arthritis, synovial membranes of the affected joints are swollen and edematous, with dense infiltration of lymphocytes and plasma cells. An autoantibody called Rheumatoid factor (RF) is present, usually of IgM type, though sometimes may be of IgG and IgA. RF acts as an antibody against F_C fragment of immunoglobulins.

RF can be detected by sensitized sheep RBC agglutination test (Rose-waaler test), Latex agglutination tests, Immunofluorescence, Radioimmunoassay.

(c) Polyarteritis nodosa

It is a necrotizing angitis involving small arteries, ending fatally due to coronary thrombosis, cerebral hemorrhage or gastrointestinal bleeding. Polyarteritis is seen as a component of serum sickness and other immune complex diseases.

(d) Sjogren's syndrome

This is a triad of conjunctivitis, sicca, dryness of the mouth with or without salivary gland enlargement and rheumatoid arthritis. This syndrome may occur in association with other collagen diseases antinuclear antibodies and rheumatoid factor occur in sera.

4. Transitory Autoimmune Diseases

Following certain infections or drug therapy certain self antigens may undergo antigenic alteration and produce anemia, thrombocytopenia or nephritis. The diseases are transient and undergo spontaneous cure.

Table 33.1 Differences Between Organ-Specific and Systemic (Non-Organ-Specific) Autoimmune Diseases

Organ-specific autoimmune diseases	*Non-organ-specific (systemic autoimmune diseases)*
1. Antigens only available to lymphoid system in low concentration and immune tolerance not firmly established.	Antigens fully accessible and tolerance established normally.
2. Antibodies organ-specific.	Antibodies non-organ-specific.
3. Clinical and serologic overlap-thyroiditis, gastritis and adrenalitis.	Overlap SLE, rheumatoid arthritis, and other connective tissue disorders.
4. Familial tendency to organ-specific autoimmunity.	Familial connective tissue disease.
5. Therapy aimed at replacing specific hormones.	Therapy aimed at inhibiting inflammation and antibody synthesis.
6. Lymphoid invasion, parenchymal destruction by autoantibodies or delayed hypersensitivity.	Lesions due to deposition of antigen-antibody complexes.
7. Tendency to cancer in organ.	Tendency to lymphoreticular neoplasia.
8. Antigens evoke antibodies in normal animals with complete Freund's adjuvant.	No antibodies produced in animals with comparable stimulation.
9. Experimental lesions produced with antigen in Freund's adjuvant.	Diseases and autoantibodies arise spontaneously in certain animals or after injection of parental lymphoid tissue into F_1 hybrids.

SIMILARITIES BETWEEN ORGAN-SPECIFIC AND SYSTEMIC AUTOIMMUNE DISEASES

1. Circulating autoantibodies react with normal body constituents.
2. Patients often have increased immunoglobulins in serum.
3. Antibodies may appear in each of the main immunoglobulin classes.
4. Greater incidence in women.
5. Disease process not always progressive, exacerbations and remissions.
6. Autoantibody tests of diagnostic value.

DIAGNOSIS OF AUTOIMMUNITY

Serum autoantibodies frequently provide valuable diagnostic markers. The most useful routine tests are CFT, agglutination tests, immunofluorescence, enzyme immunoassay and Radioimmuno assay. The tests will also prove of value in screening for people at risk and the general population.

TREATMENT OF AUTOIMMUNE DISEASES

(1) In cases of organ-specific diseases, replacement therapy is usually adequate *e.g.*, thyroxine in primary myxedema, vitamin B_{12} in pernicious anemia and so forth.

(2) In SLE and immune complex nephritis, steroids, often in high doses, help to suppress inflammatory lesions.

(3) Immunosuppressive drugs such as azathioprene, cyclophosphamide, methotrexate, and cyclosporine are used to inhibit the synthesis autoantibodies.

(4) Long-term treatment with antilymphocyte serum.

(5) Plasma exchange to lower the rate of immune complex deposition.

(6) In rheumatoid arthritis, apart from steroids, antiinflammatory drugs are widely used.

A potentially valuable approach is "switching-off" primed B cells by presenting hapten linked to a thymus-independent carrier like the copolymer of D-Glutamic and D-lysine or isologous IgG particularly when given with high cortisone doses.

QUESTIONS

Essay Question

1. Describe autoimmunity (or) Define autoimmunity. Classify autoimmune diseases. What are the mechanisms of autoimmune diseases?

Short Notes

1. Autoimmunity.
2. Mechanism of autoimmunity.
3. Rheumatoid arthritis (or) Rheumatoid factor (RF).
4. Systemic lupus erythematosus (SLE) or LE cell.
5. Name two autoimmune diseases and their autoantibodies.
6. Sequestrated antigens or hidden antigens.

34

Immunodeficiency Diseases

- *Definition*
- *Primary immunodeficiency states*
  - *Disorders of specific immune mechanisms*
    - *Humoral immunodeficiencies*
    - *Cellular immunodeficiencies*
    - *Combined immunodeficiencies*
  - *Disorders of complement*
  - *Disorders of phagocytosis*
- *Secondary immunodeficiency states*
- *Diagnosis and investigations*

DEFINITION

Immunodeficiency diseases are conditions where the defense mechanisms of the body are impaired, leading to repeated microbial infections of varying severity and sometimes enhanced susceptibility to malignancies.

Deficiencies of immune mechanisms may involve specific immune mechanisms such as humoral immunity or cell mediated immunity or both; or nonspecific immune mechanisms such as phagocytosis and complement, which promote and act in conjunction with specific immune mechanisms.

Immunodeficiency diseases may be classified into two major groups.

I. Primary immunodeficiency states – occur rarely due to defects in the development of immune mechanisms or B and T lymphocytes.

II. Secondary immunodeficiency states – occur as a consequence of malnutrition, lymphoproliferative disorders, agents such as X-rays and cytotoxic drugs and viral infections that may interfere with the effective functioning of the mature immune system e.g., HIV–1 and HIV–2 infections cause AIDS.

PRIMARY IMMUNODEFICIENCY STATES

I. Disorders of Specific Immune Mechanisms

1. *Humoral immunodeficiencies (B-cell defects)*

(*a*) **X-linked agammaglobulinemia (Bruton's disease).** Seen in male infants. All classes of immunoglobulins are absent. Recurrent pyogenic bacterial infections are common. It is due to rare X-linked mutations.

(*b*) **Transient hypogammaglobulinemia of infancy.** It is due to an abnormal delay in the initiation of IgG synthesis in some infants. Recurrent respiratory infections and otitis media may occur. Spontaneous recovery occurs.

(*c*) **Common variable immunodeficiency or late onset hypogammaglobulinemia.** It occurs only by 15–35 years of age in both males and females, clinically resembles X-linked agammaglobulinaemia.

(*d*) **Selective Immunoglobulin deficiencies.** Selective deficiency of one or more Ig classes occurs, while the other Ig classes remain normal or elevated.

Selective IgA deficiency is common accompanied by atopic allergy. Patients become susceptible to respiratory infections and steatorrhea.

Selective IgM deficiency is found to be associated with septicemia.

(*e*) **Immunodeficiency with hyper-IgM** (Hyper IgM deficiency syndrome). This disease is characterized by an increased level of IgM associated with a deficiency of IgG and IgA; It is rare and inherited in X-linked manner. Patients become susceptible to infections and autoimmune processes.

(*f*) **Transcobalamin II deficiency.** Metabolic defects like megaloblastic anemia and intestinal villous atrophy are seen due to vitamin B_{12} deficiency. The associated defects are decrease in plasma cells, consequently Ig levels and impaired phagocytosis.

Treatment with B_{12} restores hematopoietic, gastrointestinal and B-cell functions, but not phagocytic activity.

(*g*) **X-linked lymphoproliferative syndrome (Duncan's syndrome).** It is associated with Epstein-Barr virus infection. The immunodeficiency consists mainly of acquired hypogammaglobulinemia.

2. ***Cellular Immunodeficiencies (T-Cell Defects)***

(*a*) **Thymic hypoplasia (Di George's syndrome).** It is due to failure of thymic development from third and fourth pharyngeal pouches, leading to aplasia or hyperplasia of thymus and parathyroid glands. Immunodeficiency is primarily cell mediated. Transplantation of fetal thymus tissue can restore the immunological function.

(*b*) **Chronic mucocutaneous candidiasis.** Cell mediated immunity is deficient in patients with severe chronic candidiasis of the mucosa, skin and nails. Transfer factor therapy alongwith amphotericin-B is effective.

(*c*) **Purine nucleoside phosphorylase (PNP) deficiency.** An inherited disorder with decrease in cell mediated immunity and recurrent or chronic infections. A low serum uric acid may point to the diagnosis, as the enzyme degrades purines to hypoxanthine and uric acid.

3. ***Combined immunodeficiencies***

(*a*) **Nezelof syndrome.** It is a cellular immunodeficiency with abnormal Ig synthesis. Patients are susceptible to recurrent bacterial, fungal, viral and protozoan infections.

(*b*) **Ataxia telangiectasia.** It is a hereditary combined immunodeficiency with neurological defects such as cerebellar ataxia.

(*c*) **Wiskott-Aldrich syndrome.** It is an X-linked disease characterized by éczema, thrombocytopenic purpura and recurrent infections.

(*d*) **Immunodeficiency with thymoma.** Consists of benign thymic tumor, impaired cell mediated immunity and agammaglobulinemia.

(*e*) **Immunodeficiency with short-limbed dwarfism.** Ectodermal dysplasia, thymic defects; an inherited disorder.

(*f*) **Episodic lymphopenia with lymphocytotoxin.** Patients lacks immunological memory.

(*g*) **Severe combined immunodeficiencies.** *e.g.*, swiss type agammaglobulinemia; reticular dysgenesis of de vaal; Adenosine deaminase (ADA) deficiency is associated with chondrocyte abnormalities.

II. Disorders of Complement

(*a*) **Complement component deficiencies.** C3 deficiency is associated with recurrent pyogenic infections. C_6, C_7 and C_8 deficiencies are associated with neisserial infections, bacteremia and toxoplasmosis.

(*b*) **Complement inhibitor deficiencies.** Genetic deficiency of C_1 inhibitor results in hereditary angioneurotic edema. A rare deficiency of C_{3b} inactivator is associated with chronic recurrent pyogenic lesions.

III. Disorders of Phagocytosis

Phagocytosis may be impaired by either intrinsic or extrinsic defects. Intrinsic defects are within the phagocytic cell, such as enzyme deficiencies. Extrinsic disorders may be due to a deficiency of opsonic antibody, complement or other factors promoting phagocytosis or to the effects of drugs or antineutrophil antibodies.

(*a*) **Chronic granulomatous disease.** Leucocytes are unable to kill catalase positive bacteria. The decreased H_2O_2 production is responsible for bactericidal defect. Leucocytes fail to reduce nitroblue tetrazolium (NBT) during phagocytosis. This property is used as a screening method (NBT test) for the diagnosis of chronic granulomatous disease.

(*b*) **Myeloperoxidase deficiency**

(*c*) **Chediak–Higashi syndrome.** It is a genetic disorder characterized by decreased pigmentation of the skin, eyes, hair, photophobia, nystagmus and giant peroxidase positive inclusions in the cytoplasm of leucocytes.

(*d*) **Leucocyte G6 PD deficiency.** Glucose–6–phosphate dehydrogenase is deficient in leucocytes and shows decreased phagocytosis.

(*e*) **Job's syndrome.** Characterized by multiple, large 'cold' staphylococcal abscesses containing large quantities of pus, occurring repeatedly on the skin and in various organs.

(*f*) **Tuftsin deficiency.** A leucokinin, called tuftsin (discovered at Tuftsin university, Boston) which stimulates phagocytosis is deficient.

(*g*) **Lazy leucocyte syndrome.** The defect is in chemotaxis and neutrophil mobility.

(*h*) **Hyper–IgE syndrome**

(*i*) **Actin–binding protein deficiency**

(*j*) **Shwachman's disease**

SECONDARY IMMUNODEFICIENCY STATES

Deficiencies of humoral and cellular immune responses may occur secondarily during the course of many disease states such as metabolic disorders, malnutrition, malignancy, infections or after exposure to cytotoxic drugs and chemicals.

Humoral immunodeficiency results :

(1) When B cells are depleted as in lymphoid malignancy and chronic lymphoid leukemia.

(2) When immunoglobulin catabolism is increased as in the nephrotic syndrome.

(3) When excessive loss of serum protein occurs as in exfoliative skin diseases and in protein losing enteropathies.

(4) When excessive production of abnormal immunoglobulins occurs as in multiple myeloma.

Deficiency of cell mediated immunity results :

(1) Lymphoreticular malignancies as in Hodgkin's disease.

(2) Obstruction to lymph circulation or lymphorrheas.

(3) When the thymus dependent areas of lymph nodes are infiltrated with nonlymphoid cells as in lepromatous leprosy.

(4) Transiently, following certain viral infections such as measles.

Both, humoral and cellular Immunodeficiency results :

(1) Due to malnutrition

(2) Due to aging

(3) Due to administration of immunosuppressive therapy.

Table 34.1 Primary Immunodeficiency States

I. Disorders of specific immune mechanisms

1. Humoral immunodeficiencies (B cell defects)
   - (*a*) X-linked agammaglobulinemia (Bruton's disease)
   - (*b*) Transient hypogammaglobulinemia of infancy
   - (*c*) Common variable immunodeficiency
   - (*d*) Selective immunoglobulin deficiency
   - (*e*) Immunodeficiency with hyper-IgM
   - (*f*) Transcobalamin II deficiency
   - (*g*) X-linked lymphoproliferative syndrome.
2. Cellular immunodeficiencies (T cell defects)
   - (*a*) Thymic hypoplasia (Di George's syndrome)
   - (*b*) Chronic mucocutaneous candidiasis
   - (*c*) Purine nucleoside phosphorylase (PNP) deficiency
3. Combined immunodeficiencies
   - (*a*) Nezelof syndrome
   - (*b*) Ataxia telangiectasia
   - (*c*) Wiskott–Aldrich syndrome
   - (*d*) Immunodeficiency with thymoma
   - (*e*) Immunodeficiency with short-limbed dwarfism.

II. Complement immunodeficiency disorders
   - (*a*) Complement component deficiencies
   - (*b*) Complement inhibitor deficiencies

III. Disorders of phagocytosis
   - (*a*) Chronic granulomatous disease
   - (*b*) Myeloperoxidase deficiency
   - (*c*) Chediak-Higashi syndrome
   - (*d*) Leucocyte G6PD deficiency
   - (*e*) Job's syndrome
   - (*f*) Tuftsin deficiency
   - (*g*) Lazy leucocyte syndrome
   - (*h*) Hyper-IgE syndrome
   - (*i*) Actin-binding protein deficiency
   - (*j*) Shwachman's disease

DIAGNOSIS AND INVESTIGATIONS

History and a careful clinical examination often give the first clue regarding the possible nature of the deficiency. In persons with an immunodeficiency it is likely not to find any palpable lymph gland. However, some immunodeficiency patients may actually have hyperplasia of the lymph gland. Several quantitative tests are available to investigate the possible causes of immunodeficiencies. A full peripheral blood count is the first examination required. Serum level of the different immunoglobulin classes and IgG subclasses can be determined. Using monoclonal antibodies against specific surface markers of different types of lymphocytes, a full blood count for each cell type (usually the CD4+count) can be performed.

Tests for T cell function

(1) Response to intradermal test with an antigen with which person is already likely to be sensitized, *e.g.*, positive tuberculin test indicates intact T cell function.

(2) Proliferative response of the patient's T_H cells to mitogens or allogenic lymphocytes.

Tests for B cell function

(1) Level of natural antibodies *i.e.*, antibodies against common bacterial antigens such as antistreptolysin 'O' (ASO) or antibodies against bacterial toxins such as tetanus or diphtheria with which the person is already vaccinated.

(2) Pre and post immunization levels of antibodies against bacterial polysaccharide vaccine such as pneumococcal or Hib (*Haemophilus influenzae* capsular serotype b) can be measured.

Tests for phagocyte function

(1) Reduction of nitroblue tetrazolium test is done for functional effectiveness of the oxidative phase of phagocytosis. It is negative in chronic granulomatous disease.

(2) Test for neutrophil chemotaxis.

Tests for serum complement function

(1) Total hemolytic complement test

(2) Test for lytic activity.

Several tests for a functional evaluation of complement system, phagocytes and T and B cells can be performed.

QUESTIONS

Essay Question

1. What are immunodeficiency disorders ? Classify and enumerate immunodeficiency diseases.

Short Notes

1. Immunodeficiency diseases.
2. Primary immunodeficiency diseases.
3. Secondary immunodeficiency diseases.
4. Diagnosis of immunodeficiency diseases.

35

Tumor Immunology/ Immunology of Malignancy

- *Introduction*
- *Immune surveillance*
- *Tumor antigens*
- *Oncofetal antigens*
  - *Alpha foetoprotein (AFP)*
  - *Carcinoembryonic antigen (CEA)*
- *Tumor Immunotherapy*

INTRODUCTION

Cell growth and cell death are normally balanced. Occasionally, cells arise that no longer responds to the usual checks and balances for division and death. These are tumor cells.

A **tumor**, or **neoplasm**, is a collection of the clonal descendants of a cell whose growth has gone unchecked. When a tumor continues to grow and to invade healthy tissue, it is considered to be a cancer.

IMMUNE SURVEILLANCE

Burnet (1967) postulated the theory of immune surveillance, which states that the T-lymphocytes (cell mediated immunity) constantly detects and destroys malignant cells that arise by somatic mutations, so eliminating early cancers from the body. Immunologicaly surveillance is carried out by cytotoxic T-lymphocytes, macrophages and NK cells.

Malignancy results due to failure of this function. Circulating tumor antigens may act as a "smoke screen" coating the lymphocytes and prevents them from acting on tumor cells. Moreover, malignant cells proliferate at a very fast rate so that they "sneak through" before the development of immune response. Some tumors may be of low antigenicity or may form cytokines which suppress cell mediated immunity.

TUMOR ANTIGENS

Tumor antigens are antigens that are present on the membranes of malignant cells but absent in the corresponding cells of the host. Tumor cells express antigens on their surfaces that are often the targets of immune responses. Many tumor antigens are cellular peptides presented by MHC molecules that stimulate antigen-specific T cell proliferation.

1. Tumor-specific transplantation antigens (TSTAs): They are not found on normal somatic cells but result from mutations of genes and the resulting altered proteins that are expressed by the tumor cells.

2. Tumor-associated transplantation antigens (TATAs): They are not unique to tumor cells; rather their expression on tumor cells is altered. For example, the tumor antigen may be found in excessive amounts or amy be expressed on a cell type where it would not normally exist. Oncofetal antigens are expressed on tumors and on normal fetal cells.

Virus-induced tumors have common antigens. All tumors produced by one virus in different animals or species, in different tissues in one animal will have the same antigen.

Chemically induced tumors will have different antigens, eventhough induced by the same carcinogen.

ONCOFETAL ANTIGENS

They are found in embryonic and malignant cells but not in normal adult cells *e.g.*, alphafetoprotein found in hepatomas and the carcinoembryonic antigen found in colonic cancers.

Alphafetoprotein (AFP), an alphaglobulin is synthesized in the fetal liver, yolk sac and gastrointestinal tract. In normal human serum, it is present only in traces, about 5 to 25 ng/ml. In the human fetus, during 3rd to 6th month, it is present in peak level 2-3 mg/ml. Its level drops sharply after birth and is hardly detectable in adults. High levels are found in primary liver cancer (diagnostic value), cancers of stomach and pancreas, embryonal cell tumors, chronic hepatitis and cirrhosis of the liver. After surgical excision of a tumor, the persistence of an elevated alphafetoprotein or a later increase suggests that tumor cells remain or that the tumor has recurred.

Carcinoembryonic antigen (CEA) is a glycoprotein, with more carbohydrate (65%) than protein. It is found in high levels in the serum of patients with colon cancer, particularly in the presence of metastases. It is also found in other conditions such as alcoholic cirrhosis, pancreatic cancer, less frequently in cancer of other organs (breast, lungs) or with certain chronic or recurrent inflammatory conditions (*e.g.*, colitis, chronic bronchitis, heavy cigarette smokers). Many of these conditions have in common excess mucin production.

TUMOR IMMUNOTHERAPY

Immune system may be induced to mount an attack against cancer, known as tumor immunotherapy.

(1) In adoptive cellular immunotherapy, cells that have antitumor activity are injected into the blood of a cancer patient. These "adopted cells" will destroy tumour cells.

One method uses patient's own inactive cytotoxic T cells and NK cells. They are removed in a blood sample and cultured with IL-2, which activates them. Such cells are called "Lymphokine activated killer (LAK) cells". The LAK cells are then transfused back into the patient's blood. Although some tumor regression does occur with this procedure, severe complications may be seen.

(2) Cytokine therapy uses cytokines.

Interferons, particularly alpha interferon induces almost complete cure in a rare cancer called hairy cell leukemia, modest improvement in renal cell carcinoma, melanomas, lymphomas and Kaposi's sarcoma.

The most widely used interleukin is IL-2 either alone or alongwith LAK cells. It causes tumor regression by stimulating cytotoxic T cells and NK cells. It is very toxic. Hence, IL-4 is being tested which has fewer adverse side effects.

(3) Antibody therapy uses monoclonal antibodies either alone or in combination with radioactive isotopes, toxins or drugs. This method overcomes the major adverse effects of chemotherapy and radiation treatment by destroying diseased tissues only, while sparing healthy tissues.

QUESTIONS

Short Notes

1. Immunological surveillance.
2. Tumour antigens.
3. Oncofetal antigens.
4. Alphafetoprotein.
5. Carcinoembryonic antigen.
6. Tumor immunotherapy.
7. TSTA
8. TATA.

36

Immunology of Transplantation

- *Definition*
- *Classification of transplants*
- *Allograft reaction*
- *Mechanism of allograft rejection*
- *Factors surviving allograft survival*
- *Graft-versus-host (GVH) reaction*

DEFINITION

When an organ is congenitally defective or absent or when an organ or tissue is damaged due to injury or disease, grafting is done to restore the function.

The tissue or organ transplanted is known as the "**Transplant**" or "**graft**". The individual from whom the transplant is obtained is known as the "donor" and the individual to whom it is applied, the recipient.

CLASSIFICATION OF TRANSPLANTS

Transplants may be classified in several ways

1. Based on the organ or tissue transplanted, they are classified as kidney, heart, skin transplant and so on.
2. Based on the anatomical site of origin of the transplant and the size of its placement, grafts are classified as "orthotopic" or "heterotopic".

   Orthotopic grafts are applied in anatomically normal sites, as in skin grafts. **Heterotopic grafts** are placed in anatomically abnormal sites, as when thyroid tissue is transplanted in a subcutaneous pocket.
3. Transplants may be of fresh tissues or stored ones.
4. Transplants may be of living or dead tissues.

   "**Live grafts**" such as kidney and heart are expected to survive and function physiologically in the recipient and are called "**vital grafts**". Nonliving transplants like bone or artery merely provide a scaffolding on which new tissue is laid by the recipient. They are called "**static** or **structural grafts**".
5. Based on the genetic relationship (or antigenic relationship) between the donor and the recipient, transplants may be classified into many types.

Autograft – An organ or tissue taken from an individual and grafted on himself is called an autograft.

Isograft – A graft taken from an individual and placed on another individual of the same genetic constitution is called an isograft. Grafts made between identical twins or between syngeneic members of highly inbred strains of animals are examples of isografts.

Allograft or **homograft** – Grafts between two genetically nonidentical members of the same species are called allografts.

Xenograft or **heterograft** – Grafts between members of different species are called Xenografts.

ALLOGRAFT REACTION

When a skin graft from an animal is applied on a genetically unrelated animal of the same species, the graft appears to be accepted initially during first 2 or 3 days, but by 4th day, the graft is invaded by lymphocytes and macrophages, undergo ischemic necrosis, and assumes a scab like appearance and sloughs off by 10th day. These events occurring in the rejection of allograft are called as "first set response or **first set rejection (reaction)**", and brought out by T-lymphocytes (Fig. 36.1).

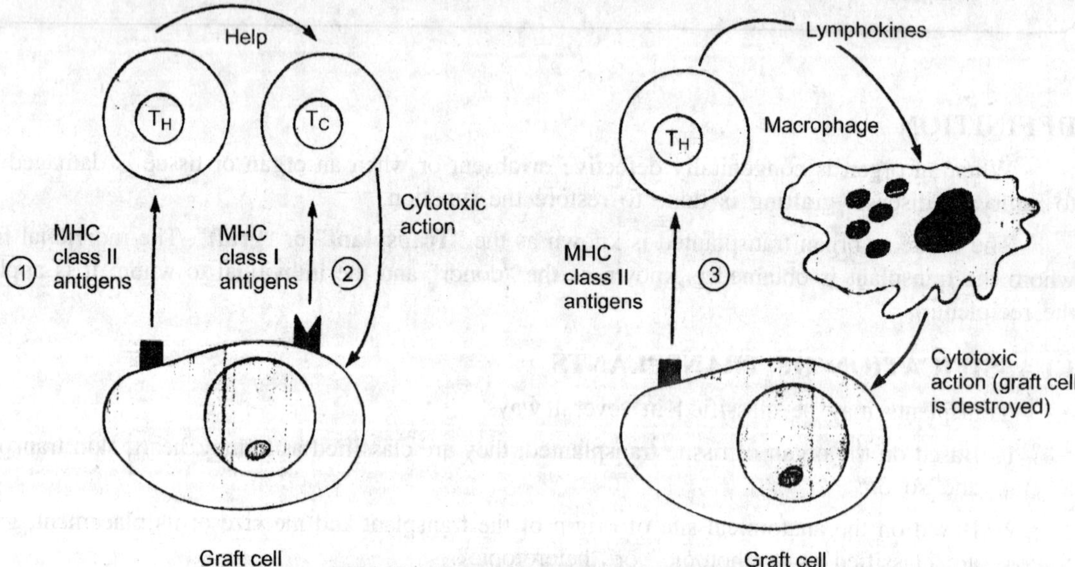

Fig. 36.1 Graft rejection mechanism.

1. Foreign MHC class II molecules on graft cells stimulate T cells.
2. Cytotoxic T cells recognize graft cell by its foreign MHC class I molecules.
3. T_H cells release lymphokines that activate macrophages to destroy the graft cells.

If, in an animal which has rejected a graft by the first set response, another graft from the same donor is applied, it will be rejected in an accelerated fashion. Necrosis sets in early and the graft sloughs off by 6th day. This accelerated allograft rejection is known as "**second set response**".

MECHANISM OF ALLOGRAFT REJECTION

Transplantation immunity is predominantly cell mediated by T-lymphocytes. Antibodies are also produced which can be detected by hemagglutination, lymphocytotoxicity, complement fixation and immunofluorescence.

Antibodies are formed more rapidly and abundantly during second set response than during first set response, and participate in second set response alongwith cell mediated immunity.

When a graft is applied to an animal possessing the specific antibodies in high titres, hyperacute rejection takes place. The graft remains pale and is rejected within hours without even an attempt at vascularization. This is known as "**white graft response**". This type of hyperacute rejection is sometimes seen in human recipients of kidney transplants, who may possess preexisting antibody as a result of prior transplantation, transfusion or pregnancy. The glomeruli in such cases are choked by platelet and leucocyte agglomerates. Donor specific blood transfusions to recipients before kidney transplantation have been found to favour graft survival.

Humoral antibodies may sometimes act in opposition to cell mediated immunity, by inhibiting graft rejection. This phenomenon is called "immunological enhancement".

FACTORS FAVOURING ALLOGRAFT SURVIVAL

Several factors contribute for allograft survival.

1. HLA compatibility, tested by HLA typing and tissue matching.
2. Immunosuppression, particularly suppression of cell mediated immunity. Clinical transplantation employs immunosuppressive drugs, steroids, cyclosporin A, repamycin and FK-506.
3. There are certain privileged sites, where allografts survive. Any site that is not invaded by immunocompetent cells is an immunologically privileged site *e.g.*, cartilage. Areas where lymphatic drainage system is absent such as brain or ineffective such as testes can accept allografts without rejection.

Lack of vascularization at the site also prevents graft rejection. This is the reason for the success of corneal transplants.

The intrauterine fetus is actually an allograft in a privileged site.

GRAFT-VERSUS-HOST (GVH) REACTION

Graft rejection is due to the reaction of the host to the graft. But sometimes the graft may initiate an immune response against the host tissues. It is known as GVH reaction. In other words, the clinical and pathological sequelae of the reactions of T-lymphocytes in a graft against the cells of the recipient is known as GVH. In humans GVH may occur following bone marrow transplantation.

GVH occurs under the following conditions :

(*i*) When graft contains T-lymphocytes.

(*ii*) When recipient possesses transplantation antigens that are absent in the graft.

(*iii*) When graft is accepted and not rejected by the recipient.

The major clinical features of GVH reactions are rash, fever, retardation of growth, emaciation, diarrhea, hepatosplenomegaly, lymphoid atrophy, anemia and terminating fatally. This condition is called "**runt disease** or **runting syndrome**".

QUESTIONS

Short Notes

1. What is a transplant or graft ?
2. Classify transplants (or) Types of transplants.
3. Define allograft or homograft.
4. Allograft reaction.
5. GVH.
6. Mechanism of allograft rejection.
7. Factors favouring allograft survival.

37

Immunohematology

- *Introduction*
- *ABO blood group system*
- *H antigen*
- *Rh (Rhesus) factor*
- *MN blood group system*
- *P system*
- *Lewis system*
- *Applications of blood groups*
- *Blood transfusion*
- *Cross matching*
- *Hazards of incompatible blood transfusion*
- *Hemolytic disease of the new born*
- *Prevention of Rh isoimmunisation*
- *ABO hemolytic disease*

INTRODUCTION

The ability to replace blood lost following surgery or trauma is a vital aspect of modern medicine. This relies on an understanding of immune reactions against RBC, since these may be fatal and must be avoided if blood from one person (the donor) is to be safely transfused into another (the recipient).

The membranes of human RBC contain a variety of blood group antigens (agglutinogens). When these antigens come into contact with antibodies (agglutinins), the RBC clump together or agglutinate. By testing for agglutination with known antibodies, the erythrocyte antigens present can be identified and this defines the "**blood group**" (Fig. 37.1).

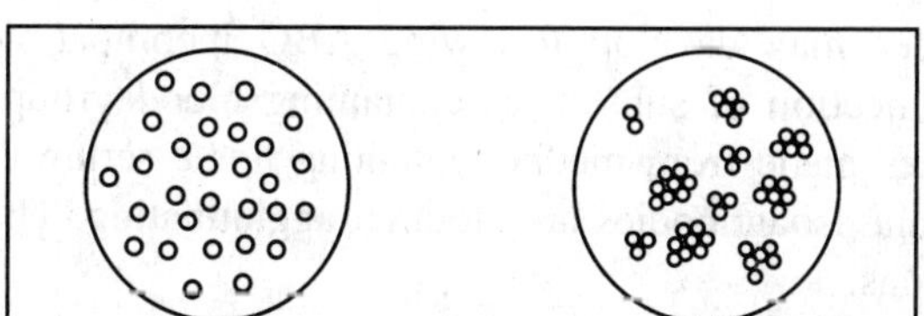

A group RBC in A group plasma

B group RBC in A group plasma. Agglutination of RBC seen

Fig. 37.1 RBC agglutination in incompatible plasma

A variety of different antigen types have been identified—ABO system, MN system, P system, Rh system, Lutheran, Lewis, Kell, Duffy, Kidd, Diego, Yt, Kg, Dombrock, Colton etc. The most important and best known of these are the ABO system and Rh system.

ABO BLOOD GROUP SYSTEM

Based on the presence or absence of A and B antigens on the surface of RBC, individuals are divided into 4 major blood groups. **Group A** individuals have the A antigen, **group B** have the B antigen, **group AB** have both A and B antigens and **group O** have neither.

These four blood groups are also distinguished by the presence or absence of two distinct isoantibodies in the serum. The serum contains the isoantibodies specific for the antigen that is absent on the surface of RBC. The serum of group A individual has anti-B antibody, group B has anti-A and group O both anti-A and anti-B, while in group AB both anti-A and anti-B are absent.

Table 37.1 Distribution of A, B Antigens on RBC and Antibodies in serum; Inheritance of A and B Antigens.

Blood group	*Antigen on RBC*	*Antibodies in plasma*	*Genotype*
A	A	anti-B	OA or AA
B	B	anti-A	OB or BB
AB	A and B	none	AB
O	none	anti-A and anti-B	OO

Subgroups of A and B groups have been described, the most important being A_1 and A_2. About 80 percent of group A blood is A_1 and 20 percent A_2. Antiserum of group A agglutinates group A_1 RBC powerfully. The recognition of group A subgroups increases the number of ABO phenotypes from 4 to 6 : A_1, A_2, B, A_1B, A_2B and O.

Blood group antigens are inherited as Mendelian dominants. Their synthesis is determined by allelomorphic genes A, B and O. Genes A and B give rise to corresponding antigens, but O is an amorph and does not produce any antigen.

In India, the ABO distribution is approximately O-40 percent, B-33 percent, A-22 percent and AB-5 percent.

Anti-A and Anti-B isoantibodies appear in the serum of infants by about the age of six months and persists thereafter. These are called natural antibodies (IgM) and arise without any antigenic stimulation. However, it is believed that they develop as a result of unidentified environmental stimuli with the blood group like antigens present in intestinal bacteria or other sources.

Immune isoantibodies may develop following ABO incompatible pregnancy or transfusion. Often, they result from injection of substances containing blood group-like antigens such as horse serum or bacterial vaccines made from media containing horse serum. Natural antibodies are saline agglutinating, while immune isoantibodies are albumin agglutinating. The latter generally cause more severe transfusion reactions.

H-ANTIGEN

RBC of all ABO groups possess a common antigen, the H antigen, which is the precursor for the formation of A and B antigens. Due to its universal distribution, H antigen is not ordinarily important in grouping or blood transfusion. However, Bhende et. al. (1952) from Mumbai reported a very rare instance in which A and B antigens as well as H antigens were absent from RBC. This is known as **"Mumbai" or "OH" blood group**. Sera of these individuals have anti-A, anti-B and anti-H antibodies, therefore, they can accept the blood only from the same rare blood group.

A, B and H antigens are glycoproteins. In addition to RBC, these antigens are also found in salivary glands, saliva, pancreas, kidney, liver, lungs, testes, semen and amniotic fluid. A and B antigens have also been extracted and purified commercially from stomach of hogs and horses. Anti-A antibodies can be obtained from the albumin gland of the snails. Because anti-A harvested from snails has a very high titre, as much as 2.5 lit of potent reagent can be prepared from one snail.

Rh (RHESUS) BLOOD GROUP

Aside from the antigens of the ABO system, those of the Rh system are of the greatest clinical importance. The "Rh factor", named for the rhesus monkey, because it was first studied using the blood of this animal, is a system composed primarily of the C, D and E antigens, although it actually contains many more. Blood is either Rh positive or Rh negative depending on whether RBC carry one of the Rh antigens or not. Unlike the ABO antigens, the system has not been detected in tissues other than RBC. D is by far the most common, and the term "Rh positive" is generally used to mean that the individual has agglutinogen D. The Rh negative individual has no D antigen and forms the anti-D antibody when injected with D-positive cells. The Rh typing serum used in routine blood typing is anti-D serum.

Among Indians approximately 93 percent are Rh positive and 7 percent are Rh negative.

Unlike the antibodies of the ABO system, there are no natural anti-Rh antibodies in the serum. They arise only as a result of Rh incompatible pregnancy or transfusion.

A variant of D is known as Du. RBC of Du subtype react with some but not all anti-D sera, but they absorb the antibody on their surface. The Du subtype can therefore be detected by reacting RBC with anti-D serum and then by Direct Coombs test. For the purpose of blood donation, Du cells are considered Rh positive. But when a Du individual requires transfusion, it is advisable to use Rh negative blood because he may be immunised by Rh positive blood.

MN BLOOD GROUP SYSTEM

Using Rabbit antisera, M and N antigens have been identified on the surface of RBC. This will classify individuals into three groups— M, N and MN. This system has expanded to include atleast 28 antigens.

P SYSTEM

Landsteiner and Levine (1927) demonstrated P^+ and P^- groups. The P factor is inherited as Mendelian dominant.

LEWIS BLOOD GROUP SYSTEM

This system consists of two antigens Le^a and Le^b. It differs from other blood group systems in that the antigens are present primarily in the plasma and saliva. RBC acquire the antigen by adsorbing them from plasma. Naturally occurring Lewis antibodies are frequently found in the sera of persons lacking the corresponding antigen.

Lutheran, Kell, Duffy, Kidd blood groups, named after those in whose blood they were first discovered (between 1946 and 1951).

Blood group systems other than ABO and Rh are of little clinical importance as they do not usually cause transfusion reactions or hemolytic disease. They have applications in paternity testing, genetics, anthropology, tissue typing and forensic medicine.

APPLICATIONS OF BLOOD GROUPS

(1) Blood transfusion
(2) Detection and diagnosis of blood diseases
(3) Paternity testing
(4) In forensic medicine
(5) Ethnological studies
(6) Anthropological studies
(7) Genetics
(8) Tissue typing
(9) Various experimental purposes.

BLOOD TRANSFUSION

In blood transfusion, the donor and recipient should belong to the same group.

It was believed that O group blood can be transfused to any other group, as they possess neither A or B antigen on the surface of RBC. Hence O group was known as "**universal donor**". The anti-A and anti-B antibodies present in O blood, do not cause any damage to RBC of A or B group recipients because they will be rendered ineffective by dilution in the recipient's plasma. But some O group plasma may contain isoantibodies in high titres (1:200 or above) so that the damage to the recipient's RBC may result. This is known as "**dangerous O group**". The anti-A antibody in the O group blood is generally more potent than the anti-B antibody. Hence the O group blood is more likely to cause reaction when given to group A recipient, than those of the group B. While O group blood may be transfused to a patient of any other group in dire emergency, this practice should never be employed as a routine.

Due to the absence of isoantibodies in plasma, AB group was designated "**Universal recipient**". AB group donors may not always be available due to their rarity and it may, on occasion, be necessary to use donors of other groups. In such cases, group A blood is safer than group B, because the anti-A antibody is usually more potent than the anti-B antibody.

Rh compatibility is important only when the recipient is Rh negative. An Rh positive person may safely receive either Rh positive or negative blood. But an Rh negative individual receiving Rh positive blood may form antibodies against the Rh antigen. A subsequent transfusion with Rh positive blood may then cause an adverse reaction. An additional risk in women is Rh sensitisation leading to **hemolytic disease** of the newborn.

CROSS MATCHING

Besides ABO grouping and Rh typing of the donor and recipient, it is necessary before transfusion to perform a "cross matching" to ensure that the donor's blood is compatible with the recipient's blood. The routine procedure used in most blood banks is a rapid cross match by the tile or slide method. This is done in two parts – (1) the major cross match where the donor RBC are tested against the recipient's serum, and (2) the minor cross match where the recipient's RBC are tested against the donor serum.

One drop of a 5% suspension of donor RBC in a saline is added to a drop of recipient's serum on a porcelain tile or a glass slide, mixed and observed for agglutination macroscopically and under low power microscope. This slide test does not detect Rh and other minor incompatibilities. The most discriminating method is the Coombs cross match where washed donor RBC and recipient serum are incubated in a water bath at 37°C for two hours and a direct Coombs test done.

HAZARDS OF INCOMPATIBLE BLOOD TRANSFUSION

(1) When mismatched blood is injected intravenously to a recipient, the RBC may undergo clumping (or agglutination) and intravascular hemoloysis or the RBC may be coated by antibodies and engulfed by phagocytes, removed from circulation and subjected to extravascular lysis.

Incompatible transfusion may be accompanied by symptoms such as shivering, tingling sensation, excruciating headache. Hypotension, cold clammy skin, cyanosis, feeble pulse and other signs of collapse may be seen.

Jaundice, hematuria, oliguria and anuria may follow.

(2) Leucocyte incompatibility may cause fever, pulmonary infiltrates, dyspnoea, cough and chest pain.

(3) Leucocyte incompatibility, platelet incompatibility, allergy and infections may also lead to fever.

(4) When recipient is allergic to some component present in donor blood; rigor, urticaria and other manifestations may develop.

(5) The most common complications following blood transfusion are of infectious origin. Transfusion of blood contaminated by bacteria may lead to endotoxic shock and septicemia.

Some important infections transmitted by blood transfusion are :

Viruses. Hepatitis B virus, Hepatitis C virus, HIV 1 and 2, HTLV I and II, cytomegalovirus.

Bacteria. *Treponema pallidum* (Syphilis)

Parasites. *Plasmodium* sp (Malaria), *Leishmania donovani* (Kala azar), *Toxoplasma gondii*, *Trypanosoma cruzi*, *Babesia* sp.

HEMOLYTIC DISEASE OF THE NEW BORN

This complication is due to "Rh incompatibility" arises when Rh negative mother carries an Rh positive fetus. Small amounts of fetal blood leak into the maternal circulation during pregnancy and at the time of delivery. During the next pregnancy, the mother's anti-Rh antibodies cross the placenta to the fetus and cause hemolysis known as "hemolytic disease of new born (erythroblastosis fetalis)". If hemolysis in the fetus is severe, the infant may die in utero or may develop anemia, severe jaundice and edema (hydrops fetalis).

PREVENTION OF Rh ISOIMMUNISATION

Rh isoimmunisation can be prevented by administration of anti-Rh IgG antibody (100–300μg) to an Rh negative woman immediately after delivery. This passively administered antibody may prevent isoimmunisation by a negative feed back mechanism.

ABO HEMOLYTIC DISEASE

Maternofetal ABO incompatibility is very common, and sometimes hemolytic disease occurs in the newborn. In persons of blood group A and B, natural antibodies are IgM in nature which do not cross the placenta. However, in persons of blood group A, the isoantibodies are predominantly IgG in nature. Hence ABO hemolytic disease is seen largely in O group mothers, bearing A or B group fetus. As ABO hemolytic disease is due to naturally occurring maternal isoantibodies, it may occur even in the first born, without prior immunisation. ABO hemolytic disease is much milder than Rh disease.

QUESTIONS

Essay Questions

1. Describe ABO and Rh blood groups and their applications.
2. Give an account of various blood groups and their clinical importance. Add a note on hazards of incompatible blood transfusion.

Short Notes

1. ABO blood groups.
2. H antigen.
3. Rh factor.
4. Applications of blood groups.
5. Blood transfusion.
6. Cross matching.
7. Hazards of incompatible blood transfusion.
8. Hemolytic disease of the new born (or) erythroblastosis fetalis.
9. ABO hemolytic disease.
10. Prevention of Rh isoimmunisation.

PART-III

SYSTEMATIC BACTERIOLOGY

38

Staphylococci

INTRODUCTION

The staphylococci are ubiquitous in nature, with some species indigenous to humans occurring as part of normal flora and on fomites. Staphylococci are classified by several ways.

(*a*) based on pigment production —

(*i*) *Staph. aureus* — produces golden-yellow pigment.

(*ii*) *Staph. albus* (*staph. epidermidis*) — forms white pigment.

(*iii*) *Staph. citreus* — forms lemon-yellow pigment.

(*b*) based on coagulase production and virulence —

(*i*) Coagulase positive staphylococci *e.g., Staph. aureus*.

(*ii*) Coagulase negative staphylococci *e.g., Staph. albus*.

Almost all isolates of virulent species of staphylococci secrete coagulase — an enzyme that causes citrated plasma to clot.

STAPHYLOCOCCUS AUREUS

Morphology

Staphylococci are Gram positive cocci, arranged in bunches like grapes. The cluster formation is due to cell division occurring in more than one plane with daughter cells remaining close together. Each coccus measure one micron in diameter approximately. They may also be found singly, in pairs and in short chains of three or four cells in smears from pus and liquid cultures. They are nonmotile, nonsporing and noncapsulated. A few strains may be capsulated. In the presence of penicillin and salt, they may be converted to L-forms.

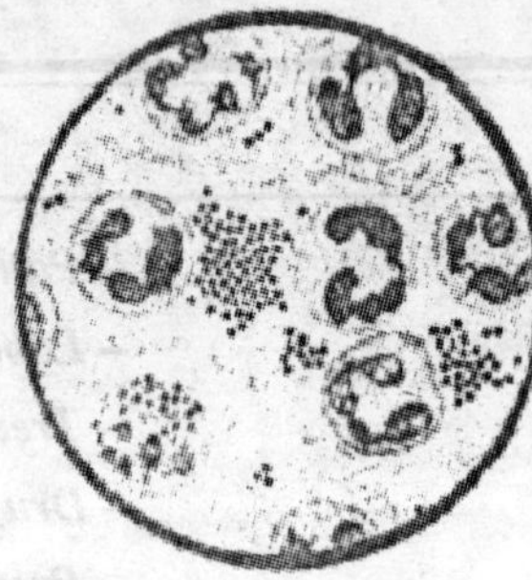

Fig. 38.1 Staphylococci in pus

Cultural characteristics

They are true facultative anaerobic organisms. The optimum temperature for growth is 37ºC and optimum pH 7.4. They grow well on ordinary media.

On Nutrient agar colonies are 2–4 mm in diameter, opaque with a smooth glistening surface and easily emulsifiable. *Staph. aureus* produces **golden-yellow pigment** and *Staph. epidermidis*, white pigment. Other species may form lemon-yellow, orange, pink and other pigments. Pigment production is best at 20ºC in aerobic cultures. The pigment is a carotenoid or its derivative located in cell membrane and therefore in the colony and does not diffuse into the medium. Pigment production is better on milk agar and when 1% glycerol monoacetate is incorporated into nutrient agar.

On blood agar, *Staph. aureus* produces **beta hemolysis**. On MacConkey agar, colonies are small and pink due to lactose fermentation.

Phenolphthalein phosphate agar is used for demonstrating *Staph. aureus* from other species in mixed cultures by demonstration of the production of phosphatase. The medium is prepared by adding sodium phenolphthalein diphosphate. When *Staph. aureus* is grown on this medium it produces phosphatase, which liberates phenolphthalein from sodium phenolphthalein diphosphate. When these colonies of *Staph. aureus* are exposed to ammonia vapor, colonies assume a bright pink color due to the presence of free phenolphthalein.

Salt broth containing 10% NaCl is used as enrichment medium. Several selective media are used for the isolation of *Staph. aureus* from mixed cultures — **salt-milk agar** containing 10% NaCl and milk; **salt agar** containing 10% NaCl in nutrient agar; **mannitol-salt agar** containing 1% mannitol, 7.5% NaCl and phenol red (0.0025%) in nutrient agar; and **Ludlam's medium** containing lithium chloride and tellurite.

Resistance

Staphylococci are among more resistant of nonsporing bacteria. They may withstand 60ºC for 30 min. Some require 80ºC for one hour to be killed. They resist 1% phenol for 15 min. Mercury perchloride 1% solution kills them in 10 min. They are sensitive to aniline dyes such as crystal violet.

Table 38.1 Properties of Virulent Staphylococci

(*i*) Coagulase positive.
(*ii*) Ferment mannitol, producing acid only.
(*iii*) Produce beta hemolysis on blood agar.
(*iv*) Produce golden-yellow pigment.
(*v*) Liquefy gelatin.
(*vi*) Produce phosphatase.
(*vii*) Produce black colonies on potassium tellurite blood agar by reducing tellurite to metallic tellurium.
(*viii*) Produce thermostable nucleases which can be demonstrated by the ability of killed cultures to degrade DNA in an agar diffusion test.
(*ix*) Majority of the strains (particularly cowan-I strain) possess protein-A in their cell wall which can bind to Fc fragment of IgG.

Toxins and enzymes (virulence factors)

The virulence of *Staph. aureus* depends on the production of several exotoxins and enzymes.

1. **Coagulase.**

2. **Cytolytic exotoxins (hemolysins or staphylolysins)** — Four antigenically distinct hemolysins called alpha, beta, gamma and delta lysins are produced. Alpha hemolysin is chromosomally encoded and causes lysis of RBC and skin destruction. Beta hemolysin destroys RBC and sphingomyelin around nerves. Gamma and delta hemolysins destroy RBC.

3. **Superantigen exotoxins** — These toxins have an affinity for the T-cell receptor — MHC class II antigen complex and stimulate enhanced T-lymphocyte response. As many as twenty percent of T-cells respond as compared to 0.01 per cent responding to the usual processed antigens. This major T-cell activation can cause toxic shock, primarily by release into the circulation of large amounts of cytokines, such as interleukin-2, interferon-γ and tumor necrosis factor-α.

(*a*) ***Enterotoxins*** — There are nine antigenic types (A, B, C, D, E, G, H, I and J) of enterotoxins, produced by approximately half of all *Staph. aureus isolates*, mostly by Group II phage type. When these bacteria contaminate food and are allowed to grow, they secrete enterotoxin, ingestion of which can cause food poisoning. The toxin stimulates the vomiting center in the brain by binding to neural receptors in the upper GI tract. Enterotoxins are superantigens that are even more heat-stable than *Staph. aureus*, therefore, organisms are not always recovered from incriminated food.

(*b*) ***Toxic shock syndrome toxin*** (***TSST-1***) — It is a super antigen *i.e.,*potent activator of T-lymphocytes resulting in the liberation of cytokines. It is associated with fever, shock and multi-system involvement of toxic shock syndrome (TSS). It is sometimes referred to as enterotoxin-F, because of similarity in molecular structure, although it does not cause food poisoning.

(*c*) ***Exfoliative toxin*** (***ET, exfoliatin***) — It is also a super antigen, causes loss of the surface layers of the skin (exfoliation) in staphylococcal scalded skin syndrome (SSSS) in children.

4. **Cell wall virulence factors**

(*a*) Protein A is a major component of *Staph. aureus* cell wall. It can bind to Fc moiety of IgG, exerting an antiopsonin and therefore strongly antiphagocytic effect.

(*b*) Fibronectin-binding protein (FnBP) and other staphylococcal surface proteins promote binding to mucosal cell and tissue matrices.

5. **Leukocidins (Panton-Valentin leucocidin)** — They destroy WBC and inhibits phagocytosis by neutrophils.

6. **Beta lactamase** — It causes break down of beta lactam ring of penicillin and thereby confers drug resistance.

7. **Catalase** — It converts H_2O_2 into H_2O and O_2 and reduces killing by phagocytosis.

8. **Hyaluronidase** — Breaks down hyaluronic acid.

9. **DNAase** — Destroys DNA.

10. **Proteinases** — Break down proteins.

11. **Lipases** — Break down lipids.

Staphylocoagulase/Staphylopathogenicity test/Coagulase test

Staph. aureus produces an enzyme called coagulase, which converts fibrinogen into fibrin, along with an activator coagulase reacting factor (CRF) and clots citrated human or rabbit plasma.

$$\text{Fibrinogen} \xrightarrow[\text{CRF}]{\text{Coagulase}} \text{Fibrin (clotting)}$$

Coagulase is of two types — free coagulase and bound coagulase.

Table 38.2 Differences between Free and Bound Coagulases

Free coagulase	*Bound coagulase*
1. Heat labile	Heat stable
2. Secreted freely into surrounding medium	Present within cell wall
3. Requires the cooperation of CRF for its action	Does not require the cooperation of CRF for its action
4. Eight antigenic types are present, designated as A-H. Most humans strains produce coagulase A	Only one antigenic type is found
5. Detected by tube test	Detected by slide test

Coagulase test is done routinely to differentiate between *Staph. aureus* and *Staph. epidermidis* or pathogenic and nonpathogenic staphylococci.

Slide test — When a saline suspension of *Staph. aureus* is mixed on a slide with a drop of plasma, the cocci are clumped.

Tube test — 0.1 ml of overnight broth culture or agar culture suspension is added to approximately 0.5 ml of citrated or oxalated or heparinised human or rabbit plasma, diluted 1 in 5 with saline in a narrow test tube. Diluted plasma in similar tube serves as control. The tubes are incubated in a water bath at 37°C for 3–6 hrs. If positive, the plasma clots and does not flow when the tube is inverted. Tube test is a confirmative test.

Functions of coagulase:

(*i*) inhibits phagocytosis and thereby promotes virulence.

(*ii*) protects cells from bactericidal substances present in tissue fluids.

(*iii*) by laying down a fibrin barrier around the cocci, it helps in walling off the lesion.

Epidemiology

Staph. aureus is carried by twenty to forty percent of healthy individuals at any one time, and by almost everyone at some time. It occurs as a part of normal flora of mucus membranes *e.g.*, anterior nares, vagina and on the skin. Immunocompromised state significantly increases the staphylococcal colonization leading to disease. Carriers serve as a source of infection to themselves and others. The organisms may be shed by patients or carriers and contaminate fomites. The mode of transmission may be through direct contact or indirect contact through fomites or by air-borne droplets. Hospital strains of staphylococci are usually resistant to antibiotics and cause postoperative wound infections and hospital acquired infections.

Pathogenicity

Staph. aureus causes diseases by infecting tissues — typically creating abscesses — and/or by producing toxins. They often cause acute, localised suppurative (pyogenic) infections. Staphylococcal diseases may be grouped as follows:

1. ***Cutaneous infections*** — These include (*i*) Styes — small, superficial abscesses involving sweat or sebaceous glands or hair follicles, (*ii*) Furuncles or boils—subcutaneous abscesses that form around foreign bodies such as splinters, (*iii*) Carbuncles — they are larger, deeper, multiloculated skin infections that can lead to bacteremia and require antibiotic therapy and debridement, (*iv*) Impetigo (pyoderma) — it is a usually localized, superficial, spreading crusty skin lesion generally seen in children. It can be caused by *Staph. aureus*, but more commonly by *Strept. pyogenes* or both organisms together.

2. ***Deep infections*** — These may be metastatic from superficial infections or skin carriage, or may result from trauma (*i*) Osteomyelitis — *Staph. aureus* is the most common cause of acute and chronic infection of the bone marrow, (*ii*) Arthritis — *Staph. aureus* is the most common cause of acute infection of the joint space in children (septic joint).

3. ***Other infections*** — (*i*) Acute endocarditis — it is generally associated with intravenous drug abuse, and is caused by injection of contaminated preparations or by needles that are contaminated with *Staph. aureus*, (*ii*) Septicemia — it is a generalized infection with sepsis or bacteremia that may be associated with a known focus.

4. ***Respiratory infections*** — Tonsillitis, pharyngitis, sinusitis, otitis, bronchopneumonia, lung abscess etc. Rarely, a severe, necrotizing pneumonia may occur as a secondary complication.

5. ***Toxic shock syndrome*** **(*TSS*)** — It is caused by *Staph. aureus* producing toxic shock syndrome toxin (TSST-1) or enterotoxin-F.

It is a multisystem illness characterized by high fever, headache, confusion, conjunctival reddening, subcutaneous edema, vomiting, diarrhea, scarlatiniform rash and fine desquamation of the hands and feet. Severe cases progress to acute renal failure, disseminated intravascular coagulation, peripheral gangrene, profound hypotensive shock and death.

Initially the disease was noted among women during menstruation associated with the use of tampons, who happened to be vaginally colonized by TSST positive strains of *Staph. aureus*. Subsequently, the disease has been reported both in males and females, associated with ordinary *Staph. aureus* infections, and many are due to a circulating enterotoxin rather than to TSST.

6. ***Staphylococcal food poisoning (gastroenteritis)*** — It results when food contaminated with enterotoxin producing *Staph. aureus* is consumed. The types of food responsible are meat, fish, eggs, milk and milk products, often contaminated by food handlers.

It is a toxic type of food poisoning — where preformed toxin is ingested with the food. The toxin induces nausea, vomiting and diarrhea within six hours of consumption of contaminated food. The incubation period is short, 2–6 hours. The toxin acts directly on autonomic nervous system to cause the illness, rather than on gastrointestinal mucosa.

Several *Staph. aureus* strains produce enterotoxins in meat, fish, egg, salad, milk and milk products, the source of infection being a carrier, usually food handler. Nine antigenic types of enterotoxin (A, B, C, D, E, G, H, I and J) are responsible for food poisoning.

7. ***Exfoliative skin diseases or staphylococcal scalded skin syndrome (SSSS)*** — This disease is produced by exfoliative toxin (ET) or exfoliatin or epidermolytic toxin of *Staph. aureus*. In this disease, the outer layer of epidermis gets separated from the underlying tissues. The toxin attacks the intercellular adhesive of the stratum granulosum, causing marked epithelial desquamation.

The severe form of SSSS is known as Ritter's disease in new born and toxic epidermal necrolysis in old patients. Mild forms of disease is known as pemphigus neonatorum and bullous impetigo.

8. ***CNS diseases*** — *Staph. aureus* may cause brain abscess and meningitis.

9. Hospital acquired cross infections, particularly post-operative wound infections.

Laboratory diagnosis

Specimens to be collected include pus from pyogenic lesions, blood from a patient with PUO, sputum from respiratory infections, feces, food remains and vomit from a case of food poisoning, urine from a urinary tract infection case. Nasal and perineal swabs may be used for the detection of carriers.

Microscopy — Examination of Gram stained smear may show Gram positive cocci in clusters and pus cells.

Culture — Specimens are inoculated on to nutrient agar, blood agar or selective media such as salt agar or salt milk agar and incubated at 37ºC for 24 hrs. The plates are inspected for pigment color. Beta hemolysis on blood agar plate should be checked. Smears are examined and tube coagulase test should be done to differentiate pathogenic staphylococci. Antibiotic sensitivity tests should be done as a guide to treatment. Phage typing may be done for epidemiological purposes.

Serological tests — Antistaphylolysin titre of more than 2 units/ml or an increase in titre may be of value in the diagnosis of deep infections.

Treatment

Benzyl penicillin is the drug of choice. If the strain is resistant to penicillin, penicillinase–resistant penicillins such as cloxacillin, oxacillin, nafcillin, flucloxacillin and methicillin are used. Patients allergic to penicillins may be given erythromycin, vancomycin or first generation cephalosporins.

Drug resistance

Resistance determinants are often present on plasmids and transposons and can be transferred among *Staph. aureus* strains, and between staphylococcal species.

(*a*) ***Penicillin resistance*** — Almost all *Staph. aureus* isolates are now resistant to penicillin-G due to penicillinase-encoding plasmids or transposons, which spread by transduction. The production of betalactamase or penicillinase, which inactivates penicillin by breaking the betalactam ring is coded by plasmid. Staphylococci produce four types of penicillinases A to D. The penicillinase plasmids may carry genes for resistance to other antibiotics.

(*b*) ***Methicillin-resistant Staph. aureus*** (***MRSA***) — The binding of betalactam antibiotics to cells is inhibited due to alteration of surface receptors. It is chromosome mediated.

In recent decades, a high percentage (about fifty per cent) of hospital *Staph. aureus* isolates has been found to be also resistant to methicillin and/or oxacillin, due to chromosomal acquisition of the gene for a modified penicillin-binding protein (PBP), PBP–2a. This protein codes for a new peptidoglycan transpeptidase with a low affinity for all currently available betalactam antibiotics, and thus renders infections with methicillin-resistant *Staph. aureus* unresponsive to betalactam antibiotic therapy. These strains may exhibit resistance to other antibiotics and heavy metals, some being sensitive only to vancomycin and cause outbreaks of hospital acquired infections. These strains are called **"Epidemic Methicillin Resistant** *Staph. aureus* **(EMRSA)"**. Methicillin resistance is tested by using oxacillin discs.

Prevention and control of nosocomial infections caused by EMRSA depend on proper hand washing and eradication of colonized sites such as the skin or nose with topical agents such as mupirocin or chlorhexidine.

(*c*) ***Vancomycin resistance*** — Several MRSAs have acquired low-level resistance to vancomycin, which is a drug of choice in the treatment of life-threatening *Staph. aureus* infections.

Prevention

No vaccine or preventive drug is available. Infection control procedures such as barrier precautions, washing of hands and disinfection of fomites are important in the control of noscomial *Staph. aureus* epidemics.

COAGULASE-NEGATIVE STAPHYLOCOCCI

They constitute the normal flora of skin and often isolated from clinical specimens. They are morphologically similar to *Staph. aureus*, but can be differentiated from them by their white pigment, absence of coagulase production.

They are opportunistic pathogens and cause infections in debilitated or immunocompromised patients. They may cause infections in patients fitted with plastic catheters, cannulae, cardiac valves, pace makers, urinary catheters and artificial joints.

The most important coagulase-negative staphylococci are *Staphylococcus epidermidis (albus)* and *Staphylococcus saprophyticus.*

Staphylococcus epidermidis (albus)

It is a coagulase-negative, nonpathogenic *Staphylococcus* and constitutes a part of normal skin flora. They are common contaminants in clinical specimens being derived from skin during collection of specimens. Hospital strains are usually multidrug resistant.

It is an opportunistic pathogen; infections are predominantly hospital acquired. It causes stitch abscesses, cystitis in urinary tract, septicemia and subacute bacterial endocarditis. The predisposing factors are instrumentation procedures such as catheterization, prosthetic heart valve implantation and immunosuppressive therapy.

Many strains of *Staph. albus* can produce polysaccharide slime, which helps the organism to adhere and form microcolonies on plastic catheters and prosthetic devices.

Staphylococcus saprophyticus

It is coagulase-negative and normally present on human skin and periurethral area.

It has become clinically important as a common cause of acute urinary tract infection in sexually active young women. It causes cystitis and pyelonephritis. Patients with this infection usually present with dysuria, pyuria and hematuria. It may also cause urethritis in both men and women, catheter associated urinary tract infections, prostatitis in elderly men, and rarely bacteremia.It tends to be sensitive to most antibiotics, even penicillin-G. It can be distinguished from *Staph. epidermidis* and most other coagulase-negative staphylococci by its natural resistance to novobiocin.

MICROCOCCI

They are Gram positive cocci found in clusters, which differ from staphylococci in attacking sugars oxidatively. They may occur in irregular clusters, in groups of four (tetrads as in *Gaffkya tetragena*) or of eight (as in *Sarcina luteum*). The cocci are of irregular size and often larger than staphylococci. Staining is also not uniform.

They are saprophytes and commensals and may cause opportunistic infections. They are catalase and oxidase positive.

To differentiate between micrococci and staphylococci, Hugh and Leifson's oxidation-fermentation test is used in which micrococci show oxidative and staphylococci show fermentative metabolism.

QUESTIONS

Essay Type Questions

1. Classify staphylococci. Describe the pathogenicity and lab. diagnosis of *Staph. aureus.*
2. Give an account of *Staphylococcus aureus.*

Short Essay Type Questions

1. Properties of pathogenic staphylococci.
2. Coagulase or staphylocoagulase

   Or

   Coagulase test or staphylopathogenicity test.
3. Toxins and enzymes of *Staphylococcus aureus.*
4. Pathogenicity of *Staph. aureus.*
5. Coagulase negative Staphylococci.

Short Answer Type Questions

1. Name 4 selective media for staphylococci.
2. Staphylococcal food poisoning.
3. TSS.
4. Drug resistance in staphylococci.
5. EMRSA.
6. *Staph. epidermidis* or *Staph. albus.*
7. *Staph. saprophyticus.*
8. Micrococci.

39

Streptococci

- ***Differences between staphylococci and streptococci***
- ***Classification***
- ***Group A streptococci (Str. pyogenes)***
  - ***Morphology***
  - ***Cultural characteristics***
  - ***Differentiation from other streptococci***
  - ***Resistance***
  - ***Antigenic structure***
  - ***Lancefield serogrouping***
  - ***Toxins and enzymes***
  - ***Epidemiology,***
  - ***pathogenicity***
  - ***Post-streptococcal sequelae***
  - ***Lab. diagnosis***
  - ***Treatment.***
- ***Group B streptococci (Str. agalactiae)***
- ***Group D streptococci***
- ***Enterococci***
- ***Viridans (alpha hemolytic) streptococci***
- ***Streptococcus MG***

Table 39.1 Differences between Staphylococci and Streptococci

Staphylococci	*Streptococci*
1. Catalase positive	Catalase negative
2. Gram positive cocci arranged in grape like clusters	Gram positive cocci arranged in chains
3. Produce localized pyogenic (suppurative) infections infections	Produce generalized (spreading) pyogenic and non-suppurative post-streptococcal compli cations
4. *Staph. aureus* produces coagulase, which converts fibrinogen to fibrin	*Strept. pyogenes* produces fibrinolysin (strep tokinase) which causes lysis of fibrin clots

CLASSIFICATION

Streptococci are first divided into facultative anaerobes and obligate anaerobes. Based on hemolysis on blood agar, Brown classified facultative anaerobes into three groups.

1. ***Alpha hemolytic streptococci*** — They produce a greenish discoloration with partial hemolysis around the colonies. The zone of lysis is small (1 or 2 mm wide), with indefinite margins and unlysed RBCs can be made out microscopically within this zone. They are known as viridans streptococci or *Streptococcus viridans* (viridans = green). They are normal commensals of throat and upper respiratory tract.

2. ***Beta hemolytic streptococci*** — They produce a sharply defined, clear, colorless zone of hemolysis, 2 to 4 mm wide, within which RBCs are completely lysed. Hemolysis is due to the production of hemolysins (streptolysins) *e.g., Strept. pyogenes.*

3. ***Gamma hemolytic streptococci*** — They do not produce hemolysis and are known as non-hemolytic streptococci *e.g., Enterococcus fecalis.*

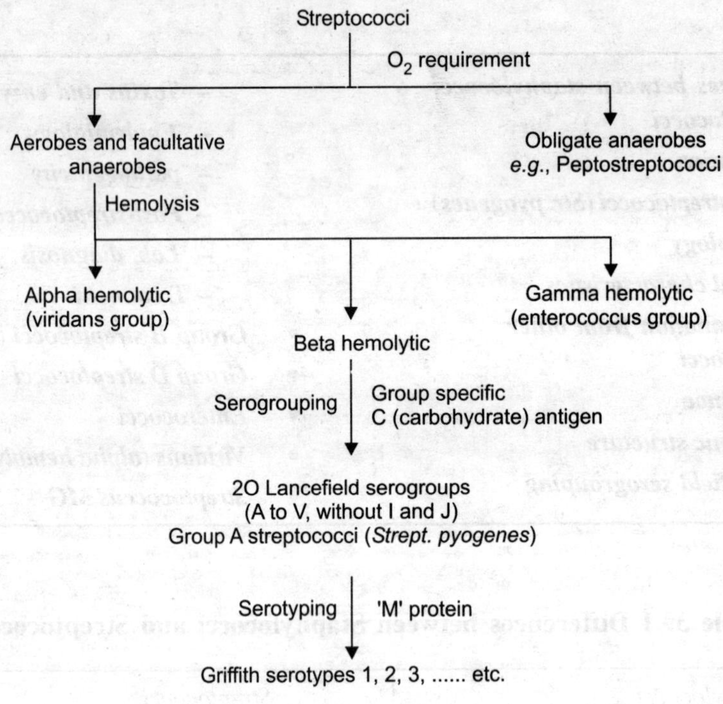

Fig. 39.1 Classification of streptococci.

GROUP A STREPTOCOCCI (*STREPTOCOCCUS PYOGENES*)

Morphology

They are Gram positive cocci arranged in chains. Individual cocci are spherical in shape, measure one micron in diameter. Chain formation is due to cocci dividing in one plane only and the daughter cells failing to separate completely (Fig. 39.2). They are nonmotile and nonsporing. Some strains possess capsule made of hyaluronic acid. Capsules are best seen in young cultures. In the presence of penicillin or salt, they may convert to protoplasts or L-forms.

Cultural characteristics

They are aerobes and facultative anaerobes. The optimum temperature is 37ºC, optimum pH is 7.2 to 7.4. It has fastidious growth requirements and growth occurs only on media enriched with blood and serum.

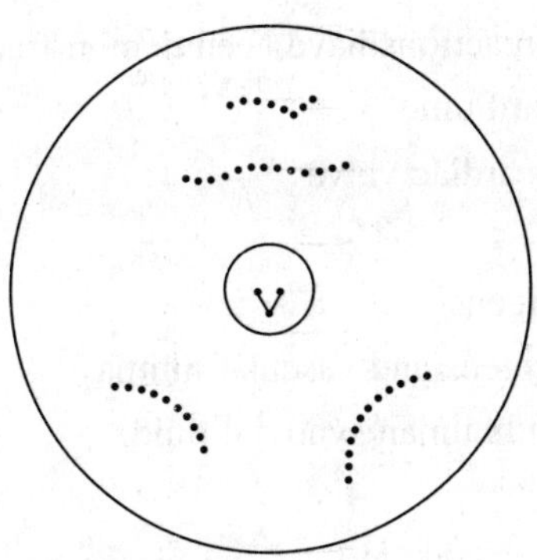

Fig. 39.2 Streptococci

On blood agar, colonies are small, circular, semitransparent, low convex discs with beta hemolysis. Growth and hemolysis are promoted by 10% CO_2. On fresh isolation, virulent strains produce a matt (finely granular) colonies and avirulent strains form glossy colonies. Capsulated strains form mucoid colonies.

Crystal violet blood agar and PNF medium (blood agar containing polymyxin-B, neomycin and fusidic acid) are selective for beta hemolytic streptococci.

Pike's medium is a transport medium for clinical specimens containing Group A streptococci.

Pike's medium is prepared by adding crystal violet (1 in 1,000,000) and sodium azide (1 in 16,000) to blood agar.

Differentiating Group A Streptococci from other Streptococci

Strept. pyogenes can be differentiated from other streptococci by their

(*i*) sensitivity to **bacitracin**

(*ii*) hydrolysis of pyrrolidonyl naphthylamide (PYR test)

(*iii*) failure to ferment ribose.

Resistance

Strept. pyogenes is a delicate organism; can be killed by heat at 54°C for 30 min. It is rapidly inactivated by antiseptics. It can survive in dust for several weeks, if protected from sunlight. It dies in a few days in cultures; therefore it is preserved in RCM broth at 4°C. It is highly resistant to crystal violet than many other bacteria, including *Staph. aureus*. Hence, crystal violet is incorporated into blood agar to make it selective for the isolation of streptococci. Unlike *Staph. aureus*, it does not develop resistance to drugs. It is sensitive to bacitracin. This property is made use of in differentiation of *Strept. pyogenes* from other hemolytic streptococci.

Antigenic Structure

Cell wall of *Strept. pyogenes* consists of

(*i*) an outer layer of protein and lipoteichoic acid, containing protein antigens (M, T, R).

(*ii*) middle layer of group specific carbohydrate (rhamnose-n-acetyl glucosamine), and

(*iii*) an inner layer of peptidoglycan.

The capsule when present is composed of hyaluronic acid.

Antigenic similarities and cross reactions have been demonstrated between

- cell wall protein and myocardium
- group A carbohydrate and cardiac valves
- M protein and glomeruli
- peptidoglycan and skin antigens
- cytoplasmic membrane antigens and vascular intima
- capsular hyaluronic acid and human synovial fluid.

Lancefield Serogrouping

Both hemolytic streptococci can be classified into 20 Lancefield serogroups, based on the carbohydrate (C) antigen present in the cell wall, by ring precipitation test.

The antigen extract and specific antisera are allowed to react in capillary tubes, where a ring like precipitation is formed between them. The 20 serogroups are named A–V (without I and J).

For extraction of C antigen, the streptococci are grown in Todd-Hewitt broth and extracted with hydrochloric acid (Lancefield acid extraction method) or formamide (Fuller's method) or by an enzyme produced by *Streptomyces albus* (Maxted's method) or by autoclaving (Rantz and Randall's method).

Toxins and Enzymes

Strept. pyogenes forms many exotoxins, enzymes and virulence factors.

1. ***Hemolysins (Streptolysins)*** — *Strept. pyogenes* produces 2 types of hemolysins — streptolysin 'O' and streptolysin 'S'.

Streptolysin 'O' is oxygen labile. It is inactive in oxidized form. It is also heat labile. Streptolysin 'O' is antigenic and antistreptolysin 'O' (ASO) appears in sera following streptococcal infections. Estimation of this antibody is used as a standard serological test for retrospective diagnosis of post streptococcal lesions.

Streptolysin 'S' is oxygen stable and responsible for hemolysis on blood agar. It is soluble in serum, hence called streptolysin 'S'. It is a protein but not antigenic.

2. ***Erythrogenic or Dick or Scarlatinal toxin or Pyrogenic exotoxin*** — It is responsible for scarlatiniform rash of scarlet fever. It is heat stable and antigenic and is neutralized by antibodies. This property is used in susceptibility tests and diagnostic tests for scarlet fever—Dick test and Schultz-Charlton reaction.

Three types of streptococcal pyrogenic exotoxins (SPE) are identified. Type A and C are coded by phage genes, while type B is chromosomal. These toxins are superantigens.

3. ***Streptokinase or Fibrinolysin*** — It promotes the lysis of human fibrin clots by activating plasminogen, which facilitates the spread of infection by breaking the fibrin barrier around lesions. It is an antigenic protein and neutralizing antibodies appear, which may be estimated for retrospective diagnosis of streptococcal infections. Streptokinase may be given intravenously for treatment of pulmonary emboli and venous thrombosis.

4. ***Deoxyribonucleases or Streptodornase*** — It causes depolymerisation of DNA, which is responsible for thin serous character of streptococcal pus or exudates. Four antigenically distinct streptodornases A, B, C, D have been recognized.

5. ***NADase*** — It acts on coenzyme NAD and liberates nicotinamide. It is a antigenic and specifically neutralized by antibody in convalescent sera.

6. ***Hyaluronidase*** — This enzyme breaks down hyaluronic acid of tissues, which favours the spread of infection along intercellular spaces.

7. Many strains also produce proteinase, phosphatase, esterase, amylase, neuraminidase, N-acetyl glucosaminidase etc.

8. ***Serum opacity factor (SOF)*** — It is a lipoproteinase, produces opacity when applied to agar gel containing horse and swine serum. Hence, this enzyme is known as serum opacity factor (SOF). It is produced by Group a streptococci of certain M types.

9. ***C 5a peptidase*** — It degrades C 5a, thus interfering with mobilization of WBC to sites of strept. pyogenes infection.

Epidemiology

The streptococci are normally present in the upper respiratory tract—throat, nasopharynx or nose of patients and carriers. Asymptomatic infection is common and helps to maintain the organism in the community. Transmission of infection is either by direct contact or through contaminated fingers, dust or fomites. Crowding is an important factor in the transmission of infection. Respiratory droplets or skin contact spread infection from person to person, especially in crowded environments such as classrooms or children's play areas.

Pathogenicity

Strept. pyogenes cells, perhaps in an inhaled droplet, attach to the pharyngeal mucosa via actions of protein F, lipoteichoic acid and M protein. The bacteria may colonize, grow and secrete toxins, causing damage to surrounding cells, invading the mucosa, and eliciting an inflammatory response with influx of WBC, fluid leakage and pus formation. The patient then has streptococcal pharyngitis. The bacterial hyaluronic acid capsule and M protein inhibit phagocytosis, and C5a peptidase interfers with attraction of more WBC. Streptokinase, streptodornase and hyaluronidase tend to decrease the viscosity of the pus, and to enhance spread through the tissues. Occasionally blood stream is invaded, resulting in septicemia.

Thus, *Strept. pyogenes* produces generalized (spreading) or rapidly progressive pyogenic infections. Strept. pyogenes is a major cause of **cellulitis**—diffuse spreading skin and subcutaneous soft tissue inflammation. More specific syndromes include the following.

1. ***Acute pharyngitis or pharyngotonsilittis*** — *Strept. pyogenes* is the most common bacterial cause of **sore throats,** and pharyngitis is the most common type of *Strept. pyogenes* infection. A special variety of sore throat, characterized by fever and sunburn—like rash due to the release of pyrogenic exotoxin without antibody formation is known as **scarlet fever.**

Streptococcal sore throats are mild and many sore throats of other etiologies (for example, viral or mycoplasmal) are severe. Hence, laboratory confirmation is important.

2. ***Impetigo*** — Although *Staph. aureus* causes impetigo, *Strept. pyogenes* is the classic cause of this syndrome. The disease begins on any exposed surface (most commonly the legs). It usually affects children and can cause severe and extensive lesions on the face and limbs.

3. ***Erysipelas*** — It is characaterized by fiery red, advancing erythema, especially on the face or lower limbs and affects all age groups.

4. ***Puerperal sepsis*** — This infection is initiated during or following soon after, the delivery of a new born. It can occur due to exogenous transmission (for example, by nasal droplets from an infected carrier or from contaminated instruments) or endogenously, from the patient's vaginal flora. This is the

disease of a uterine endometrium in which patients suffer from a purulent vaginal discharge, and are systemically very ill.

5. ***Invasive group A streptococcal disease*** — It is characaterized by deep local invasion without necrosis (cellulitis) or with it (necrotizing fascitis/myositis). The disease often spreads rapidly, even in otherwise healthy individuals, leading to bacteremia and sepsis. Symptoms include a toxic shock-like syndrome, fever, hypotension, multi-organ involvement, a sunburn-like rash, or a combination of these symptoms.

6. ***Strept. pyogenes*** may produce abscesses in internal organs such as brain, liver, lungs and kidneys and septicemia and pyemia.

Post-Streptococcal Sequelae

Strept. pyogenes infections lead to two important non-suppurative complications or sequelae known as acute rheumatic fever and acute glomerulonephritis. These complications set in 1–3 weeks after the acute infection so that the organism is no longer detectable when sequelae set in.

1. ***Acute rheumatic fever*** — It is an autoimmune disease characterized by inflammatory lesions involving the heart valves, joints, subcutaneous tissues and CNS. It occurs two to three weeks after the initiation of streptococcal pharyngitis. The disease occurs most frequently among children. The lesions are due to antigenic cross reactions between antigens of the heart and joint tissues, and the streptococcal antigen (particularly M protein). It is characterized by fever, rash, **carditis** and arthritis. The essential lesion is carditis including connective tissue degeneration of the heart valves and inflammatory myocardial lesions characterized by Aschoff nodules. Rheumatic fever follows persistent or repeated streptococcal infections of throat (respiratory tract) with strong antibody response. Rheumatic fever is preventable if the patient is treated within the first ten days following initiation of acute pharyngitis.

2. ***Acute glomerulonephritis (Bright's disease)*** — It is an immune complex disease (Type III hypersensitivity) due to antigenic cross reaction between glomerular antigen and streptococcal 'M' protein. The damage to renal glomeruli is due to the deposition of antigen-antibody complexes on the basement membrane of the glomerulus. Clinically, the affected person exhibits edema, fever, hypertension, hematuria. The disease occurs primarily among children. The disease occurs as soon as one week after impetigo or pharyngitis ensues, due to a few "nephritogenic" strains of group A streptococci.

Post-streptococcal lesions can be prevented by prophylactic antibiotic therapy with penicillin G and erythromycin.

3. ***Erythema nodosum*** — It is due to hypersensitivity to cell wall fragments and characterized by small red nodules under the surface of the skin.

Laboratory Diagnosis

Specimens collected are pus, sputum, genital swabs, blood and CSF. Specimens can be transported in Pike's medium.

Microscopy — The presence of Gram positive cocci in chains alongwith pus cells is indicative of streptococcal infections. But smears from throat and genitalia are of no value, where streptococci form part of normal flora. The fluorescent antibody technique has been employed for rapid identification of Group A streptococci.

Culture — The specimen is inoculated on blood agar and incubated at 37ºC, under 5–10% CO_2 both aerobically and anaerobically. The growth is identified by beta hemolysis, Gram's staining and bacitracin sensitivity.

Strept. pyogenes is sensitive to bacitracin. A disc of bacitracin is applied on the surface of an inoculated blood agar. After incubation, a wide zone of inhibition is seen with *Strept. pyogenes*, but not with other streptococci. Hemolytic streptococci are grouped by Lancefield method.

ASO test — It is used for retrospective diagnosis of post streptococcal complications—acute rheumatic fever, and acute glomerulonephritis. Estimation of this antibody (anti streptolysin-O) is used as a standard serological test. ASO titres higher than 160 or 200 Todd units are indicative of post streptococcal complications.

Following certain chemical treatments or bacterial contamination, sera may develop inhibitory activity, due to some changes in lipoproteins. Such sera are unfit for ASO test.

ADNaseB Test — Antideoxyribonuclease-B (ADNase B) estimation is also employed. Titres higher than 300 or 350 are taken as significant.

Streptozyme test is a passiive hemagglutination test using RBC sensitized with crude extracellular antigens of streptococci. It is a convenient, specific, sensitive screening test. It becomes positive in all types of streptococcal infections.

Treatment

Penicillin is the drug of choice. Resistance to penicillin is not observed. When patient is allergic to penicillin, erythromycin or cephalexin or clarithromycin or azithromycin is the preferred drug.

Penicillin or erythromycin is also used prophylactically to control post streptococcal complications and to prevent recurrence of streptococcal infections.

GROUP B STREPTOCOCCI (*STREPT. AGALACTIAE*)

Group B streptococci, represented by the pathogen *Streptococcus agalactiae*, are Gram positive, catalase-negative organisms. They possess a polysaccharide capsule that is antiphagocytic, and thus allows the bacterium to infect tissue, and induce an inflammatory response. *Strept. agalactiae* is found in the vaginocervical tract of female carriers, and the urethral mucus membranes of male carriers, as well as in the GI tract, especially the rectum. Transmission occurs from an infected mother to her infant at birth, and venereally (propagated by sexual contact) among adults.

The group B streptococci are a leading cause of meningitis and septicemia in neonates with high mortality rate. Neonatal meningitis is of two types — (*i*) Early onset type—occurring within a week of birth and presents as septicemia, meningitis or pneumonia, and is often fatal. Infection is acquired from maternal vagina during birth, (*ii*) Late onset type—developing between the second and twelfth weeks of life. Infection is more often obtained from the environment or hospital personnel.

They are also an occasional cause of infections in post-partum women (endometritis), and individuals with impaired immune systems, in whom the organism may cause septicemia or pneumonia. They are also associated with lower extremity infections in diabetics. Other group B streptococcal infections in neonates include arthritis, osteomyelitis, conjunctivitis, peritonitis, respiratory infections and endocarditis. In cattle, it causes mastitis (bovine).

Samples of blood, cervical swabs, sputum or CSF can be obtained for culture on blood agar. Group B streptococci are β-hemolytic, with larger colonies and less hemolytic than group A. ELISA test can be used to detect the antigen from samples.

Group B streptococci can be identified by:

(*i*) ***Hippurate hydrolysis*** — *Strept. agalactiae* produces hippuricase, which hydrolyzes sodium hippurate to form sodium benzoate and glycine. This hydrolysis can be detected by adding ninhydrin, which reacts with alpha amino groups to form a purple color.

(*ii*) ***CAMP reaction*** — Group B streptococci can be identified by CAMP (Christie, Atkins and Munch-Peterson) reaction.

Strept. agalactiae is inoculated on blood agar perpendicular to the streak of *Staph. aureus* (plazan strain). The two streak lines must not touch each other and there should be a space of about 1 cm between them. Then the plate is incubated at 37ºC for 24 hrs aerobically in the presence of 10% CO_2. A prominent zone of hemolysis appears at the junction of the two organisms, which assumes the shape of an arrow-head.

Group B streptococci are sensitive to penicillin G and Ampicillin and are the drugs of choice. In life-threatening infections, an aminoglycoside can be added to the regimen.

GROUP D STREPTOCOCCI

They are divided into two groups :

(*i*) Enterococcus group (enterococci or fecal streptococci) classified into genus *Entercoccus e.g., E. fecalis, E. fecium, E. durans.*

(*ii*) Non-enterococcal group — *e.g., Str. bovis, Str. equinus.* They can be differentiated from enterococci — (*a*) failure to grow on nutrient broth with 6.5% NaCl, (*b*) PYR (pyrrolidonyl naphthylamide) test negative, (*c*) sensitive to penicillin, (*d*) hydrolyze hippurate, (*e*) alpha hemolytic or nonhemolytic on blood agar.

They may cause endocarditis, urinary tract infections, septicemia, abscesses and wound infections.

Both enterococci and nonenterococcal group D streptococci can grow in the presence of 40% bile and can hydrolyze aesculin to aesculein and glucose.

ENTEROCOCCI (FECAL STREPTOCOCCI)

Enterococci contain a C-carbohydrate that reacts with group D streptococci. But DNA analysis and other properties have placed them in their own genus *Enterococcus*. The most important species are *E. fecalis, E. fecium, E. durans, E. avium.* They can be differentiated by biochemical properties.

They are Gram positive cocci, present in pairs or short chains. They are nonmotile and noncapsulated. The cocci are oval shaped, typically arranged at right angles to each other.

They constitute normal flora of intestine and genital tract. They can also colonize oral mucus membranes and skin, especially in hospital environment. They are highly resistant to environmental and chemical agents, and can persist on fomites. Enterococci have become an important cause of nosocomial infections due to their multiple antibiotic resistance.

Under conditions, where host resistance is lowered, or where the integrity of GI or genitourinary tract has been disrupted, for example by instrumentation, the enterococci can spread to normally sterile sites, causing urinary tract infections, bacteremia and septicemia, subacute bacterial endocarditis, biliary tract infections or intra-abdominal abscesses.

On blood agar, enterococci can be alpha, beta or nonhemolytic. On MacConkey agar tiny, deep pink colonies are formed due to lactose fermentation. They can grow in the presence of 6.5% NaCl, 40% bile, at pH 9.6. They are relatively heat resistant, surviving 60ºC for 30 minutes.

Enterococci are distinguished from nonenterococcal group D streptococci by their ability to grow in 6.5% NaCl, yield a positive PYR test, and inability to hydrolyze hippurate.

Enterococci can grow in the presence of 40% bile and to hydrolyze the polysaccharide esculin.

Enterococci are naturally resistant to penicillins, sulphonamides, cephalosporins. Judicious use of antibiotics is an important factor in controlling these infections.

VIRIDANS STREPTOCOCCI/ALPHA HEMOLYTIC STREPTOCOCCI/ ORAL STREPTOCOCCI

They are commonly found in human throat and mouth as commensals. They produce alpha hemolysis (greenish discoloration) on blood agar. Based on biochemical reactions, 5 species have been identified—*Str. salivarius, Str. mutans*, *Str. sanguis*, *Str. mitior* (mitis) and *Str. milleri*.

They are normally nonpathogenic, but in persons with predisposing conditions such as valvular disease of the heart, they produce **subacute bacterial endocarditis** (Infective endocarditis). Tooth extraction and injury of the oral cavity in such persons is dangerous and should be done under antibiotic cover. Other organisms such as enterococci, *Staph. aureus*, coagulase-negative staphylococci, *Coxiella burnettii* and some fungi also cause infective endocarditis.

Diagnosis of subacute bacterial endocarditis is established by repeated blood cultures. Alpha hemolytic streptococci can be identified by their alpha hemolysis on blood agar, their sensitivity to penicillin and failure to grow on MacConkey's agar. When isolated from mouth or respiratory tract, they are regarded as harmless commensals. But, when isolated from blood or a closed lesion, they may be pathogenic.

Str. mutans causes **dental caries.** It breaks down dietary sucrose, producing acid and a tough adhesive dextran. The acid damages dentine and the dextran bind together food debris, epithelial cells, mucus and bacteria to form dental plaques, which lead to caries. *Str. mutans* is so called because it assumes a bacillary form in acid environment.

STREPTOCOCCUS MG

It is an alpha hemolytic group F streptococci. It may be present in the sputum of normal persons. It is isolated from the cases of primary atypical pneumonia. Demonstration of antibodies to *Streptococcus* MG has been used as a diagnostic serological test for primary atypical pneumonia.

QUESTIONS

Essay Type Questions

1. Describe the morphology, cultural characteristics and lab. diagnosis of *Strept.pyogenes* or Group A streptococci.
2. Classify streptococci. Describe the pathogenesis and lab. diagnosis of post-streptococcal complications.

Short Essay Type Questions

1. Classification of streptococci.
2. Toxins and enzymes of streptococci.
3. Pathogenicity of streptococci.
4. Post–streptococcal complications.
5. Lab. diagnosis of streptococcal infections.
6. Group B streptococci.
7. Enterococci (or) fecal streptococci.
8. Alpha hemolytic streptococci.

Short Answer Type Questions

1. How do you differentiate staphylococci and streptococci?
2. Lancefield serogrouping.
3. How do you differentiate Group A streptococci from other streptococci?
4. Pike's medium.
5. Streptolysins.
6. Streptokinase.
7. Streptodornase.
8. Acute rhenumatic fever.
9. Acute glomerulonephritis.
10. ASO test.
11. CAMP reaction.
12. Subactue bacterial endocarditis.
13. Lab. diagnosis of subacute bacterial endocardititis.
14. Dental caries.
15. Streptococcus MG.

40

Pneumococci (Streptococcus pneumoniae) (Formerly Diplococcus pneumoniae)

- *Morphology*
- *Cultural characteristics*
- *Resistance*
- *Bile solubility test*
- *Optochin sensitivity*
- *Differences between streptococci and pneumococci*
- *Epidemiology*
- *Pathogenicity*
- *Laboratory diagnosis*
- *CRP*
- *Prophylaxis*
- *Treatment*
- *Drug resistant pneumococci*
- *Causative agents of typical pneumonia.*

Morphology

Pneumococci are Gram positive diplococci. Cocci are small, slightly elongated, with one end broad or rounded and the other pointed, presenting a flame shape or lanceolate appearance. They occur in pairs with broad ends in opposition (Fig. 40.1). The cell wall contains a 'C' antigen similar to carbohydrate (C antigen) antigen of streptococci. They are capsulated; the capsule enclosing each pair. The capsule is composed of polysaccharide. There are 90 antigenically distinct capsular types but only 23 are associated with human diseases. Since, capsular polysaccharide diffuses into infective tissues and exudates and culture medium, it is also known as specific soluble substance (SSS). Capsules can be demonstrated by various methods.

(*i*) ***Negative staining*** — When capsulated bacteria are mixed with Indian ink or Nigrosin and spread on a glass slide and examined under microscope, capsules are seen unstained clear halos against a uniformly black stained background.

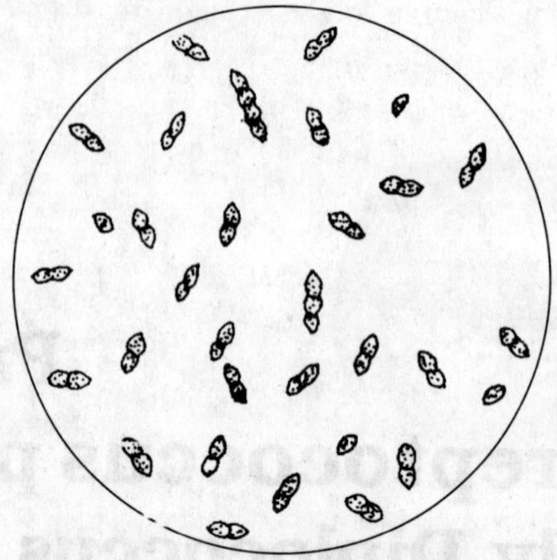

Fig. 40.1 *Streptococcus pneumoniae.*

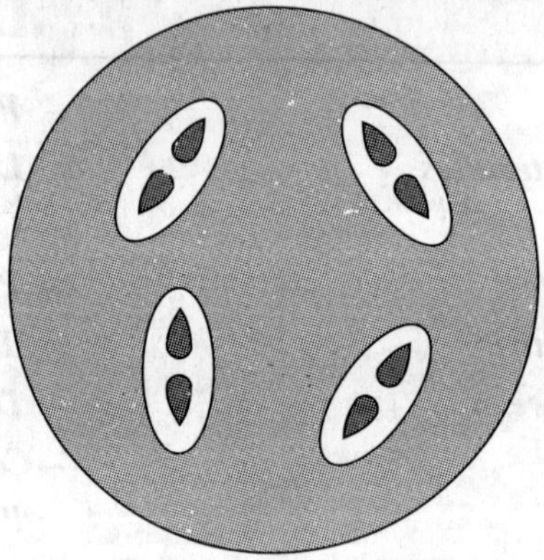

Fig. 40.2 Negative staining.

(*ii*) ***Capsule swelling reaction* (*Quellung reaction*)** — It was first described by Neufeld (1902). It was widely employed for typing of pneumococci.

When a suspension of pneumococci is mixed on a slide with a drop of type specific antiserum and loopful of methylene blue solution, and examined under microscope; in the presence of homologous antiserum, the capsular antigen reacts with it and becomes swollen, refractile and sharply delineated. The quellung test can be done directly with sputum from acute pneumonia cases.

(*iii*) ***Hiss stain*** — It is a special stain used to demonstrate bacterial capsules, where copper salts are used as mordants.

Cultural characteristics

They are aerobes and facultative anaerobes. Optimum temperature is 37ºC and optimum pH 7.4. It has fastidious (complex) growth requirements and grows only on enriched media. Growth is better in the presence of 5–10% CO_2.

On blood agar, upon overnight incubation, the colonies are small, glistening and dome shaped with an area of greenish discoloration (**alpha hemolysis**) around them. On prolonged incubation, the colonies become flat with central depression (umbonation) and raised edges, so that concentric rings are seen on the surface giving a carrom coin or **draughtsman appearance**. Under anaerobic conditions, colonies may show beta hemolysis due to oxygen labile hemolysins 'O'.

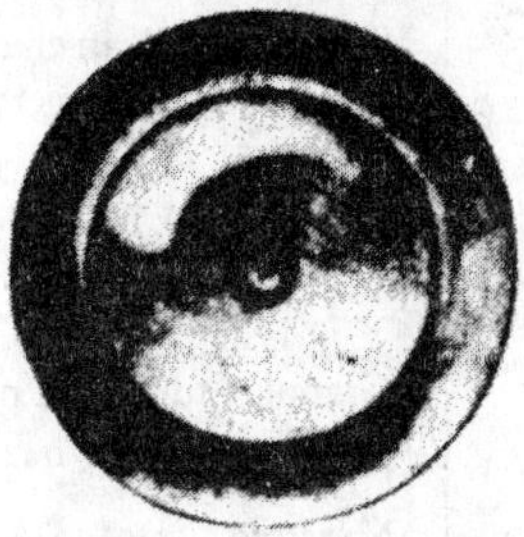

(*a*) View from above to show concentric rings.

(*b*) Side view.

Fig. 40.3 Draughtsman appearance of pneumococcus colonies.

Some strains form large, mucoid colonies because of the production of abundant capsular material. The cocci readily undergo autolysis in cultures due to the activity of intracellular enzymes. Heat killed cultures do not undergo autolysis. Transformation is frequent among pneumococci. On repeated sub-cultures, S → R variation occurs.

Fermentation is tested in Hiss's serum water or serum agar slopes.

Resistance

Pneumococci are delicate organisms and readily killed by heat at 55°C in 10 min and antiseptics. In cultures, they die on prolonged incubation. Strains may be maintained on blood agar or preferably by lyophilisation.

Bile Solubility Test

Pneumococci are bile soluble. When a few drops of 10% sodium deoxycholate solution are added to 1 ml of an overnight broth culture, the culture clears due to the lysis of cocci. Alternatively, when a loopful of 10% deoxycholate solution is placed on a pneumococcal colony on blood agar the colony lyses within a few minutes. The test should be carried out at neutral pH using deoxycholate and live young culture in saline suspension.

The test is of diagnostic importance and used to differentiate pneumococci from streptococci. The test is based on the presence of an autolytic amidase in the pneumococci that cleaves the bond between alanine and muramic acid in the peptidoglycan. The amidase is activated by surface active agents such as bile or bile salts, resulting in the lysis of organisms.

Optochin Sensitivity

The sensitivity of pneumococci to optochin (ethyl hydrocuprcin) is useful in differentiating them from streptococci. When an optochin disc is applied on blood agar plate inoculated with pneumococci, a wide zone of inhibition appears on incubation.

Table 40.1 Differences between Streptococci and Pneumococci

	Pneumococcus	*Str. viridans*
1. Morphology	Lanceolate diplococci, capsulated	Spherical cells in chains, non-capsulated
2. Quellung test	Positive	Negative
3. Colonies	Initially dome shaped, later 'draughtsman' colonies	Dome shaped
4. Growth in liquid media	Uniform turbidity	Granular turbidity, powdery deposit
5. Bile solubility	Positive	Negative
6. Inulin fermentation	Positive	Negative
7. Optochin sensitivity	Positive	Negative
8. Intraperitoneal inoccu-lation in mice	Fatal infection	Non-pathogenic

Epidemiology

Pneumococci are obligate human parasites, and found in the nasopharynx of many healthy individuals. Pneumococcal infections can be either exogenous or endogenous. In exogenous infections, the organisms are transmitted from one to another by fingers or by inhalation of contaminated droplets or droplet nuclei. The dissemination is facilitated by overcrowding. Endogenous infection involves the spread of pneumococci from nasopharynx to lungs or brain. The predisposing conditions are general debilitation caused by malnutrition or alcoholism, viral respiratory diseases, immunodeficiency and patients with sickle cell anemia or those who have had their spleens removed.

Pathogenicity

Pneumococci colonizes nasopharynx of 5–10% normal adults and 20 to 40% children. Infection spreads by air-borne droplets. Mode of transmission is by inhalation.

Virulence factors

1. ***Capsule*** — The pneumococcal polysaccharide capsule is both antiphagocytic and antigenic. Antibodies to it are opsonic. The capsule inhibits phagocytosis, facilitating the growth of bacteria prior to the appearance of anticapsular antibodies.

2. ***Autolysin*** — This peptidoglycan hydrolase, present in the bacterial cell wall is normally inactive. However, it is readily triggered (by surface active agents, beta lactam antibiotics or aging), resulting in cell lysis, releasing intracellular virulence factors such as pneumolysin.

3. ***Pneumolysin*** — Once released, it attacks mammalian cell membranes causing lysis.

4. Cell wall components such as teichoic acid and peptidoglycan fragments causes tissue destruction by activating alternative complement pathway.

5. Pneumococci produce IgA proteases, H_2O_2, pneumolysin and a protein adhesin.

Clinical Syndromes

1. ***Acute pneumococcal pneumonia*** — It is rarely a primary infection and results only when the normal defence barriers of the respiratory tract are disturbed. Chilling, general anaesthesia, convulsions,

cerebrovascular accidents, epilepsy, morphine, alcoholic intoxication and head injury predispose to pneumococcal pneumonia. These factors impair epiglottal reflex, mucociliary escalator and cough reflex, thus facilitating aspiration of pneumococci in the infected secretions from the nasopharynx to lower respiratory tract. A prior virus infection (*e.g.*, Influenza) causing increased volume and viscocity of bronchial secretions, and inhibition of the action of the bronchial cilia is a major contributory cause of penumococcal pneumonia. Pneumococci present in the nasopharynx proliferate in the viral-modified environment and are carried down into the alveoli by the thin bronchial secretions. Aspiration of small quantities of oropharyngeal secretions can also be demonstrated in healthy individuals during sleep.

Other predisposing conditions of acute pneumococcal pneumonia are congestive heart failure, diabetes mellitus, chronic renal failure, cirrhosis of liver, hypogammaglobulinemia, multiple myeloma and HIV infection.

In adults, most of the pneumococcal infections are caused by serotypes 1–8 and 18. In children, commonest prevalent types are 6, 14, 19 and 23. The pneumonia may be either lobar pneumonia or bronchopneumonia. Lobar pneumonia is exclusively a disease of the age group 10–50 years, whereas bronchopneumonia is characteristically a disease of young children and older adults over 50 years. Other pneumococcal lesions are acute bronchitis and sinusitis.

2. ***Otitis media*** — The most common bacterial infection of children, characterized by ear ache is most frequently caused by pneumococcus, followed by *Haemophilus influenzae* and *Moraxella catarrhalis*.

3. ***Bacteremia/sepsis*** — In the absence of a focus of infection it is commonly due to pneumococcus, especially in splenectomized individuals.

4. ***Pneumococcal meningitis*** — Pneumococcus is the second most important cause of pyogenic meningitis next to meningococci. It is most common and serious in children. It occurs as a complication of lobar pneumonia or otitis media. Pneumococci may spread from pharynix through blood stream (bacteremia) or follwing head trauma and dural tear, particularly with CSF leak.

5. Pneumococci also produces suppurative lesions such as empyema, pericarditis, conjunctivitis, septic arthritis, peritonitis, endocarditis and osteomyelitis.

Laboratory Diagnosis

Specimens collected are nasopharyngeal swabs, blood, pus, sputum, pleural exudate and CSF.

Microscopy — (*i*) The demonstration of lanceolate shaped Gram positive diplococci with plenty of pus cells in Gram stained smear establishes the diagnosis.

(*ii*) Pneumococcal capsules can be demonstrated by quelling reaction and negative staining.

Culture — The specimen is inoculated on to blood agar plates with an optochin disc and incubated overnight at 37ºC in the presence of CO_2 (in a candle jar). Alpha hemolytic colonies that are sensitive to optochin are presumptively identified as pneumococcus. Bile solubility test is done for further identification and serotyping is done by mixing with appropriate antisera. Blood cultures in glucose broth are also useful.

Demonstration of antigen — Pneumococcal capsular polysaccharide antigen in serum or CSF can be detected by latex agglutination, coagglutination, counterimmunoelectrophoresis and ELISA.

Animal pathogenicity test — Specimens or the isolates may be injected intraperitoneally into mice and the animal develops a fatal pneumonia and dies within one to three days. Pneumococci may be demonstrated in the peritoneal exudate and heart blood.

Demonstration of antibodies — Antibodies in patient's serum can be demonstrated by agglutination, precipitation, mouse protection tests and bactericidal tests with the whole blood. Indirect hemagglutination, indirect fluorescent-antibody test and RIA are also employed.

C-Reactive Protein

It is an abnormal protein (beta globulin) that precipitates with the somatic "C" antigen of pneumococci, appears in acute phase sera of cases of pneumonia but disappears during convalescence. It also occurs in some other pathological conditions. It is an antibody produced as a result of pneumococcal infection.

It is an **acute phase substance** produced in hepatocytes. Its production is stimulated by bacterial infections, inflammation, malignancies and tissue destruction. It disappears when inflammatory reactions subside. The CRP is used as an index of response to treatment in rheumatic fever and certain other conditions. The CRP is tested by capillary precipitation of the patient's sera with antisera prepared in rabbits against purified CRP, or by passive agglutination using latex particles coated with anti-CRP antibody.

Prophylaxis

A polyvalent antipneumococcal capsular polysaccharide vaccine that immunizes against 23 serotypes of *Streptococcus pneumoniae* is indicated for the protection of high-risk individuals such as asplenic, sickle cell anemic individuals with renal failure, nephrotic syndrome, chronic heart or lung diseases, immunodeficiency, immunosuppression and diabetes mellitus, over two years of age. The vaccine should always be given before splenectomy or starting an immunosuppressive therapy. Immunity persists for about five years and revaccination is required every 3–5 years. Response to vaccine is poor in children below the age of two and immunosuppressed or immunodeficient patients. This vaccine protects against the pneumococcal strains responsible for 85 to 90 per cent of infections, including penicillin-resistant strains.

The heptavalent pneumococcal conjugate vaccine (PCV-7), effective in young children, is made up of seven pneumococcal antigens conjugated to CRM197 — a mutant nontoxic diphtheria toxin. Three doses of vaccine are given at two, four and six months of age. The PCV-7 provides serotype and serogroup cross protection.

Treatment and Drug Resistance

Penicillin G or amoxycillin is the drug of choice. But strains with intermediate and high level of resistance to penicillin are increasing in many parts of the world. They do not form penicillinase. The resistance is chromosome mediated and may be due to the changes in the penicillin-binding proteins (PBPs) in the cell wall.

Highly penicillin resistant strains are usually also resistant to chloramphenicol, tetracycline and trimethoprim-sulphamethoxazole. A third generation cephalosporins are effective in intermediate penicillin resistant strains, but may not be effective against highly penicillin-resistant strains.

Vancomycin or rifampicin has to be combined with a third generation cephalosporins in severe infections with highly penicillin-resistant strains.

CAUSATIVE AGENTS OF TYPICAL PNEUMONIA

(*i*) *Streptococcus pneumoniae*

(*ii*) *Haemophilus influenzae*

(*iii*) *Staphylococcus aureus*

(*iv*) Influenza virus types A and B

(*v*) Parainfluenza viruses

(*vi*) Respiratory syncytial viruses.

QUESTIONS

Essay Type Questions

1. Describe the morphology, cultural characters, pathogenicity and lab. diagnosis of pneumococci.

Short Answer Type Questions

1. Morphology of *Streptococcus pneumoniae.*
2. Negative staining.
3. Quellung reaction.
4. Bile solubility test.
5. Optochin sensitivity.
6. Differences between streptococci and pneumococci.
7. Pneumococcal pneumonia.
8. Laboratory diagnosis of pneumococcal infections.
9. Prophylaxis of pneumococcal infections.
10. C-reactive protein.
11. Drug resistant *Str. pneumoniae*.
12. List out the causative agents of typical pneumonia.

41

Gonococci (Neisseria gonorrhoeae)

INTRODUCTION

The genus *Neisseria* consists of Gram negative aerobic cocci. Two *Neisseria* species are pathogenic for humans—*Neisseria gonorrhoeae* (commonly called gonococcus), the causal agent of gonorrhea; and *Neisseria meningitidis* (commonly called meningococcus), a frequent cause of meningitis.

Morphology

Gonococci are **Gram negative diplococci**. The cocci are typically kidney or bean seed shaped with the adjacent sides being concave. They are intracellular parasites, abundantly found in neutrophils (pus cells). Gonococci possess pili on their surface which act as virulence factor and help in their adhesion to mucosal surfaces.

Piliated gonococci can agglutinate human RBC, but not RBC from other mammals. This hemagglutination is not inhibited by mannose.

Based on the specificity of "Por" protein, gonococci are classified into 16 serotypes by coagglutination tests. Nutritionally, gonococci are classified into several auxotypes.

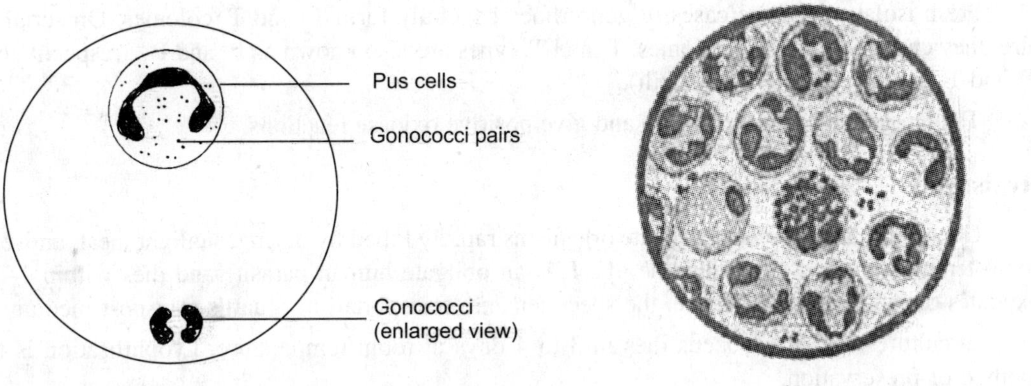

(a) (b)

Fig. 41.1 Gonococci in urethral pus

Cultural characteristics

They are aerobic but may grow anaerobically also. Growth occurs best at pH 7.2–7.6 and at a temperature of 35–36ºC.

Gonococci are difficult to grow than meningococci. They have fastidious growth requirements and grows best on enriched media containing substances such as heated blood, hemin and animal proteins, preferably in the presence of 5 to 10 per cent CO_2, provided by incubating inside a candle jar.

The media used for cultivation are:

Enriched media — Chocolate agar,
Mueller-Hinton agar,
Chacko-Nair egg medium.

Selective medium — **Thayer-Martin medium** (chocolate agar containing vancomycin, colistin and nystatin).

The colonies are small, round translucent, glistening, elevated, convex or slightly umbonate, with finely granular surface and lobate margins. They are soft and easily emulsifiable.

Based on colony morphology, autoagglutinability and virulence, gonococci are divided into four types – T_1 to T_4. Types 1 and 2 form small brown colonies. The cocci are fimbriated, autoagglutinable and virulent. Types 3 and 4 form larger, granular, nonpigmented colonies. Cocci are nonfimbriated, autoagglutinable and avirulent.

Table 41.1 Differences between meningococci and gonococci

meningococci	*gonococci*
1. Ferments glucose and maltose	Ferments glucose only
2. Diplococci – cocci are oval shaped; opposite ends are flat	Diplococci – cocci are kidney shaped; opposite ends are concave
3. Causes meningitis and septicemia	Causes gonorrhoea, arthritis, conjunctivits
4. Septicemia is common	Septicemia is rare

Fresh isolates of acute cases of gonorrhoea generally form T_1 and T_2 colonies. On serial subculture, they change to T_3 or T_4 colonies. T_1 and T_2 types are also known as P^+ and P^{++}, respectively, while T_3 and T_4 are known as P^- (P for pili).

The neisseriae produce oxidase and give positive oxidase reactions.

Resistance

Gonococci are extremely delicate organisms rapidly killed by drying, sunlight, heat, antiseptics, at room temperature and at an alkaline pH. It is an obligate human parasite and dies within 1–2 hrs in exudates outside the body. Hence, the specimens are transported in Stuart's transpost medium.

In cultures, the gonococcus dies in 3 to 4 days at room temperature. Lyophilisation is the best method of preservation.

Virulence factors

(*i*) ***Pili*** — They enhance attachment of the organism to host epithelial and mucosal cell surfaces, and confer resistance to phagocytosis. Gene conversion and phase variation are two mechanisms by which the gonococcus can avoid the host's immune response, and thereby cause repeated infections in the same individual.

(*ii*) ***Outer Membrane Proteins (OMPs)*** — OMP I functions as a porin in complex with OMP III, also known as Reduction modifiable protein (Rmp). OMP II is referred to as opacity associated protein (Opa), because its presence renders gonococcal colonies less translucent. OMP II, along with the pili, mediates attachment of the organism to a host cell.

(*iii*) ***Lipooligosaccharide (LOS)*** — It is different from lipopolysaccharide (LPS) of Gram negative bacilli only in lacking O-antigenic side chain. The bactericidal antibodies in normal human serum are IgM molecules directed against the LOS antigens.

(*iv*) ***Other Proteins*** — Other proteins such as Lip (H8), Fbp (iron-binding protein) and IgA1 protease may contribute to virulence.

Epidemiology

Gonorrhoea is an exclusively human disease. A higher proportion of females than males are generally asymptomatic and act as reservoirs for maintaining and transmitting gonococcal infections. The mode of transmission is exclusively venereal.

Pathogenicity

Gonococci are obligate human pathogens. It causes gonorrhoea, a venereal disease transmitted by sexual contact. Gonococci adhere to the epithelial cells of urethra or cervix with the help of pili and outer membrane proteins and multiply. Adhesion is rapid and firm so that micturition cannot flushout organisms from urethra. Incubation period is usually about 2 days, but can be 1–10 days. Most of the female cases are asymptomatic, inspite of active infection in the cervix.

Clinical features in males —

(*i*) **Urethritis** with a yellow mucopurulent discharge containing gonococci in large numbers with painful urination and dysuria is seen among males.

(*ii*) Proctitis (rectal gonorrhoea) prevalent in male homosexuals, is characterized by constipation, painful defecation and purulent discharge.

(*iii*) Pharyngitis is contracted by oral-genital contact. Infected individuals may show a purulent exudate, and the condition may mimic and mild viral or a streptococcal sore throat.

(*iv*) Prostatitis and epididymitis.

(*v*) Bacteremia may occur which leads to fever, erythematous or maculopapular lesions on the skin, painful and purulent arthritis, endocarditis, meningitis which together constitute "Disseminated gonococcal infection (DGI)".

(*vi*) Conjunctivitis due to self-inoculation by fingers.

Clinical features in females —

(*i*) The infection occurs in the endocervix and extends to the urethra and vagina. A greenish-yellow cervical discharge is most common, often accompanied by intermenstrual bleeding.

(*ii*) The disease may progress to the uterus, causing inflammation of fallopian tubes (salpingitis), ovary and pelvic tissues, known as **pelvic inflammatory disease (PID)**. The long term sequelae of PID include fibrosis (tubal scarring) so that infertility or ectopic pregnancy may result.

(*iii*) Proctitis (rectal gonorrhoea) due to anal sex.

(*iv*) Pharyngitis due to oral sex.

(*v*) Bartholinitis (abscesses in bartholin glands).

(*vi*) Bacteremia may occur which leads to fever, erythematous or maculopapular lesions on the skin, septic arthritis, endocarditis, meningitis, which together constitute "Disseminated gonoccoal infection (DGI)".

(*vii*) Conjunctivitis due to self-inoculation by fingers.

Ophthalmia neonatorum is an infection of the conjunctival sac that is acquired by a newborn during passage through the birth canal of a mother infected with gonococcus. If untreated, acute conjunctivitis may lead to blindness. For many years, routine prevention was performed immediately after birth by the instillation of a dilute solution of silver nitrate into the eye. Today, clinicians prefer the use of erythromycin in place of silver nitrate, because the antibiotic also eradicates *Chlamydia trachomatis*, if present.

Laboratory Diagnosis

Specimens collected are urethral discharge, cervical swabs, pus, secretions from urethra, cervix etc. Specimens may be collected by charcoal-coated swabs and transported immediately to laboratory in Stuart's transport medium.

Microscopy — In the male, the finding of numerous neutrophils containing Gram negative diplococci in a Gram stained smear of urethral exudate permits a provisional diagnosis of gonococcal infection, and indicates that the individual should be treated. But this finding is unreliable in females as normal genital flora may have similar morphology. For microscopic examination, fluorescent antibody techniques are more sensitive and specific.

Cultutre — To diagnose gonococcal infection in the female, or at other sites in the male, a positive culture is needed. If disseminated gonococcal infection is suspected, appropriate cultures should be set up as indicated, for example, of skin lesions, joint fluid and blood.

The specimens are plated on to **Thayer-Martin medium** and incubated at 35–36°C, in the presence of 5–10% CO_2 (in candle jar) for 1–2 days. The culture is confirmed as gonococcal by Gram's staining, sugar fermentation tests and specific fluorescent antibody tests.

Blood cultures should be done from suspected cases of arthritis, PID and skin manifestations of disseminated gonococcal disease.

Serology — Specific antibodies in patient's serum can be detected by CFT, passive agglutination, RIA and ELISA. Serum and genital fluid contain IgG and IgA antibodies against gonococcal pili, outer membrane proteins and LPS.

Molecular methods — Ligase chain reaction (LCR) is highly sensitive and specific nucleic acid based detection test using urine samples.

Treatment

Many strains of gonococci are resistant to penicillin, tetracycline, and spectinomycin. Penicillin-resistant organisms are called PPNG — penicillinase producing *Neisseria gonorrhoeae*. These strains contain plasmids that carry the gene for betalactamase.

However, gonococci are sensitive to several antibiotics such as ceftriaxone, ciprofloxacin, ofloxacin or azithromycin and are used in the treatment of gonococcal infections.

Prophylaxis

Prevention of gonorrhoea consists of early detection and treatment of cases and contacts, health education, safe sex and use of physical barriers, and by applying erythromycin ointment or silver nitrate for conjunctivitis.

NON-GONOCOCCAL URETHRITIS/NON-SPECIFIC URETHRITIS

Chronic urethritis caused by organisms other than gonococci is called non-gonococcal or non-specific uretheritis. In some of these, urethritis forms part of a syndrome consisting of conjunctivitis and arthritis (Reiter's syndrome). Some of these cases may be due to gonococcal infection, the cocci persisting as L-forms and hence undetectable by routine tests. The majority of cases are, however, caused several organisms such as *Chlamydia trachomatis*, *Ureaplasma urealyticum*, *Mycoplasma hominis*, *Gardnerella vaginalis*, *Acinetobacter*, herpes virus, cytomegalovirus, *Candida albicans*, *Trichomonas vaginalis* or even by mechanical or chemical irritation.

COMMENSAL NEISSERIAE

Several species of *Neisseria* constitute the normal flora of respiratory tract, particularly nasopharynx. They are *Neisseria sicca*, *N. subflava*, *N. cinera*, *N. mucosa* and *N. flavescens*. They have been reported occasionally as having caused meningitis.

N. lactamica, frequently found in nasopharynx is closely related to meningococci, but avirulent. It ferments lactose, unlike other Neisseriae and differs from pathogenic neisseriae in being positive in the ONPG test for beta galactosidase. Nasopharyngeal colonization by *N. lactamica* in young children may induce antibodies protective against meningococcal infections.

N. cinera sometimes resembles *N. gonorrhoeae* in sugar fermentation patterns.

QUESTIONS

Short Essay Type Questions

1. Describe the morphology, cultural characteristics, pathogenicity and lab. diagnosis of *Neisseria gonorrhoeae*.

Short Answer Type Questions

1. Morphology of *N. gonorrhoeae.*
2. Cultivation of gonococci.
3. Differences between meningococci and gonococci.
4. Virulence factors of gonococci.
5. Pathogenicity of *N. gonorrhoeae.*
6. Lab. diagnosis of gonorrhoea.
7. Lab. diagnosis of gonorrhoea in a male patient.
8. Non-gonococcal urethritis (or) Non-specific urethritis.
9. Commensal *Neisseria*.

42

Meningococci (Neisseria meningitidis)

- *Morphology*
- *Cultural characteristics*
- *Biochemical properties*
- *Antigenic classification*
- *Resistance*
- *Epidemiology*
- *Virulence factors*
- *Pathogenicity*
- *Laboratory diagnosis*
- *Treatment*
- *Prophylaxis*

Morphology

Meningococci are **Gram negative intracellular diplococci**. The cocci are oval or spherical with adjacent sides flattened. The long axis of the coccus is at right angles to a line joining the two cocci in a pair. They are nonmotile and possess pili. They are typically seen in large numbers inside neutrophils. When meningococcus is isolated from blood or spinal fluid it is invariably encapsulated. The capsule is made of polysaccharide that can be demonstrated by quellung reaction. The characteristics of capsule are as follows:

(*i*) It is antiphagocytic thereby enhances virulence

(*ii*) It is the antigen detected in the CSF of meningitis patients

(*iii*) It is the antigen that defines the serogroups

(*iv*) It is the antigen in the vaccine.

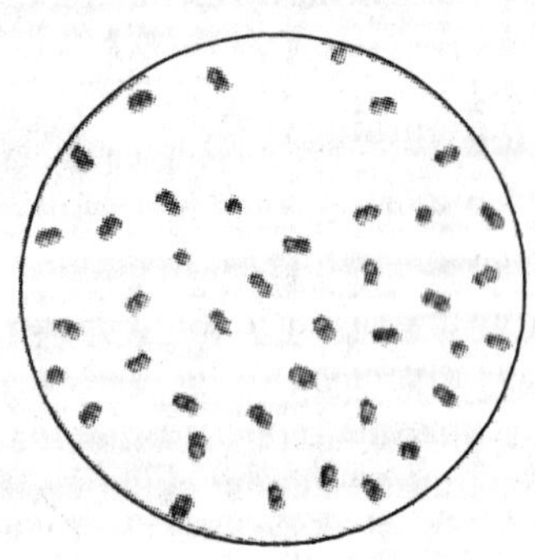

Fig. 42.1 *Neisseria meningitidis*

Cultural characteristics

It is an obligate aerobe. The optimum temperature for growth is 37ºC and optimum pH 7.4–7.6. Growth is best in the presence of 5–10% CO_2, provided by incubating in a candle jar.

Meningococci have fastidious growth requirements and do not grow on ordinary media. Growth occurs on media enriched with blood, serum or ascitic fluid. These substances are believed to promote growth by neutralizing certain inhibitory substances found in culture media rather than by providing additional nutrients. However, they grow well on trypticase-soy agar and Muller-Hinton agar medium without the addition of blood or serum.

On solid media, after 24 hours incubation, the colonies are small, translucent, round, convex, bluish-grey, with a smooth glistening surface and with entire edges. The colonies are typically lenticular in shape, butyrous in consistency and easily emulsifiable. Weak hemolysis occurs on blood agar. On chocolate agar the colonies are slightly larger than on blood agar. Modified Thayer-Martin medium (with antibiotics vancomycin, colistin, amphotericin) is a useful selective medium, particularly for samples obtained from a skin lesion or nasopharyngeal swab, in order to eliminate contaminating organisms.

Growth is poor in liquid media, producing a granular turbidity with little or no surface growth.

Biochemical Reactions

Meningococci are catalase and oxidase positive. Meningococci utilize glucose and maltose by oxidative method with the production of acid but no gas. They do not attack sucrose or lactose. Indole and H_2S are not produced and nitrates are not reduced.

Resistance

Meningococci are very delicate organisms. In cultures they die out in a few days. They are killed by heating at 55ºC in 5 minutes or less. They are highly susceptible to heat, desiccation, alterations in pH and to disinfectants.

Antigenic Classification

Meningococci are classified into 13 serogroups, based on their capsular polysaccharide antigens. Most infections are due to serogroups A, B, C, W and Y, although approximately ninety per cent of cases of meningococcal disease are caused by serogroups A, B and C. Serogroup A is usually responsible for massive epidemics in developing countries. Groups W-135 and Y also frequently cause meningitis. Groups X, Z and 29E are only rarely associated with some form of immune deficiency. Serogroups H, I, K and L have been isolated from carriers and have not been associated with disease. Organisms that do not have a capsule are called "ungrouped".

Based on outer membrane proteins (OMPs) and lipo-oligosaccharides (LOS), meningococci are classified into 20 (1, 2, 3 ...) serotypes.

Epidemiology

Meningococci are normally present in the human nasopharynx (asymptomatic carriers). The carriage rate is highest in children, institutions such as schools and military camps and in places of overcrowding. Transmission occurs through inhalation of respiratory droplets from a carrier or a patient in the early stages of the disease. In addition to contact with a carrier, risk factors include recent viral or mycoplasmal upper respiratory tract infection, active or passive smoking and complement deficiency. The transmission rate among family members of an infected individual is thousand-fold higher than in the general population.

Virulence Factors

(*i*) Capsular polysaccharide aid in the maintenance of infection by inhibiting phagocytosis.

(*ii*) Pili allow attachment of the organism to the nasopharyngeal mucosa where it is harbored both in carriers and in those with meningococcal disease.

(*iii*) Endotoxins or lipopolysaccharides released during autolysis and bacterial cell division are responsible for many of the toxic effects found in disseminated meningococcal disease.

(*iv*) Meningococci make an IgA protease, that cleaves IgA_1, and thus helps the pathogens to evade immunoglobulins of this class. (The non pathogenic neisseriae do not make this IgA protease).

(*v*) Outer membrane proteins (OMPs) help in the attachment to the host cell.

Pathogenicity

Meningococci initially colonizes the nasopharynx, resulting in a largely asymptomatic meningococcal pharyngitis. In young children and other susceptible individuals, the organism can cause disseminated disease by spreading through the blood, leading to meningitis and/or fulminating septicemia. Deficiency of C6–C9 components favors meningococcal disease.

Meningococci penetrate the epithelial lining of nasopharynx, and enter the blood stream where they rapidly multiply (meningococcemia). Meningococci can cause a life-threatening septicemia in a healthy individual in less than twelve hours. In patients with fulminating septicemia, meningococci can be detected in blood smears — an unusual occurrence. Up to thirty per cent of patients with meningitis go on to fulminant septicemia. In this condition, the clinical presentation is one of severe septicemia and shock for which the bacterial endotoxin is largely responsible. If not severe, the patient may have only a fever and other nonspecific symptoms.

An acute fulminating meningococcal septicemia seen mainly in very young children is referred to as **Waterhouse-Friderichsen syndrome.** It is characterized by large, blotchy skin hemorrhages, vomiting and diarrhea, circulatory collapse, necrosis of the adrenals and death within ten to twelve hours.

The organism can seed from the blood to other sites. It crosses blood-brain barrier and infect the meninges. There they multiply and induce an acute inflammatory response, accompanied by an influx of neutrophils, resulting in a **purulent meningitis** or **pyogenic meningitis.** Joint symptoms are also commonly seen in meningococcal infections, and a petechial rash is commonly observed. Within several hours, the initial fever and malaise can evolve into severe headache, a rigid neck, vomiting and sensitivity to bright lights—symptoms characteristic of meningitis. Coma can occur within a few hours. Meningococci may also spread along the perineural sheath of the olfactory nerve, through the cribriform plate to the subarachnoid space and cause meningitis.

Laboratory diagnosis

Specimens collected may include CSF, blood, aspirates from skin lesions, pus from infected joint and throat, nasopharyngeal swabs. Swabs should be transported in **stuart's transport medium**. All specimens should be transported immediately to the laboratory.

Examination of CSF — The CSF fluid will be under pressure and turbid. For bacteriological examination, the CSF is divided into three portions.

One portion of CSF is centrifuged and Gram's stained smears are prepared from the sediment. Meningococci will be seen intracellularly inside the polymorphs but often extracellularly also. This presumptive diagnosis is sufficient to start antibiotic treatment. The supernatant will contain meningococcal antigens, which may be demonstrated by latex agglutination or counter immunoelectrophoresis using meningococcal antisera. Antigen detection is particularly useful in partially treated patients in whom smear and culture tests may be negative.

The second portion of the CSF is inoculated on blood agar or chocolate agar plates and incubated at 35–36ºC, under 5 to 10% CO_2. Colonies appear after 18–24 hrs and may be identified by morphology and biochemical reactions. The isolated meningococcus strains may be grouped by using appropriate antisera.

The third portion of CSF is incubated overnight, either as it is or after adding an equal volume of glucose broth and then subcultured on chocolate agar. This method may succeed where direct plating fails.

Blood culture — In meningococcemia and in early cases of meningitis, blood culture is often positive. Cultures should be incubated for 4–7 days, with daily subcultures. Meningococcal antigens can be found in the blood in active disease.

Nasopharyngeal swabs — Demonstration of meningococci in the nasopharynx helps in the detection of carriers. Sampling should be done without contamination with saliva.

Aspirates from skin lesions — Meningococci may sometimes be demonstrated in petechial lesions by microscopy and culture.

Serology — Specific antibodies in patient's serum may be demonstrated.

Treatment

Penicillin G or ampicillin are the drugs of choice given intravenously, both of which can pass through inflamed blood-brain barrier. Chloramphenicol is equally effective. One of the later cephalosporins ceftriaxone or ceftazidime or cefotaxime are now preferred.

Prophylaxis

Chemoprophylaxis–Rifampin is usually used to treat family members of an infected individual. The drug is efficiently secreted into saliva, (in contrast to penicillin G) and effective in eliminating the carrier state.

Immunization — The meningococcal vaccine containing group specific polysaccharide capsule of A, C, Y and W-135 strains is used for reducing the carrier state and also to prevent epidemics of meningitis especially in military personnel or during an outbreak in civilian population. The vaccine does not contain the group B capsular polysaccharide, which is poorly immunogenic in humans.

QUESTIONS

Essay Type Questions

1. Describe the morphology, pathogenicity and lab. diagnosis of meningococcal meningitis.
2. Enumerate the causative agents of pyogenic or purulent meningitis. Describe the lab. diagnosis of pyogenic meningitis.

Short Answer Type Questions

1. Morphology of *Neisseria meningitidis.*
2. Cultivation of meningococci.
3. Pathogenicity of meningococci.
4. Lab. diagnosis of pyogenic meningitis.

43

Moraxella, Acinetobacter and Kingella

Moraxella

Members of the genus *Moraxella* are nonmotile, Gram negative coccobacilli that are generally found in pairs. They are related to the neisseriae, and the two organisms can be confused on Gram stain (Fig. 1). Moraxella are aerobic, oxidase-positive, fastidious organisms that do not ferment carbohydrates. The genus *Moraxella* includes a variety of organisms that are part of the normal human flora, particularly the respiratory and genital tracts. Disease most commonly occurs in immunocompromised hosts.

Moraxellae can be differentiated from Neisseriae by the following characteristics.

(*i*) Moraxellae cannot grow on the selective media used to isolate pathogenic neisseriae.

(*ii*) Moraxellae can grow on ordinary media such as nutrient agar and MacConkey agar, whereas neisseriae cannot.

(*iii*) *Moraxella* cannot ferment carbohydrates.

(*iv*) *Moraxella* hydrolyzes butyrate.

M. Catarrhalis

The most important pathogen in the genus *Moraxella* is *Moraxella catarrhalis*, which was previously classified as *Neisseria catarrhalis* and then as *Branhamella catarrhalis*. It is a commensal in the upper respiratory tract and female genital tract. It may cause primary infection in the pediatric age group. It can cause opportunistic infections of respiratory system (trachitis, laryngitis, pneumonia), middle ear (otitis media), eye (keratitis, ophthalmia neonatorum), CNS (meningitis), joints (septic arthritis) and endocarditis in immunocompromised hosts and hospitalized patients.

These organisms can be cultured on blood agar or chocolate agar and identified by a battery of biochemical tests. Treatment depends on clinical presentation and results of sensitivity testing. Most strains are resistant to penicillin due to the production of betalactamase. They are sensitive to cephalosporins, chloramphenicol, tetracycline and aminoglycosides.

Acinetobacter

Members of the genus *Acinetobacter* are nonmotile, Gram negative coccobacilli that are frequently confused with neisseriae under Gram stain. They look like Gram negative diplococci and mimic

Neisseriae, hence named as "Mimeae". They are generally encapsulated, oxidase negative, obligately aerobic and do not ferment carbohydrates.

Acinetobacter are widely distributed in nature and are commonly found in soil, water, food stuff, on fomites, and as part of the normal flora of humans and other animals, particularly on the skin and in pharynx. They can cause a similar range of opportunistic infections as caused by enteric Gram negative bacilli. They are capable of infecting virtually any body site, organ system or tissue in immunocompromised hosts. They have been responsible for meningitis, septicemia, urinary, genital, respiratory and wound infections. They are important opportunistic pathogens causing nosocomial infections, particularly iatrogenic meningitis.

The organisms may be cultured on a variety of laboratory media and frequently resistant to a variety of antibiotics. The treatment of choice depends on clinical presentation and the results of antibiotic sensitivity testing.

Kingella

Kingella species are plump, Gram negative, nonmotile bacilli or coccobacilli occurring in pairs or short chains. They produce β-hemolysis on blood agar. They constitute the normal flora of oropharynx. *K. kingae* has been reported to cause endocarditis and infections of bones, joints and tendons. *K. denitrificans* has been reported from endocarditis, septicemia and abscesses. They are oxidase positive and unlike *Neisseria* and *Moraxella* species, catalase positive.

QUESTIONS

Short Answer Type Questions

1. *Moraxella catarrhalis.*
2. *Acinetobacter.*
3. *Kingella.*

44

Diphtheria bacilli (Corynebacterium diphtheriae)

– Introduction	*– Schick test*
– Morphology	*– Corynebacterium ulcerans*
– Cultural characteristics	*– C. pseudotuberculosis*
– Biochemical reactions	*– C. minutissimum*
– Resistance	*– C. jeikeium*
– Epidemiology	*– C. xerosis*
– Pathogenicity	*– C. pseudodiphtheriticum,*
– Diphtheria toxin	*– C. bovis*
– Laboratory diagnosis	*– Diphtheroids*
– Treatment	*– Arcanobacterium hemolyticum*
– Prophylaxis	

Introduction

Corynebacterium is a large genus of diverse habitat. The genus includes *Corynebacterium diphtheriae*, the cause of the prototypic toxin-mediated disease, diphtheria, as well as several usually harmless human commensals. The diphtheria bacillus was first observed and described by Klebs (1883) but was first cultivated by Loeffler (1884), hence known as Klebs-Loeffler bacillus.

Morphology

Corynebacteria are small, slender, pleomorphic, Gram positive bacilli that tend to stain unevenly but do not form spores. They frequently show club shaped swellings and hence the name corynebacteria (from coryne, meaning club). The bacilli are pleomorphic, and measure approximately 3–6 μm × 0.6–0.8 μm. They are nonmotile and noncapsulated.

They occur in characteristic clumps that look like Chinese characters or picket fence patterns presumably created by the snapping motion with which the cells complete their division. The bacilli in smears, appear in pairs, pallisades (parallel rows of 3–4 bacilli) or small groups, the bacilli being at various angles to each other, resembling the letters V or L. This has been called **Chinese letter pattern** or **cuneiform arrangement.** This is due to the incomplete separation of the daughter cells after binary fission.

They contain bipolar bodies called as **metachromatic granules** or **volutin granules** or Babes-Ernst granules. The name volutin refers to *Spirillum volutans* in which these granules were first found. They appear reddish purple when stained with Loeffler's methylene blue (stain red with blue dye) and therefore called metachromatic granules. They are composed of polymetaphosphate and are considered to be reserve sources of energy. They can be demonstrated by special stains:

(*i*) Albert's stain — volutin granules appear bluish black and diphtheria bacilli light green

(*ii*) Neisser's stain — granules appear deep blue and bacilli pink color

(*iii*) Ponder's stain — granules appear dark blue and the bacilli pale blue color

(*iv*) Pugh's stain — granules take up reddish-purple color and the bacilli light blue

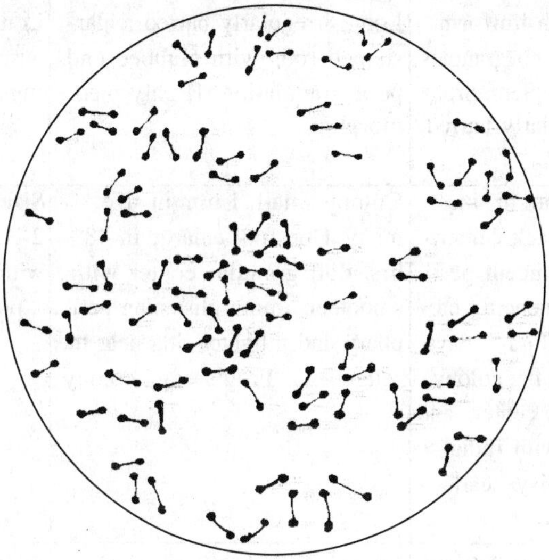

Fig. 44.1 *Corynebacterium diphtheriae* with volutin granules.

The presence of metachromatic granules in thin, slender bacilli helps to distinguish *Corynebacterium diphtheriae* from short, thick, plumpy nonpathogenic diphtheroids which lack granules. The granule formation is best seen on Loeffler's serum slope.

Cultural characteristics

C. diphtheriae is an aerobe and facultative anaerobe. Optimum temperature for growth is 37ºC and optimum pH 7.2–7.4. It can grow on ordinary media such as nutrient agar, but growth is best in the presence of blood, serum or egg.

Loeffler's serum slope and potassium tellurite blood agar are usually employed for the cultivation of diphtheria bacilli.

Diphtheria bacilli grow very rapidly on Loeffler's serum and colonies can be seen in 6–8 hours, long before other bacteria grow. The colonies are at first small, white, opaque discs but enlarge on continued incubation and may acquire a distinct yellow tint.

Potassium tellurite blood agar is a selective medium, devised by McLeod (hence McLeod's medium) with heated rabbit's blood and potassium tellurite (0.04%) and was called chocolate tellurite agar. Potassium tellurite acts as a selective agent inhibiting the growth of other organisms, particularly commensals of throat. Diphtheria bacilli reduce tellurite to metallic tellurium, which gets incorporated in the colonies giving them a black or grey color. The growth may be slow and colonies appear on two days of incubation.

Based on colony morphology on potassium tellurite blood agar, McLeod classified diphtheria bacilli into three **biotypes**: gravis, intermedius and mitis. The characteristics of these biotypes listed in Table 44.1.

Table 44.1 Characteristics of three biotypes of *C. diphtheriae*

	Gravis	*Intermedius*	*Mitis*
Morphology	Short rods, with uniform staining, few or no granules. Some degree of pleomorphism, with irregularly barred tear-drop forms.	Long, irregularly barred, cigar-shaped rods with clubbed ends, poor granulation. Highly pleomorphic.	Long, curved, pleomorphic, wispy rods with terminal swellings. Prominent granulation.
Colonies on tellurite blood agar after 18–24 hr incubation	Colony is 1–2 mm in size, with greyish black center, paler, semitranslucent periphery and commencing crenation of edge. In 2–3 days, 3–5 mm in size, flat colony with raised dark center and crenated edge with radial striation — "daisy head" colony.	Colony small, 1 mm in size, misty. Does not enlarge in 48 hrs, dull granular center with smoother, more glistening periphery and a lighter ring near the edge — "Frog's egg" colony.	Size variable, shiny black. In 2–3 days, colonies become flat, with a central elevation — "poached egg" colony.
Consistency of colonies	Like "cold margarine", brittle on the plate, not easily picked out or emulsifiable.	Intermediate between gravis and mitis.	Soft buttery, easily emulsifiable.
Hemolysis	Variable	Nonhemolytic	Beta hemolytic
Growth in broth	Surface pellicle, granular deposit, little or no turbidity	Turbidity in 24 hrs, clearing in 48 hrs, with fine granular sediment	Diffuse turbidity with soft pellicle later
Glycogen and starch fermentation	Positive	Negative	Negative
Phase types	14	3	4
Serotypes (based on agglutination)	13	4	40
Toxigenic strains	Almost 100%	95–99%	80–85%

Biochemical reactions

Diphtheria bacilli ferment glucose, galactose, maltose and dextrin with the production of acid, but no gas. Lactose, sucrose, mannitol are not fermented. Some virulent strains may ferment sucrose. Hiss's serum water is employed for testing fermentation. They are H_2S positive and reduces nitrates to nitrites. They cannot liquefy gelatin or hydrolyze urea.

Resistance

Diphtheria bacilli may be killed by heat 58°C for 10 min. It is easily destroyed by antiseptics. It is more resistant to light, desiccation and freezing than most nonsporing bacilli. It remains fully virulent in blankets and floor dust for five weeks.

Diphtheria toxin

All virulent strains of diphtheria bacilli produce a powerful exotoxin, known as diphtheria toxin. It is a heat labile protein and consists of two fragments A and B. The toxin is released in inactive form because the active site on fragment 'A' is masked. It is activated by proteases present in tissues or culture media. Diphtheria is caused by the local and systemic effects of a single exotoxin that inhibits eukaryotic protein synthesis.

Fragment B binds to susceptible cell membranes and mediates the delivery of fragment A to its target. Inside the cell, fragment A separates from fragment B, and catalyzes a reaction between nicotine adenine dinucleotide (NAD^+) and the eukaryotic polypeptide chain elongation factor (EF–2). The resulting ADP-ribosylation of EF–2 inactivates it and blocks the translocation of a polypeptidyl-tRNA from the acceptor site (A site) to the donor site (P site) on the ribosome.

$$\text{EF–2} + \text{NAD}^+ \xrightarrow[\text{fragment A}]{} \text{EF–2–ADP ribose} + \text{nicotinamide}$$

A single molecule of diphtheria toxin can inhibit all protein synthesis in a eukaryotic cell within hours of its introduction. Recent genetic studies have identified the cell receptor for diphtheria toxin as being identical to the receptor for a heparin–binding epidermal growth factor.

The structural gene for diphtheria toxin (tox) is encoded in the genome of a corynebacterial bacteriophage, beta phage. Only those strains of *C. diphtheriae* that are lysogenic for beta phage can produce toxin and are therefore virulent. The phage's tox gene is regulated by a host bacterium-encoded repressor, Dt_xR, which itself is repressed under conditions of limited iron. In other words, low intracellular concentrations of iron allow maximum expression of the tox gene.

The toxin can be converted into toxoid by prolonged storage, incubation at 37°C for 4–6 weeks, treatment with 0.2 to 0.4 per cent formalin or by acid pH. Toxoid is toxin that has lost its toxicity but not its antigenicity. The toxin is antigenic, and is capable of inducing antitoxin formation, with which it reacts specifically. The strain used for toxin production (as a source of diphtheria toxoid for vaccine) is Park-Williams (PW8) strain.

Epidemiology

C. diphtheriae is found in the throat and nasopharynx of carriers and patients with diphtheria. The disease is a local infection, usually of the throat. Therefore, the organism is primarily spread by respiratory droplets, usually by convalescent or asymptomatic carriers. It is less frequently spread by contaminated fomites. The infection may spread through the milk of infected cows.

Pathogenicity

The disease is known as **diphtheria**, an **air-borne** infection.

(*i*) ***Upper respiratory tract infection*** — Diphtheria consists of a strictly local infection, usually of the throat. The infection produces a distinctive, thick, greyish, adherent exudate called a pseudomembrane, which is tough and leathery (**diphtheros = leathery**) and composed of fibrinous exudates together with disintegrating epithelial cells, leucocytes, RBC and bacteria, which is a characteristic of diphtheritic infection. It coats the throat and may extend into the nasal passages or downward in the respiratory tract, where the exudate sometimes obstructs the airways, even leading to suffocation (asphyxia). As the disease progresses, generalized symptoms occur due to production and absorption of toxin. Although, all human cells are sensitive to diphtheria toxin, the major clinical effects involve the heart and peripheral nerves. Cardiac conduction defects and myocarditis may lead to congestive heart failure and permanent heart damage. Neuritis of cranial nerves and paralysis of muscle groups, such as those that control movement of the palate or the eye, are seen late in the disease.

(*ii*) ***Cutaneous diphtheria*** — A puncture wound or cut in the skin can result in the introduction of *C. diphtheriae* into the subcutaneous tissue. Rarely, colonization and exotoxin production lead to tissue degeneration and death.

Laboratory diagnosis

The initial diagnosis and decision to treat for diphtheria must be made based on clinical observation. The widespread immunization beginning in early childhood has made the disease rare. Early presumptive diagnosis is critical, but few present-day clinicians have seen a case of the disease.

Specimen collected is swab from lesions, for example, one or two throat swabs may be collected from lesions, under vision using a tongue depressor. Laboratory diagnosis consists of microscopic demonstration, isolation of the bacillus and its toxigenicity testing.

Microscopy — Diphtheria bacilli and their metachromatic granules can be demonstrated in clinical specimens by staining with methylene blue or special stains such as Albert's stain or immunofluorescence. The metachromatic granules are often seen in thin, sometimes club-shaped rods that appear in clumps, suggestive of Chinese characters or picket fences. This method of visual identification is not very useful, however, for a diagnostic microbiologist who has never before seen a specimen of *C. diphtheriae* — a situation that is increasingly common due to decreasing incidence of diphtheria.

Culture — Swabs are inoculated on Loeffler's serum slope, potassium tellurite blood agar and ordinary blood agar, the last for differentiating streptococcal or staphylococcal pharyngitis, which may simulate diphtheria. All these media are incubated at 37ºC. The Loeffler's serum slope may show growth in 4–8 hours, but if it is negative it must be examined after 6–12 hrs and after 18–24 hrs. Tellurite plates will have to be incubated for atleast two days before being considered negative, as growth may sometimes be delayed. Smears are prepared from growth and stained with methylene blue or by special stains such as Albert's or Neisser's method and examined for characteristic metachromatic granules and typical cuneiform arrangement.

Toxigenicity tests or virulence tests — The identification of an isolate as *C. diphtheriae* does not mean that the patient has diphtheria. Diagnosis of diphtheria depends on demonstration of the production of toxin by isolate. This can be done by two methods:

I. *In vivo* methods — rarely used; subcutaneous tests and intradermal tests.

II. *In vitro* methods — reliable, less expensive, no need of animal; Elek's gel precipitation test and tissue culture test.

***In vivo* tests:**

(*i*) ***Subcutaneous test*** — The growth from an overnight culture on Loeffler's serum slope is emulsified in 2–4 ml broth and 0.8 ml of the emulsion injected subcutaneously into two guinea pigs, one of which has been protected with 500 units of diphtheria antitoxin 18–24 hours previously. If the strain is virulent, the unprotected animal will die within four days showing the autopsy appearance of:

(*i*) gelatinous hemorrhagic oedema at the site of inoculation.

(*ii*) blood stained pleural and peritoneal exudates.

(*iii*) hemorrhagic inflammation of adrenal glands.

This method is usually not employed as it is wasteful of animals.

(*ii*) ***Intradermal test*** — 0.1 ml of the broth emulsion of the culture is inoculated intracutaneously into two guinea pigs (or rabbits). One animal acts as the control and should receive 500 units of the antitoxin, the previous day. The other animal is given 50 units of antitoxin intraperitoneally four hours after the skin test, in order to prevent death. Toxigenicity is indicated by inflammatory reaction at the site of injection, progressing to necrosis in 48–72 hours in the test animal and no change in the control animal. An advantage in the intracutaneous test is that the animals do not die. As many as 10 strains can be tested at a time on a rabbit.

***In vitro* tests:**

(*i*) ***Elek's gel precipitation test*** — A rectangular strip of filter paper impregnated with the diphtheria antitoxin (1000 units/ml) is placed on the surface of a 20% normal horse serum agar in a petri dish while the medium is still in molten state. Instead of horse serum, sheep or rabbit serum may be used. When the medium has set, the surface is dried and narrow streaks of the strains are made at right angles to the filter paper strip. A positive and negative control should be put up. The plate is incubated at 37ºC for 24–48 hours. Toxins produced by the bacterial growth will diffuse in the agar and where it meets the antitoxin at optimum concentration will produce a line of precipitation. The formation of such arrow-head lines of precipitates indicates that the strain is toxigenic. No precipitate will form in the case of nontoxigenic strains. This test is very convenient and economical.

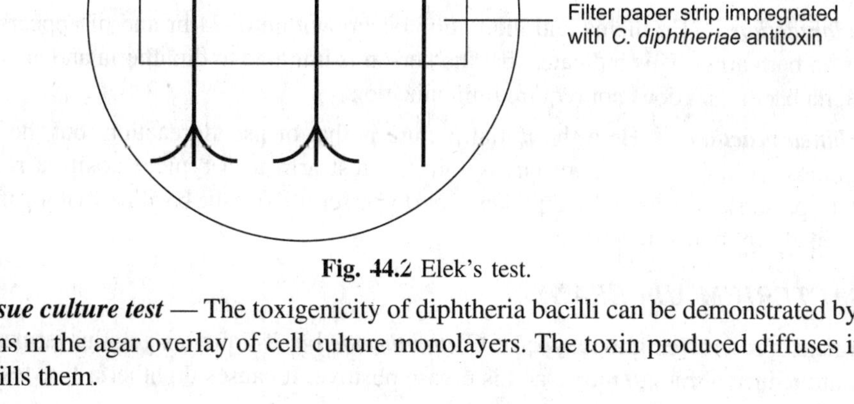

Fig. 44.2 Elek's test.

(*ii*) ***Tissue culture test*** — The toxigenicity of diphtheria bacilli can be demonstrated by incorporating the strains in the agar overlay of cell culture monolayers. The toxin produced diffuses into the cells below and kills them.

Treatment

Treatment of diphtheria requires prompt neutralization of toxin, followed by eradication of the organism by antitoxic and antibiotic therapy. A single dose of horse serum diphtheria antitoxin inactivates any circulating toxin, although it does not affect toxin that is already bound to cell-surface receptor. *C. diphtheriae* is sensitive to several antibiotics, such as erythromycin and pencillin.

Prophylaxis

Diphtheria can be controlled by immunization. Three methods of immunization are available — active, passive and combined. Of these, only active immunization can lead to eradication of the disease. Passive and combined immunization can only provide emergency protection to susceptible individuals exposed to risk.

(*i*) ***Active immunization*** — Formol toxoid or adsorbed toxoid is usually given in children as triple antigen containing diphtheria toxoid, pertussis bacilli (killed) and tetanus toxoid, known as DPT vaccine.

(*ii*) ***Passive immunization*** — Diphtheria antitoxin or antidiphtheritic serum (ADS), prepared by immunization of horses, is used as a emergency measure when susceptibles are exposed to infection.

(*iii*) ***Combined immunization*** — This consists of administration of the first dose of adsorbed toxoid on one arm, while ADS is given on the other arm, to be continued by the full course of active immunization. Ideally, all cases that receive ADS prophylactically should receive combined immunization.

Schick test

Schick test is used to differentiate between susceptible and immune persons to diphtheria. A test dose of diphtheria toxin (0.2 ml containing 1/50 minimal lethal dose) is injected intradermally on the left forearm and a similar dose of toxin inactivated by heating at 70ºC for 30 minutes is injected on the right forearm. Readings are taken after 1, 4 and 7 days. Four types of reaction may occur.

1. ***Positive reaction*** — An area of erythema and swelling at the site of injection of the toxin, appears in 1–2 days reaching its maximum between fourth and seventh days, when it measures 1–5 cm with superficial scaling and persistent brownish pigmentation. The control area injected with heated toxin will show no reaction. A positive test indicates that the person is susceptible to diphtheria and needs immunization.

2. ***Negative reaction*** — There is absence of any reaction on either arm. It indicates that the toxin has been neutralized by the circulating antitoxin and the person is immune to diphtheria and does not require immunization.

3. ***Pseudoreaction*** — Erythema and induration occurs within 6–24 hr and disappears completely within 4 days on both arms. This indicates that the person is immune to diphtheria and also hypersensitive to diphtheria bacilli and does not require immunization.

4. ***Combined reaction*** — Here the initial picture is that of pseudoreaction, but the erythema in control arm fades within 4 days. It progresses in the test arm to a typical positive reaction. This indicates that the person is susceptible to diphtheria and hypersensitive to the bacillus, making immunization necessary but likely to induce reaction.

CORYNEBACTERIUM ULCERANS

This organism resembles gravis type of *C. diphtheriae* but it liquefies gelatin, ferments trehalose slowly, does not reduce nitrate to nitrite and is urease positive. It causes diphtheria-like lesions particularly in immunocompromised hosts. It produces two types of toxins, one probably identical with the diphtheria toxin and the other resembling the toxin of *C. pseudotuberculosis*. It is pathogenic to guinea pigs, the lesions produced resembling those caused by *C. diphtheriae*. It has been found to cause infection in cows, and human infections may be transmitted through cow's milk. Diphtheria antitoxin is protective. It is sensitive to erythromycin.

CORYNEBACTERIUM PSEUDOTUBERCULOSIS

It is also known as Preisz-Nocard bacillus, which causes pseudotuberculosis in sheep and suppurative lymphadenitis in horses.

CORYNEBACTERIUM MINUTISSIMUM

It causes erythrasma, a localized infection of the stratum corneum usually affecting the axilla and groin, particularly in immunocomprcmised hosts. It is a lipophilic corynebacterium and can be grown readily in media containing 20% fetal calf serum.

C. JEIKEIUM

It is normal commensal found on the human skin and muscosal surfaces. It has been isolated from blood, tissues and CSF in patients with neutropenia, after cardiac surgery, patients with intravenous cannulae and patients with hematological malignancy receiving cytotoxic chemotherapy. It exhibits a high degree of drug resistance but responds to vancomycin.

C. XEROSIS

It is a commensal of nasopharynx, conjunctiva and skin. It is usually nonpathogenic but can cause opportunistic infections such as pneumonia and endocarditis in immunodeficiency states.

C. PSEUDODIPHTERITICUM (C. HOFFMANII)

It is a normal commensal of nasopharynx. It can cause several opportunistic infections including respiratory and urinary tract infections, cutaneous wound infections and endocarditis in immunosuppressed patients and in AIDS.

C. BOVIS

It is a commensal of bovine udder which may cause bovine mastitis. In humans it may cause infections of CNS and prosthetic heart valves.

DIPHTHEROIDS

Corynebacteria resembling *C. diphtheriae* that occur as normal commensals in the throat, skin, conjunctiva, urinary tract and other areas, mistaken for diphtheria bacilli are called diphtheroids. Diphtheroids stain more uniformly than diphtheria bacilli, possess a few or no metachromatic granules and tend to be arranged in parallel rows (pallisades) rather than cuneiform pattern. However, some diphtheroids may be indistinguishable from diphtheria bacilli microscopically. Differentiation is by biochemical reactions and more reliably by virulence tests. The common diphtheroids are *C. pseudodiphtheriticum* and *C. xerosis*.

ARCANOBACTERIUM HAEMOLYTICUM

It was formerly known as *Corynebacterium haemolyticum*. It is a slender, Gram positive bacillus resembling *C. diphtheriae* but it does not possess metachromatic granules. It produces betahemolysis on blood agar. It may cause pharyngitis, skin ulcers, peritonsillar abscesses, cervical lymphadenitis, cellulitis, osteomyelitis and brain abscess. When isolated from pharyngitis, it must be distinguished from *C. diphtheriae*, *C. ulcerans* and *Strept. pyogenes*. It is catalase negative whereas *C. diphtheriae* and *C. ulcerans* are catalase positive. Erythromycin, penicillin and tetracycline are used for treatment.

QUESTIONS

Essay Type Questions

1. Describe the morphology, cultural characters and pathogenicity of diphtheria bacilli.
2. Describe the pathogenicity, lab. diagnosis and prophylaxis of diphtheria.

Short Answer Type Questions

1. Morphology of *C. diphtheriae*.
2. Metachromatic granules. Or Volutin granules. Or Babes-Ernst granules.
3. Albert's stain.
4. Cuneiform arrangement.
5. Cultivation of *C. diphtheriae*.
6. Loeffler's serum slope.
7. Potassium tellurite blood agar. Or McLeod's medium.
8. Biotypes of *C. diphtheriae* Or McLeod's classification.
9. Diphtheria toxin.
10. Pathogenicity of *C. diphtheriae*.
11. Complications of diphtheria.
12. Cutaneous diphtheria.
13. Lab. diagnosis of diphtheria.
14. Toxigenicity testing of diphtheria bacilli.
15. Elek's test.
16. Prophylaxis against diphtheria.
17. Schick test.
18. DPT vaccine. Or Triple vaccine.
19. *Corynebacterium ulcerans*.
20. Diphtheroids.

45

Listeria monocytogenes

– *Morphology*	– *Pathogenicity*
– *Cultural characters*	– *Lab. diagnosis*
– *Biochemical reactions*	– *Treatment*
– *Antigenic properties*	– *Prevention*
– *Epidemiology*	– *Erysipelothrix rhusiopathiae*
– *Virulence factors*	

Morphology

Listeria species are slender, short, Gram positive rods or coccobacilli, diphtheroid like and pleomorphic. They are nonsporing, noncapsulated and nonacid fast. Sometimes they occur as diplobacilli or in short chains, and are avid intracellular parasites they may be seen within host cells in tissue samples. They display a distinctive tumbling motility in liquid medium, which is most active after growth at 25°C.

Cultural characteristics

They are aerobes and facultative anaerobes. They grow over a wide range of temperature 0–50°C, and a pH of 5.5–9.5 and at upto12% NaCl concentration. However, the optimum temperature for growth is 37°C. They can grow on ordinary media but growth is better on blood agar or tryptose phosphate agar. On blood agar, they produce betahemolysis, that may be confused with groupt B streptococci. After 24 hr incubation, at 37°C. The colonies are 1–2 mm in diameter, round, smooth, translucent, easily emulsifiable and nonpigmented. It produces a characteristic "Umbrella pattern" in mannitol motility agar medium, when incubated at 25°C, but not at 37°C.

Biochemical reactions

Based on biochemical properties, the genus *Listeria* is classified into 8 species. *Listeria monocytogenes* is responsible for most of the human infections. It gives a positive CAMP reaction, whereas other species are CAMP negative. It is catalase positive.

L. monocytogenes can be differentiated from group B streptococci (catalase negative) and *Corynebacterium* (nonmotile) by a positive catalase test, tumbling motility at 25°C and a negative hippurate hydrolysis test.

Antigenic properties

L. monocytogenes has an endotoxin, which is usually present in Gram negative bacilli. Based on 'O' and 'H' antigenic specificity, *L. monocytogenes* is further serologically typed into several serotypes. Serotypes 1/2a, 1/2b, and 4b are responsible for most human infections.

Epidemiology

Listeriae are ubiquitous in the environment as a saprophyte in soil, water, sewage, mud and vegetation.

They are widespread among animals in nature, particularly birds, fish, ticks and crustaceans. Human infections are zoonotic due to contact with infected animals or inhalation of contaminated dust or ingestion of contaminated milk.

Listeria infections are often food-borne. The organisms can multiply at 4ºC in refrigerated foods such as poultry, meat, dairy products like icecream and cheese. Healthy humans may serve as asymptomatic intestinal carriers of these organisms.

Listeria infections are most common in pregnant women, their fetuses or newborns, and in immunocompromised individuals such as the older adults or AIDS patients.

Virulence factors

L. monocytogenes is a facultative intracellular parasite, and has been used extensively to study phagocytosis and immune activation of macrophages.

The organism attaches to and enters a variety of mammalian cells, apparently by normal phagocytosis, and once internalized, escapes from the phagocytic vacuole by elaborating a membrane – damaging toxin called **listeriolysin 'O'.** This is a sulfhydryl-activated, poreforming cytolysin with amino acid sequence similarities to streptolysin 'O' and pneumococcal pneumolysin. Mutants lacking a functional listeriolysin 'O' are avirulent.

The organisms induce a reorganization of cellular actin such that short filaments and actin-binding protein cohere to the bacteria, creating a comet-like "tail". This complex appears to propel the organisms through the cell to psuedopods in contact with adjacent cells.

The organisms produce phospholipases, which cause membrane degradation, then mediate the passage of the organism directly to a neighbouring cell.

Pathogenicity

L. monocytogenes infection is called **listeriosis.** The organism is an intracellular pathogen and resides mainly within the macrophages. Monocytosis is a characteristic feature of listeriosis.

Maternal listeriosis — Infection in pregnant women leads to abortion or still birth. Asymptomatic carriage of female genital tract may cause infertility.

Neonatal listeriosis — Pregnant women, usually in the third trimester, may have a milder "flu-like" illness. In this, as well as in asymptomatic vaginal colonization, the organism can be transmitted to a new born. The early onset disease, within first week after birth is manifested as sepsis and granulomatous skin lesions. Granulomatous infantisepticum, a syndrome manifested as disseminated abscesses in the liver, lungs, adrenal glands and other organs. The late onset disease occurs usually as meningitis or meningoencephalitis, *L. monocytogenes* is a relatively common cause of neonatal meningitis.

Adult listeriosis — In adults, listeriosis may lead to meningitis, meningoencephalitis, encephalitis, brain abscess, spinal abscess, septicemia and endocarditis. The elderly and patients with AIDS, malignancies, diabetes mellitus, chronic renal and liver diseases and prolonged steroid therapy are at an increased risk.

Laboratory diagnosis

Specimens — Blood, CSF, pus, cervical or vaginal secretions, meconium, cord blood etc.

Microscopy — Peripheral blood film shows leucocytosis. Rarely, Gram stained films of CSF show Gram positive bacilli either intra or extracellularly.

Culture — Specimens are inoculated on to blood agar, chocolate agar and tryptose phosphate agar and incubated at 37°C for 1–3 days. On blood agar the colonies are small, with a narrow zone of beta hemolysis.

Specimens are stored in glucose broth at 4°C and subcultures are done at weekly intervals for 1–6 months, known as **"cold enrichment".**

The isolate is identified by morphological, biochemical and serological properties. *Listeria* species can be distinguished from streptococci and corynebacteria by positive motility and the production of catalase.

Molecular methods — *L. monocytogenes* DNA can be detected by PCR in CSF.

The leucocytes and protein content of CSF is raised in listeriosis.

Anton's test — When *L. monocytogenes* culture is instilled into eye of rabbits, it produces kerato conjunctivitis. This test is known as Anton's test.

Treatment

A variety antibiotics including ampicillin and trimethoprim—sulfamethoxazole are used to treat *L. monocytogenes* infections.

Prevention

Prevention of *L. monocytogenes* infections can be accomplished by proper food preparation and handling.

ERYSIPELOTHRIX RHUSIOPATHIAE

It is a slender, filamentous, Gram positive rod. It is nonmotile, nonsporing and noncapsulated. It is an aerobe and facultative anaerobe. It grows on ordinary media. It forms black colonies on media containing tellurite.

E. rhusiopathiae occurs in soil, food and water. It has a wide range of pathogenicity in animals — swines, mice, rabbits, birds, fish and crustaceans. In humans, rarely, it causes a skin infection called **erysipeloid** in people who commonly handle animal products, for example, butchers, veterinarians and fishermen. The organisms are believed to enter the skin through minor abrasions. The lesions are painful, edematous and erythematous, usually involving the local lymph nodes and joints. Occasionally it can cause septicemia and endocarditis.

The bacillus is sensitive to penicillin, erythromycin and tetracycline.

QUESTIONS

Short Answer Type Questions

1. *Listeria monocytogenes.*
2. Listeriosis.
3. Anton's test.
4. *Erysipelothrix rhusiopathiae.*
5. Erysipeloid.

46

Actinomycetes

INTRODUCTION

Actinomycetes (Actino = ray; mycetes = fungus) are a group of filamentous, branching, Gram positive organisms that easily fragment into slender rods. They are free-living mostly soil organisms that are related to corynebacteria and mycobacteria, as well as to the streptomycetes that are sources of important antibiotics. Actinomycetes were thought to be transitional forms between bacteria and fungi. Like bacteria, they — (*i*) possess cell walls containing muramic acid, (*ii*) possess prokaryotic nuclei, and (*iii*) are susceptible to antibiotics. Though they superficially resemble fungi on morphologic grounds, they are prokaryotes of bacterial size and are considered as true bacteria.

Actinomycetes include many genera of medical interest such as *Actinomyces*, *Arachnia*, *Actinomadura*, *Nocardia* and *Streptomyces*. Thermophilic actinomycetes such as *Micropolyspora* and *Thermoactinomyces* species present in moldy hay cause allergic alveolitis (farmer's lung disease) on repeated inhalation, leading to chronic obstructive pulmonary disease.

ACTINOMYCES

Actinomyces israelii, *Arachnia propionica* are part of the normal oral and intestinal flora in humans. *Actinomyces naeslundii* and *Actinomyces viscosis* are normal mouth commensals. Most of the infections are caused by *A. israelii*.

Morphology

Actinomyces are Gram positive nonmotile, nonsporing, nonacid fast, branching filaments that often break up into coccoid or bacillary forms. They were first discovered by Bollinger (1877) and known as Bollinger bodies. In lesions, the organism appears like sun ray (Actino = ray) in the granules.

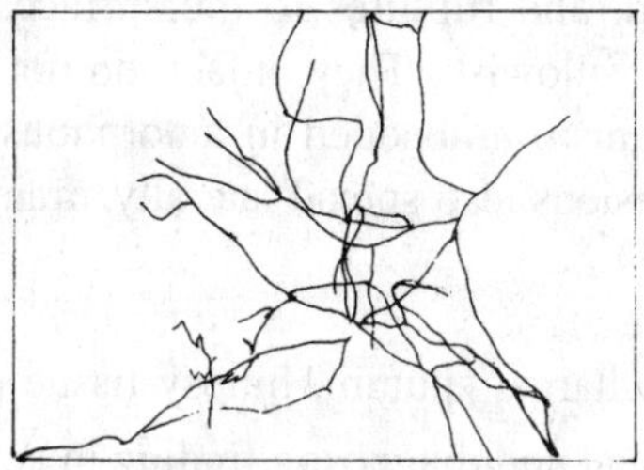

Fig. 46.1 *Actinomyces.*

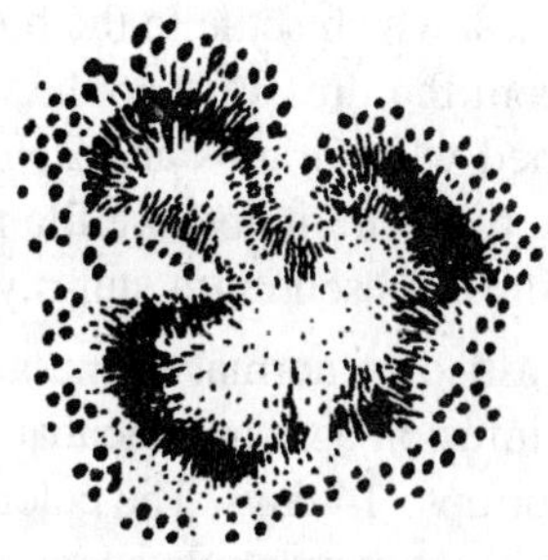

Fig. 46.2 Sun ray appearance of *Actinomyces*

Cultivation

They are strict anaerobes. Growth is best in the presence of 5–10% CO_2. They can be grown anaerobically on blood agar, brain-heart infusion agar and thioglycollate broth. Growth is slow, often requiring ten to fourteen days for visible colonies.

Epidemiology

The disease occurs throughout the world. Actinomycosis is more common in rural areas and in agricultural workers. Young males of 10–30 year old are most commonly affected. About 60% of cases are cervicofacial and some 20% abdominal. Pelvic actinomycosis is seen mainly among women using intrauterine contraceptive devices.

Pathogenicity

The *Actinomyces* species are normally present in mouth, intestine and female genital tract as commensals. The infection is known as **"Actinomycosis"**. It is an endogenous opportunistic infection, in which a chronic suppurative abscess leads to scarring and disfigurement. Trauma, foreign bodies or poor oral hygiene may favour tissue invasion. The infection is probably initiated by accidental introduction of organisms into the underlying soft tissues, where the organisms grow and multiply when anaerobic conditions prevail.

Important sites of actinomycotic infection are (*i*) cervicofacial (lumpy jaw) — with indurated lesions on the cheek and submaxillary region and are associated with poor dental hygiene and/or tooth extraction, (*ii*) thoracic — with lesions in the lung that may involve pleura and pericardium and spread outwards through chest wall, (*iii*) abdominal — around the caecum, appendix and abdominal wall are involved, (*iv*) pelvic — pelvic organs or female genital tract may be involved, particularly common in association with the use of intrauterine contraceptive devices.

The lesion, known as **mycetoma** begins as a hard, red, relatively nontender swelling that develops slowly, becomes filled with liquid, and ruptures to the surface, discharging pus, which consists of "sulfur granules" that are white to yellowish. They, infact, do not contain sulfur, but are microcolonies composed of filaments of the organism embedded in amorphous, eosinophilic material thought to be antigen-antibody complexes. The lesions also spread laterally, draining pus through several sinus tracts.

Laboratory diagnosis

Specimens — Pus, sinus discharge, sputum, biopsy tissue etc.

Microscopy — The most typical and diagnostic finding in actinomycosis is the presence of "sulfur granules" in the draining pus. The granules are, in fact, bacterial colonies.

The specimen is taken in a test tube alongwith sterile water or normal saline and allowed to stand after a thorough shaking. Sulfur granules, which settle to the bottom may be collected by pasteur pipette. The granules can also be obtained from the dressings applied over draining sinus tracts. Granules are crushed between two slides and stained with Gram's and ZN methods and are examined for the presence of Gram positive or nonacid fast, thin, Gram positive filaments, surrounded by a peripheral zone of swollen radiating club shaped structures, presenting a sun-ray appearance.

Culture — The granules are washed in normal saline and inoculated into thioglycolate broth or streaked on blood agar or brain-heart infusion agar and incubated at 37°C, both anaerobically and aerobically in the presence of 5–10% CO_2 for upto 14 days. The colonies of *Actinomyces israelii* are 0.5–2 mm in diameter, white to grey-white, smooth, entire or lobulated resembling molar tooth (molar tooth colonies). The identity of isolate may be confirmed by direct fluorescence, microscopy and biochemical tests.

Treatment

Penicillin G is the drug of choice for actinomycosis, although a number of antibiotics such as clindamycin, erythromycin and tetracycline have been shown to have clinical effect. Treatment must be sustained for weeks to months, and may be accompanied by surgical debridement and/or drainage. No significant resistance to penicillin G has been reported.

Prevention

Good oral hygiene is an important preventive measure.

NOCARDIA

Nocardia species are saprophytes in soil. Medically important species are *N. asteroides* and *N. brasiliensis*.

Morphology

Nocardiae are Gram positive, but irregularly staining, branched filaments. They do not form sulfur granules. They are acid fast under ZN stain, when 1% sulphuric acid is used for decolorization. The cell wall contains specific lipids such as mycolic acids and a large amount of meso-diaminopimelic acids. They are nonmotile.

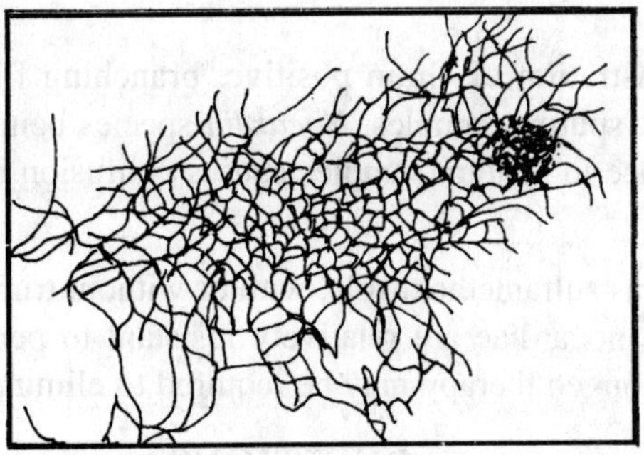

Fig. 46.3 *Nocardia.*

Cultivation

Nocardiae are strictly aerobic. They grow on a variety of simple media such as fungal media without antibiotics (Sabouraud's dextrose agar) and on blood agar. The inoculated plates should be incubated at 37ºC for upto three weeks. Nocardiae form white, yellow, pink or brown colonies, which are dry, granular and wrinkled.

Pathogenicity

The infection is known as **nocardiosis.** It causes opportunistic infections in humans and animals. The infection is acquired by inhalation of nocardiae from soil dust or are acquired by contamination of skin wounds. The most common presentation of human nocardiosis is a **pneumonia** of rather chronic course with abscesses, extensive necrosis and cavity formation resembling TB. The organisms may metastasize, with the brain and kidneys as the most common secondary locations. Common predisposing conditions are the immunosuppression associated with lymphoma or other malignancy, or with drugs. Systemic nocardiosis occurs more often in immunodeficient persons.

Cutaneous or subcutaneous nocardiosis may occur through contamination of skin wounds or by traumatic implantation. It usually involves feet and hands. The infection begins as a localized subcutaneous abscess that is invasive and quite destructive of the tissues and underlying bone. This lesion is known as **mycetoma,** characterized by swelling, draining sinuses, discharging pus.

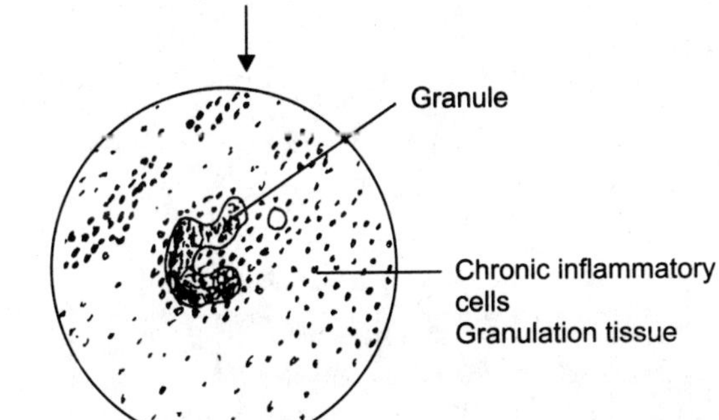

Mycetoma (or) Maduramycosis (Madura foot)

Granules white to yellow coloured

Filaments if seen in actinomycetoma are thin » 1μ

Agents causing actinomycetoma

Actinomyces israeli
Actinomyces bovis
Nocardia asteroides
Nocardia brasilienses
Nocardia carlae
Actinomadura madurae
Actinomadura pelletierii
Streptomyces somaliensis

Treatment

Responds to prolonged antibiotic and chemotherapeutic agents (Penicillin, tetracycline, contrimoxazole). Surgical debridement may be required.

Fig. 46.4 *Actinomycotic mycetoma* (Subcutaneous actinomycotic infection).

Laboratory diagnosis

Diagnosis is by demonstration of Gram positive, branching filaments microscopically and by isolation in culture from pus, sputum samples. *Nocardia* species being acid fast, can be demonstrated by ZN staining. Their presence in sputum samples causes confusion in the diagnosis of tuberculosis.

Treatment

The sulfonamides such as sulfamethoxazole, with or without trimethoprim are the drugs of choice for treating nocardiosis. The nocardiae are relatively resistant to penicillin. Surgical drainage of the lesions is important, and prolonged therapy may be required to eliminate the infection.

QUESTIONS

Short Answer Type Questions

1. What are actinomycetes? Name two actinomycetes.
2. Actinomycosis.

   Or

   Pathogenicity of *Actinomyces.*
3. *Actinomyces.*
4. Bollinger bodies.
5. Sulfur granules.
6. Laboratory diagnosis of actinomycosis.
7. *Nocardia.*
8. Nocardiosis.
9. *Nocardia asteroides.*
10. *Nocardia brasiliensis.*

47

Mycobacterium tuberculosis

(Tubercle bacillus, Koch's bacillus)

- *Mycobacteria*
- *Myco. tuberculosis*
  - *Morphology*
  - *Cultural characteristics*
  - *Biochemical tests*
  - *Differences between Myco. bovis and Myco. tuberculosis*
  - *Resistance*
  - *Antigenic structure*
  - *Mycobacteriophages*
  - *Virulence factors*
  - *Epidemiology*
  - *Pathogenicity*
  - *Immunity*
  - *Tuberculin test*
  - *Laboratory diagnosis*
  - *Prophylaxis*
  - *Treatment*

MYCOBACTERIA

Mycobacteria are slender, Gram positive rods, that sometimes show branching filamentous forms resembling fungal mycelium. In liquid cultures, they form a mold-like pellicle. Hence the name *Mycobacterium* (fungus-bacterium).

Mycobacteria possess lipid-rich cell walls that are resistant to penetration by chemical dyes, such as those used in the Gram stain. They, therefore stain poorly, but once stained, cannot be easily decolorized by treatment with acidified organic solvents. Hence they are termed "acid-fast".

Table 47.1 Classification of Mycobacteria

TUBERCLE BACILLI		
Human	–	*M. tuberculosis*
Bovine	–	*M. bovis*
Murine	–	*M. microti*
Avian	–	*M. avium*
Cold blooded	–	*M. marinum*

LEPRA BACILLI Human – *M. leprae* Murine – *M. lepraemurium*
ATYPICAL MYCOBACTERIA Photochromogens Scotochromogens Nonphotochromogens Rapid growers
MYCOBACTERIA CAUSING SKIN ULCERS *M. ulcerans* *M. balnei*
JOHNE'S BACILLUS *M. paratuberculosis*
SAPROPHYTIC MYCOBACTERIA *M. smegmatis* *M. butyricum* *M. phlei* *M. stercoris*

MYCOBACTERIUM TUBERCULOSIS

(Tubercle bacillus; Koch's bacillus)

Morphology

M. tuberculosis are long, slender rods, that are straight or slightly curved, measure about 3 µm × 0.3 µm, occurring singly, in pairs or in small clumps. *M. bovis* is usually straighter, shorter and stout bacillus. They are nonmotile, noncapsulated and nonsporing.

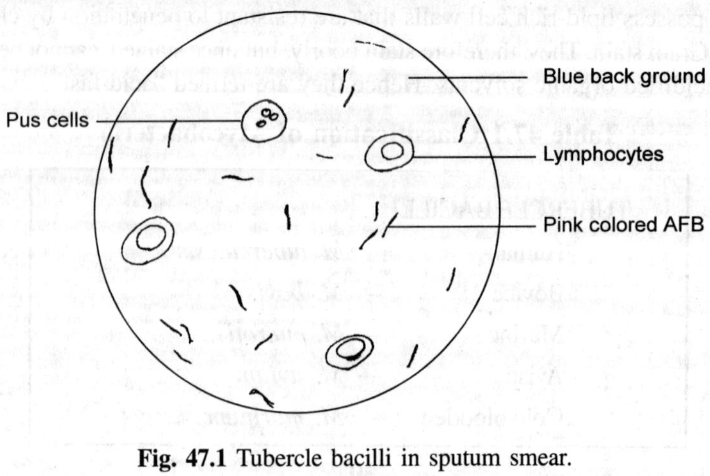

Fig. 47.1 Tubercle bacilli in sputum smear.

Mycobacterial cell walls are unusual in that they are approximately sixty percent lipid, including a unique class of very long chain (75 to 90 carbons), β-hydroxylated fatty acids called **mycolic acids.** These complex with a variety of polysaccharides and peptides, creating a waxy cell surface that makes mycobacteria strongly hydrophobic and accounts for their acid-fastness; impervious to many chemical disinfectants, and offer resistance to the corrosive action of strong acids or alkalies as well. This fact is made use of in decontaminating clinical specimens such as sputum, where nonmycobacterial organisms are digested by such treatments (with acid or alkali) (Table 47.2).

Table 47.2 Properties of Mycobacteria conferred by Lipid-Rich Cell Walls

1. Acid-fastness
2. Resistance to penetration by stains
3. Resistance to the corrosive action of strong acids or alkalies
4. In liquid media, the organisms tend to adhere to each other and float on the surface due to their hydrophobic character, unless dispersed by detergents or wetting agents
5. Slow growth by inhibiting the entry of nutrients into the cells
6. Resistance to the bactericidal action of antibodies and complement
7. Cellular tissue reactions of the body

It is an acid-fast bacillus and also alcohol-fast. The Ziehl-Neelsen acid-fast stain is used for staining organisms from clinical specimens and cultures. Under this stain, the tubercle bacilli appear bright pink, whereas the tissue cells and other organisms are stained blue. Organisms, often stain irregularly and have a beaded or barred appearance, probably due to the presence of vacuoles and polymetaphosphate. *M. bovis* usually shows uniform staining.

Tubercle bacilli may also be stained with auramine 'O' (and rhodamine) and smears are examined by fluorescence microscope. Tubercle bacilli appear as brightly luminous yellow rods against a dark-field.

Tubercle bacilli are Gram positive, but it is difficult to stain them with the Gram stain. This is because the lipid-rich cell walls are resistant to the penetration of dyes.

Much (1907) demonstrated the Gram positive granules in cold abscess pus where there was no evidence of acid-fast bacilli, but could produce tuberculosis when injected into susceptible animals. Much suggested that these granules were non-acid-fast forms of tubercle bacilli, and are known as **Much's granules.**

Cultural Characteristics

M. tuberculosis is an obligate aerobe, whereas *M. bovis* is microaerophilic on primary isolation, becoming aerobic on subculture. Optimum temperature for growth is 37°C and optimum pH is 7.0–7.2.

Several enriched media, both solid and liquid have been described for the cultivation of tubercle bacilli. The solid media used are Lowenstein—Jensen (LJ) medium, Dorset's egg medium and Petrgnini medium containing egg, Tarshis medium containing blood, Loeffler's serum slope containing serum and Pawlowsky's medium containing potato. The solid medium most widely employed for routine cultivation is Lowenstein–Jensen (LJ) medium containing hen's egg, mineral salt solution, asparagine, malachite green, glycerol or sodium pyruvate. The medium is solidified and sterilized simultaneously by inspissation. Malachite green acts as a selective agent inhibiting the growth of other bacteria and provides a color contrast against which colonies of mycobacteria can be easily seen.

Among the liquid media Dubo's medium, Middlebrook's medium, Proskauer and Beck's medium, Sula's medium and Sauton's media are commonly employed. Liquid media are not generally employed for routine cultivation, but are used for sensitivity testing, chemical analyses and preparation of antigens and vaccines.

The addition of 0.5% glycerol improves the growth of *M. tuberculosis*, but has no effect or may even impair the growth of *M. bovis*. Sodium pyruvate helps the growth of both types.

Mycobacteria grow slowly with generation times of 8 to 24 hours, in part because of their hydrophobic surface promotes clumped growth and slow uptake of nutrients. Colonies appear in about two weeks and may sometimes take up to eight weeks.

M. tuberculosis grows luxuriantly in culture as compared to *M. bovis* which grows sparsely. They are therefore termed "eugonic" and "dysgonic" respectively.

On solid media, *M. tuberculosis* forms dry, rough, raised, irregular colonies with a wrinkled surface. They are creamy white, becoming yellowish or buff colored on further incubation. They are tenacious and not easily emulsified. In comparison, the colonies of *M. bovis* are flat, smooth, moist, white and break up easily when touched.

In liquid media without dispersing agents the growth begins at the bottom, creeps up the sides and forms a prominent whitish, wrinkled surface pellicle which may extend along the sides above the medium. Diffuse growth is obtained in Dubo's medium containing Tween–80 (polyoxyethylene sorbitan monnucleate). It wets the surface, deters aggregation of cells and permits them to grow diffusely.

When tubercle bacilli are grown in a liquid medium such as Dubo's medium, virulent strains often grow as twisted rope-like colonies, in which bacilli aggregate with their long axes parallel, which appear like serpentine cords. This is due to a **"cord factor"**. Chemically it is a trehalose dimycolate (two mycolic acids linked to a trehalose). It is correlated with virulence.

Mycobacterial species are differentiated by rate of growth, optimal temperature of growth, production of pigments and other biochemical tests.

Biochemical tests

Several biochemical tests are used in identifying and differentiation of mycobacterial species.

Niacin test — The test is positive with human tubercle bacilli, *M. simiae* and a few strains of *M. cheloneii*, but negative with bovine tubercle bacilli. When 10% cyanogen bromide and 4% aniline in 96% ethanol are added to a suspension of the culture, a canary yellow color indicates a positive reaction.

Aryl sulphatase test — The test is positive only with atypical mycobacteria. The organisms are grown for two weeks in a medium containing 0.001 M tripotassium phenolphthalein disulphate. If aryl sulphatase is produced, it will split free phenolphthalein from tripotassium phenolphthalein disulphate, which can be detected by adding 2N NaOH dropwise to the culture. A pink color indicates a positive reaction.

Neutral red test — Virulent strains of tubercle bacilli are able to bind neutral red in alkaline buffer solution, while avirulent strains are unable to do so.

5 ml of ethyl alcohol is placed in a test tube and inoculated with one or two colonies from LJ medium, and incubated at 37ºC for 1 hour. Supernatant alcohol is carefully removed with a pipette and 5 ml of distilled water and 0.2 ml of 0.05% aqueous solution of neutral red are added. The fluid is rendered alkaline by adding N/100 NaOH drop by drop till the color is just amber. The tube is further incubated in the water bath at 37ºC for another one hour with frequent shaking. Appearance of red staining of the colonies suspended in the amber fluid constitutes a positive test.

Catalase-peroxidase tests — These tests help in differentiating tubercle bacilli from atypical mycobacteria and provide an indication of the sensitivity of the strain to isoniazid. Most atypical mycobacteria are strongly catalase positive, while tubercle bacilli are only weakly positive. On the other hand, tubercle bacilli are peroxidase positive, but not atypical mycobacteria. Catalase and peroxidase activities are lost when tubercle bacilli become INH resistant. Catalase negative strains of tubercle bacilli are not virulent for guinea pigs.

A mixture of equal volumes of 30% H_2O_2 and 0.2% catechol in distilled water is added to 5 ml of the tests culture and allowed to stand for few minutes. Effervescence indicates catalase production and browning indicates peroxidase activity.

Amidase tests — Mycobacteria can be differentiated by their ability to split amides. The amides commonly used are acetamide, benzamide, carbamide, nicotinamide and pyrazinamide. A 0.00164 M solution of the amide is incubated with bacillary suspension at 37°C. To this is added 0.1 ml of $MnSO_4.4H_2O$, 1 ml of phenol solution and 0.5 ml of hypochlorite solution. The tubes are placed in boiling water bath for 20 minutes. Development of blue color in the tube indicates a positive test. *M. tuberculosis* produces nicotinamidase and pyrazinamidase.

Nitrate reduction test — *M. tuberculosis, M. kansasii, N. fortuitum, M. chelonei, M. szulgai, M. flavescens, M. terrae* and *M. triviale* produce enzyme nitroreductase and reduce nitrate to nitrite. *M. bovis* and *M. avium* cannot produce this enzyme and therefore cannot reduce nitrate to nitrite.

The test organism is suspended in a buffer solution containing nitrate and incubated at 37°C for 2 hours. Then sulphanilamide and n-naphthylethylene diamine dihydrochloride solution is added. Positive reaction is indicated by the development of pink or red color within 30–60 seconds.

Tween-80 hydrolysis — Certain mycobacteria possess a lipase that splits tween-80 into oleic acid and polyoxyethylated sorbitol which modifies the optical characteristics of the test solution from a straw yellow to pink. Place a loopful of culture in a mixture of Tween-80-buffer-neutral red. Incubate at 37°C. The reaction is read at every 3–6 hours for 3 days and daily thereafter for ten days. Formation of pink color indicates hydrolysis of Tween 80. *M. kansasii* produces a positive reaction within 3 to 6 hours, whereas *M. gordonae, M. flavescens* and *M. smegmatis* are positive in 3–10 days. *M. bovis, M. avium, M. africanum, M. ulcerans, M. scrofulaceum* and *M. xenopi* are negative for Tween 80 hydrolysis test.

Susceptibility to pyrazinamide — *M. tuberculosis* is sensitive to 50 μg/ml pyrazinamide, while *M. bovis* and other mycobacteria are resistant.

Susceptibility to thiophen-2-carboxylic acid hydrazide (TCH) — *M. bovis* is usually susceptible to 10 μg/ml of TCH, while *M. tuberculosis* is usually resistant.

Table 47.3 Differentiating features of *M. tuberculosis* and *M. bovis*

	M. tuberculosis	*M. bovis*
1. Microscopic morphology	Slender, straight or slightly curved rods with barred or beaded appearance	Straight, stout, short uniformly stained rods
2. Colony morphology	Dry, rough, raised, wrinkled, white to buff colored and not easily emulsifiable (rough, buff and tough)	Moist, smooth, flat, friable and white
3. Average duration of time for growth	12–25 days	20–40 days
4. Growth at 37°C	Growth is eugonic (luxuriant)	Growth is dysgonic (sparse)

5. Effect of glycerol	0.75% concentration enhances the growth However, a concentration of 0.5 % has no effect	At 0.75% concentration, growth is inhibited.
6. Susceptibility to pyrazinamide (50 µg/ml)	Sensitive	Resistant
7. Susceptibility to thiophen 2-carboxylic acid hydrazide (10µg/ml)	Resistant	Sensitive
8. Biochemical properties		
– Niacin test	Positive	Negative
– Nitrate reduction test	Positive	Negative
9. Oxygen requirement	Obligate aerobe	Microaerophilic on primary isolation but becomes aerobic on subculture
10. Animal pathogenicity test		
– Guinea pig	Positive	Positive
– Rabbit	Negative	Positive

Resistance

Tubercle bacilli are highly resistant to drying. When exposed to direct sunlight, organisms from culture are killed in 2 hours, but bacilli contained in sputum require an exposure of 20–30 hours. In dried sputum, protected from sunlight, they survive for as long as 6 months. The tubercle bacillus is generally more resistant to chemical disinfectants than other nonsporing bacilli, especially in sputum. It can survive exposure to 5% phenol, 15% H_2SO_4, 3% nitric acid, 5% oxalic acid and 4% NaOH. It is destroyed by tincture of iodine in 5 minutes and by 80% ethanol in 2–10 minutes.

Antigenic structure

Mycobacteria possess cell wall (insoluble) antigens and cytoplasmic (soluble) antigens. Cell wall antigens include arabinomannan, arabinogalactan and lipoarabinomannan. Group specificity is due to polysaccharide and type specificity to protein antigens.

Following infection by tubercle bacilli, delayed hypersensitivity is developed to the bacillary protein (tuberculin). Tuberculins from human, bovine and murine bacilli appear to be same and indistinguishable. There is also some antigenic relationship between tubercle and lepra bacilli.

Antibodies against polysaccharide, protein and phosphatide antigens of tubercle bacilli can be demonstrated by serological tests, but they are not much useful in diagnosis or relevant in immunity.

Mycobacteriophages

Several mycobacteriophages have been isolated from soil, human excreta, polluted water and biopsy specimens of sarcoid and lung cancer patients. Mycobacteriophages are double-stranded DNA phages with G+C content similar to that of the host bacterium. Most of them have an hexagonal or oval head and a long non-contractile tail. An exception is phage 13, a temperate phage of *M. smegmatis*, which has a contractile tail. Many mycobacteria infected with phages are not truly lysogenic. The phage DNA appears to exist as an independent plasmid (instead of being integrated into the chromosome) and is only transmitted to some of the daughter cells. This is known as pseudolysogeny.

M. tuberculosis is divided into four phage types A, B, C and I. Type A is commonest and has a world wide distribution. Type B mainly occurs in Europe, Middle East and North America and type C is rarely seen. Type I is intermediate between A and B and is frequently encountered in India and neighbouring countries. Phage 33D can lyse *M. tuberculosis*, *M. bovis*, *M. africanum* and *M. microti* but not BCG.

Virulence factors

1 Cord factor, 2. Sulpholipids may contribute to virulence by inhibiting phagosome-lysosome fusion within the macrophages thus allowing them to multiply within them.

Epidemiology

The source of infection is a patient with active pulmonary tuberculosis, who sheds large numbers of organisms by coughing (open case), thus creating aerosol droplet nuclei. Because of resistance to dessication, the organisms can remain viable in the environment for a long time. The principal mode of contagion is person-to-person transmission by inhalation of the aerosol, and repeated or prolonged contact is usually required for transmission of infection. Transmission is facilitated by crowding and poor ventillation. Individuals in nursing homes, homeless shelters, and prisons are among those particularly at risk. A single infected person can pass the organism to numerous people in an exposed group such as family, a classroom, or a hospital ward.

M. bovis infection in humans is zoonotic acquired through direct contact or by ingestion of raw milk from animals.

Tuberculosis has increasingly become a cause of special concern in immunodeficiency cases. A close association exists between AIDS and tuberculosis.

Racial differences in susceptibility to tuberculosis has been noticed. Dark-skinned races and groups are more susceptible. Studies of disease frequency in twins demonstrate a genetic component as well. When one twin is infected, the attack rate in the other is 75 per cent for identical pairs, but only 25 per cent in fraternal twins.

Pathogenicity

The incubation period is about 4 to 12 weeks, and the disease develops slowly. The symptoms of TB are fever, fatigue and weight loss. A cough, which is characteristic of pulmonary involvement, may result in expectoration of bloody sputum.

After being inhaled, mycobacteria reach the alveoli where they multiply in the pulmonary epithelium or in macrophages. Within two to four weeks, many bacilli are destroyed by the immune system, but some survive, and are spread by the blood to extrapulmonary sites. The virulence of *M. tuberculosis* resists with its ability to survive and grow within host cells. The organism produces no demonstrable toxins. However, when engulfed by macrophages, bacterial sulfolipids inhibit the fusion of phagocytic vesicles with lysosomes. The ability of the organism to grow even in immunologically activated macrophages, and to remain viable in a dormant form within the host for decades, are keys to the unique character of tuberculosis. Tuberculous lesions are of two types — productive and exudative.

Primary tuberculosis — Once in the lungs, the bacteria are phagocytosed by macrophages and a hypersensitivity response forms a productive (granulomatous) lesions, characterized by small, hard nodules called **tubercles,** which are characteristic of tuberculosis and give the disease its name. It consists of large, multinucleate giant cells (macrophage syncytia) containing tubercle bacilli, a mid zone of pale epitheloid cells, and a peripheral collar of fibroblasts and mononuclear cells.

The disease process usually stops at this stage, but the bacteria often remain alive within macrophage phagosomes. In time the tubercle may change to a cheeselike consistency and is then called a **caseous lesion.** If such lesions calcify, they are termed **Ghon complexes** (exudative lesion), which show up prominently in a chest X-ray. The Ghon focus with the hilar lymph nodes that undergo calcification is known as **Ranke complex.**

In case of *M. bovis,* which enters orally, as in milk-borne bovine tuberculosis, the primary complexes involve the tonsil and cervical lymph nodes or the intestine, often the ileocaecal region, and the mesenteric lymph nodes.

Miliary tuberculosis — Sometimes the tuberculous lesions break down, the caseous material is discharged, and a cavity is created known as **tuberculous cavities,** that can facilitate the spread of infection. The organisms are dispersed by the lymph and the blood stream, and can seed the lungs, the regional lymph nodes, or various distant tissues, such as liver, spleen, kidneys, bone or meninges. In progressive disease, one or more of the resulting tubercles may expand leading to destruction of tissue and clinical illness, for example, chronic pneumonitis, tuberculous osteomyelitis or tuberculous meningitis. Tuberculosis of the spine is called **pott's disease.** In the extreme instance, active tubercles develop throughout the body, a serious condition known as **miliary (disseminated) tuberculosis.**

Reactivation tuberculosis — This is usually caused by *M. tuberculosis* that has survived in a dormant primary tubercle lesion. (Note : Resistance and hypersensitivity induced in the host by the first infection with tubercle bacilli normally prevent reinfection from external sources). Any of the preexisting tubercles may be involved, but pulmonary sites are most common, particularly the lung apices where high oxygen tension favours mycobacterial growth. Bacterial populations in such lesions often become quite large, and many organisms are shed in sputum. The patient thus again becomes capable of exposing others to the disease. Reactivation is apparently due to an impairment in immune status, often associated with malnutrition, alcoholism, advanced age or severe stress. Immunosuppressive medication, or diseases such as diabetes and, particularly AIDS are common predisposing conditions.

The relationship between the tubercle bacillus and the human host is complex, the outcome of their encounter presenting a wide spectrum of possibilities. The majority of individuals exposed to tubercle bacilli, suffer a recognizable primary infection. The course of this infection is variable. One person develops only a small limited primary complex which never gives rise to illness, whilst another rapidly extensive progressive disease.

Immunity

M. tuberculosis stimulates both a humoral and cell mediated immune response. Although circulating antibodies appear, they do not offer resistance to the organism. Instead, cell mediated immunity and the accompanying delayed hypersensitivity, directed against a number of bacterial protein antigens, develop in the course of infection, and contribute to both the pathology of and immunity to the disease. Tubercle bacilli are excellent immunogens; their cell wall products, particularly a muramyl dipeptide fragment of the peplidoglycan, enhance immunologic responsiveness nonspecifically. Consequently, they have been used as adjuvants.

The tuberculin reactivity was first demonstrated in guinea pigs by Robert Koch (1890-91), that led to the discovery of **Koch's phenomenon.** When a healthy guinea pig is inoculated subcutaneously with tubercle bacilli, the puncture site heals quickly and there is no immediate visible reaction. But after 10–14 days a hard nodule appears which soon breaks down to form an ulcer that persists till the animal dies of progressive tuberculosis. The regional lymph nodes are enlarged and become caseous.

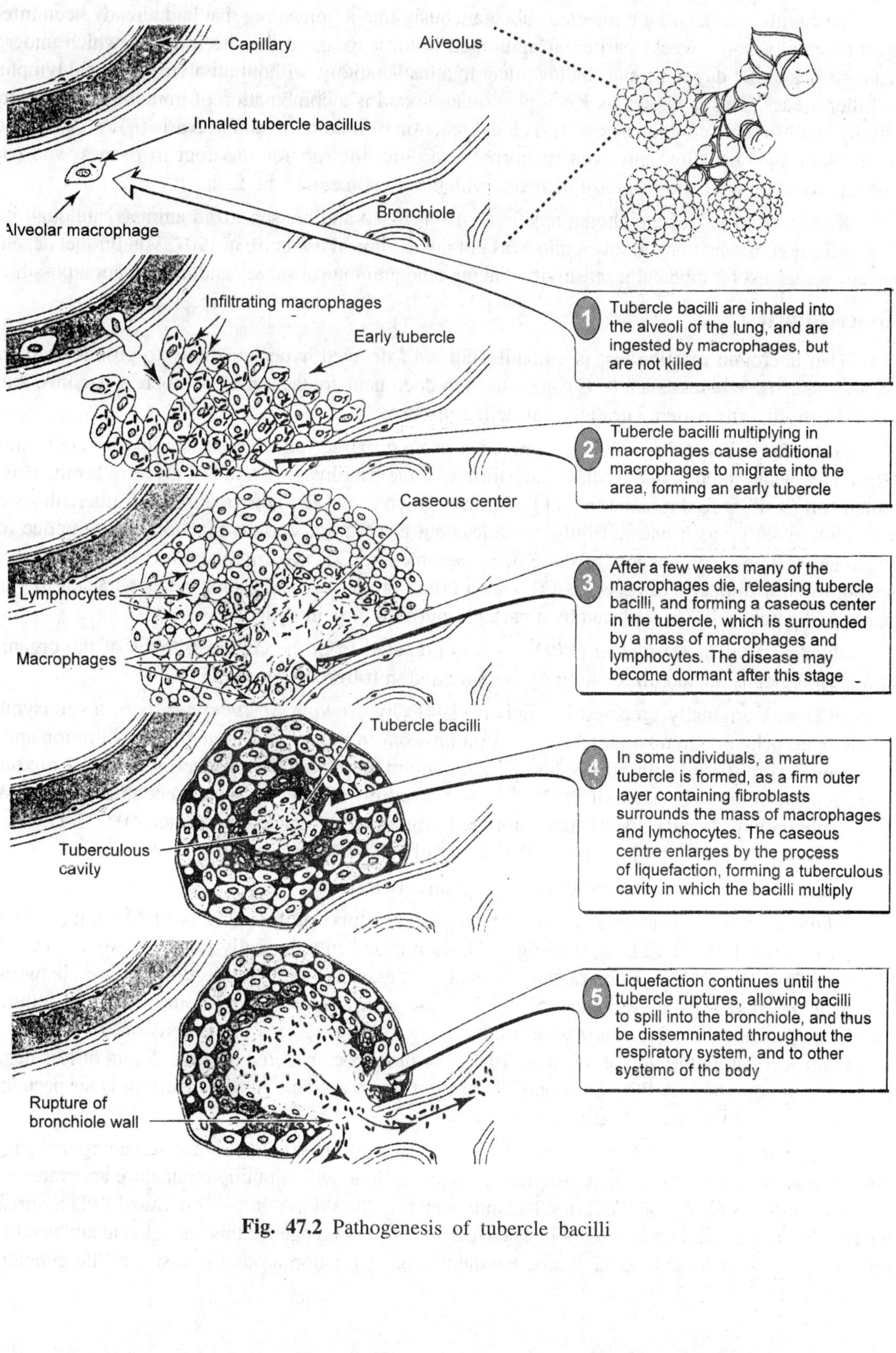

Fig. 47.2 Pathogenesis of tubercle bacilli

When tubercle bacilli are injected subcutaneously into a guinea pig that had already been infected with tuberculosis 4–6 weeks earlier, an indurated lesion appears at the site in a day which undergoes necrosis in another day to form a shallow ulcer that heals rapidly, without involving regional lymphatics or other tissues. This is known as Koch phenomenon and is a combination of immunity and hypersensitivity and has three components — (*i*) A local reaction of induration and necrosis (*ii*) A focal response manifested as congestion and even hemorrhage around the tuberculous foci in tissues, and (*iii*) A constitutional or systemic response of fever, which may sometimes be fatal.

Koch's discovery of the altered reactions in sensitized and nonsensitized animals, although it was first indication of sensitivity to tuberculin, was not put to clinical use until, in 1907, Von Pirquet developed his cutaneous test for tuberculin sensitivity making epidemiological survey and investigation possible.

Tuberculin test

The tuberculin reaction test is a manifestation of delayed hypersensitivity to protein antigens of *M. tuberculosis*. Whereas such tests can be used to document contact with the tubercle bacillus, they do not confirm that the patient currently has active disease.

Old tuberculin (OT) — Koch prepared a protein extract of tubercle bacillus by concentrating tenfold by evaporation, a 6–8 week culture filtrate of the bacillus grown in 5% glycerol broth. This was called "original" or "old tuberculin (OT)". Initially Koch used OT in the treatment of tuberculosis but it was soon given up as it was not only of useless but also caused serious reactions in some due to the focal and systemic components of the Koch phenomenon. OT was first used for allergic (tuberculin) testing by Von Pirquet. However, as OT was a crude product and different batches tended to vary in purity and potency, it was replaced by a partially purified protein antigen.

Purified Protein Derivative (PPD) — It is prepared from the culture filtrates of the organisms, and is biologically standardized. Activity is expressed in **tuberculin units (TU).**

PPD was originally prepared by Siebert (1941) by growing *M. tuberculosis* in a semisynthetic medium, autoclaving, removing debris by filtration, concentrating the filtrate by ultrafiltration and precipitating several times with 50% saturated ammonium sulphate. The product is mostly a mixture of small proteins. One large batch of PPD made by Seibert in 1939 (PPD-S) was recognized by the WHO as the international standard PPD-tuberculin and arbitrarily designated to contain 50,000 TU per mg. One TU is equal to 0.01 ml of OT or 0.00002 mg of PPD-S.

Many methods have been described for tuberculin testing.

Mantoux test — The routinely used technique for tuberculin testing is of Mantoux (1910). In Mantoux test, 0.1 ml of PPD containing 5 TU is injected intradermally on the flexor aspect of the forearm with a tuberculin syringe raising a wheal. It is essential that the injection be given between the layers of the skin and not subcutaneously. The site is examined 48–72 hours later and induration (hardening) measured at its widest point transversely to the long axis of the forearm. Erythema is not taken into account. Induration of diameter 10 mm or more is considered positive, 5 mm or less negative and 6–9 μm equivocal. A PPD dose one TU is used when extreme hypersensitivity is suspected; and doses of 10 or 100 when 5 TU test is negative.

Heaf test — This test involves multiple puncturing and is satisfactory for screening and surveys, but not accurate enough as a diagnostic test. The test is done with a multiple puncture apparatus with 6 needles, known as Heaf gun, that prick 1–2 mm deep into the skin. A drop of undiluted PPD is spread on the area of skin selected for inoculation. The Heaf gun is pressed against this area of skin and needles are released. The test is read after 72 hours. Erythema and induration around atleast 4 of the punctures is regarded as positive. The Heaf gun has to be sterilised between tests to prevent cross infections.

Tine test — This test utilizes disposable prongs carrying dried PPD. The test is not quantitative and is therefore useful for population screening, but not for individual diagnosis.

A positive reaction usually develops four to six weeks after initial contact with the organism. It remains positive for life, although it may wane after some years. A positive tuberculin test indicates delayed (Type IV) hypersensitivity to tuberculoprotein denoting infection with tubercle bacillus or BCG immunization, recent or past, with or without clinical disease. In endemic areas the allergy is maintained by repeated contact with the bacilli.

Persons who have never had contact with tubercle bacilli are tuberculin negative. False negative tests (anergy) may be seen in certain conditions like miliary tuberculosis, convalescence from some viral infections like measles, lymphoreticular malignancy, sarcoidosis, severe malnutrition, immunosuppressive therapy or defective cell mediated immunity. False positive reactions may be seen in infections with related mycobacteria (atypical mycobacteria).

Conditions affecting the tuberculin reaction — Active tuberculosis is often associated with conditions of suppressed cell mediated immunity. Under these circumstances, loss of delayed hypersensitivity and a state of anergy (absence of sensitivity), may develop; the tuberculin reaction will then be attenuated or negative. Finally, cross-reaction is occasionally observed with other pathogens in the genus mycobacterium.

Uses of Tuberculin test — Tuberculin test is used as an aid

(*i*) to diagnose active infection in infants and young children

(*ii*) to measure prevalence of infection in an area

(*iii*) to select susceptibles for BCG vaccination, and

(*iv*) indication of successful vaccination.

Tuberculin testing of cattle has been of great value in the control of bovine tuberculosis.

Laboratory diagnosis

In pulmonary tuberculosis, the specimen tested is sputum. Sputum is best collected in the morning before any meal. If sputum is scanty, a 24-hour sample may be tested. Clean, sterile wide-mouthed containers may be used for sputum collection. Sputum sampling on three consecutive days increases chances of detection. Some clinicians prefer to collect three sputum specimens over a period of 14 days, before the case is declared as sputum-negative. Where sputum is not available, laryngeal swabs or bronchial washings may be collected. In small children, who tend to swallow the sputum, gastric lavage can be examined.

In tuberculous meningitis, CSF is collected by lumbar puncture, which often develops a spider web clot on standing, examination of which may be more successful than of the fluid.

Bone marrow and liver biopsy specimens from miliary tuberculosis and blood from those with HIV coinfection are useful. Pus may be collected from tuberculous abscesses. Pleural effusion and other exudates may be collected with citrate to prevent coagulation.

In renal tuberculosis, the urinary excretion of bacilli is intermittent. Hence it is advisable to test 3–6 morning samples of urine.

Concentration methods — Several methods have been described for homogenization, decontamination and concentration of sputum and other specimens.

Table 47.3 Identification of Tubercle Bacilli and Related Mycobacteria.

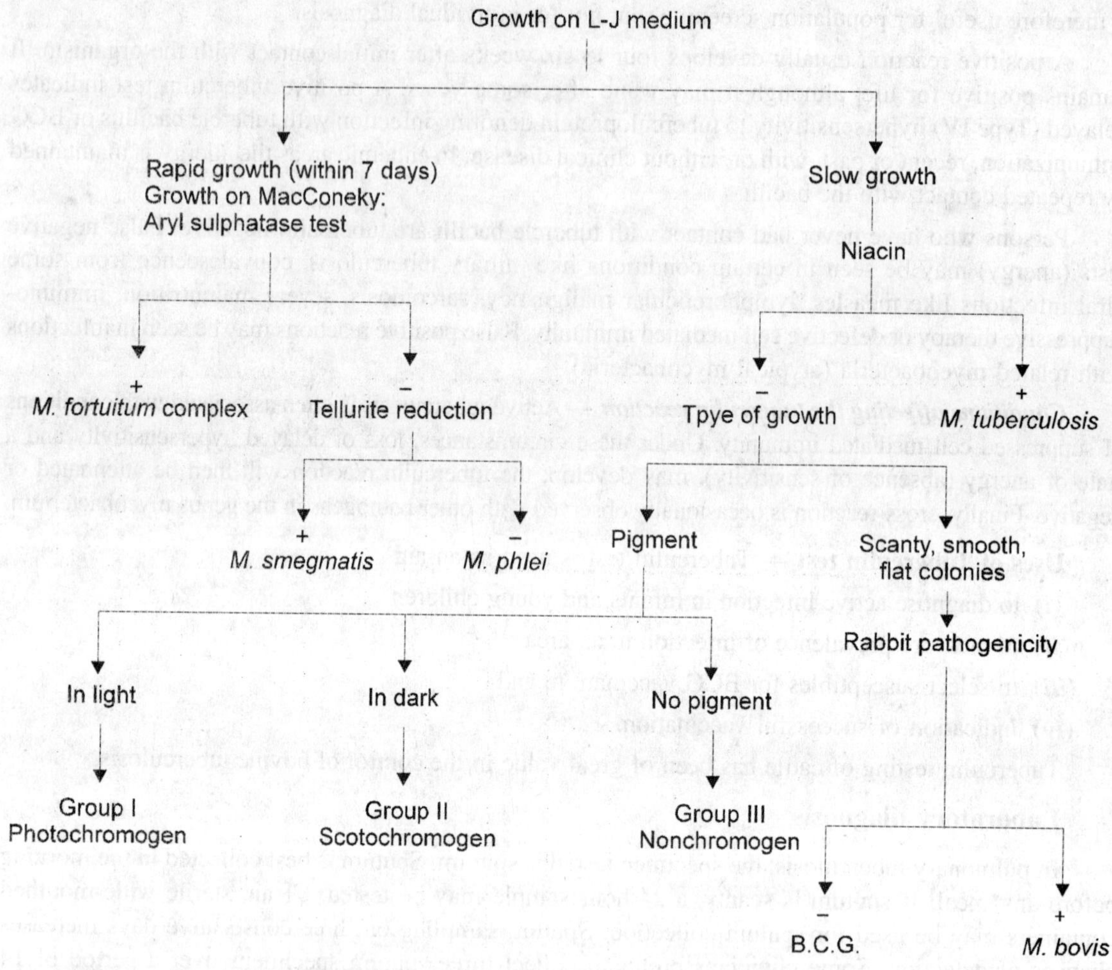

Petroff's method — It is a simple and widely used method of concentration. Sputum is incubated with an equal volume of 4% NaOH (alkali) solution at 37ºC with frequent shaking till it becomes clear, on an average for 20–30 minutes. It is then contrifuged at 3000 rpm for 20–30 minutes. The supernatant is discarded and the sediment is neutralized with N/10 HCl and used for smear, microscopy and culture.

Instead of alkali, homogenization can be achieved by treatment with dilute acids such as 6% H_2SO_4, 3% HCl or 5% oxalic acid or mucolytic agents such as N-acetyl L-cysteine with NaOH and pancreatin.

The methods of laboratory diagnosis include microscopy, culture, animal inoculation, molecular techniques, serological techniques and tuberculin test.

Microscopy — A microscopic search for acid-fast bacilli, using Ziehl-Neelsen stain is the most rapid test for mycobacteria. Smears can be made from various specimens-sputum, bronchial washings, urine, CSF, biopsy material-either directly or after concentration. New slides should be used for smears and they should not be reused, as acid-fast bacilli may not always be removed from slides by cleaning. Smears should be prepared from thick purulent part or blood-tinged part of the sputum. Smears are dried, heat fixed and stained by Ziehl-Neelsen technique.

Table 47.4 Laboratory Diagnosis of Tuberculosis.

CLINICAL SPECIMEN

Sputum/Laryngeal Swab/Gastric lavage
CSF
Aspirate/pleural/peritoneal
Biopsy from lesions, at operation
Pus from cold abscess, Urine

Mantoux (tuberculin) intradermal test.
Delayed hypersensitivity reaction
Not diagnostic in adults
Diagnostic significance only in early paediatric age group

→ DIRECT MICROSCOPY

Examination of Smear

1. Stained by Z-N method (50,000-1 lakh bacilli must be present in 1 ml. of sputum for positive finding)
2. Examination under fluorescent microscope after staining with Auramine

→ CONCENTRATION OF SPECIMEN

Different methods
Eg. Petroff's

Advantages :

1. Liquefy
2. Destroy other bacteria
3. Concentration of *M. tuberculosis*

→ MOLECULAR TECHNIQUES

1. PCR
2. Nucleic acid probes

Concentration of specimen →

CULTURE
L-J MEDIUM

4–12 Weeks

Growth within 10 days - atypical mycobacterium
Colonies of *M. tuberculosis* - rough, tough, buff
Confirmation of microscopy and Niacin test

↓

Drug sensitivity tests

ANIMAL INOCULATION
GUINEA PIG

IM into thigh 4–8 weeks

Autopsy findings :

1. Caseous local lesions
2. Caseous draining lymph nodes
3. Tuberculous lesions in different organs except kidney

NOTE : RENAL TUBERCULOSIS :

Centrifuged urine sediment of 24 hours sample or early morning sample on three successive days for microscopy. (Both acid fast and alcohol fast, culture on L-J medium and animal inoculation).

The smear is covered with strong carbol fuchsin and gently heated to steaming for 3–5 minutes, without allowing the stain to boil, evaporate and dry. The slide is then washed with water and decolorized with 20% H_2SO_4 till no more stain comes off and then with 95% ethanol for two minutes. Decolorisation may be carried out as a single step with acid-alcohol (3% HCl in 95% ethanol). After washing, the smear is counterstained with Loeffler's methylene blue, 1% picric acid or 0.2% malachite green for one minute. Under the oil immersion objective, acid-fast bacilli are seen as bright pink rods while the background is blue, yellow or green depending on the counterstain used.

It has been estimated that over 10,000 acid-fast bacilli per ml must be present for them to be readily demonstrable in direct smears. A negative report should not be given till atleast 100 fields have been examined, taking about 10 minutes. A positive report can be given only if two or more typical bacilli are seen. Smears are graded depending on the number of bacilli seen : 1+ when 3–9 bacilli are seen in the entire smear, 2+ when 10 or more bacilli are seen in the smear, and 3+ when 10 or more bacilli are seen in most oil immersion fields.

When several smears are to be examined daily, it is more convenient to use fluorescent microscopy. Smears are stained with auramine phenol or auramine rhodamine fluorescent dyes and when examined under UV illumination, the bacilli will appear as bright rods against a dark background. Because of the contrast, the bacilli can be seen even under the high dry power objective, enabling large areas of the smear to be screened rapidly.

Microscopic demonstration of acid-fast bacilli provides only presumptive evidence of tuberculosis. *M. tuberculosis* cannot be reliably distinguished on morphologic grounds from the occasional pathogens in the genus, from saprophytic mycobacteria or from those mycobacteria that may be part of the normal flora. Therefore, a definitive identification of *M. tuberculosis* can only be obtained by culturing the organism or by the molecular methods. However, most saprophytic species stain uniformly without appearing barred or beaded and are usually only acid-fast without being alcohol-fast. As saprophytic mycobacteria may be present in tap water, rubber tubes, cork or bark, they can get into clinical materials or may contaminate glassware and reagents in the laboratory.

Culture — Cultural method is very sensitive diagnostic technique for tubercle bacilli than direct microscopy and sputa which are negative by microscopy may become positive on culture, detecting as few as 10 to 100 bacilli per ml. Moreover, isolation of the organism is essential for determining its antibiotic sensitivity, in addition to confirming the specific identity of the bacillus by growth and biochemical characteristics. If the specimen is positive, a direct drug sensitivity test may also be set up.

The concentrated specimen is inoculated into atleast two bottles of LJ medium and incubated at 37ºC. Cultures are examined for growth for four days (for contaminant bacteria, fungi and rapid growing mycobacteria) and atleast twice weekly thereafter. A negative report is given if no growth occurs after 8–12 weeks. The medium should not be allowed to dry out during prolonged incubation. Therefore, screw-capped bottles are used.

Any growth seen is smeared and tested by ZN staining. For routine purposes, a slow growing, nonpigmented, niacin positive acid-fast bacillus is taken as *M. tuberculosis*. Confirmation is by detailed biochemical studies. When the isolate is niacin negative, a battery of tests may be needed for identification, including growth at 25ºC and 45ºC, animal pathogenicity and biochemical tests (Table 47.3).

Bactec-460 — It is a radiometric method based on the release of radioactive CO_2 from a labelled precursor by bacterial metabolism. The released gas is detected by periodic sampling of the air space over the medium by special instrument. The sensitivity testing is done by incorporation of drugs in the same media. It is a rapid, reliable but expensive method. Mycobacteria can be isolated from clinical samples by radiometric respirometry using the Bactec-460 TB instrument. The procedure utilizes vials containing ^{14}C-labelled palmitic acid substrate, which during microbial growth releases $^{14}CO_2$ into the atmosphere above the medium. The $^{14}CO_2$ is detected by the instrument and converted proportionally to a quantitative growth index (GI) on a scale of 0–999.

For mycobacterial isolation, the vial is inoculated with a specimen (decontaminated, concentrated and neutralized) and incubated and read at regular intervals on the instrument. By this method mycobacteria can be isolated in 2 weeks as opposed to 6 to 8 weeks by conventional egg media.

Bactec-460 TB instrument also allows the antibiotic sensitivity results to be produced in 1–2 weeks.

Sensitivity tests — As drug resistance is an important problem in tuberculosis, it is desirable to have sensitivity of isolates tested as an aid to treatment. Sensitivity tests for tubercle bacilli are mainly of three types.

(*i*) ***Absolute concentration method*** — In this method a number of media containing serial concentrations of the drugs are inoculated and the MIC is determined.

(*ii*) ***Resistance ratio method*** — In this method two sets of media containing graded concentrations of the drugs are inoculated, one set with the test strain and the other with a standard strain (H37RV strain of *M. tuberculosis*) of known sensitivity. The result is expressed as resistance ratio *i.e.,* the ratio of the MIC of the test strain to the MIC of strain with known sensitivity.

(*iii*) ***Proportion method*** — This method indicates the average sensitivity of the strain, taking into account the fact that any population will contain cells with varying degrees of sensitivity to a drug. In this method, the number of colonies growing from a standard inoculum on a drug-containing medium is compared with the colony count from same sized inoculum on a drug-free medium. The strain is regarded as resistant when more than 1% of the bacteria grow in the presence of the drug.

Animal Inoculation — The concentrated material is inoculated intramuscularly into the thigh of two healthy guinea pigs about 12 weeks old. Subcutaneous inoculation is not recommended as it leads to a local ulcer which may be infectious. The animals are weighed before inoculation and at intervals thereafter. Progressive loss of weight and a positive tuberculin skin reaction are indications of development of tuberculosis. One animal is killed after 4 weeks and if it shows no evidence of tuberculosis at autopsy, the other is killed after 8 weeks.

At autopsy, a positive animal will show a caseous lesion at the site of inoculation. Sometimes the local lesion may contain pus under tension, which may spurt on incision. The draining and internal lymph nodes are enlarged and caseous. The spleen is enlarged with irregular necrotic areas. Tubercles are seen in the peritoneum and sometimes in the lung, but the kidneys are unaffected. The autopsy lesions have to be confirmed as tuberculous by acid-fast staining of smears, to exclude *Yersinia pseudotuberculosis* and other bacterial and fungal infections which may resemble the lesions of tuberculosis.

Guinea pig inoculation was a popular method for the diagnosis of tuberculosis, but it is now seldom resorted to because it is cumbersome, expensive and less sensitive than culture. Moreover, the excretion of *M. tuberculosis* in the urine and feces of infected animals creates a health hazard. However, guinea pig inoculation is superior to culture for the isolation of *M. bovis* from clinical material.

Nucleic Acid Amplification — Molecular techniques are important in the diagnosis of tuberculosis, because they can detect and identify *M. tuberculosis* in clinical specimens, within a short time.

(*i*) The amplified *M. tuberculosis* direct test utilizes enzymes that rapidly make copies of *M. tuberculosis* 16S ribosomal RNA, which can be detected using nucleic acid probes. The sensitivity of the test ranges from 75 to 100 per cent, with a specificity of 95 to 100 per cent.

(*ii*) The polymerase chain reaction (PCR) amplifies a small portion of a predetermined target region of the *M. tuberculosis* DNA. Using human sputum, commercial PCR kits can confirm the diagnosis of tuberculosis within eight hours. In addition, PCR analysis facilitates DNA fingerprinting of specific strains, allowing studies of the progress of epidemics.

Serological tests — Serological tests are not useful in diagnosis, though antibodies to many bacillary antigens have been demonstrated in the sera of patients. Detection of antibody to mycobacterial lipoarabinomannan has been reported to be of some value. ELISA and latex agglutination tests are used.

Tuberculin test — Demonstration of delayed hypersensitivity to tuberculous protein by intradermal test is often used in the diagnosis.

Gas liquid chromatography — In tuberculous meningitis, detection of tuberculostearic acid by gas liquid chromatography in CSF is sensitive and specific.

Prophylaxis

General measures such as adequate nutrition, good housing and health education and public health measures such as tuberculin tests, chest X-rays, case registries and contact tracing, early detection and treatment of cases are important in the prevention of tuberculosis.

Immunoprophylaxis — Immunoprophylaxis is by intradermal injection of BCG vaccine developed by Calmette and Guerin (1921). It is a live attenuated vaccine. This is a strain of *M. bovis* attenuated by 239 serial subcultures in a glycerine-bite-potato medium over a period of 13 years. Injection of BCG in guinea pigs induces self-limited infection, with multiplication and dissemination of the bacillus in different organs and production of small tubercles.

The vaccine is given soon after birth or during the first year of life. It induces immunity and delayed hypersensitivity. Following BCG vaccination, a tuberculin negative recipient is converted to positive. The immunity may last for 10–15 years and is similar to the immunity following natural infection. BCG induces a nonspecific stimulation of the immune system providing some protection against leprosy and leukemia. The consenus opinion is that BCG may not protect from the risk of tuberculosis infection, but gives protection to infants and young children against the more serious type of the disease, such as meningitis and disseminated tuberculosis.

The complications of BCG vaccination are:

(*i*) Local — Abscess, indolent ulcer, keloid, tuberculides

(*ii*) Regional — Lymphadenitis

(*iii*) General — Fever, erythema nodosum

BCG vaccine is contraindicated in patients of tuberculosis, AIDS, measles, pertussis, eczema and patients on steroids and tuberculin positive individuals.

Chemoprophylaxis — For individuals who are tuberculin positive but asymptomatic, chemotherapy is indicated, usually with a single antibiotic, isoniazid. For example, tuberculin positive patients who need immunosuppressive therapy for another illness, can be protected from active tuberculosis by this treatment.

Treatment

Several chemotherapeutic agents are effective against *M. tuberculosis*. The antituberculous drugs rifampin, isoniazid, pyrazinamide, streptomycin, ethambutol and thiacetazone are the "first line" drugs because of their efficacy and acceptable degree of toxicity. Other drugs ethionamide, cycloserine, capreomycin, kanamycin and p-aminosalicylic acid are less often used.

In clinical practice, mutational drug resistance is a major problem in chemotherapy. Drug resistance may be 'primary' (before treatment) when the patient is infected with a strain of tubercle bacillus which is already resistant, or "acquired" (secondary, after treatment), when the infecting strain initially sensitive becomes resistant, usually as a result of inadequate treatment. This type of resistance is more common. A serious consequence of unchecked drug resistance has been the emergence and spread of "multidrug resistant tuberculosis (MDR-TB)". The term multidrug resistance, in the context of tuberculosis, specifically refers to resistance to rifampin and isoniazid, two first-line drugs. The presence of MDR-TB in those with concomitant HIV infection makes it more dangerous.

Multiple drug therapy is employed to delay or prevent the emergence of resistance. A combination of four drugs rifampin, pyrazinamide, isoniazid and ethambutol are given. MDR-TB can be treated with ethambutol, pyrazinamide and streptomycin (amikacin, if resistant to streptomycin).

"**Directly observed therapy under supervision (DOTS)**" strategy is at present implemented by WHO to control and prevent tuberculosis. This treatment is fully supervised to comply with the treatment regimen. DOTS can prevent deterioration of resistance problem in TB patients by ensuring the patient's compliance.

QUESTIONS

Essay Type Questions

1. Describe the morphology, cultural characteristics and pathogenicity of *Myco. tuberculosis*. Mention the lab. diagnosis of pulmonary tuberculosis.
2. Classify mycobacteria. Describe briefly *Myco. tuberculosis.*
3. Classify mycobacteria. Describe the lab. diagnosis of pulmonary tuberculosis.

Short Answer Type Questions

1. Classification of Mycobacteria.
2. Morphology of *Myco. tuberculosis.*
3. Much granules.
4. Z-N staining.
5. Cultivation of *Myco. tuberculosis.*
6. LJ medium.
7. Cord factor.
8. Niacin test.
9. Differences between *Myco. bovis* and *Myco. tuberculosis.*
10. Pathogenicity of tuberculosis.
11. Koch's phenomenon.
12. Tuberculin test.
13. Old tuberculin.
14. PPD.
15. Mantoux test.
16. Lab. diagnosis of pulmonary tuberculosis.
17. Petroff's method.
18. Bactec-460.
19. Sensitivity tests for Myco. tuberculosis.
20. BCG vaccine.
21. DOTS.

48

Atypical Mycobacteria

- *Introduction*
- *Classification*
- *Group-I Photochromogens*
- *Group-II Scotochromogens*
- *Group-III Non-chromogens*
- *Group-IV Rapid growers*
- *Differences between M. ulcerans and M. marinum*

INTRODUCTION

Several species of mycobacteria other than human or bovine tubercle bacilli and leprae bacilli, which are acid-fast and normally exist as saprophytes in soil and water and occasionally cause opportunistic chronic granulomatous disease, often resembling tuberculosis and produce a delayed hypersensitivity reaction that may or may not cross-react with tuberculoprotein are grouped together and referred to as atypical or environmental or opportunistic or nontuberculous mycobacteria or **MOTT** (Mycobacteria other than typical tubercle bacilli). They produce **aryl sulphatase** enzyme. In general, these species are not transmitted from human to human. Most are found in the soil and water, although they may have mammalian or avian reservoirs. They are sensitive to the same range of chemotherapeutic agents as is *M. tuberculosis*, but, in some cases they require higher doses and more aggressive treatment schedules.

Infections are usually asymptomatic, though it may result in sensitization, causing weak positive tuberculin reaction, due to cross reaction with tubercle bacillus protein. Tuberculins prepared from different environmental mycobacteria induce reactions of appropriate specificity. Sensitization with a typical mycobacteria is believed to influence the protective response to BCG vaccination. This may be one of the reasons for the wide variation in protective effect of the BCG vaccine.

An inverse relation seems to exist between tuberculosis and disease caused by environmental bacteria. Where tuberculosis is endemic, opportunistic mycobacterial disease is rare. Where tuberculosis is rare, environmental mycobacterial disease is more common.

Some species may colonize tap water *e.g., M. avium*, *M. kansasii*, *M. xenopi.* These may cause problems in the laboratory where they may to mistaken for tubercle bacilli.

CLASSIFICATION

Based on rate of growth and pigment production Runyon (1959) classified atypical mycobacteria in four groups (Table 48.1).

(*i*) Group-I Photochromogens

(*ii*) Group-II Scotochromogens

(*iii*) Group-III Non-chromogens

(*iv*) Group-IV Rapid growers

Table 48.1 Atypical Mycobacteria

Runyon group	*Name*	*Species*
Group-I	Photochromogens	*M. kansasii, M. marinum, M. simiae*
Group-II	Scotochromogens	*M. scrofulaceum, M. gordonae, M. szulgai*
Group-III	Non-chromogens	*M. avium, M. intracellulare, M. xenopi, M. ulcerans, M. malmoense*
Group-IV	Rapid growers	*M. chelonei, M. fortuitum*

GROUP-I PHOTOCHROMOGENS

They form colorless colonies (no pigment) when incubated in the dark, but when the young culture is exposed to light for one hour in the presence of air (cap of the culture bottle loosened) and reincubated for 24–48 hours, they develop a bright yellow or orange pigment (beta carotene). They are slow growing, though growth is faster than that of tubercle bacilli.

Photochromogenesis can be tested by inoculating the test organism on two slopes of LJ medium. One of them is wrapped in aluminium foil to exclude light from it and the other is left unwrapped and incubated at 37ºC in the presence of light for two weeks. If unwrapped culture shows a bright yellow or orange pigment, which is absent in wrapped culture, the test organism is photochromogenic.

The important species in this group are *M. kansasii*, *M. marinum* and *M. simiae.*

M. kansasii is a photochromogen that causes chronic pulmonary, lymph node and other systemic diseases, resembling tuberculosis, particularly in old persons with pre-existing lung disease. Infections are more common in cities and industrial areas. The bacilli have been isolated from soil, milk and piped water supplies. It grows well at 37ºC on LJ medium and produces a good growth within two weeks. It reduces nitrate to nitrite. The bacterial cells are usually elongated and have a distinct beaded appearance. The delayed hypersensitivity that develops is strongly cross-reactive with standard PPD, and the organism is susceptible to rifampin and other standard antituberculous drugs.

M. marinum is a natural pathogen of cold blooded animals, causing tuberculosis in fish and amphibia. It may also occur as a saprophyte in fresh or salt water. Human infection originates from contaminated swimming pools or fish tanks, known as "*swimming pool granuloma*" or "fish tank granuloma", characterized by a warty skin lesion. The lesion begins as a papule and breaks down to form an indolent ulcer following abrasions, that occur particularly on prominences — elbows, knees, ankles, nose, fingers or toes. The organism is widely distributed in temperate areas. It is not pathogenic for guinea pigs but intradermal inoculation in rabbits leads to a superficial granulomatous lesion. Foot pad inoculation in mice leads to a more severe lesion, with local inflammation being followed by a purulent ulcer formation. Infection with *M. marinum* may cause a low grade tuberculin reaction.

M. marinum closely resembles *M. kansasii* but can be differentiated by its poor growth at 37ºC (grows well at 30ºC), failure to reduce nitrate, and failure to produce catalase and positive pyrazinamide hydrolase and L-fucosidase activities.

M. simiae was originally isolated from monkeys, have been associated with pulmonary disease in humans. It grows well at 37ºC. They produce niacin and may be falsely identified as *M. tuberculosis*.

GROUP-II SCOTOCHROMOGENS

They form pigmented colonies (yellow-orange-red) when incubated in the dark. They are widely distributed in the environment and sometimes contaminate cultures of tubercle bacilli.

M. scrofulaceum is a common cause of chronic cervical lymphadenitis (scrofula) in children, and a rare cause of other granulomatous conditions. It tends to be resistant to antituberculous drugs like isoniazid, but sensitive to cycloserine and ethionamide. Surgical excision of infected cervical nodes is curative. The bacilli may be short or long and filamentous.

M. gordonae, often found in tap water (hence called "the tap water scotochromogen") is a common contaminant in clinical specimens and a rare cause of pulmonary disease. It differs from *M. scrofulaceum* in failing to hydrolyze urea, nicotinamide and pyrazinamide.

M. szulgai is a scotochromogen when incubated at 37ºC and photochromogen at 25ºC. It may occasionally cause pulmonary disease and bursitis.

GROUP-III NON-CHROMOGENS

They do not form pigment even on exposure to light. The medically important species are *M. avium*, *M. intracellulare*, *M. xenopi*, *M. malmoense* and the skin pathogen *M. ulcerans*.

M. intracellulare is commonly known as "**Battey bacillus**", because it was first identified as a human pathogen at the Battey state hospital for tuberculosis, Georgia, USA. The infection with this organism is common in south-east USA, where the organism occurs in soil and water. It infects a variety of mammals including humans.

M. avium causes tuberculosis in birds and lymphadenopathy in pigs. It cannot infect humans. It can grow best at 41°C (thermophile). Colonies of both these species are smooth, non-pigmented and easily emulsifiable. Both are common as opportunistic human pathogens.

M. avium and *M. intracellulare* are so closely similar that they have been grouped together as ***M. avium-intracellulare (MAI)*** or ***M. avium complex (MAC),*** which can be divided into a number of serotypes with variable ecologies. Based on agglutination, this complex is divided into 28 serotypes. Types 1, 2, and 3 are regarded as *M. avium* and the others as *M. intracellulare*. MAC causes pulmonary disease resembling tuberculosis, lymphadenitis and disseminated (miliary) disease, now recognized as a common opportunistic infection in AIDS patients. Extensive pulmonary MAC infections are sometimes superimposed on chronic bronchitis or emphysema, cervical lymphadenitis, chronic osteomyelitis and renal or skin infections occur, usually following some compromise of the tissues. Diseases caused by MAC are particularly refractory to chemotherapy. The usual practice is to treat with four or more drugs, regardless of sensitivity determinations. Relapses are common.

M. xenopi was first isolated from a skin lesion in a South African toad (*Xenopus laevis*). It is a thermophile and grows well at 45ºC. It may cause chronic pulmonary lesions in man. Though it is a nonchromogen, it may form scotochromogenic yellow colonies. It has been isolated from water taps, mostly hot water taps in hospitals.

M. ulcerans, the causative agent of Buruli ulcer, was originally isolated from ulcerative skin lesions in Australia in 1948. The name Buruli ulcer is derived from the Buruli district of Uganda, where a large outbreak of the disease occurred. Ulcers are usually seen on the legs or arms and are believed to follow infection through minor injuries. After an incubation period of a few weeks, indurated nodules appear, which break down forming indolent ulcers, which slowly extend under the skin. Initially, smears from the edge of the ulcer show large clumps of bacilli which are acid-fast and alcohol-fast. Later, the immunoreactive phase sets in and the bacilli disappear. The ulcers then heal with disfigurement.

M. ulcerans grows slowly in 4–8 weeks on LJ medium at 30–33°C but not at 25°C or 37°C. Inoculation into the foot pad of mice leads to edema of the limb though ulceration is infrequent. *M. ulcerans* produces an exotoxin, a high molecular weight phospholipoprotein-lipopolysaccharide complex, which causes inflammation and necrosis when injected into the skin of guinea pigs. This is the only known instance of toxin produced by any *Mycobacterium* species.

M. malmoense causes pulmonary disease and lymphadenitis. It was first isolated from patients at Malmo in Sweden. It is a very slow growing and colonies may appear after ten weeks incubation. It is resistant to standard antituberculous drugs such as rifampin, isoniazid and sometimes to streptomycin and ethambutol.

M. terrae, *M. triviale* and *M. chromogenicum* are rare pathogens of Group-III (nonchromogens) and are referred to as *Mycobacterium terrae-triviale-nonchromogenicum* group.

GROUP-IV RAPID GROWERS

It is a heterogenous group of mycobacteria capable of rapid growth, colonies appearing within seven days of incubation at 37°C or 25°C. Within the group, photochromogenic, scotochromogenic and nonchromogenic species occur. All the chromogenic rapid growers are saprophytes *e.g.*, *M. smegmatis, M. phlei.*

M. smegmatis forms rough colonies, white to buff in color. The bacilli are slender rods, which may be curved and beaded. Since they are normally present in smegma, a whitish secretion around the orifice of urethra, it is frequently encountered as a contaminant in urine specimens. Some strains are acid-fast but not alcohol-fast. Therefore, they are not seen in ZN smears when acid-alcohol is used as decolorizer. Other strains are both acid-fast and alcohol-fast. They can be differentiated from *M. tuberculosis* by their rapid growth on LJ medium and animal pathogenicity test by guinea pig inoculation. M. smegmatis has been implicated in rare cases of pulmonary, skin, soft tissue and bone infections.

M. phlei is a non-pathogen and rarely encountered. They form rough colonies, which are buff colored at first and become yellow to orange later. It can be differentiated from *M. smegmatis* by its ability to grow at 52°C and survive heating at 60°C for 4 hours.

The medically important rapid growers are *M. fortuitum* and *M. chelonei* (chelonae), both of which can cause chronic abscesses in human beings. Outbreaks of abscesses following injection of vaccines and other preparations (drug abusers) contaminated by these mycobacteria have been reported. They are found in the soil and infection usually follows some injury. They occasionally cause pulmonary or disseminated disease. They form white to cream colored colonies and do not produce any pigment. Both of them are coccoid to filamentous. *M. chelonae* grows better at 25°C than at 37°C. M. fortuitum can further be differentiated from *M. chelonei* in reducing nitrate and assimilation of iron from ferric ammonium citrate. *M. chelonie* was originally identified as turtle tubercle bacilli and *M. fortuitum* as frog tubercle bacilli. Pulmonary lesions caused by *M. fortuitum* cannot be distinguished radiologically from typical tuberculosis. No effective chemotherapy is available.

A rapid grower, ***M. vaccae*** is an immunomodulator and acts as an adjuvant stimulating protective immune responses in tuberculosis and inhibits hypersensitivity reactions.

Some noncultivable or poorly growing mycobacteria identified from the blood of AIDS patients have been characterized by their 16S RNA base sequence. They grow sparsely in some liquid media *e.g., M. genevense, M. confluentis* and *M. intermedium*.

DIFFERENCES BETWEEN *M. ULCERANS* AND *M. MARINUM*

Two species of mycobacteria, *M. ulcerans* and *M. marinum* are exclusively skin pathogens, causing chronic ulcers and granulomatous lesions on the skin. Systemic invasion does not occur and the regional lymph glands are not involved. Cutaneous localization is because they multiply optimally at skin temperature.

	M. ulcerans	*M. marinum*
Distribution	Tropics	Temperate areas
Clinical course	Chronic progressive ulcer	Self-limited ulcer
Bacilli in ulcer	Abundant	Scanty
Rate of growth	Slower, 4–8 weeks	Faster, 1–2 weeks
Growth at 25°C	–	+
Growth at 37°C	–	+
Culture film	Bacilli in cords	No cord formation
Pigment in light	–	+
Mouse foot pad inoculation	Edema, rarely ulcer	Marked inflammation-purulent ulcer

QUESTIONS

Essay Type Questions

1. Classify mycobacteria. Give a brief account of atypical mycobacteria.

Short Answer Type Questions

1. Atypical mycobacteria.
2. Photochromogens or Group-I atypical mycobacteria.
3. *M. marinum* or Swimming pool granuloma.
4. Scotochromogens or Group-II atypical mycobacteria.
5. Non-chromogens or Group-III atypical mycobacteria.
6. MAC or *M. avium-intracellulare* complex.
7. Battey bacillus.
8. *M. ulcerans.*
9. Rapid growers or Group-IV atypical mycobacteria.
10. Mycobacteria causing skin ulcers.
11. *M. smegmatis.*

49

Mycobacterium leprae
(Hansen's bacillus)

- *Introduction*
- *Morphology*
- *Cultivation*
- *Antigenic structure*
- *Resistance*
- *Epidemiology*
- *Pathogenicity*
- *Immunity*
- *Lepromin test*
- *Laboratory diagnosis*
- *Prophylaxis*
- *Treatment*
- *M. lepraemurium*

INTRODUCTION

Mycobacterium leprae, the causative agent of leprosy was discovered by Hansen (1874) in Norway. Though this was the first bacterial pathogen of humans to be described, it remains one of the least understood. This is because, the leprae bacilli cannot grow on artificial laboratory media.

MORPHOLOGY

M. leprae is a straight or slightly curved slender bacillus, measuring 3 × 0.3 μm size (average). Polar bodies and other intracellular elements may be present. They have pointed, rounded or club-shaped ends. It is Gram positive and stains more readily than the tubercle bacillus. It is acid-fast but less than tubercle bacillus. Hence 5% H_2SO_4 is employed for decolorisation in ZN staining.

The bacilli are seen singly and in groups intracellularly or lying free outside the cells. Inside the host cells, they are usually present in parallel bundles of 50 or more organisms, known as "agglomerates", the bacilli being bound together by a lipid-like substance, the glia. These masses of bacteria are known as "globi" which are seen inside the histiocytes which have a foamy appearance and are known as **"lepra cells"**. The parallel rows of bacilli in the globi present a "cigar bundle" appearance. In tissue sections, the clumps of bacilli resemble cigarette ends.

Live bacilli in the smear appear solid and uniformly stained, while dead or dying bacilli appear fragmented, beaded and granular. The percentage of uniformly stained bacilli in tissues is known as "morphological index (MI)". This provides a method for assessing the progress of patients on chemotherapy and is more meaningful than the old criterion, the "bacteriological index (BI)". BI is the total number of acid-fast bacilli seen under oil immersion field in a smear. It is expressed 1+ to 6+ by Ridley's scale. A continuing decrease in the MI is encouraging but a decrease followed by rise indicates development of drug resistance.

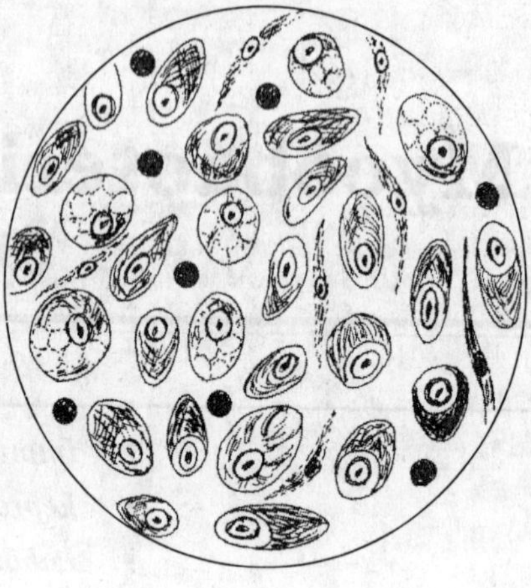

Fig. 49.1 Leprae bacilli.

CULTIVATION

Leprae bacilli cannot grow either in bacteriological media or in tissue culture. Shepard (1960) reported that leprae bacilli could multiply in the foot pads of mice kept at a low temperature (20ºC). Following intradermal inoculation into the foot pads of mice, a granuloma develops at the site in 1–6 months.

Leprae bacilli are able to produce a generalized infection simulating lepromatous leprosy in nude mice. **Nude mice** are those in which cell mediated immunity is suppressed either by thymectomy or by administration of antilymphocyte serum (ALS). These nude mice are used to propagate leprae bacilli.

The nine-banded armadillo (*Dasypus novemcinctus*) is highly susceptible to infection with leprae bacilli. Following inoculation into armadilloes, a generalized infection occurs with extensive multiplication of the bacilli and production of lesions typical of lepromatous leprosy. Some wild armadilloes in captivity have been observed to be naturally infected with a *Mycobacterium* resembling the lepra bacillus. Natural disease has also been identified in chimpanzees and mangabey monkeys from West Africa but it is not known whether they have any relevance to human infection.

In animal experiments, the generation time of the lepra bacillus has been found to be exceptionally long. 12–13 days on the average but may vary from 8–42 days, in comparison with about 14 hours in the case of tubercle bacilli and about 20 minutes in the case of coliform bacilli.

ANTIGENIC STRUCTURE

M. leprae genome has been mapped and the genes for its major protein antigens cloned and sequenced.

Lipoarabinomannan-B (LAM-B), present in cell wall is a dominant antigen of *M. leprae.* It is strongly antigenic and is used in the serodiagnosis of leprosy. It is distinct from lipoarabinomannan of *M. tuberculosis* from which it can be differentiated by monoclonal antibodies.

Pheonlic glycolipid-1 (PGL-1), a major component of outermost layer of cell wall protects the organism against host cell enzymes. It suppresses CMI. Patients with *M. leprae* infection develop antibodies against polysaccharide component of PGL-1. The latter and synthetic trisaccharide attached to bovine serum albumin have been used for the serodiagnosis of leprosy.

RESISTANCE

Leprae bacilli are able to remain viable in a warm humid environment for 9–16 days and in moist soil for 46 days. They survive exposure to direct sunlight for two hours and UV light for 30 minutes.

EPIDEMIOLOGY

Leprosy is an exclusively human disease and the only source of infection is the patient. Very large numbers of bacilli are shed in the nasal secretions and in discharges from superficial lesions of the lepromatous leprosy cases. The mode of entry may be either through the respiratory tract or through the skin.

Leprosy is not highly communicable. *M. leprae* is transmitted from human to human through prolonged contact, for example, between exudates of a leprosy patient's skin lesions, and the abraded skin of another individual. The infectivity of *M. leprae* is low, and the incubation period is very long (average 2–5 years but vary from a few months to as long as 30 years), so that clinical disease may develop years or even decades after initial contact with the organism.

PATHOGENICITY

Leprosy (Hansen's disease) is a chronic granulomatous disease of humans primarily involving the skin, peripheral nerves and nasal mucosa but capable of affecting and tissue or organ.

The disease may be classified into four types (Madrid, 1953) — lepromatous, tuberculoid, dimorphous and indeterminate.

Ridley and Jopling (1966) have introduced a scale for classifying the spectrum of leprosy into five groups, based on clinical, histopathological and immunological findings — tuberculoid (TT), borderline tuberculoid (BT), borderline (BB), borderline lepromatous (BL) and lepromatous (LL).

The type of disease is a reflection of the immune status of the host, and therefore not permanent and varies with chemotherapy and alterations in host resistance.

The bacilli invades peripheral nerves and skin cells and becomes an obligate intracellular parasite. It is most frequently found in Schwann cells that surround peripheral nerve axons and in mononuclear macrophages. The earliest symptom of leprosy is slightly pigmented skin eruption (several cms in diameter). Approximately, 75% of all individuals with this early solitary lesion heal spontaneously because of the CMI to *M. leprae*. However, in some CMI may be so weak that the disease progresses. The two extreme or polar forms of the disease are the lepromatous and tuberculoid types.

Lepromatous leprosy — The course of the disease is slow, but progressive. It is seen in persons whose resistance is low. The bacilli are seen in large numbers or as globi inside lepra cells or extracellularly. Superficial nodular lesions (lepromata) develop, ulcerate, become secondarily infected and cause distortion and mutilation. Bacilli invade the mucosa of the nose, mouth and upper respiratory tract and are shed in large numbers in nasal and oral secretions. The reticuloendothelial system, eyes, testes, kidneys and bones are also involved. Bacteremia is common. The lepromatous type is more infective than other types. The prognosis is poor. Cell mediated immunity is deficient and the lepromin test is negative. There is an exaggerated and broad humoral immune response. Antibodies in high titres are seen against mycobacterial as well as other antigens. Autoantibodies are common. Most cases show biological false positive reaction in standard serological tests for syphilis.

Tuberculoid leprosy — At the other end of the spectrum is tuberculoid leprosy, seen in patients with high degree of resistance. Lesions occur as large maculae (spots) in cooler body tissues such as skin (especially nose and outer ears, testicles), and in superficial nerve endings. Skin lesions are a few and consist of sharply demarcated, nonelevated hypo- or hyperpigmented macular anaesthetic patches involving the face, trunk and limbs. Neural involvements occurs and may be pronounced, leading to deformities in hands and feet. Bacilli are scanty in the lesions and infectivity is minimal. CMI is adequate and lepromin test is positive. Antimycobacterial and autoantibodies are rare. The prognosis is good.

Table 49.1 Differences between Lepromatous and Tuberculoid Types

Lepromatous leprosy	*Tuberculoid leprosy*
1. Seen in persons whose resistance is low.	Seen in persons whose resistance is high.
2. The bacilli are seen in large numbers. Multibacillary disease.	The bacilli are scanty in lesions. Paucibacillary disease.
3. Highly infectious. Bacilli invade mucosa of nose, mouth and upper respiratory tract and are shed in large numbers in nasal and oral secretions.	Less infectious.
4. Superficial nodules (lepromata) develop on skin, which may ulcerate become secondarily infected causing distortion and mutilation.	Skin lesions are a few, consisting of macular anaesthetic patches. Neural involvement occurs and may be pronounced leading to deformities in hands and feet.
5. CMI is deficient.	CMI is adequate.
6. Lepromin test is negative.	Lepromin test is positive.
7. Antibodies are present in high titres.	Antibodies are rare.
8. Autoantibodies are common.	Autoantibodies are rare.
9. Prognosis is poor.	Prognosis is good.

Borderline or dimorphous leprosy — It refers to lesions possessing characteristics of both tuberculoid and lepromatous types. It may shift either to the lepromatous or tuberculoid type depending on chemotherapy and alterations in host resistance.

Indeterminate leprosy — It is an early, unstable tissue reaction, which is not characteristic of either the lepromatous or the tuberculoid type. In many persons, these lesion may undergo spontaneous healing. In some, the lesions may progress to tuberculoid or lepromatous types.

Though leprosy is a chronic disease, its course is sometimes interspersed with acute exacerbations which are of an allergic nature due to immune reactions. These are of two types.

Type 1 (Reversal reaction) — This occurs in borderline cases (BT, BB, BL) who develop cell mediated immunity and consequently shift towards tuberculoid type. There is erythema and swelling skin lesions which may undergo ulceration. The lesions are infiltrated with lymphocytes and epitheloid cells with reduction in number of bacilli. It may rapidly cause severe and permanent nerve damage.

Type 2 (Erythema nodosum leprosum) — This is usually seen in lepromatous leprosy patients undergoing chemotherapy. Crops of red nodules appear in the skin, lasting for 1 or 2 days, with intense neutrophilic infiltration and the blood vessels in the dermis show acute fibrinoid necrosis. Fever, arthritis, iridocyclitis, orchitis and painful neuritis are common.

When bacilli die, mycobacterial antigens may be released into the circulation, which may combine with antibodies present in blood leading to an immune complex disease similar to Arthus phenomenon.

IMMUNITY

A high degree of innate immunity against leprae bacilli seems to exist in humans so that only a minority of those infected develop clinical disease. *M. leprae* infection induces both humoral and cellular immune responses. Of these, CMI is protective. The type of leprosy in an individual is determined by the status of CMI in that person. When it is adequate, the lesions are of tuberculoid type. The patient exhibits a strong delayed type hypersensitivity to lepromin. The macrophages phagocytose the bacilli and destroy them. Specific humoral antibodies are not prominent. There is no increase in the Ig level and the albumin:globulin ratio in the serum is not altered.

When CMI is deficient, the lepromatous type of disease develops. Delayed hypersensitivity is absent. The macrophages phagocytose the bacilli but instead of being destroyed, the bacilli proliferate inside the cells. The albumin:globulin ratio in the serum is altered. In lepromatous leprosy, there is extensive polyclonal B cell activation with large amounts of antibodies being produced, both antimycobacterial and autoimmune. The antimycobacterial antibodies are not beneficial.

The deficiency in CMI is specific to the antigens of leprae bacilli. Lepromatous patients are not susceptible to viruses, parasites and other intracellular pathogens against which CMI is important. Tuberculin reactivity may be suppressed in untreated lepromatous patients, but it becomes positive following treatment, unlike the lepromin response which remains negative.

Lepromatous patients have large numbers of CD8+ lymphocytes in circulation, which can be specificially activated by antigens of leprae bacilli. The lymphocytes present in skin granulomas are almost exclusively CD8+ cells, in contrast to tuberculoid lesions which contain predominantly CD4 + cells.

There is evidence of genetic effect in the pattern of response to leprae bacillus infection. HLA-DRZ is seen in persons with tuberculoid type, whereas HLA-MT1 and HLA-DQ1 are associated with leptomatous type.

LEPROMIN TEST

It was first described by Mitsuda in Japan 1919. The lepromins used as antigen in lepromin test may be of human origin (lepromin-H) or of Armadillo origin (lepromin-A) and are of two types.

(*i*) ***Integral lepromin (Mitsuda lepromin)*** — This was the original antigen developed by Mitsuda (1919). It is a boiled, emulsified, lepromatous tissue rich in leprae bacilli. Standard Mitsuda lepromin contains 4×10^7 leprae bacilli per ml and has a shelf life of 2 years at 4°C. Mitsuda lepromin is increasingly being prepared from Armadillo-derived leprae bacilli (lepromin-A), replacing human derived lepromin.

(*ii*) ***Bacillary lepromin*** — It contains more of bacillary components and less of tissue. *e.g.*, Dharmendra antigen, which is prepared by floating out the bacilli from finely ground lepromatous tissue with chloroform, evaporating it dry and removing the lipids by washing in ether. The antigen is made up in phenol saline for use.

The response to the intradermal injection of 0.1 ml of lepromin is typically biphasic, consisting of two separate events.

(*i*) ***Early reaction of Fernandez*** — It consists of erythema and induration developing in 24–48 hours and usually remaining for 3–5 days. This is analogous to tuberculin reaction. This reaction indicates that the patient has been infected at some time in the past and is a measure of pre-existing delayed hypersensitivity. Therefore, it carries no significance.

(*ii*) ***Late reaction of Mitsuda*** — It starts in 1–2 weeks, reaching a peak in 3–4 weeks after the injection, in the form of a nodule that may undergo central necrosis and ulceration, and gradually subsides in the next few weeks. This reaction does not indicate preexisting delayed hypersensitivity but is a measure of the CMI induced by the injected lepromin itself. It thus distinguishes between persons who can mount a CMI response against leprae bacillus antigens and those who cannot. Therefore, this test is more meaningful to determine lepromin positivity.

The lepromin test is not used to diagnose leprosy, nor does it indicate prior contact with the leprae bacilli. Healthy persons in nonendemic areas with no change of contact with the bacillus may give a positive lepromin test. The test is employed for the following purposes.

1. To classify the lesions of leprosy patients. The lepromin test is positive in tuberculoid, negative in lepromatous and variable in dimorphous and indeterminate types of disease.
2. To assess the prognosis and response to treatment. A positive reaction indicates good prognosis and a negative one bad prognosis. Conversion to lepromin positivity during treatment is evidence of improvement.
3. To assess the resistance of individuals to leprosy. It is desirable to recruit only lepromin positive persons for work in leprosaria as lepromin negative persons are more prone to develop the disease.
4. To verify the identity of candidate *M. Leprae*. Cultivable acid-fast bacilli claimed to be *M. leprae* should give matching results when tested in parallel with standard lepromin.

LABORATORY DIAGNOSIS

Specimens are collected from the nasal mucosa, skin lesions and ear lobules by "slit and scrape method". A blunt, narrow scalpel is introduced into the nose and the internal septum scraped sufficiently to remove a piece of mucous membrane, which is transferred to a slide and teased out into an uniform smear. Samples from the skin should be obtained from the edges of the lesion, rather than from the centre. The skin is pinched up tight to minimise bleeding and a cut about 5 mm long made with a scalpel, deep enough to get into the infiltrated layers. After wiping off blood or lymph that may have exuded, the scalpel blade is turned transversely to scrape the sides and bottom of the cut so as to obtain a little tissue pulp which is smeared uniformly on a slide. About 5–6 different areas of the skin should be sampled, including the skin over the buttocks, forehead, chin, cheeks and ears. Biopsy of nodular lesions and thickened nerves, and lymph node puncture may be necessary in some cases.

Microscopy — The diagnosis consists of a demonstration of acid-fast bacilli in the lesions. The smears are stained by Ziehl-Neelsen's technique using 5% H_2SO_4, instead of 20% H_2SO_4 for decolorisation. The smears are examined under the microscope. Based on the number of bacilli, the smears are graded and Bacteriological Index (BI) and Morphological Index (MI) are determined.

In tuberculoid leprosy, organisms are extremely rare, and diagnosis depends on clinical findings and the histology of biopsy material.

Animal inoculation — Mouse foot pad inoculation has been reported to be more sensitive than skin slit smears for detection of leprae bacilli in tissues. Injection of ground tissue from lepromatous nodules into the foot pads of mice produces typical granuloma at the site of inoculation in 1–6 months. But this is unsuitable for routine diagnosis and feasible only for drug potency or resistance testing and research studies.

Table 49.2 Bacteriological Index (Ridley's scale)

Bacteriological Index	*No. of Acid-fast bacilli*
1+	1–10 bacilli per 100 oil immersion fields
2+	1–10 bacilli per 10 oil immersion fields
3+	1–10 bacilli per oil immersion field
4+	10–100 bacilli per oil immersion field
5+	100–1000 bacilli per oil immersion field
6+	More than 1000 bacilli, clumps per oil immersion field

Nine-banded Armadillo is highly susceptible to leprosy. Following inoculation of ground tissue from lepromatous nodules and nasal scrapings from leprosy patient, develops generalized infection with extensive multiplication of bacilli and the lesions produced resemble lepromatous leprosy. The lesions which develop in the mouse and armadillo can be identified by histopathological examination and ZN staining.

Serology — Detection of antibodies against phenolic glycolipid –1 antigen by latex agglutination test, ELISA has been claimed to be a specific diagnostic test.

PROPHYLAXIS

Case finding, early diagnosis and treatment and long term chemoprophylaxis in child contacts of infectious cases are the methods employed for prophylaxis. The vaccination with BCG has shown some protective effect in leprosy.

TREATMENT

Several drugs are effective in the treatment of leprosy, including sulfones such as dapsone, rifampin and clofazamine. Treatment is prolonged, and combined multiple drug therapy is necessary to ensure the suppression of resistant mutants. Thalidomide, an inhibitor of TNF-α, is being distributed under tight restrictions for use as treatment for erythema nodosum leprosum, a serious and severe skin complication of leprosy (Note: Thalidomide, originally marketed in the late 1050s as a sedative for pregnant women, was linked to severe limb deformities in their offspring, and was removed from the market).

MYCOBACTERIUM LEPRAEMURIUM

It is a causative agent of rat leprosy and was first described by Stefansky in 1901 at Odessa. The disease exists in two forms — the glandular type and the musculocutaneous type. In the glandular type, one or more groups of subcutaneous lymph nodes such as inguinal, axillary and cervical are enlarged. In the musculocutaneous type, there is emaciation, ulceration and loss of hair.

Acid-fast bacilli resembling lepra bacilli are found in the lesions in large numbers in the mononuclear cells of the subcutaneous tissues, lymph nodes and nodules in the liver and lungs. However, the disease differs from human leprosy in that the nerves are not affected. DNA studies revealed that *M. leprae* and *M. lepraemurium* are not related species but there is a relatedness between *M. avium* and *M. lepraemurium*.

M. lepraemurium is not easily cultivated *in vitro*. It is grown on Ogawa's egg-yolk medium, pH 5.8–6.3 at 37°C, by using large inocula. It is also grown on rat fibroblast cell culture.

QUESTIONS

Essay Type Questions

1. Describe mycobacteria. Discuss the aetiology, pathogenesis and lab. diagnosis of leprosy.

Short Answer Type Questions

1. Morphology of *M. leprae.*
2. Cultivation of leprae bacilli.
3. Nude mice.
4. Armadillo.
5. Pathogenicity of *Myco. leprae.*
6. Lepromatous leprosy.
7. Tuberculoid leprosy.
8. Differences between lepromatous and tuberculoid leprosy.
9. Lepromin test.
10. Lab. diagnosis of leprosy.
11. *M. lepraemurium.*

50

Bacillus

INTRODUCTION

Species of the genus *Bacillus* are Gram positive, aerobic and form endospores. They are ubiquitous, being found in soil, water, dust and air and are usually encountered in the medical laboratory as airborne contaminants. The genus includes psychrophilic, mesophilic and thermophilic species. *Bacillus anthracis*, the cause of the disease anthrax is an important pathogen. *B. cereus* can cause food-borne gastroenteritis. Some species may produce opportunistic infections. *Bacillus stearothermophilus* spores are used to check the efficiency of autoclaving.

BACILLUS ANTHRACIS (Anthrax bacilli)

It was the first pathogenic bacterium to be observed under the microscope by Pollender (1849). It was the first communicable disease shown to be transmitted by inoculation of infected blood by Davaine (1850). It was the first bacillus to be isolated in pure culture and shown to possess spores by Robert Koch (1876). It was the first bacterium used for the preparation of an attenuated vaccine by Louis Pasteur (1881).

Morphology

It is Gram positive and largest pathogenic bacillus measuring 3–10μ in length and 1–1.5μ in diameter. In tissues, it is found singly, in pairs or in short chains, the entire chain being surrounded by a capsule. The capsule is polypeptide in nature, being composed of a polymer of d (–) glutamic acid. Capsules are not formed under ordinary conditions of culture but only on media containing serum or bicarbonate in the presence of excess (10–25%) CO_2. When blood films containing anthrax bacilli are stained with polychrome methylene blue for a few seconds and examined under the microscope, an amorphous purplish material is noticed around the bacilli. This represents the capsular material and is characteristic of the anthrax bacillus. This is called the **M'Fadyean's reaction** and is employed for the presumptive diagnosis of anthrax in animals.

The anthrax bacillus is nonmotile, unlike most other species of the genus. In cultures, the bacilli are arranged end to end in long chains. The ends of the bacilli are truncated or often concave and somewhat swollen so that a chain of bacilli presents a **"bamboo stick"** appearance. It is nonacid-fast.

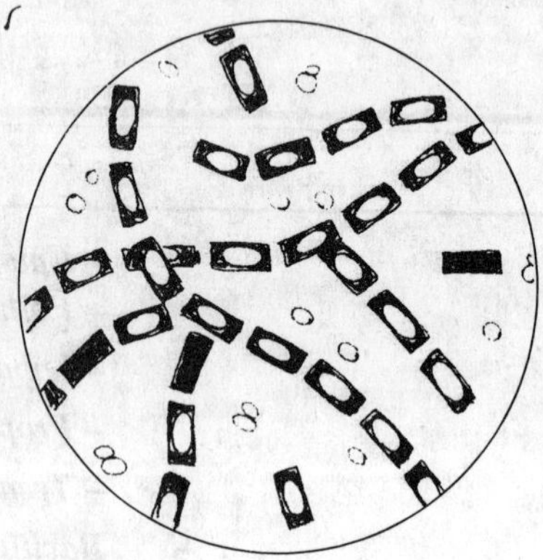

Fig. 50.1 Anthrax bacilli showing bamboo stick appearance.

Spores are formed in culture or in the soil but never in the animal body during life. Sporulation occurs under unfavourable conditions for growth and is encouraged by distilled water, 2% NaCl or growth in oxalated agar. Oxygen is required for sporulation, but not for germination. Sporulation is inhibited by calcium chloride. Spores are central, elliptical or oval in shape, and are of same width as the bacillary body so that they do not cause bulging of the vegetative cell.

When stained with Giemsa's satin, the bacillus stains purple and capsule red.

Cultural characteristics

It is an aerobe and facultative anaerobe. The optimum temperature for growth is 37ºC, but growth occurs over a wide temperature range of 12–45ºC. Optimum pH for growth is 7.0–7.4. Good growth occurs on ordinary media.

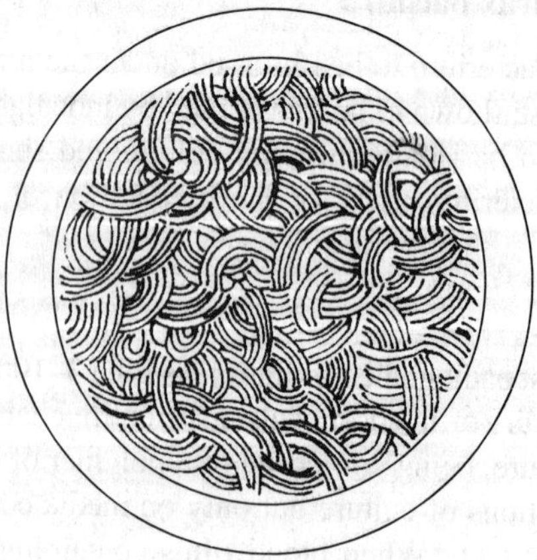

Fig. 50.2 Medusa head colony of anthrax bacillus.

On nutrient agar, the colonies are 2–3 mm in diameter raised, opaque, greyish-white, with an irregular fringe-like edge with a frosted glass appearance. Under low power of the microscope, the edge of the colony is composed of long, interlacing chains of bacilli, resembling locks of matted hair. This is called the **"Medusa head"** appearance. Virulent capsulated strains form rough colonies, while avirulent or attenuated strains form smooth colonies.

On blood agar, weak hemolysis may be produced. In gelatin stab cultures, a characteristic **"inverted fir tree"** appearance is seen, with slow liquefaction commencing from the top. In broth, growth occurs, as floccular deposit, with little or no turbidity.

When *B. anthracis* is grown on the surface of agar medium containing penicillin (0.05–0.5 units/ml), the cells become large, spherical and occur in chains on the surface of the agar within 3–6 hours, resembling a **"string of pearls"**. This string of pearls reaction differentiates *B. anthracis* from *B. cereus* and other aerobic spore bearers. Another useful test to differentiate between the two is the susceptibility of *B. anthracis* to gamma phage.

A selective medium called PLET medium consisting of polymyxin, lysozyme, ethylene diamine tetra acetic acid (EDTA) and thallous acetate, added to heart infusion agar, has been used to isolate *B. anthracis* from mixtures containing other spore-bearing bacilli.

Biochemical reactions

B. anthracis ferments glucose, sucrose, maltose and dextrin, with the production of acid but no gas. Nitrate is reduced to nitrite, catalase is produced and VP test is positive.

Resistance

The vegetative bacilli are destroyed at 60°C in 30 minutes. In the animal carcass, died of anthrax, the bacilli remain viable in the bone marrow for a week and in the skin for two weeks. Normal heat fixation of smears may not kill the bacilli in blood films.

The spores are highly resistant to adverse physical and chemical conditions. In the soil, in dry state, the spores can remain viable for many years, sometimes for decades and serve as a source of infection for long periods of time. They resist dry heat at 140°C for 1–3 hours and boiling for 10 minutes. With moist heat, spores are killed at 100°C in 10 minutes. Four per cent potassium permanganate kills spores in 15 minutes.

Destruction of the spores in animal products is achieved by "duckering" in which formaldehyde is used as 2% solution at 30–40°C for 20 minutes for disinfection of wool and as 0.25 per cent at 60°C for six hours for animal hair and bristles.

Antigenic structure

Two virulence factors have been identified – the capsular polypeptide and the anthrax toxin, each of which is encoded by a separate plasmid.

(*i*) ***Capsular polypeptide*** — It contains D (–) glutamic acid. It inhibits phagocytosis. Antibody to capsular polypeptide is not protective. Loss of the plasmid which controls capsule production leads to loss of virulence. This is how the live attenuated anthrax spore vaccine from sterne strain was obtained.

(*ii*) ***Anthrax toxin*** — It is a complex exotoxin, responsible for the clinical manifestations of anthrax disease. This protein toxin is a complex of three fractions — the edema factor (EF or Factor I), the protective antigen factor (PA or Factor II) and the lethal factor (LF or Factor III). They are not toxic individually, but act synergistically to produce the characteristic systemic effects of anthrax. PA is capable of inducing protective antibody. PA fraction binds to the surface receptors on the target cell, and in turn provides attachment sites for EF or LF, facilitating their entry into the cell. EF is a clamodulin-dependent adenyl cyclase, which is activated only inside the target cells, leading to intracellular accumulation of cyclic AMP, leading to edema. Entry of LF into the target cell causes cell death but the mechanism of action is not known.

(*iii*) ***Somatic polysaccharide*** — It is a component of cell wall. It is made up of N-acetylglucosamine and D-galactose. It cross-reacts with blood group A antigen and with capsular polysaccharide of type 14 pneumococcus. The antibody against this antigen is not protective.

Epidemiology

Anthrax is a zoonosis. Anthrax affects principally domestic herbivores — cattle, sheep, goats, swine and horses — and is transmitted to humans by contact with infected animal products or contaminated dust. Infection is usually initiated by the subcutaneous inoculation of spores through incidental skin abrasions. Less frequently, the inhalation of spore-laden dust causes a pulmonary form of anthrax. Animals are infected by ingestion of the spores present in the soil. Direct spread from animal to animal is rare. Infected animals shed large numbers of bacilli in the discharges from mouth, nose and rectum, which sporulate in soil, and serve as the source of infection.

Pathogenicity

Based on the mode of infection, human anthrax is of three types — cutaneous anthrax, pulmonary anthrax and intestinal anthrax, all types leading to fatal septicemia. The disease may be seen as an occupational hazard in veterinarians, butchers and farmers.

Cutaneous anthrax (***Malignant pustule, hide-porter's disease***) — Infection is acquired through small cuts or abrasions in the skin. About 95 per cent of human cases of anthrax are of the cutaneous form. Upon introduction of organisms or spores that germinate, a papule develops within 1–3 days. It becomes vesicular, containing fluid which may be clear or blood stained. It rapidly evolves into a painless, black (anthrax = cold), severely swollen (edematous) **"malignant pustule",** which eventually crusts over. The whole area is congested and edematous, and several satellite lesions filled with serum or yellow fluid are arranged around a central necrotic lesin which is covered by a black eschar. The organisms may invade regional lymph nodes, and then the general circulation, leading to a fatal septicemia. Although some cases remain localized and heal, the overall mortality in untreated cutaneous anthrax is about twenty per cent. The disease used to be common in dock workers carrying loads of hides and skin on their bare backs and hence was known as **"hide porter's disease".**

Pulmonary anthrax (***Wool sorter's disease***) — It is caused by inhalation of spores. It used to be common among workers in wood factories, due to inhalation of dust from infected wool. It is characterized by progressive hemorrhagic pneumonia and hemorrhagic lymphadenitis (inflammation of lymph nodes), and has a mortality rate approaching 100 per cent if left untreated. Hemorrhagic meningitis may occur as a complication.

Intestinal anthrax — This unusual form of anthrax is caused by the ingestion of spores, for example, by eating raw or inadequately cooked meat containing *B. anthracis* spores. A violent enteritis with bloody diarrhea occurs, with a high fatality rate.

Laboratory diagnosis

B. anthracis is easily recovered from clinical materials, where it is often present in massive numbers.

In case of malignant pustule, specimen collected is fluid aspirated from the vesicles surrounding black eschar or material beneath the edge of the black eschar. Sputum from pulmonary anthrax; gastric aspirates, feces or food in intestinal anthrax and blood in the septicemic stage are commonly used clinical specimens.

Anthrax may be diagnosed by microscopy, culture, animal inoculaion and serology. When an animal is suspected to have died of anthrax, autopsy is not permissible, as the split blood will lead to contamination of the soil. An ear may be cut off from the carcass and sent to the laboratory. Alternatively, swabs soaked in blood or several blood smears may be sent. Suspected anthrax should be handled with extreme caution, particularly to prevent transmission via aerosols.

Microscopy — The demonstration of Gram positive bacilli with bamboo-stick apperance, that occur singly, in pairs or frequently in long chains in Gram stained smears and a positive M'fadyeans reaction constitute the presumptive diagnosis. A direct immunofluorescence assay aids in the identification of the organism.

Culture — The specimens are inoculated on to nutrient agar, blood agar, PLET medium and incubated at 37°C for 24 hours. The colonies may be examined for medusa head appearance, and growth is identified by examination of Gram stained smears. Tangled chains of large Gram positive bacilli some of which have oval, central oval, nonbulging spores can be seen. The identity of the culture may be confirmed by biochemical reactions and animal inoculation.

Animal inoculation — Broth culture (0.1 ml) is injected subcutaneously into guinea pigs. Alternatively, the tissues from an animal, suspected to be died of anthrax, are applied over the shaven skin of a guinea pig. It is able to penetrate through minute abrasions and produce fatal infection. Autopsy of animal reveals hemorrhagic edema at the site of inoculation, petechial hemorrhages in the peritoneum and an enlarged dark red spleen. Smears from heart blood and spleen are examined by Gram staining and M'fadyeans methods.

Serology — If the sample received is putrid so that viable bacilli are unlikely, diagnosis may be established by **Ascoli's thermoprecipitation test**. The tissue is grinded in saline, boiled for 5 minutes, filtered and layered over antianthrax serum in a narrow test tube. If the tissues contain anthrax antigens, a well-marked ring (ring test) of precipitation appears at the junction of two layers within 5 minutes at room temperature.

Prophylaxis

Carcasses of animals suspected to have died of anthrax are buried deep in quicklime or cremated to prevent soil contamination.

Pasteur's vaccine was the anthrax bacillus attenuated by growth at 42–43°C. Spore vaccines have been extensively used in animals. They provide protection for a year following single injection. The sterne vaccine contained spores of a noncapsulated a virulent mutant strain. The Mazucchi vaccine contained spores of stable attenuated carbazzoo strain in 2% saponin.

Alum precipitated toxoid prepared from the protective antigen has been shown to be safe and effective vaccine for human use. The anthrax vaccine consists of a noninfectious sterile filtrate from the culture of an attenuated strain of *B. anthracis* that contains no dead or viable bacteria. The filtrate is adsorbed to an adjuvant, aluminium hydroxide. The vaccine is recommended for goat hair and woolen mill workers, veterinarians, laboratory workers and live-stock handlers who are at risk due to occupational exposure. Three doses intramuscularly at intervals of six weeks between first and second, and six months between second and third doses induce good immunity. Safety and efficacy of the vaccine are supported by studies in nonhuman primates where efficacy was close to 100 per cent.

Because of the resistance of endospores to chemical disinfectants, autoclaving is the most reliable means of decontamination.

Treatment

B. anthracis is sensitive to penicillin, doxycycline and ciprofloxacin.

BACILLUS CEREUS

It is widely distributed in nature and is commonly found in soil, water, milk, vegetables, cereals, meat and poultry. It is an aerobic, sporeforming, large Gram positive bacillus resembling *B. anthracis* except that it is motile and lacks the glutamic acid capsule. Colonies are large, grey with frosted glass appearance resembling those of *B. anthracis*. On blood agar, *B. cereus* produces a large zone of beta hemolysis, while those of *B. anthracis* do not. It is not susceptible to gamma phage and does not react with anthrax fluorescent antibody conjugate.

Bacillus cereus produces two patterns of food poisoning. Food poisoning by *B. cereus* is most likely far more frequent than is diagnosed.

1. One form of food poisoning is associated with a wide range of foods including meat, poultry, vegetables such as potatoes and various soups. It is characterised by profuse diarrhea and abdominal pain, 8–16 hours after ingestion of contaminated foods. Vomiting is rare. *B. cereus* is not found in large numbers in feces of these patients. It is mostly caused by serotypes 2, 6, 8, 9, 10 or 12, which produce an heat-labile enterotoxin resembling cholera toxin and labile toxin of *E.coli*. It causes fluid accumulation in ligated rabbit illeal loop test. It acts on the epithelial cells of small intestine, stimulating cell-bound adenyl cyclase, which leads to increased levels of cyclic AMP resulting in active secretion of large volumes of fluid into the intestinal lumen.
2. The second type of food poisoning known as emetic illness is associated almost exclusively with the consumption of cooked rice, usually fried rice from Chinese restaurants. The illness is characterized by nausea and vomiting, 1–5 hours after the meal. Diarrhea is not common. *B. cereus* is present in large numbers in the cooked rice and fecal samples from these patients. This disease is caused by serotypes 1, 3 or 5, which produce a heat-stable emetic toxin.

Both types of food poisoning are mild and self-limited, requiring no specific treatment.

Table 50.1 Differences between *B. anthracis* and *B. cereus*

	B. anthracis	*B. cereus*
Motility	–	+
Hemolysis on sheep blood agar	–	+
Resistance to penicillin	–	+
Salicin fermentation	–	+/–
Gelatin hydrolysis	–	+
Lecittinase production	+	+
Pathogenicity ior mice	+	–

A special **mannitol-egg yolk-phenol red-polymyxin agar (MYPA) medium** is useful in isolating *B. cereus* from feces and other sources. *B. cereus* produces lecithinase and ferments glucose but not mannitol.

Prevention is best accomplished by the prompt refrigeration of boiled rice and other foods.

ANTHRACOID BACILLI

Many nonpathogenic aerobic spore bearing bacilli appearing as common contaminants in culture and having a general resemblance to anthrax bacilli have been collectively called as anthracoid bacilli *e.g., B. subtilis, B. licheniformis* and *B. mycoides*. Unlike anthrax bacilli, anthracoid bacilli are generally motile, noncapsulated, grow in short chains, do not produce medusa head colonies, produce beta hemolysis on blood agar and are not pathogenic to laboratory animals. They are implicated in opportunistic lesions, following trauma or the placement of artificial devices and catheters.

B. subtilis, which is ubiquitous in nature and a common laboratory contaminant may occasionally cause eye infection and septicemia. The colonies of *B. subtilis* are large may be pigmented from pink and yellow to orange or brown.

Table 50.2 Differences between Anthrax and Anthracoid bacilli

Anthrax bacilli	*Anthracoid bacilli*
1. Non motile	Motile
2. Capsulated	Noncapsulated
3. Grow in long chains	Grow in short chains
4. Medusa head colony	Not present
5. No growth in penicillin agar (10 units/ml)	Grow usually
6. Haemolysis is absent or weak	Well marked hemolysis
7. Slow gelatin liquefaction and inverted fir tree growth	Rapid liquefaction
8. No turbidity in broth	Turbidity produced in broth
9. Salicin fermentation negative	Positive
10. No growth at 45°C	Grows usually
11. Susceptible to gamma phage	Not susceptible to gamma phage
12. Growth inhibited by chloral hydrate	Not inhibited
13. Pathogenic to lab. animals	Not pathogenic

QUESTIONS

Essay Type Question

1. Describe the morphology, cultural characters and pathogenicity of *Bacillus anthracis*. Outline the procedure in the lab. diagnosis of infection caused by organism.

Short Answer Type Questions

1. Morphology of anthrax bacillus.
2. M'fadyeans reaction.
3. Medusa head.
4. Anthrax in man or pathogenicity of B. anthracis or human anthrax.
5. Cutaneous anthrax or malignant pustule or hide porter's disease.
6. Pulmonary anthrax or wool sorter's disease.
7. String of pearls reaction.
8. Lab. diagnosis of anthrax.
9. Ascoli's thermoprecipitation test.
10. *Bacillus cereus.*
11. Anthracoid bacilli.
12. *Bacillus subtilis.*

51

Clostridium tetani

- ***Clostridia***
- ***Clostridium tetani***
  - ***Morphology***
  - ***Cultural characteristics***
  - ***Biochemical reactions***
  - ***Resistance***
  - ***Classification***
  - ***Toxins***
  - ***Epidemiology***
  - ***Pathogenicity***
  - ***Laboratory diagnosis***
  - ***Prophylaxis***
  - ***Treatment***

CLOSTRIDIA

Clostridia are anaerobic, Gram positive, spore-forming bacilli of greatest clinical importance. The spores are wider than the bacillary bodies, giving the bacillus a swollen appearance, resembling a spindle. Hence the name *Clostridium* (kloster = spindle). Most are saprophytes found in soil, water and decomposing plant and animal matter. Some species are found in the large intestine of humans and animals as normal commensals. Many species are pathogenic. They produce some of the most potent exotoxins known. Some are of industrial importance used for the production of acetone and butanol (*e.g., Cl. acetobutyricum*).

Clostridia are all obligate anaerobes. They obtain energy exclusively by fermentation, because they cannot utilize molecular oxygen for the production of energy. They are also, in varying degrees, damaged by free oxygen, which limits the conditions under which these organisms can colonize the human body or cause disease.

Clostridia are classified — based on shape and position of spores, based on biochemical properties and based on the diseases they produce.

I. **Classification based on the shape and position of spores —**

(*i*) Oval and terminal *e.g., Cl. tertium, Cl. difficle* and *Cl. cochlearum*

(*ii*) Spherical and terminal *e.g., Cl. tetani, Cl. tetanomorphum* and *Cl. sphenoides*

(*iii*) Subterminal and oval *e.g., Cl. welchii, Cl. botulinum, Cl. histolyticum* and *Cl. novyi*

II. **Classification based on biochemical reactions —**

(*i*) Predominantly proteolytic *e.g., Cl. bifermentans, Cl. histolyticum, Cl. botulimum*A, B, F, *Cl. sordelli* and *Cl. sporogenes.*

(*ii*) Predominantly saccharolytic *e.g., Cl. welchii, Cl. septicum, Cl. novyi, Cl. difficle*

(*iii*) Slightly proteolytic but not saccharolytic *e.g., Cl. tetani*

(*iv*) Saccharolytic but not proteolytic *e.g., Cl. fallax, Cl. tertium, Cl. tetanomorphum, Cl. sphenoides* and *Cl. botulinum*C, D, E.

(*v*) Neither proteolytic nor saccharolytic *e.g., Cl. cochlearum.*

III. **Classification based on the diseases they produce —**

(*i*) The gas gangrene group *e.g., Cl. welchii (perfringens), Cl. septicum, Cl. novyi, Cl. histolyticum, Cl. fallax, Cl. bifermentans, Cl. sporogenes*

(*ii*) Tetanus — *Cl. tetani*

(*iii*) Food poisoning group

1. Gastroenteritis *e.g., Cl. welchii* (type A)
2. Necrotising enteritis *e.g., Cl. welchii* (type C)
3. Botulism *e.g., Cl. botulinum*

(*iv*) Acute colitis *e.g., Cl. difficle.*

Clostridia cannot use free oxygen as the terminal electron acceptor in energy production as do aerobic organisms. Instead, they use a variety of small organic molecules such as pyruvate as the final electron acceptors in the generation of energy.

CLOSTRIDIUM TETANI

Morphology

Cl. tetani is a Gram positive, slender bacillus, about 4–8 μ × 0.5 μ in size with a straight axis, parallel sides and rounded ends. The spores are spherical, terminal and bulging giving the bacillus the characteristic '**drum stick**' appearance. It is noncapsulated and motile by peritrichate flagella. Type VI strains are nonflagellated and nonmotile. Young cultures are strongly Gram positive but older cells are Gram variable and may even be Gram negative.

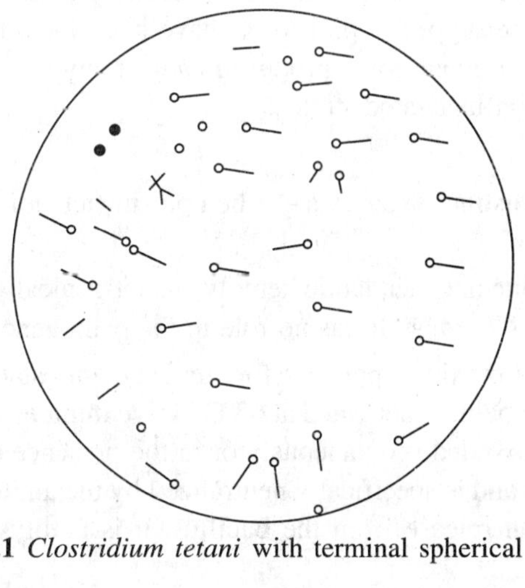

Fig. 51.1 *Clostridium tetani* with terminal spherical spores.

Cultural characteristics

It is an obligate anaerobe. The optimum temperature for growth is 37ºC and pH 7.4. It grows well on ordinary media. Growth is improved by blood and serum. It produces characteristic swarming growth with an extremely fine, translucent film of growth, which is practically invisible, except at the delicately filamentous advancing edge. This property enables the separation of *Cl. tetani* from mixed cultures. If the water of condensation at the bottom of a slope of nutrient agar is inoculated with mixed culture, subcultures from the top of the tube will yield a pure growth of the tetanus bacillus (Filde's technique).

On blood agar, alpha hemolysis is produced, which later develops into beta hemolysis, due to the production of hemolysin (tetanolysin). It grows well in RCM broth and the meat is turned black (proteolytic) on prolonged incubation.

In deep agar shake cultures, the colonies are spherical fluffy balls, 1–3 mm in diameter, made up of filaments with a radial arrangement. In gelatin stab cultures, a fir tree type of growth occurs, with slow liquefaction. A greenish fluorescence is produced on media containing neutral red (as on MacConkey's agar).

Biochemical reactions

Cl. tetani has slightly proteolytic activity but no saccharolytic activity. It does not attack any sugar. It is indole positive, MR and VP negative. H_2S is not formed. Nitrates are not reduced, gelatin is liquefied very slowly.

Resistance

Spores are highly resistant and are able to survive in soil for years. They are not destroyed by 5% phenol or 0.1% mercuric chloride solution in two weeks, but are killed by Iodine (1% aqueous solution), hydrogen peroxide (10 volumes) and glutaraldehyde (2%) within a few hours.

Spores of strains of *Cl. tetani* are killed by boiling for 10–15 minutes, but some resist boiling for upto three hours and dry heat at 160ºC for one hour. They can, however, be killed by autoclaving at 121ºC for 15 minutes.

Classification

Cl. tetani contains flagellar (H) and somatic (O) antigens. Based on agglutination tests with type specific flagellar antigens, 10 serotypes (type I to X) have been identified. All the types produce the same toxin, which is neutralized by antitoxin produced against any one type. All types carry same 'O' antigen. Type VI consists of nonflagellated strains.

Toxins

Cl. tetani produces two distinct exotoxins – a hemolysin (tetanolysin) and a neurotoxin (tetanospasmin).

Tetanolysin is oxygen labile and heat labile hemolysin, antigenically related to streptolysin 'O' and θ toxin of *Cl. perfringens* and *Cl. novyi.* It has no role in the pathogenesis.

Tetanospasmin is the neurotoxin responsible for clinical manifestations of the disease. It is oxygen stable but relatively heat labile, being inactivated at 65ºC in five minutes. It is plasmid coded exotoxin of single antigenic type. It gets toxoided spontaneously or in the presence of low concentrations of formaldehyde. It is a strong antigen and is specifically neutralized by the antitoxin. The toxin is composed of a single polypeptide chain. On release from the bacillus, it is autolysed to form two chains joined through a disulphide bond. Tetanus and botulinum toxins resemble each other in their amino acid sequence. It is an extremely powerful exotoxin second in potency only to the exotoxin of *Cl. botulinum.*

Epidemiology

Cl. tetani is widely distributed in the soil and in the intestines of humans and animals. *Cl. tetani* spores are common in backyard, garden, and other soils. The spores have been recovered from a wide variety of other sources, including street and hospital dust, cotton wool, plaster of paris, bandages, catgut, talc, wall plaster and clothing.

The most typical focus of infection in tetanus is a puncture wound caused, for example, by a splinter. Introduced foreign bodies or small areas of cell killing create a nidus of devitalized material in which tetanus spores can germinate and grow. Special circumstances may also lead to infection, for example after severe burns or surgery or abortion or child birth. Illicit drugs often contain spores that are introduced by injection. In less developed countries, tetanus is a common complication of birth, where the umbilical wound becomes infected from unclean cutting instruments or dressings.

When the wound is devitalized and/or infected with aerobic organisms the redox potential in the local wound environment may reduce sufficiently to allow germination of the spores. Subsequently, toxin is produced by vegetative bacteria.

Pathogenicity

Cl. tetani is noninvasive. The spores implanted in a wound can germinate and multiply, when anaerobic conditions exist, such as presence of devitalized tissues, foreign bodies, blood clots and reduced oxidation-reduction potential.

The vegetative bacteria multiply and remain localized in the wound and elaborate an extremely potent toxin, called tetanospasmin. It is transported from an infected locus by retrograde neuronal flow or by blood. Tetanospasmin is produced as a single polypeptide that is cleaved to generate the mature toxin of two chains held together by a disulfide bond. The heavy fragment (B, binding) mediates binding to a receptor on peripheral motor neuron terminals, and penetration of light fragment (A, active) into axons by "receptor mediated endocytosis" and transported to the nerve cell body in the brain stem and the spinal chord by "retrograde axonal transport". The toxin migrates across the synapses to the presynaptic terminals, where it blocks release of inhibitory neurotransmitters such as glycine and GABA. The A fragment is a protease, which cleaves a small synaptic vesicle protein, synaptobrevin, and abolishes the flow of inhibitory neurotransmitters. The abolition of presynaptic inhibition causes uncontrolled spread of impulses initiated anywhere in the CNS, resulting in muscle rigidity and spasms. Tetanospasmin resembles strychnine in its effect. The toxin acts presynaptically, unlike strychnine which acts postsynaptically.

Tetanus has an incubation period varying from four days to several weeks. A shorter incubation period is usually associated with more severe disease and wounds closer to the brain. Tetanus presents as a spastic paralysis, in which muscle spasms often first involve the site of infection. In the early stages of the disease, the jaw muscles are affected, so that the mouth cannot open (Trismus or lock-jaw). Gradually other voluntary muscles become involved — facial muscles (Risus sardonicus) and back muscles (opisthotonos; "arched back"). Any external stimulus, for example bright light or noise, precipitates a painful spasm, and sometimes convulsions. Death, which occurs in fifteen to sixty per cent of cases is usually the result of paralysis of chest muscles leading to respiratory failure.

Laboratory diagnosis

Because treatment must be initiated immediately, the diagnosis of tetanus is based largely on clinical findings. Specimens are usually wound swabs, pus or necrotic material or excised bits of tissue from necrotic depth of the wound. Laboratory diagnosis may be made by microscopy, culture or by animal inoculation.

Microscopy — Gram stained smears may be examined for long, slender, Gram positive bacilli with terminal, spherical spores with drumstick appearance. Microscopy is unreliable and the demonstration of the typical "drumstick" bacilli in wounds itself is not diagnostic of tetanus. The bacilli may be present in some wounds without tetanus developing. It may not also be possible to distinguish by microscopy between *Cl. tetani* and morphologically similar bacilli such as *Cl. tetanomorphum* and *Cl. sphenoides*.

Culture — Diagnosis by culture is more dependable. Isolation is more likely from excised bits of tissue from the necrotic depths of wounds than from wound swabs. The material is inoculated on one half of a blood agar plate. *Cl. tetani* produces a swarming growth which may be detected on the opposite half of the plate after 1–2 days incubation anaerobically.

The material is also inoculated into three tubes of RCM broth, one of which is heated to 80ºC for 15 minutes, the second for five minutes, and the third left unheated. The purpose of heating for different periods is to kill vegetative bacteria, while leaving undamaged tetanus spores, which vary widely in heat resistance. The RCM tubes are incubated at 37ºC and subcultured on one half of blood agar plates daily for upto four days. *Cl. tetani* may be isolated in pure culture by subculturing from the swarming edge of the growth. The incorporation of polymyxin B, to which clostridia are resistant, makes the medium more selective.

***Toxigenicity testing — In vitro* method** — This method is used for identification and toxigenicity testing. Blood agar plates with 4% agar to inhibit swarming, having tetanus antitoxin (1500 units per ml) spread over one half of the plate are used. The *Cl. tetani* strains are stab-inoculated on each half of the plate, which is then incubated anaerobically for two days. Toxigenic *Cl. tetani* strains show hemolysis around the colonies, only on the half without the antitoxin. Hemolysis is inhibited by the antitoxin on the other half. This may help in identification of the culture as *Cl. tetani* but is unreliable as a test of toxigenicity since it indicates the production only of tetanolysin and not necessarily of tetanospasmin, which is the pathogenic toxin.

***In vivo* method** — Toxigenicity is best tested in animals. 0.2% ml of two to four day old cooked meat culture is inoculated into the root of the tail of two mice. One animal is protected by injecting 1000 units tetanus antitoxin an hour earlier serves as the control. Symptoms develop in the test animal in 12–24 hours, beginning with stiffness of the tail. Rigidity proceeds to the leg on the inoculated side, the opposite leg, trunk and forelimbs, in that order. The animal dies within two days but may be killed earlier as the appearance of ascending tetanus is diagnostic.

When the toxin is injected intramuscularly in one of the hind limbs, muscles spasms of the inoculated limb appear first. This is known as **"local tetanus"** and is due to the toxin acting on the segment of the spinal cord containing the motor neurons of the nerve supplying the inoculated area. Subsequent spread of the toxin up the spinal cord causes **"ascending tetanus"**. The opposite hindlimb, trunk and forelimbs are involved in an ascending fashion. If the toxin is injected intravenously, spasticity develops first in the muscles of the head and neck and then spreads downwards known as **"descending tetanus"**. This type resembles the naturally occurring tetanus in humans.

Prophylaxis

The methods of prophylaxis are — (*i*) Surgical, (*ii*) Antibiotic, and (*iii*) Immunization — active, passive and combined.

Surgical prophylaxis — It aims at removal of foreign bodies, necrotic tissue and blood clots, to prevent an anaerobic environment favorable for the growth of tetanus bacilli. The extent of surgery may vary from cleansing to radical excision depending on the type of wound.

Antibiotic prophylaxis — It aims at destroying tetanus bacilli and pyogenic bacteria in wounds so that the production of toxin is prevented. Antibiotics may be started before starting surgical treatment. Penicillin is the drug of choice. An alternative is erythromycin. Bacitracin or neomycin may be applied locally also. Antibiotics have no action on the toxin. Hence, antibiotic prophylaxis does not replace immunisation but serves as a useful adjunct.

Active immunisation — Active immunisation with tetanus toxoid (formalin-inactivated toxin) prevents tetanus. The tetanus toxoid is available either as "plain toxoid" or adsorbed on aluminium hydroxide or aluminium phosphate. The adsorbed toxoid is a better antigen, because aluminium hydroxide acts as an adjuvant. A course of immunisation consists of three doses of tetanus toxoid given intramuscularly, with an interval of 4–6 weeks between the first two injections and the third dose 6 months later. A full course of immunisation confers immunity for a period of at least ten years. Recent studies have confirmed that circulating antibody levels gradually decline and many older individuals lose protec-tion. Therefore booster immunisations of tetanus toxoid given every ten years throughout life are recommended.

The tetanus toxoid (adsorbed) is usually administered to children as a triple vaccine with diphtheria toxoid and pertussis bacilli, called DPT or triple vaccine, in which killed pertussis bacilli act as an adjuvant. The currently recommended regimen calls for injections of infants at two, four, six and eighteen months of age, followed by a booster upon entering school, at about age five years.

Passive immunization — Tetanus antitoxin (antitetanus serum; ATS) can be used to give immediate passive immunity to injury victims with no history of immunization. ATS is useful not only in reducing the incidence of tetanus but also in prolonging the incubation period and reducing the mortality when it did not prevent the disease. The usual prophylactic dose 1500 IU given intramuscularly. ATS is prepared by immunization of horses with tetanus toxoid. This equine ATS carries two disadvantages implicit in the use of any heterologous serum-**immune elimination** and hypersensitivity. The half-life of ATS in humans is normally about seven days, but in persons with prior injections of horse serum, it is eliminated much more quickly by combination with pre-existing antibodies. Prior sensitization also leads to hypersensitivity reactions which may range from mild local reactions to **serum sickness,** and even fatal anaphylaxis. It is, therefore, obligatory that a test for hypersensitivity should invariably be made before administration of ATS. For this, a dose of 0.5 ml of ATS is given subcutaneously and the patient observed for atleast half an hour for general reactions. Since even this dose may lead to anaphylaxis in some individuals, a syringe loaded with adrenaline (1/1000) must be kept ready.

Passive immunity without risk of hypersensitivity can be obtained by the use of human antitetanus immunoglobulin (TIG). This is effective in smaller doses (250 units) and has a longer half-life (3–5 weeks). Since, TIG is prepared by immunization of human volunteers, its availability is limited.

Combined immunization — It consists of administering ATS or TIG and adsorbed tetanus toxoid in different areas of the body, given simultaneously to a nonimmune person exposed to the risk of tetanus, followed by second and third doses of tetanus toxoid to built up active immunity. Ideally, combined immunisation should be employed whenever passive immunization is called for.

Treatment

Prompt administration of antitoxin to neutralize any toxin not yet bound to neurons is the first order of treatment. Treatment with human hyperimmune globulin (TIG) or horse ATS is used. Vigorous treatment with sedatives and muscle relaxants to minimize spasms, and attention to maintenance of ventilation, are important. The organism is sensitive to penicillin, and this drug can be used to eradicate the infection.

QUESTIONS

Essay Type Questions

1. Enumerate various pathogenic clostridia. Describe the pathogenesis, lab. diagnosis and prophylaxis of tetanus.
2. Classify clostridia. Describe the etiology and pathogenesis of tetanus.
3. Mention the anaerobes. Describe the pathogenesis and prophylaxis of tetanus.

Short Answer Type Questions

1. Classification of clostridia.
2. Morphology of *Cl. tetani.*
3. Toxins of *Cl. tetani.*
4. Pathogenicity of *Cl. tetani.*
5. Lab. diagnosis of tetanus.
6. Prophylaxis of tetanus.
7. Immunoprophylaxis of tetanus.
8. ATS.
9. Immune elimination.
10. DPT vaccine.

52

Clostridium perfringens (Cl. welchii)

– *Morphology*	– *Laboratory diagnosis*
– *Cultural characteristics*	– *Prophylaxis*
– *Biochemical reactions*	– *Treatment*
– *Resistance*	• *Cl. septicum*
– *Classification*	• *Cl. novyi (Cl. oedematiens)*
– *Toxins*	• *Cl. histolyticum*
– *Epidemiology*	• *Cl. sordelli*
– *Pathogenicity*	

MORPHOLOGY

Cl. perfringens is a large, nonmotile, Gram positive, encapsulated bacillus with straight, parallel sides and rounded or truncated ends (box-car appearance), about 4–6μ × 1μ in size, usually occurring singly or in chains or small bundles. Its spores are found in soil. Spores are oval shaped, central or terminal in position. Spores are rarely seen in the body and materials from pathological lesions or following *in vitro* cultivation.

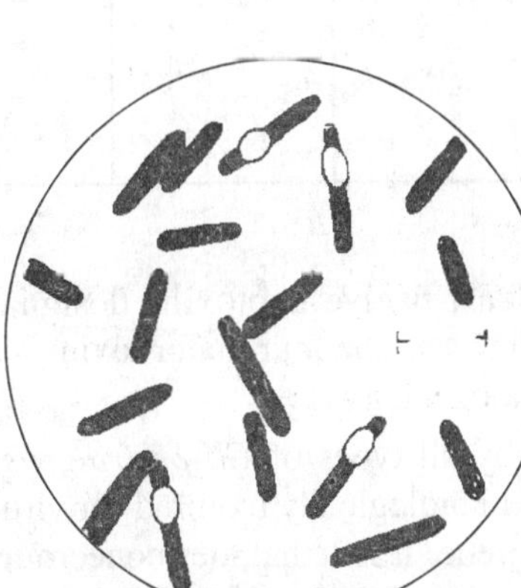

Fig. 52.1 *Clostridium welchii* with subterminal oval spores

Cultural characteristics

It is an anaerobe but can also grow under microaerophilic conditions. It grows over a pH range of 5.5–8.0 and temperature range of 20ºC–50ºC. Optimum temperature for growth is 37ºC. It grows best on media containing carbohydrates such as glucose agar or glucose blood agar. Good growth occurs in RCM broth. The meat is turned pink (saccharolytic) but not digested.

On blood agar, a double zone of hemolysis is produced, with a narrow zone of complete hemolysis due to theta toxin, surrounded by a much wider zone of incomplete hemolysis due to alpha toxin.

Biochemical reactions

It is actively saccharolytic and ferments glucose, maltose, lactose and sucrose with the production of acid and gas. It is indole negative, MR positive and VP negative and forms H_2S abundantly. Most strains reduce nitrates.

In litmus milk medium, fermentation of lactose leads to formation of acid, which is indicated by the change in the color of litmus from blue to red. The acid coagulates the casein (acid clot) and the clotted milk is disrupted due to the vigorous gas production. The paraffin plug is pushed up and shreds of clot are seen sticking to the sides of the tube. This is known as **"stormy fermentation".**

Resistance

Spores are resistant to the antiseptics and disinfectants in common use except formaldehyde and glutaraldehyde. Spores are usually destroyed within five minutes by boiling but those of the food poisoning strains of Type A and certain Type C strains resist boiling for 1–3 hours. Autoclaving at 121ºC for 15 minutes is lethal.

Classification

Cl. perfringens strains are classified into five types (A to E) based on the production of four major toxins. Typing is done by neutralization tests with specific antitoxins by intracutaneous injections in guinea pigs or intravenous injection in mice.

Table 52.1 Typing of *Cl. perfringens*

Type	*Toxin produced*			
	α	β	ε	*i*
A	+	–	–	–
B	+	+	+	–
C	+	+	–	–
D	+	–	+	–
E	+	–	–	+

Toxins

Cl. perfringens elaborates at least twelve exotoxins designated by Greek letters and several enzymes and biologically active substances. The four major toxins – alpha, beta, epsilon (ε) and iota (*i*) are predominantly responsible for pathogenicity.

Alpha toxin — It is produced by all types of *Cl. perfringens* and most abundantly by Type A strains. This is the most important toxin biologically required for virulence in tissues, and is responsible for the profound toxemia of gas gangrene. It is lethal, dermonecrotic and hemolytic. It is a phospholipase (lecithinase C) which, in the presence of Ca^{++} and Mg^{++} ions, splits lecithin into phosphoryl choline and diglyceride.

$$\text{Lecithin} \xrightarrow[\text{Ca}^{++} \text{ and Mg}^{++}]{\text{Lecithinase}} \text{Phosphoryl choline + Diglyceride}$$

This reaction is seen as an opalescence on serum or egg yolk media and is specifically neutralized by the antitoxin. When *Cl. perfringens* is grown on a medium containing 6% agar, 5% Filde's peptic digest of sheep blood and 20% human serum, with the antitoxin spread on one half of the plate. The plate is then inoculated with the test organism and incubated anaerobically at 37°C for overnight. The colonies, on the half without antitoxin, are surrounded by a zone of opacity. There will be no zone of opacity on the half with the antitoxin, due to neutralization of the alpha toxin. This specific lecithinase effect, known as the **Nagler reaction,** is a useful test for the rapid detection of *Cl. perfringens* in clinical specimens. The incorporation of neomycin sulphate, makes it more selective, inhibiting coliforms and aerobic spore bearers. Human serum may be replaced by 5% egg yolk. This Nagler reaction is also produced by other lecithinase forming bacteria such as *Cl. novyi, Cl. bifermentans*, some vibrios and some aerobic spore bearers. In the case of these bacteria, the reaction is not neutralized by *Cl. perfringens* antitoxin, except with *Cl. bifermentans* which produces a serologically related lecithinase.

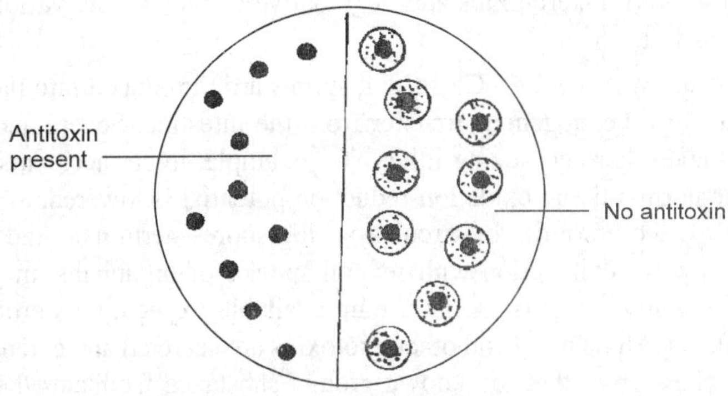

Fig. 52.2 Nagler's reaction

Alpha toxin is relatively heat stable and is only partially inactivated by boiling for five minutes. The alpha toxin is hemolytic for RBC of most animals except horse and goat, due to its action on the phospholipids on RBC membranes.

The clear zone of hemolysis seen on around colonies of Type A strains grown on blood agar are produced by theta toxin and not by alpha toxin. It is a hot-cold hemolysin, and the lysis is of hot-cold variety, being best seen after incubation at 37°C followed by chilling at 4°C.

Beta (β), epsilon (ε) and iota (ι) toxins have lethal and necrotising properties. Gamma (γ) and eta (η) toxins have minor lethal actions. The delta (δ) toxin has a lethal effect and is hemolytic for the RBC of even-toed ungulates (sheep, goats, cattle, pigs). The theta (θ) toxin is an oxygen labile hemolysin, antigenically related to streptolysin 'O'. It is also a lethal and a general cytolytic toxin. The kappa (κ) toxin is a collagenase. The lambda (λ) toxin is a proteinase and gelatinase. The mu (μ) toxin is a hyaluronidase and nu (ν) toxin is a deoxyribonuclease. All these degradative hydrolytic enzymes liquefy tissue and promote the spread of infection.

Cl. perfringens Type A strains produce an enterotoxin, acts in the lower portion of the small intestine. The molecule binds to receptors on the epithelial cell surface and alters the cell membrane, disrupting ion transport, primarily in the ileum, and leading to loss of fluid and intracellular proteins. Enterotoxin-producing strains are unusually heat-resistant, the spores remaining viable for over an hour at 100°C, thus enhancing their threat as enteropathogens.

Epidemiology

Cl. perfringens is a normal inhabitant of the large intestine of humans and animals. Clostridia may also be present on the normal skin, especially on the perineum and thighs. Thus, infection may at times be endogenous.

The spores are widely distributed in soil, dust and air. Clostridia usually enter the wounds alongwith implanted foreign particles such as soil, dust, bits of clothing or shrapnel. When the wound is devitalized and/or infected with aerobic organisms the redox potential in the local wound environment may reduce sufficiently to allow germination of the spores followed by multiplication of vegetative bacteria with the production of toxins and enzymes.

Type A strains of *Cl. perfringens* cause food poisoning, usually associated with meat, chicken, fish and their byproducts by consumption of undercooked food that fails to inactivate spores.

Pathogenicity

The disease processes initiated by *Cl. perfringens* result from a combination of infection with the production of exotoxins and/or enterotoxins and degradative enzymes. The various diseases produced by *Cl. perfringens* are as follows:

(*a*) ***Myonecrosis* (*gas gangrene*)** — Clostridial spores are introduced into tissue, for example, by contamination with dirt, or by endogenous transfer from the intestine. Severe and open wounds, such as compound fractures and other necrotizing injury (for example, in car accidents) are a prime predisposing condition. If the normal tissue oxidation-reduction potential is lowered, as occurs when there is considerable cell injury or compromise of circulation, the spores germinate and grow rapidly. These lesions almost always involve coinfection with several species of organisms, including clostridia and other anaerobes, and facultative organisms that use up available oxygen, thus protecting the anaerobes from oxygen's toxic effects. Alpha toxin and other exotoxins are secreted and extensive cell killing takes place. The production of enzymes that breakdown ground substance facilitates the spread of infection. Fermentation of tissue carbohydrates yields gas and an accumulation of gas bubbles in the subcutaneous spaces produces a crinkling sensation on palpation (crepitation), hence the name gas gangrene. The exudates are copious and foul smelling. As the disease progresses, increased capillary permeability leads to the exotoxins being carried by the circulation from damaged tissue to other organs, resulting in systemic effects such as shock, renal failure and intravascular hemolysis. Untreated clostridial myonecrosis is uniformly fatal within days of the initiation of the gangrene.

Clostridia most often involved in gas gangrene are *Cl. perfringens* (80 per cent) and *Cl. novyi* and *Cl. septicum* being the next common (20 to 40 per cent) and *Cl. histolyticum* and *Cl. sordelli* occasionally. Other clostridia usually found are *Cl. sporogenes*, *Cl. fallax*, *Cl. bifermentans*, *Cl. aerofoetidum* and *Cl. tertium*. Anaerobic streptococci and facultative anaerobes such as *E. coli*, *Proteus* and staphylococci are also commonly encountered in gas gangrene.

(*b*) ***Anaerobic cellulitis*** — This is a clostridial infection of connective tissue in which the spread of bacterial growth along fascial planes (fascitis) does not involve invasion of muscles. Necrotic processes play a more limited role, but surgical intervention is generally unsuccessful because of the rapidity of spread of the infection.

(*c*) ***Food poisoning*** — Some strains *Cl. perfringens* Type A can produce food poisoning. They are characterized by the marked heat resistance of their spores and the feeble production of alpha and theta toxins. They produce a heat labile enterotoxin which, like the enterotoxins of *V. cholerae* and ETEC (enterotoxigenic *E. coli*) leads to fluid accumulation in the rabbit illeal loop.

Meat, chicken, fish and their by products are the most common vehicles for clostridial food poisoning, and the occurrence of clinical symptoms requires a large inoculum of 10^8 organisms or greater. Therefore a typical episode of clostridial enterotoxin food poisoning involves cooking that fails to inactivate spores, followed by holding the food for several hours under conditions (cold or warmed up) that allow bacterial germination and several cycles of growth. Typically, the onset of nausea, abdominal cramps and diarrhea occurs 8–18 hours after eating contaminated food. Fever is absent and vomiting rare. The attack is usually self-limited, with recovery within one to two days. Diagnosis is made by isolating the organism from suspected food and patient's feces.

(*d*) ***Enteritis necroticans*** **(necrotising enteritis)** — Outbreaks of a necrotizing bowel disease with high mortality (greater than fifty per cent) caused by *Cl. perfringens* Type C have been sporadically reported. The disease is known as pigbel in New Guinea and darmbrand in Germany and also reported from East Africa, Thailand and Nepal. *Cl. perfringens* Type C strains with heat resistant spores which germinate in the intestine producing beta toxin causing mucosal necrosis. The evocative name "pigbel" is New Guinea pidgin for abdominal pain and diarrhea following unaccustomed feasting on pig meat along with trypsin inhibitors like sweet potatoes. Immunisation with Type C toxoid has been shown to protect this condition.

(*e*) ***Clostridial endometritis*** — This condition is a grave complication of incomplete abortion, or the use of inadequately sterilized instruments. Gangrenous infection of uterine tissue is followed by toxemia and bacteremia.

(*f*) ***Urinary tract infections*** may occasionally follow surgery such as nephrectomy.

(*g*) ***Thoracic infections*** commonly seen in battle casualties, follow penetrating wounds of the thorax.

(*h*) ***Panophthalmitis*** due to *Cl. perfringens* may occur ocassionally following penetrating eye injuries.

(*i*) ***Brain abscess*** and meningitis have been reported rarely.

(*j*) ***Biliary tract infections*** — Acute emphysematous cholecystitis and postcholecystectomy speticemia may occur rarely.

(*k*) ***Gas gangrene of abdominal wall*** has been reported as a rare complication of abdominal surgery. The infection is endogenous, the organism being derived from the intestine and infect the abdominal wall during surgery. Gas gangrene of the thigh as a result of infection tracking from the abdomen has also been reported.

Laboratory diagnosis

Diagnosis of gas gangrene or cellulitis rests largely on clinical impression. The presence of clostridia in clinical materials may be due to an accidental contamination.

The specimens to be collected include necrotic tissue, exudates from the depth of wounds or edges of necrotic muscle fragments. These specimens from diseased tissue, when Gram-stained, usually show vegetative clostridial forms (large, Gram positive bacilli) accompanied by other bacteria and cellular debris. Because of the extensive necrosis, intact host cells, including inflammatory cells, are rare in exudates. Gram stained smears give presumptive idea about the species of clostridia present and their relative numbers. The presence of large numbers of regularly shaped Gram positive bacilli without spores is strongly suggestive of *Cl. perfringens* infection. "Citron bodies" and boat or leaf shaped pleomorphic bacilli with irregular straining suggest *Cl. septicum.* Large bacilli with oval, subterminal spores indicate *Cl. novyi*. Slender bacilli with round, terminal spores may be *Cl. tetani* or *Cl. tetanomorphum.*

Aerobic and anaerobic cultures are made on blood agar and chocolate agar, preferably with 5–6 per cent agar to prevent swarming. A plate of serum or egg yolk agar, with *Cl. perfringens* antitoxin spread on one half is used for the "Nagler reaction". Four tubes of RCM broth are inoculated and heated at 100ºC for 5, 10, 15 and 20 minutes, incubated and subcultured on blood agar plates after 1–2 days, to differentiate the organisms with heat resistant spores. Blood cultures are often positive, especially in *Cl. perfringens* and *Cl. septicum* infections. However *Cl. perfringens* bacteremia may occur without gas gangrene. The isolates are identified based on sugar fermentation, organic acid production and the production of toxins.

In food poisoning, the organism can be isolated from suspected food and patients feces. Quantitative cultures are required to show heavy growth, greater than 10^5 organisms/gram of food or feces, which suggests causal significance. The isolate can be tested for enterotoxin production.

Prophylaxis and Treatment

The key to both prevention and treatment of gas gangrene is immediate and thorough removal of foreign material and devitalized tissue, and exposure of the wound to hyperbaric O_2, which increase the O_2 tension of tissues in the affected part, and probably inhibit the pathologic process. If debridement is unable to control the progression of the gangrene, amputation, when anatomically possible, is still mandatory in gangrene. Supplementary to this is the administration of antibiotics in high dose. *Cl. perfringens* is sensitive to penicillins and tetracyclines. Since clostridial infections usually involve a mixture of species, a broad-spectrum approach is important. The administration of antitoxin has not proven to be clinically useful, and such antisera are not presently available.

Clostridial food poisoning is almost always self-limited, and requires only supportive care. Prevention is a matter of appropriate food handling practice. The food may be kept hot or refrigerated.

CLOSTRIDIUM SEPTICUM

It is found in the soil and in the intestine of animals and humans. It is associated with gas gangrene in humans, usually with other clostridia. It also causes "braxy" in sheep and "malignant edema" in cattle and sheep.

It is an anaerobic, Gram positive, pleomorphic bacillus. Spores are readily formed. They are oval, central or subterminal and bulging. It is motile by peritrichate flagellae. Growth occurs anaerobically on ordinary media at 37ºC. The colonies are irregular and transparent initially, turning opaque on continued incubation. It produces hemolysis on blood agar. Growth is promoted by glucose. It is saccharolytic and produces abundant gas. Based on somatic and flagellar antigens, six groups have been identified. *Cl.septicum* produces atleast four distinct toxins and a fibrinolysin. The alpha toxin is hemolytic, dermonecrotic and lethal. The beta toxin is leucotoxic deoxyribonuclease. The gamma toxin is a hyaluronidase and the delta toxin an oxygen labile hemolysin.

CLOSTRIDIUM NOVYI (*CLOSTRIDIUM OEDEMATIENS*)

It is widely distributed in soil. It is a large, pleomorphic, Gram positive bacillus with large, terminal, oval spores. It is an obligate anaerobe, readily inactivated by exposure of cultures to air. Based on the producton of toxins, four types A to D are recognised. Only Type A is of medical importance, as it causes gas gangrene. Gas gangrene caused by *Cl. novyi* is characterised by high mortality and large amounts of edema fluid with little or no observable gas in infected tissues. Other types produce veterinary diseases.

CLOSTRIDIUM HISTOLYTICUM

It is a long, slender, Gram positive bacillus with oval, subterminal, bulging spores. It is aerotolerant and some growth may occur aerobically, but growth is best anaerobically. It is actively proteolytic. It forms atleast five distinct toxins — alpha toxin (lethal and necrotising), beta toxin (collagenase and gelatinase), gamma toxin (proteinase and gelatinase), delta toxin (elastase and gelatinase) and epsilon toxin (oxygen labile haemolysin).

Cl. histolyticum is widely distributed in the soil and intestine of humans and animals. It has been associated with gas gangrene in man, but less often.

CLOSTRIDIUM SORDELLI

It is found in soil and as normal flora of intestine of humans and animals and is responsible for gas gangrene occasionally. It is a Gram positive bacillus with rounded end, may occur in chains, possessing large, oval, central nonbulging spores. It produces hemolysis on blood agar. It is both proteolytic and saccharolytic. It ferments glucose and maltose but not lactose and sucrose. It liquefies gelatin and decomposes milk protein. It produces a lecithinase that is serologically related to the alpha toxin of *Cl. perfringens* and is therefore partially neutralised by *Cl. perfringens* antitoxin.

QUESTIONS

Essay Type Questions

1. Describe the morphology, cultural characteristics of *Cl. welchii*. Enumerate toxins of importance in the pathogenesis of organism.
2. Describe the lab. diagnosis and prophylaxis of gas gangrene.

Short Answer Type Questions

1. Morphology of *Cl. perfringens.*
2. Stormy fermentation.
3. Toxins of *Cl. welchii.*
4. Alha toxin.
5. Nagler reaction.
6. Pathogenicity of *Cl. welchii.*
7. Gas gangrene.
8. Enumerate various organisms causing gas gangrene.
9. How do you diagnose gas gangrene.
10. Prophylaxis of gas gangrene.
11. *Cl. novyi. Or Cl. oedematiens.*
12. *Cl. histolyticum.*
13. *Cl. septicum.*

53

Clostridium botulinum and Clostridium difficile

- *Cl. botulinum*
  - *Morphology*
  - *Cultural characteristics*
  - *Biochemical reactions*
  - *Resistance*
  - *Classification*
  - *Toxins*
  - *Epidemiology*
  - *Pathogenicity*
  - *Laboratory diagnosis*
  - *Prophylaxis*
  - *Treatment*
- *Cl. difficile*

CLOSTRIDIUM BOTULINUM

Morphology

It is a Gram postive bacillus, measuring about 5μ × 1μ in size. It is noncapsulated, motile by peritrichate flagellae. Spores are oval, subterminal and bulging.

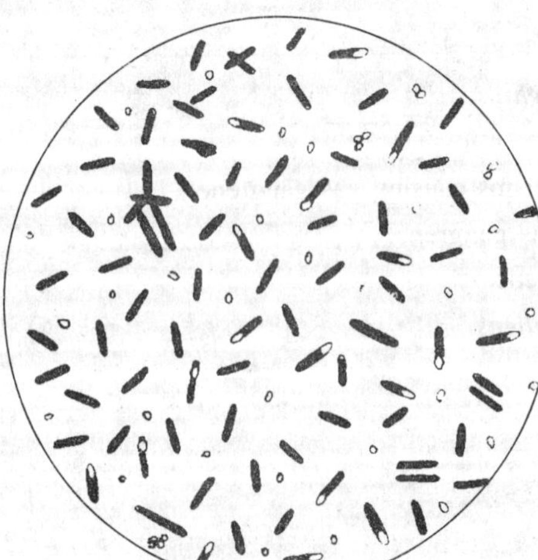

Fig. 53.1 *Clostridium botulinum*

Cultural characteristics

It is an obligate anaerobe. Optimum temperature for growth is 35°C, but some strains may grow even at 1–5°C. Good growth occurs on ordinary media. Colonies are large, irregular, semitransparent, with fimbriate border. Spores are produced consistently when grown in alkaline glucose gelatin media at 20–25°C. They are not produced at higher temperatures.

Biochemical reactions

Table 53.1 Biochemical Reactions Vary in Different Types

Types	*Acid from*				*Gelatinase*	*Indole*	*digestion of*	*Lecithinase C*	*lipase*
	G	*M*	*L*	*S*	*activity*	*production*	*milk protein*	*activity*	*activity*
A, B, F	+	+	–	+	+	–	+	–	+
C, D, E	+	+	–	V	+	–	–	–	+
G	–	–	–	–	+	–	+	–	–

G = Glucose; M = Maltose; L = Lactose; S = Sucrose; V = Variable

Resistance

Spores of *Cl. botulinum* are highly resistant, surviving several hours at 100ºC and for up to 10 minutes at 120ºC. Therefore proper canning is very important in the preservation of food. Spores of nonproteolytic types of B, E and F are much less resistant to heat. Spores are also resistant to radiation, UV light, alcohols, phenolics and quaternary ammonium compounds. They are, however, relatively susceptible to hypochlorite, ethylene oxide and formaldehyde.

Classification

Based on the antigenic differences in the toxins produced, *Cl. botulinum* is classified into eight types – A, B, C1, C2, D, E, F, G. The toxins produced by different types are identical in their pharmacological activity but are neutralized only by the homologous antiserum. An exception is C2 toxin, which is a cytotoxin of unknown significance, while all others are neurotoxins.

Toxins

Cl. botulinum produces a powerful exotoxin (**neurotoxin**), that is one of the most potent poisons known. It is chemically a protein with 19 aminoacids and a molecular weight of about 1,50,000 daltons. Minimum lethal dose of this toxin for mice is 0.03 ng and for humans one microgram. It is a neurotoxin and acts slowly taking several hours to kill.

The toxin is relatively stable, being inactivated after 30–40 minutes at 80ºC and 10 minutes at 100°C. Food suspected to be contaminated with **botulinum toxin** can be rendered completely safe by pressure cooking or boiling for 20 minutes. It resists digestion and is absorbed through the small intestine in active form. The botulinum toxin can be toxoided. It is a good antigen and is specifically neutralized by antitoxin. Toxin production appears to be determined by the presence of **bacteriophages**.

The toxin acts by blocking the production or release of **acetyl choline** at the synapses and neuromuscular junctions. The onset is marked by diplopia, dysphagia and dysarthria due to involvement of cranial nerves, causing flaccid paralysis, ending in death by respiratory failure.

Epidemiology

Cl. botulinum is found worldwide in soil and aquatic sediments, and the sproes frequently contaminate vegetables, meat or fish. Under appropriate conditions, including a strictly anaerobic environment at neutral or alkaline pH, the spores germinate, and toxin is produced during vegetative growth. Because the toxin is often elaborated in food, outbreaks frequently occur in families or other eating groups.

Pathogenicity

Cl. botulinum causes botulism, a paralytic disease usually presenting as a form of **food poisoning**. The name **botulism** is derived from "Sausage" (botulus, latin for sausage) formerly associated with this type of food poisoning. *Cl. botulinum* is noninvasive and noninfectious. Its pathogenicity is due to the action of its toxin. The disease is a pure **intoxication**.

Botulinum toxin and tetanus toxin constitute a homologous set of proteins whose neurotoxicity arises from proteolytic cleavage of specific synaptic vesicle peptides, causing subsequent failure of neurotransmission. In contrast to tetanus toxin, which causes constant contraction (spasms), botulinum toxin affects peripheral cholinergic synapses by blocking the neuromuscular junction and inhibiting release of the neurotransmitter, acetyl choline, thus preventing contraction and causing flaccid paralysis (Note – In minute doses, botulinum toxin preparations have been used therapeutically to relieve spastic conditions such as post-stroke spasticity and strabismus).

Botulism is of three types – Foodborne (classic) botulism, infant botulism and wound botulism.

Foodborne botulism — It is due to the ingestion of preformed toxin present in the contaminated food. Different commercial preparations *e.g.*, canned foods are implicated. The spores survive the heating process in the food, and subsequently germinate, if a suitable anaerobic environment is generated inside the container, and the vegetative bacteria produce the toxin. Proteolytic varities of *Cl. botulinum* can digest food, which then appears spoiled. The cans are often inflated and show bubbles on opening. Nonproteolytic varities leave food unchanged.

The patient first begins to experience difficulties in focusing vision (diplopia), in swallowing (dysphagia) and in other cranial nerve functions, 12–36 hours after ingesting toxin–containing food but not necessarily viable organisms. There is no fever or sepsis. A progressive paralysis of striated muscle groups develops. A symmetric descending paralysis of the striated muscles of head, neck, arms, thorax, abdomen and lower extremities is the characteristic pattern. Mortality rate is about 25–70%. Recovery is protracted, lasting several weeks. Death is due to respiratory paralysis.

Infant botulism (floopy baby syndrome) — It is a *toxico-infection. Cl. botulinum* spores are ingested in food, get established in the large intestine of infants, 3 to 24 weeks of age, and the toxin produced is slowly absorbed. Honey has been incriminated as a likely food item through which the bacillus enters the gut. Constipation, feeding problems, lethargy and poor muscle tone are common early signs. Eventually the baby appears "floppy", hence this disease is known as "*floppy baby syndrome*". The condition is possibly a cause of sudden infant death syndrome, but recovery is the usual outcome, following symptomatic treatment, that may be prolonged. Patients excrete toxin and spores in their feces.

Wound botulism — A rare form of botulism occurs when a wound becomes contaminated with the organism, and toxin absorbed from that site.

Laboratory diagnosis

Diagnosis may be confirmed by demonstration of the bacillus or toxin in suspected food or feces. Gram positive bacilli with oval, bulging, subterminal spores can be demonstrated in smears made from food. *Cl. botulinum* may be identified by direct immunofluorescence.

Cl. botulinum may be isolated by inoculating food or feces on to blood agar, incubated anaerobically. The specimens may be inoculated into RCM broth and incubated at 37ºC for 3–5 days. The growth may be identified by fluorescent antibody test.

The food is macerated in sterile saline, and the filtrate inoculated into mice or guinea pigs intraperitoneally. Control animals are protected by polyvalent antitoxin. Typing is done by passive protection with type specific antitoxin.

The toxin may occasionally be demonstrable in the patient's blood. A retrospective diagnosis may be made by detection of antitoxin in the patient's serum, occasionally.

Prophylaxis

Non-acid, canned foods are the best known sources of botulinal food poisoning, with most cases associated with home processing. Other methods of food preservation, such as smoking, have also been implicated. The toxin is inactivated by boiling temperature and the killing of spores requires autoclaving.

Treatment

Antitoxin, which neutralizes unbound botulinum toxin, should be administered as soon as possible in suspected botulinal intoxication. A variety of supportive measures, including mechanical ventilation, may be required. In wound botulism, the infection can be treated with penicillin or other anitbiotics to which the organism is sensitive.

CLOSTRIDIUM DIFFICLE

It was so named because of the unusual difficulty in isolating it. It is a long, slender Gram positive bacillus with oval and terminal spores. It is nonhemolytic, saccharolytic and weakly proteolytic.

Cl. difficle is a minor component of the normal flora of the large intestine. In hospitalized patients, however, the organism is much more common. After its introduction to a site, the environment – dust, bedding, toilets – becomes persistently contaminated with spores, and new residents are easily colonized. When antimicrobial treatment suppresses predominant species of normal flora of large intestine, *Cl. difficle* proliferates. Pathogenic strains produce two toxic polypeptides, designated A and B. Toxin A is an **enterotoxin** that causes excessive fluid secretion, but also stimulates an inflammatory response and has some cytopathic effect in tissue culture. Toxin B is a *cytotoxin*; in tissue culture it disrupts protein synthesis and causes disorganization of the cytoskeleton. Both toxins are encoded by linked chromosomal genes.

Cl. difficle causes **pseudomembranous colitis (PMC)** and **antibiotic associated diarrohea (AAD),** as a complication of antimicrobial or antineoplastic drug treatment. The three drugs most commonly implicated are clindamycin, ampicillin and the cephalosporins. The severity of the disease varies widely from mild diarrhea through varying degrees of inflammation of the large intestine to a fulminant PMC. The pseudomembranous exudate composed of mucus, fibrin, inflammatory cells and cell debris overlying an ulcerated epithelium, is best demonstrated by endoscopy. Milder disease often lasts some time after cessation of drug treatment, or may reoccur.

Diagnosis can be made by demonstration of toxin in feces by ELISA or by its characteristic effect on tissue cultures such as Hep-2 and human diploid cell lines (tissue culture cytotoxicity tests). *Cl. difficle* can be isolated from stools by routine anaerobic procedures.

Discontinuance of the predisposing drug, and fluid replacement, usually lead to resolution of the symptoms. In severe cases, oral administration of metronidazole or vancomycin are the drugs of choice.

QUESTIONS

Essay Type Questions

1. Describe the morphology, cultural characteristics, pathogenicity and lab. diagnosis of *Cl. botulinum.*

Short Answer Type Questions

1. *Cl. botulinum.*
2. Botulism.
3. Botulinum toxin.
4. Foodborne botulism.
5. *Cl. difficle.*
6. Pseudomembranous colitis.
7. Antibiotic associated colitis (diarrhea).

54

Nonsporing Anaerobes

- *Introduction*
- *Anaerobic infections*
- *Laboratory diagnosis*
- *Classification*
- *Peptococcus*
- *Peptostreptococcus*
- *Sporosarcina*
- *Veillonella*
- *Lactobacillus*
- *Propionibacterium*
- *Eubacterium*
- *Bifidobacterium*
- *Mobilincus*
- *Bacteroides*
- *Prevotella*
- *Porphyromonas*
- *Fusobacterium*
- *Leptotricha*

INTRODUCTION

Nonsporing anaerobes constitute an important cause of human and animal infections. They are generally neglected in diagnostic laboratories. They are normal commensals of mouth, skin, large intestine, genitourinary tract of humans and animals. Indeed, they outnumber aerobic bacteria in many habitats. Anaerobic bacteria are ten to thirty times more frequent than aerobes in the mouth and on the skin. In the large intestine, they outnumber aerobes a thousand fold. They are important **opportunistic pathogens**, particularly when body resistance is lowered. If they gain access to internal tissues through wounds, bowel surgery, dental extraction, during abortion severe infections occur. Several anaerobes occur in soil and water, which may be of agricultural and industrial importance *e.g.*, methanobacteria, butyrivibrios.

Anaerobic bacteria differ widely in the degree of anaerobiasis required for their growth. Some of them are **obligate anaerobes**, and the presence of oxygen is toxic to them, while others are **aerotolerant** and may grow sparsely on the surface of aerobic plates. Anaerobic bacteria form certain volatile fatty acids as metabolic products. These are characteristic for different species and can be detected by gas liquid chromatography.

ANAEROBIC INFECTIONS

Anaerobic bacteria constitute a part of the normal flora of skin, mouth, nasopharynx, upper respiratory tract, large intestine and genitourinary tract. Anaerobic infections are usually endogenous and are caused by tissue invasion by normal resident bacteria, and generally follow some precipitating factor such as trauma, tissue necrosis, impaired circulation, hematoma formation or the presence of foreign bodies. Diabetes, malnutrition, malignancy or prolonged aminoglycoside antibiotic theropy may act as predisposing conditions. Anaerobic infections are typically polymicrobial, more than one anaerobe being responsible besides aerobic bacteria. The infections are usually localized, but general dissemination may occur by bacteremia.

The pus produced in anaerobic infections is characteristically putrid, with a pervasive, nauseating odor. However, there may be exceptions; infections due solely to bacteroides fragilis may be free of this smell. Pronounced cellulitis is a common feature of anaerobic wound infections. Toxemia and fever are not marked.

LABORATORY DIAGNOSIS

As anaerobes form part of the normal flora of skin and mucus surfaces, their isolation from specimens has to be interpreted cautiously. The mere presence of an anaerobe does not prove its causal role. Specimens should be collected in such a manner as to avoid resident flora. For example, the sputum is unsatisfactory for culture from a suspected case of lung abscess; only material collected by aspiration would be acceptable.

As obligate anaerobes die on exposure to oxygen care, should be taken to minimize contact with air during collection, transport and handling of specimens. The best method of collection is to aspirate the specimen into an airtight syringe, plunge the needle into a sterile rubber cork to seal it and send it immediately to the laboratory. Pus and other fluids may be collected in small bottles with airtight caps and transported immediately, ensuring that the specimens fill the bottles completely. Swabs are generally unsatisfactory but where they are to be used, they should be sent in **Stuart's transport medium**.

In the laboratory, specimens should be handled in anaerobic glove boxes to prepare smears and to inoculate culture plates. Examination of Gram stained smear is useful. Pus in anaerobic infection usually shows a large variety of different organisms and numerous pus cells. Rarely, as in brain abscess, a single type of organism alone may be seen. Examination of the specimen under UV light may show the bright red fluorescence of Prevotella melaninogenica. **Gas liquid chromatography** may be used to detect characteristics fatty acids, and therefore the type of anerobes present.

Several special media have been described for anaerobes, but for routine diagnostic work, freshly prepared blood agar with neomycin, yeast extract, hemin and vitamin K is adequate. Inoculated plates are incubated at 37ºC, in an anaerobic jar, with 10% CO_2. The **Gas-Pak** system provides a convenient method for routine anaerobic cultures. Plates are examined after one to two days. Some anaerobes, such as Fusobacteria require longer periods of incubation. Parallel aerobic cultures should always be put up. This is necessary as a control for the growth on anaerobic plates and also because in most anaerobic infections, aerobic bacteria are also involved.

CLASSIFICATION

Current classification of anaerobes is based on DNA base composition and analysis of the fatty acid and products of metabolism. However, on the basis of morphology and staining characters, medically important nonsporing anaerobes can be classified as follows.

I. Cocci		
	A. Gram postive	1. *Peptococcus*
		2. *Peptostreptococcus*
		3. *Sporosarcina*
	B. Gram negative	1. *Veillonella*
II. Bacilli		
	A. Gram positive	1. *Lactobacillus*
		2. *Propionibacterium*
		3. *Eubacterium*
		4. *Bifidobacterium*
		5. *Mobilincus*
		6. *Actinomyces*
	B. Gram negative	1. *Bacteroides*
		2. *Prevotella*
		3. *Porphyromonas*
		4. *Fusobacterium*
		5. *Leptotricha*
III. Spirochetes		1. *Treponema*
		2. *Borrelia*

PEPTOCOCCUS

They are Gram positive, nonsporing, anaerobic cocci, that occur singly or in pairs or in clusters. They produce black colonies on blood agar on prolonged incubation due to the production of H_2S. They occur as normal flora of skin, intestine and genitourinary tract. They may cause pyogenic infections of wounds, puerperal sepsis and urinary tract infections. *P. niger* is the important species.

PEPTOSTREPTOCOCCUS

They are Gram positive cocci, arranged in chains. **Anaerobic streptococci** are more properly designated as members of the genus *Peptostreptococcus*. They are normally present on mucus membranes of the genitourinary and GI tracts, and are particularly abundant among the normal oral, especially periodontal flora. Relatively avirulent, they contribute to mixed anaerobic infections of soft tissues, where they are involved in wound infections, abscesses, pneumonia, and genital tract disease (puerperal sepssis). *P. anaerobius* and *P. magnus* are commonly isolated from wound infections. *P. anaerobius* is commonly associated with puerperal sepsis.

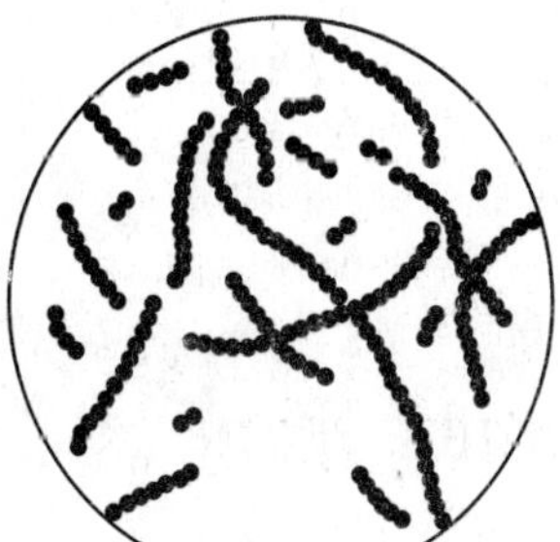

Fig. 54.1 *Peptostreptococcus*

SPOROSARCINA

They are large, spherical Gram positive cocci occurring in packets of eight or more. They were formerly known as *Sarcina*. They form heat resistant spores. They are flagellated and motile. The organisms are nonpathogenic and are found in soil and occur as normal flora in GI tract.

VEILLONELLA

They are Gram negative cocci occurring in pairs, short chains and clumps. They are obligate anaerobes, oxidase negative and catalase negative. They are present in the mouth, GI tract and genital tract as part of normal flora. *V. parvula* has been reported from clinical specimens, but its pathogenic role is uncertain.

Veillon and Zuber (1898) isolated a strictly anaerobic coccus from bartholiniits and perinephric abscess of patients which emitted foul smell and the organism was named *Micrococcus fetidus* by them. It was later named *Veillonella*, in their honour.

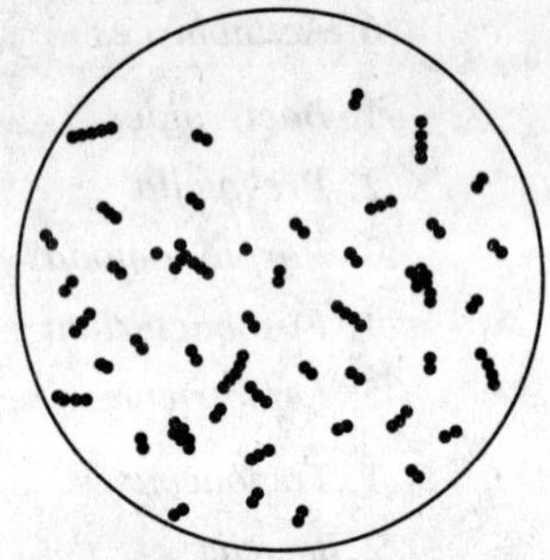

Fig. 54.2 *Veillonella*

LACTOBACILLUS

They are Gram positive bacilli, straight or slightly curved. Like corynebacteria, they frequently show bipolar bodies due to the presence of metachromatic granules. They are nonsporing and nonmotile, while a few strains are motile by peritrichous flagellae. These organisms are usually long and slender with squared ends, and frequently occur in chains.

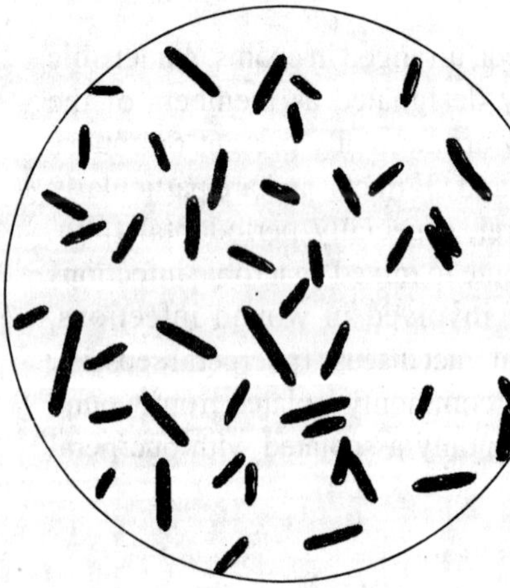

Fig. 54.3 *Lactobacillus*

Lactobacilli are normally present in the mouth and ferment sucrose to produce lactic acid, which dissolves the mineral components of enamel and dentine causing **dental caries**.

Some species are normal commensals of large intestine, the most common being *L. acidophilus*. Intestinal lactobacilli are beneficial in synthesizing vitamins such as biotin, vitamin B_{12} and vitamin K, which may be absorbed by the host.

They constitute the normal flora of vagina and ferment the glycogen deposited in the vaginal epithelial cells, forming lactic acid, which accounts for the highly acidic pH of vaginal mucus epithelia. Lactobacilli of several species occur in vagina and are collectively called as **Doderlein's bacilli**. In prepubertal and postmenopausal vagina, lactobacilli are scanty.

It is generally nonpathogenic. *L. catenaforme* has been associated with bronchopulmonary infections. Lactobacilli are acidophilic and grow best at acidic pH. Some species have strict growth requirements and are used for the microbiological assay of growth factors (vitamins).

PROPIONIBACTERIUM

They are anaerobic or microaerophilic, Gram positive bacilli of diphtheroid-like morphology. They are common inhabitants of skin, and, in rare instances, have been reported as causes of endocarditis or infections of plastic implants. *P. acnes*, often a strict anaerobe, has been implicated as a contributing cause of **acne**. It occurs as common contaminant in blood and CSF cultures.

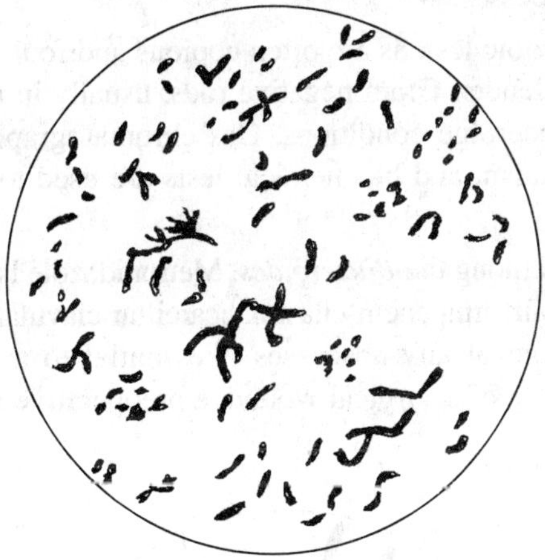

Fig. 54.4 *Propionibacterium*

EUBACTERIUM

They are Gram positive bacilli, strictly anaerobic and grow very slowly. They are part of normal flora of mouth and GI tract. Some species such as *E. brachy*, *E. timidum*, *E. nodatum* are commonly seen in the **periodontitis**. *E. lentum* is commonly isolated from nonoral clinical specimens.

BIFIDOBACTERIUM

They are nonmotile, nonsporing and pleomorphic Gram positive bacilli, showing true and false branching. The name is derived from the frequent bifid Y-shaped cells. Most species are obligate anaerobes, but a few are aerotolerant. They occur as normal flora of mouth, GI tract and genitourinary tract. They are usually nonpathogenic. *B. bifidium* is commonly found in the feces of infants and adults.

MOBILINCUS

They are motile, curved, anaerobic Gram positive bacilli that may appear as Gram variable. *M. mulieris* and *M. curtisii* have been isolated from the vagina in bacterial vaginosis, along with *Gardnerella vaginalis*. *Bacterial vaginosis* is a polymicrobial infection characterised by a thin, malodorous vaginal discharge. Its "rotten fish smell" is accentuated by mixing it with a drop of KOH solution. "*Clue cells*" (epithelial cells with adherent bacilli on the surface) are seen in stained and unstained smears from vaginal discharge.

BACTEROIDES

They are Gram negative pleomorphic slender rods, branching forms or coccobacilli seen singly, in pairs or in short chains. They possess polysaccharide capsule, which is an important virulence factor, conveying resistance to phagocytosis and antibodies to them can be demonstrated in patient's sera. Cell wall lipopolysaccharide has no endotoxic activity.

They are predominant anaerobes found in the colon. They may be transmitted to blood or peritoneum following abdominal trauma or surgery. The major disease causing species is *B. fragilis*, which is divided into five subspecies, referred to *B. fragilis* group. It elaborates several enzymes (heparinase, collagenase etc.) that contribute to tissue destruction. When released from colon into the blood, *B. fragilis* multiplies rapidly, causing bacteremia. If introduced into the abdominal cavity, *B. fragilis* causes peritonitis and/or abdominal abscesses.

Exudates from mixed anaerobic lesions are often copious and foul smelling. A Gram stain of such exudates show numerous faint, slender, Gram negative rods, usually in mixed flora. *B. fragilis* can be cultured on blood agar under anaerobic conditions. Gas chromatography can be used to identify the fatty acids produced by the organism and biochemical tests are used to determine sugar fermentation pattern.

Drug resistance is common among the *Bacteroides*. Metronidazole is the drug of choice. Alternative choices include ampicillin-sulbactam, imipenem-cilastin, ticarcillin-clavulanate, chloramphenicol, cefoxitin or clindamycin. Surgical drainage of any abscesses is essential to assure penetration of drugs. To prevent *Bacterioides* contamination of a surgical wound, a preoperative antibiotic such as cefoxitin can be administered.

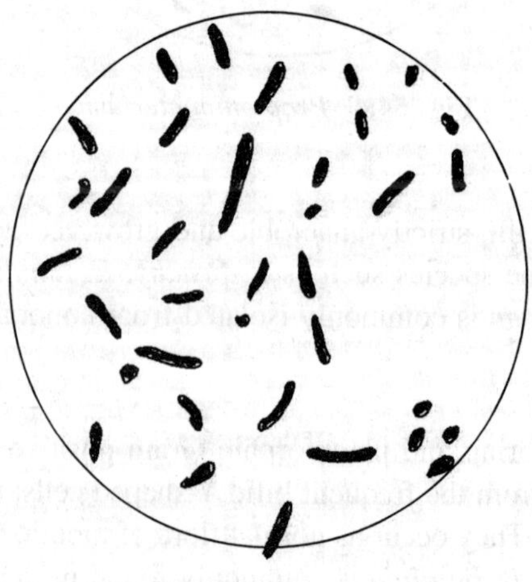

Fig. 54.5 *Bacteroides*

PREVOTELLA

Prevotella melaninogenica is part of the normal flora of the mouth and upper alimentary and respiratory tracts. Its cell wall contains a strong **endotoxin**. *Prevotella* infections are usually associated with the upper respiratory tract, causing dental and sinus infections, pulmonary infections and abscesses, brain abscesses, and infections caused by a human bite. The source of these infections is generally the oral flora. *P. melaninogenica* forms black colonies on blood agar, a characteristic from which its name was derived. It is usually sensitive to penicillin and exhibits less drug resistance than *Bacteroides*. *Prevotella* species are moderately saccharolytic, inhibited by 20% bile.

PORPHYROMONAS

They are anaerobic Gram negative bacilli, asaccharolytic, pigmented. They are normal commensals of mouth. *P. gingivalis* causing periodontal disease, *P. endodontalis* causing dental root canal infections are important species.

FUSOBACTERIUM

Fusobacteria are spindle-shaped, Gram negative bacilli with pointed ends. They are found as part of the normal flora of the mouth, female genital tract and colon. They grow slowly *in vivo*, and are therefore of limited virulence. These organisms are involved in a great variety of clinical presentations, for example, in peritonitis and abdominal abscesses, and can cause pelvic inflammatory disease, empyema (accumulation of pus in a cavity such as thoracic cavity), bronchiectasis, a necrotizing aspiration pneumonia, brain abscesses, osteomyelitis, and periodontal disease. *F. necrophorum* produces a wide range of exotoxins.

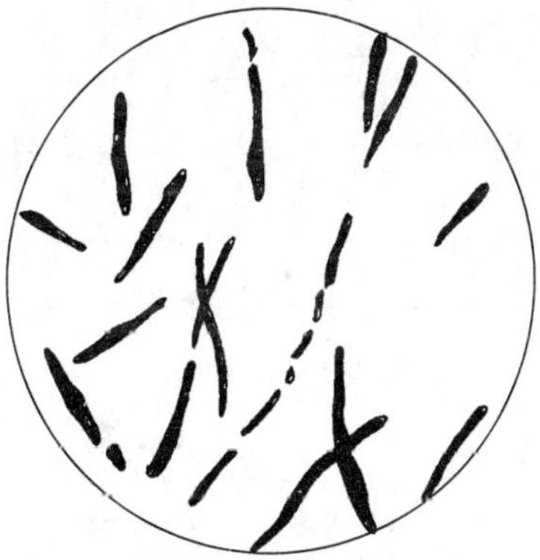

Fig. 54.6 *Fusobacterium*

LEPTOTRICHA

The genus *Leptotricha* contains the single species, *L. buccalis* which was formerly known as *Fusobacterium fusiforme* or vincent's fusiform bacillus. They are long, straight, curved Gram negative rods with pointed ends. They are part of the normal oral flora and are seen in acute necrotising lesions in the mouth. It is associated with *Borrelia vincentii* in "**vincent's angina**".

QUESTIONS

Essay Type Questions

1. Give an account of infections caused by nonsporing anaerobes.

Short Answer Type Questions

1. Nonsporing anaerobes.
2. Anaerobic cocci.
3. *Lactobacillus.*
4. *Bacteroides.*
5. *Fusobacterium.*
6. What is the natural habitat of *Bacteroides fragilis*? What infections do they cause?
7. Enumerate nonsporing anaerobes.

55

Family: Enterobacteriaceae

- *General features*
- *Classification*

GENERAL FEATURES

1. Normal flora of large intestine of humans and animals (constitute only a minor fraction of the total microbial flora of the GI tract. Most of the bowel organisms are either Gram positive or Gram negative anaerobes).
2. Aerobes and facultative anaerobes.
3. Gram negative bacilli.
4. Nonsporing and nonacid fast.
5. May or may not be capsulated.
6. Motile by peritrichate flagellae (*E. coli*, *Proteus*, *Salmonella*) or nonmotile (*Klebsiella*, *Shigella*).
7. Ferment glucose producing acid and gas or acid only.
8. Reduce nitrates to nitrites.
9. Oxidase negative (lack cytochrome oxidase).
10. Catalase positive (an exception is *Shigella shiga*, which is catalase negative).
11. Genetic recombination such as conjugation, transduction and transformation are frequent.
12. Contain lipopolysaccharide (LPS), which is both antigenic and a potential virulence factor (endotoxin).

Note : 1. *Yersinia pestis*, a causative agent of plague is included in enterobacteriaceae family, as it is oxidase negative.

2. *Vibrio cholerae* and *Pseudomonas*, though live in the intestine, are not included in enterobacteriaceae family, as they are oxidase positive.

CLASSIFICATION

The oldest method was to classify enterobacteriaceae into three groups based on lactose fermentation, usually tested in **MacConky agar**.

1. Lactose fermenters (LF) *e.g., E. coli, Klebsiella.*
2. Late lactose fermenters (LLF) *e.g., Shigella sonnei*, Paracolons.
3. Nonlactose fermenters (NLF) *e.g., Salmonella, Shigella.*

The majority of the commensal intestinal bacilli are lactose fermenting. As the most common member of this group is the colon bacillus, or *E. coli*, all lactose fermenting, enteric bacilli are called "coliform bacilli" (*e.g., E. coli, Klebsiella, Citrobacter* and *Enterobacter*).

The current method of classification is to group together bacteria that possess a number of common morphological and biochemical properties and similar DNA base composition. The three widely used systems — Bergey's manual, Kauffmann, and Edwards-Ewing, for the classification of enterobacteriaceae, have certain differences, but the general approach is the same. The family is first classified into its major subdivision — group or tribe. Each tribe consists of one or more genera and each genus one or more subgenera and species. The species are classified into biotypes, serotypes, phage types, colicin types etc.

Table 55.1 Enterobacteriaceae

Tribes	*Genera*
Tribe I : Escherichieae	1. *Escherichia* 2. *Edwardsiella* 3. *Citrobacter* 4. *Salmonella* 5. *Shigella*
Tribe II : Klebsielleae	1. *Klebsiella* 2. *Enterobacter* 3. *Hafnia* 4. *Serralia*
Tribe III : Proteeae	1. *Proteus* 2. *Morganella* 3. *Providencia*
Tribe IV : Erwineae	1. *Erwinia*
Tribe V : Yersineae	1. *Yersinia*

The various biochemical properties used to classify enterobacteriaceae members are lactose fermentation, ONPG (Orthonitrophenyl-β-D-galactopyranoside) test, IMViC tests, phenyl alanine deaminase test, urease test, H_2S production, gelatin liquefaction, growth in the presence of KCN and malonate utilization.

Table 55.2 Enterobacteriaceae : Important distinguishing Features of the different Genera

	Escherichia	*Edwardsiella*	*Citrobacter*	*Salmonella*[1]	*Shigella*[2]	*Klebstella*	*Enterobacter*	*Hafnia*	*Serratia*	*Proteus*	*Morganella*	*Providencia*
Motility	+	+	+	+	−	−	+	+	+	+	+	+
Gas from glucose	+	+	+	+	−	+	+	+	d	d	+	+
Acid from lactose	+	−	+	−	−	+	+	−	−	−	−	−
Acid from sucrose	d	−	d	−	−	+	+	−	+	d	−	d
Growth in KCN	−	−	+	d	−	+	+	+	+	+	+	+
Indole	+	+	d	−	d	−	−	−	−	d	+	+
MR	+	+	+	+	+	−	−	−	−	+	+	+
VP	−	−	−	−	−	+	+	+	+	−	−	−
Citrate	−	−	+	+	−	+	+	+	+	d	d	d
H_2S	−	+	+	+	−	+	−	−	−	+	−	−
Urease	−	−	−	−	−	+	d	−	−	+	+	d
Phenylalanine deaminase (PPA)	−	−	−	−	−	−	−	−	−	+	+	+
Arginine dehydrolase	d	−	d	+	−	−	d	−	−	−	−	−
Lysine decarboxylase	+	+	−	+	−	d	d	+	+	−	−	−
Ornithine decarboxylase	d	+	d	+	d	−	+	+	+	d	+	−

(d = results different in different species or strains).

Important exceptions:

1. *S. typhi* does not produce gas from sugars.
2. *Sh. sonnei* ferments lactose and sucrose late.

QUESTIONS

Essay Type Questions

1. Describe the general properties and classification of family enterobacteriaceae.

Short Answer Type Questions

1. General properties of enterobacteriaceae.
2. Classification of enterobacteriaceae.

56

Escherichia coli

- *Introduction*
- *Morphology*
- *Cultural characteristics*
- *Biochemical reactions*
- *Antigenic structure (virulence factors)*
- *Toxins*
- *Epidemiology*
- *Pathogenicity*
  - *intestinal diseases*
  - *extraintestinal diseases*
- *Laboratory diagnosis*
- *Prevention*
- *Treatment*

INTRODUCTION

The genus "*Escherichia*" is named after Escherich who first described this colon bacillus under the name bacterium coli commune (1885). *E. coli* is part of the normal flora of the colon in humans and other animals, but can be pathogenic both within and outside of the GI tract. Voided in feces, it remains viable in the environment only for a few days. Therefore, the presence of *E. coli* in drinking water is taken as evidence of recent pollution with human or animal feces.

MORPHOLOGY

It is a Gram negative bacillus. The bacillus is straight, measures 1–3×0.4–0.7 μm in size. It is motile by peritrichate flagellae, but some strains are nonmotile. It is noncapsulated, but a polysaccharide capsule is found in some strains. It has chromosomally determined fimbriae or pili of type I *i.e.*, hemagglutinating and mannose-sensitive. It is nonsporing.

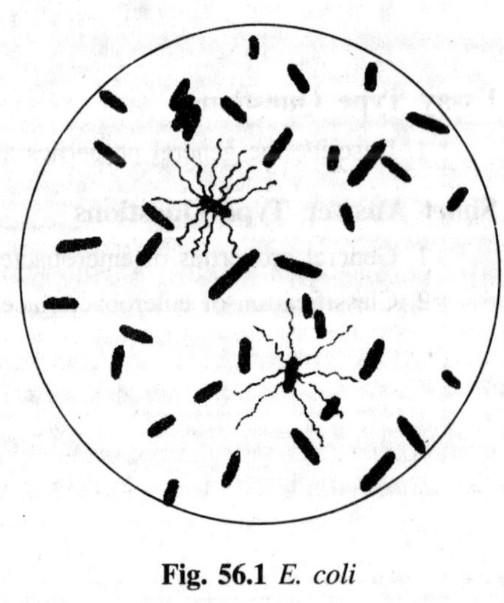

Fig. 56.1 *E. coli*

CULTURAL CHARACTERISTICS

It is an aerobe and facultative anaerobe. Optimum temperature for growth is 37ºC and optimum pH is 7.2–7.6. Good growth occurs on ordinary media.

On **nutrient agar**, the colonies are large, thick, greyish white, moist, smooth, opaque or partially translucent on overnight incubation. Some strains may occur in mucoid form due to the presence of capsule. On repeated subcultures, the colonies undergo S → R (smooth to rough) variation, associated with loss of surface antigens and virulence. Smooth (S) form is seen on fresh isolation, which is easily emulsifiable in saline. The rough (R) form colonies will have an irregular dull surface and are autoagglutinable in saline.

On **blood agar**, the strains isolated from pathological specimens show betahemolysis. On **Mac Conkey's agar**, colonies are bright pink due to lactose fermentation. Growth is largely inhibited on selective media such as DCA or SS agar (Salmonella-shigella agar) used for the isolation of *Salmonella* and *Shigella*.

In nutrient broth, growth occurs as general turbidity and a heavy deposit, which disperses completely on shaking.

BIOCHEMICAL REACTIONS

E. coli produces both acid and gas during fermentation of carbohydrates such as glucose, lactose, mannitol, maltose, sucrose etc. Typical strains do not ferment sucrose. *E. coli* is indole and methyl red tests positive and Voges Proskaner and citrate utilization tests are negative. (*IMViC* + + – –). Gelatin is not liquefied. H_2S is not formed, urea is not hydrolysed and growth does not occur is KCN medium.

ANTIGEN STRUCTURE/VIRULENCE FACTORS

Serotyping *of E. coli* strains is based on differences in three structural antigens : O, H and K. So far some 170 types of O antigens, 100 K antigens and 75 H antigens have been recognized. The antigenic pattern of a strain is recorded as the number of the particular antigen it carries, as for example O 111 : K 58 : H 2.

The **O antigens** (somatic antigens or cell wall antigens) are found on the polysaccharide portion of the LPS. The **H antigens** are associated with flagellae. The **K antigen** is the acidic polysaccharide antigen located in the capsule. It encloses the O antigen and renders the strain inagglutinable by the O antiserum. It may also contribute to virulence by inhibiting phagocytosis. Several different serotypes of *E. coli* are found in the GI tract.

A number of filamentous protein structures resembling fimbriae which are plasmid coded (The differences in the degree of virulence of different *E. coli* strains are caused by the individual plasmid and integrated prophage repertoire associated with each strain) and mediate mannose-resistant hemagglutination have been described in *E. coli*. These include K88, K99 and colonization factor antigens (CFAS). They probably play a significant role in the pathogenesis of diarrhea and urinary tract infection.

TOXINS

E. coli produces two kinds of exotoxins-hemolysins and **enterotoxins**. Three distinct types of *E. coli* enterotoxins have been identified – heat labile toxin (LT), heat stable toxin (ST) and verotoxin (VT) also known as shiga-like toxin (SLT).

Hemolysins are responsible for hemolysis of RBC on blood agar and are produced more commonly by virulent strains, particularly from extra-intestinal infections.

Heat labile toxin (LT) can be destroyed by heating at 65°C for 30 minutes. It resembles the cholera toxin in its structure, antigenic properties and mode of action. It is a complex of one polypeptide A (active) subunit and five identical B (binding) subunits. The B subunit binds to the Gm_1 ganglioside receptor on intestinal epithelial cells, which facilitates the entry of subunit A into the cell, following which the subunit A is activated to yield two fragments — A_1 and A_2. The A_1 fragment activates **adenyl cyclase** in the enterocyte, which catalyses the conversion of ATP to cyclic AMP (cAMP). The accumulation of **cAMP** in the intestinal mucosa leads to increased outflow of water and electrolytes into the intestinal lumen, resulting in a **watery diarrhea**. Though the mechanism of action of LT and cholera toxin (CT) is the same, the latter is about a hundred times more potent than the former.

LT is a powerful antigen and can therefore, be detected by a number of serological as well as biological tests such as **ligated rabbit illeal loop** (read at 18 hours), adult rabbit skin (vascular permeability factor), steroid production in Y1 mouse adrenal cell culture, morphological changes in Chinese hamster ovary cells, gel diffusion, reverse passive latex agglutination test and ELISA.

Heat stable toxin (ST) is a low molecular weight polypeptide and poorly antigenic. Two types of ST are known. ST_A (or ST-I) and ST_B (or ST-II). ST_A acts by activation of **cyclic GMP** in the intestine. It acts very rapidly and induces fluid accumulation in the intestines of infant mice within four hours of intragastric administration. This **infant mouse intragastric test** is the standard method for demonstration of ST_A. It also induces fluid accumulation in the intestinal loops of neonatal but not weaned piglets. ST_A is methanol soluble. ST_B causes fluid accumulation in young piglets (upto nine weeks) but not in infant mice. The mode of action of ST_B is not known but it is not through cAMP or cGMP. ST_B is not methanol soluble. ST genes are carried on plasmids which may also carry other genes, such as for LT and drug resistance. However, ST_A and ST_B genes are not seen to be carried on the same plasmid.

Verotoxin (VT) or verocytotoxin was so named because it was first detected (1977) by its cytotoxic effect on vero cells, a cell line derived from African green monkey kidney cells. It is also known as **shiga-like toxin (SLT)** as it is similar to the *Shigella dysenteriae* type 1 toxin in its physical, antigenic and biological properties. VT also shows enterotoxicity in rabbit illeal loops and mouse paralytic-lethality as does the shiga toxin. VT is also composed of A and B subunits. VT genes appear to be phage encoded. An antigenically different VT, known as VT_2 has been identified, which is not neutralized by the shiga antitoxin, unlike VT_1.

EPIDEMIOLOGY

Transmission of intestinal disease is commonly by the fecal-oral route, with contaminated food and water serving as vehicles for transmission.

The source of infection for extraintestinal disease is frequently the patient's own flora, where the individual's own *E. coli* is nonpathogenic in the intestine, but causes disease in that individual, when the organism is found in the bladder or blood stream (normally sterile sites).

E. coli is excreted in feces of man and animals in very large numbers and contaminate soil and water.

PATHOGENICITY

E. coli can cause both intestinal and extraintestinal diseases.

Intestinal disease (diarrhea) — Atleast five types of intestinal infections that differ in their pathogenic mechanisms have been identified.

1. Enterotoxigenic *E. coli* (ETEC) — These strains produce **enterotoxins** — LT or ST or both. They are associated with diarrhea in infants and adults in tropical and subtropical climates, especially in developing countries, where it is one of the major causes of **infantile diarrhea.** ETEC are a common cause of **traveller's diarrhoea** seen in persons from developed countries visiting endemic developing countries. Transmission occurs through food and water contaminated with human waste, or by person-to-person contact. ETEC colonize the small intestine. Pili or colonization factor antigens facilitate the binding of the organism to the intestinal mucosa. In a process mediated by enterotoxins (see toxins), ETEC cause prolonged hypersecretion of chloride ions and water by the intestinal mucosal cells, while inhibiting the reabsorption of sodium. The gut becomes full of fluid, resulting in significant watery diarrhea that continues over a period of several days. Common serogropus of ETEC are O 6, O 8, O 15, O 25, O 27, O 63, O 78, O 115, O 148, O 153, O 159 and O 167.

2. Enteropathogenic *E. coli*, (EPEC) — They are an important cause of diarrhea in infants (infantile enteritis), especially in locations with poor sanitation. The new born becomes infected during birth, or *in utero*. The EPEC attach to mucosal cells in the small intestine, causing destruction of microvilli and development of characteristic lesions. Watery diarrhea results, which on rare occasions may become chronic. The name **enteroadherent *E. coli*** (EAEC) has been proposed for these strains, which can be identified by their adhesion to HE_{P-2} cells. Common serogroups of EPEC are O 26, O 55, O 86, O 111, O 114, O 119, O 125, O 126, O 127, O 128 and O 142.

3. Enterohemorrhagic *E. coli* (EHEC) or **Verotoxigenic E. coli (VTEC)** — EHEC binds to cells in the large intestine, where they produce an exotoxin (**verotoxin**, VT), or shigalike toxin (SLT), causing a severe form of copious, bloody diarrhea, known as **hemorrhagic colitis** in the absence of mucosal invasion or inflammation. Serotype O157:H7 is the most common strain of *E. coli* that produces verocytotoxin. This strain is also associated with outbreaks of a potentially life-threatening, acute renal failure, known as **hemolytic uremic syndrome (HUS).** The primary target for VT appears to be the vascular endothelial cells. This may explain the pathogenesis of HUS, in which a characteristic renal lesion is capillary microangiopathy. The primary reservoir of EHEC is cattle. Therefore the possibility of infection can be greatly decreased by thoroughly cooking ground beef and pasteurizing milk.

4. Enteroinvasive *E. coli* (EIEC) — They cause a dysentery like syndrome with fever and blood stools. **Sereny test** is used for laboratory diagnosis of EIEC, where instillation of a drop of EIEC suspension (or *Shigella*) into the eyes of guinea pigs (or mice) leads to mucopurulent conjunctivitis and severe keratitis. Cell penetration of HeLa or HEP_{-2} cells in culture is a more humane diagnostic test. This ability to penetrate cells is determined by a large plasmid, detection of which can also be a diagnostic test. The plasmid codes for outer membrane antigens called the "virulence marker antigens (VMA)", which can be detected by ELISA.

EIEC resemble *Shigella* in many respects. Many of these strains are nonmotile, do not ferment lactose or ferment it late with acid, but without producing any gas and do not form lysine decarboxylase. Many of these show O antigen cross reaction with Shigellae. Besides these "**atypical strains**" many typical *E. coli* strains can also cause clinical illness resembling shigellosis. They have been termed EIEC because they have the capacity to invade intestinal epithelial cells *in vivo* and penetrate HeLa cells in tissue culture (*in vitro*). Common serogroups of EIEC are O 28, O 112, O 124, O 136, O 143, O 144, O 152 and O 164.

5. Enteroaggregative *E. coli* (EAEC) — These strains are so named because they appear aggregated in a "stacked brick" formation on HEP_{-2} cells or glass. They have been associated with persistent diarrhea, by adhering to the mucosal surface of the intestine, especially in developing countries. Most of them are O-untypable but may are H-typable. In animal experiments they cause shortening of villi, hemorrhagic necrosis and mild edema with mononuclear infiltration of the submucosa. They form a low molecular weight heat stable enterotoxin called **enteroaggregative heat stable enterotoxin-1 (EAST-1)**.

Extraintestinal diseases — *E. coli* can cause various extraintestinal infections such as urinary tract infections, neonatal meningitis, pyogenic infections and speticemia.

1. Urinary tract infections (UTI) — *E. coli* is the most common cause of UTI, including cystitis and pyelonephritis. Women are particularly at risk for infection. **Uncomplicated cystitis** (the most commonly encountered UTI) is caused by uropathogenic strains of *E. coli*, characterized by P fimbriae (an adherence factor) and, frequently, hemolysin, colicin V, and resistance to the bactericidal activity of complement. The P fimbriae are so named because they attach to the receptor on epithelial cells of urinary tract, which is a part of P blood group antigen. **Complicated UTI (pyelonephritis)** typically occur in settings of obstructed urinary flow, and may be caused by nonuropathogenic strains.

E. coli that cause UTI often originate in the gut of the patient. The bacteria may gain access to the urinary tract by the ascending or the hematogenous route. The ascending route of infection is believed to be common. The bacteria from the fecal flora spread to the perineum and from there they ascend into the bladder. The high incidence of UTI in pregnant women can be attributed to impairment of urine flow due to pressure on the urinary tract and due to hormonal changes. Pregnant women will have urinary tract infections, without any clinical symptoms, known as **"asymptomatic bacteriuria".** When it is undetected and untreated, may lead to symptomatic infection later in pregnancy, such as pyelonephritis, hypertension in women, prematurity and perinatal death of the fetus. Other conditions predisposing to UTI include enlarged prostrate, urinary caliculi, congenital malformations and neurological disorders. Catheterization and cystoscopy may introduce endogenous or exogenous bacteria into the bladder leading to UTI.

UTI may be defined as the presence and multiplication of bacteria in urine within the urinary tract. Kass (1956) gave a criterion of active bacterial infection of urinary tract according to which a count exceeding 10^5 (one lakh) bacteria/ml denotes **significant bacteriruria** and indicates active UTI. Counts of 10^4 (10,000) bacteria/ml or less per ml are due to contamination during voiding and are of no significance. This count is, however, not applicable to tuberculosis of urinary tract because of slow generation time of *Mycobacterium tuberculosis*. Bacterial counts in urine are, however, influenced by various factors such as high fluid intake, use of alkalinizing or acidifying agents and inadequate chemotherapy. Therefore, a low bacterial count should be considered significant in patients with symptoms and pyuria.

Most frequently encountered O serotypes of *E. coli* in UTI include O1, O2, O4, O6, O7, O18 and O 75.

2. Neonatal meningitis — *E. coli* is a major cause of this disease occurring within the first month of life. The K1 (capsular) antigen is particularly associated with such infections.

3. Pyogenic infections — *E. coli* is the most common cause of intra-abdominal infections, such as peritonitis and abscesses resulting from spillage of bowel contents.

4. Septicemia — Blood stream invasion by *E. coli* may lead to fatal conditions like septic shock and systemic inflammatory response syndrome.

5. Nosocomial infections — These include sepsis/bacteremia, endotoxic shock and pneumonia.

LABORATORY DIAGNOSIS

Lab. diagnosis of diarrheas — A sample of feces is collected and plated on blood agar and MacConkey agar. After overnight incubation, the bacterial growth has to be identified by biochemical reactions and slide agglutination tests with appropriate antisera.

The fluorescent antibody method can be used for the detection of some specific serotypes.

EPEC are identified by slide agglutination tests with polyvalent and monovalent antisera against EPEC serotypes.

Enterotoxins of ETEC can be detected by various methods. Labile toxin (LT) can be detected by ligated rabbit illeal loop test, adult rabbit skin test, steroid production in Y1 mouse adrenal cell culture, morphological changes in chinese hamster ovary cells, gel diffusion, reverse passive latex agglutination test and ELISA.

EHEC, unlike most other strains of *E. coli*, ferment sorbitol slowly if at all, and may be detected on MacConkey sorbitol agar.

EIEC can be demonstrated by **Sereny test**. When EIEC is instilled into the eyes of guinea pigs, they cause keratoconjunctivitis. EIEC are also identified by their ability to invade HeLa tissue culture.

Laboratory diagnosis of UTI

Collection of specimen — Normal urine is sterile, but during voiding may get contaminated with commensal flora. Therefore, clean-voided **midstream sample** of urine is employed for culture. The normal flora of anterior urethra must be adequately flushed out by discarding some urine before the specimen is obtained. In case of male, retract the prepuce, clean it with sterile normal saline and collect midstream sample. In case of female, anogenital toilet is more important. Wash perineum and periurethral area with soap and water. Then clean with nonirritant antiseptic such as chlorhexidine. Separate apart labia with fingers of one hand and collect midstream portion of urine into a wide mouthed sterile container.

Urine is an excellent culture medium, therefore, it should be transported to the laboratory without delay. If there is a delay of 1—2 hrs, it should be refrigerated.

Microscopic examination — The direct microscopic examination of urine is done to detect the presence of increased number of polymorphs (pyuria) which is an indication of UTI. The deposit of the centrifuged urine can be examined under microscope to find out the presence of pus cells, RBC and bacteria in it. Presence of more than 3 pus cells per high power field is suggestive of infection. Presence of RBC indicate damage to urinary tract.

Culture — Measured quantity of urine (0.004 ml or 1/250 ml) is inoculated on blood agar and MacConkey agar with the help of standard wire loop (internal diameter 3.26 mm) of nichrome wire of SWG 28, and incubated overnight at 37°C. The number of colonies is counted and multiplied by 250 to get the bacterial count per ml. On the basis of this result, it can be reported whether the patient has significant bacteriuria or not. Quantitative estimation of bacterial counts can be carried out by pour-plate method and surface viable count. The isolate is identified by cultural characteristics, biochemical reactions and slide agglutination tests. The isolate is subjected to antibiotic sensitivity testing.

Lab. diagnosis of pyogenic infections and septicemia — The specimens collected are pus, wound swabs, blood and CSF and inoculated on to blood agar, MacConkey agar and incubated at 37°C for one to two days. The growth is identified by cultural characteristics, biochemical reactions and slide agglutination tests.

PREVENTION

Intestinal disease can best be prevented by care in selection, preparation, and consumption of food and water.

TREATMENT

Maintenance of fluid and electrolyte balance is of primary importance in treatment. Antibiotics may shorten duration of symptoms; however, resistance is widespread. Extraintestinal diseases require antibiotic treatment. Antibiotic sensitivity testing of isolates is necessary to determine the appropriate choice of drugs.

QUESTIONS

Essay Type Questions

1. Enumerate the organisms causing UTI. Outline the steps in the lab. diagnosis of a case of UTI.
2. Mention the bacteria causing diarrhoeas. Describe the lab. diagnosis of bacterial diarrheas.

Short Answer Type Questions

1. List out the causative organisms of UTI.
2. Describe significant bacteriuria or Kass concept.
3. Enterotoxins.
4. ETEC.
5. Traveller's diarrhea.
6. Asymptomatic bacteriruria.
7. EPEC.
8. EIEC.
9. Sereny test.
10. EHEC or VTEC.
11. LT.
12. Hemolytic uremic syndrome.

57

Salmonella

INTRODUCTION

The genus *Salmonella* is named after D.E. Salman, an American microbiologist and consists of bacilli that parasitise the intestines of a large number of vertebrate species and infect human beings, leading to enteric fever, gastroenteritis, septicemia, with or without focal suppuration and the carrier state.

The genus *Salmonella* comprises more than 2300 serotypes. A recent classification scheme based on DNA relatedness recognizes only two species *S. enterica* and *S. bongori*. Organisms causing human disease belong to *S. enterica*, whereas *S. bongori* is a nonhuman pathogen.

S. enterica is further classifed into six subspecies. Each of the subspecies, in turn, contains multiple serovars. *S. enterica* subspecies *enterica* includes almost all the human pathogenic serovars, the most important of which is *S. enterica* subsp. *enterica* (subspecies I) which includes the typhoid and paratyphoid bacilli and most other serotypes responsible for causing disease in mammals. Salmonellae are named as, for example, *S. enterica* subsp. *enterica* serotype *enteritidis*. For convenience it is usual to abbreviate this to *S. enteritidis*. Serotype names should be given in Roman (not in italics).

MORPHOLOGY

Salmonellae are Gram negative bacilli, about 1–3 × 0.5 μm in size. They are motile with peritrichate flagellae, except for one type, *S. gallinarum-pullorum*, which is always nonmotile. Nonmotile mutants of other types may sometimes be found *e.g.,* 901–O strain is a stable nonmotile mutant of *S. typhi.* Salmonellae are noncapsulated and nonsporing but may possess fimbriae of type 1 (mannose-sensitive and hemagglutinating).

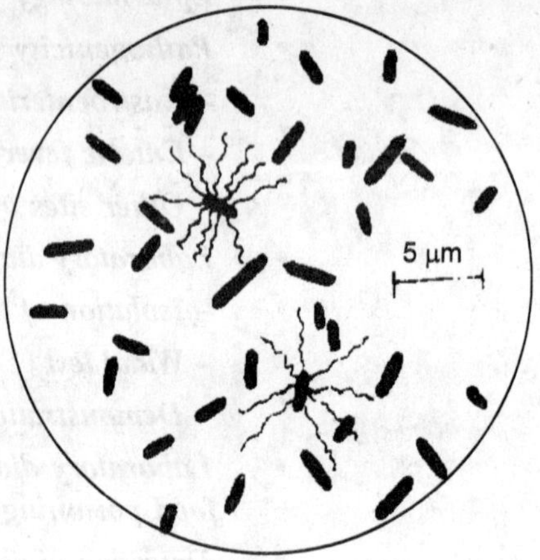

Fig. 57.1 *Salmonella*

CULTURAL CHARACTERISTICS

Salmonellae are aerobes and facultative anaerobes. Optimum temperature for growth is 37°C and optimum pH 7.2. They can grow readily on ordinary media.

On nutrient agar or blood agar the colonies are large, 2–3 mm in diameter, circular, low convex, greyish-white and translucent. On MacConkey and DCA media, colonies are colorless due to the absence of lactose fermentation. **Wilson and Blair bismuth sulphite agar** medium is a selective medium, on which jet black colonies with a metallic sheen are formed due to the production of H_2S. *S. paratyphi A, S. cholerae-suis* and other species that do not form H_2S produce green colonies. **Selenite F broth** and tetrathionate broth are commonly employed as enrichment media.

BIOCHEMICAL REACTIONS

Salmonellae ferment glucose, mannitol, maltose, forming both acid and gas. An important exception is *S. typhi* which is **anaerogenic** *i.e.,* produces acid only without gas. Lactose, sucrose and salicin are not fermented. Indole is not produced. They are MR positive, VP negative and citrate positive. *S. typhi* and a few other salmonellae do not grow in Simmon's citrate agar medium, as they need tryptophan as the growth factor. Urease negative. H_2S is produced, except by *S. paratyphi A*, *S. cholerae-suis* and some other species. They decarboxylate lysine, ornithine and arginine but not glutamic acid. However, *S. typhi* and *S. paratyphi* A do not decarboxylate ornithine and lysine respectively.

RESISTANCE

The bacilli are killed at 55°C in one hour or at 60°C in 15 minutes. Boiling or chlorination of water and pasteurization of milk destroy the bacilli. In polluted water and soil, they survive for weeks and in ice for months. Cultures may be viable for years if prevented from drying. They are killed within five minutes by mercuric chloride (1 : 500) or 5% phenol.

ANTIGENIC STRUCTURE

Salmonellae possess three main types of antigens on the basis of which they are serologically typed and classified: 1. Flagellar (H) Antigens, 2. Somatic (O) antigens, and 3. A surface antigen, known as Vi antigen.

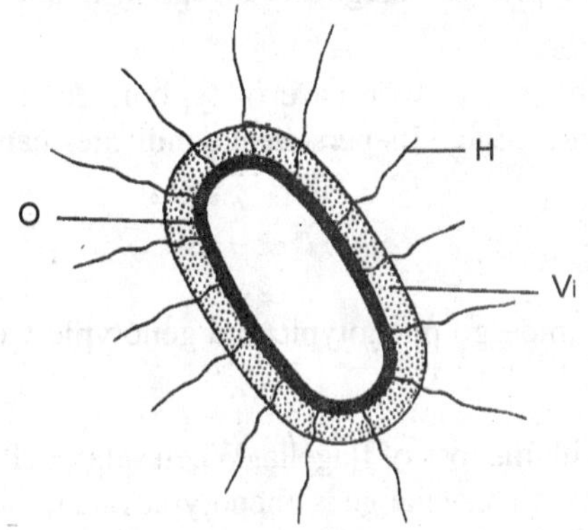

Fig. 57.2 Antigens of *salmonella*

H antigen

H antigen is present in flagellae. It is a heat labile protein. It can be destroyed by boiling or by treating with alcohol, but not by formalin. It is a strong antigen and induces antibody formation rapidly and in high titre following infection or immunisation. When mixed with antisera, H agglutination produces large, loose, fluffy clumps and takes place best at 37°C.

H antigen is of dual nature and exist in one of the two phases:

(*i*) Phase 1 antigen is either specific for a species or shared by a few species; hence, called as a "specific phase" and are designated a, b, c, d etc. and after Z, Z_1 and Z_2 etc.

(*ii*) Phase 2 antigens are fewer and are designated 1, 2, 3 etc. They are widely shared among salmonellae species; hence, called "nonspecific phase".

O antigen

O antigen is an integral part of cell wall, also called as endotoxin or Boivin antigen. It is relatively heat stable. It is a phospholipid-protein-polysaccharide complex. It can be extracted from the cell by treatment with trichloroacetic acid. It is not affected by boiling, alcohol or weak acids. O antigen is less antigenic than H antigen and the titre of antibody induced after infection or immunization is lower than that of H antibody. When O antigen is mixed with antisera, O agglutination takes place more slowly and optimally at 50–55°C and forms compact, chalky, granular clumps.

O antigen is not a single factor, but a mosaic of two or more factors, known as O antigenic factors, based on which, the genus salmonellae is classified into a number of groups, designated as A, B, C etc.

Vi antigen

Vi antigen was first described by Felix and Pitt and believed that it was related virulence. It is analogous to K antigen. Many strains of *S. typhi* fail to agglutinate with the O antiserum on fresh isolation due to the presence of a surface antigen, enveloping the O antigen. They become agglutinable after heating at 60°C for one hour.

Vi antigen is not affected by alcohol or 0.2% formalin. This antigen is present in *S. typhi*, *S. paratyphi C*, *S. dublin* and in certain strains of *Citrobacter* (Ballerup-Bethesda group). Vi antigen tends to be lost on serial subculture.

Vi antigen is a weak antigen, and only low titres of antibodies are produced following infection. Detection of Vi antibody is not helpful for diagnosis of cases; hence Vi antigen is not employed in widal test.

Total absence of Vi antibody in a proven case of typhoid fever indicates poor prognosis. The antibody disappears early in convalescence. Its persistence indicates carrier state. Vi antigen is used for epidemiological typing.

ANTIGENIC VARIATIONS

The antigens of salmonellae undergo phenotypic and genotypic variations.

H → O variation

This variation is associated with the loss of flagella. When salmonellae are grown on agar containing phenol (1:800) flagellae are inhibited. This change is phenotypic and temporary. Flagellae reappear when the strain is subcultured on agar without phenol. Rarely, salmonellae may lose flagellae by mutations. A stable nonmotile mutant of *S. typhi* is 901-0 strain, used for preparation of O antigen. Generally, the loss of flagellae is not total and flagellated cells are found in small numbers. To obtain Flagellated cells in such cultures, selection is done by Craigie's tube.

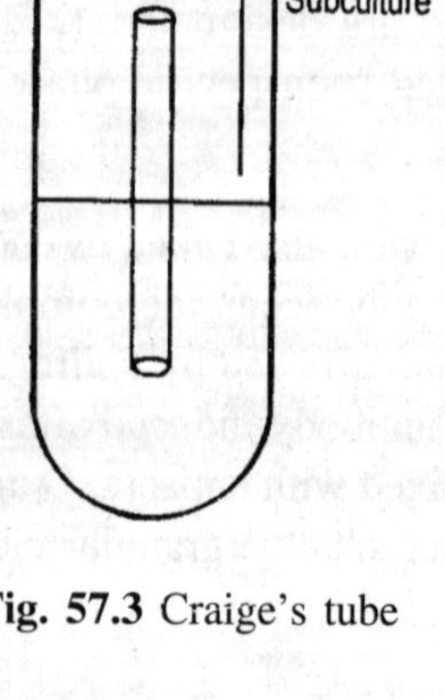

Fig. 57.3 Craige's tube

Craigie's tube consists of wide tube containing soft agar (0.2%) in the center of which is embedded a short, narrow tube open at both ends, in such a way that it projects above the surface of agar. The strain is inoculated into the inner tube. After incubation, subcultures withdrawn from the top of the agar, outside the central tube, will yield a population of motile cells. Instead of Craigie's tube, a U-tube can be used; inoculation being made into one limb and subculture taken from the other limb.

Phase variation

Flagellar (H) antigen is of dual nature and occur in any one of two phases – phase 1 antigen (specific phase) and phase 2 antigen (nonspecific phase).

Strains that possess both phases are called diphasic. Some strains like *S. typhi* occur only in one phase and are called monophasic. In some species phase 1 may occur as phase 2 antigens and this is called phase variation.

A culture will contain cells with flagellar antigens of both phases; but one or the other phase will predominate and the culture is agglutinated by that specific phase antisera.

V → W variation

Fresh isolates of *S. typhi* carry a surface layer of Vi antigen that completely masks the O antigen. Such bacilli are agglutinable with Vi antiserum but not with O antiserum. This is called V form.

After a number of subcultures, the Vi antigen is completely lost. Such cultures are not agglutinable with Vi antiserum, but agglutinable with O antiserum. This is called W form.

Intermediate stages during the loss of Vi antigen, when the bacilli are agglutinable with both Vi and O antisera, are called VW forms.

Other Vi-containing bacilli such as *S. paratyphi* C and *S. dublin* seldom have the O antigen completely masked by the Vi antigen.

S → R variation

The smooth to rough variation is associated with the change in the colony morphology and loss of the O antigen and of virulence. The colony becomes large, rough and irregular. Suspensions in saline are autoagglutinable. Conversion into R forms occurs by mutation. R forms occur rarely in nature but is common in strains maintained through serial subcultures. S → R variation may be prevented to some extent by maintaining cultures on Dorset's egg media or by lyophilisation.

Variations in O antigen

A change in structural formulae of O antigen may be brought about by lysogenization with some phages resulting in the alternation of the bacterial serotype. Thus *S. anatum* (serotype 3, 10 : e, h : 1, 6) is converted by phage 15 into *S. newington* (serotype 3, 15 : e, h : 1, 6) and the latter into *S. minneapolis* (serotype 3, 15, 34, : e, h : 1, 6) by phage 34. It is likely that such changes occurring in nature contribute to the abundance of *Salmonella* serotypes.

KAUFFMAN-WHITE SCHEME OF CLASSIFICATION

This scheme (1934) classifies salmonellae into different O serogroups, each of which contains a number of serotypes possessing a common O antigen not found in other O serogroups. Formerly O serogroups were designated by capital letters A-Z and those discovered later by the number 51–67. Some serogroups were subdivided into subserogroups ($C_1 – C_4$; $E_1 – E_4$). Serogroups A to Z and 51–67 represent O antigens 2 to 50 and 51–67 respectively.

Each serogroup is named by its common O antigen. Therefore, these numbers are not continuous. Within each O serogroup, the different serotypes are distinguished by their particular H antigen or combination of H antigens.

The antigenic structure of a *Salmonella* serotype is expressed as an antigenic formula which has three parts describing the O antigens, the phase 1 H antigens and phase 2 H antigens in that order. The three parts are separated by colons and the component antigens in each part by commas. More than 2,300 serotypes have so far been described in Kauffman-white scheme.

Table 57.1 Kauffman-White Scheme – Illustrative examples

Serogroups	*Serotype*	*Antigen*		
		O	H	
		Phase I	**Phase II**	
2–A	*S. paratyphi A*	1, 2, 12	a	–
4–B	*S. paratyphi B*	1, 4, 5, 12	b	1.2
	S. typhimurium	1, 4, 5, 12	i	1.2
	S. chester	4, 5, 12	e, h	e, n, x
7–C_1	*S. paratyphi C*	6, 7, (Vi)	c	1.5
	S. cholerae-suis	6, 7	c	1.5
8–C_2	*S. muenchen*	6, 8	d	1.2
9D	*S. typhi*	9, 12, (Vi)	d	–
	S. enteritidis	1, 9, 12	g, m	–
	S. gallinarum	1, 9, 12	–	–
10–E_1	*S. anatum*	3, 10	e, h	1.6

EPIDEMIOLOGY

Salmonellae are widely distributed in nature. Serotype *typhi* is the exclusively human pathogen, whereas other strains are associated with animals and foods (for example, eggs and poultry). Water becomes polluted by the feces from humans or animals excreting salmonellae. Man acquires infection by ingestion of contaminated water or food (fecal-oral transmission). Infection by food usually results either from ingestion of contaminated meat or by way of the hands of the carrier.

The source of infection is a patient or a carrier. Convalescent carriers and chronic carriers are important in the transmission of the disease. Food handlers or cooks who become carriers are particularly dangerous.

Young children and the elderly are particularly susceptible to *Salmonella* infection. Individuals in crowded institutions may also sustain *Salmonella* epidemics. The rate of clinical typhoid is about twenty five times higher in the HIV infected than in others.

PATHOGENICITY

Salmonella infection can cause both intestinal and extraintestinal diseases. Salmonellae invade epithelial cells of the small intestine. Disease may remain localized or become systemic, sometimes with desseminated foci. The organisms are facultative, intracellular parasites that survive in phagocytic cells. Development of clinical symptoms include depends on : (*i*) **the infectious dose,** which is strain dependent; (*ii*) **bacterial factors** including proteins that induce the intestinal epthelial cells to endocytose the organisms and promote survival within phagocytic cells, and (*iii*) **host factors** including achlorhydria, sickle cell disease and reduced cell mediated immunity (immunodeficiency).

Salmonellae cause gastroenteritis or food poisoning, enteric fever and septicemia with or without local suppurative lesions.

Gastroenteritis or food poisoning

It is generally a **zoonotic** disease, the source of infection being animal products. It is caused by ingestion by foods like meat, egg, milk and sweets contaminated by certain serotypes of Salmonellae, which are primarily animal pathogens. It is a localized disease, caused primarily by serotypes *enteriditis* and *typhinurium*. Other common serotypes include newport, dublin, heidelberg and indiana. The disease is characterized by nausea, vomiting and diarrhea (usually nonbloody), which develop generally within 48 hours of ingesting contaminated food or water. Fever and abdominal cramping are common. In uncompromised patients, disease is generally self-limiting and heals within 48–72 hours, although convalescent carriage of organisms may persist for a month or more.

Enteric fever

This is a severe, life-threatening systemic illness. It is most usually caused by serotype *typhi* (**typhoid fever**) or *paratyphi A*, *B* and *C* (**paratyphoid fever**), but other serotypes can also cause this disease.

On reaching the gut, the bacilli attach themselves to microvilli of the ileal mucosa and penetrate to the lamina propria and submucosa, where they are phagocytosed by neutrophils and macrophages. The resist intracellular killing and multiply within these cells. These cells enter the mesenteric lymph nodes, where after a period of multiplication, the bacilli invade the blood stream via thoracic duct and a transient bacteremia follows. During this period, the bacilli are seeded in the liver, gall bladder, spleen, bone marrow, lymph nodes, lungs and kidneys, where further multiplication takes place. After multiplicaton in these organs, bacilli pass into the blood, causing a second and heavier bacteremia, heralding the onset of clinical illness. As bile is a good culture medium for the bacillus, it multiplies abundantly in the gall bladder and is discharged continuously into the intestine where it involves the peyer's patches and lymphoid follicles of the ileum. These become inflamed, undergo necrosis and slough off, leaving behind characteristic typhoid ulcers. (**Note:** Infected gall bladders are the main source of fecal contamination.)

The incubation period varies from 5 to 21 days. The disease is characterized by fever and, frequently, abdominal symptoms. Nonspecific symptoms may include chills, sweats, headache, anorexia, weakness, sorethroat, cough and myalgias. About thirty percent patients have a faint maculopapular rash on the trunk (**rose spots**). Untreated, mortality is approximately fifteen percent; among survivors, the symptoms generally resolve in three to four weeks. Timely and appropriate antibiotic therepy reduces mortality to less than one percent, and speeds resolution of the fever. Complications can include intestinal hemorrhage and, rarely, focal infections and endocarditis. A small percentage of patients become chronic carriers. Such carriage leads to cholecystitis.

Other sites of *Salmonella* infection

Sustained bacteremia is often associated with vascular *Salmonella* infections that occur when bacteria seed atherosclerotic plaque. *Salmonella* can also cause abdominal infections (often of the hepatobiliary tract and spleen), osteomyelitis, septic arthritis, and rarely, infections of other tissues or organs. Chronic carriage may, rarely, develop.

LABORATORY DIAGNOSIS OF ENTERIC FEVER

The lab. diagnosis of enteric fever consists of (*i*) isolation of the bacillus from patient's specimen, (*ii*) demonstration of antibodies in patient's serum by widal test, and (*iii*) demonstration of bacillary antigen in blood or urine.

I. Isolation of the bacillus. In patients with diarrhea, *Salmonella* can typically be isolated from stools on MacConkey agar or selective media. For patients with enteric fever, appropriate specimens include blood, bone marrow, urine and tissue from typical rose spots.

(*i*) Blood culture — About 5–10 ml blood is collected by venepuncture and inoculated into a culture bottle containing 50–100 ml of 0.5 percent bile broth (glucose broth or brain heart infusion broth can also be used). Blood contains substances that inhibit the growth of the bacilli and hence it is essential that the broth be taken in sufficient quantity to provide atleast fourfold dilution of blood. The addition of liquoid (sodium polyanethol sulphonate) counteracts the bactericidal action of blood. It should be incubated for 10 days, during which subcultures are done every other day till growth is obtained; if there is no growth after 10 days, the cultures should be declared negative. Bacteremia occurs early in the disease and blood cultures are positive in approximately 90 percent of cases in the first week of fever, 75 percent of cases in the second week, 60 percent in the third week and 25 percent thereafter.

Subcultures are done on MacConkey's agar, and incubated for overnight. Pale nonlactose fermenting colonies that may appear on this medium are picked out for biochemical tests and motility. Salmonellae will be motile, indole and urease negative and ferment glucose, mannitol and maltose, but not lactose or sucrose. *S. typhi* is anaerogenic, while paratyphoid bacilli form acid and gas. The isolate is identified by slide agglutination test. Fresh isolates of *S. typhi* are in the V-form, do not agglutinate with O-antiserum; it should be heated and then tested for slide agglutination with O-antiserum. For identification of unusual serotypes, it should be sent to National Salmonella Reference Centre at Central Research Institute, Kasauli.

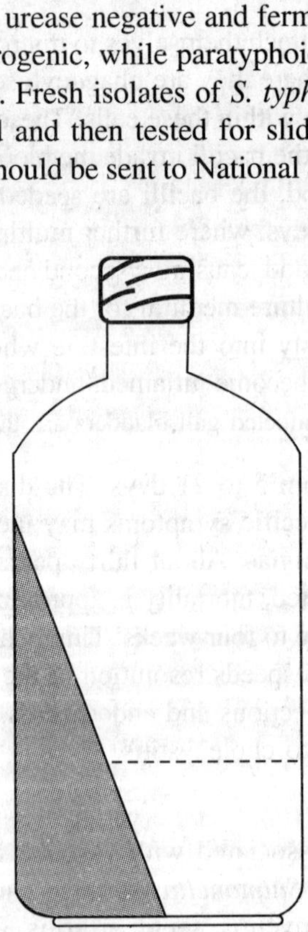

Fig. 57.4 Blood culture bottle containing biphasic (Castaneda's) medium.

To avoid the risk of contamination during subcultures, and also for economy and safety, **Castaneda's biphasic medium** containing bile broth and agar slant on one side in the same bottle is used. After inoculation of blood, for subculture, the bottle is tilted so that the broth runs over the surface of the agar and incubated in upright position and if salmonellae are present, the colonies will appear on slant.

An alternative to blood culture is the clot culture. Here, 5 ml of blood is taken from the patient into a sterile test tube and allowed to clot. The clot may be broken up with a sterile glass rod or lysed by the addition of streptokinase and inoculated into bile broth. Clot cultures yield a higher rate of isolation than blood cultures as the bactericidal action of the serum is eliminated, and a sample of serum also becomes available for widal test.

***(ii)* Feces culture** — Salmonellae are excreted in feces throughout the course of the disease and during convalescence, with varying frequency. Hence, fecal cultures are almost as valuable as blood cultures in diagnosis. However, fecal cultures are positive both in patients and as well as carriers. Fecal cultures are more valuable when patient is on antibiotics, as drug cannot eliminate bacilli from gut. Fecal samples are inoculated directly on MacConkey agar, DCA and Wilson and Blair's agar (selective medium). For enrichment, specimens are inoculated into **selenite F broth** or tetrathionate broth and incubated overnight before subculturing on to MacConkey agar.

***(iii)* Other specimens for culture** — Salmonellae may be isolated from several other specimens such as urine, bone marrow, bile obtained by duodenal aspiration, pus from suppurative lesions, CSF, sputum, and biopsy tissue from rose spots, bile cultures may be employed for detection of carriers.

II. Widal test. It is a tube agglutination test used for the measurement of O and H antibodies for typhoid and paratyphoid bacilli in the patient's sera for the serodiagnosis of enteric fever.

Two types of tubes are generally used for the test — a short, round bottomed tube, known as Felix tube for O agglutination and a narrow tube with a conical bottom, known as Dreyer's tube for H agglutination. Equal volumes of doubling dilutions of the patient's serum (from 1/20 to 1/640) and the H and O antigens are mixed in Dreyer's and Felix tubes, respectively, and incubated in a water bath at 37°C overnight. Control tubes containing antigen and normal saline are put up to check autoagglutination. The antigens used in the test are H and O antigens of serotype *typhi* and the H antigens of serotypes *paratyphi A* and *B*. The paratyphoid C antigens are not employed as they cross react with the typhoid O antigen due to sharing of O antigenic factor 12. O agglutination forms compact, chalky, granular clumps seen as a disk like pattern. H agglutination forms large, loose, fluffy, cotton woolly clumps. The highest dilution of the patient's serum showing agglutination indicates the titre of the antibody.

Interpretation — 1. Antibodies appear by seventh to tenth day of the illness, so that blood taken earlier will be negative. The antibody titre increases till third or fourth week, after which it declines gradually.

2. Demonstration of a rise in titre of antibodies, by testing two or more serum samples is more meaningful than a single test, preferably between first and third week.

3. The titres of 1/100 or more for O agglutinins and 1/200 or more for H agglutinins are significant (may vary from place to place).

4. Antibodies may be present on account of prior disease, subclinical infection or immunisation. Serum from immunised person will have antibodies to all serotypes *typhi*, *paratyphi A* and *B*, while in case of infection antibodies will be seen against infecting species.

5. Persons who have prior infection or vaccination may develop an **anamnestic response** during an unrelated fever. This may be differentiated by repetition of the test after a week. The anamnestic response shows only a transient rise, while in enteric fever the rise is sustained.

6. Cases treated with chloramphenicol may show a poor anitbody response.

III. Demonstration of bacillary antigen. The bacillary antigens are consistently present in the blood in the early phase of the disease, and also in the urine of patients. Therefore the bacillary antigen can be detected in blood and urine by ELISA, counter immunoelectrophoresis and coagglutination.

Staph. aureus (cowan I strain), which contains protein A, is stabilised with formaldehyde and coated with antibody to serotype *typhi*. When 1% suspension of such sensitised staphylococcal cells is mixed with serum from typhoid fever patients, the typhoid antigen present in serum combines with antibody attached to staphylococcal cells and produces visible agglutination. This is called **coagglutination**. The test is rapid, sensitive and specific.

LABORATORY DIAGNOSIS OF GASTROENTERITIS OR FOOD POISONING

The specimens collected are feces, vomitus and suspected food. Examination of stained smears of specimens is useful to demonstrate heavy contamination with *Staphylococcus*, *Bacilus cereus* and *Clostridium welchii*. The specimen can be directly inoculated on to MacConkey agar and Wilson and Blair's agar medium or inoculated into enrichment media such as selenite F broth or tetrathionate broth before subculturing on to MacConkey agar. The growth has to be identified by biochemical reactions and slide agglutination tests with appropriate antisera. Paired serum samples help to demonstrate serological diagnosis of infection. In case of death of patient, samples of intestinal contents, spleen, liver and heart blood may be collected.

DETECTION OF CARRIERS

The detection of carriers is important for epidemiological and public health purposes. It is also useful for screening food handlers and cooks. The identification of fecal carriers is carried out by isolation of the bacillus from the feces or from bile. In majority of the cases, there is intermittent shedding of the organisms. Therefore, it is essential to test repeated samples.

The widal test is of no value in detection of carriers in endemic countries. The demonstration of Vi antibodies (1:10 or more) has been claimed to indicate the carrier state. While this is useful as a screening test, confirmation should be made by culture.

The tracing of carriers in cities may be accomplished by the "sewer-swab" technique. Gauze pads left in sewers and drains are cultured, and by tracing positive swabs, the house harbouring carrier can be traced.

PROPHYLAXIS

Prevention of *Salmonella* infection is accomplished by proper sewage disposal, correct handling of food, provision of protected water supply and good personal hygiene.

TAB vaccine

Heat killed, phenol (0.5%) preserved, whole cell vaccines containing a mixture of cultures of serotypes *typhi*, 1,000 million and *paratyphi A* and *B*, 750 million each per ml, has been used in endemic areas. The vaccine is injected in 2 doses of 0.5 ml each at an interval of 4–6 weeks followed by a booster dose every three years. It confers protection against typhoid fever with an efficacy of 70–90% for 3–7 years. However, there has always been doubt about the value of paratyphoid components as well as concern about the unpleasant side effects such as fever, local discomfort etc., associated with large antigenic load of the triple vaccine.

In civilian practice, protection is mainly required against typhoid fever. Since only one of the *paratyphi A* or *B* is found in an area, either A or B may be added. Hence, in India, instead of the TAB vaccine a divalent typhoid-paratyphoid A vaccine (eliminating paratyphoid B which is very rare in the country) or the monovalent typhoid vaccine is used.

Vaccine of purified Vi antigen

The injectable vaccine (typhim-Vi) contains purified Vi polysaccharide antigen in a dose of 25 μg from serotype *S. typhi* strain *Ty 2*. It is a given as a single subcutaneous or intramuscular injection, which causes only minimal local reaction.

Oral vaccine

The live oral vaccine (typhoral) is a stable mutant of *S. typhi* strain *Ty 21a*, lacking the enzyme UDP galactose-4-epimerase (Gal E mutant). On ingestion, it initiates infection but undergoes "self destruction" after four or five cell divisions, and therefore cannot induce any illness. The vaccine is an enteric coated capsule containing 10^9 viable lyophilised mutant bacilli. Three doses of the vaccine are given on alternate days to children. No antibiotic should be given during this period.

TREATMENT

For gastroenteritis in uncompromised hosts, antibiotic therapy is often not needed, and may prolong the convalescent carrier state. For enteric fever chloramphenicol has been the drug of choice since its discovery. Ampicillin, amoxycillin, furazolidine and cotrimoxazole are other drugs used in the treatment. But there is a development of plasmid-mediated drug resistance to chloramphenicol and emergence and spread of multidrug resistant salmonellae, which have now become important agents of hospital cross infections. Such nosocomial salmonellosis manifests particularly in neonates as septicemia, meningitis and suppurative lesions. At present, the drugs useful in treatment of such multidrug resistant cases are the third generation cephalosporins (ceftriaxone, cefotaxime, ceftazidime) and fluoroquinolones (ciprofloxacin, oflaxacin, pefloxacin).

QUESTIONS

Essay Type Questions

1. Describe the lab. diagnosis of enteric fever.
2. Describe the pathogenesis and lab. diagnosis of enteric fever.
3. Enumerate the salmonellae causing enteric fever and describe the pathogenesis and lab. diagnosis of enteric fever.
4. Describe the salmonella gastroenteritis or food poisoning.

Short Answer Type Questionsd

1. Flagellar antigen or H antigen.
2. Somatic antigen or O antigen.
3. Vi antigen or surface antigen.
4. H → O variation.
5. V → W variation.
6. Phase variation.
7. S → R variation.
8. Craigie's tube.
9. Lab. diagnosis of enteric fever.
10. Blood culture.
11. Castaneda type of blood culture.
12. Widal test.
13. Coagglutination.
14. TAB vaccine.
15. *Salmonella* gastroenteritis.
16. Multidrug resistant salmonellae.
17. Wilson and Blair's media.
18. Enrichment media.
19. Selenite F broth.
20. Tetrathionate broth.

58

Shigella

- *Introduction*
- *Morphology*
- *Cultural characteristics*
- *Resistance*
- *Biochemical reactions*
- *Antigenic structure*
- *Classification*
  - *Sh. dysenetriae*
  - *Sh. flexneri*
  - *Sh. boydii*
  - *Sh. sonnei*
- *Epidemiology*
- *Pathogenicity*
- *Laboratory diagnosis*
- *Prophylaxis*
- *Treatment*

INTRODUCTION

The genus *Shigella* is named after Kiyoshi Shiga, who isolated the first member of the genus in 1896 from the feces of a dysentery patient. It was then called *Sh. shiga* and is now known as *Sh. dysenteriae* serotype 1.

Dysentery is a clinical condition of multiple etiology, characterised by the frequent passage of blood stained, mucopurulent feces. The three types of dysentery are: 1. bacillary dysentery caused by *Shigella* sp., 2. amoebic dysentery caused by *Entamoeba histolytica*, and 3. ciliate dysentery caused *Balantidium coli*. Some other bacilli such as EIEC, *Vibrio parahaemolyticus* and Compylobacter can also cause dysentery.

By DNA homology studies, it is evident that *Shigella* species are closely related to *E. coli.*

MORPHOLOGY

Shigellae are short Gram negative bacilli measuring 1–3 × 0.5 μm in size. Shigellae are nonmotile, unencapsulated and nonsporing. Fimbriae may be present.

CULTURAL CHARACTERISTICS

Shigellae are aerobes and facultative anaerobes. The optimum temperature required for growth is 37°C and optimum pH 7.4. It grows on ordinary media. On nutrient agar, after overnight incubation, colonies are small, about 2–3 mm in diameter, circular, convex, smooth and translucent. Some colonies may be of rough type on repeated subcultures and occasionally on primary isolation. Colonies on

MacConkey agar are colorless due to the absence of lactose fermentation. An exception is *Sh. sonnei* which ferments lactose late and forms pale pink colonies. **Deoxycholate agar (DCA)**, Salmonella-Shigella (SS) agar and xylose lysine deoxycholate (XLD) agar are used as selective media. No growth occurs on Wilson and Blair's bismuth sulphite agar medium.

RESISTANCE

Shigellae are killed at 56°C in one hour and by 1% phenol in 15 minutes. In feces they die within a few hours due to the acidity produced by the growth of coliforms, but can survive for several days in feces kept non-acid in buffered glycerol saline or preserved at 4°C. In general, *Sh. sonnei* is more resistant than other species.

BIOCHEMICAL REACTIONS

Shigellae are MR positive and reduce nitrates to nitrites. They cannot utilise citrate, do not form H_2S, and are inhibited by KCN. Catalse is produced, except by *Sh. dysenteriae* type 1. Glucose is fermented with the production of acid, without gas, except for the Newcastle and Manchester biotypes of *Sh. flexneri* type 6, which form both acid and gas. Lactose and sucrose are not fermented, except by *Sh. sonnei* which ferments them late. Adonitol, inositol and salicin are not fermented.

Fermentation of mannitol is of importance in classification and *Shigellae* have traditionally been classified into mannitol fermenting and nonfermenting species. *Sh. flexneri*, *Sh. boydii* and *Sh. sonnei* ferment mannitol, while *Sh. dysenteriae* does not.

Table 58.1 Differentiation of *Shigella* Species

Species	*Acid produced in fermentation of*					*Indole*	*Lysine decar-boxylase*	*Ornithine decar-boxylase*	*No. of sero-types*
	Lactose	*Sucrose*	*Mannitol*	*Dulcitol*	*Xylose*				
Sh. dysenteriae	–	–	–	–	–	V	–	–	12
Sh. flexneri	–	–	+	–	–	V	–	–	6+2 variants
Sh. boydii	–	–	+	V	V	V	–	–	18
Sh. sonnei	–*	–*	+	–	V	–	–	+	2 phases 26 colicin types

* = negative at 24 hrs, late positive at 2–8 days; V = variable

ANTIGENIC STRUCTURE

All Shigellae species possess O antigens and some strains may possess K antigens. K antigens are not relevant in typing, but may interfere with agglutination by O antisera. Fimbrial antigens are also present. There is considerable antigenic sharing between some members of the genus as well as between Shigellae and *E. coli*. The identification of Shigellae should be made by a combination of antigenic and biochemical properties and not by slide agglutination alone.

CLASSIFICATION

Shigellae are classified into four species or subgroups based on a combination of biochemical reactions and serological relatedness of their polysaccharide O antigens. Serotypes (about 40) are distinguished within the species. *Sh. sonnei* is serologically homogenous and is classified by colicin typing.

1. *Sh. dysenteriae* (subgroup A) —This species is **mannitol nonfermenting** and consists of twelve serotypes.

Type 1 is ***Sh. shigae,*** originally described by Shiga. It is Indole negative and is the only member of the family that is always catalase negative. It is responsible for most severe form of dysentery. It produces a powerful exotoxin, which is heat labile and can be toxoided when the exotoxin is injected intravenously into rabbits, it leads to diarrhea and paralysis. It acts as enterotoxin and neurotoxin. As enterotoxin, it acts on the intestinal mucosa causing transudation of fluid in the lumen and can be demonstrated by induction of fluid in the ligated rabbit illeal loop. As neurotoxin, it damages endothelial cells of small blood vessels of the central nervous system which results in neurological complications like polyneuritis, coma and meningism.

Type 1 serotype of *Sh. dysenteriae* also produces a cytotoxin which is active on Vero cells and is known as verotoxin (VT). A similar cytotoxic action of VT has been shown on human colon and ileal cells in tissue cultures. There are two distinct verotoxins, known as VT 1 and VT 2. The VT 1 appears to be same as VT 1 (shiga like toxin) produced by VTEC.

Tpye 2 is called ***Sh. schmitzi.*** It is indole positive and ferments sorbitol and rhamnose.

Serotypes 3–7 were described by Large and Sachs in India and hence used to be known as the **Large-Sachs group**. Five serotypes (8–12) further have been described making a total of 12.

2. *Sh. flexneri* (subgroup B) — This species is named after Flexner, who reported it from Philippines (1900). It is mannitol fermenting. This group is biochemically heterogenous and antigenically the most complex among Shigellae. Based on type specific (I to VI) and group specific (1–8) antigens, they have been classified into 6 serotypes (1–6) and several subtypes (1a, 1b, 2a, 2b, 3a, 3b, 3c, 4a, 4b, 5a, 5b). In addition, two antigenic variants called X and Y are recognized which lack the type specific antigens. Setotype 6 is always indole negative and can be subdivided into three biotypes: Boyd 88, Manchester and Newcastle.

Table 58.2 Antigens of *Sh. flexneri* Serotypes

Serotype	*Subtype*	*Type and specific antigen*	*Group specific antigen*
1	1a	I	1, 2, 4
		1b	I 1, 2, 4, 6
2	2a	II	1, 3, 4
		2b	II 1, 7, 8
3	3a	III	1, 6, 7, 8
		3b	III 1, 3, 4, 6, 7, 8
		3c	III 1, 6
4	4a	IV	1, 3, 4
		4b	IV 1, 3, 4, 6
5	5a	V	1, 3, 4
		5b	V 1, 7, 8
6		VI	1, 2, 4
X variant		–	1, 7, 8
Y variant		–	1, 3, 4

Table 58.3 Biotypes of *Sh. flexneri* type 6

Biotype	*Fermentation of*	
	Glucose	*Mannitol*
Boyd 88	Acid	Acid
Manchester	Acid and gas	Acid and gas
Newcastle	Acid or Acid and gas	–

3. *Sh. boydii* (subgroup C) — This group is named after Boyd who first described these strains from India (1931). This group resembles *Sh. flexneri* biochemically but not antigenically. Eighteen serotypes have been identified in this group. *Sh. boydii* are isolated least frequently from cases of bacillary dysentery.

4. *Sh. sonnei* (subgroup D) — This species was first described by Sonne (1915) in Denmark, which ferments lactose and sucrose late. It is indole negative. It is antigenically homogenous but may occur in two forms — Phase I and Phase II. The former gives rise to smooth (S) colonies while the colonies of the latter are larger, flatter and irregular (R). Cultures often contain a mixture of both forms, but the colonies of one form can be selected by the addition of the other form to the culture medium since both forms are antigenically different. Organisms in phase II are more common in convalescents and carriers.

Sh. sonnei has been classified into 26 colicin types. It causes the mildest form of dysentery. The infection is more common in developed countries.

EPIDEMIOLOGY

Shigellosis is worldwide in distribution. The only source of infection are human beings — patients or carriers. Shigellosis has a low infectious dose (fewer than 200 viable organisms are sufficient to cause disease). Hence secondary cases within a household are common, particularly under conditions of crowding and/or poor sanitation. Malnutrition and immunodeficiency (AIDS) may serve as predisposing factors. Shigellae are typically spread from person to person, with contaminated stools serving as a major source of organisms. The modes of transmission may be as follows:

1. Through contaminated water or food as food poisoning.
2. Through contaminated fingers —'hand-to-mouth' infection.
3. Through fomites such as door handles, water taps, lavatary seats.
4. Through flies which may transmit the infection as mechanical vectors.
5. Shigellosis may occur in young male homosexuals as part of the gay bowel syndrome.

PATHOGENICITY

Shigellae cause classic bacillary dysentery, characterized by diarrhea with blood, mucus and painful abdominal cramping and tenesmus. Fever and vomiting may be present. The disease is generally most severe in the very young and elderly, and among malnourished individuals, in whom shigellosis may lead to severe dehydration, and sometimes death. Among uncompromised populations, untreated dysentery commonly resolves in a week, but may persist longer.

Infection occurs by ingestion. The bacilli invade and multiply in the mucosa of the large intestine, spreading laterally to infect adjacent epithelial cells and penetrating into the lamina propria. Inflammatory reaction develops with capillary thrombosis, leading to necrosis of patches of epithelium, which slough off, leaving behind transverse superficial ulcers. Infection rarely penetrates to deeper layers of the intestine, and does not lead to *Shigella* bacteremia. Bacteremia may occur in severe infections, particularly in malnourished children and AIDS cases. The toxigenicity of exotoxin of *Sh. dysenteriae* type 1 may play a secondary role in the development of intestinal lesions.

The severity of the disease may vary from acute fulminating dysentery to mild diarrhea. Complications are most often seen in infection with **Sh. dysenteriae** type 1 and include arthritis, toxic neuritis, conjunctivitis, parotitis and in children intussusception. Hemolytic uremic syndrome may occur as a complication in severe cases. The term "**bacillary dysentery**" refers only to the intestinal disease, whereas the term "**shigellosis**" has been employed to include the whole spectrum of disease caused by Shigellae.

LABORATORY DIAGNOSIS

Specimens collected are fresh feces or direct swab of an ulcer taken by sigmoidoscopy.

Microscopic examination of the feces or mucus shows numerous RBC and neutrophils (pus cells) and a few macrophages. The fluorescent antibody technique is used for the direct identification of Shigellae from feces.

Table 58.4 Identification of *Shigellae* by Biochemical Reactions

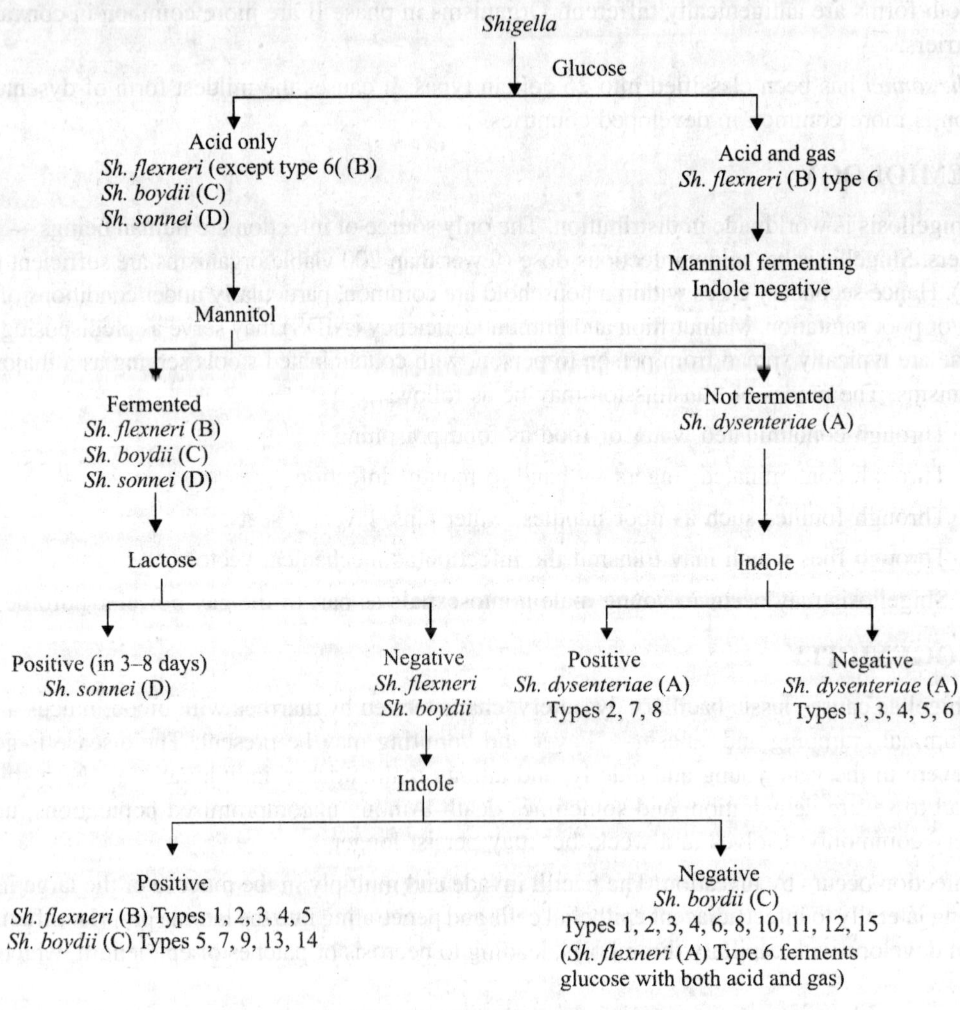

During acute illness, organisms can be cultured from stools using differential, selective or other media specific for intestinal pathogens. Fresh feces should be inoçulated without delay or transported in a suitable medium such as Sach's buffered glycerol saline, pH 7.0–7.4. Feces, preferably mucus flakes, if present, should be inoculated on MacConkey's agar and DCA, SS agar and XLD medium and incubated overnight at 37°C. The plates are inspected for pale, nonlactose fermenting colonies on MacConkey agar and DCA, and red colored colonies without black centres on XLD agar and colorless colonies with no blackening on SS agar, which are tested for motility, biochemical reactions and by slide agglutination tests. Any nonmotile bacillus that is urease, citrate, H_2S and KCN negative should be further investigated by biochemical tests. Identification is confirmed by slide agglutination with polyvalent and monovalent antisera.

PROPHYLAXIS

Protection of the water and food supply, and personal hygiene are crucial for preventing *Shigella* infections. Vaccine development is currently experimental.

TREATMENT

Most of the cases of bacillary dysentery are self-limited in which the patient recovers spontaneously in a few days and do not require antibiotic therapy. Oral rehydration is adequate in most cases. However, in acute cases, particularly in infants, young children, the aged and debilitated, intravenous replacement of fluids and electrolytes plus antibiotic therapy is necessary. The choice of the antibiotic should be based on the sensitivity of the prevailing strain. Ampicillin, cotrimoxazole, tetracycline, azithromycin, nalidixic acid and ciprofloxacin can reduce the duration of illness and the period of shedding organisms, but usage is controversial because of widerspread antibiotic resistance. Multiple drug resistance plasmids are widely prevalent in Shigellae. Indiscriminate antibiotic treatment may enhance the problem of drug resistance among intestinal bacteria.

QUESTIONS

Essay Type Questions

1. Enumerate the various causes of bacillary dysentery in tropics. Describe in detail the lab. diagnosis of bacillary dysentery.

Short Answer Type Questions

1. Lab. diagnosis of bacillary dysentery.
2. *Sh. shiga* or *Sh. dysenteriae* type 1.
3. *Sh. dysenteriae.*
4. *Sh. flexneri.*
5. Enumerate the causative agents of dysentery.
6. *Sh. sonnei.*
7. *Sh. boydii.*
8. Pathogenesis of bacillary dysentery.

59

Citrobacter, Edwardsiella, Hafnia, Serratia and Erwinia

- ***Citrobacter***
- ***Edwardsiella***
- ***Hafnia***
- ***Serratia***
- ***Erwinia***

CITROBACTER

Citrobacter is a normal inhabitant of human intestine and may cause urinary tract, gall bladder and middle ear infections. Genus *Citrobacter* has three species: *C. freundii*, *C. koseri* (formerly *C. diversus*) and *C. amalonaticus*. *C. koseri* may occasionally cause neonatal meningitis. They grow well on ordinary media. They are motile Gram negative bacilli which utilise citrate, grow in KCN medium, produce H_2S and ferment lactose late or not at all. They produce β-galactosidase (ONPG positive). They do not decarboxylate lysine but most strains decarboxylate ornithine. They exhibit extensive antigenic sharing with Salmonellae, which may lead to confusion in the diagnosis. Some strains (*e.g.*, Bhatnagar strain) possess a Vi antigen, serologically identical to the Vi antigen of *S. typhi* and *S. paratyphi* C. *C. freundii* strains were formerly classified as the **"Ballerup-Bethesda group"**.

EDWARDSIELLA

E. tarda is the only recognised human pathogen and the term tarda refers to slow or weak fermentation of sugars by the organism. It is a normal intestinal inhabitant of snakes and other cold blooded animals and their environment, particularly fresh water. It is pathogenic for eels, cat fish and other animals. It is an occasional pathogen of man causing wound infection. It has rarely been found in the feces of healthy people. A higher isolation rate of *E. tarda* has been found in patients with diarrhea. However, its pathogenic role is uncertain. It is a motile, noncapsulated, Gram negative bacillus and ferments only glucose and maltose with the production of acid and some gas. It is indole and MR positive, and VP and citrate negative. It produces H_2S but it is negative for urease test, gelatin liquefaction and malonate utilization. No growth occurs in the presence of KCN. Genus *Edwardsiella* is separated from *Escherichia* by its ability to produce H_2S in triple sugar iron agar.

HAFNIA

Genus *Hafnia* has only one species *H. alvei*. It is found in human and animal feces, sewage, soil and water. It has been recovered from wounds, abscesses, sputum, urine, blood and other sites. Since it is often associated with other bacterial species, its role in pathogenesis is uncertain. It is believed that it may be an opportunistic pathogen. It is a motile, nonlactose fermenting Gram negative bacillus which is indole and MR negative and VP and citrate positive. Biochemical reactions are evident best at 22°C; at 37°C, they may be negative or irregular. *H. alvei* can be distinguished from *Serratia* species by its inability to produce lipase or deoxyribonuclease.

SERRATIA

It is a saprophyte found in water, soil and food. The species of *Serratia* that most frequently causes human infection is *S. marcescens*. It is pleomorphic, with minute coccobacillary and normal bacillary forms. It forms a pink, red or magenta colored, nondiffusible pigment called prodigiosin optimally best at room temperature. *Serratia* can cause extraintestinal infections such as meningitis, endocarditis, urinary tract infections, septicemia, peritonitis, respiratory infections especially among hospitalized patients. Nosocomial infections particularly in the new born, the debilitated or the patients receiving immunosuppressive drugs due to *S. marcescens* are being reported with increasing frequency. *Serratia* are commonly resistant to cephalosporins. Multiple drug resistance is common in hospital strains.

ERWINIA

They are usually found in soild and cause plant diseases. *E. herbicola* has occasionally been isolated from respiratory tract infections and urinary tract infections in predisposed and hospitalized patients. They are anaerogenic Gram negative bacilli and form a yellowish pigment.

QUESTIONS

Short Answer Type Questions

1. Citrobacter.
2. Serratia.

60

Klebsiella and Enterobacter

- *Klebsiella pneumoniae*
  - *Introduction*
  - *Classification*
  - *Morphology*
  - *Cultural characteristics*
  - *Biochemical reactions*
  - *Antigenic structure*
  - *Pathogenicity*
  - *Laboratory diagnosis*
  - *Treatment*
- *Klebsiella ozaenae*
- *Klebsiella rhinoscleromatis*
- *Enterobacter*

KLEBSIELLA PNEUMONIAE (Freidlander's bacillus)

Introduction

This bacillus was first isolated by Freidlander (1883) from pneumonia cases. Klebsiellae are widely distributed in nature, occurring both as commensals in the intestines and as saprophytes in soil and water. They possess *nif* genes responsible for nitrogen fixation that improves soil fertility. It is the second most populous member of the aerobic bacterial flora of the intestine. It also occurs in the respiratory tract as a normal commensal.

Classification

Based on biochemical properties, *Klebsiella pneumoniae* has been classified into 4 subspecies. The most frequently encountered, biochemically typical form is *K. pneumoniae* subsp. *aerogenes*. Other subspecies are *ozaenae*, *pneumoniae* and *rhinoscleromatis*. Indole positive strains that are similar to *K. pneumoniae* subsp. *aerogenes* in other respects are classified in a separate species *K. oxytoca*.

Morphology

They are plump, straight and short Gram negative bacilli, about 1–2 × 0.5–0.8 μm in size. It is nonmotile and nonsporing fimbriae may be present. It contains a large, luxurious polysaccharide capsule, which can be demonstrated by negative staining in Indian ink preparations and quellung reaction. The capsule is so prominent that it can be made out even in Gram stained smears as halo around the bacilli. The bacilli may occur singly or in pairs.

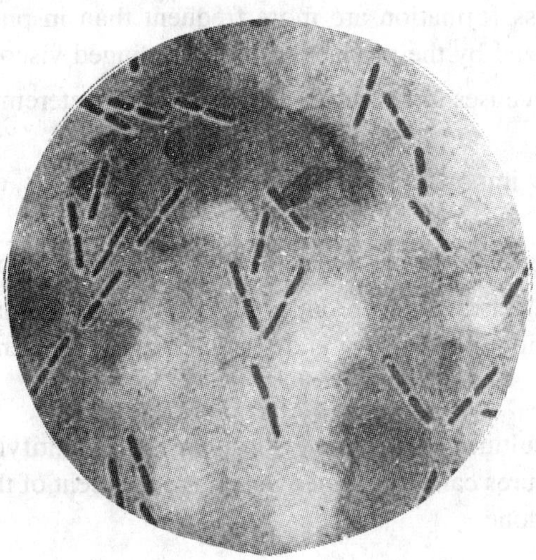

Fig. 60.1 *Klebsiella pneumoniae*

Cultural characteristics

It is an aerobe and facultative anaerobe. Optimum temperature required for growth is 37°C and optimum pH 7.4. It grows well on ordinary media forming **large, dome shaped, mucoid colonies** of varying degrees of stickness. On MacConkey agar colonies are large, mucoid with red color due to lactose fermentation.

Biochemical reactions

It ferments sugars such as glucose, lactose, sucrose, mannitol, maltose with the production of abundant acid and gas. It is indole and MR negative and VP and citrate positive (IMViC – – + +). Biochemically variant strains are common. It forms urease.

Table 60.1 Differences between *E. coli* and *Klebsiella*.

Character	*E. coli.*	*Klebsiellae*
Motility	+	–
Indole	+	–
Methyl red	+	–
Voges-Proskauer	–	+
Citrate utilization	–	+
Urease production	–	+

Antigenic structure

Klebsiellae possess five O antigens (O 1 – O5). On the basis of capsular (K) antigens, the Klebsiellae have been differentiated into over 90 serotypes. Type 2 is antigenically related to type 2 pneumococcus. Human respiratory tract infection is mostly caused by capsular types 1–6.

Pathogenicity

1. *K. pneumoniae* and *K. oxytoca* cause a necrotizing lobar pneumonia in middle aged or older persons compromised by alcoholism, diabetes, or chronic obstructive pulmonary disease.

Necrosis and abscess formation are more frequent than in pneumococcal pneumonia. The disease is characterized by the production of blood tinged viscous sputum.

2. *K. pneumoniae* also causes urinary tract infections and bacteremia, particularly in hospitalized patients.
3. It has become a very important cause of nosocomial infections, even replacing *E. coli* in some centres.
4. It also causes pyogenic infections such as abscesses, meningitis and septicemia.
5. Some strains cause diarrhea and produce an enterotoxin similar to the heat stable toxin of *E. coli*. The production of this toxin is determined by the presence of a plasmid.

Laboratory diagnosis

Diagnosis is made by culturing appropriate specimens and identifying the isolate by biochemical reactions. Positive blood cultures can be obtained in about 25 percent of the cases. Antibiotic sensitivity testing should invariably be done.

Treatment

Many strains carry plasmids determining multiple drug resistance. The drug for treatment should be selected based on antibiotic sensitivity pattern.

KLEBSIELLA OZAENAE

This bacillus causes ozaena, a disease characterized by foul smelling nasal discharge. Identification is difficult due to wide variations in the biochemical reactions of individual strains. *K. ozaena* belongs to capsular types 3–6.

KLEBSIELLA RHINOSCLEROMATIS

It causes rhinoscleroma, a chronic granulomatous hypertrophy of the nose prevalent in India, Central America and Southeastern Europe. The bacilli are seen intracellularly in lesions. It can be identified by biochemical reactions. It belongs to capsular type 3.

Table 60.2 Differentiation of species and subspecies of *Klebsiella*.

Property	*K. pneumoniae subspecies*				*K. oxytoca*
	aerogenes	*ozaenae*	*pneumoniae*	*rhinoscleromatis*	
Indole	–	–	–	–	+
MR	–	+	+	+	V
VP	+	–	–	–	V
Citrate	+	V	+	–	+
Urease	+	–	+	–	+
Gelatin liquefaction	–	–	–	–	V
Lactose (acid)	+	+	+	–	+
ONPG	+	+	+	–	+
Lysine decarboxylase	+	V	+	–	+
Ornithine decarboxylase	–	–	–	–	–
Growth in KCN medium	+	+	–	+	+

ENTEROBACTER

It is a saprophyte, widely distributed in water, sewage, soil and on vegetables. It also occurs as a commensal in the intestine and occasionally in the respiratory tract. It is a motile, lactose fermenting bacillus which is indole and MR negative and VP and citrate postive. It is encapsulated but less heavily than *Klebsiella*. Therefore, the colonies of *Enterobacter* are less mucoid. The genus *Enterobacter* has 12 species, but two species are clinically relevant, *E. aerogenes* and *E. cloacae*.

They rarely cause primary disease in humans, but frequently colonize hospitalized patients, especially in association with antibiotic treatment, indwelling catheters, or invasive procedures. These organisms may infect burns, wounds, the respiratory tract (causing pneumonia) or the urinary tract. Aminoglycosides are often effective in the treatment.

Table 60.3 Differentiation between *E. aerogenes* and *E. cloacae*.

	E. aerogenes	*E. cloacae*
Gas from glycerol	+	–
Aesculin hydrolysis	+	–
Lysine decarboxylase	+	–
Arginine dihydrolase	–	+

QUESTIONS

Short Answer Type Questions

1. *Klebsiella pneumoniae.*
2. Pathogenicity of *Klebsiella.*
3. What are the properties which differentiate *E. coli* from *Klebsiella.*
4. *Enterobacter.*

61

Proteus, Morganella and Providencia

- ***Proteus***
  - ***– Introduction***
  - ***– Morphology***
  - ***– Cultural characteristics***
  - ***– Dienes phenomenon***
  - ***– Biochemical reactions***
  - ***– Antigenic structure***
  - ***– Pathogenicity***
  - ***– Laboratory diagnosis***
  - ***– Treatment***
- ***Morganella***
- ***Providencia***

PROTEUS

Introduction

Proteus bacilli are widely distributed in nature as saprophytes, being found in decomposing animal matter, in sewage, in manured soil, human and animal feces. They are also normal commensals of intestines of humans and animals and are found in human and animal feces. They are frequently present on the moist areas of the skin. Genus *Proteus* has four species: *Pr. mirabilis*, *Pr. vulgaris*, *Pr. myxofaciens* and *Pr. penneri.*

Morphology

They are Gram negative, unencapsulated bacilli. They are actively motile with peritrichate flagellae. They exhibit pleomorphism and may exist as short coccobacillary forms or long filamentous forms. The name "*Proteus*" refers to their pleomorphism, after the Greek god Proteus who could assume any shape. Nonflagellated, nonmotile variants are also encountered. They possess more than one type of fimbriae.

Cultural characteristics

It is an aerobe and facultative anaerobe. Optimum temperature required for growth is 37°C and optimum pH 7.4. They can grow on ordinary media like nutrient agar. The cultures emit a putrefactive (fishy or seminal) odor. *Pr. mirabilis* and *Pr. vulgaris* **swarm** (spread) on the surface of solid culture media in successive waves to form a thin filmy layer in concentric circles. Swarming can be inhibited by increasing the concentration of agar to 6%, incorporation of chloralhydrate (1 : 500), sodium azide (1 : 500), alcohol (5–6%), sulphonamides, surface active agents or boric acid (1 : 1000) so that discrete colonies can be obtained. Swarming does not occur on MacConkey's agar, on which smooth colorless colonies are formed.

Dienes phenomenon

When two identical strains of *Proteus* are inoculated at different points of the same culture plate (without any substance to inhibit swarming), the resulting swarms of growth coalesce without any sign of demarcation. When two different strains of *Proteus* species are inoculated, the spreading films of growth fail to coalesce and remain separated by a narrow but easily visible furrow. This is known as Dienes phenomenon. Thus, it can be used to determine the identity or nonidentity of various strains of *Proteus.*

Biochemical reactions

Table 61.1 Differentiation of *Proteus* and *Morganella*.

Property	*Proteus*				*M. morganii*
	mirabilis	***vulgaris***	***penneri***	***myxofaciens***	
Motility	+	+	+	+	+
Swarming growth	+	+	–	–	–
Indole	–	+	–	–	+
Methyl red	+	+	+	+	+
Voges-Proskauer	V	–	–	+	–
Citrate	V	V	–	V	–
Phenyl alanine deaminase test	+	+	+	+	+
Urease	+	+	+	+	+
Ornithine decarboxylation	+	–	–	–	+
H_2S	+	+	–	+	–
Gelatin liquefaction	+	+	V	+	–
Lipase production	+	+	V	+	–
Gas from glucose	+	+	V	+	+
Acid from mannose	–	–	–	–	+
Acid from maltose	–	+	+	+	–
Acid from xylose	+	+	+	–	–
Acid from trehalose	+	V	V	+	–

All species of *Proteus* produce acid from glucose and no acid from lactose, mannose, mannitol, adonitol, inositol, rhamnose, dulcitol, sorbitol, raffinose and arabinose. They cannot utilize malonate and reduce nitrates to nitrites. They are MR positive and VP negative. They do not form arginine or lysine decarboxylase and betagalactosidase. They degrade tyrosine. A characteristic feature of tribe proteeae is the presence of enzyme, **phenyl alanine deaminase** which converts phenyl alanine to phenyl pyruvic acid (PPA reaction). It produces a powerful **urease** which rapidly hydrolyses urea to ammonia and CO_2.

Antigenic structure

Motile strains of *Proteus* possess both O (somatic) antigens and H (flagellar) antigens. Certain nonmotile strains of *Pr. vulgaris* OX2, OX19 and *Pr. mirabilis* OXK and Rickettsiae share the alkali stable fraction of O antigen. This forms the basis of **Weil-Felix reaction**, an heterophile agglutination test, where *Proteus* strains are used as antigens for the serodiagnosis of Rickettsial infections.

Pathogenicity

Proteus species are relatively common causes of uncomplicated as well as nosocomial urinary tract infections. Other extraintestinal infections such as wound infections, pneumonias and septicemias are associated with compromised patients. UTI caused by *Proteus* tends to be more serious than that caused by *E. coli* and other coliforms, because these organisms are usually confined to the bladder, whereas *proteus* has a predilection for the upper urinary tract. It produces urease, which liberates ammonia from urea. Ammonia inactivates complement, damages renal epithelium and makes the urine alkaline. The alkaline conditions lead to the precipitation of phosphates and the formation of calculi in the urinary tract. It may also lead to hyperammonemic encephalopathy and coma.

Laboratory diagnosis

The diagnosis consists of culture of the specimen on MacConkey agar and DCA and the identification of isolate by biochemical reactions and slide agglutination tests.

Treatment

Proteus bacilli are resistant to many of the common antibiotics. The treatment should be guided by antibiotic sensitivity testing.

MORGANELLA

The genus *Morganella* has only one species, *M. morganii* (formerly *Pr. morganii*). It is motile, but does not swarm on solid media. It is frequently found in human and animal feces. It has also been isolated from diarrheic stools in the absence of other known bacterial enteropathogens. It may cause nosocomial urinary tract infections, pneumonia and wound infections. Occassionally, it is isolated from blood.

PROVIDENCIA

The genus *Providencia* (formerly known as *Proteus inconstans*) has five species – *P. rettgeri*, *P. alcalifaciens*, *P. stuartii*, *P. rustigianii* and *P. heimbachae*. They are motile but do not swarm on solid media. The colonies emit "fruity" smell and on DCA they form yellow or orange – centred colonies because the ferric hydroxide in the medium is precipitated at the alkaline pH which is formed during growth. All the species deaminate phenyl alanine, but only *P. rettgeri* hydrolyzes urea consistently.

Prov. rettgeri is part of the normal fecal flora of reptiles and amphibians and sometimes causes nosocomial infection of the urinary tract, wounds, burns and blood. *Prov. alcalifaciens* is sometimes seen in normal human feces but far more frequently in diarrheal stools. *Prov. stuartii* may occasionally cause hospital-associated urinary tract infection, particularly in patients undergoing long-term catheterization and in those with urinary tract abnormalities. It may also cause infection of burns and pneumonia. In aged and immunodeficient patients, it may lead to septicemia.

QUESTIONS

Short Answer Type Questions

1. Pathogenicity of *Proteus* species.
2. Swarming growth.
3. Dienes phenomenon.
4. *Morganella.*
5. *Providencia.*
6. Nonmotile strains of *Proteus.*

62

Yersinia

- *Yersinia pestis*
  - *Introduction*
  - *Morphology*
  - *Cultural characteristics*
  - *Biochemical reactions*
  - *Resistance*
  - *Antigens, toxins and virulence factors*
  - *Epidemiology*
  - *Pathogenicity*
  - *Laboratory diagnosis*
  - *Prophylaxis*
  - *Treatment*
- *Yersinia pseudotuberculosis*
- *Yersinia enterocolitica*

YERSINIA PESTIS (Plague bacillus)

Introduction

The genus *Yersinia* is a member of the family enterobacteriaceae. The most clinically notorious member of this genus is *Yersina pestis*, which causes plague rather than enteric disease, and therefore, generally discussed separately from the rest of the family. The plague bacillus was discovered independently and simultaneously by Yersin and Kitasato (1984) in Hong Kong at the beginning of the last pandemic of the disease. Therefore, the genus was so named after Alexandre Yersin, who discovered it.

Morphology

Y. pestis is a short, plump, ovoid Gram negative bacillus, about 1.5 µm × 0.7 µm in size, with rounded ends and convex sides, arranged singly, in short chains or in small groups. In smears stained with methylene blue (simple staining) or Giemsa, it shows bipolar staining, with the two ends densely stained and the central area clear, giving a "**safety pin appearance**". Pleomorphism is very common and in old cultures, involution forms are seen-coccoid, club shaped, filamentous and giant forms. Pleomorphism is characteristically enhanced in media containing 3% NaCl. The bacillus is surrounded by a slime layer (capsule or envelope). It is nonmotile, nonsporing and nonacidfast.

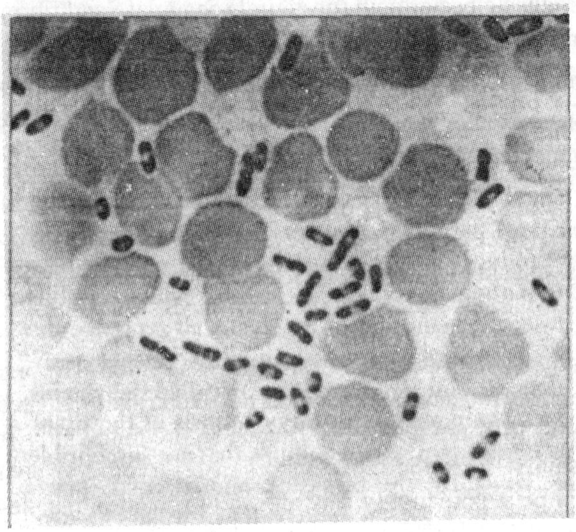

Fig. 62.1 *Yersinia pestis* organisms exhibit a bipolar, or "safety pin", appearance in this smear of mouse blood. The large round objects are red blood cells

Cultural characteristics

It is an aerobe and facultative anaerobe. Optimum temperature required for growth, unlike most pathogens is 27°C and optimum pH 7.2. It grows on ordinary media. On nutrient agar, colonies are small, delicate, transparent discs, becoming opaque on prolonged incubation. Colonies on blood agar are dark brown due to absorption of hemin pigment. Colorless colonies (nonlactose fermenters) are formed on MacConkey agar. In broth, a flocculent growth occurs at the bottom and along the sides of the tube, with little or no turbidity. A delicate pellicle may form later. When grown in an oil broth or ghee broth in a flask, a characteristic **stalactite growth** occurs, which hangs down from the surface into the broth, resembling stalactites.

Biochemical reactions

It ferments glucose, maltose, mannitol with the production of acid but no gas. Lactose, sucrose or rhamnose are not fermented. Indole is not produced. It is MR positive and VP and citrate negative, catalase positive, aesculin positive, oxidase and urease negative. Gelatin is not liquefied.

Resistance

It is destroyed by heat 55°C or by 0.5% phenol in 15 minutes. It remains viable for long periods in cold, moist environments. It can survive for several months and even multiply in the soil of rodent burrows.

Antigens, toxins and virulence factors

Plague bacillus has a complex antigenic structure and about 20 antigens have been identified. Most of them are virulence factors.

1. A heat labile protein envelope antigen known as Fraction I (FI). It is formed *in vivo* and in cultures grown at 37°C. It inhibits phagocytosis and is generally present only in virulent strains and is considered to be virulence determinant. It is plasmid encoded. The antibody to this antigen is protective in mice.
2. Two protein antigens designated V and W are also formed by virulent strains of *Y. pestis* at 37°C. These virulence factors inhibit phagocytosis and intracellular killing of the bacillus. Their production is palsmid mediated.

3. Virulent strains produce a bacteriocin (pesticin I) coagulase and fibrinolysin, whose production is under the control of a plasmid.
4. It possesses an endotoxin, a lipopolysaccharide similar to the endotoxins of enteric bacilli.
5. A surface component of the bacillus which absorbs hemin and basic aromatic dyes in culture media to form pigmented colonies.
6. Murine toxins or plague toxins are pathogenic in mice and rats but their role in natural human disease is not clear.
7. Virulence is also associated with the ability to synthesize purines.

Epidemiology

Plague is predominantly a **zoonosis** with world-wide distribution. The organism can infect a variety of mammals. For example, rats (rodents) are common reservoirs in urban areas, responsible for **urban plague** or **domestic plague.** In some countries, plague is predominantly found in the wild, where prairie dogs and ground squirrels are the most important reservoirs, responsible for **wild plague** or **sylvatic plague.** Household pets, particularly cats allowed to roam in plague-endemic areas, may also become infected.

Plague is characteristically transmitted by fleas, which serve to maintain the infection within the animal reservoir. Humans are generally accidental and dead-end hosts. Several species of fleas may act as vectors, the most important being *Xenopsylla cheopis*, *X. astia* and *Ceratophyllus fasciatus*. Plague can also be transmitted by ingestion of contaminated animal tissues or via the respiratory route, causing **pneumonic plague.** This pneumonic plague occurs either when organisms reach the lung and establish a secondary pneumonia, or following exposure to respiratory secretions from a patient or animal with plague pneumonia.

Pathogenicity

Plague is a zoonotic disease. The plague bacillus is a natural pathogen of rats and rodents. Infection is transmitted among them by **rat fleas**. Humans may acquire the disease when an infected flea bites them.

Organisms are carried by the lymphatic system from the site of inoculation to regional lymph nodes, where they are ingested by phagocytes. However, the organisms are resistant to intracellular killing by phagocytes, and instead may multiply within these cells. Furthermore, the bacteria released from lysed phagocytes have synthesized a new envelope antigen that confers increased resistance to phagocytosis. The affected lymph nodes display hemorrhagic necrosis accompanied by high concentration of both polymorphonuclear leucocytes and extracellular bacteria. Hematogenous spread of bacteria to other organs or tissues, resulting in additional hemorrhagic lesions at these sites.

In human beings plague may present several clinically different pictures.

1. Bubonic plague — The infectious cycle begins when a flea ingests a blood meal from an animal that is infected and bacteremic. *Y. pestis* produces a coagulase that causes the blood to clot in the flea's foregut. The organism multiplies in this environment. When the flea next attempts to feed, it regurgitates these bacteria from its foregut into the new animal's skin. The incubation period (from flea bite to development of symptoms) is generally two to eight days. Onset of nonspecific symptoms, such as high fever, chills, headache, myalgia and weakness that proceeds to prostration, is characteristically sudden. Within a short time, a characteristic, painful **bubo** develops. Pronounced swellings comprised of one or more infected nodes and surrounding edema that led to the name "bubonic plague". Buboes are typically located in the groin, but may also occur in axillae or on the neck. As the disease proceeds, blood pressure generally drops, potentially leading to septic shock and death. Mortality of untreated bubonic plague generally exceeds fifty percent. Other manifestations associated with bubonic plague include pustules or vesicles containing leucocytes and *Y. pestis.*

2. Pneumonic plague — It is highly contagious, and the organisms cause pneumonic plague directly when inhaled. If plague bacilli reach the lungs they cause a purulent pneumonia that being invariably fatal unless rapidly treated. Pneumonic plague may occur sometimes during epidemics of bubonic plague.

3. Septicemic plague — Septicemic plague is a variation in which the patient is overwhelmed by massive bacteremia before the characteristic buboes develop. Purpura and necrosis of extremities may occur during systemic disease. Septicemic plague is usually the terminal event in the bubonic or pneumonic plague but may sometimes occur primarily.

4. Plague meningitis — It is typically a secondary focus resulting from hematogenous dissemination of organisms to the meninges. It may cccur following inadequately treated bubonic plague or, like septicemic plague, may occur without or prior to development of a bubo. Organisms can be demonstrated in the CSF.

5. Pharyngitis — Ingestion of contaminated meat or exposure to air-borne bacilli can result in primary lesions in the pharynx. These produce a severe tonsillitis and cervical buboes.

6. Cutaneous plague — It is acquired by handling contaminated animal tissues.

Laboratory diagnosis

Diagnosis of *Y. pestis* infection may be made on the basis of clinical presentation. Laboratory identification can be initiated by microscopy and culture of aspirate (pus) from bubo, sputum, blood and CSF.

Microscopy — The smears are stained by Methylene blue (**simple staining**) and observed for ovoid, short bacilli with bipolar bodies resembling safety pin. The smears are also stained by Gram's method and observed for Gram negative, ovoid coccobacilli with bipolar bodies. The fluorescent antibody technique may be of use in identifying plaguqe bacilli.

Culture —The specimens are inoculated on to blood agar, MacConkey agar, nutrient agar and ghee broth and incubated at 27°C. The colonies grow somewhat more slowly than do those of other enterobacteriaceae. The growth is identified by biochemical tests and slide agglutination tests. Colonies on blood agar are dark brown due to absorption of hemin pigment. Colonies on MacConkey agar are colorless. In ghee broth, a characteristic stalactite growth is produced.

Animal inoculation — When the specimen (or broth culture) is rubbed on the shaven abdomen of guinea pig, the plague bacillus can penetrate through the minute abrasions caused by shaving and cause lethal infection.

Serology — The antibodies to F-I antigen can be demonstrated in patient's serum by passive hemagglutination test and CFT.

Diagnosis of plague in rats — A rat died of plague may carry infected fleas and should be disinfected by pouring 3% lysol. Necropsy reveals enlargement of lymph nodes with periglandular inflammation and edema. Buboes are usually present in the cervical region. They are hard and can be moved under the skin. On section, the bubo may show congestion, hemorrhagic points or grey necrosis. Smears from the bubo stained with methylene blue show the bipolar stained bacilli, with considerable pleomorphism. The liver is mottled withr red, yellow or grey stippling. The spleen is enlarged and moulded over the stomach. A characteristic feature is pleural effusion which may be clear, abundant and straw colored or less often blood stained. The fluorescent antibody technique may be of use in identifying plague bacilli in the impression films of the tissues. Cultures may be made from the buboes, spleen and heart blood and particularly from bone marrow in decomposed carcasses.

Prophylaxis

For individuals in enzootic areas, efforts to minimize exposure to rodents and fleas is important. A formalin-killed vaccine is available for those at high risk of acquiring plague. A virulent strain of the plague bacillus is grown in casein hydrolysate broth for 2–4 weeks at 32°C and killed by 0.05 percent formaldehyde and preserved with phenyl mercuric nitrate (Sokhey's modification of Haffkine's vaccine). Standardisation is by immunogenic potency rather than by bacterial counts. The vaccine is given subcutaneously, two doses at an interval of 1–3 months, followed by a third six months later vaccination gives some protection against bubonic plague but not against pneumonic plague. The vaccine is recommended only in those exposed occupationally or otherwise to infection, such as laboratory or hospital personnel and troops deployed in known plague areas. It is of no value in plague outbreaks and mass vaccination is not advised.

Live attenuated vaccines prepared from two avirulent strains of *Y. pestis*, Otten's Tjiwidez strain from Indonesia and Girard's EV 76 strain from Malagasy cause severe reactions and are not in use now.

Treatment

Streptomycin is the drug of choice; gentamicin and tetracycline are acceptable alternatives. For plague meningitis, chloramphenicol offers good penetration into the CSF. Because of the potential for overwhelming septicemia, rapid institution of antibiotic therapy is crucial. Supportive therapy is essential for patients with signs of shock.

YERSINIA PSEUDOTUBERCULOSIS

It is a small, ovoid , bipolar stained Gram negataive bacillus resembling plague bacillus closely but can be distinguished by its relatively poor growth on MacConkey's agar, **motility at 22°C (but not at 37°C)**, productin of urease, fermentation of rhamnose and melibiose and failure to be lysed by the antiplague bacteriophage at 22°C. On the basis of somatic and flagellar antigens, six serogroups and several serotypes have been identified. It shows antigenic cross relationship with *Y. pestis* as well as salmonellae.

It causes pseudotuberculosis, a zoonotic disease. The natural mode of infection in animals is through GI tract. In infected guinea pigs, the liver, spleen and lungs show multiple nodules resembling tubercles; hence the name psuedotuberculosis. Most of the human infections are caused by serogroup-I. Humans acquire infection either through skin contact with contaminated water or through the ingestion contaminated vegetables or other foods. Human infection occurs rarely and may present as a fatal typhoid like illness with hepatosplenomegaly and purpura or as mesenteric lymphadenitis simulating acute appendicitis. It has also been reported to cause erythema nodosum and gastroenteritis.

Laboratory diagnosis may be made by isolating the organisms from an excised mesenteric lymph node or blood and/or demonstration of antibodies in patient's serum by tube agglutination tests during acute phase of the illness. Ampicillin and tetracycline are used for treatment.

YERSINIA ENTEROCOLITICA

It is a Gram negative coccobacillus showing pleomorphism in older cultures. It resembles *Y. pseudotuberculosis* in being **motile at 22°C**, but differs from it in fermenting sucrose and cellobiose and decarboxylating ornithine. It does not ferment rhamnose or melibiose. Many strains are indole and VP positive. It is an aerobe and facultative anaerobe. Optimum temperature for growth is 22–29°C. On Mac Conkey agar, it forms pinpoint colonies. On blood agar the colonies are nonhemolytic and translucent after incubation at 22°C. Six biotypes have been identified based on cultural and biochemical characateristics. Based on O and H antigens, more than 60 serotypes have been reported. O 3, O 8, O 9 serotypes account for majority of human infections.

Y. enterocolitica has been isolated from a wide range of domestic and wild animals and, in recent years, is increasingly being reported from human infections. It produces three types of disease in humans.

1. Gastroenteritis or enterocolitis, which is self limited and occurs in young children. It may be either inflammatory noninflammatory.
2. Mesenteric adenitis and inflammatory terminal ileitis in older children that may mimic appendicitis, and
3. Systemic disease typically seen in adults, of characterized by septicemia, meningitis, arthralgia or erythema nodosum. Persons belonging to HLA-B 27 group are prone to develop reacative arthritis.

QUESTIONS

Essay Type Questions

1. Name the diseases spread by rats. Describe the pathogenesis and lab. diagnosis of plague bacillus.

Short Answer Type Questions

1. *Yersinia pestis.*
2. Morphology of plague bacillus.
3. Ghee broth or stalactite broth
4. Pathogenesis of plague.
5. Bubonic plague.
6. Pneumonic plague.
7. Lab. diagnosis of plague.
8. Prophylaxis of plague.
9. *Y. pseudotuberculosis.*
10. *Y. enterocolitica.*

63

Vibrios

VIBRIO CHOLERAE

Introduction

Members of the genus *Vibrio* are short, curved, rod shaped organisms. They are actively motile by means of a single polar flagellum. Vibrios are closely related to family enterobacteriaceae, but not included in this family as they are oxidase positive. O and H antigens are both present but only O antigens are useful in distinguishing strains of vibrios that cause epidemics. Vibrios are facultative anaerobes. The growth of many *Vibrio* strains either requires or is stimulated by NaCl. Pathogenic vibrios include: (1) *V. cholerae*, serogroup O 1 strains that are associated with epidemic cholera, (2) Non-O 1 *V. cholerae* and related strains that cause sporadic cases of cholera-like and other illnesses, and (3) *V. parahaemolyticus* and other halophilic vibrios, which cause gastroenteritis and extraintestinal infections.

V. cholerae, the causative agent of cholera, was first isolated by Robert Koch (1883), though it was first described by Pacini (1854).

Morphology

The *V. cholerae* is a short, curved or comma shaped rod with rounded or pointed ends, about 1.5 µm × 0.2 – 0.4 µm in size. The cell is typically comma shaped, hence the old name *V. comma*. S. shaped or spiral forms may be seen due to two or more cells lying end to end. Pleomorphism is frequent in old cultures. In stained films of mucus flakes from acute cholera cases, the vibrios are seen arranged in parallel rows, resembling "fish in stream" appearance. It is actively motile, with a single polar flagellum (**monotrichous**). The motility is of **darting** type, and when acute cholera stool or young culture is examined under microscope by hanging drop preparation, the actively motile vibrios suggest a "swarm of gnats". They are Gram negative, nonsporing, noncapsulated and non-acid fast.

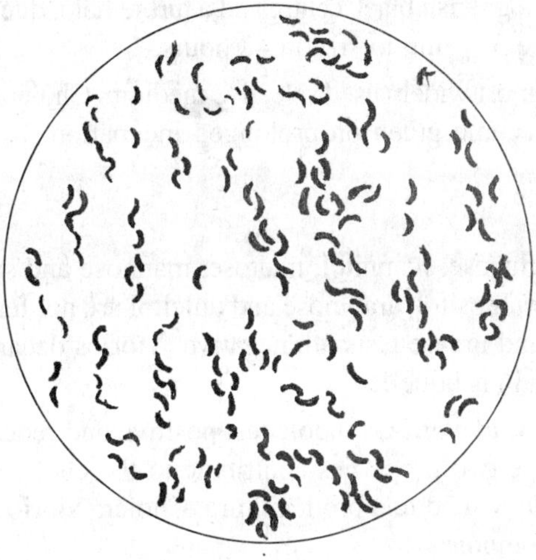

Fig. 63.1 *Vibrio cholerae*

Cultural characteristics

It is strongly aerobic, the growth being scanty and slow anaerobically. The optimum temperature required for growth is 37°C. The optimum pH required for growth is 8.2 (**alkaline pH**). NaCl of 0.5 – 1% is required for optimum growth, though high concentrations (6% and above) are inhibitory.

It grows well on ordinary media. On nutrient agar, colonies are moist, translucent, round disks, about 1–2 mm in diameter, with a bluish tinge in transmitted light. The growth has a distinctive odour. On MacConkey's agar, the colonies are colorless at first, but become reddish on prolonged incubation due to the late fermentation of lactose. On blood agar classical biotype does not produce hemolysis although some strains produce greenish discoloration surrounding the colonies, which later becomes clear due to hemodigestion. Colonies of El Tor biotype are hemolytic. In gelatin stab culture, infundibuliform (funnel shaped) or napiform (turnip shaped) liquefaction occurs in three days at 22°C. In peptone water, growth occurs in about six hours as a fine surface pellicle, which on shaking breaks up into membranous pieces.

Several special media have been employed for the cultivation of *V. cholerae*:

Transport (holding) media — *V. cholerae* is quite sensitive to drying, exposure to sunlight and extreme changes in pH. It is also inhibited by normal intestinal flora. Therefore, the cholera stool samples are transported in transport (holding) media.

1. Venkatraman-Ramakrishnan (VR) medium — It is prepared by dissolving 20 gm crude sea salt and 5 gm peptone in one litre of distilled water and adjusting the pH to 8.6–8.8. It is dispensed in screw-capped bottles in 10–15 ml amounts. About 1–3 ml stool is to be added to each bottle. In this medium vibrios do not multiply but remain viable for several weeks.

2. Cary-Blair medium — This is a buffered solution of NaCl, sodium thioglycholate, disodium phosphate and calcium chloride at pH 8.4. It is a suitable transport medium for *Salmonella*, *Shigella* as well as for vibrios.

Enrichment media — (1) **Alkaline peptone water** at pH 8.6, (2) Monsur's taurocholate tellurite peptone water at pH 9.2. Both these are good transport as well as enrichment media.

Plating media — 1. Alkaline bile salt agar (BSA) pH 8.2. The colonies are similar to those on nutrient agar.

2. Monsur'a gelatin taurocholate trypticase tellurite agar (GTTA) pH 8.5. Cholera vibrios produce small, translucent colonies with a greyish black centre and a turbid halo, due to hydrolysis and denaturation of gelatin. The colonies become 3–4 mm in size in 48 hours.

3. **TCBS agar** — It is the most widely used selective medium. Cholera vibrios produce large, yellow, convex colonies which may become green on prolonged incubation. It contains thiosulphate, citrate, bile and sucrose.

Biochemical reactions

Cholera vibrios ferment glucose, mannitol, maltose, mannose and sucrose producing acid, but no gas. It is a late lactose fermenter. Inositol, arabinose and dulcitol are not fermented. Catalase and oxidase tests are positive. Methyl red and urease tests are negative. Vibrios decarboxylate lysine and ornithine but do not utilise arginine. Gelatin is liquefied.

Cholera red reaction — *V. cholerae* is indole test positive and reduces nitrates to nitrites (Nitrate reduction test is positive). These two properties contribute to the cholera red reaction, which is tested by adding a few drops of sulphuric acid to a broth culture. Cholera vibrios produce a reddish pink color due to the formation of nitroso-indole.

String test — Vibrio colonies can be identified by string test. When a loopful of growth is mixed with a drop of 0.5% sodium deoxycholate in saline on a slide; the suspension loses its turbidity, becomes mucoid and forms a "string", when the loop is drawn slowly away from the suspension.

Resistance

Cholera vibrios are destroyed at 55°C in 15 minutes. They are sensitive to common disinfectants and acids. They die within minutes when exposed to normal gastric juices. They survive for 1–2 weeks in clean, nonacid fresh sea water. They can survive for 30 days in clean tap water. On fruits, they survive for 1–5 days at room temperature and for a week in the refrigerator. In grossly contaminated water, such as the Ganges water in India, the vibrios do not survive for any length of time apparently due to the presence of vibriophages.

Classification

Heiberg (1934) classified vibrios into six groups based on the fermentation of mannose, sucrose and arabinose. Two more groups were added later. **Serological (antigenic) classification** was introduced by **Gardner and Venkatraman** (1935). Cholera vibrios and biochemically similar vibrios, possessing a common flagellar (H) antigen were classified as Group A vibrios and the rest as Group B vibrios.

Based on the major somatic (O) antigen, Group A vibrios were classified into subgroups (also called O serogroups or serovars). All isolates from epidemic cholera (till 1992) belonged to serogroup O-1. Therefore, Group O 1 antiserum is used in the diagnostic laboratory for identifying pathogenic cholera vibrios, referred to as "**agglutinable vibrios**". Other vibrio, isolates which were not agglutinated by the O 1 antiserum came to be called "**nonagglutinable (NAG) vibrios**". They were considered nonpathogenic, but some of them can cause cholera. The NAG vibrios resemble *V. cholerae* but are unrelated biochemically and antigenically to O1 subgroup. They are commonly isolated from environmental sources and healthy human intestines. The NAG vibrios have been classified into many serogroups, currently upto 139.

Table 63.1 Gardner and Venkatraman's classification

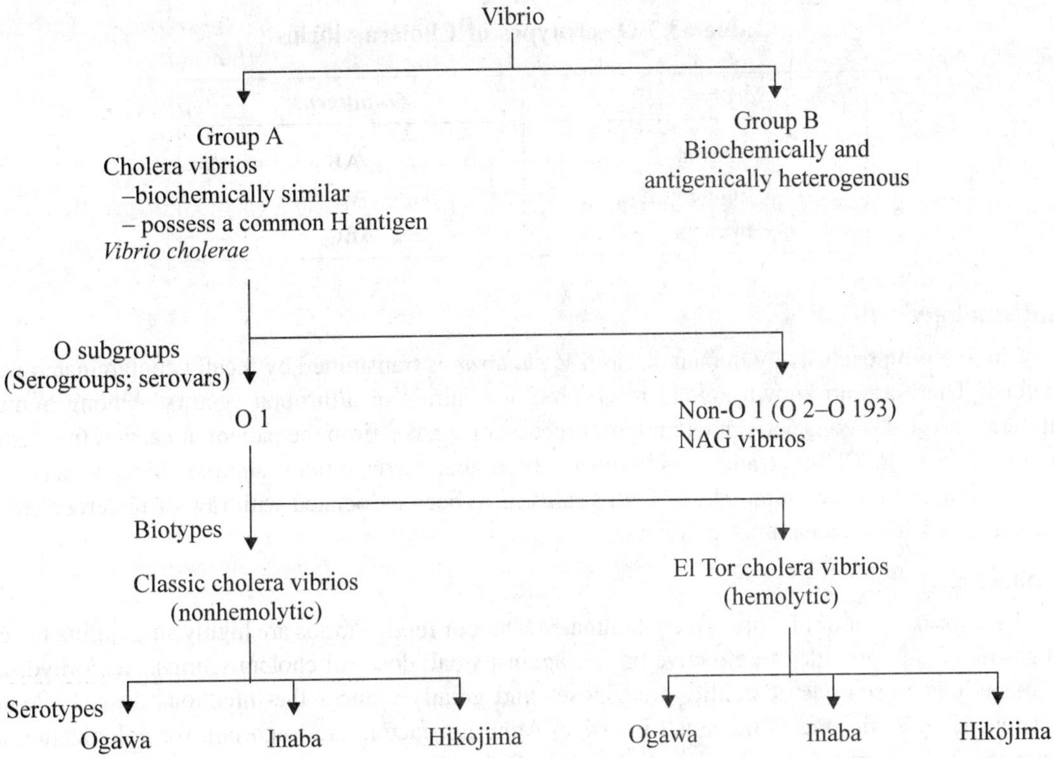

Based on biochemical reactions, cholera vibrios are classified into two biotypes — Classic and El Tor. **El Tor vibrios** were first isolated from Haj pilgrims who died of dysentery or gangrene of the colon at the Tor quarantine station at Sinai Peninsula. Hence the name El Tor. They are similar to **classical cholera vibrios** in all respects. Except that they were hemolytic and VP positive. In contrast to the classic strain, the El Tor strain is distinguished by the production of hemolysins, higher carriage rates, and the ability to survive in water for longer periods, increased virulence and invasiveness.

Table 63.2 Differences between Classic and El Tor vibrios

Test	*ClassicEl Tor*	
Hemolysis	–	+*
Voges-Proskauer	–	+*
Chick RBC agglutination	–	+
Polymyxin B sensitivity	+	–
Group IV phage susceptibility	+	–
El Tor phage 5 susceptibility	–	+

* Strains isolated after 1961 gave variable results.

Based on minor surface antigenic characteristics both classic and El Tor biotypes were classified into three serotypes — Ogawa, Inaba and Hikojima. The **Ogawa** and **Inaba** strains are agglutinated by their own respective specific antisera only, while the **Hikojima** strains are agglutinated by both Ogawa and Inaba antisera. Serotyping is only of epidemiological significance and there is no difference in pathogenicity between the three serotypes.

Table 63.3 O serotypes of Cholera vibrios

Serotypes	*O antigens*
Ogawa	AB
Inaba	AC
Hikojima	ABC

Epidemiology

Cholera is an exclusively human disease. *V. cholerae* is transmitted by fecally contaminated water and food. There are no known animal reservoirs, nor animal or arthropod vectors. Among humans, long-term carriage is considered uncommon. Infection originates from the patient or carrier. In constrast to classic strain, the El Tor strain is distinguished by higher carriage rates, and the ability to survive in water for longer periods. Outbreaks of both strains have been associated with raw or undercooked sea food harvested from contaminated waters.

Pathogenicity

The vibrios enter orally through contaminated water or food. Vibrios are highly susceptible to acids and gastric acidity provides an effective barrier against small doses of cholera vibrios. Achlorhydria or treatments that lessen gastric acidity predisposes and greatly reduces the infectious dose. Following ingestion, *V. cholerae* infects the small intestine. Adhesion factors are important for colonization and virulence. The organism is noninvasive and causes disease through the action of an enterotoxin, known as choleragen, **cholera toxin**, which is similar to LT of *E. coli.* The cholera toxin production is determined by a filamentous phage integrated with the bacterial chromosome. Cholera toxin is a protein. It can be toxoided. It can be destroyed by heating at 56°C for 30 minutes.

Cholera toxin is a multimeric protein composed of an A and a B subunit. The B (binding) subunit, consisting of five identical monomers, binds to GM_1 ganglioside receptor of cells lining the intestine. The A (active) subunit has two components A_1 and A_2. A_2 fragment facilitates penetration of the cell membrane and links the biologically active A_1 to the B subunit. A_1 fragment is an ADP-ribosyl transferase that ADP-ribosylates the membrane-bound Gs protein. As a result, Gs protein activates **adenylate cyclase**, which produces elevated levels of intracellular **cAMP**. This in turn causes an outflowing of ions and water to the lumen of the intestine. The fluid secreted is isotonic with plasma but contains much more of potassium and bicarbonate.

Full-blown cholera is characterized by massive loss of fluid and electrolytes from the body. After an incubation period ranging from hours to a few days, profuse **watery diarrhea (rice-water stools)** and vomiting begins. Untreated, the death from severe dehydration causing hypovolemic shock may occur in hours to days. The outpouring of bicarbonate-rich isotonic electrolyte solution leads to decrease in extracellular fluid volume, hemoconcentration, hypokalemia, base-deficit acidosis and shock. The common complications are muscular cramps, renal failure, pulmonary edema, cardiac arrythmias and paralytic ileus.

Laboratory diagnosis

Specimens collected are feces and rectal swabs. Feces is best collected by introducing a rubber catheter Nos. 24–26 into the rectum and letting the liquid stool flow directly into a sterile screw-capped container. The specimens are preserved in appropriate holding media such as VR fluid or Cary Blair medium. If the specimen can reach the laboratory in a few hours, it may be transported in enrichment media such as alkaline peptone water or Monsur's medium, thus saving the time required for isolation. If transport media are not available, strips of blotting paper may be soaked in the watery stool and sent to the laboratory packed in plastic envelopes.

Microscopy

For rapid diagnosis, the characteristic **darting motility** of *V. cholerae* in hanging drop preparations and its inhibition by specific antiserum can be demonstrated under the dark field or phase contrast microscope, using cholera stool from acute cases, or more reliably after enrichment for six hours. Cholera vibrios can be directly identified by direct immunofluorescence in stools.

Culture

The specimens sent in holding media should be inoculated into enrichment media and incubated for 6–8 hours. The specimens sent in enrichment media should be incubated for 6–8 hours including transit time. The specimens should be plated, before and after enrichment, into standard media such as nutrient agar, blood agar and MacConkey agars, and also into selective media such as TCBS agar, and incubated overnight at 37°C. The organism is oxidase positive, but further biochemical testing is necessary for specific identification of *V. cholerae*.

The colonies should be tested by slide agglutination with O1 antisera. If positive, the test is repeated using monospecific Ogawa and Inaba antisera. Hikojima strains will agglutinate with both Ogawa and Inaba antisera. If agglutination is negative by O1 antisera, it should be tested for agglutination with H antisera. Any vibrio which is agglutinated by H antisera and not by O1 antisera is considered to be serogroup O 2 – O 193, as H antigen is shared by all serogroups of *V. cholerae*.

To differentiate the biotypes (classic and El Tor) of O 1 serogroup, biochemical tests such as VP test, chick RBC agglutination test, hemolysis, polymyxin B sensitivity and Group IV phage susceptibility are used.

Prophylaxis

Prevention relies primarily on public health measures that reduce fecal contamination of water supplies and food. Adequate cooking of foods can minimize transmission. Vaccination is the most widely used method of prevention in endemic areas.

Killed cholera vaccine — It is a killed suspension containing 8000 million *V. cholerae* per ml, composed of equal numbers of Ogawa and Inaba serotypes. Classic and El Tor biotypes are included in equal numbers. The concentration of the vaccine may be increased to 12,000 million *V. cholerae* cells per ml, in order to improve the antigenic stimulus. The vaccine is given subcutaneously or intramuscularly in two doses with 1–4 week intervals.

Killed oral B subunit-whole cell vaccine — This vaccine contains cholera toxin B subunit, 2.5×10^{10} heat killed vibrios of Ogawa and Inaba serotypes of classic biotype and equal number formalin killed vibrios each of Ogawa and Inaba serotypes of El Tor biotype.

Live oral vaccine — Recombinant DNA vaccine with expression of *V. cholerae* O 1 in attenuated strain of *S. typhi Ty 21a* as a carrier bacterium has been developed. The live salmonellae colonize the peyer's patches of small intestine and induce IgA response by local immunity. Live attenuated oral vaccine against *V. cholerae* O 139 is also available.

Treatment

Replacement of fluids and electrolytes is crucial in preventing shock and does not require bacteriologic diagnosis. Antibiotics can shorten the duration of diarrhea and excretion of the organism. Tetracycline is the drug of choice.

HALOPHILIC VIBRIOS

These organisms are characterized by a requirement for higher-than-usual concentrations of NaCl, and their ability to grow in ten percent NaCl. They are common in coastal waters. *V. parahemolyticus*, *V. alginolyticus* and *V. vulnificus* are three important species of halophilic vibrios.

Vibrio parahemolyticus

It is an enteropathogenic halophilic vibrio, associated with gastroenteritis, as an important cause of food poisoning that result from ingestion of contaminated and inadequately cooked seafood, especially shellfish and crustaceans. The disease is self-limiting, and antibiotics do not alter the course of infection. Neither human carriers nor mammalian reservoirs have been identified. It was named as *V. parahemolyticus* because of the true hemolysis produced by this organism on blood agar.

Morphologically, it resembles *V. cholerae*, except that it is capsulated, shows bipolar staining and exhibits pleomorphism, especially when grown on 3% salt agar and in old cultures. It produces peritrichate flagellae on solid media and polar flagellae in liquid cultures. It grows well on media with NaCl upto eight percent. On TCBS agar, the colonies are green with an opaque, raised centre and flat translucent periphery. The string test is positive.

Strains of *V. parahemolyticus* associated with gastroenteritis produce hemolysis on **Wagatsuma agar** (a special high salt blood agar) due to the production of a heat stable hemolysin. This is known as **Kanagawa phenomenon.** Kanagawa positive strains are considered pathogenic for humans and negative strains nonpathogenic. It is oxidase, catalase, nitrate, indole and citrate positive. Glucose, maltose, mannitol, mannose and arabinose are fermented producing acid only. Lactose, sucrose, salicin, xylose, adonitol, inositol and sorbitol are not fermented.

It can be destroyed at 60°C in 15 minutes. It does not grow at 4°C but can survive refrigeration and freezing. It dies in distilled water or vinegar in a few minutes. Three antigens — Somatic (O), Flagellar (H) and Capsular (K) antigens have been identified. Serotyping is based O and K antigens.

Vibrio vulnificus

It resembles *V. parahemolyticus*, in forming green, nonsucrose fermenting colonies on TCBS medium. The ability of *V. vulnificus* to ferment lactose (lactose fermenters) is a characteristic feature. It can grow in the presence of polymyxin (300 units). It has a high salt tolerance of less than eight percent. It causes wound infections, septicemia and soft tissue infections (in compromised patients with liver disease) resulting either from contact of wounds with contaminated sea water or from ingestion of contaminated seafood. For soft tissue infections, prompt administration of anitbiotics such as tetracycline or cefotaxime is important, and surgical debridement/drainage may be required.

Vibrio alginolyticus

It is an halophilic vibrio, grow in the presence of 10% NaCl. On TCBS agar, it grows well and forms large, yellow (sucrose fermenting) colonies. It is widely found in sea water and sea fish. It is an opportunistic pathogen causing wound infections or otitis media and otitis externa (swimmer's ear) in humans exposed to sea water.

AEROMONAS

The genus *Aeromonas* belongs to the family vibrionaceae. Several species of Aeromonas are associated with human disease. They are ubiquitous in fresh and brackish water, and infection results from ingestion of contaminated food and water. *A. hydrophila*, found in water, is the causative agent of "red leg disease" of frogs, from which it was originally isolated. It may also infect other cold-blooded animals like fish and reptiles. It may cause diarrhea and pyogenic wound infections (mainly skin and soft tissues) in man.

PLESIOMONAS

The genus *Plesiomonas* belongs to the family vibrionaceae. Only one species *P. shigelloides* has been described, which is taxonomically related to *Proteus* species and serologically related to *Shigella sonnei*. It is ubiquitous in surface waters and soil and commonly infects cold-blooded animals like frogs, snakes and other reptiles. It causes gastroenteritis and rarely extraintestinal infections such as septicemia, meningitis. Man is primarily infected by ingestion of contaminated water or food.

Both *Aeromonas* and *Plesiomonas* are oxidase positive, polar flagellated, Gram negative rods. Since they are not agglutinated by *V. cholerae* O1 antisera, they may be mistaken for non-O1 *V. cholerae* (NAG). They may be differentiated from vibrios by biochemical tests such as utilisation of aminoacids.

QUESTIONS

Essay Type Questions

1. List the bacterial agents which cause diarrhoeal disease in man. Describe the pathogenesis and lab. diagnosis of cholera.
2. Describe the pathogenesis, lab. diagnosis and immunoprophylaxis of cholera.

Short Answer Type Questions

1. Morphology of *V. cholerae*.
2. Culture media for *V. cholerae*.
3. V–R fluid.
4. Cary-Blair medium.
5. Cholera red reaction.
6. String test.
7. TCBS agar.
8. Transport media for *V. cholerae*.
9. Enrichment media for *V. cholerae*.
10. Classification of vibrios.
11. Antigenic or serological classification of vibrios. *Or* Gardner and Venkatraman's classification of vibrios.
12. Classic vibrios.
13. El Tor vibrios.
14. Differences between classic and El Tor vibrios.
15. Pathogenesis of cholera.
16. Cholera toxin.
17. Lab. diagnosis of cholera.
18. Cholera vaccine.
19. Halophilic vibrios.
20. *V. parahemolyticus*.
21. Kanagawa phenomenon.

64

Campylobacter and Helicobacter

• ***Campylobacter***	• ***Helicobacter***
– ***Morphology***	– ***Morphology***
– ***Cultural characteristics***	– ***Cultural characteristics***
– ***Biochemical reactions***	– ***Biochemical reactions***
– ***Epidemiology***	– ***Epidemiology***
– ***Pathogenicity***	– ***Virulence factors***
– ***Laboratory diagnosis***	– ***Pathogenicity***
– ***Prevention***	– ***Laboratory diagnosis***
– ***Treatment***	– ***Treatment and prevention***

CAMPYLLOBACTER

Morphology

Members of the *Campylobacter* (Greek, meaning curved rod) are slender, curved, spiral, or S-shaped Gram negative rods that microscopically resemble vibrios. A single polar flagellum provides the organism with its characteristic **darting motility**. They are nonsporing. Old cultures are coccoid and pleomorphic. Somatic, flagellar and capsular antigens all contribute to the numerous serotypes.

The genus *Campylobacter* possess ten species out of which *C. jejuni*, *C. coli*, *C. lari*, *C. fetus*, *C. concisus*, *C. sputorum, C. hyointestinalis* are medically important.

Cultural characteristics

Most campylobacters are microaerophilic, that is, they require oxygen, but at lower concentrations than found in air. Optimum temperature required for growth is 37°C, but many pathogens are thermophilic, grow well at 42°C. Colonies are circular and convex but those of thermophilic group, particularly *C. jejuni*, are flat and tend to swarm on moist agar. The selective media used for isolation are Butzler's medium, Skirrow's medium and Blaser's (Campy-BAP) medium.

Biochemical reactions

Campylobacters do not ferment carbohydrates and utilize a respiratory (oxidative) pathway. They are strongly oxidase positive. They are catalase positive and reduce nitrates to nitrites. *C. jejuni* has the ability to hydrolyze sodium hippurate.

Epidemiology

Campylobacter are widely distributed in nature as commensals of GI tract of many different vertebrate species, including mammals and fowl, both wild and domestic. These serve as reservoirs of infection. *Campylobacter* can be transmitted to humans primarily via the fecal-oral route-through direct contact, exposure to contaminated meat (especially poultry), raw milk or contaminated water supplies. Therefore, the infection is **zoonotic**. *C. jejuni* alongwith ETEC and rotaviruses are the major cause of diarrhea world-wide.

Pathogenicity

Campylobacter infect the intestine and can cause ulcerative, inflammatory lesions in the jejunum, ileum or colon. In otherwise healthy individuals it typically causes an **acute enteritis** following one to seven days incubation. The disease lasts days to several weeks, and generally is self–limiting. Symptms may be both systemic (fever, headache, myalgia) and intestinal (abdominal cramping and diarrhea, which may or may not be bloody). *C. jejuni* is a cause of both **traveler's diarrhea** and **pseudo-appendicitis.** Bacteremia (often transient) may occur, most often in infants and the elderly. In compromised hosts, **campylobacteriosis** is more likely to result from infection with *C. fetus* than with *C. jejuni.* Complications include septic abortion, reactive arthritis and Guillain-Barre syndrome. *C. fetus* particularly causes infection of vascular sites, but may also infect the CNS and other local sites.

Laboratory diagnosis

Presumptive diagnosis can be made on the basis of finding curved organisms with rapid, darting motility in a wetmount of feces by direct microscopic examination under phase contrast or dark field microscopy.

Campylobacter can be isolated from feces or rectal swabs using special selective media — Skirrow's, Campy-BAP and Butzler's and microaerophilic conditions. The inoculated plates are incubated at 42°C in an atmosphere of 5% oxygen, 10% CO_2 and 85% nitrogen. Colonies appear usually by 48 hours. They are nonhemolytic, grey or colorless, moist and flat or convex. The growth is identified by Gram's staining, motility and oxidase tests. Confirmation is by further biochemical tests, including positive catalase and nitrate reduction tests.

In case of delay in culturing, transport media can be used. Campylobacters survive for 1–2 weeks at 4°C in **Cary-Blair transport medium**.

Prevention

Thorough cooking of potentially contaminated foods (for example, poultry) and pasteurisation of milk and milk products is essential to prevention of campylobacteriosis.

Treatment

Diarrhea should be treated symptomatically with fluid and electrolyte replacement. For patients with more severe symptoms for example, high fever, bloody diarrhea, worsening illness or illness of more than a week's duration, or for patients with systemic illness, antibiotics should be administered. For *C. jejuni*, ciprofloxacin is the drug of choice. Other antibiotics such as erythromycin, penicillin, tetracycline and aminoglycosides are also effective. For *C. fetus*, ampicillin or third-generation cephalosporins are effective.

HELICOBACTER

The genus *Helicobacter* contains several species. Of these *H. pylori* is the species of human significance. *H. cinnaedi* and *H. fennelliae* are associated with proctitis in the HIV infected cases.

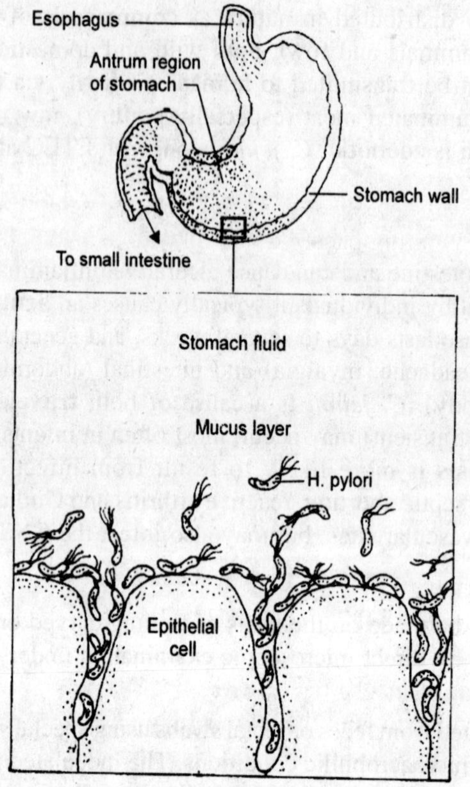

Fig. 64.1 *Helicobacter pylori* growing on the surface of epithelial cells lining the antrum of the stomach and in the overlying mucus layer

Morphology

Members of the genus *Helicobacter* are curved or spiral shaped Gram negative bacteria. They have a rapid, corkscrew motility due to a tuft of unipolar sheathed flagellae (**lophotrichous**).

Cultural characteristics

It is microaerophilic. It grows best in the presence of high humidity and 10% CO_2. It grows on cholocate agar and Skirrow's campylobacter selective medium in 3–7 days at 37°C (but not at 42°C) forming circular, convex and translucent colonies.

Biochemical reactions

A distinctive feature of *Helicobacter* is the production of a abundant **urease**, which is exceptionally powerful, about 100 times more powerful than that produced by *Proteus vulgaris*. This property has been used as a rapid diagnostic test in gastric biopsy samples. It does not metabolize carbohydrates or reduce nitrates. It produces oxidase, catalase, phosphatase and H_2S.

Epidemiology

H. pylori infections are relatively common, and world-wide in distribution. *H. pylori* are unusual in their ability to colonize the stomach, whose acidic pH normally protects against bacterial infection. The source of infection is human gastric mucosa. Transmission of *H. pylori* is thought to be from person to person; the organism has not been isolated from food and water. Untreated, infections tend to be chronic and life long. Lower socioeconomic status appears to be a risk factor of *H. pylori* infections.

Virulence factors

1. *H. pylori* produces a cytotoxin causing vacuolation of gastric mucosa. Its production is determined by Cag A Gene.
2. Urease released by *H. pylori* produces ammonia ions that neutralize stomach acid in the vicinity of the organism, thus favouring bacterial multiplication. Ammonia may also both cause injury and potentiate the effects of a cytotoxin produced by *H. pylori.*
3. The bacterial antigens cross-react with antran gastric antigens stimulating an autoimmune response.
4. Protease produced by the organism degrades gastric mucosa.
5. *H. pylori* infected patients show hypergastrinemia that upsets gastrin–HCl homeostasis.

Pathogenicity

H. pylori colonizes gastric mucosal (epithelial) cells in the stomach, and metaplastic gastric epithelium in the duodenum or esophagus, but does not colonize the rest of the intestinal epithelium. The organism survives in the mucus layer that coats the epithelium, and causes a chronic inflammation of the mucosa. *H. pylori* penetrates the mucous layer lining the stomach's epithelium, attracted to the chemotactic substances hemin and urea. Although the organism is noninvasive, it recruits and activates inflammatory cells. It also releases urease that cleaves urea, producing NH_3 that neutralizes stomach acid in its vicinity. *H. pylori* cytotoxin, and the ammonia produced by its urease, cause destruction of the mucus-producing cells, exposing the underlying connective tissue to stomach acid.

Initial infection with *H. pylori* causes **acute gastritis,** sometimes with **diarrhea** that lasts about one week. The infection usually becomes chronic, with diffuse superficial gastritis that may be associated with epigastric discomfort. Both **gastric ulcers** and **duodenal ulcers** are closely correlated with infection by *H. pylori. H. pylori* infection is found in over 95 percent of duodenal ulcer patients, and in nearly all patients with gastric ulcers who do not use aspirin or other nonsteroidal anti-inflammatory drugs, both risk factors for gastric ulcers. *H. pylori* infection appears to be a risk factor for development of **gastric carcinoma** and **gastric B-cell lymphoma.** In *H. pylori* infected persons, gastrin production is increased which contribute to an increased parietal cell mass.

Laboratory diagnosis

Diagnosis can be made either by invasive techniques or noninvasive means.

Invasive tests involve gastric biopsy specimens obtained by endoscopy. *H. pylori* can be detected in such specimens histologically by microscopy, by culture or by a test for urease. The biopsy specimen can be examined by microscopic examination of Gram's staining, silver staining, H and E staining, Giemsa staining or immunofluorescence for the presence of bacteria. The specimen may be cultured in a selective medium (**Skirrow's medium**) and nonselective medium such as chocolate agar. Plates are incubated for 2–7 days in a moist, microaerophilic atmosphere at 35–37°C in the presence of 5–10% CO_2. Colonies can be identified by the typical morphology of the bacteria in the Gram stain, motility, biochemical properties and positive urease tests. The biopsy urease test can be performed by crushing biopsy tissue in 0.5 ml urea solution with an indicator and incubated at 37°C. If *H. pylori* is present, the pH changes within a few minutes to 2 hours due to the production of ammonia.

Noninvasive diagnostic tests include serologic tests such as ELISA for demonstration of serum antibodies to *H. pylori* and breath tests for urease. **Urea breath test** detects the urease activity in the stomach. The test involves administering radioactively labeled (C_{13} or C_{14}) urea by mouth. If *H. pylori* are present in the patient's stomach, the urease produced by the organism will split the urea to CO_2 (radioactively labeled) and NH_3. The radioactively labeled CO_2 which is exhaled is detected in the patient's breath if the test is positive. The patient has to fast overnight before the test.

Treatment and Prevention

Elimination of *H. pylori* requires combination therapy with two or more antibiotics. Although *H. pylori* is innately sensitive to many antibiotics, resistance readily develops. A typical regimen includes metronidazole, tetracycline and bismuth. An alternative schedule employs a proton pump inhibitor (ant-acid) like omeprazole and clarithromycin (or amoxycillin).

QUESTIONS

Short Answer Type Questions

1. *Campylobacter jejuni.*
2. *Campylobacter* infections
3. *Campylobacter.*
4. *Helicobacter pylori.*
5. Urea breath test.
6. *Helicobacter pylori* infections.

65

Pseudomonas, Burkholderia and Stenotrophomonas

PSEUDOMONAS

Introduction

The genus *Pseudomonas* belongs to the family pseudomonadaceae comprising over 200 species. *Pseudomonas aeruginosa*, the primary human pathogen in the genus *Pseudomonas*, is widely distributed in nature. It is found in soil, water, plants and animals. It may colonize healthy humans without causing disease, but is also a significant opportunistic pathogen, and a major cause of nosocomial infections.

Based on molecular analysis, pseudomonads have been reclassified and many former *Pseudomonas* species reallocated to new genera such as *Burkholderia*, *Stenotrophomonas* and others.

Morphology

It is a slender Gram negative bacillus measuring 1.5–3.0 μm × 0.5 μm; actively motile by a polar flagellum. Occasionally some strains may possess two or three flagellae. Clinical isolates are often fimbriated. It is noncapsulated, but some strains particularly from cystic fibrosis cases possess abundant extracellular polysaccharide slime composed of alginate polymers, known as glycocalyx capsule.

Cultural characteristics

It is an obligate aerobe, but can grow anaerobically if nitrate is available (chemoautotroph). Nutritional requirements are minimal, and the organism can grow on a wide variety of organic substrates.

It can grow over a wide range of temperature 5–42°C, the optimum being 37°C. It grows well on ordinary media, producing large, opaque, irregular colonies with a distinctive, musty, earthy smell. It grows on MacConkey and DCA media, forming nonlactose fermenting colonies. Many strains are hemolytic on blood agar. In broth, it forms a dense turbidity with a surface pellicle.

P. aeruginosa produces a number of diffusible **pigments**.

1. Pyocyanin is a bluish green phenazine pigment soluble in water and chloroform. It is produced only by *P. aeruginosa* and not by other species; therefore, its detection is diagnostic of *P. aeruginosa*.

2. Pyoverdin (fluorescein) is a greenish yellow pigment soluble in water but not in chloroform. In old cultures, it may be oxidised to a yellowish brown **pigment**.

3. Pyorubin (red) is a bright red water soluble phenazine pigment that is insoluble in chloroform.

4. Pyomelanin is a brown to black pigment. Some of the pigments, particularly pyocyanin, inhibit the growth of many other bacteria and may therefore contribute to *P. aeruginosa* emerging as a dominant bacterium in mixed infections.

Biochemical reactions

The metabolism is oxidative and *Pseudomonas* does not ferment carbohydrates. For this, special media such as the O-F medium of Hugh and Leifson must be used. It utilizes glucose oxidatively with the production of acid only. Lactose and maltose are not utilized. Indole, MR, VP and H_2S tests are negative. All strains are oxidase positive within 30 seconds. Nitrates are reduced to nitrites and further to gaseous nitrogen. It is catalase, arginine dihydrolase and gelatinase positive and lysine decarboxylase and aesculin hydrolysis negative.

Resistance

It is resistant to many commonly used antiseptics and disinfectants such as quarternary ammonium compounds, chloroxylenol and hexachlorophene and may even grow profusely in bottles of such antiseptic lotions kept for use in hospitals. Therefore, dettol or cetrimide can be incorporated in selective media for isolation of *Pseudomonas*. It is sensitive to glutaraldehyde (cidex), silver salts and strong phenolic disinfectants. *Ps. aeruginosa* possesses innate mechanisms of antibiotic resistance, in addition to rapid development of resistance mutations.

Epidemiology

The members of *Pseudomonas* are widely distributed in nature, found in soil, water, plants and animals. It may colonize healthy humans without causing disease, but is also a significant opportunistic pathogen, and a major cause of nosocomial infections. The nutritional requirements are minimal and the organism can grow on a wide variety of organic substrates. In fact, *P. aeruginosa* can even grow in laboratory water baths, hot tubs, wet IV tubing, disinfectant solutions and other water-containing vessels. This explains why the organism is responsible for so many nosocomial infections. Transmission is via hands of the hospital personnel or fomites. Individuals most at risk include those with impaired immune defenses. It is resistant to many commonly used antiseptics and disinfectants, and antibiotics. A prior treatment with antibiotics that eliminate normal flora can also provide *P. aeruginosa* with increased access for colonizing tissue. It occasionally colonizes the skin, external ear, respiratory tract and the large bowel of healthy humans.

Pathogenesis

P. aeruginosa disease begins with attachment to and colonization of host tissue. Pili on the bacteria mediate adherence, and a glycocalyx capsule reduces the effectiveness of normal clearance mechanisms. Host tissue damage facilitates adherence and colonization. *P. aeruginosa* produces numerous toxins and extracellular products that promote local invasion and dissemination of the organism. These include extracellular proteases (*e.g.,* elastase, alkaline protease), cytotoxin (formerly called leucocidin), hemolysins (phospholipase C and rhamnolipid) and pyocyanin. Systemic disease is promoted by an antiphagocytic capsule, endotoxin, exotoxin-A (an inhibitor of mammalian protein synthesis that ADP-ribosylates elongation factor) and exotoxin-S (that ADP-ribosylates specific GTP-binding proteins).

P. aeruginosa causes both localized and systemic illness. Virtually any tissue or organ system may be affected. Individuals most at risk include those with impaired immune defenses. A prior antibiotic therapy that eliminate normal flora can also provide *P. aeruginosa* with increased access for colonizing tissue. *P. aeruginosa* is regularly a cause of nosocomial pneumonia, nosocomial urinary tract infections, surgical site infections, infections of severe burns and infections of patients undergoing either chemotherapy for neoplastic diseases or antibiotic therapy.

Localized infections have the potential to lead to disseminated infections and may occur in the

1. Eye – keratitis and endophthalmitis, following trauma.

2. Ear – external otitis or swimmer's ear; invasive and necrotizing otitis externa, particularly in elderly diabetic or trauma patients.

3. Skin – wound sepsis, purulent rashes occuring in epidemics associated with use of contaminated whirlpools, hot tubs and swimming pools.

4. Urinary tract – particularly in hospitalized patients who have been subjected to catheterization, instrumentation, surgery or renal transplantation.

5. Respiratory tract – pneumonia in individuals with chronic lung disease, congestive heart failure, or cystic fibrosis and particularly in patients who have been intubated or are on ventilators.

6. Gastrointestinal tract – infections range from relatively mild diarrheal illness in children to severe, necrotizing enterocolitis in infants and neutropenic cancer patients.

7. CNS – meningitis and brain abscesses, particularly in association with trauma, surgery or tumors of the head or neck.

Systemic infections include

1. Bacteremia – most common in patients whose immune system has been compromised by hematologic malignancies, congenital or acquired immunodeficiencies, neutropenia, severe burns or diabetes mellitus.

2. Secondary pneumonia – particularly in patients with hematologic malignancies.

3. Bone and joint infections – in IV drug users and patients with urinary tract or pelvic infections.

4. Endocarditis – in IV drug users and patients with prosthetic heart valves.

5. CNS – in immunocompromised patients.

6. Skin/soft tissue infections (erythematous necrotic lesions known as ecthyma gangrenosum) abscesses, cellulitis, bullae and necrotizing fascitis.

Laboratory diagnosis

The specimens to be collected include pus, wound swab, urine, sputum, CSF or blood. The organism can be isolated by plating on blood agar and MacConkey agar. It may be necessary to use selective media such as **cetrimide agar** for isolation of *P. aeruginosa* from feces or wound swabs or other samples with mixed flora. Identification is based on colony morphology, biochemical tests and other diagnostic tests. As *P. aeruginosa* is a frequent contaminant, isolation of the bacillus from a specimen should not always be taken as proof of its etiological role. Serotyping and pyocin typing is used in the investigation of a cluster of cases, which may originate from exposure to a common source.

Treatment and prevention

Specific therapy varies with the clinical presentation and the antibiotic sensitivity pattern of the isolate. It is difficult to find antibiotics that are effective against *P. aeruginosa*, due to its rapid development of resistance mutations and its own innate mechanisms of antibiotic resistance. *Pseudomonas* infections typically occur in patients with impaired defenses. Therefore aggressive antimicrobial therapy, often a combination of two bactericidal antibiotics such as an aminoglycoside, antipseudomonal penicillins or a quinolone is generally required.

BURKHOLDERIA

B. Mallei (formerly *P. mallei*)

It differs from genus *Pseudomonas* in being nonmotile. It is the etiologic agent of **glanders,** a serious infection that affects primarily horses, donkeys and mules, but occasionally infects other animals and rarely humans. Human infection is usually occupational and infection is acquired via skin abrasions or wounds which come in contact with the discharges of a sick animal (zoonotic). Human-to-human transmission can occur. In humans, the clinical presentation depends on the route of infection. For example, it may be:

1. an acute, localized, suppurative infection of the mucous membranes leading to mucopurulent discharge and ulcerating granulomatous lesions, typically of the eyes, nose or lips.
2. an acute pulmonary infection characterized by lung abscesses, or lobar or bronchopneumonia.
3. an acute septicemic infection, which is nearly always fatal; or
4. a chronic suppurative infection characterized by multiple subcutaneous or intramuscular abscesses, often of the arms and legs.

The natural disease in equines occurs in two forms:

1. Glanders – In glanders, the respiratory system is affected, with the formation of firm, round nodules and a profuse catarrhal discharge from the nose. Later, the nodules may breakdown to form ulcers.

2. Farcy – This follows infection through the skin with involvement of lymph vessels and nodes, which stand out as hard cords under the skin.

Intraperitoneal inoculation of small amounts of a pure culture in male guinea pigs causes swelling of the testes, inflammation of tunica vaginalis and ulceration of the scrotal skin due to bacterial invasion. This is known as **Strauss reaction**.

Culture and serologic tests are useful diagnostically. Treatment depends on presentation and the results of sensitivity testing.

B. PSEUDOMALLEI (formerly *P. pseudomallei*)

It differs from B. mallei in being motile, hydrolyzing aesculin and utilizes lactose oxidatively. It is a normal inhabitant of soil and water. This is the causative agent of **melioidosis,** a glanders-like disease, epizootic in rodents in Southeast Asia, India, North Australia, as well as parts of Africa and Middle East. Transmission occurs when the organism is introduced into wounds or abrasions of the skin, and may also occur through inhalation or ingestion. Rare instances of human-to-human transmission have been described. Although exposure to the organism in endemic areas may be common (based on seroconversion rates), the disease is much less common.

The human disease may take different forms. It may be an acute septicemia, a subacute typhoid like disease, or pneumonia and hemoptysis resembling tuberculosis. In chronic form, there may be multiple caseous or suppurative foci, with abscess formation in the skin and subcutaneous tissues, bones and internal organs.

Diagnosis may be made by demonstration of the bacillus in exudates by microscopy, isolation by culture from sputum, pus, blood or urine, by serological tests such as ELISA and indirect hemagglutination to detect IgG and IgM antibodies. A PCR test has also been developed. The organism appears as small, irregularly staining Gram negative bacilli; showing typical bipolar "safety pin" appearance with methylene blue stain.

Ceftazidime is the drug of choice, alongwith cotrimoxazole, tetracycline, amoxycillin, clavulanate or chloramphenico).

B. CEPACIA (formerly *P. cepacia*)

It is ubiquitous in the environment. It is an opportunistic pathogen occasionally implicated in nosocomial outbreak. Colonization of various body sites precedes infections. It can cause pneumonia, UTI, meningitis, peritonitis, surgical, wound and burn infections, bacteremia and endocarditis in IV drug users. It is nutritionally very versatile. It can grow in many common disinfectants and can even use penicillin G as a sole source of carbon. It is oxidase positive. It is inherently resistant to most antibiotics.

STENOTROPHOMONAS MALTOPHILA (formerly *P. maltophila*)

It is a free-living saprophytic Gram negative bacillus, ubiquitous in nature. It is motile, aerobic and oxidase negative (or weakly positive). It is an opportunistic pathogen causing pneumonia, UTI, wound infections, peritonitis, meningitis, bacteremia, cholangitis and endocarditis in hospitalized patients, particularly in an intensive care setting.

It is resistant to many antibiotics effective against *P. aeruginosa* by virtue of reduced outer membrane permeability and production of inducible betalactamase. For this reason, it is an emerging nosocomial pathogen under the selective pressure of the antibiotics in the hospital environment. Trimethoprim-sulphamethoxazole is often effective in the multi-drug resistant strains. Alternative agents are ciprofloxacin, tetracycline, and tricarcillin + clavulanate. Sensitivity testing is of utmost importance for an appropriate therapy.

QUESTIONS

Essay Type Questions

1. Describe the morphology, cultural characteristics, pathogenicity and lab. diagnosis of *Pseudomonas aeruginosa.*

Short Answer Type Questions

1. *Pseudomonas.*
2. Pathogenicity of *Pseudomonas aeruginosa.*
3. Pigments of *Pseudomonas.*
4. Drug resistance in *Pseudomonas sp.*
5. Why *Pseudomonas aeruginosa* is an important nosocomial pathogen?
6. *Burkholderia mallei.*
7. *Stenotrophomonas maltophila.*

66

Hemophilus

- *Hemophilus influenzae*
  - *Morphology*
  - *Cultural characteristics*
  - *Biochemical reactions*
  - *Resistance*
  - *Antigenic structure*
  - *Epidemiology*
  - *Pathogenicity*
  - *Laboratory diagnosis*
  - *Prophylaxis*
  - *Treatment*
- *Hemophilus aegypticus*
- *Hemophilus ducreyi*
- *Hemophilus parainfluenzae*
- *Hemophilus aprophilus*
- *HACEK*

HEMOPHILUS INFLUENZAE

Morphology

It is a small, Gram negative, nonmotile, nonsporing bacillus, exhibiting pleomorphism. In sputum, it usually occurs as clusters of coccobacillary forms, while in the CSF from meningitis cases, long, bacillary and filamentous forms predominate. Cells from young cultures are usually coccobacillary, while older cultures are distinctly pleomorphic. Virulent strains are often capsulated, which can be demonstrated by negative staining or quellung reaction. The capsule is antiphagocytic. The bacilli are relatively difficult to stain. Staining for 5–15 minutes with Loeffler's methylene blue or dilute carbol fuchsin gives good results.

Cultural characteristics

It is an aerobe and facultative anaerobe. The optimum temperature for growth is 37°C and optimum pH 7.6. Some strains require 5–10% CO_2. It has fastidious growth requirements. It requires two growth factors X (hemin) and V (NAD^+) for growth. The **X factor** is required for the synthesis of cytochromes, catalase and peroxidase involved in aerobic respiration. The **V factor** is present inside the RBC. Therefore, the growth is scanty on blood agar. **Chocolate agar** (heated blood agar) is superior to blood agar for the growth of *H. influenzae*, because V factor is released from RBC during heating (80–90°C) of blood agar.

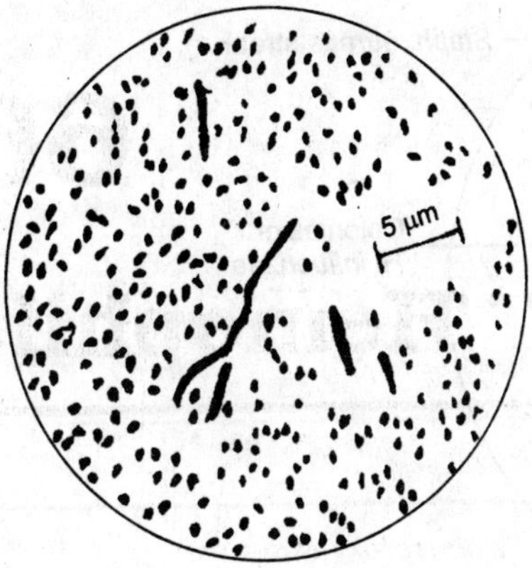

Fig. 66.1 *Hemophilus influenzae*

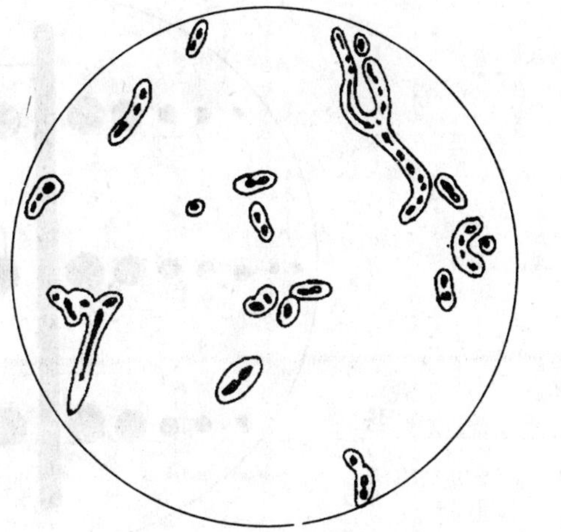

Fig. 66.2 *Hemophilus influenzae* by capsular swelling

Table 66.1 Growth Characteristics of *Hemophilus sp.*

Species	*Requires*		*Hemolysis*
	X	*Y*	
H. influenzae	+	+	−
H. aegypticus	+	+	−
H. parainfluenzae	−	+	−
H. ducreyi	+	−	−
H. hemolyticus	+	+	+
H. parahemolyticus	−	+	+
H. aprophilus	+	−	−
H. paraprophilus	−	+	−

Satellite phenomenon — The V factor (NAD^+) is present inside the RBC. It is synthesized by some fungi and bacteria such as *Staph. aureus* in excess of their requirements and released into the surrounding medium. When *Staph. aureus* is streaked across a plate of blood agar, on which a specimen containing *H. influenzae* has been inoculated, after overnight incubation, the colonies of *H. influenzae* will be large and well developed alongside the streak of *Staphylococcus*, and smaller away from it. This phenomenon is called **"satellitism"**, which demonstrates the dependence of *H. influenzae* on the V factor, which is available in higher concentrations near the staphylococcal growth and in smaller quantities away from it. This is a routine test in clinical bacteriology for the presumptive identification of *H. influenzae* from specimens.

Biochemical reactions

It ferments glucose and xylose with the production of acid, but not lactose, sucrose and mannitol. Catalase and oxidase reactions are positive. It reduces nitrates to nitrites. Based on the production of indole, urease and ornithine decarboxylase, *H. influenzae* is divided into eight (I to VIII) biotypes. Biotype I is most frequently responsible for meningitis.

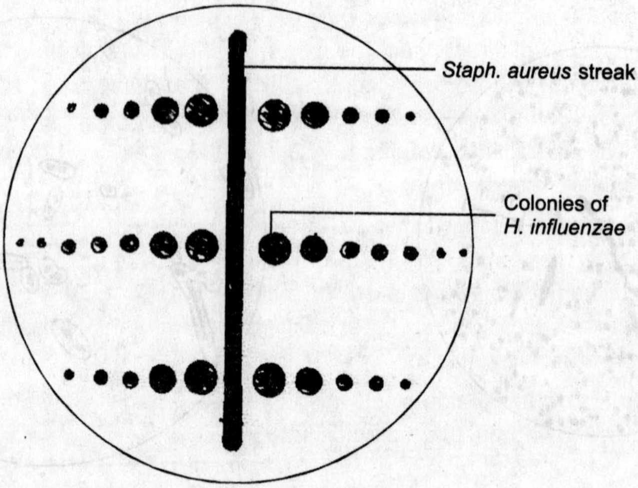

Fig. 66.3 Satellitism

Resistance

H. influenzae is a delicate organism. It is destroyed by heating at 55°C for 30 minutes, refrigeration, drying and disinfectants. In cultures, the cells die within two or three days due to autolysis. On chocolate agar, the cultures may be preserved for about a month. For long term preservation, the cultures may be lyophilised.

Antigenic structure

The major antigen is capsulated polysaccharide present in encapsulated *H. influenzae*. Based on antigenic differences, *H. influenzae* strains have been classified into six types (a–f). The capsular antigen of *H. influenzae* type b (Hib) is a **polyribose ribitol phosphate (PRP)**. Type b is the only one of the six capsular types that contains a pentose (ribose), rather than a hexose. Encapsulated *H. influenzae* can be typed by a capsule swelling test with specific antiserum. Hib antigens induces the formation of antibodies, which are protective. Hib PRP is therefore employed for immunization.

The other antigens present in *H. influenzae* include outer membrane proteins (OMP) and lipooligosaccharides (LOS).

The DNA extracted from a given type of *H. influenzae* is capable of transferring that type specificity to other cells by genetic transformation.

Epidemiology

H. influenzae is an indigenous normal component of the upper respiratory tract flora in humans, and may also colonize the conjunctiva and genital tract. Humans are the only natural hosts, and colonization begins shortly after birth, with unencapsulated strains and capsular type b being carried most frequently. *H. influenzae* illnesses are usually sporadic in occurrence.

Pathogenicity

H. influenzae is transmitted air-borne respiratory droplets. Capsular polysaccharide and IgA proteases produced by the organism are important virulence factors. IgA protease degrades secretory IgA, thus facilitating colonization of the upper respiratory tract mucosa. From this site, *H. influenzae* can enter the blood stream and disseminate to distant sites. Diseases caused by *H. influenzae* therefore fall into two categories. First, non-invasive disorders such as otitis media, sinusitis, epiglottitis, and bronchopneumonia result from contiguous spread of the organism from its site of colonization in the respiratory tract. Second, invasive disorders such as meningitis, septic arthritis and cellulitis result from invasion of the blood stream, followed by localization of *H. influenzae* in other areas of the body. Contiguous spread is more commonly associated with unencapsulated strains in a setting where there has been a breakdown in natural host defenses, whereas severe, invasive disease is more commonly associated with encapsulated type b strains.

H. influenzae has been a leading cause of **bacterial meningitis,** primarily in infants and very young children, frequently in conjunction with an episode of otitis media. Clinically, *H. influenzae* meningitis is indistinguishable from other purulent meningitis cases, and may be gradual in onset or fulminant (sudden onset with great severity). Mortality is high in untreated patients. Survivors may be left with permanent neurologic sequelae.

Epiglottitis (cellulitis of the epiglottis and surrounding tissues) is a rare but life threatening condition, primarily of younger children, for whom death may result from either airway obstruction or sepsis.

Other presentations include **bacteremia** (which may result in **cellulitis** or **spetic arthritis** or may occur without localized disease), **otitis media, pneumonia, empyema, chronic bronchitis** and **conjunctivitis.**

Laboratory diagnosis

The specimens to be collected depends upon the type of lesion and include CSF, blood, throat swab, sputum, pus, aspirates from joints, middle ears or sinuses. The methods of diagnosis consists of microscopy, culture and serology. Rapid diagnosis is crucial because of the potentially fulminant course of type b infections.

Microscopy — In Gram stained smears, the presence of pleomorphic Gram negative bacilli that do not stain well should arouse suspicion of *H. influenzae* infection. Type b capsule may be demonstrated directly in CSF, either by the **capsular swelling (quellung) reaction** or by immunofluorescent staining.

Culture — Isolation from normally sterile sites and fluids (for example blood, CSF or synovial fluid) is significant, whereas isolation from pharyngeal cultures is inconclusive.

CSF should be inoculated on to blood agar or chocolate agar. A strain of *Staph. aureus* should be streaked across the plate. Then the plate is incubated at 37°C with 5–10% CO_2, overnight. The growth is identified by colony morphology, Gram staining, satellite phenomenon, biochemical reactions and serotyping.

Blood cultures are often positive in cases of epiglottitis and pneumonia. Culture may be done in nutrient broth, as it will be enriched with X and V factors from the blood sample itself. For early results, culture may be examined after 4–6 hrs by quellung reaction. After overnight incubation, subcultures are done on chocolate agar and processed further as above.

Isolation from sputum or throat swab requires special care. Sputum should be homogenized by treatment with the pancreatin or by shaking with sterile water and glass beads for 10–15 minutes. Culturing several samples of sputum from the patient increases the rate of isolation.

Serology — Capsular antigen may be detected in CSF or other body fluids using serological tests such as latex agglutination, coagglutination, counter current immunoelectrophoresis, RIA and ELISA.

Prophylaxis

Active immunization against Hib is effective in preventing invasive disease, and also reduces respiratory carriage. Children aged two months or older can be immunized with **Hib PRP conjugate vaccine** with appropriate booster doses. The vaccine is conjugated with one of two carriers — toxoid of *Corynebacterium diphtheriae* CRM_{197} mutant or *Neisseria meningitidis* outer membrane complex.

Rifampin is given prophylactically to individuals in close contact with a patient infected with *H. influenzae*.

Treatment

Most strains are susceptible to chloramphenicol and essentially all strains are susceptible to the newer cephalosporins. When invasive *H. influenzae* is suspected, a suitable antibiotic (for example, a third-generation cephalosporin such as ceftriaxone or cefotaxime) should be started as soon as appropriate specimens have been taken for culture. Antibiotic sensitivity testing is necessary because of emergence of strains resistant to antibiotics commonly used to treat *H. influenzae* (for example, strains with β-lactamase-mediated ampicillin resistance). Sinusitis, otitis media and other upper respiratory tract infections are treated with trimethoprim-sulfamethoxazole or ampicillin plus sulbactam.

HEMOPHILUS AEGYPTICUS

It is sometimes called *H. influenzae* biotype III. It was first observed by Koch (1883) and first cultivated by Weeks (1887), hence formerly known as **Koch-Weeks bacillus**. It is closely associated with outbreaks of highly communicable form of **purulent conjunctivitis.** It may also cause a life threatening bacteremia, **Brazilian purpuric fever,** a disease of children characterized by fever, purpura, shock and death.

HEMOPHILUS DUCREYI

It was first demonstrated by Ducreyi (1890). It causes **chancroid** or **soft sore,** a sexually transmitted disease. It is characterised by tender, nonindurated, painful, irregular ulcers on genital organs. The regional lymph nodes are enlarged and painful. The disease must be differentiated from syphilis, herpes simplex infection, and lymphogranuloma venereum.

It is a short, ovoid, Gram negative coccobacillus may show bipolar staining. In the lesions, they occur in strands resembling a "school of fish" or "rail road track appearance", usually in association with other pyogenic microorganisms.

H. ducreyi requires X factor but not V factor. It is grown best from scrapings of the ulcer base on chocolate agar containing 1% IsoVitaleX and 3 μg/ml vancomycin, and incubated in 10% CO_2 at 33 to 35°C. It can also be cultivated on fresh clotted rabbit blood and on chorioallantoic membrane of the chick embryo.

Treatment with intramuscular ceftriaxone, oral trimethoprim-sulfamethoxazole, or oral erythromycin often results in healing in two weeks.

HEMOPHILUS PARAINFLUENZAE

H. parainfluenzae resembles *H. influenzae*, and is a normal inhabitant of the human respiratory tract. It has been encountered occasionally in infective endocarditis and in urethritis. It differs from *H. influenzae* in requiring only the V factor and not the X factor.

HEMOPHILUS HEMOLYTICUS

H. hemolyticus is the most markedly hemolytic organism of the group *in vitro*; it occurs both in the normal nasopharynx and in association with rare upper respiratory tract infections of moderate severity in childhood. It requires both X and V factors. Colonies on blood agar may be mistaken for those of hemolytic streptococci.

HEMOPHILUS APROPHILUS

It is sometimes encountered in infective endocarditis and pneumonia. It is present in the normal oral and respiratory tract flora. It is related to *Actinobacillus (Hemophilus) actinomycetemcomitans*. It requires X factor but not the V factor. Its name refers to its high CO_2 requirement for optimal growth. Similar strains requiring the V factor but not the X factor have been termed *H. paraphrophilus*.

HACEK GROUP OF BACTERIA

The acronym "**HACEK**" stands for *Hemophilus* species (*parainfluenzae*, *aprophilus*, *paraphrophilus*), *Actinobacillus actinomycetemcomitans*, *Cardiobacterium hominis*, *Eikenella corrodens* and *Kingella kingae*. This group includes fastidious, Gram negative bacteria, normally resident in the oropharynx and urogenital tract, which can sometimes cause severe infections, particularly endocarditis.

They are slow growing and blood cultures from HACEK patients take 7–30 days to become positive. They grow better in blood or chocolate agar and does not grow in ordinary media. Antibiotic sensitivity tests are essential for effective therapy as drug resistance is very common.

QUESTIONS

Short Answer Type Questions

1. *Hemophilus influenzae.*
2. Cultivation of *H. influenzae.*
3. X and V factors.
4. Satellitism.
5. Pathogenicity of *H. influenzae.*
6. What are the two methods of preventing *H. influenzae* meningitis.
7. *H. aegypticus* or Koch-Weeks bacillus.
8. *H. ducreyi* or Chancroid or Soft sore.

67

Bordetella

- *Introduction*
- *Bordetella pertussis*
  - *– Morphology*
  - *– Cultural characteristics*
  - *– Biochemical reactions*
  - *– Resistance*
  - *– Antigenic structure and virulence factors*
  - *– Variation*
  - *– Epidemiology*
  - *– Pathogenicity*
  - *– Laboratory diagnosis*
  - *– Prophylaxis*
  - *– Treatment*
- *Bordetella parapertussis*
- *Bordetella bronchiseptica*

INTRODUCTION

Bordetellae are small, Gram negative coccobacilli. The genus contains four species.

1. *Bordetella pertussis*, a highly communicable and important pathogen of humans, causing whooping cough (pertussis). It was first observed by Bordet and Gengou (1900).
2. *Bordetella parapertussis* can cause a similar disease and was isolated from mild cases of whooping cough by Bradford and Slavin (1937).
3. *Bordetella bronchiseptica* (*Bordetella bronchicanis*) causes diseases in animals, and occasionally causes a pertussis-like illness in humans.
4. *Bordetella avium* causes turkey coryza and is not known to infect humans.

B. pertussis, *B. parapertussis* and *B. bronchiseptica* are closely related with 72–94% DNA homology.

BORDETELLA PERTUSSIS

Morphology

The organisms are minute Gram negative coccobacilli resembling *H. influenzae*. With toulidine blue, bipolar metachromatic granules can be demonstrated. A capsule is present. It is nonmotile and nonsporing. Freshly isolated strains may possess flagellae.

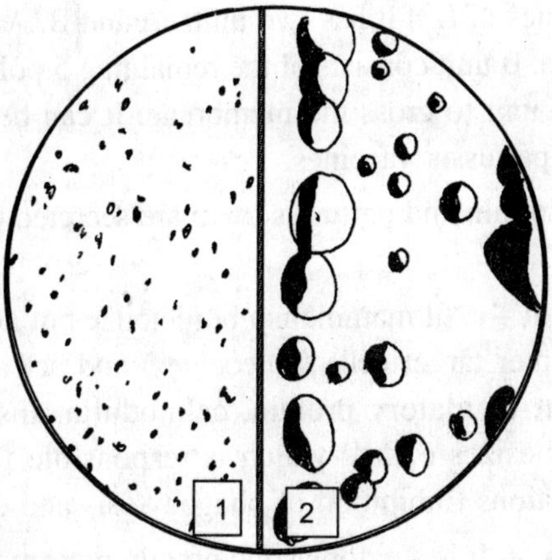

Fig. 67.1 *Bordetella pertussis.* **Fig. 67.2** Colonies of *Bordetella pertussis.*

Cultural characteristics

It is an obligate aerobe. It grows best at 35–36°C and 7.6 pH. It does not require X and V factors for its growth. Primary isolation of *B. pertussis* requires enriched media. **Bordet-Gengou medium** (potato-blood-glycerol agar) that contains penicillin G (0.5 μg/ml) can be used. The addition of charcoal, ion-exchange resins or 15–20% blood neutralizes the growth-inhibiting effects. Charcoal blood agar is a useful medium. The plates are incubated at 35–36°C for 3–7 days in a moist environment (*e.g.*, a sealed plastic bag). Colonies are small, dome shaped, smooth, opaque, viscid, greyish white, refractile and glistening, resembling "**bisected pearls**" or "**mercury drops**". Colonies are surrounded by hazy zone of hemolysis. The small, faintly Gram negative rods are identified by immunofluorescence staining.

Biochemical reactions

It does not ferment sugars. Metabolism is oxidative and forms acid but not gas from glucose and lactose. It forms indole, reduces nitrates, utilizes citrate and splits urea. It is oxidase and catalase positive.

Resistance

It is a delicate organism, being killed readily by heat (55°C for 30 minutes), drying and disinfectants. Outside the body, *Bord. pertussis* can survive for five days on glass, three days on cloth and a few hours on paper.

Antigenic structure and virulence factors

B. pertussis produces a number of factors that are involved in the pathogenesis of disease.

1. Pili probably play a role in adherence of the bacteria to the ciliated epithelial cells.

2. Filamentous hemagglutinin — It mediates adhesion to ciliated epithelial cells. Antibodies against filamentous hemagglutinin are protective.

3. Pertussis toxin — It promotes lymphocytosis, sensitization to histamine and enhanced insulin secretion and ADP-ribosylating activity, with an A/B structure and mechanism of action similar to that of cholera toxin. Antibody to pertussis toxin is also protective. Pertussis toxin is made up of 6 polypeptide chains ($S_1 - S_5$, with 2 copies of S_4). It has two units, A and B. A unit is made up of S_1 polypeptide chain. It is enzymatically active. B unit consists of the remaining 5 polypeptide chains. It binds the toxin to the target cells and helps A unit to cross the membrane. It can be toxoided. Pertussis toxoid is the major component of acellular pertussis vaccines.

The filamentous hemagglutinin and pertussis toxin are secreted proteins and are found outside the *B. pertussis* cells.

4. Adenylate cyclase toxin — All mammalian bordetellae but not *Bord. avium* produce adenylate cyclase. It has the ability to enter target cells (leucocytes) and act as a toxin. It can be activated by eukaryotic calcium–dependent regulatory protein, calmodulin. Inside the cell, after activation by calmodulin, this enzyme synthesizes cAMP which is responsible for the biological effects such as interfering with leucocyte functions (inhibition of phagocytosis and chemotaxis).

5. Dermonecroting toxin — It is a cytoplasmic protein present in all bordetellae. It is inactivated in 30 minutes at 56°C. It may be responsible for vasoconstriction and inflammatory reaction in the respiratory tract. This toxin in conjunction with endotoxin may be responsible for rhinorrhoea, sneezing and mild cough in the catarrhal stage of whooping cough. This toxin causes ischemic necrosis when injected intradermally into suckling mice.

6. Hemolysin — It is produced by all mammalian bordetellae, but not by *B. avium.* It is responsible for the hemolysis around colonies on Bordet-Gengou medium.

7. Tracheal cytotoxin — It is a low molecular weight peptidoglycan produced by all bordetellae. It induces ciliary damage in hamster tracheal ring cultures and inhibition of DNA synthesis in the ciliated respiratory epithelial cells, resulting in accumulation in the lungs of mucus, bacteria and inflammatory debris leading to severe cough. The disruption of ciliary function may also contribute to the secondary bacterial infections.

8. Lipopolysaccharide in the cell wall may also be important in causing damage to the epithelial cells of the upper respiratory tract.

9. Agglutinogens — Bordetellae possess 14 agglutinogens associated with fimbriae or capsular K antigens. Factor 7 is common to all three mammalian species of bordetellae. Agglutinogens 1–6 are found only in *Bord. pertussis*, all of which carry factor I and one or more of the other factors. Agglutinogens 14 and 12 are specific for *Bord. parapertussis* and *Bord. bronchiseptica* respectively. Agglutinogens promote virulence by helping bacteria to attach to respiratory epithelial cells. They are useful in serotyping strains and in epidemiological studies.

Variation

Bord. pertussis undergoes a smooth to rough variation. All fresh isolates are in the smooth form—hemolytic, toxin producing virulent phase (phase I). On subculture, they undergo progressive loss of surface antigens, and pass through phases II and III, and finally becoming phase IV which is the rough, avirulent form.

Epidemiology

Bord. pertussis survives for only brief periods outside the human host. There are no vectors. The source of infection is the patient in the early stage of the disease or carriers. The major mode of transmission is via droplets spread by coughing and fomites contaminated by oropharyngeal secretions.

The incidence of the disease among different age groups can vary susbstantially, depending on whether or not active immunization of young children is widespread in the community. In the absence of an immunization program, disease is most common among young children (ages one to five). Widespread immunization markedly reduces the incidence of disease overall, but shifts the age distribution to adults who have lost the protection conferred by childhood immunization, and to young infants who have not yet been vaccinated. The disease is commoner in the female than in the male at all ages. It is worldwide in distribution.

Pathogenicity

Bord. pertussis causes the syndrome called "**pertussis**" or "**whooping cough**". The organism binds to and multiplies rapidly on the epithelial surface of the trachea and bronchi and interferes with ciliary action. The blood is not invaded. The bacteria liberate the toxins and substances that irritate surface cells, causing coughing and marked lymphocytosis. Later, there may be necrosis of parts of the epithelium and polymorphonuclear infiltration, with peribronchial inflammation and interstitial pneumonia. Secondary invaders like staphylococci or *H. influenzae* may give rise to bacterial pneumonia. Obstruction of the smaller bronchioles by mucus plugs results in delectasis and diminished oxygenation of the blood. This probably contributes to the frequency of convulsions in infants with whooping cough.

The incubation period for pertussis generally ranges from one to three weeks. The disease can be divided into three phases: catarrhal, paroxysmal and convalescent.

1. Catarrhal stage — This phase begins with relatively nonspecific symptoms such as sneezing and mild coughing. During this stage, large numbers of organism are sprayed in droplets, and the patient is highly infectious but not very ill. Clinical diagnosis in this stage is difficult.

2. Paroxysmal stage — During the paroxysm, the patient is subjected to violent spasms of continuous coughing, followed by a long inrush of air into the almost empty lungs, with a characteristic "whoop" upon inhalation (hence the name). Large amounts of mucus may be produced. The paroxysms of coughing may be so severe that cyanosis, vomiting and convulsions follow, completely exhausting the patient. The disease usually lasts 6–8 weeks, though in some it may very protracted. The white blood count is high 16,000–30,000/μL (normal range = 4500–11,000 WBC/μL) with an absolute lymphocytosis.

3. Convalescent stage — Following the paroxysmal phase, convalescence requires atleast an additional three to four weeks, during which the frequency and severity of the coughing gradually decrease.

Complications that occur during the course of the disease include.

1. pressure effects due to violent spasms of coughing-sub conjunctival hemorrhage, subcutaneous emphysema, lung collapse.

2. secondary infections such as otitis media and pneumonia.

3. CNS dysfunction (for example encephalopathy or seizures).

Several types of adenoviruses and *Chlamydia pneumoniae* can produce a clinical picture resembling that caused by *Bord. pertussis*. Rarely, whooping cough is followed by the serious and potentially fatal complications of encephalihs.

Laboratory diagnosis

Presumptive diagnosis may be made on clinical grounds once the paroxysmal phase of classic pertussis begins.

A saline nasal wash is the preferred specimen. Specimens may be collected by different methods.

1. Cough plate method — A culture plate is held about 10–15 cm infront of the patient's mouth during a paroxysm, so that droplets of respiratory exudates impinge directly on the medium. This has the advantage that specimens are directly inoculated at bedside. The medium employed is glycerine-potato-blood agar of Bordet and Gengou or Lacey's DFP (diamidine fluoride, penicillin) medium.

2. West's post nasal swab — Secretions from the posterior pharyngeal wall are collected with a calcium alginate swab on a bent wire passed through the mouth. Salivary contamination should be avoided.

3. Pernasal swab — A calcium alginate swab on a flexible nichrome wire is passed along the floor of the nasal cavity and material is collected from the pharyngeal wall. This method yields the highest percentage of isolation.

Cotton swabs should not be used as cotton is inhibitory to the organisms.

Microscopic diagnosis depends on demonstration of the bacilli in respiratory secretions by the Direct fluorescent antibody (DFA) technique.

The swabs should be plated without delay. In case of delay, the swab should be transported in casamino acid solution (0.5 ml) at pH 7.2, in modified Stuart's medium or Mischulow's charcoal agar. The medium employed is the glycerine-potato-blood agar of Bordet and Gengou. Incorporation of diamidine fluoride and penicillin (Lacey's DFP medium) makes it more selective. Plates are incubated in high humidity at 35–36°C. Pin point colonies are produced in three to six days of incubation. Identification is confirmed by microscopy, slide agglutination and direct fluorescent antibody technique.

Serologic tests are of little diagnostic help, because a rise in antibody titre does not occur until the third week of illness.

Prophylaxis — During the first year of life, every infant should receive three intramuscular injections of pertussis vaccine. Two forms of vaccine are currently available that have had a significant effect on lowering the incidence of whooping cough.

One form is killed whole cells of smooth phase I strain, detoxicated with 0.2% merthiolate during several months storage at 4°C. The second form is acellular, containing proteins purified from *Bord. pertussis*. Both are formulated in combination with diphtheria and tetanus toxoids (triple vaccine/DPT vaccine). The advantage of **triple vaccine** is it minimizes the number of injections and improves the immune response because the pertussis bacilli acts as an adjuvant for toxoids.

Treatment

Erythromycin is the drug of choice for infections with *Bord. pertussis* both as chemotherapy, and as chemoprophylaxis for household contacts. For erythromycin treatment failures, trimethoprim-sulfamethoxazole is an alternative choice. Chloramphenicol, ampicillin are also useful. Supportive therapy is also very important during the paroxysmal phase. Oxygen inhalation and sedation may prevent anoxic damage to the brain.

BORDETELLA PARAPERTUSSIS

It may produce a disease similar to whooping cough. The infection is often subclinical. *Bord. parapertussis* grows more rapidly than typical *Bord. pertussis* and produces larger colonies. It also grows on blood agar.

BORDETELLA BRONCHISEPTICA

It inhabits the respiratory tracts of canines. It has been found to cause a very small proportion of cases of whooping cough. It is motile by peritrichate flagellae.

QUESTIONS

Short Answer Type Questions

1. *Bord. pertussis.*
2. Cultivation of *Bord. pertussis.*
3. Bordet-Gengou potato medium.
4. Pathogenicity of *Bord. pertussis* ***Or*** Pertussis ***Or*** Whooping cough.
5. Lab. diagnosis of whooping cough.
6. Specimen collection for diagnosis of pertussis.
7. Cough plate.
8. West's post nasal swab.
9. Pernasal swab.

68

Legionella pneumophila

- *Morphology,*
- *Cultural characteristics*
- *Antigenic structure*
- *Epidemiology,*
- *Pathogenicity,*
- *Laboratory diagnosis*
- *Prophylaxis,*
- *Treatment*

MORPHOLOGY

L. pneumophila are Gram negative, pleomorphic bacilli, appearing as coccobacilli (short rods) in clinical specimens and longer in culture. They are motile and noncapsulated and stain better by silver impregnation methods and immunofluorescence.

CULTURAL CHARACTERISTICS

It is aerobic and fastidious with a growth requirement for L-cysteine. It grows on **Buffered Charcoal Yeast Extract (BCYE)** enriched with L-cysteine, iron and α-ketoglutarate. Colonies appear in two to three days at 37°C.

ANTIGENIC STRUCTURE

L. pneumophila possesses both flagellar and somatic antigens. It is classified into 14 serogroups.

It possesses an endotoxin and produces hemolysin, cytotoxin and a protease. Protease appears to be an important virulence factor.

EPIDEMIOLOGY

L. pneumophila's normal habitats are water and soil, and the organism can colonize cooling towers, humidifiers, air conditioners and water distribution systems. The organism is chlorine tolerant, and thus survives water treatment procedures.

Humans acquire infection by inhalation of aerosols containing pathogens. Both sporadic cases and localized outbreaks may occur. One famous outbreak occured in 1976 during a convention of American Legion members (hence the name Legionella).

PATHOGENICITY

The organism gains entry to the upper respiratory tract by inhalation of a contaminated aerosol or by aspiration of water containing the organism. Macrophages phagocytose the *L. pneumophila*, but the phagosome fails to fuse with a lysosome. Instead, the organisms multiply within this protected environment, until the cell ruptures, releasing a new crop of increased numbers of infectious bacteria.

L. pneumophila primarily cause respiratory tract infections. There are two distinctly different presentations : Legionnaire's disease and Pontiac fever.

1. **Legionnaire's disease:** This is an acute lobar pneumonia with multisystem symptoms. Predisposing conditions include immunocompromise, heavy smoking, alcoholism, diabetes, chronic lung disease, old age and debilitation. Pneumonia associated with cough (that is only slightly productive) is the predominant symptom. Watery, nonbloody diarrhea occurs in 25 to 50 percent of cases. Nausea, vomiting and neurologic symptoms may also occur.
2. **Pontiac fever:** This is an influenza-like illness that characteristically infects otherwise healthy individuals. Recovery is usually complete within one week.

Occasionally, *L. pneumophila* causes wound infections following immersion of a wound in contaminated water and infection of extrapulmonary sites due to spread by blood circulation in a patient with Legionnaire's disease.

LABORATORY DIAGNOSIS

It consists of :

1. Legionellae can be detected in sputum, bronchial aspirates, lung biopsy by direct fluorescent antibody (DFA) test. Although the organisms can be Gram stained, the Giminez stain is more useful for visualization.
2. The definitive method of diagnosis involves the culturing of *Legionella* from respiratory secretions, using buffered (pH 6.9) charcoal yeast extract (BCYE) agar enriched with L-cysteine, iron and α-ketoglutarate. Visible colonies form in three to five days on incubation at 37ºC.
3. Bacterial antigens in the urine can be detected by ELISA, RIA and latex agglutination tests.
4. Antibodies in patient's serum can be demonstrated by ELISA or indirect immunofluorescent technique.
5. DNA probe for hybridization with *Legionella* ribosomal RNA.

PROPHYLAXIS

No vaccine is available. Measures such as flushing the water supply with extremely hot water decrease the chance of contamination.

TREATMENT

Macrolides such as erthyromycin or azithromycin are the drugs of choice for legionnaire's disease. Fluoroquinolones are also effective. No specific therapy is required for pontiac fever.

QUESTIONS

Short Notes

1. *Legionella pneumophila*
2. Legionnaire's disease or Legionellosis.

69

Brucella

- *Morphology*
- *Cultural characteristics*
- *Biochemical reactions*
- *Resistance*
- *Antigenic structure*
- *Classification*
- *Epidemiology*
- *Pathogenicity*
- *Laboratory diagnosis*
- *Prophylaxis*
- *Treatment.*

MORPHOLOGY

Brucellae are Gram negative small coccobacilli arranged singly or in pairs. They are nonmotile, noncapsulated and nonsporing. (Fig. 69.1.).

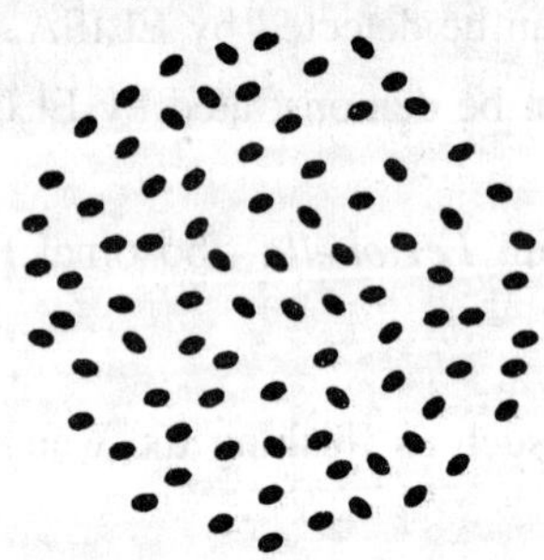

Fig. 69.1 *Brucella*

CULTURAL CHARACTERISTICS

Brucellae are obligate aerobes. *Br. abortus* is capnophilic, requiring 5–10% CO_2 for growth. The optimum temperature for growth is 37ºC and optimum pH 6.6–7.4. They grow on nutrient agar, though growth is slow and scanty. Growth is improved by the addition of serum or liver extract. The media used for the cultivation are **serum dextrose agar**, **serum potato infusion agar**, **trypticase soy agar**. The addition of bacitracin, polymyxin and cycloheximide to the above media makes them selective. On serum dextrose agar, Brucellae produce small, low convex, circular, smooth, transparent colonies on incubation at 37ºC in four or five days. Erythritol has a specially stimulating effect on the growth of brucellae.

BIOCHEMICAL REACTIONS

The metabolism is oxidative and not fermentative. They are catalose positive, oxidase positive (except *Br. neotomae* and *Br. ovis* which are oxidase negative) and urease positive. Nitrates are reduced to nitrites. citrate is not utilised. Indole is not produced and MR and VP tests are negative.

RESISTANCE

Brucellae are destroyed by heating at 60ºC for 10 minutes, hence in milk, they are killed by pasteurization. They may survive in soil and manure and in meat for several weeks. They are sensitive to direct sunlight and acid. They may remain viable for 10 days in refrigerated milk. They can be killed by 1% phenol in 15 minutes.

ANTIGENIC STRUCTURE

Lipopolysaccharide is the major virulence factor and major somatic antigen.

CLASSIFICATION

Brucellae are classified into six species based on CO_2 requirements, H_2S production, sensitivity to dyes, agglutination by monospecific antisera, phage lysis and oxidative metabolic tests.

1. *Br. melitensis* is the classical species of the genus and is usually pathogenic for sheep and goats but other animals like cattle may also be infected. Humans are also susceptible to infection with this organism.
2. *Br. abortus* infects cattle, usually causing abortions. It may also infect other animals including sheep, goats, horses and dogs. It can also infect humans.
3. *Br. suis* is a natural parasite of pigs but other animals and humans may also be infected.
4. *Br. canis* causes abortion in dogs. Occasionally, it may produce mild fever in humans.
5. *Br. ovis* causes sexually transmitted epididymitis in rams.
6. *Br. neotomae* causes infection of wood rats.

Br. ovis and *Br. neotomae* do not cause disease in humans. *Br. suis* strains that produce H_2S are known as "American" strains and those that do not as "Danish" strains.

EPIDEMIOLOGY

Brucellosis is a chronic, life-long infection in animals such as sheep, goats, cattle, pigs, dogs etc. Organisms localize in reproductive organs (male and female), and are shed in large numbers in milk, urine, and the placenta and other tissues discharged during delivery or spontaneous abortion. The primary manifestations of infection in animals are sterility and abortion. Transmission to humans is **zoonotic**, characteristically occurs as a result of either direct contact with infected animal tissues or ingestion of unpasteurized milk or milk products. Brucellosis is also an occupational risk for laboratory personnel and veterinarians. Because few organisms are found in muscle, meat products are rarely sources of infection.

PATHOGENICITY

The infection is known as brucellosis (undulant fever, malta fever). Brucellae typically enter the body through cuts and abrasions in the skin, or through the GI tract. Inhalation of infected aerosols can also lead to disease.

The organism is a facultative intracellular parasite and multiplies in the macrophages of reticuloendothelial system. Once the organism gain entry, they are transported via the lymphatic system to the regional lymph nodes, where they multiply. The organisms are then carried by the blood to organs that are involved in the reticuloendothelial system, including the liver, spleen, kidneys, bonemarrow and other lymph nodes.

The incubation period range from five days to several months, but typically lasts several weeks. Symptoms are nonspecific and include malaise, fever, sweats, anorexia and GI symptoms, headache, back pains and may also include depression. Their onset may be abrupt or insidious. Untreated, patients may develop an undulating pattern of fever, the temperatures repeatedly rise then fall, hence the name "**undulant fever**" as the traditional name for brucellosis. Subclinical infections occur. Manifestations of brucellosis may involve any of a variety of organ systems including the GI tract, and the skeletal, neurologic, cardiovascular and pulmonary systems.

LABORATORY DIAGNOSIS

Although the nonspecific symptoms may not point to a diagnosis of brucellosis, a detailed history is often crucial, including the patient's occupation, exposure to animals, travel to countries where the brucellosis is prevalent or ingestion of contaminated foods. Laboratory diagnosis consists of culture and serology.

(i) Culture

The organism can be cultured from blood and other body fluids, or from tissue specimens. Multiple blood specimens should be cultured. For plated materials, colonies may appear in four to five days ; however, longer times are required for blood cultures, and these are routinely examined for up to two months before being declared negative.

Five to ten ml of blood or biopsy material is inoculated into 50-100 ml of serum dextrose broth and incubated at 37°C in air enriched with 5-10% CO_2. Subcultures are made every 3-5 days for eight weeks on serum dextrose agar or chocolate agar. The **Castaneda** method of **blood culture** has several advantages. Here both liquid and solid media are available in the same bottle. The blood is inoculated into the broth and the bottle incubated in the upright position. For subculture, it is sufficient the bottle is tilted so that the broth flows over the surface of the agar slant. It is again incubated in an upright position. Colonies appear on the slant. This method minimises materials and manipulation, reducing the chances of contamination and risk of infection.

(*ii*) Serology

As blood cultures are positive only in about 30 - 50 per cent of cases, serological methods are important in diagnosis. The standard **tube agglutination** test is employed, in which equal volumes of serial dilutions of the patient's serum and the standardised antigen (killed suspension of a *Br. abortus* strain) are mixed and incubated at 37°C for 24 hours. A titre of 160 or more is considered significant. In brucellosis, IgM antibodies appear in 7-10 days after the onset of clinical infection. However, IgG and IgA antibodies are formed during the course of the infection, which may bind with antigen, thus preventing agglutination by larger IgM. These IgG and IgA antibodies are therefore known as blocking or nonagglutinating antibodies.

The blocking effect can be eliminated by prior heating of the serum at 56°C for 30 minutes or by using 4% saline as the diluent for the test. The blocking antibodies can be detected by coombs test. As the prozone phenomenon to high titres, up to 1/640, is very frequent, it is essential that several serum dilutions be tested.

Other serological tests such as CFT, RIA and ELISA are also used.

(*iii*) Intradermal test (brucellin test)

Protein extract of the organism, known as brucellin is injected intradermally. In positive cases, erythema and induration appears within 6–24 hrs. The test is not useful for the diagnosis of acute brucellosis.

LABORATORY DIAGNOSIS OF ANIMAL INFECTION

The methods employed for the human brucellosis may also be employed for the diagnosis of animal infection. In addition, several rapid methods such as rapid plate agglutination test and Rose bengal card test are employed for the detection of brucellosis in cattle.

For the detection of infected animals in diaries, pooled milk samples may be tested for bacilli by culture and for antibodies by several techniques. In the **Milk Ring test**, a sample of whole milk is mixed well with a drop of the stained brucella antigen (a concentrated suspension of killed *Br. abortus* stained with hematoxylin) and incubated in a water both at 70°C for 40-50 minutes. If antibodies are present in the milk, the bacilli are agglutinated and rise with the cream to form a blue ring at the top, leaving the milk unstained. If antibodies are absent, no colored ring is formed and the milk remains unformly blue.

PROPHYLAXIS

Prevention consists of checking brucellosis in dairy animals and by pasteurisation of milk.

Br. abortus strain 19 vaccine is used in cattle.

TREATMENT

Combination therapy involving doxycycline and gentamycin is recommended. Prolonged treatment may be necessary to prevent relapse, and to reduce the incidence of complications.

QUESTIONS

Short Notes

1. Classify Brucellae.
2. Pathogenicity of *Brucella* (or) Brucellosis (or) undulant fever.
3. Acute brucellosis.
4. Lab. diagnosis of brucellosis.
5. Castaneda method of blood culture.

70

Francisella tularensis

- *Morphology*
- *Cultural characteristics*
- *Epidemiology*
- *Pathogenicity*
- *Laboratory diagnosis*
- *Prophylaxis*
- *Treatment.*

MORPHOLOGY

It is a small, Gram negative, pleomorphic coccobacillus that possess a lipid-rich capsule, which may be a virulence factor. It is nonsporing and nonmotile. It resembles *Mycoplasma* in being filterable and in multiplying by filament formation and budding, besides binary fission. It is a facultative intracellular parasite that can survive and multiply within host macrophages as well as in other types of cells.

CULTURAL CHARACTERISTICS

The organisms are strict aerobes, and nutritionally fastidious, requiring a sulfhydryl source such as cysteine. **Francis blood dextrose cystine agar** is employed for its isolation. Minute transparent colonies appear after incubation for 3-5 days at 37ºC. The organism is highly infectious, and laboratories must take special precautions to avoid transmission of infection.

EPIDEMIOLOGY

The organism is the causative agent of **Tularemia**, a disease of rabbits and other rodents, originally described in Tulare county, California, and hence the name. The host range of *F. tularensis* is broad and includes wild and domestic animals and birds. Several biting and blood sucking arthropods such as ticks, lice, and mites can serve as vectors. Ticks can also serve as reservoirs of the organism, passing the bacteria to progeny via their eggs (transovarian transmission). Infection of humans occurs as a result of contact with infected animal tissues or the bite of an infected arthropod. Tularemia is an occupational risk for veterinarians, live stock workers and meat handlers.

PATHOGENICITY

F. tularensis is primarily a pathogen of animals. Thus tularemia is a **zoonosis**. Tularemia varies in severity from mild to fulminant and fatal. In two to six days an ulcerating papule develops. The organisms spread to the regional lymph nodes, where they cause enlarged, tender nodes that may suppurate. The organisms spread via the lymphatic system to various organs and tissues, including lungs, liver, spleen, kidneys and the CNS. Onset of symptoms is usually abrupt. The most common symptoms are chills, fever, headache, malaise, anorexia, and fatigue (flu-like), although respiratory and gastrointestinal symptoms may also occur. The most common presentation of tularemia is ulceroglandular. Tularemia characterized by lymphadenopathy without evidence of ulceration is known as glandular tularemia. In oculoglandular tularemia, the organism gains entry through the conjuctiva, which becomes inflamed. In pharyngeal tularemia, the organism gains entry through the pharynx, and causes a severe sore throat. In pneumonic tularemia, the pneumonia may be primary, a result of inhalation of infectious aerosols, or secondary, a result of hematogenous dissemination of the organisms from a primary site elsewhere in the body to the lungs.

LABORATORY DIAGNOSIS

Clinical presentation and history consistent with possible exposure is of primary importance in diagnosis. Laboratory diagnosis can be established by isolating and identifying the organisms from ulcer scrapings, lymph node biopsies, gastric washings and sputum, but rarely from blood or by inoculation into guinea pigs or mice. Antibodies to *Francisella* can be readily detected by agglutination or ELISA tests.

PROPHYLAXIS

An attenuated vaccine is available which can be administered by scarification to persons who are subject to high risk.

TREATMENT

The drug of choice for treatment of tularemia is streptomycin or gentamycin.

QUESTIONS

Short Notes

1. *Francisella tularensis.*
2. Tularemia.

71

Pasteurella

- *Morphology*
- *Cultural characteristics*
- *Epidemiology*
- *Pathogenicity*
- *Laboratory diagnosis*
- *Treatment*

MORPHOLOGY

Pasteurellae are Gram negative, nonmotile coccobacilli that often exhibit bipolar staining. Some strains are encapsulated virulence factors include the organism's capsule and endotoxin.

CULTURAL CHARACTERISTICS

Pasteurellae are aerobes and facultative anaerobes. They grow on blood agar and chocolate agar. It resembles *Yersinia* but differs in being oxidase positive, producing indole and failing to grow on MacConkey agar.

EPIDEMIOLOGY

Members of the genus *Pasteurella* primarily colonize in the upper respiratory tract of mammals and birds. The majority of Pasteurellae infections in humans are soft tissue infections that follow an animal bite or a cat scratch. Thus, Pasteurella infections are considered **zoonoses**. Though more than 17 species are known, the major human pathogen in this genus is *Pasteurella multocida*, which can cause either disease or asymptomatic infections.

PATHOGENICITY

P. multocida infection should be suspected in cases of acute, painful cellulitis that develop within 24 hours of an animal bite or cat scratch, if an infected animal licking an open wound. Soft tissue infections are characterized by the rapid onset of acute local inflammation within hours of the bite or scratch. Lesions often begin to drain within one to two days. Manifestations of *P. multocida* infection can include lymphangitis, lymphadenitis, fever and local complications such as osteomyelitis or arthritis. It can cause respiratory infections such as sinusitis, bronchitis and pneumonia, meningitis or appendicitis.

LABORATORY DIAGNOSIS

Laboratory diagnosis can be accomplished by culturing the organism on blood agar, and performing appropriate biochemical tests.

TREATMENT

Penicillin is the drug of choice. Tetracyclines and streptomycin are also effective. For soft tissue infections, wounds should be cleansed, irrigated and debrided. Deep-seat infections require surgical drainage and prolonged antibiotic treatment.

QUESTIONS

Short Notes

1. *Pasteurella*
2. Pasteurellosis
3. *Pasteurella multocida*

72

Treponema pallidum

- *Introduction to Spirochetes*
- *Treponema pallidum - Morphology, Cultivation, Resistance, Antigenic structure, Pathogenicity, Laboratory diagnosis, Prophylaxis, Treatment.*
- *Other Treponemal infections-Bejel, Yaws, Pinta.*

INTRODUCTION

Spirochetes (Spiera = Coil; Chaite = hair) are long, slender, motile, flexible, undulating Gram negative bacilli that have a characteristic corkscrew or helical shape. Some species are free-living and some are part of the normal flora of humans and animals. A characteristic feature is the presence of endoflagellae, between the outer membrane and cell wall, wound along the helical protoplasmic cylinder, responsible for motility.

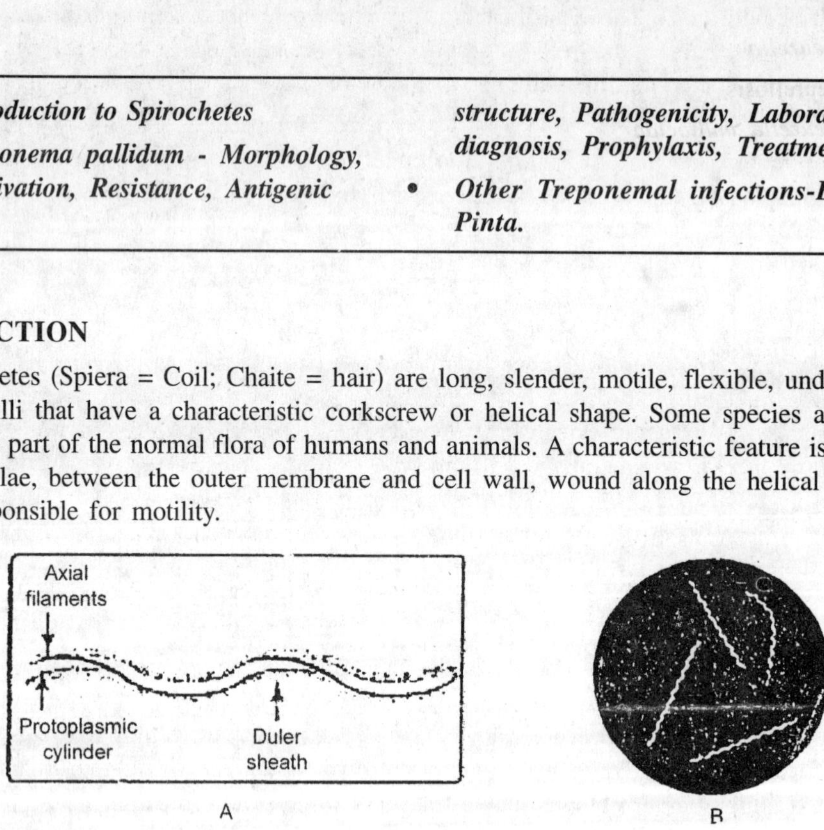

Fig. 72.1 *Treponema pallidum*
A = Gross morphology, B = Dark ground illumination

Spirochetes that are important human pathogens are confined to three genera: *Treponema* (*T. pallidum* is the cause of syphilis), *Borrelia* (*B. recurrentis* causes relapsing fever, *B. vincenti* causes vincent's angina and *B. burgdorferi* causes Lyme disease), and *Leptospira* (*L. interrogans* causes leptospirosis).

Spirochetes belong to the order spirochetales comprising two families : (*i*) Spirochetaceae containing the genera *Spirocheta*, *Cristispira*, *Treponema* and *Borrelia*; and (*ii*) Leptospiraceae containing the genus *Leptospira*.

MORPHOLOGY

Treponema (Trepos = to turn; nema = thread) is a thin, delicate Gram negative spirochete with tapering ends, about 10 μm long and 0.1-0.2 μm wide. It has about ten regular spirals, which are sharp and angular, at regular intervals of about one μm.

It is actively motile, exhibiting rotation around the long axis (cork-screw motility), backward and forward movements, and flexion of the whole body. Spirochetes have a unique structure that is responsible for their motility. The spirochete cell has a central protoplasmic cylinder bounded by a plasma membrane and a typical Gram negative cell wall. Unlike other bacilli, this cylinder is enveloped by an outer sheath composed of glycosaminoglycans. Between the cell wall and the outer sheath are located multiple **periplasmic flagella** that do not protrude from the cell but are oriented axially. Bundles of these endoflagella, called **axial filaments,** span the entire length of the cell and are anchored at both ends. These periplasmic flagellae rotate like external flagellae of other motile bacteria, thereby propelling the cell in a cork-screw like manner. Spirochetes can move through highly viscous solution so that the pathogen can penetrate and invade host tissue, just as a corkscrew penetrates cork.

Its morphology and motility can be seen under the Dark ground or phase contrast microscope. In wet films, it can be made out by negative staining with Indian ink. It can be stained by silver impregnation methods. Fontana's method is useful for staining wet films and Levaditi's method for tissue sections.

CULTIVATION

Nonpathogenic treponemes (Reiter strain) are cultivable under strictly anaerobic conditions in Smith-Noguchi medium or in digest broth enriched with serum. The Reiter strain is now classified as *T. phagedenis*. Pathogenic (virulent) treponemes, known as **Nichol's strain** do not grow in artificial culture media. It is maintained, in rabbit testes, by serial passage for several decades. It can be maintained for 1-6 days in a complex anaerobic medium (Nelson medium) that contains rabbit serum, reducing agents (such as cysteine, thioglycolate and glutathione), vitamins, cofactors, amino acids and salts, *in vitro*.

RESISTANCE

T. pallidum is very delicate, being readily inactivated by drying or by heat at 41-42°C in one hour. This was the basis of "**fever therapy**" for syphilis. It is killed in 1-3 days at 0-4°C, so that **transfusion syphilis** can be prevented by storing blood for atleast four days in the refrigerator before transfusion. It is inactivated by contact with oxygen, distilled water, soap, arsenicals, common antiseptics and antibiotics. It remains viable for years when stored frozen at –70°C in 10% glycerol, or in liquid nitrogen at –130°C.

ANTIGENIC STRUCTURE

Treponemal infection induces atleast three types of antibodies. The first is the "**reagin**" antibody that reacts with a lipid hapten extracted from beef (ox) heart. The hapten is known as cardiolipin and is chemically a diphosphatidyl glycerol. It is not certain whether cardiolipin (nonspecific antigen) is present in *T. pallidum* itself or a product of damaged tissue caused by infection.

The second is a group specific protein antigen found in *T. pallidum* as well as nonpathogenic cultivable treponemes like Reiter's strain.

The third is a species specific polysaccharide antigen present only in *T. pallidum.*

PATHOGENICITY

Transmission of *T. pallidum* is almost always by sexual contact (or transplacentally-congenital syphilis). The organism enters the body through a break in the skin or by penetrating mucus membranes, such as those of the genitalia. Clinical disease sets in after an incubation period of 10-90 days (average incubation period is three weeks). The disease syphilis occurs in three stages: primary, secondary and tertiary.

PRIMARY SYPHILIS

The first symptom of primary stage syphilis is a painless, indurated, hard ulcer, known as chancre. Most chancres are on the genitals, but may also develop in or on the mouth or on the breasts. Rectal chancres are common in male homosexuals. In females, chancres may develop in the vagina or on the cervix. In syphilis acquired nonvenereally, as occupational hazard in doctors and nurses, the chancres may on the fingers (extragenital).

It is known as **hard chancre** to differentiate it from painful, nonindurated **soft sore** produced by *Hemophilus ducreyi*.

The chancre contains a thick, glairy exudate rich in spirochetes. The regional lymph nodes are enlarged and swollen, rubbery and nontender. Chancres heal spontaneously in about 1-5 weeks. From lymph nodes, treponemes spread to the blood stream.

SECONDARY SYPHILIS

Syphilis enters its second stage between 6 weeks and 6 months after contracting the infection. Chancres may still be present but are usually self-healing. Thus, both primary and secondary stages teem with *T. pallidum* and are extremely infectious.

Secondary stage is characterised by the appearance of a red, maculopapular rash on almost any part of the body, including on the palms of the hands and soles of the feet. Also present are pale, moist papules seen primarily in the anogenital region (where they are called condylomas), the armpits and the mouth. The secondary stage may be accompanied by systemic involvement, causing hepatitis, meningitis, nephritis or chorioretinitis. Lesions of secondary syphilis usually heal spontaneously and may take as long as 4-5 years.

LATENT SYPHILIS

Upon healing of the secondary lesions, the disease enters a latent period that can last for many years. The disease is characterized by relative absence of clinical symptoms and can be detected only by serological means.

Some cases of latent syphilis get cured spontaneously, whereas approximately one third of patients with Latent syphilis develop the signs and symptoms of Tertiary syphilis.

TERTIARY SYPHILIS

The tertiary stage is characterized by granulomatous inflammatory lesions known as **gummas**, in the liver, skin and bones ; cardiovascular lesions such as aneurysms ; and degeneration of the nervous system (**Neurosyphilis**). Tabes dorsalis or general paralysis of the insane may develop several years after the syphilitic infection. AIDS appears to increase the severity of syphilis and speeds up the development of neurosyphilis.

CONGENITAL SYPHILIS

T. pallidum can be transmitted through the placenta to a fetus after the first ten to fifteen weeks of pregnancy. Infection can cause death and spontaneous abortion of the fetus, or cause it to be stillborn. Infected infants that live develop a condition similar to secondary syphilis, including a variety of CNS and structural abnormalities. Treatment of the pregnant mother with appropriate antibiotics prevents congenital syphilis.

LABORATORY DIAGNOSIS

History and physical examination of the patient prelude to laboratory tests. Laboratory tests are necessary both for the diagnosis and for assessing cure after treatment. Laboratory diagnosis consists of (*i*) demonstration of *T. pallidum* by microscopy, and (*ii*) serological tests to demonstrate antibodies in the serum or CSF.

MICROSCOPY

Diagnosis by microscopy is done in primary and secondary stages and congenital syphilis with superficial lesions. Specimens should be collected with care as the lesions are highly infectious. The chancre is cleaned with a gauze soaked in warm saline and the margins gently scraped so that the superficial epithelium is abraded. Gentle pressure is applied to the base of the lesion and the serum that exudes is collected. Wet films are prepared with exudates and after applying coverslips, are examined. *T. pallidum* is so thin that it cannot be observed by conventional light microscopy, but requires dark-field microscope. *T. pallidum* can be recognized by its slender structure, regularity of spirals and slightly pointed ends. The direct fluorescent antibody test (DFA-TP) for *T-pallidum* is a better method of microscopic diagnosis. Silver impregnation method is also used to detect treponemes.

SEROLOGY

T. pallidum cannot be cultured on conventional bacteriological media and hence the diagnosis of syphilis is primarily based on serology. Serodiagnosis of syphilis is carried out by using two types of tests.

1. Non-Treponemal Tests (or) Standard Tests for Syphilis

These tests use **cardiolipin**, a phospholipid derived from beef (ox) heart as antigen. Since the antigen is not derived from the Treponemal organisms, these tests are known as Nontreponemal tests. During syphilis, the host forms antibodies (IgG and IgM) to the lipoidal material released from the host cells. These antibodies are known as "antilipoidal antibodies" or "**Reagins**". These reagins are different from IgE antibodies. Cardiolipin used in Nontreponemal tests reacts with these antilipoidal antibodies to give a flocculation. To the cardiolipin, lecithin and cholesterol are added to improve test sensitivity. These cardiolipin-based tests are less specific, and are liable to give more false positives. They are nevertheless useful in screening and for monitoring therapy, because tests for reagin become negative about a year after successful treatment.

2. Treponemal Tests

These tests use Treponemal organisms as antigens to detect the antibodies formed to Treponemal antigens. Treponemal tests are generally used to confirm the results of Nontreponemal tests that conflict with clinical findings. These antitreponemal antibody tests are more specific than reagin-based tests, but remain positive during successful treatment, and are thus not useful for monitoring therapy. Treponemal tests are of two types :

(*a*) Those using cultivable treponemes, such as Reiter treponemes (*T. phagedenis*) as the antigen, and

(*b*) Those in which virulent *T. pallidum* is the antigen employed. These tests may further be classified according to whether the antigen employed is live, killed or extracts of the treponemes.

Table 72.1 : Major Serological Tests for Syphilis

I. Nontreponemal tests or **reagin antibody tests** or **Nonspecific tests** or **Standard tests for Syphilis** using cardiolipin antigen :
(*i*) Wassermann reaction (CFT)
(*ii*) Kahn flocculation test
(*iii*) VDRL (Venereal diseases research laboratory) test
(*iv*) RPR test
II. Treponemal tests :
A. Those using cultivable treponemes such as Reiter strain as antigen
(*i*) Reiter protein CFT (RPCFT)
B. Specific tests using pathogenic treponemes (*T. pallidum*) as antigen
(*i*) Tests using live *T. pallidum*
(*a*) *T. pallidum* immobilisation test (TPI)
(*ii*) Tests using killed *T. pallidum*
(*b*) *T. pallidum* agglutination (TPA) test
(*c*) *T. pallidum* immune adherence (TPIA) test
(*d*) Fluorescent treponemal antibody (FTA) test
(*iii*) Tests using *T. pallidum* extract
(*e*) *T. pallidum* hemagglutination test (TPHA)
(*f*) Enzyme immunoassay (EIA)

Nontreponemal tests or Standard tests (Nonspecific) (STS) for Syphilis

The nonspecific standard tests for syphilis that can be employed are Wassermann, Kahn, VDRL and RPR tests. The antigen used is an alcoholic extract of ox heart tissue, known as cardiolipin lecithin and cholesterol are added.

VDRL TEST

It is the most widely used serological test and is a microscopic **slide flocculation test.** In VDRL test inactivated patient's serum (heated at 56ºC for 30 minutes) is mixed with freshly prepared cardiolipin antigen on a special glass slide (VDRL slide) and rotated for four minutes at 180 rpm on a VDRL rotator and flocculation can be observed under a low power objective of a microscope. The cardiolipin remains as uniform crystals when the test is nonreactive but forms visible clumps (flocculation) on combining with reagin antibody, when the test is reactive. In reactive (positive) cases, the antibody titre can be determined by testing serial dilutions of patient's serum.

Though VDRL test is used as a screening test for syphilis, the major disadvantages of the test are the need to prepare fresh antigen every day and inactivation of sera and to use microscope to read the results.

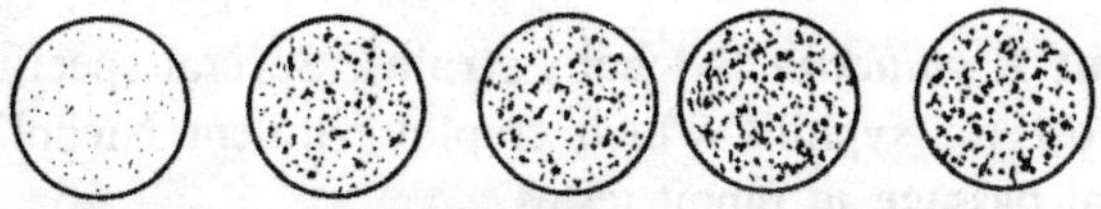

Non reactive Weakly reactive Reactive

Non reactive - Free needle like particles, no clumps
Weakly reactive - Small clumps with free particles
Reactive - Medium and large clumps on a clear background

Fig. 72.2 VDRL test (microscopic view)

RPR (RAPID PLASMA REAGIN) CARD TEST

In this test the cardiolipin antigen coated with fine carbon particles is used. It makes the test results more clear and evident to the naked eye and there is no need of microscope. RPR test can be done with unheated serum or plasma. A drop of patient's serum or plasma and a drop of antigen is added on a card in the circle and rotated for a few minutes. If black particles are aggregated in the centre, the test is nonreactive; if the black particles are seen throughout the circle, the test is reactive.

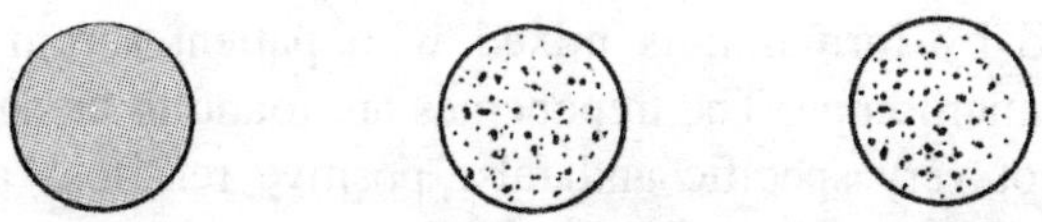

Non reactive Weakly reactive Reactive

Non reactive - No floccules, even light greay mat on the reaction circle.
Weakly reactive - Small black floccules against white background
Reactive - Large and medium black foccules against white background

Fig. 72.3. RPR card test (microscopic view)

BIOLOGICAL FALSE POSITIVE (BFP) REACTIONS

The major disadvantage of standard tests is that the antigen is nonspecific and may react with the sera of patients who may not have syphilis. This occurence of false positive reactions, for inherent reasons and not due to any technical error, is known as biological false positive (BFP) reactions.

The reagin antibody reacting with cardiolipin may occur in a wide variety of infections like leprosy, malaria, relapsing fever, infectious mononucleosis, hepatitis, tropical eosinophilia and certain autoimmune conditions like systemic lupus erythematosus, rheumatoid arthritis ; and in coronary disease, severe trauma, vaccination, pregnancy, repeated blood loss and menstruation.

BFP reactions may be acute or chronic. In acute BFP, the reagin antibodies disappear within six months whereas in chronic BFP reactions, they persist indefinitely. To eliminate BFP reactions, tests have been developed using treponemal antigens.

TREPONEMAL TESTS

(*a*) **Tests using Cultivable Reiter's Treponemes:** Reiter's Protein Complement fixation test (RPCFT) is same as Wassermann test, but the antigen used is protein derived from *Treponema phagedenis* (Reiter treponeme), used to detect group-specific antibody.

(*b*) **Tests using virulent *T. pallidum* (Nichol's strain):** Several specific tests are available for the accurate diagnosis of syphilis which employ virulent Nichol's strain of *T. pallidum* maintained by serial passage in rabbit testes.

(i) Tests using live *T. pallidum*

***Treponema pallidum* immobilization (TPI) test:** This test determines the ability of patient serum to immobilize motile virulent *T. pallidum.* The test serum is incubated anaerobically with a suspension of the treponemes and complement. If antibodies are present in the serum, the treponemes will be immobilized, when examined under dark-ground microscope. The test is considered reactive if more than 50% of the treponemes are immobilized, and nonreactive if less than 20% are immobilized. The test is doubtful if 20-50% treponemes are immobilized.

Presence of traces of penicillin can interfere with the test. The TPI test is the most specific test available for syphilis. However, the test is reactive in other treponemal infections like yaws.

(*ii*) Tests using killed *T. pallidum*

***Treponema pallidum* agglutination (TPA) test:** In this test, a suspension of *T. pallidum* (Nichol's strain), inactivated by formalin, is mixed with patient serum and incubated and then examined under darkground microscope. The treponemes are found to be agglutinated in the presence of antibodies. This test is not very specific and false positive reactions are common.

***Treponema pallidum* immune adherence (TPIA) test:** When a suspension of inactivated treponemes is mixed with patient serum, complement and fresh heparinised blood from a normal person and incubated, the treponemes will be found to adhere to erythrocytes in the presence of antibodies. In the absence of antibodies, immune adherence will not occur.

Fluorescent treponemal antibody (FTA) test: It is an indirect immunofluorescence test, using smears prepared with Nichol's strain of *T. pallidum* as the antigen. Smears can be stored in deep freeze for several months. The patient serum is added on the smear and incubated for the antibody to react with the treponemes. The excess serum is then washed off and the antibodies that bind to the fixed organisms are detected by treating the smear with fluorescein labelled antihuman immunoglobulin. After incubation and washing off the unfixed conjugate, the slide is examined under Fluorescent microscope. In a positive test, treponemes fluoresce.

Originally patient serum was used in a dilution of 1 in 5. At this dilution, the test has high sensitivity and poor specificity. Therefore, the dilution of the serum was raised to 1 in 200. In this test, called FTA-200, the specificity was improved but sensitivity was decreased. Therefore, this test was further modified to fluorescent treponemal antibody absorption **(FTA-ABS)** test. Here the patient serum is first absorbed with an extract of nonpathogenic Reiter treponeme (*T. phagedenis*) to remove group-specific antibody. FTA-ABS test has high specificity and sensitivity. It is almost as specific as the TPI test. Another modification of this test, the IgM FTA-ABS test, can detect IgM antibodies in congenital syphilis.

(*iii*) Tests using *T. pallidum* extract

***Treponema pallidum* hemagglutination (TPHA) test:** In this test, an extract *T. pallidum* is adsorbed on to the surface of RBC. When these RBCs are mixed with patient serum, specific antibody, if present, causes hemagglutination. As in FTA-ABS test patient serum is preabsorbed with an extract of Reiter treponeme to remove group-specific antibody.

TPHA is very simple to perform, therefore, it was the first of the specific tests suitable for routine screening. TPHA may be performed in microtitre plates. This is referred to as microtitre hemagglutination—*T. pallidum* (MHA-TP) test.

Enzyme immunoassay (EIA): Ultrasonicate of *T. pallidum* antigen is coated on tubes or ferrous metal beads as a solid phase carrier for antigen, which can be used to detect antibody in patient serum by enzyme immunoassay.

Prophylaxis: There is no vaccine against *T. pallidum*, and prevention depends on safe sexual practices.

Treatment: A single treatment with penicillin is curative for primary and secondary syphilis, and no antibiotic resistance has been reported. In cases patient sensitive to penicillin, alternate therapy with erythromycin or tetracyclines may also be effective.

OTHER TREPONEMAL INFECTIONS

Three geographically localized treponemal diseases closely mimic syphilis. The causative organisms are *Treponema* species or subspecies that are morphologically and antigenically indistinguishable from *T. pallidum*, and the diseases exhibit primary, secondary and tertiary stages similar to those of syphilis. However, unlike syphilis, direct skin contact, crowded living conditions, and poor hygiene contribute to the spread of these diseases. Sexual contact is usually not the mode of transmission. Congenital infections are absent. All three diseases are curable with penicillin.

1. **Bejel** (endemic syphilis) found in hot, arid areas of Africa, South east Asia and the Middle East. The etiologic agent is *T. endemicum*.
2. **Yaws** found in humid, tropical areas of Africa, Asia and America. In India cases have been reported from Andhra Pradesh, Orissa and Madhya Pradesh. The disease is caused by *T. pertenue*.
3. **Pinta** found in South and Central America, Mexico and the Philippines. It is caused by *T. carateum.*
4. **Oral Treponemes:** T. denticola, T. macrodentium, T. oralis, T. Socranskii and T. pectinovorum are normal mouth commensals.

QUESTIONS

Essay Questions

1. Classify spirochetes. Describe the lab. diagnosis of syphilis.
2. Describe the serodiagnosis of syphilis.

Short Notes

1. *Treponema pallidum.*
2. Morphology of *T. pallidum.*
3. Cultivation of *T. pallidum.*
4. Nichol's strain.
5. Cardiolipin.
6. Pathogenesis of syphilis.

7. Primary syphilis.
8. Chancre.
9. Hard chancre.
10. Latent syphilis.
11. Congenital syphilis.
12. Neurosyphilis.
13. Tertiary syphilis.
14. Quaternary syphilis.
15. Lab. diagnosis of primary syphilis.
16. STS (or) Standard tests for syphilis (or) Nonspecific tests for syphilis.
17. VDRL test.
18. RPR card test.
19. BFP (or) Biological false positive reactions.
20. FTA-ABS.
21. FTA - 200.
22. Fluorescent treponemal antibody test.
23. TPI (or) *T. pallidum* immobilisation test.
24. TPHA (or) *T. pallidum* hemagglutination test.
25. Endemic syphilis (or) Bejel.
26. Yaws.
28. *Treponema pertenue.*
29. Pinta.
30. *T. carateum.*
31. Nonpathogenic treponemes.

73

Borrelia

- *Introduction*
- *Relapsing fever - Types of relapsing fever and causative agents, morphology, cultural characteristics, antigenic structure, pathogenicity, Epidemiology, Laboratory diagnosis, prophylaxis, Treatment.*
- *Borrelia vincentii (vincent's angina)*
- *Borrelia burgdorferi (Lyme disease)*

INTRODUCTION

Members of the genus *Borrelia* are relatively large spirochetes with irregular, wide open coils, which like the *Treponema* have endoflagella that make them highly motile. *Borrelia* species are unusual among bacteria in that they have linear rather than circular plasmid and chromosomal DNA. Several species of *Borrelia* occur as commensals on the buccal and genital mucosa. Borrelia of medical importance are those causing relapsing fever, *B. vincenti* and *B. burgdorferi.*

RELAPSING FEVER

Relapsing fever is of two types : i). epidemic or louse-borne relapsing fever, transmitted from person to person by body lice, caused by *Borrelia recurrentis* ii). endemic or tick-borne relapsing fever is caused by over ten species of *Borrelia* : *B. duttoni*, *B. hermsii*, *B. parkeri* etc. These species live in their natural hosts-rodents or other mammals on which the vector ticks feed. Human infection occurs by infected tick bite and is only an accidental event. The *Borrelia* are transmitted from mother tick to her progeny.

The borreliae causing relapsing fever are indistinguishable and DNA homology studies indicate that all of them may belong to single species, with separate arthropod host adaptation. The description that follow apply to all of them.

MORPHOLOGY

B. recurrentis is a large irregular spiral with one or both ends pointed. It is Gram negative and stains well with Giemsa. It is 8-20 μm long and 0.2-0.4 μm wide. It possesses 5 to 10 loose spiral coils at intervals of about 2μm (Fig. 73.1).

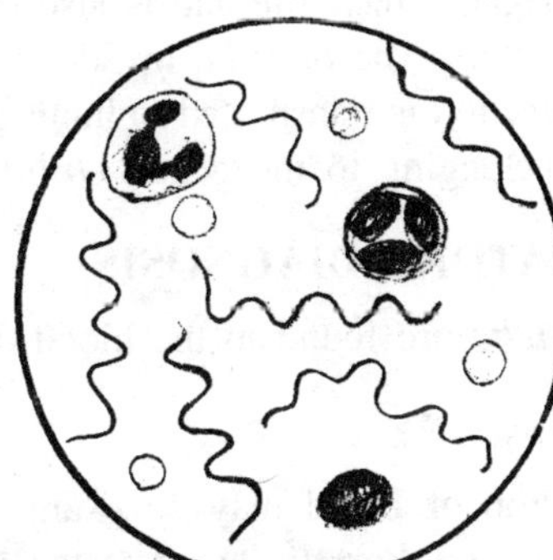

Fig. 73.1 *Borrellia recurrentis* from a peripheral blood smear

CULTURAL CHARACTERISTICS

Borrelia are microaerophilic. Optimum temperature for growth is 28-30ºC. The organism is culturable on complex media containing serum, blood or tissues (**Noguchi medium** containing ascitic fluid with rabbit kidney tissues). Growth occurs on chorioallantoic membrane of chick embryos. For primary isolation, the best method is to inoculate mice or rats intraperitoneally.

ANTIGENIC STRUCTURE

A most striking property of *B. recurrentis* is its ability to change its surface protein antigens, which accounts for the relapsing nature of the disease, because with each relapse a new antigenic variant arises. These **antigenic variations** are due to DNA rearrangement in linear plasmids present in *Borrelia*.

PATHOGENICITY

The organism is responsible for the disease known as **relapsing fever**, which is characterized by several cycles of apparent recovery, each followed by a relapse.

The first symptoms of relapsing fever appear three to ten days after exposure to an infected arthropod. These symptoms include an abrupt onset of high fever accompanied by severe headache, muscle pain and general malaise. During this febrile period, which lasts three to five days, abundant spirochetes are present in the blood. The fever abates along with the number of spirochetes, and apparent recovery is experienced for a period of four to ten days, but is followed by a recurrence of the initial symptoms. There may be as many as ten such recurrences, generally with decreasing severity. In fatal cases, the spirochete invades many organs of the body (heart, spleen, liver, kidney), with death generally due to myocarditis.

EPIDEMIOLOGY

Louse-borne relapsing fever occurs as epidemics wherever poverty, overcrowding and lack of personal hygiene encourage louse infestation. The louse-borne disease presents a more severe clinical picture than the tick-borne disease. In lice, the borreliae are confined to hemolymph and is not shed in excreta. So the infection is not by the bite of lice but by their being crushed and rubbed into abraded skin. The organism is not transmitted transovarially in lice.

Tick-borne relapsing fever occurs sporadically in endemic areas. The disease is milder but relapses are more frequent than in louse-borne fever. The borrelia persists in the body of infected ticks throughout their life and is also transmitted transovarially so that the ticks act as reservoirs as well as vectors. The *Borrelia* invade all parts of the body of the tick and is shed in saliva and feces. So the infection is transmitted to humans through the bite of ticks or their discharges. Several species of ticks belonging to the genus *Ornithodorus* act as vectors.

LABORATORY DIAGNOSIS

Borrelia are found in the blood during fever but never in the apyrexial intervals.

MICROSCOPY

A drop of blood may be examined as a wet film under the dark ground or phase contrast microscope and *Borrelia* are detected by their lashing movements. Diagnosis is also based on the appearance of loosely coiled spirochetes in the blood smears stained by Giemsa or Leishman or Wright stains or dilute carbol fuchsin.

Isolation: One to two ml of patient's blood is inoculated into mice intraperitoneally. The borreliae multiply in the animals and appear in large numbers in peripheral blood within two days. Smears are prepared from blood collected from the tail vein and examined daily for two weeks.

Prophylaxis: No vaccines are available and protection is best accomplished by protecting against ticks and lice.

Treatment: Tetracyclines, erythromycin and penicillin have proven effective treatments.

BORRELIA VINCENTII (*Treponema vincentii*)

Borrelia vincentii is an actively motile spirochete with 3-8 coils. It is Gram negative. It is an obligate anaerobe. It is a normal mouth commensal. Under certain predisposing conditions like malnutrition or viral infections, gives rise to a disease known as **vincent's angina** or **ulcerative gingivostomatitis** or **oropharyngitis**. In this disease, *B. vincentii* is always associated with fusiform bacilli (*Fusobacterium fusiforme*). This symbiotic infection is known as **fusospirochetosis**. (Fig.73.2).

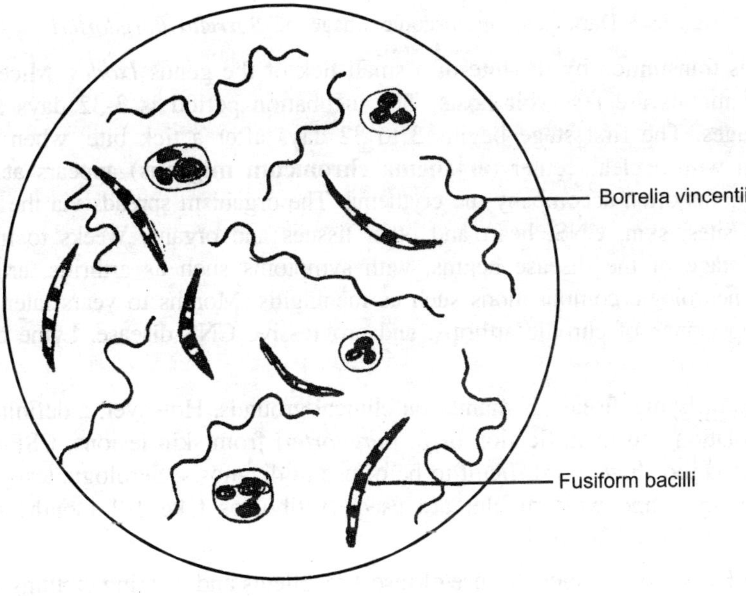

Fig. 73.2 *Borrelia vincentii* and fusiform bacilli in a throat swab smear from a case of vincent's angina

A large number of spirochetes and fusiform bacilli may also be demonstrated in some cases of lung abscesses, skin ulcers which may be opportunistic diseases in devitalised tissues.

Diagnosis may be made by demonstrating spirochetes and fusiform bacilli in stained smears of exudates from lesions.

Penicillin and metronidazole are effective for treatment.

BORRELIA BURGDORFERI (Lyme disease)

Lyme disease was first identified in 1975 in Lyme, Connecticut, USA, hence the name. It is caused by a spirochete, *Borrelia burgdorferi.* It is Gram negative and microaerophilic (Fig. 73.3). It can be cultivated on modified **kelley's (BSK) medium** on incubation for 2-3 weeks at 33°C.

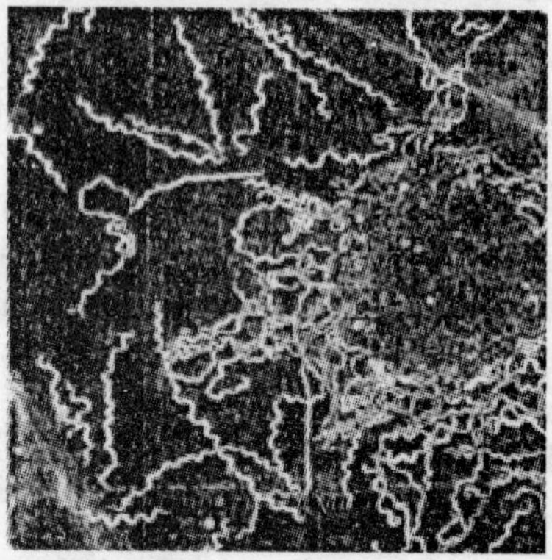

Fig. 73.3 Dark-field microscopic image of *Borrelia burgdorferi*

The disease is transmitted by the bite of a small tick of the genus *Ixodes.* Mice, other rodents, Deer and other mammals are reservoir hosts. The incubation period is 3-32 days and the disease occurs in three stages. The first stage begins 3 to 32 days after a tick bite, when a characteristic red, circular lesion with a clear center (**erythema chronicum migrans**) appears at the site of the bite. Flu-like symptoms often accompany the erythema. The organism spreads via the lymph or blood to musculoskeletal sites, skin, CNS, heart and other tissues and organs. Weeks to months after the onset, the second stage of the disease begins, with symptoms such as arthritis, arthralgia, cardiac complications and neurologic complications such as meningitis. Months to years later, the third stage begins with the appearance of chronic arthritis, and progressive CNS disease. Lyme disease is rarely fatal.

The diagnosis of Lyme disease is mainly on clinical grounds. However, a definite diagnosis can be made by the isolation and identification of *B. burgdorferi* from skin lesions, CSF or blood of the patients, but culture is too slow and difficult to be of use in diagnosis. Serologic tests such as ELISA and Immunofluorescence and western blot are used. Antibodies take 1-2 months to appear, with initial IgM response followed by IgG.

Prevention of Lyme disease includes use of insect repellents and wearing clothing that sufficiently protects the body from tick bites.

Tetracyclines, penicillin, newer macrolides and cephalosporins are useful for treatment.

QUESTIONS

Short Notes

1. Relapsing fever
2. *Borrelia recurrentis*
3. Lab. diagnosis of relapsing fever
4. *Borrelia vincentii* (or) vincent's angina (or) fusospirochetosis.
5. *Borrelia burgdorferi* (or) Lyme disease
6. Name four oral commensal treponemes

74

Leptospira interrogans

- *Introduction*
- *Morphology*
- *Cultural characteristics*
- *Resistance*
- *Pathogenicity*
- *Epidemiology*
- *Laboratory diagnosis*
- *prophylaxis*
- *Treatment.*

INTRODUCTION

The genus is included in the family Leptospiraceae under order spirochetales and comprises two species. (*i*) *L. biflexa* comprise free living saprophytes found in surface waters, and (*ii*) *L. interrogans* containing pathogenic leptospires. *L. interrogans* is further classified into 22 serogroups (e.g., *icterohemorrhagiae*). Within each serogroup, several serotypes or serovars are known and are specific to distinct geographic locales. So far over 200 serotypes have been identified.

MORPHOLOGY

Leptospires are very slender (lepto = slender) and delicate spirochetes about 6-20 μm long and 0.1 μm thick. They are actively motile. They contain numerous tightly coiled coils set so close together that they can be distinguished only under dark ground illumination in the living state or by electron microscopy. Their ends are hooked and resemble umbrella handles. They possess a single, thin axial filament. They stain poorly with aniline dyes but can be demonstrated by fluorescent antibody technique and silver impregnation methods. (Fig. 74.1).

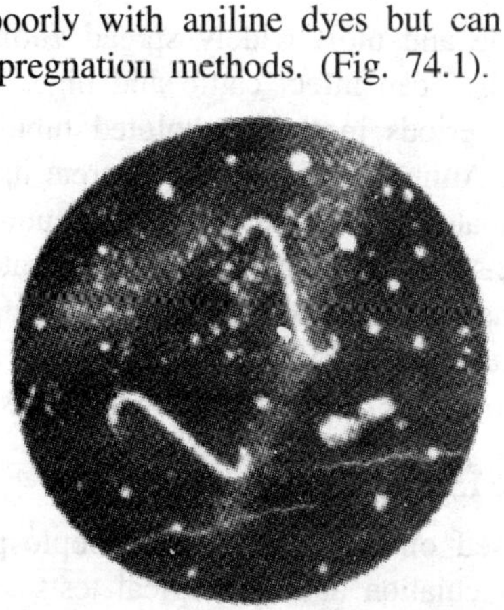

Fig. 74.1. *Leptospira* under darkground illumination

CULTURAL CHARACTERISTICS

Leptospires are aerobic and microaerophilic. Optimum temperature for growth is 28-32°C and pH 7.2–7.4. Leptospires can be grown in medium enriched with rabbit serum. Several liquid and semisolid media, such as Korthof's medium, Stuart's medium and Fletcher's medium are used. EMJH (Ellinghausen, Mc Cullough, Johnson, Harris) medium is now commonly used. Leptospires may be grown on the chorioallantoic membrane of chick embryos.

Bacterial contamination is a serious problem in isolating and maintaining leptospires in culture. The use of 5-fluorouracil inhibits contamination of bacteria in cultures.

RESISTANCE

L. interrogans is sensitive to drying and to a broad range of disinfectants. It can survive for weeks in slightly alkaline (pH 6.8-8.0) water.

PATHOGENICITY

The organism causes a disease known as **Leptospirosis**. The disease occurs worldwide and is known with various local names, such as **Weil's disease**, infectious jaundice, marsh fever and Swineherd's disease.

Leptospirosis is essentially an animal disease, seen in rodents (Rats), dogs, pigs and cattle. Leptospires localize in the convoluted tubules and are continuously shed in the urine of some infected animals. The disease is transmitted to humans zoonotically–primarily by water or food contaminated with animal urine or feces. Entrance to the body can also occur via small skin abrasions or via the conjunctiva or through the mucus membranes of nose and mouth.

Fever occurs one to two weeks after infection, at which spirochetes appear in the blood. These symptoms decrease after about one week.

However, in cases of biphasic disease (that is, the disease having two stages), spirochetes reappear, accompanied by invasion of the liver, kidneys and CNS. This results in **jaundice**, hemorrhage, tissue necrosis, and/or aseptic meningitis. **Albuminuria** is a constant feature. This second stage of the disease, which lasts three or more weeks, involves a rise in circulating IgM antibodies. In severe cases, the mortality can be as high as ten percent.

EPIDEMIOLOGY

Leptospirosis is worldwide and most widely spread **zoonoses**. Several animals such as rats, field mice act as reservoirs. They can infect cattle and pigs. Humans are 'end' hosts. Pathogenic treponemes survives for long periods in the convoluted tubules of the kidneys in natural hosts, multiply and are shed in urine. Animal carriers often excrete upto 100 million leptospires per ml of urine. When this urine contaminates water or mud that is neutral or slightly alkalilne, the leptospires survive for weeks. When humans come in contact with such water, leptospires enter the body through abraded skin, mucus membranes or conjunctiva. Certain occupational groups such as agricultural workers in rural areas are more often exposed to infection. In recent times, the disease is observed in urban areas in developing countries due to overcrowding, insanitation, increasing rat population.

LABORATORY DIAGNOSIS

Diagnosis is usually based on demonstration of leptospires in blood or CSF or urine by microscopy, culture, animal inoculation and serological tests.

(*i*) **Microscopy:** Leptospires are present in the blood during first week and appear in urine in the second week of the disease and intermittently thereafter for 4-6 weeks. A drop of blood or centrifuged deposit of fresh urine may be examined by dark field microscope or immunofluorescence.

(*ii*) **Culture:** Specimen is inoculated into Stuart's or Korthof or EMJH medium and incubated at 37ºC for two days and left thereafter at room temperature in dark for two weeks. Samples from cultures are examined every third day under dark ground illumination.

(*iii*) **Animal inoculation:** The blood or fresh urine of the patient is inoculated intraperiteneally into young guinea pigs. The infection in guinea pigs will have to be identified by demonstration of leptospires in the peritoneal fluid, blood obtained by cardiac puncture by dark ground illumination and by culture. The identification of serovar is by agglutination tests.

(*iv*) **Serology:** Antibodies appear at the end of first week of disease and increase till fourth week. Two types of serological tests are available.

(*a*) Genus specific tests or broadly reactive screening tests detects antibodies to the antigen prepared from nonpathogenic *L. biflexa patoc 1* strain. These tests include CFT, sensitised erythrocyte lysis, hemagglutination test and ELISA.

(*b*) Type specific tests identify the infecting serovar by demonstrating specific antibodies. Macroscopic and microscopic agglutination tests are widely used. In macroscopic agglutination, formalinised suspensions of prevalent *Leptospira* serovars are tested with serial dilutions of the patient serum. The microscopic agglutination test generally uses live cultures of different serotypes and agglutination is observed under the low power dark field microscope.

PROPHYLAXIS

Prevention of exposure to contaminated water and food helps control the transmission of the disease. Rodent control, disinfection of water contribute to the prevention of the disease. No vaccine is available.

TREATMENT

Penicillin, tetracyclines are effective for treatment.

QUESTIONS

Essay Question

1. Name the diseases spread by rats. Describe the pathogenicity and lab. diagnosis of leptospirosis.

Short Notes

1. *Leptospira interrogans.*
2. *Leptospira icterohemorrhagiae.*
3. Morphology of *Leptospira.*
4. Weil's disease (or) Leptospirosis.
5. Lab. diagnosis of Weil's disease.
6. Cultivation of *Leptospira.*

75

Miscellaneous Bacteria

- *Alcaligenes fecalis*
- *Chromobacterium violaceum*
- *Flavobacterium meningosepticum*
- *Gardenerella vaginalis*
- *Calymmatobacterium granulomatis*
- *Streptobacillus moniliformis*
- *Spirillum minus*

ALCALIGENES FECALIS

They are commensals in the small intestine of humans and animals and occurs as a saprophyte in soil and water contaminated with decaying organic matter. They have been isolated from a variety of clinical specimens such as urine, pus and blood and may cause urinary tract infections, wound infections, typhoid like fever, infantile gastroenteritis and suppuration in various parts of the body.

Alcaligenes is a small Gram negative, nonsporing, noncapsulated bacillus. It is actively motile by peritrichate flagella. It is an obligate aerobe and cannot ferment any sugars but produces an alkaline reaction in the litmus milk. It is catalase and oxidase positive. It is indole, H_2S, urease, deamination of phenyl alanine and nitrate reduction test negative. It can grow on MacConkey agar and can tolerate 6.5% NaCl.

CHROMOBACTERIUM VIOLACEUM

It occurs as a saprophyte in soil and water. Human infections are common in tropical areas and include skin lesions with pyemia and multiple abscesses, intestinal and genitourinary tract infections and septicemia with pneumonia.

It is a Gram negative, nonsporing bacillus, motile by means of a single polar flagellum and lateral flagellae. It occurs singly or in pairs. It is an aerobe and facultative anaerobe. It grows well on ordinary media producing a nondiffusible violet pigment soluble in ethanol and insoluble in chloroform and water. It is catalase and oxidase positive and indole and urease negative.

FLAVOBACTERIUM MENINGOSEPTICUM

It occurs as a saprophyte in soil, water, foodstuffs and moist environments. It causes opportunistic infections. In adults, it may cause a mild febrile illness or pneumonia. It is highly pathogenic for newborn infants and may cause neonatal meningitis.

It is a Gram negative, nonmotile, nonsporing bacillus. It grows well on nutrient agar, producing smooth, circular glistening colonies on incubation for 24 hours at 37ºC. It forms a yellow nondiffusible pigment. It is oxidase positive. Sugars are oxidized and acid is produced. It is proteolytic. It is usually sensitive to cotrimoxazole, novobiocin, rifampicin and clindamycin.

GARDNERELLA VAGINALIS

It is a small, Gram negative, pleomorphic bacillus which shows metachromatic granules. It is nonmotile, noncapsulated and nonsporing. It was formerly known as *Hemophilus vaginalis* or *Corynebacterium vaginale.*

It is an aerobe and facultative anaerobe and grow best in the presence of 5-10% CO_2. It is nutritionally fastidious and grows on blood agar or chocolate agar. Minute colonies appear in one to two days and show betahemolysis on blood agar. Catalase, oxidase and urease tests are negative.

It is a member of normal flora of female genital tract. It causes **bacterial vaginosis** characterised by foul smelling discharge and the presence of "**clue cells**", which are vaginal epithelial cells covered with numerous Gram negative bacilli. Bacterial vaginosis is associated with a mixed bacterial flora consisting of *Mobiluncus* sp. particularly. Metronidazole is effective in treatment.

CALYMMATOBACTERIUM VAGINALIS

It is a small, capsulated, nonmotile, Gram negative coccobacillus. They show bipolar condensation of chromatin giving rise to "safety pin" appearance. In the infected tissues, it can be best stained by Wright-Giemsa method, in which bacillus appears blue and the capsule pink. It is an intracellular parasite, present within the cytoplasmic vacuoles (phagosomes) of macrophages and are known as "**Donovan bodies**". They are sometimes seen inside polymorphonuclear leucocytes or lying free outside the cells. It can be cultured readily in the yolksac of embryonated hen's egg and with difficulty on media containing egg-yolk. It is morphologically and antigenically related to *Klebsiella.*

It causes a sexually transmitted, chronic granulomatous disease known as **granuloma inguinale** or granuloma venereum or **donovanosis**. The incubation period ranges from 1 to 12 weeks. It begins as a painless papule on the genitalia, which leads to a slowly progressive, autoinoculable ulcers. The disease runs a chronic course pathogenicity is restricted to human beings. Tetracycline, cotrimoxazole, chloramphenicol, gentamycin, quinolones and the newer macrolides are effective for treatment.

STREPTOBACILLUS MONILIFORMIS

It is a Gram negative, nonmotile, noncapsulated, pleomorphic bacillus, forming chains of various length, with beaded or fusiform swellings (hence the name moniliformis), readily developing into L-forms.

It is an aerobe and facultative anaerobe. It is nutritionally fastidious and grows on media enriched with blood, serum or ascitic fluid. Growth is improved by addition of 5 – 10% CO_2 and a moist atmosphere. It is catalase, oxidase, urease, nitrate and indole negative. It ferments glucose and a few other sugars forming acid but no gas.

It is a normal inhabitant of the nasopharynx of wild and laboratory rats. In humans, it causes streptobacillary **rat-bite fever** following the bite of a rat or occasionally a mouse. The organisms enter the body through the wound caused by rat bite. The disease also occurs due to ingestion of food, water and water contaminated by rats. This condition, first observed Haverhill, USA, is called **Haverhill fever** or **erythema arthriticum epidemicum**.

After an incubation period of 2 to 10 days, there is an abrupt onset of chills, fever, headache, myalgia, followed by a petechial rash and arthritis. Relapses are common in untreated cases.

Laboratory diagnosis of streptobacillary rat-bite fever or Haverhill fever may be made by the isolation of bacilli from blood, pus and joint fluids. Smears of the joint fluid may show pleomorphic, Gram negative bacilli. Mice are highly susceptible to intraperitoneal inoculation of infected material. Agglutination, CFT and fluorescent antibody tests are used for serological diagnosis.

Penicillin is effective for treatment. Cephalosporins erythromycin, clindamycin, tetracycline and aminoglycosides are also useful. L-phase variant is resistant to penicillin but sensitive to tetracycline.

SPIRILLUM MINUS

It is a Gram negative spiral organism with two to three regular rigid spirals. It is actively motile with the help of 1 - 7 amphitrichous flagellae. It exhibits darting motility similar to *V. cholerae*. The organisms can be better visualised in fresh specimens, with the dark ground microscope or by staining with Giemsa or Leishman or fontana methods. It has not been cultivated in laboratory media and is best isolated by intraperitoneal inoculation of blood and infected tissues into guinea pigs, mice and rats.

It is a natural parasite of rats and other rodents. In humans, it causes one type of rat-bite fever, called "**Soduku**" ; transmitted by rat bite. The incubation period is 1 - 4 weeks. The rat bite wound which may have healed, suppurates at the onset of fever, with regional lymphadenopathy. The subsequent course is similar to that of streptobacillary type. Endocarditis, meningitis, hepatitis, nephritis are rare complications.

Diagnosis is by intraperitoneal inoculation of blood or material from lymph node into guinea pigs or mice and by demonstration of Spirilla in their blood and peritoneal fluid. *Spirillum minus* may be demonstrated directly in exudates from the lesions or lymph node biopsies or blood of the patient Penicillin and tetracycline are effective for treatment.

QUESTIONS

Short Notes

1. *Calymmatobacterium granulomatis*.
2. Granuloma inguinale.
3. Rat bite fever.
4. *Streptobacillus moniliformis*.
5. *Spirillum minus*.
6. *Gardenerella vaginalis*.

76

MYCOPLASMA (PPLO, EATON's agent)

- *Introduction,*
- *Classification*
- *Morphology*
- *Resistance*
- *Cultivation*
- *Mycoplasmas of humans*
- *T-strains*
- *Pathogenicity*
- *Laboratory diagnosis*
- *Treatment*

INTRODUCTION

Mycoplasmas are the smallest, cell wall deficient, prokaryotic microorganisms found in man, animals, plants, insects, soil and sewage, that can grow on bacteriological media.

The first member that was first isolated by Nocard and Roux (1898) was *Mycoplasma mycoides* from cattle suffering from pleuropneumonia. A similar organism was found to cause contagious agalactia in sheep. Later, many similar organisms were isolated from humans, animals, plants and environmental sources ; they were together known as **"Pleuropneumonia Like Organisms (PPLO)"**.

Eaton (1944) found that this was filterable, and was considered to be a virus, became known as **"Eaton's agent"**.

Now, the name "*Mycoplasma*" is coined for this group of organisms (Myco = fungus like form of branching filaments ; Plasma = plasticity of shape).

Classification: Mycoplasmas have been placed in the class **Mollicutes** (meaning soft skin), order **Mycoplasmatales**, which contains the following families and genera.

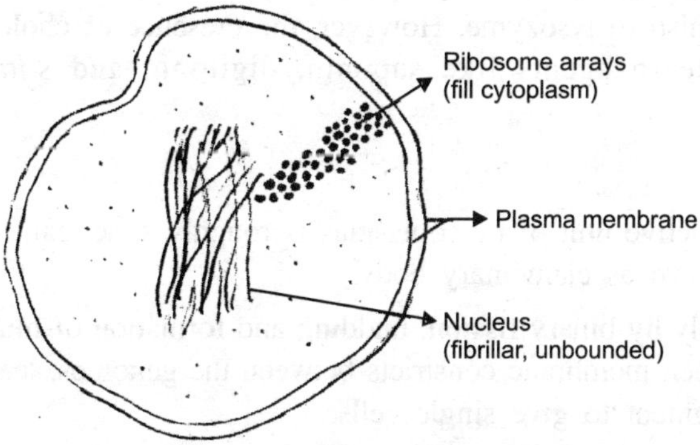

Fig. 76.1. *Mycoplasma* cell

1. Family **Mycoplasmataceae** includes parasitic mycoplasmas requiring cholesterol or other sterols as essential growth factors.

   e.g., Genus *Mycoplasma* : It can utilize glucose or arginine ; but cannot produce urease, consequently cannot split urea.

   Genus *Ureaplasma* : It produces urease enzyme and hydrolyzes urea.

2. Family **Acholeplasmataceae** includes saprophytic mycoplasmas. They do not require sterols as growth factors. e.g., ; Genus *Acholeplasma*.

3. Family **Spiroplasmataceae** includes helical or spiral shaped mycoplasmas. They are parasites of plants and arthropods. They require sterols e.g., Genus *Spiroplasma*.

4. Family Anaeroplasmataceae includes obligate anaerobes found in rumen of cattle and sheep. e.g., Genus *Anaeroplasma.*

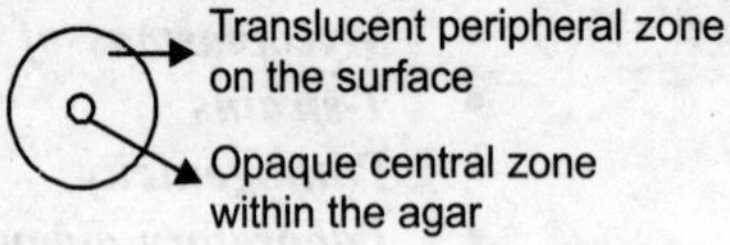

Fig. 76.2 Colony of *Mycoplasma* with "Fried-Egg" appearance.

MORPHOLOGY

Mycoplasmas are smallest, Gram negative bacteria. They lack cell wall and therefore possess the property of plasticity and are filterable and exhibit pleomorphism. Their shape ranges from spherical through coccoid, coccobacillary, ring and dumb-bell forms to short and long branching, beaded or segmented filaments. Some mycoplasmas have specialized structures at one or both ends by which they attach to suitable host cells such as respiratory or genital mucosa possessing neuraminic acid receptors. They may be responsible for hemadsorption property.

Though, they are Gram negative, they are better stained by Giemsa stain. They are nonmotile and nonsporing and do not possess flagellae and fimbriae. Some species may exhibit gliding motility.

The cytoplasm is packed with ribosomes and the nuclear material is in fibrillar form, placed centrally or dispersed. The genome has smallest molecular weight and the DNA content ranges from 1.5 to 4% of their dry weight. The G+C content ranges from 23 to 41%.

RESISTANCE

Because of the absence of cell wall, Mycoplasmas are resistant to antibiotics such as penicillins that act on cell wall and also to lysozyme. However, the presence of cholesterol in cell membrane renders them susceptible to agents like saponin, digitonin and some polyene antibiotics (amphotericin-B).

Reproduction

The minimal reproductive unit of mycoplasmas is roughly spherical, measuring 200 - 250 nm in diameter. It is also known as elementary body.

Mycoplasmas multiply by binary fission, budding and formation of multinucleate filaments due to genome replication. When membrane constricts between the genomes, leads to formation of chain of beads, which later fragment to give single cells.

CULTIVATION

Mycoplasmas are facultative anaerobes. They grow over a temperature range of 20–41°C ; The parasitic species grow best at 35 to 37°C and saprophytes at lower temperatures 20–30°C. Because of small genomic size, they have limited biosynthetic ability, so that they need a rich growth medium, and are fastidious in growth requirements.

The most widely used media are beef heart infusion peptone broth (PPLO broth) and beef heart infusion agar (PPLO agar), which contains heart infusion (or meat infusion), yeast extract to which 30% human ascitic fluid or animal (horse, rabbit) serum is added as a source of cholesterol ; penicillin and thallium acetate may be added as selective agents. Cultures are incubated at 37°C for two to six days, preferably in the presence of CO_2.

The colonies appear after an incubation for two to six days and are typically biphasic, with a "fried egg" appearance, consisting of a central, opaque granular area of growth extending into the depth of the medium, surrounded by a flat, translucent peripheral zone.

The colonies cannot be picked up by inoculation wire loop. Subculture is done by cutting out an agar block with colonies and rubbing it on fresh plates. Colonies may be seen with a handlens but are best studied by staining with Giemsa stain or Dienes method. For this, a block of agar containing the colony is cut and placed on a slide, and stained with alcoholic solution of methylene blue and azure (Diene's stain) and examined under microscope. Such slides can also be stained with specific fluorescent antibody.

MYCOPLASMAS OF HUMANS

Mycoplasmas may be saprophytic, parasitic or pathogenic. About sixteen species are found in human beings.

Pathogens

M. pneumoniae causes primary atypical pneumonia.

M. hominis causes genital infections.

Ureaplasma urealyticum causes genital infections.

Nonpathogens (Commensals)

In oropharynx	*M. orale, M. buccale, M. salivarium, M. faucium.*
In genital tract	*M. fermentans, M. genitalium, M. penetrans, M. primatum M. spermatophilum.*
On skin and mouth	*Acholeplasma laidlawii*

T-STRAINS

Some strains of mycoplasmas isolated from genital infections of humans and animals form very tiny colonies. They were called T-strains or T-form mycoplasmas (T for tiny). They are peculiar in their ability to hydrolyze urea, which is an essential growth factor in addition to cholesterol. They have been named as *Ureaplasma urealyticum*. They are highly susceptible to erythromycin and are more susceptible to thallium acetate than other mycoplasmas.

PATHOGENICITY

Three species of *Mycoplasma – M. pneumoniae, M. hominis* and *Ureaplasma urealyticum* cause human diseases. They cause respiratory and urogenital infections.

Respiratory infections – *M. pneumoniae* causes **primary atypical pneumonia (walking pneumonia**), by infecting lower respiratory tract and adhering to respiratory mucosal cells. The disease spreads by air-borne droplets of nasopharyngeal secretions and by close contact. The onset is insidious with malaise, myalgia, sore throat with paroxysmal dry cough. The disease is found among all age groups and is world-wide in distribution. The organism can cause infections in CNS (meningoencephalitis, aseptic meningitis) and joints (arthritis).

M. hominis and *Ureaplasmas* may occasionally cause respiratory disease in the newborn, being acquired in utero.

Urogenital infections—*M. hominis* and *U. urealyticum* can cause **nonspecific urethritis (nongonococcal urethritis**) transmitted by sexual contact. *M. hominis* causes acute pyelonephritis and pelvic inflammatory disease (PID). Urease produced by *Ureaplasma* may lead to the formation of calculi or stones.

U. urealyticum also causes surgical wound infections, arthritis in agammaglobulinemic persons and respiratory and CNS infections in neonates.

Mycoplasmas cause more severe and prolonged infections in immunodeficiency cases.

LABORATORY DIAGNOSIS

The specimens collected in respiratory infections are throat swabs, respiratory secretions or sputum. In genital infections urethral swabs, vaginal swabs or centrifuged deposit of urine are used. Lab. diagnosis consists of culture, serology and molecular methods.

Culture

The specimens are inoculated into Mycoplasma medium containing glucose and phenol red and incubated at 37ºC, for three weeks. Growth is slow and indicated by acid production. (see cultivation). Mycoplasmas form distinct colonies with a fried egg appearance.

Serology

The antibodies in patient sera can be demonstrated by two types of serological tests.

1. *Specific tests:* Where mycoplasmal antigens are employed to detect antibodies. e.g., Immunofluorescence, hemagglutination inhibition (HI), metabolic inhibition, indirect hemagglutination (IHA) and CFT.
2. Nonspecific tests are those in which antigens other than mycoplasmal are employed and are termed as heterophile agglutination tests e.g., *Streptococcus* MG agglutination test and cold agglutination test.

Streptococcus MG agglutination test

It is a **heterophile tube agglutination test** used for serodiagnosis of primary atypical pneumonia, caused by *Mycoplasma.* The test is based on the presence of heterophile antigens among *M. pneumoniae* and *Streptococcus* MG.

The test is done by mixing serial dilutions of patient's serum and a heat-killed suspension of *Streptococcus*MG and incubated at 37ºC overnight. A titre of 1:20 or over is significant.

Cold agglutination test

It is a **heterophile tube agglutination test** used for the serodiagnosis of primary atypical pneumonia caused by *M. pneumoniae.*

The test is done by mixing serial dilutions of patient's serum with an equal volume of 0.2% washed human 'O' group RBC and incubated overnight at 4ºC (cold temperature) and examined for clumping of RBC. A titre of 1:32 or over is significant.

The test is based on the presence of heterophile antigens among *M. pneumoniae* and human 'O' group RBC and the ability of antibodies to react with human 'O' group RBC at cold temperature.

Molecular Methods like DNA probes and PCR are used to detect mycoplasmas from the clinical specimens.

TREATMENT

Erythromycin, alternatively doxycycline is the drug of choice. Newer macrolides azithromycin and clarythromycin are also highly active. Quinolones (ciprofloxacin) can be used as second line agents.

QUESTIONS

Essay Question

1. Classify Mycoplasmas. Describe the morphology, cultivation pathogenicity and Lab. diagnosis of Mycoplasmas.

Short Notes

1. Morphology of *Mycoplasma.*
2. Cultivation of *Mycoplasma* (or) PPLO agar.
3. Dienes method.
4. Pathogenicity of *Mycoplasma.*
5. Primary atypical pneumonia.
6. Lab. diagnosis of Mycoplasmal diseases.
7. Streptococcus MG agglutination test.
8. Cold agglutination test.
9. *Mycoplasma pneumoniae* or PPLO or Eaton's agent.
10. *Ureaplasma* or T-strains.
11. *Acholeplasma.*

77

Rickettsiaceae

- ***Introduction, Classification***
- ***Rickettsiae—Morphology, Cultivation, Antigenic structure, Pathogenesis, Typhus fevers, Spotted fevers.***
- ***Orientia - Scrub typhus***
- ***Lab. diagnosis—Neill-Mooser reaction, Weil-felix test***
- ***Ehrlichia***
- ***Coxiella burnetii***
- ***Bartonella***

INTRODUCTION

Rickettsiae are primarily parasites of arthropod Insects such as lice, fleas, ticks and mites, in which they are found in alimentary canal. In vertebrates including humans, they infect the vascular endothelium and Reticuloendothelial cells.

Rickettsiae resemble viruses in several properties. Like viruses –

1. They are obligate intracellular parasites.
2. Cannot be cultivated in bacteriological media and grow only in cell cultures and embryonated eggs.
3. Different in genetic properties.

But, Rickettsiae are considered to be true bacteria, adapted to obligate intracellular parasitism. Like bacteria –

1. They are Gram negative bacilli.
2. Possess cell wall.
3. Multiply by binary fission.
4. Susceptible to antibiotics.
5. Possess both RNA and DNA.
6. Held back by bacterial filters.

CLASSIFICATION

Rickettsiae have been placed in volume I, section 9 of Bergey's Manual. The order "Rickettsiales" have been classified into 3 families – Rickettsiaceae. Bartonellaceae and Anaplasmataceae.

The family Rickettsiaceae is named after Howard Taylor Ricketts for discovery of spotted fever Rickettsiae and died of typhus fever acquired during his research.

In the 2nd edition of Bergey's Manual, the genus *Rickettsia* is placed in the order Rickettsiales, whereas *Coxiella* is in the order Legionallales and family Coxiellaceae.

The family Rickettsiaceae has 3 genera: 1. *Rickettsia*, 2. *Orientia*, and 3. *Ehrlichia.*

The 16S rRNA sequencing has suggested that Rickettsiae can be grouped with purple bacteria, more specifically with the plant pathogen *Agrobacterium tumefaciens.*

RICKETTSIAE

Morphology

Rickettsiae are Gram negative coccobacilli. For staining these organisms Giminez, Macchiavello and Giemsa stains are used. They appear deep red with Giminez and Macchiavello and purple with Giemsa stain. The bacteria are pleomorphic being rod shaped or coccoid. They are nonmotile and nonsporing. They possess a trilaminar plasma membrane.

They lack the glycolysis and do not use glucose as energy source and generate ATP by oxidation of aminoacids such as glutamate and Kreb's cycle intermediates such as succinate. They obtain the ATP from host cells. The Rickettsiae plasma membrane has carrier mediated transport systems and host cell nutrients and coenzymes are absorbed directly.

Cultivation

Rickettsiae cannot grow on cell-free bacteriological media

1. Rickettsiae can be cultivated in **yolk sac** of developing chick embryos. The inoculated eggs are incubated at 33-35ºC for 8 days.
2. They can be cultivated in mouse fibroblast, HeLa, HEp-2, Detroit-6 and other continuous cell lines but tissue cultures are not satisfactory for primary isolation.
3. Laboratory animals such as Guinea Pigs and mice are useful for the isolation of rickettsiae from patients. They may also be propagated in insect vectors.

Antigenic Structure

Rickettsiae possess 3 types of antigens:

1. A group specific soluble antigen present on the surface of the organisms. This can be separated from the organisms by repeated washing and centrifugation.
2. A species specific, and in case of scrub typhus strain specific antigen associated with the cell wall of the organism.
3. An alkali stable polysaccharide found in some Rickettsiae and in some strains of *Proteus vulgaris* OX19 and OX2 and *Proteus mirabilis* OX K. This sharing of antigen between Rickettsiae and *Proteus* is the basis of **weil-felix reaction** used for the diagnosis of rickettsial infections, by the demonstration of antibodies to the proteus strains.

Pathogenesis

Rickettsiae are transmitted to man by the bite or feces of an infected arthropod vector. Following inoculation into the dermis, the organisms spread via the lymphatics and blood stream. It binds to the vascular endothelial cells by means of the outer membrane protein-A (OMP-A) and induces its uptake by the endothelial cells in a vesicle. Subsequently, it escapes from the vesicle and multiplies in the cytoplasm by binary fission and spreads from cell to cell. This leads to the damage of vascular endothelial cells resulting in increased permeability, inflammation, hemorrhage and necrosis. Incubation period is about one week.

Various Rickettsial diseases are listed in the Table.

TYPHUS FEVERS (typhos = smoke or cloud)

This group consists of epidemic typhus, Brill-Zinsser disease and endemic typhus.

Epidemic typhus (Classical typhus, Gaol fever, louse-borne typhus) – It is caused by *R. prowazekii.* The organisms are transmitted to man by body louse (*Pediculus humanus corporis*) and head louse (*Pediculus humanus capitis*). Lice become infected by ingesting the blood from rickettsemic patients. The Rickettsiae multiply in the gut of the lice and appear in the feces. Lice defecate while feeding. Infection is transmitted when the louse feces is rubbed through the minute abrasions caused by scratching. Lice, being temperature sensitive, leave the febrile patient and parasitise other host.

The disease starts with fever and chills with maculopapular rash first appearing on the body trunk and progresses to the extremities, but sparing face, palms and soles.

Brill-Zinsser disease (Recrudescent typhus)

In some patients who recover from epidemic typhus, the Rickettsiae may remain latent in the lymphoid tissues or organs for many years. Such latent infections may at times be reactivated leading to recrudescent typhus, first noticed by Brill and Zinsser.

Lice that feed on a patient with recrudescent typhus can become infected and if conditions are favorable epidemics may occur due to louse-human-louse transmission.

It is a mild disease. Patients develop severe headache, malaise and myalgia.

Table 77.1 Rickettsial Diseases of Man

Group	*Disease*	*Causative Agent*	*Insect Vector*	*Mode of transmission*
I. Typhus fevers	1. Epidemic typhus (Gaol fever)	*R. prowazekii*	human body louse	louse feces scratched into skin.
	2. Recrudescent typhus (Brill-Zinsser disease)	*R. prowazekii*	–	–
	3. Endemic (murine) typhus	*R. typhi* (*R. mooseri*)	Rat flea	flea bite or flea feces scratched into skin
II. Spotted fevers.	1. Rocky mountain spotted fever	*R. rickettsii*	*Ixodid* ticks	tick bite
	2. Boutonneuse fever	*R. conorii*	*Ixodid* ticks	tick bite
	3. Australian tick typhus	*R. australis*	*Ixodid* ticks	tick bite
	4. Siberian tick typhus	*R. siberica*	*Ixodid* ticks	tick bite
	5. Rickettsial pox	*R. akari*	Mites	Mite bite
III. Scrub typhus	Scrub typhus	*O. tsutsugamushi*	Trombiculid mites	Mite bite

Endemic typhus (Murine typhus)

It is milder than epidemic typhus. It is caused by *R. mooseri* (*R. typhi*), which is maintained in nature as a mild infection of Rats through Rat fleas (*Xenopsylla cheopis*) and the Rat louse (*Polypus spinulosa*).

Humans acquire infection through 1. Flea bite, 2. Ingestion of food contaminated with infected Rat urine or flea feces, 3. Inhalation of dried flea feces, and 4. Contamination of conjunctiva with flea feces.

The disease is characterized by mild fever, persistent headache and maculopapular rash. Often the recovery is spontaneous.

Spotted Fevers

Rickettsiae of spotted fevers possess a common soluble group antigen and grow both in the nucleus and the cytoplasm of infected cells. These diseases include Rocky mountain spotted fever, Boutonneuse fever, Australian tick typhus, Siberian tick typhus and Rickettsial pox. These infections are transmitted by ticks, except rickettsial pox, which is transmitted by mite. Rickettsiae are transmitted transovarially in ticks and mites, which act both as reservoirs and vectors. Infection occurs by the bite of an infected tick or mite or by ingestion contaminated with their feces. An eschar frequently develops at the site of tick bite in spotted fevers.

Rocky mountain spotted fevers

It is caused by *R. rickettsii*, transmitted by ticks of the genera *Amblyomma* and *Dermacentor*. The hall marks of this disease are a high fever lasting for many days and a skin rash reflecting damage to the small blood vessels. The rash begins as pink spots called Macules, and progresses to pink-red pimple like spots known as papules. Where the spots fuse, they form a maculopapular rash, which becomes dark red and then fades without scarring. The rash generally begins on the palms of the hands and soles of the feet and progressively spreads to the body trunk.

Other spotted fevers

Boutonneuse fever caused by *R. conorii*, Australian tick typhus caused by *R. australis* and siberian tick typhus caused by *R. siberica* resemble Rocky mountain spotted fever but are milder. These organisms are maintained in nature in *Ixodid* ticks and wild animals. The disease is transmitted by tick bite. A black spot with a necrotic center (eschar) develops at the site of tick bite.

Rickettsial pox

It is a self-limited, nonfatal, vesicular exanthema resembling chicken pox. It is also called vesicular or varicelliform rickettsiosis. The causative agent is *R. akari.* The vector is mite (*Allodermanyssus sanguineus*), in which the organism undergoes transovarial transmission. Common house mouse (*Mus musculus*) is the reservoir host.

The patient develops a papulovesicular lesion at the site of bite and the enlargement of regional lymph nodes, followed by fever, chills, headache, malaise and myalgia. A generalized papulovesicular rash appears. The disease lasts for 10-14 days, followed by recovery.

ORIENTIA

Scrub Typhus

It is caused by *Orientia tsutsugamushi* (tsutsuga = disease and mushi = mite), transmitted by trombiculid mites.

The disease is so named because it occurs in scrubland. When man trespasses into this scrubland, where mite larval stages are present, he may be bitten by mite larvae (chiggers). Hence, also called **chigger-borne typhus**.

The disease sets in with fever, headache, chills, conjunctivitis and a characteristic eschar at the site of bite. A maculopapular rash appears by fifth day.

O. tsutsugamushi contains three major antigenic types – Karp, Gilliam and Kato.

LABORATORY DIAGNOSIS

It consists of (1) Demonstration of organism or antigen (2) Isolation of organisms (3) Serology.

Demonstration of Organism or antigen

Biopsy specimens from the rash, chronic hepatitis, impression smears from the organs of infected animals and endolymph from ticks may be stained with Giemsa, Macchiavello, Giminez stains and with direct or indirect immunofluorescence techniques. In tissue smears Rickettsiae are usually seen as bipolar rods in the cytoplasm of infected cells. *R. rickettsii* may also be seen in the nuclei of infected cells.

Isolation of Rickettsiae

Rickettsiae are highly infectious and their isolation should be attempted with utmost care.

Blood clot ground in skimmed milk or brainheart infusion broth is inoculated intraperitoneally in male guinea pigs or mice. The animals are observed for 3–4 weeks. In Rocky mountain spotted fever, guinea pigs develop fever, scrotal necrosis and may die. In *R. typhi*, *R. conori* and *R. akari*, guinea-pigs develop fever and tunica reaction.

R. prowazekii produces only fever without any testicular inflammation. Smears from the peritoneum, tunica and spleen of infected animals may be stained by Giemsa or Giminez methods to demonstrate Rickettsiae.

Rickettsiae can also be grown in the embryonated hen's egg and cell cultures.

Tunica reaction or Neill-Mooser reaction

When male guinea-pigs are inoculated intraperitoneally with blood from a case of endemic typhus or with a culture of *R. typhi* (*R. mooseri*), they develop fever and scrotal inflammation. The scrotum becomes enlarged and the testes cannot be pushed back into the abdomen because of inflammatory adhesions between the layers of tunica vaginalis. This is known as Neill-Mooser reaction or tunica reaction. This is negative with *R. prowazekii* or with blood from epidemic typhus.

Serology

Serological diagnosis of rickettsial diseases may be done by weil-felix reaction, CFT, Immunofluorescence, Latex agglutination test, ELISA.

Weil-Felix reaction

It is a **heterophile tube agglutination test** used in serodiagnosis of typhus fever caused by Rickettsial species. The test is negative in Rickettsial pox, trench fever, Q fever.

Patients with rickettsial infection develop antibodies in their blood, which react with *Proteus vulgaris* OX 19 and OX 2 and *Proteus mirabilis* OX K due to sharing of an alkali stable carbohydrate antigen. Sera from epidemic and endemic typhus and tick-borne spotted fever agglutinates *Proteus vulgaris* OX 19 and OX 2. Sera from scrub typhus agglutinates *Proteus mirabilis* OX K.

The antibodies appear rapidly and reaches a peak titre upto 1:1000 or 1:5000 by the second week and declines rapidly in convalescence.

TREATMENT

Rickettsial diseases may be treated with tetracyclines or chloramphenicol.

EHRLICHIA

They are small, Gram negative, obligate intracellular bacilli, that multiply within phagosomes of phagocytes as mulberry like clusters, called morula. They are tick-borne. Three *Ehrlichia* species cause human diseases.

1. ***E. Sennestu*:** It causes sennestu ehrlichiosis, resembling glandular fever (sennestu = glandular fever). Patient develops lymphoid hyperplasia and atypical lymphocytosis. It is suspected to be caused by ingestion of raw fish. The disease occurs in Japan and South East Asia.
2. ***E. Chaffeensis*:** It causes human monocytic ehrlichiosis, transmitted by ticks (*Ambylomma*). Deer and rodents are reservoir hosts. Human, disease is characterized by leucopenia, thrombocytopenia and increased levels of liver enzymes. It occurs in USA, Europe and Africa.
3. ***E. Phagocytophila*:** It causes human granulocytic ehrlichiosis. The causative organism *E. phagocytophila* is almost identical to equine pathogen *E. equi.* The disease is transmitted by *Ixodid* ticks. Deer, cattle and sheep are suspected to be reservoir hosts. Leucopenia and thrombocytopenia are seen. It occurs in USA and Europe.

Ehrlichiosis can be diagnosed by

1. demonstration of bluish intracytoplasmic inclusions (morula) in neutrophils of blood films stained by Giemsa.
2. specific antibodies may be demonstrated by indirect immunofluorescence.
3. PCR.

Doxycycline is used for the treatment of ehrlichiosis.

COXIELLA BURNETII

It is a pleomorphic, filterable Gram negative bacillus, but appears Gram positive when alcoholic Iodine is used as mordant. It is relatively resistant to physical and chemical agents and survives the holder method in pasteurisation. It grows well in yolksac of chick embryos and cell cultures. It exhibits phase variation. Fresh isolates are phase I on repeated passage into yolksac, become phase II.

It causes Q fever (Q refers to Query). It is worldwide in distribution. It is primarily a disease of cattle, sheep and poultry. Wild animals act as reservoir hosts. It is transmitted among them, and to cattle, sheep and poultry by *Ixodid ticks*. Transovarial transmission occurs in ticks. *Coxiella* are abundant in tick feces and survive in dried feces for long periods. They are shed in the milk of infected animals and conception products.

Human infection is **zoonotic** and acquired by consumption of raw milk, handling of infected wool or hides or meat, soil contaminated with animal feces. *Coxiella* may enter through abraded skin, mucosa, lungs or intestine. The human disease is an acute systemic infection characterized by an interstitial pneumonia. The bacilli spread throughout the body and may cause hepatitis, meningoencephalitis or endocarditis. Recovery is Spontaneous. The organisms may remain latent in the tissues for many years. Asymptomatic infections are common.

Laboratory diagnosis is by serological demonstration of antibodies by CFT and indirect immunofluorescence. Weil-felix reaction is negative. *Coxiella burnetii* can be isolated from clinical specimens by intraperiteneal inoculation of guinea pigs, mice and embryonated hen's eggs.

Doxycycline, tetracycline in combination with rifampicin is used for treatment.

BARTONELLA

They are Gram negative bacilli, which invade mammalian endothelial cells and erythrocytes. They are mainly arthropod-borne. Human pathogenic species are *B. bacilliformis*, *B. quintana* and *B. henselae*.

Bartonella bacilliformis

It causes *oroya fever*, spread by sandflies. It is characterized by fever, anemia due to invasion of erythrocytes. Survivors develop nodular ulcerating skin lesions as a late sequel, known as verruga peruana.

It is a pleomorphic Gram negative bacillus, motile with a tuft of polar flagellae. It can be cultivated on semisolid agar with Rabbit or human blood. It is an intracellular parasite living inside RBC. Inoculation of cultures into monkeys leads to verruga peruana but not oroya fever.

Bartonella quintana

It was formerly known as *Rochalimaea quintana.* It is a small Gram negative bacillus and differs from *Rickettsia* in following respects –

1. Occurs extracellularly in vectors.
2. Grows poorly in yolksac of chick embryos.
3. It does not cause experimental infection in any animal except monkeys.
4. Can grow on bacteriological media like blood agar.
5. Sera from patients cannot react with Rickettsial antigens or *Proteus* antigens.

It causes **trench fever** or five-day fever, transmitted by body louse. Infection is acquired when infected lice feces are scratched into the skin. Recovery is usually followed by relapses occuring at five day intervals. *B. quintana* can be detected in the tissues by PCR.

Bartonella henselae

It is a small, slightly curved Gram negative bacillus and grows on blood agar, chocolate agar, brain heart infusion agar supplemented with blood. It produces white, dry, cauliflower-like colonies embedded in the agar.

It causes **cat-scratch disease,** characterized by lymphadenopathy and fever resulting from contact, scratch or bite of an infected cat. It may also cause endocarditis.

In AIDS and immunodeficiencies, it may cause – (1) bacillary angiomatosis – vascular nodules or tumors appear on the skin, mucosa and other locations, resembling kaposi's sarcoma (2) bacillary peliosis–involves liver and spleen.

Diagnosis is established by demonstration of clusters of bacilli in lymph node biopsy sections with the Warthin–Starry silver impregnation stain.

QUESTIONS

Essay Question

1. Give an account of Rickettsiae.

Short Essay Questions

1. Typhus fevers
2. Spotted fevers
3. *Coxiella burnetii* or Q fever
4. *Ehrlichia*

Short Answer Questions

1. Epidemic typhus or Gaol fever
2. Endemic typhus or murine typhus
3. Brill-Zinsser disease
4. Rocky mountain spotted fever
5. Rickettsial pox or Rickettsia akari
6. Scrub typhus or Orientia tsutsugamushi
7. Weil-felix reaction
8. Tunica reaction or Neill-Mooser reaction
9. Q fever
10. Oroya fever
11. Cat scratch disease

78

Chlamydiae

- *Introduction*
- *Morphology*
- *Growth cycle/Life cycle*
- *Classification*
- *Pathogenicity*
  - *Trachoma*
  - *Inclusion conjunctivitis*
  - *Non-gonococcal (Non-specific) urethritis*
  - *LGV*
  - *Psittacosis*
  - *Acute respiratory disease.*
- *Laboratory diagnosis*
  - *Specimens*
  - *Demonstration of inclusion bodies under light microscope.*
  - *Demonstration of antigen.*
  - *Cultivation*
  - *Demonstration of antibodies by serological tests.*
  - *DNA probes.*
  - *Intradermal test (Frei's test)*
- *Treatment*

INTRODUCTION

Chlamydiae are small Gram negative bacteria, which are obligate intracellular parasites of mammals and birds. Based on the human diseases they cause, they were called **"psittacosis-lymphogranuloma-trachoma (PLT) viruses"** or **"PLT agents"**. In recognition of the pioneering studies of Sir Samuel Bedson on psittacosis, the name **"Bedsonia"** was proposed for this group. However, they are now officially by International committee, classified as bacteria belonging to the genus *Chlamydia*, in the chlamydiaceae, the only family of the order chlamydiales.

Chlamydiae were originally thought to be viruses, because they were filterable and unable to grow in bacteriological media. But, now Chlamydiae are considered as true bacteria, as they differ from viruses.

1. They possess both DNA and RNA
2. Possess cell walls
3. Possess ribosomes
4. They are Gram negative under Gram's staining

5. Replicate by binary fission
6. Susceptible to antibiotics

However, they differ from true bacteria in that they do not have peptidoglycan in their cell wall and lack the ability to produce their own ATP because of absence of flavoprotein and cytochrome electron transport chain carriers. They have therefore been called **"energy parasites"**.

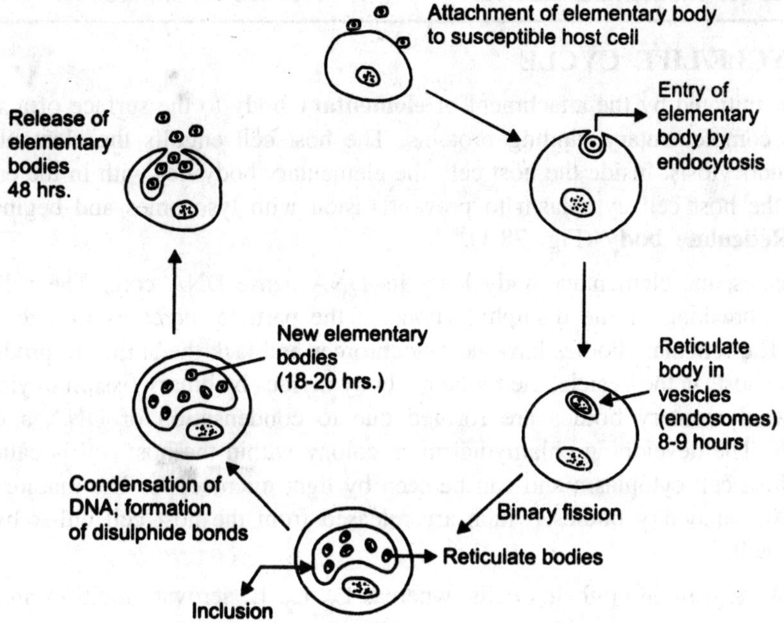

Fig. 78.1 The growth cycle of chlamydiae

MORPHOLOGY

Chlamydiae are small, nonmotile Gram negative bacteria. They stain poorly with Gram's stain, However, they can be stained with Giemsa, Machiavello, Castaneda and Giminez stains.

Chlamydiae occur in two forms – the elementary body and the reticulate body or initial body.

The **elementary body** is extracellular, infective form that is metabolically inert and measures 200-300 nm in diameter. It is a spherical particle with a rigid trilaminar cell wall similar to the cell walls of Gram negative bacteria, and an electron dense nucleoid.

The **reticulate body** is intracellular, growing and replicative form that is metabolically active and measures 500-1000 nm in diameter. It is circular in shape. No peptidoglycan is found in cell wall. The cell wall is fragile and pliable, leading to pleomorphism.

Table 78.1 Differences between Elementary and Reticulate Bodies

Elementary body	*Reticulate body*
1. Size about 200-300 nm	1. Size about 500-1000 nm.
2. Cell wall is rigid	2. Cell wall is fragile.
3. Relatively resistant to sonication	3. Sensitive to sonication
4. Resistant to trypsin	4. Lysed by trypsin

5. Subunit in cell envelope	5. No subunit in cell envelope
6. RNA:DNA content 1:1	6. RNA:DNA content 3:1
7. Toxic for mice	7. Nontoxic for mice
8. Isolated organisms are infectious	8. Isolated organisms are not infectious
9. Adapted for extracellular survival	9. Adapted for intracellular growth.

GROWTH CYCLE/LIFE CYCLE

Infection is initiated by the attachment of **elementary body** to the surface of a susceptible host cell by specific complementary binding proteins. The host cell engulfs the elementary body by a process called endocytosis. Inside the host cell, the elementary body lies with in the endosome, being separated from the host cell cytoplasm to prevent fusion with lysosomes and begins to reorganize itself to form **Reticulate body** (Fig. 78.1).

In the vesicles, the elementary body loses its DNA dense DNA core. The cell wall becomes less rigid due to breaking of the disulphide bonds ; the particle increases in size and becomes a reticulate body. The reticulate bodies have no cytochromes and lack the ability to produce ATP, which is supplied by the host. In the vesicle, the reticulate body divides by binary fission to yield pleomorphic organisms. New elementary bodies are formed due to condensation of DNA and formation of disulphide bonds. The developing chlamydial microcolony within the host cell is called "**inclusion**", which fills the host cell cytoplasm and can be seen by light microscope. The mature inclusion body contains 100-500 elementary bodies, which are released from the host cell either by exocytosis or autolysis of the cell.

TRIC serovars grow in epithelial cells, whereas L_1, L_2, L_3 serovars multiply in regional lymph nodes.

During the active intracellular growth, the *Chlamydia*-specific lipopolysaccharides are formed on the host cell surface, contributing to pathogenesis by inflammatory and immunological responses.

CLASSIFICATION

The genus *Chlamydia* is classified into 4 species, based on growth characters, nucleic acid profile, antigens and nature of the inclusion body.

1. *Chlamydia trachomatis.*
2. *Chlamydia psittaci.*
3. *Chlamydia pneumoniae.*
4. *Chlamydia peccrum.*

Chlamydia trachomatis is classified into two biological variants (biovars).

1. TRIC agents – classified into 12 serovars.
   – A, B, Ba and C cause Trachoma disease.
   – D, E, F, G, H, I, J, K (D – K) cause inclusion conjunctivitis, genital infections.
2. LGV biovar comprises L_1, L_2 and L_3 serovars and are associated with Lymphogranuloma venereum, a sexually transmitted disease.

Table 78.2 Classification of Chlamydiae

Species	*Serotype*	*Disease*
C. trachomatis	A, B, Ba, C	Trachoma
	D, E, F, G, H, I, J, K	Inclusion conjunctivitis genital chlamydiasis (non-specific urethritis)
		Infant pneumonia
	L_1, L_2, L_3	Lymphogranuloma venereum
C. psittaci	Many serotypes	Psittacosis
C. pneumoniae	TWAR strain	Acute respiratory disease

C. trachomatis strains form compact inclusions with glycogen matrix, are sensitive to sulphonamides and are natural parasites of humans, usually causing localised infections of eyes and genital organs.

C. psittaci strains form diffuse vacuolated inclusions without the glycogen matrix, are resistant to sulphonamides and are natural parasites of birds and animals causing pneumonia and generalised infections.

C. pneumoniae is an exclusive human pathogen and a common cause of acute respiratory disease.

C. pecorum includes strains affecting ruminants.

PATHOGENICITY

Chlamydiae strains cause several diseases in humans, animals and birds.

Trachoma

It is caused A, B, Ba and C serotypes of *C. trachomatis.* It spreads either direct by contact through fingers, hand to hand contact or indirectly by fomites such as towels, soaps. Flies may transmit infection mechanically. Infection may also spread by dust particles.

Trachoma is keratoconjunctivitis begins abruptly with inflammatory cell exudate and follicular hypertrophy. The disease usually heals spontaneously. In reinfection, vascularization of cornea or pannus formation occurs that may lead to blindness.

The characteristic inclusions formed in conjunctiva are called **Halberstaedter Prowazek** or **HP bodies**. They possess glycogen matrix.

The disease is worldwide in distribution and common in developing countries because of overcrowding and unhygienic conditions. Control of the disease involves mass education and chemotherapy.

Inclusion Conjunctivitis

It is caused by serotypes D – K of *C. trachomatis.* Their natural habitat is genital tract of both males and females.

Adult inclusion conjunctivitis (paratrachoma) is most prevalent in sexually active young people and is spread from genitalia to eye. It was known as "**swimming pool conjunctivitis**" as infection was associated with bathing in community swimming pools which get contaminated with *Chlamydia* from the genital secretions of bathers. The disease is characterized by follicular hypertrophy with mucopurulent discharge. The disease is usually self-limited and do not lead to blindness.

Chlamydial **ophthalmia neonatorum** (inclusion blenorrhoea) develops in infants, characterized by swelling of eyelids, hyperemia and a purulent infiltration of the conjunctiva. In untreated cases secondary bacterial infections may cause damage to eyes and may develop pneumonia. The source of infection is the infected genital tract of mother, and the child is infected during passage through the birth canal.

Non-genococcal (nonspecific urethritis)

In men, *C. trachomatis* is a common cause of non-gonococcal urethritis, a term used to describe urethral inflammation that is caused by a microorganism other than *Neisseria gonorrhoeae*. Symptoms of non-genococcal urethritis are similar to gonorrhoea–painful urination and mucopurulent discharge from urethra.

Lymphogranuloma venereum (LGV)

It is a sexually transmitted disease caused by *C. trachomatis* serotypes L_1, L_2 and L_3. It has a world wide distribution but is more common in tropical areas.

LGV proceeds through three phases—(1) The primary lesion is a painless ulcer on external genitalia, which heals quickly and leaves no scar. (2) The secondary phase begins two to six weeks after exposure due to spread and multiplication of chlamydiae in regional lymph nodes, which become enlarged and tender, called "**buboes**". (3) In untreated cases, fibrotic changes and abnormal lymphatic drainage occurs that produces fistulas, urethral and rectal strictures.

Psittacosis

It is a worldwide infectious disease of psittacine birds (parrots) that is transmissible to humans. Now, the disease is recognized in other birds–pigeons, chickens, ducks and turkeys – and the general term "**ornithosis**" is used.

It is caused by *Chlamydia psittaci*. Humans acquire this infection either by handling infected birds or by inhalation of dried aerosols of birds feces or nasal droppings. Thus ornithosis may be seen as an occupational hazard.

After entering the respiratory tract, chlamydiae spread to liver and spleen. They multiply within these cells and then invade the lungs causing inflammation, hemorrhage and pneumonia.

Acute Respiratory disease

It is caused by *Chlamydia pneumoniae* TWAR strain. It is first isolated from Taiwan (TW) from a case of acute respiratory (AR) disease and therefore designated as TWAR strain. It appears to be a common cause of respiratory disease in older children and adults world-wide.

LABORATORY DIAGNOSIS

The specimens collected are conjunctival scrapings, sputum, throat swab, bubo pus, genital swabs and blood.

(1) Demonstration of inclusion bodies—smears may be prepared from conjunctival scrapings or bubo pus and stained by Giemsa, Castaneda, Machiavello or Giminez stains to demonstrate

characteristic inclusion bodies under light microscope. *C. trachomatis* inclusions can be stained with iodine, as they possess a glycogen matrix.

(2) Demonstration of antigen—Chlamydial antigens may be detected in smears by staining with Fluorescent-antibody technique. ELISA test can also detect chlamydial antigens.

(3) Cultivation—

(*i*) Chlamydiae can be isolated by inoculating specimens into the yolksac of 6-8 day old embryonated eggs.

(*ii*) Chlamydiae can be propagated in experimental animals such as mice. Chlamydiae differ in their infectivity to mice. *C. psittaci* strains infect mice by intracerebral, intranasal, intraperitoneal and subcutaneous routes. Among *C. trachomatis* strains, only the LGV serotypes infect mice when injected intracerebrally. The TRIC serotypes do not infect mice by any route, though they can kill mice injected intravenously due to toxic effect.

(*iii*) The most widely used method of cultivation is by the use of tissue cultures. Monkey kidney cell lines, McCoy and HeLa cell lines are commonly used. Cell cultures used for isolation are pretreated by irradiation or chemicals such as 5-iodo-2-deoxyuridine or cycloheximide to enhance replication of chlamydiae. The viral growth is detected by demonstration of inclusion bodies.

(4) Demonstration of antibodies by serological tests—*C. psittaci* produces high levels complement fixing antibody in serum from patients. To detect species-specific and serotype-specific antibody, the micro-immunofluorescence (micro-IF) test is used with antigens from all chlamydial strains.

(5) DNA probes—In certain chlamydial infections, it may not be possible to isolate viable organisms. In such cases either an antigen detection method or a DNA probe has to be used for diagnosis. DNA probes are highly valuable in trachoma and chlamydial infections of the rectum.

(6) Intradermal test (**Frei's test**)—It was widely used for the diagnosis of Lymphogranuloma venereum to detect delayed hypersensitivity. The antigen (**Lygranum**) is prepared from infected yolksac, purified by fractional centrifugation and inactivated by heat or phenol.

The antigen is inoculated intradermally on the forearm (0.1 ml) and a control from uninfected yolksac on the other forearm. A positive reaction is indicated by an inflammatory nodule appearing at the test site in 2 days and reaching a maximum in 4-5 days, measuring atleast 7 mm in diameter. Frei test becomes positive 2-6 weeks after infection and remains positive for several years perhaps for life. The antigen is group specific and false positive reactions occur in other chlamydial infections.

TREATMENT

The antibiotics of choice are tetracycline in adults and erythromycin in babies. Penicillin should not be used as it is chlamydiastatic.

QUESTIONS

Essay Questions

1. Give an account of Chlamydiae.

Short Notes

1. Classify chlamydiae
2. Life cycle of chlamydiae
3. HP bodies/Inclusion bodies
4. LGV
5. TRIC agents
6. Trachoma
7. Inclusion conjunctivitis
8. Frei's test
9. Cultivation of chlamydiae
10. Morphology of chlamydiae

PART-IV

MEDICAL VIROLOGY

79

General Properties of Viruses

- *Introduction*
- *Structure, Shape, Size*
- *Hemagglutination, HI, Elution*
- *Viral replication*
- *Virus purification*
- *Virus assays*
- *Viral genetics*
- *Cultivation of viruses—Animals, Embryonated eggs, Tissue cultures*
- *Detection of virus growth in cell cultures*
- *Classification of viruses–DNA viruses, RNA viruses*
- *Unconventional viruses—Viroids, Prions*

INTRODUCTION

The term **"virus"** is a latin word for poison or venom. Viruses do not have cellular organization and contain only one type of nucleic acid, either DNA or RNA but never both. They are obligate intracellular parasites. They lack the enzymes necessary for protein and nucleic acid synthesis and are dependent on host cells for replication. They have no metabolic activity outside the living cells. They replicate by a complex process and not by binary fission. They are not affected by antibacterial antibiotics. They cannot grow in inanimate media. Viruses occupy an intermediate position between the living and nonliving.

STRUCTURE

Structurally mature, infections virus particle is called "**virion**". The virion consists of a nucleic acid core, surrounded by a protein coat, the **capsid**. The capsid with the enclosed nucleic acid is known as **nucleocapsid**. The capsid protects the nucleic acids from nucleases and other harmful agents in the environment. The capsid is composed of a large number of capsomers, composed of polypeptide molecules. The capsomers are arranged symmetrically to form a shell around the nucleic acid corc. Three types of symmetry are encountered in the capsid, **icosahedral (cubical)**, helical and complex (Fig. 79.1).

An icosahedron is a polygon with 12 vertices or corners and 20 triangular facets or sides *e.g.*, Adenovirus. Two types of capsomers constitute the icosahedral capsid. They are the pentagonal capsomers at the vertices, known as pentons and the hexagonal capsomers making up the facets, called hexons. There are always 12 pentons but the hexons may vary.

In **helical symmetry**, the **capsomers** and nucleic acid are wound together to form a helical or spiral tube. The tube may be rigid as in the tobacco mosaic virus but in the case of animal viruses, the tubular nucleocapsid may be coiled on itself.

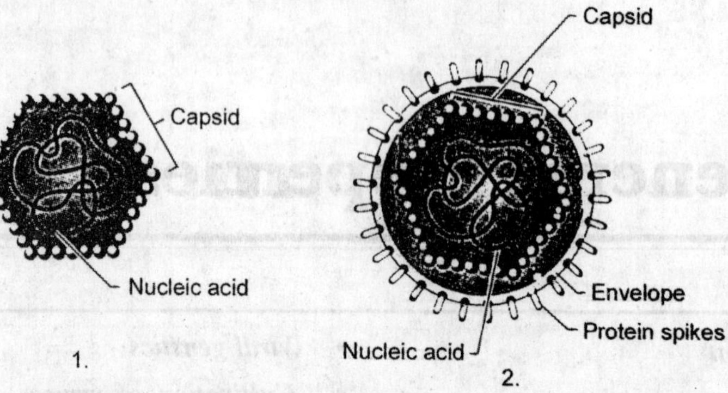

Fig. 79.1 General structure of virus 1 nonenveloped virus, 2 enveloped virus

Some virus particles do not exhibit icosahedral or helical symmetry and exhibit a complex symmetry as in poxviruses.

Virions may be enveloped or nonenveloped. **Envelope** is lipoprotein in nature. The lipid portion of envelope is derived from host cell membrane when the progeny virus is released by budding, while the protein is virus coded.

On the surface of the envelope, protein subunits may be present as projecting spikes, called **peplomers**. A virus may possess more than one type of peplomer. Influenza virus carries two types of peplomers—the triangular **hemagglutinin** spike and mushroom shaped **neuraminidase.**

Envelopes confer chemical, antigenic and biological properties on viruses. Enveloped viruses are susceptible to the action of lipid solvents like ether, chloroform and bile salts. Antibodies to the surface antigens can cause specific neutralization of virus infectivity. Biological properties such as adsorption to host cell surface or hemagglutination depend on the cell envelope.

Some viruses possess additional structural features. For example, fibrils protrude from the vertices of adenovirus particles.

Viruses contain only one type of nucleic acid, either single or double stranded DNA or RNA. Viral nucleic acids may be extracted by treatment with detergents or phenol.

The overall shape of the virus particle varies in different viruses. Most animal viruses are roughly spherical. The rabies virus is bullet shaped, poxviruses are brick shaped and Ebola virus is filamentous, the tobacco mosaic virus is rod shaped.

Viruses vary widely in size. The smallest viruses (Parvovirus) measure 20 mm and largest virus (Poxvirus) measure 300 nm. Small size and ability to pass through filters that hold bacteria are classic attributes of viruses. The following methods are used for determining the sizes of viruses.

1. Electron microscopy is the most widely used method for estimating virus size.
2. By passing viruses through membrane filters of graded porosity; the average pore diameter of the filter that permits the passage of the virion gives an approximate estimate of its size.
3. By ultracentrifugation, the virus particle size can be calculated from the rate of sedimentation by using stoke's law.

HEMAGGLUTINATION

Several viruses agglutinate erythrocytes from different species (Table 79.1). Hemagglutination by the influenza virus is due to the presence of hemagglutinin spikes on the surface of the virus. Hemagglutination can be used for the detection and assay of influenza virus in cultural fluids. Since the inactivated virus also hemagglutinates, hemagglutination can also be used for titration and assay of killed influenza vaccines. When erythrocytes are added to serial dilutions of viral suspension, the highest dilution that produces hemagglutination provides **hemagglutination titre**. The test can be carried out in test tubes or special plastic trays. Erythrocytes which are not agglutinated settle at the bottom in the form of a "button", while the agglutinated cells are seen spread into a shield-like pattern.

Table 79.1 Characteristics of Hemagglutination by Viruses

Virus	*Erythrocyte species and other conditions*
Influenza virus	Fowl, human, guinea pig, others; Elution at 37°C
Parainfluenza, mumps, NDV	Fowl, human, guinea pig, others; Elution at 37°C: Hemolysin present
Measles	Monkey, 37°C
Togavirus—several groups of Arbovirus	Goose, pigeon, one day old chick; pH and temperature critical
Rubella	Goose, pigeon, one day old chick: 4°C
Enterovirus, some Coxsackie and ECHO serotypes	Human; 4°C and 37°C
Rhinovirus, some serotypes	sheep; 4°C
Rabies	Goose: 4°C, pH 6.2
Reovirus	Human: 37°C

Hemagglutination can be inhibited by its specific antibody. This is known as **Hemagglutination Inhibition (HI)**. This HI test can be used for detection and quantitation of antibody to virus.

The influenza virus also carries on its surface another peplomer, the enzyme neuraminidase which acts on the receptor and destroys it. Neuraminidase is, therefore, called, "Receptor Destroying Enzyme (RDE)". Destruction of the receptor leads to the reversal of hemagglutination and the release of the virus from the red cell surface. This is known as "**elution**". This is an enzymatic reaction and takes place optimally at 37°C. RDE is produced by many microorganisms (*e.g.*, cholera vibrios) and is also present in many vertebrate cells. Hemagglutination and elution help in purifying and concentrating the virus.

VIRAL MULTIPLICATION (REPLICATION)

The genetic information necessary for viral replication is contained in the viral nucleic acid, but lacks biosynthetic enzymes and therefore depends on the synthetic machinery of the host cell for replication. The viral multiplication proceeds in six sequential phases.

1. Adsorption

Virions may come in contact with the cells by random collision and virus attaches on specific receptor sites on susceptible host cells. In the case of Influenza virus, the hemagglutinin gets attached to glycoprotein receptors on respiratory epithelium. Destruction of the receptor sites by RDE prevents adsorption. In AIDS, the human immunodeficiency virus attaches to CD4 receptor on host cells with surface gp120.

2. Penetration

After adsorption virus particles may be engulfed by a mechanism resembling phagocytosis, a process known as "**viropexis**". In the case of enveloped viruses, the viral envelope may fuse with the plasma membrane of the host cell and release the nucleocapsid into the cytoplasm.

3. Uncoating

The process of stripping the virus of its outer layers and capsid so that the nucleic acid is released into the cells is known as uncoating. With most viruses, uncoating is effected by the action of lysosomal enzymes of the host cell.

4. Biosynthesis

This phase includes the synthesis of viral nucleic acid, capsid protein and enzymes required in the various stages of viral synthesis, assembly and release. Biosynthesis consists of the following steps.

(*i*) Transcription of mRNA form the viral nucleic acid.

(*ii*) Translation of the mRNA into "**early proteins**" or enzymes which initiate and maintain synthesis of virus components. They may also induce shutdown of host protein and nucleic acid synthesis.

(*iii*) Replication of viral nucleic acid.

(*iv*) Synthesis of "**late proteins**" or "structural proteins, which are the components of daughter virion capsids.

Baltimore classified viruses into six classes based on their replication mechanisms (Table 79.2).

Table 79.2 Baltimore Classification of Viruses based on Replication

Class	*Characteristics*
I	Viruses have double-stranded DNA genome. In this class the designation of (+) and (–) is not meaningful, since different *m*RNA species may be synthesized from either strand.
IIa	Viruses have a single-stranded DNA genome of the same sequence as *m*RNA
IIb	Viruses have DNA complementary to *m*RNA. Before the synthesis of *m*RNA can proceed, the DNA must be converted to a double stranded form.
III	Viruses have a double-stranded RNA genome. All known viruses of this type have segmented genomes, but *m*RNA is synthesized on only one strand of each segment.
IV	Viruses have a single-stranded RNA genome of the same sequence as *m*RNA. Synthesis of a complementary strand precedes synthesis of *m*RNA.
V	Viruses have a single-stranded RNA genome which is complementary in base sequence to the *m*RNA
VI	Viruses have a single-stranded RNA genome and have a DNA intermediate during replication.

5. Maturation

The viral nucleic acid and capsid components assemble to form daughter virions. The assembly takes place in either the nucleus (herpes and adenoviruses) or cytoplasm (picorna and pox viruses). At this stage, the nonenveloped viruses are present intracellularly as fully developed virions but in the case of enveloped viruses, only the nucleocapsid is complete. Envelopes are derived form the host cell membrane during the process of budding and with the incorporation of virus coded proteins.

6. Release

In the case of bacterial viruses, the daughter virion are released by the lysis of the host bacterium. But in animal viruses, release occurs without host cell lysis, by budding from the cell membrane over a period of time. The exception is poliovirus, which is released by host cell lysis and causes damage to the host. Progeny virions are released into the surrounding medium and may infect other cells.

From the stage of penetration till the appearance of mature daughter virions, the virus cannot be demonstrated inside the host cell. This period is known as "**eclipse phase**".

Abnormal Replicative Cycles

1. Incomplete viruses

Some daughter virions that are produced may not be infective due to defective assembly. They are known as "incomplete viruses" usually seen in large numbers when cells are infected with a high dose of the influenza virus. The virus yield will have a high hemagglutinin titre but low infectivity. This is known "**Von Magnus phenomenon**".

2. Abortive infection

Virus infection in some cells does not lead to production of infectious progeny. In such cell, the viral components may be synthesized but maturation or assembly is defective, and either no release occurs or the progeny is noninfectious. This is known as abortive infection.

3. Defective viruses

Viruses which are genetically deficient and therefore incapable of producing infectious daughter virions without the helper activity of another virus are known as "defective viruses". *e.g.*, Hepatitis D virus and adeno-associated satellite viruses which replicate only in the presence of their helper viruses-hepatitis B and adenoviruses respectively. Similarly, Rous Sarcoma viruses (RSV) replicates only in the presence of helper virus avian leukosis virus.

VIRUS PURIFICATION

Pure viruses are necessary to study their properties and molecular biology. The starting material is usually large volumes of tissue culture medium, body fluids or infected cells. The first step frequently involves concentration of the virus particles by precipitation with ammonium sulfate, ethanol or polyethylene glycol or by ultrafiltration. Hemagglutination and elution can be used to concentrate orthomyxoviruses. Once concentrated, virus can then be separated from host materials by differential centrifugation, density gradient centrifugation, column chromatography and electrophoresis.

VIRAL ASSAYS (QUANTITATION OF VIRUSES)

The quantity of viruses in a sample can be determined either by counting particle numbers or by measurement of the infectious unit concentration.

(*i*) *Counting virus particles (physical methods).* Virus particles can be counted directly in the electron microscope by comparison with a standard suspension of latex particles. Hemagglutination assay is an accurate and rapid method for determining the quantity of viruses such as Influenza virus.

(*ii*) *Assay of infectivity (Biological methods).* Infectivity assays are of two types—quantitative and quantal assays.

Quantitative Assays

They measure the actual number of infectious particles in the inoculum. The most widely used assay is **plaque assay**. Monolayers of host cells are inoculated with suitable dilutions of virus and after adsorption are overlaid with medium containing agar or carboxymethyl cellulose to prevent virus spreading throughout the culture. After several days, each infectious virus particle produces a small area of infection, known as "plaque" or "**plaque forming unit (PFU)**", which can be counted macroscopically (Fig. 79.2). Therefore, a count of plaques produced at a particular dilution will give the number of infectious virions or PFUs, and the concentration of infectious units in the original sample can be calculated.

$$\text{PFU/ml} = \frac{\text{Average number of plaques}}{\text{Volume of inoculum} \times \text{dilution}}$$

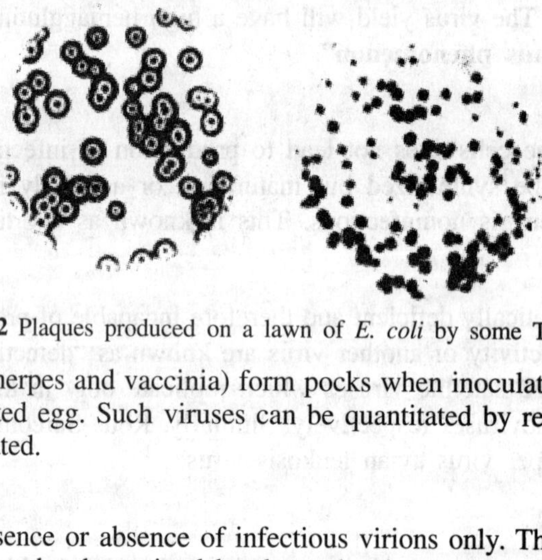

Fig. 79.2 Plaques produced on a lawn of *E. coli* by some T phages

Certain viruses (*e.g.*, herpes and vaccinia) form pocks when inoculated on to the chorioallantoic membrane of an embryonated egg. Such viruses can be quantitated by relating the number of pocks to the viral dilution inoculated.

Quantal Assays

They indicate the presence or absence of infectious virions only. The amount of virus required to cause disease or death can be determined by the end point method. Cell cultures or animals are inoculated with serial dilutions of a virus suspension. The titer is expressed as the 50% infectious dose (ID_{50}), which is the reciprocal of the dilution of virus that produces the effect in 50% of the cells or animals inoculated.

VIRAL GENETICS

Viruses are continuously changing as a result of genetic selection. They undergo subtle genetic changes through mutation and major genetic changes through recombination.

Mutations

The mutation rates of DNA viruses approximate those of eukaryotic cells (10^{-8} to 10^{-11}), yielding one mutant virus in several hundred to many thousand genome copies. RNA viruses have much higher mutation rates, perhaps one mutation per virus genome copy. Mutations can be lethal, neutral or favorable. Only mutations that do not interfere with essential virus functions can persist in a virus population.

Mutations can produce viruses with new antigenic determinants. The appearance of an antigenically novel virus through mutation is called **antigenic drift**. Antigenically altered viruses may be able to cause disease in previously resistant or immune hosts.

Mutations can produce viruses with a reduced pathogenicity, altered host range, or altered target cell specificity but with intact antigenicity. Such viruses can sometimes be used as vaccine strains.

Recombination. Recombination involves the exchange of genetic material between two related viruses during coinfection of a host cell.

Recombination by independent assortment can occur among viruses with segmented genomes. Genes that reside on different pieces of nucleic acid are randomly assorted. This can result in the generation of viruses with new antigenic determinants and new host ranges. Development of viruses with new antigenic determinants through independent assortment is called **antigenic shift**.

Recombination also occurs between genes residing on the same piece of nucleic acid. Genes that generally segregate together are called linked genes. If recombination occurs between them, the linkage is said to be incomplete. Recombination of incompletely linked genes occurs in several viruses.

Development of viruses with new antigenic determinants by either type of recombination may allow viruses to infect and cause disease in previously immune hosts.

Vaccine strains of viruses can be used to create recombinant viruses that carry extra genes coding for a specific immunogen.

Non Genetic Interaction Among Viruses

When two or more viruses infect the same host cell, they may interact in a variety of ways.

1. Complementation

It refers to the interaction of viral gene products in cells infected with two viruses, one or both of which may be defective. It results in the replication of one or both under conditions in which replication would not ordinarily occur. The basis for complementation is that one virus provides a gene product in which the second is defective, allowing the second virus to grow. The genotypes of the two viruses remain unchanged. If both mutants are defective in the same gene product, they will not be able to complement each other's growth.

2. Phenotypic mixing

When two different viruses multiply in a cell, some "mix up" may take place during assembly, so that the nucleic acid of one virus may be surrounded by a capsid belonging partly or entirely to other virus. This is known as "phenotypic mixing". In phenotypic mixing, when the nucleic acid of one virus is surrounded by the entire capsid of the other virus, it is known as "phenotypic masking" or "**transcapidation**". Such mixing is not a stable variation, because, upon replication, the phenotypically mixed parent will yield progeny encased in the capsids homologous to the genotype.

3. Interference

Infection of cell cultures (or whole animals) with two viruses often leads to an inhibition of multiplication of one of the viruses, an effect called interference. Several mechanisms have been postulated as causes of infection

(*i*) One virus may inhibit the ability of second virus to adsorb to the cell, either by blocking its receptors (retroviruses, enteroviruses) or by destroying its receptors (orthomyxoviruses).

(*ii*) One virus may compete with the second for components of the replication apparatus.

(*iii*) The first virus may cause the infected cell to produce an inhibitor (interferon) that prevents replication of the second virus.

When interference occurs between unrelated viruses, it is called heterologous interference. When it occurs between related viruses, it is called homologous interference.

Interference has been used as a basis for controlling outbreaks of infection with virulent strains of poliovirus by introducing into the population an attenuated poliovirus that interferes with the spread of the virulent virus.

4. Genotypic mixing

It occurs when more than one complete genomes are incorporated and surrounded by a single virus capsid. Since, there is no recombination between the different genomes, two kinds of viral progeny are formed on cultivation.

CULTIVATION OF VIRUSES

Viruses are cultivated in order to isolate and produce them in quantity for study or for the production of vaccines. As viruses are obligate intracellular parasites, they cannot be grown on inanimate culture media. There are three main ways of cultivating animal viruses: in living animals, in embryonated chicken (duck) eggs, and in cell cultures.

(i) Animals

Animal inoculation is a good diagnostic tool to determine whether a virus will cause infection. The animal will exhibit typical disease symptoms, and sections of infected tissue can be examined microscopically for evidence of infection. Studies of host immune responses to a viral infection also demand the use of living animals.

In the laboratory, mice, rabbits guinea pigs, ferrets and nonhuman primates are usually used. **Infant (suckling) mice** are very susceptible to Coxsackie and Arboviruses. The animals may be inoculated by several routes—subcutaneous, intraperitoneal, intracerebral or intranasal. The growth of the virus in inoculated may be indicated by death, disease or visible lesions.

Using animals for the cultivation of viruses has disadvantages immunity may interfere with viral growth and animals may harbor several latent viruses and bacteria.

(ii) Embryonated Eggs

The most economical and convenient methods for cultivating viruses is the use of the fertilized, embryonated chicken (duck) eggs (incubated for 6 to 8 days after laying). The discovery that viruses could be cultivated by this simple technique was made by Good pasture (1931). The shell surface of embryonated chicken eggs is first disinfected with iodine. The virus can be inoculated using a needle and syringe, through a hole drilled in the shell. After inoculation, the drill hole is sealed with gelatin or transparent tape and the eggs are incubated at 36°C for 2 to 3 days to allow the viruses multiply.

Chick embryos contain several kinds of cells and tissues in which various viruses will replicate. By using embryos of different ages, different methods of inoculation into different tissues within the egg (Fig. 79.3), it is possible to cultivate the type of virus desired.

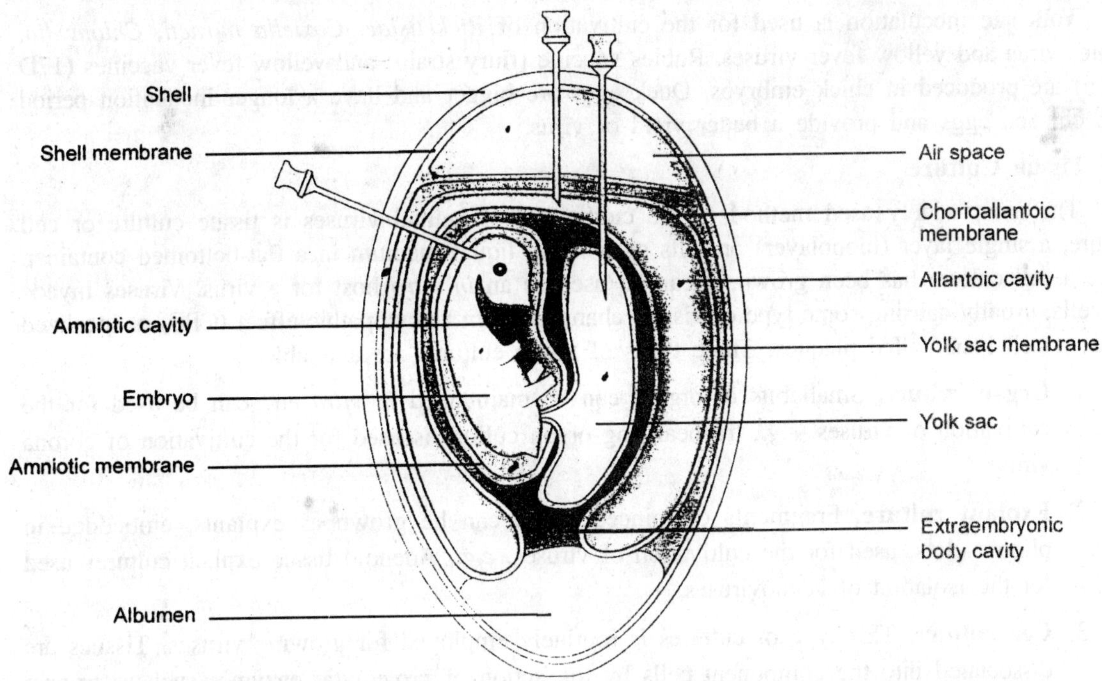

Fig. 79.3 Diagrammatic representation of a section through an embryonated hen's egg 10 to 12 days old. The hypodermic needles show the routes of inoculation of the yolk sac, allantoic cavity, and embryo (head)

Inoculation on to **chorioallantoic membrane (CAM)** can be used to cultivate herpesvirus, smallpoxvirus (variola), vaccinia, myxoma virus, Rous sarcoma virus and eastern equine encephalitis virus. The viruses such as variola, vaccinia and herpes produce a very distinct type of lesions on CAM called "**pocks**" due to their multiplication. Different viruses produce pocks with different morphology. Under optimal conditions, each infectious virus particle can form one pock. Therefore, pock counting can be used for the assay of pock-forming viruses (Fig. 79.4).

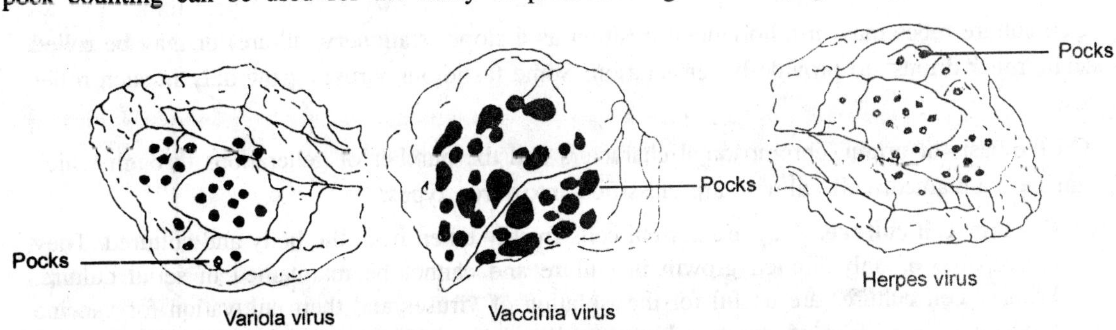

Fig. 79.4 Pock lesions on chorioallantoic membrane

Inoculation into **amniotic cavity** is used for the primary isolation of Influenza virus and mumps virus.

Inoculation into **allantoic cavity** is used for the cultivation of influenza virus for vaccine production. Most viruses that can replicate in amniotic cavity can also multiply in allantoic cavity after adaptation.

Yolk sac inoculation is used for the cultivation of *Rickettsiae, Coxiella burneti, Chlamydia*, Rabies virus and yellow fever viruses. Rabies vaccine (flury strain) and yellow fever vaccines (17D strain) are produced in chick embryos. Duck eggs are bigger and have a longer incubation period than chicken eggs and provide a better yield of virus.

(iii) Tissue Culture

The most widely used method of the cultivation of animal viruses is tissue culture or cell culture, a single layer (monolayer) or cells growing in liquid medium in a flat-bottomed container. Once a cell culture has been grown, it can be used as an *in vitro* host for a virus. Viruses invade the cells, usually causing some type of visible change known as cytopathic effect (CPE) or localized areas of cell lysis called plaques. Three types of tissue cultures are available.

1. **Organ culture.** Small bits of organs can be maintained *in vitro* and can be used for the cultivation of viruses. *e.g.*, tracheal ring organ culture is used for the cultivation of corona virus.
2. **Explant culture.** Fragments of minced tissue can be grown as explants, embedded in plasma clots, used for the cultivation of viruses. *e.g.*, Adenoid tissue explant cultures used for the isolation of adenoviruses.
3. **Cell culture.** This type of cultures is routinely employed for growing viruses. Tissues are dissociated into the component cells by the action of proteolytic enzymes such as trypsin and mechanical shaking. The cells are washed, counted and suspended in a growth medium. The growth medium consists of essential amino acids, vitamins, salts, glucose, buffer (bicarbonate in atmosphere containing about 5% carbondioxide) in physiological quantities and supplemented with 5% fetal calf serum. Antibiotics are added to prevent bacterial contamination and phenol red as indicator. This growth medium will enable most cell types to multiply. The cell suspension is dispensed in bottles, tube or petri dishes. The cells adhere to the glass surface and on incubation, divide to form a confluent monolayer sheet of cells within a week.

Cell culture tubes may in a horizontal position as a slope (stationary culture) or may be rolled in special "roller drums" to provide better aeration. Some fastidious viruses grow only in such roller cultures.

On the basis of origin, chromosomal characters and the number of generations through which they can be maintained, cell cultures are classified into three types.

(*a*) **Primary cell culture.** They are normal cells freshly taken from the body and cultured. They are capable of only limited growth in culture and cannot be maintained in serial culture. Primary cell cultures are useful for the isolation of viruses and their cultivation for vaccine production. *e.g.*, Rhesus monkey kidney cell cultures, Human amnion cell culture, chick embryo fibroblast cell culture.

(*b*) **Diploid cell strains.** They are cells of a single type that retain the original diploid chromosome number and Karyotype during serial subcultivation for a limited number of times. After about fifty serial passages, they undergo "senescence". Diploid strains developed form human fibroblasts are susceptible to a wide range of human viruses and very useful for the isolation of some fastidious pathogens. They are also used for the production of viral vaccines. *e.g.*, Human embryonic lung cell strain (WI-38), Rhesus embryo cell strain (HL-8).

(*c*) **Continuous cell lines.** They are cells of a single type, usually derived from cancer cells, capable of continuous serial cultivation indefinitely. Cell lines derived from human cancers have been used for many years. These cell lines may be maintained by serial subcultivation or stored in the cold (–70°C) for use when necessary. Some cell lines are now permitted to prepare vaccines (vero cell line for rabies vaccine).

e.g., HeLa (human carcinoma of cervix cell line)

HEP-2 (human epithelioma of larynx cell line)

KB (human carcinoma of nasopharynx cell line)

McCoy (human synovial carcinoma cell line)

Detroit-6 (sternal marrow cell line)

Vero (vervet monkey kidney cell line)

BHK-21(Baby Hamster kidney cell line)

Change C/I/L/K (Human conjunctiva (C), Intestine (I), Liver (L) and Kidney (K) cell line).

DETECTION OF VIRUS GROWTH IN CELL CULTURES

Virus growth in cell cultures may be detected by following methods.

. Cytopathic effect (CPE)

Viruses when grown in cell cultures cause visible morphological changes, called the cytopathic effect. These changes can be readily observed by microscopic examination of the cultures (Fig.79.5). Viruses producing CPE are known as cytopathogenic viruses, those that do not produce CPE are called noncytopathogenic viruses. The CPE may have different appearances, depending on the particular virus and the type of cells in the culture and help the presumptive identification of viruses.

e.g., Measles virus and Respiratory syncytial virus produce syncytium with multinucleated gaint cells.

Enteroviruses produce rapid CPE with crenation of cells and degeneration of the entire cells sheet.

Adenoviruses produce large granular clumps resembling bunches of grapes.

Herpesviruses produce discrete focal degeneration.

SV_{40} produces prominent cytoplasmic vacuolation.

Picornavirus growth leads to nuclear pyknosis, rounding, refractile and degeneration.

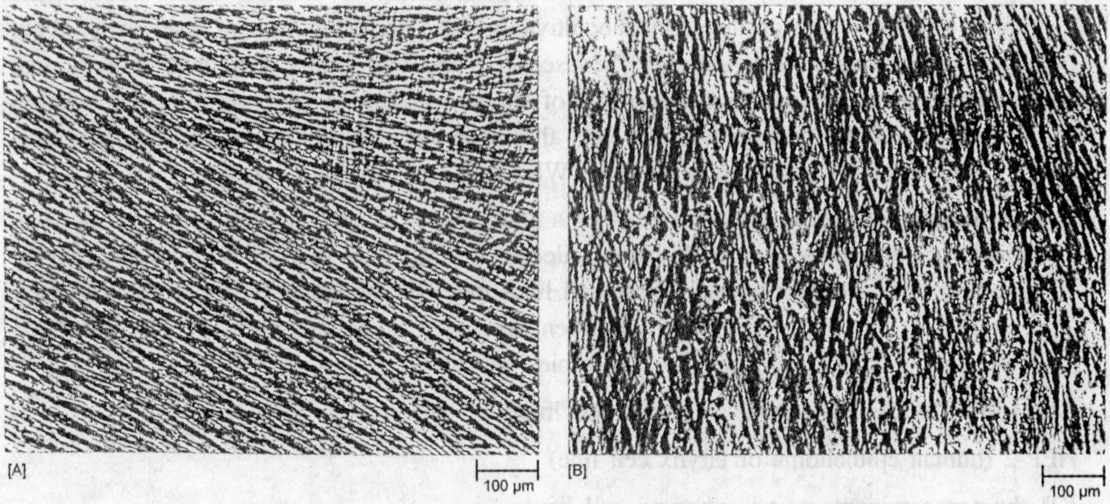

Fig. 79.5 Light-microscopic view of tissue culture used for the cultivation of viruses. [A] Normal human lung fibroblast cell culture. [B] Human lung fibroblast cell culture infected with adenovirus type 3. Note the characteristic cytopathic effect (CPE): rounded and enlarged cells

2. Hemadsorption

Ceratin viruses, when they infect cells in a culture, render the surface of those cells adsorptive for red blood cells, known as hemadsorption. This hemadsorption phenomenon is particularly helpful in the case of parainfluenza and mumps viruses which cause little or no CPE. Hemadsorption may be specifically inhibited by antiserum and can be of value in identification of certain myxoviruses. Influenza virus produces a CPE with hemadsorption in chick embryo fibroblast monolayer cell culture.

3. Interference

The growth of a noncytopathogenic virus in cell culture can be tested by subsequent challenge with a known cytopathogenic virus. The growth of the first virus (noncytopathogenic) will inhibit infection by second virus (cytopathogenic) by interference *e.g.*, Rubella virus infection in HeLa is detected by using a challenge virus ECHO 11. Interference is used as basis to control poliomyelitis with virulent strains by introducing attenuated strains.

4. Transformation

Oncogenic viruses induce cell transformation and loss of contact inhibition so that growth appears in a piled-up fashion producing microtumours.

5. Immunofluorescence

Cells from virus infected cultures can be stained with fluorescent conjugated antibody and examined under the UV microscope for the presence of virus antigen. This method gives positive results earlier than other methods and, therefore finds wide application in diagnostic virology.

6. Electron Microscopy

Viruses can be detected by electron microscopic examination of ultra thin sections of infected cells.

CLASSIFICATION OF VIRUSES

The oldest classification of viruses is based on the diseases they produced and the site affected. Thus human viruses were classified as

(*i*) Dermotropic viruses producing skin lesions *e.g.*, smallpox, chickenpox, measles.

(*ii*) Neurotropic viruses affecting central nervous system *e.g.*, rabies, poliomyelitis.

(*iii*) Pneumotropic viruses affecting the respiratory tract *e.g.*, Influenza, common cold.

(*iv*) Viscerotropic viruses affecting visceral organs *e.g.*, hepatitis, yellow fever.

The International committee for Taxonomy of viruses has developed a uniform classification system based on physical, chemical and biological characteristics (nucleic acid type, nucleic acid strandedness, the sense-positive or negative of ssRNA genomes, presence or absence of an envelope, and the host virus family names and in *viridae*; subfamily names, in *virinae*; and genus (and species) names, in *virus*. Based on the nucleic acid type viruses are classified into riboviruses containing RNA and Deoxyriboviruses containing DNA (Fig. 79.6).

DNA Viruses

1. Family Poxviridae

Large, brick shaped or ovoid viruses containing dsDNA and envelope. Multiplication and maturation takes place in the cytoplasm. They possess complex structure enclosing one or two lateral bodies and a biconcave core with all enzymes required for mRNA synthesis. All poxviruses tend to produce skin vision *e.g.*, smallpox (variola) viruses, vaccinia virus, molluscum contagiosum.

2. Family Herpesviridae

A large family of medium sized viruses containing linear dsDNA. The nucleocapsid has icosahedral symmetry with 162 capsomers and is surrounded by a lipid containing envelope. Multiplication takes place in the nucleus and maturation by budding though the nuclear membrane. Latent infections may lost for the life span of the host. Some are oncogenic, *e.g.*, Herpes simplex virus type 1 and 2, varicella-zoster virus, Epstein-Barr virus, cytomegalovirus and human herpes viruses 6, 7 and 8.

3. Family Adenoviridae

They are medium sized, nonenveloped viruses exhibiting icosahedral (cubic) symmetry, with 252 capsomers. Fibers protrude from the vertex capsomers. The genome is linear, double-stranded DNA. Replication occurs in the nucleus *e.g.,* Adenovirus.

4. Family Papovaviridae

They are small (40–55 nm), nonenveloped, icosahedral particles with 72 capsomers. It contains covalently closed, circular dsDNA. Replicates and assembles in the nucleus. They are oncogenic. *e.g.,* Papilloma virus, polyomavirus, Simian vacuolating virus (SV_{40}), JC virus, BK virus.

5. Family Parvoviridae

They are very small (18–26 nm) viruses. They are nonenveloped particles with icosahedral symmetry having 32 capsomers. The genome is linear, single-stranded DNA. Replication occurs in the nucleus. *e.g.,* Parvovirus, B19 virus (Erythrovirus), Adeno-associated virus.

6. Family Hepadnaviridae

They are small (40–48 nm), enveloped viruses containing a 27 nm icosahedral nucleocapsid. The envelope contains lipid and the viral surface antigen. The surface protein is characteristically overproduced during replication of the virus, which takes place in the liver, and is shed into the blood stream. They contain a circular dsDNA, which contains a large single-stranded gap. Replication involves repair of the single-stranded gap in the DNA, transcription of RNA and reverse transcription of the RNA to make genomic DNA. *e.g.*, Hepatitis B virus.

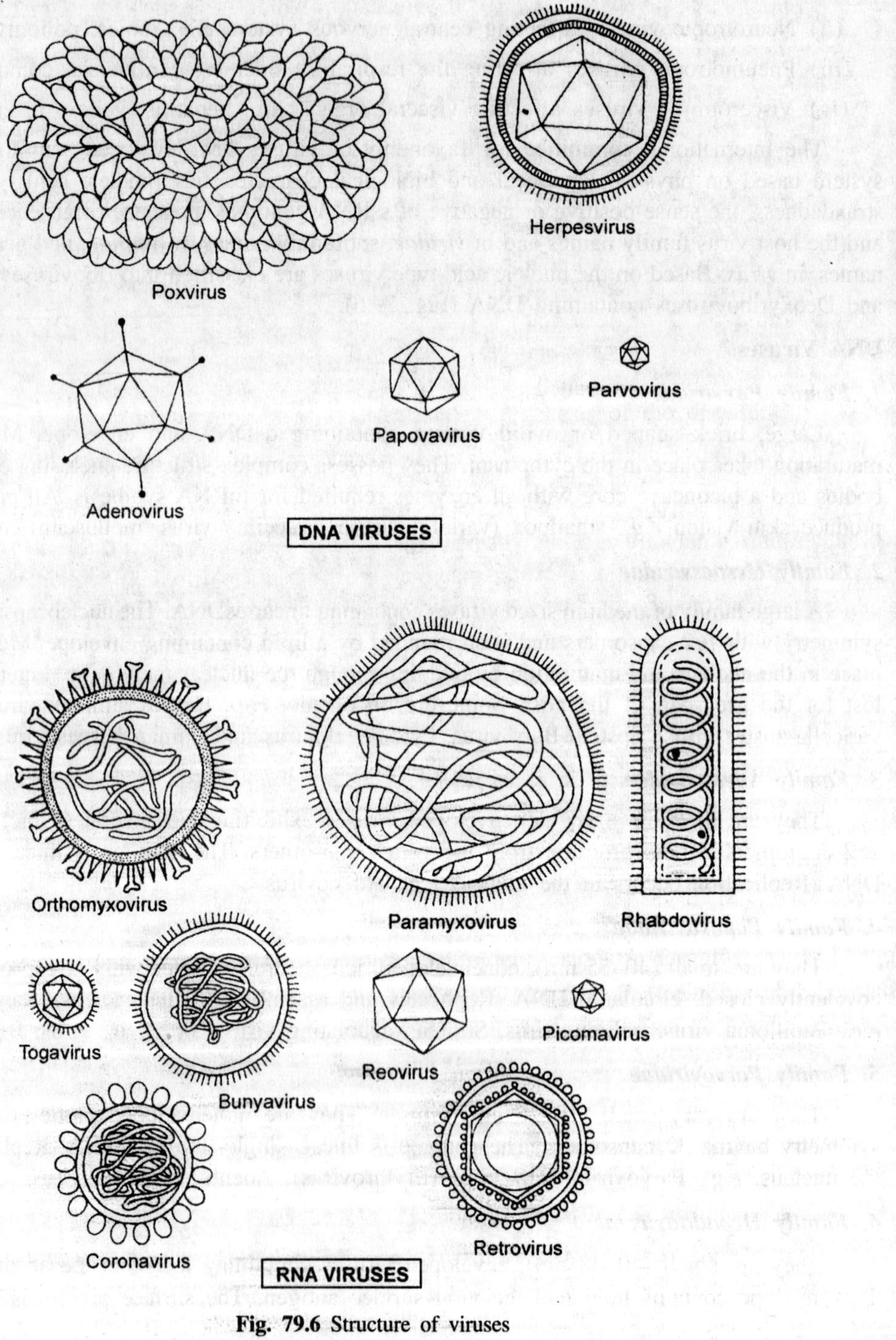

Fig. 79.6 Structure of viruses

RNA Viruses

All RNA viruses, except calicivirus are enveloped, and except reoviridae, all have a single stranded genome.

1. Family Picornaviridae

They are small (28–30 nm), ether-resistant viruses exhibiting icosahedral symmetry. The RNA genome is single-stranded and positive sense *i.e.*, it can serve as an mRNA *e.g.*, Enteroviruses (Poliovirus, Coxsackievirus and Echovirus), Rhinoviruses, and *Hepatovirus* (Hepatitis A virus).

2. Family Orthomyxoviridae

They are medium sized (80–120 nm), spherical or elongated enveloped viruses carrying hemagglutinin and neuraminidase peplomers. The genome is linear, segmented (8 pieces), negative sense, ssRNA. During replication, the nucleocapsid is assembled in the nucleus, whereas the hemagglutinin and neuraminidase accumulate in the cytoplasm. The virus matures by budding at the cell membrane. All orthomyxoviruses are Influenza viruses that infect humans or animals.

3. Family Paramyxoviridae

Similar to but larger (150–300 nm) than orthomyxoviruses. Particles are pleomorphic and enveloped. Envelope carries surface projections (spikes). The internal nucleocapsid measures 13–18 nm and contains linear, single stranded, nonsegmented, negative sense RNA. Both the nucleocapsid and hemagglutinin are formed in the cytoplasm. In contrast to orthomyxoviruses, paramyxoviruses are genetically stable. *e.g.*, Genus *Paramyxovirus* consisting of New Castle disease virus, mumps virus and parainfluenza virus; Genus *Morbilivirus* containing measles virus; Genus *pneumovirus* containing respiratory syncytial virus.

4. Family Togaviridae

They are spherical viruses, 40–70 nm in size, with a lipoprotein envelope and are ether sensitive. Their genome is single-stranded, positive sense RNA. They replicate in cytoplasm and mature by budding from host cell membranes. *e.g.*, Many Arboviruses, called Alphaviruses (Eastern, Western, Venezuelan equine encephalitis viruses, Ross river virus, Sindbis virus, Semiliki forest virus and Rubella virus, which has no arthropod vector belong to this group.

5. Family Flaviviridae

Enveloped viruses, 45–60 nm in diameter, containing single-stranded, positive sense RNA. Mature virions accumulate within cisternae of the endoplasmic reticulum and bud from ER. This group of Arboviruses includes yellow fever virus and dengue viruses. Most members are transmitted by blood sucking arthropods. Hepatitis C virus has no vector.

6. Family Bunyaviridae

They are spherical or pleomorphic, 80 to 120 nm enveloped particles. The genome is made up of a triple-segmented, circular, single-stranded, negative sense RNA. Virion particles contain three circular, helically symmetric nucleocapsids about 2.5 nm in diameter. Replication occurs in the cytoplasm and an envelope is acquired by budding from the Golgi membranes. Majority of these are Arboviruses and are transmitted to vertebrates by arthropods. *e.g.*, Bunyavirus, Hantavirus, Nairovirus, Phlebovirus.

7. Family Arenaviridae

Spherical or pleomorphic, enveloped viruses, 50–300 nm, containing a number of host cell ribosomes which gives the particles a "sandy" appearance. (Hence the name arena meaning sand in

Latin). Replication occurs in the cytoplasm and buds from plasma membrane. The genome is circular, segmented, single-stranded RNA that is negative sense. All Arenaviruses pathogenic for humans cause chronic infections in rodents *e.g.,* Lymphocytic choriomeningitis (LCM) virus, Lassa fever virus, tacaribe virus and Junin virus.

8. Family Rhabdoviridae

Enveloped virions resembling a bullet, flat at one end and round at the other, measuring about 75×180 nm. It has 5–10 nm spikes. The genome is linear, single-stranded, nonsegmented, negative sense RNA. Replicate in cytoplasm and buds from plasma membrane. *e.g.,* Vesiculovirus (vesicular stomatitis virus), Lyssavirus (Rabies virus).

9. Family Reoviridae

They are medium sized (60–80 nm), ether-resistant, nonenveloped viruses having icosahedral symmetry. Particles have two or three protein shells (capsids) with channels extending from the surface to the core. The genome is linear, double-stranded, segmented (10 to 12 pieces) RNA. Replication occurs in the cytoplasm; genome segment reassortment occurs readily. *e.g.,* Rotavirus, colorado tick fever virus (Orbivirus) and Reovirus.

10. Family Coronaviridae

Spherical or pleomorphic, enveloped, 80–130 nm particles containing positive sense, unsegmented ssRNA. The nucleocapsid is helical. They have petal or club shaped surface projections arranged in a fringe like a solar corona (Hence the name). Replication takes place in the cytoplasm and buds from Golgi apparatus and Endoplasmic reticulum. *e.g.,* Coronavirus, Torovirus.

11. Family Retroviridae

(Re = reverse; tr = transcriptase) They are spherical, enveloped viruses, 80–100 nm in diameter. The genome contains two copies of linear, positive-sense, ssRNA of the same polarity as viral mRNA. Particles have an icosahedral capsid. The virion contains a reverse transcriptase enzyme that produces a DNA copy of the RNA genome. This DNA becomes circularized and integrated into host chromosomal DNA. The virus is then replicated from the integrated "provirus" DNA copy. Virion assembly occurs by budding on plasma membranes. Three subfamilies are recognized: (*a*) Oncovirinae—the RNA tumor virus group (*b*) Spumivirinae—the foamy virus group, and (*c*) Lentivirinae—Visna and Maedi viruses, HIV1 and 2.

12. Family Caliciviridae

They are nonenveloped, icosahedral, 35 to 40 nm particles having 32 cup shaped (calyx like) depressions. The genome is positive sense, ssRNA. *e.g.,* Norwalk virus, Hepatitis E virus.

13. Family Filoviridae

They are enveloped, pleomorphic viruses that may appear very long and thread-like. They are 80 nm width and about 1000 nm long. The envelope contains large peplomers. The genome is linear, negative sense ssRNA. The nucleocapsid is helical. This family contains the Marburg and Ebola viruses causing human hemorrhagic fevers.

UNCONVENTIONAL VIRUSES (DEFECTIVE VIRUSES)

Viroids

Viroids are small nucleic acid (RNA) molecules without a protein coat. Viroids are agents that do not fit the definition of classic viruses. They are small infectious agents that cause diseases of plants. Viroids are single-stranded, covalently closed circular RNA molecules consisting of about 360 nucleotides and comprising a highly base-paired rod like structure and are sensitive to nucleases.

Prions

Prions are proteinaceous infectious particles. They possess a small protein particle without any nucleic acid and are sensitive to proteases. Degenerative neurologic disorders such as kuru or cruetzfeldt-Jakob disease or scrapie of sheep have been shown to be caused by these unconventional slow viruses called prions.

QUESTIONS

Essay Questions

1. Describe the general characters of viruses.
2. Describe the isolation and identification of viruses.
3. Describe the classification of viruses.
4. Give an account of cultivation of viruses.

Short Notes

1. Nucleocapsid.
2. Capsid.
3. Viral hemagglutination.
4. Hemagglutination inhibition reaction.
5. Elution.
6. Neuraminidase.
7. Enumerate the stages in viral replication.
8. Name four methods of virus purification.
9. What is plaque assay ? List two uses of it.
10. Phenotypic mixing.
11. Define viral interference and give one example.
12. Cultivation of viruses.
13. Suckling mice.
14. Tissuc cultures.
15. Cell cultures.
16. Diploid cell lines.
17. Continuous cell lines.
18. HeLa cell lines.
19. Cytopathic effect.
20. Hemadsorption.
21. Interference.
22. Unconventional viruses.
23. Prions.
24. Viroids.

80

Virus-Host Interactions

- *Effects of Viral Infection on Host Cells*
- *Pathogenesis of Viral Infections*
- *Host Responses to Viral Infections*

EFFECTS OF VIRAL INFECTION ON HOST CELLS

Virus-host interactions may cause different effects, ranging from no apparent cell damage to rapid cell destruction.

(*i*) Cytocidal Infections

Virus-host cell interactions may produce cytocidal or cytolytic infection, in which production of progeny virus kills (lysis) the host cell. The first effects of the replication of cytocidal viruses are morphological changes known as **cytopathic effect (CPE)**. Some viruses cause characteristic cytopathic effects which may help in the identification of viruses as a diagnostic tool. *e.g.*,

Table 80.1 Cytopathic Effects of Some Viruses

Cytopathic Effect	*Examples*
Cell rounding	Most viruses, Adenoviruses
Syncytium (multinucleated giant cells)	Herpesviruses, parainfluenza viruses
Pyknotic (cells shrivel up)	Polioviruses
Ballooning of cells	Herpesviruses
Nuclear chromatic changes	Adenoviruses, Herpesviruses
Vaculoization of cytoplasm	Measles (rubeola) virus

A characteristic histological feature in virus infected cell is the appearance of **inclusion bodies.** These inclusion bodies are intracellular structures (crystalline aggregates of virions) with distinct size, shape, location and staining properties that can be demonstrated in virus infected cells under the light microscope (Fig. 80.1). They may be situated in the cytoplasm (*e.g.*, Rabies virus, Poxviruses), nucleus (*e.g.*, herpesviruses) or both (*e.g.*, Measles virus). They are generally acidophilic (stained by eosin) and appear as pink structures. Some are basophilic (stained by hematoxylin) and appear as purple colored structured (*e.g.*, Adenoviruses). Demonstration of inclusion bodies often helps in the diagnosis of some viral infections. For example, the presence of intracytoplasmic eosinophilic inclusions (Negri bodies) in the brain cells of animals confirms presumptive diagnosis of rabies. Vaccinia infected cells show rather smaller, multiple inclusions known as Guarnieri bodies. In fowl pox, large inclusions called Bollinger bodies are found. In molluscum contagiosum, inclusion bodies (molluscum) bodies are very large and can be seen under the low power microscope. Cowdry (1934) classified **intranuclear inclusions** into two types. Cowdry type A inclusions are of variable size and granular appearance (*e.g.,* Herpes virus, Yellow fever virus), while type B inclusions are more circumscribed and often multiple (*e.g.,* Adenovirus, poliovirus).

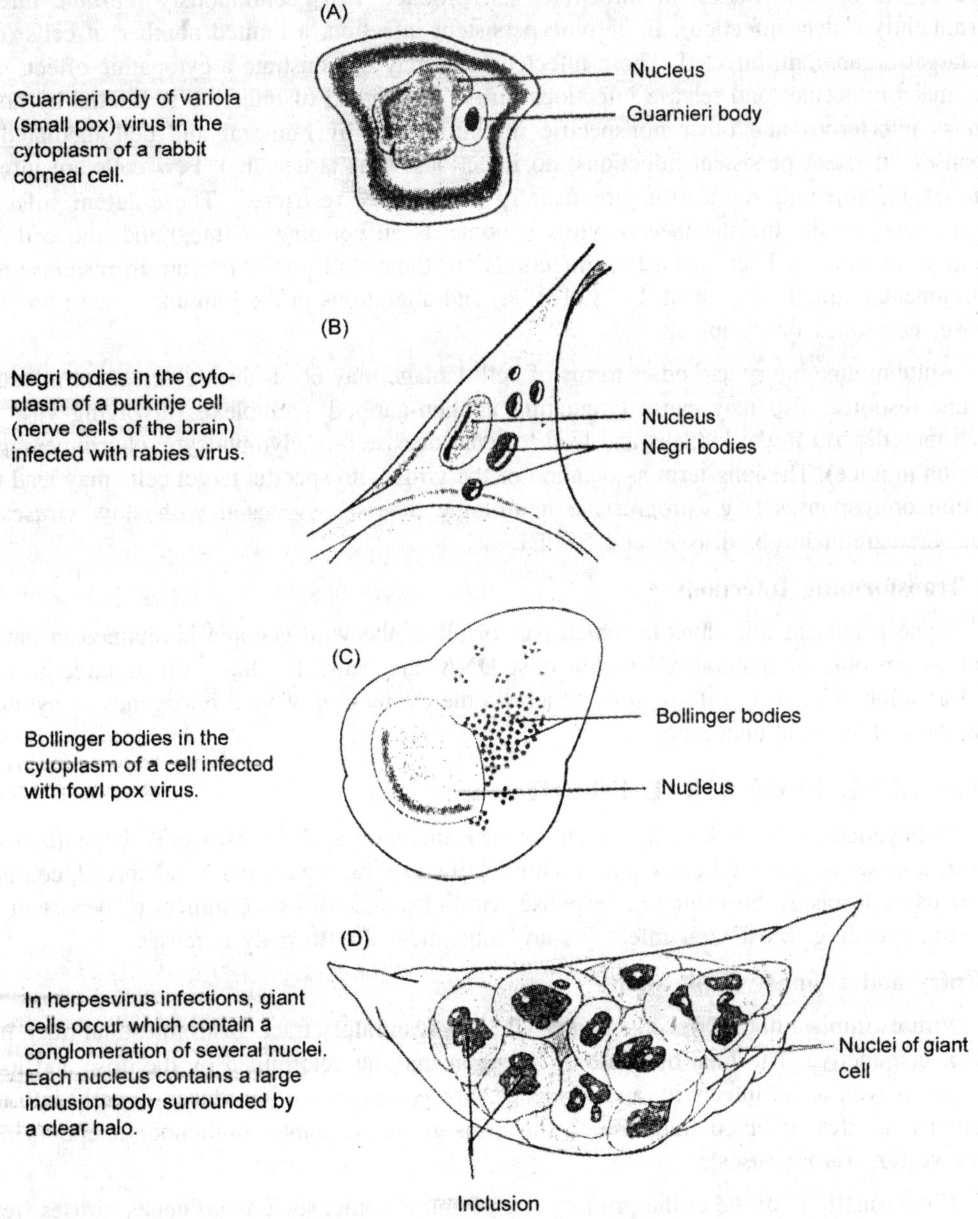

Fig. 80.1 Viral inclusion bodies

The interaction of virus and host cell may result in rapid changes in the cell membranes, including movement of ions and the metabolism of cyclic nucleotides such as cAMP and cGMP. Viruses often inhibit the synthesis of host cell macromolecules including DNA, RNA and proteins. Expression of viral genes may alter the biologic functioning of infected cells. Alterations of cellular genetic material occur following some viral infections including chromosome damage.

(*ii*) Persistent Infections

In a persistent infection the virus is not eliminated from all of the host tissues after the acute phase of the disease. Persistent infections can produce virus continuously (chronic infection) or intermittently (latent infection). In chronic persistent infection, a limited number of cells (often in a few target organs) are infected. These infected cells may demonstrate a cytopathic effect, synthesize virus macromolecules and release infectious virus. The spread of infection is limited by host factors such as interferons and other nonspecific inhibitors and by humoral and cell mediated immune responses. In latent persistent infections, no infectious virus is detected. Few cells are infected, and virus expression and replication are usually completely restricted. These latent infections are characterized by the maintenance of virus genome as an episome or integrated into cellular DNA. Important features of latent persistent infections are their ability to reactivate in response to various environmental stimuli (*e.g.*, heat, UV radiation) and alterations in the immune system brought on by disease, hormones or chemicals.

Autoimmune injury and other forms of cell damage may occur during persistent infections. The immune response also may cause circulating antigen-antibody complexes involving viral antigens, which may deposit in the kidneys and lead to renal disease (*e.g.*, lymphocytic choriomeningitis virus infection in mice). The long-term association of the virus with specific target cells may lead to altered function or responses (*e.g.*, progressive neurologic disease associated with slow viruses such as Kuru, Creutzfeldt-Jacob, disease and SSPE).

(*iii*) Transforming Infections

Some persistent infections in which part or all of the viral genome is retained in the host cell either as episome or integrated into the host DNA can cause the host cell to undergo oncogenic transformation. Viruses transform cells either via the expression of viral oncogenes or by altering the expression of cellular oncogenes.

PATHOGENESIS OF VIRAL INFECTIONS

Pathogenesis is the process by which the virus infection leads to disease. Pathogenic mechanisms of viral disease include viral entry into the host, primary viral replication, viral spread, cellular injury, cell or tissue tropisms, host immune response, viral clearance or establishment of persistent infection and viral shedding. Most viral infections are subclinical due to body defenses.

(*i*) Entry and Primary Replication

Viruses implant onto host cells mainly via skin, respiratory tract, gastrointestinal tract, urogenital tract or conjunctiva. The final outcome of infection may be determined by the dose and location of the virus as well as its infectivity and virulence. Some viruses are introduced directly into the blood stream by needles or blood transfusions (hepatitis B virus, human immunodeficiency virus or by insect vectors (arboviruses).

Virus usually replicate at the primary site of entry. Some, such as influenza viruses (respiratory infections) and rotaviruses (gastrointestinal infections), produce disease at the portal of entry.

(*ii*) Viral Spread and Cell Tropism

After primary replication at the site of entry, viruses spread within the host via the blood stream or lymphatics. The presence of virus in the blood is called viremia. Virions may be free in the plasma or associated with a particular cell types. Viruses may enter target organs by multiplying in endothelial cells or fixed macrophages or diffusing through gaps and being carried in leukocytes. Dissemination via nerves usually occurs with rabies virus and sometimes with herpesvirus and poliovirus infections.

The incubation period is the time between exposure to virus and onset of disease. During this, usually asymptomatic period, implantation, local multiplication and spread occur.

Most viruses display tissue specificity or tropism, which is determined by cell receptors for virus, the ability of cell to support virus replication, physical barriers, local temperature, pH and oxygen tension, and digestive enzymes and bile in the gastrointestinal tract that may inactivate some viruses. Viral spread may be determined in part by specific viral genes.

(*iii*) Cell Injury and Clinical Illness

Destruction of virus-infected cells in the target tissues and physiologic alterations produced in the host by the tissue injury are responsible for the development of disease or death. Direct cell damage and death may result from disruption of cellular macromolecular synthesis, diversion of the cell's energy and competition of viral mRNA for cellular ribosomes. Clinical illness from viral infection is the result of a complex series of events. Inapparent (subclinical) infections by viruses are very common.

(*iv*) Recovery from Infection

The host either succumbs or recovers from viral infection. Recovery mechanisms involve humoral and cell-mediated immunity, interferon and other cytokines, and other host defense factors.

(*v*) Virus Shedding

The last stage in pathogenesis is the shedding of infectious virus into the environment, for the maintenance of viral infection among host population. Shedding occurs usually through respiratory tract and digestive tract. For Arboviruses blood and lymph are shedding sites. Saliva is the primary source of shedding for rabies virus. The genital tract is a common site of shedding for herpesvirus type 2.

(*vi*) Congenital Infections

Infection of the fetus as a target organ is special case of infection. The immune and interferon systems of the young fetus are immature. The rapidly developing fetal organs are highly vulnerable especially during the first trimester or pregnancy. Susceptibility to virus replication may be modulated by the fetal cells and by hormonal changes during pregnancy. The virus multiplication in the fetus may lead to congenital anomalies or fetal death, but the mother may have only a mild or inapparent infection. Cytomegalovirus and Rubella viruses are the most common causing congenital anomalies.

HOST RESPONSES TO VIRAL INFECTION

The outcome of a virus infection is influenced by the virulence of the infecting strain and the resistance offered by the host. Immunity to viral infection is caused by a variety of nonspecific or specific mechanisms.

Nonspecific Defenses

Most viral infections are limited by nonspecific defenses, which act sooner than specific defenses.

(i) Anatomic Barriers

Anatomic barriers are located at body surfaces (skin and mucosa) or within the body (endothelial cells and basement membranes). They are partly effective in preventing virus spread but may be breached by large numbers of virus, by trauma, by increased permeability, by replication of virus in endothelial cells or by transportation of virus in leukocytes.

(ii) Nonspecific Inhibitors

Body fluids and tissues normally contain soluble viral inhibitors. They vary chemically and include lipids, polysaccharides, proteins, lipoproteins and glycoproteins. These nonspecific inhibitors may act by preventing viral attachment or by inactivating viruses and some act intracellularly. In the gastrointestinal tract, some susceptible viruses are inhibited by acid, bile salts and enzymes.

(iii) Phagocytosis

Viruses may be phagocytosed to different degrees by neutrophils and macrophages. The effect of phagocytosis may be virus inactivation, persistence or multiplication. Consequently, the result may be clearance of virus, transportation to distant sites or enhanced infection.

(iv) Fever

Replication of most viruses is reduced by even a modest rise in temperature. During viral infection, fever can be induced by atleast three endogenous pyrogens: interleukin-1, interferon and tumor necrosis factor. Fever also augments the generation of cytotoxic T lymphocytes.

(v) Inflammation

The local inflammation resulting from viral infection activates several metabolic, physicochemical changes which may interfere with virus multiplication through elevated local temperature, reduced oxygen tension, metabolic alterations and acid production.

(vi) Viral Interference and Interferon

Generally, infection by one virus renders host cells resistant to other, superinfecting viruses. This phenomenon is known as interference. Interference is usually mediated by the host cell protein interferon. Usually, interferon is produced at about the same time as the viral progeny are released by the infected cell, thus protecting neighboring cells from the spreading virus. Secreted interferon binds to cells and causes them to block various stages of viral replication. Interferon also inhibits growth of some normal and tumor cells and many intracellular parasites such as rickettsiae and protozoa. It also modulates the immune response and promotes cell differentiation. There are three main types of interferon—alpha, beta and gamma which differ both structurally and antigenically. Alpha interferon is produced mainly by leucocytes other than T lymphocytes, beta interferon by epithelial cells and fibroblasts and gamma interferon by T lymphocytes.

Specific Immune Defenses

Both humoral and cell mediated immune responses are involved in control of viral infections. The activation, duration and magnitude of the immune response depend on how the virus interacts with host cells and on how the virus spreads

Viruses and/or virus-infected cells can stimulate B lymphocytes to produce antibody, specific for viral antigens that neutralizes virus either by direct binding with the virus or by lysis of infected cells by complement. Antibody neutralization is most effective when virus is present in large fluid spaces (*e.g.*, serum) or on moist surfaces (*e.g.*, the gastrointestinal and respiratory tracts). Humoral immunity protects and host against reinfection by the same virus. This is the basis for viral vaccine programs.

Virus-infected or virally transformed cells activate strong cell mediated immune responses. For some viral infections, cell mediated immune reactions may be more important than antibody in early termination of viral infection and prevention of dissemination within the host. The cell mediated immune response involves the recognition and/or killing of virus and virus-infected cells by cytotoxic T lymphocytes, natural killer (NK) cells and macrophages, and the production of cytokines by these cells when stimulated by virus or virus-infected cells.

Some viruses infect and damage cells of the immune system (*e.g.,* HIV). Adverse effects of the immune response to viral infection are also known. Immune mediated disease may develop in certain virus infections in which hypersensitivity to viral antigens persist for a long period. Another potential adverse effect of the immune response is the development of autoantibodies. Another type of immunopathologic disorder was observed in humans immunized with killed measles vaccine.

Viruses have evolved a variety of ways that serve to suppress or evade the host immune response and thus avoid being eradicated.

Thus, the early nonspecific responses limit virus multiplication during the acute phase of virus infections. The later specific immune responses eliminate virus at the end of the acute phase, and subsequently to maintain specific resistance to reinfection.

QUESTIONS

Short Notes

1. Viral inclusions.
2. Virus-host interactions.

81

Laboratory Diagnosis, Prophylaxis and Chemotherapy of Viral Diseases

- ***Lab. diagnosis of Viral Infections***
  - ***— Microscopy***
  - ***— Demonstration of Virus Antigen***
  - ***— Isolation of Virus***
  - ***— Detection of Specific Antibody***
  - ***— Molecular Techniques***
- ***Prophylaxis of Viral Diseases (Viral Vaccines)***
  - ***— Killed Virus Vaccines***
  - ***— Live Attenuated Virus Vaccines***
- ***Antiviral Chemotherapy***
- ***Interferons***

LABORATORY DIAGNOSIS OF VIRAL INFECTIONS

The following methods are employed in the laboratory for the diagnosis of viral diseases.

1. Microscopy
2. Demonstration of virus antigen
3. Isolation of virus
4. Detection of specific antibody
5. Molecular techniques

It is necessary that the appropriate specimens should be collected and transported to the laboratory. Specimens can be refrigerated for up to 24 hours or frozen (at – 60°C) if there is a delay in processing. However, in case of blood sample, the serum must be separated before freezing.

Table 81.1 Types of Specimens collected and Associated Viruses

Specimens	*Viruses present*
Nasopharyngeal aspirates, throat swab, sputum	Influenza virus, Rhinoviruses, Respiratory syncytial virus, Parainfluenza viruses, Adenoviruses
Feces	Poliovirus, Coxsackievirus, Echoviruses, Hepatitis A virus, Rotavirus, Adenoviruses

Urine	Cytomegalovirus, Measles virus, Mumps virus, Adenovirus
Conjunctival swabs/scrapings	Adenoviruses
Corneal swabs	Rabies virus
Ulcer/pustular scrapings	Herpes simplex virus, Varicella-zoster virus, Molluscum contagiosum
CSF	Arboviruses (encephalitis), Rubella virus, Herpes simplex virus, Rabies virus
Blood	Hemorrhagic fever viruses, Cytomegalovirus, Lymphocytic choriomeningitis (LCM) virus, Lassa fever virus

1. Microscopy

(a) Light Microscopy

Inclusion bodies in tissue sections may be detected by light microscope. *e.g.,* Negri bodies in Rabies, molluscum bodies (Henderson-Peterson) in molluscum contagiosum, Guarnieri bodies in small pox, owl's eye inclusions in cytomegalovirus infections, Torres bodies in yellow fever.

(b) Electron Microscope

The detection of virus by electron microscopy is being used increasingly. *e.g.,* the detection of Rotavirus and Hepatitis A virus in fecal samples.

(c) Immune Electron Microscopy

The sensitivity of electron microscopy can be increased by mixing specific antiserum with specimen to aggregate the virus particles. These aggregates (antigen-antibody complexes) can be sedimented by centrifugation, negatively stained and observed under electron microscope.

(d) Fluorescent Microscopy

Direct or indirect fluorescent antibody technique can be used to detect viruses or viral antigens in vesicle fluid, in cell cultures, or in frozen tissue sections. Fluorescence microscopy of brain biopsy can be used for the diagnosis herpes simplex encephalitis, subacute sclerosing panencephalitis (SSPE) and for the diagnosis of rabies in the brain smears of animals suspected to be rabid. This method is also useful for the rapid diagnosis of respiratory infections caused by paramyxoviruses, orthomyxoviruses, adenoviruses and herpesviruses.

2. Demonstration of Virus Antigen

In cases where virus antigen is abundant in the lesions, it can be demonstrated by serological tests such as ELISA, RIA, CIEP, immunofluorescence and precipitation in gel.

3. Isolation of Virus

Viruses can be isolated from clinical samples in laboratory animals, embryonated chicken eggs and cell cultures. The methods of cultivation and their identification are described in the first chapter of virology. Demonstration of rise in titre of antibodies to the viral isolate in the patient during the course of the disease reinforces the significance of the isolation.

4. Detection of Specific Antibodies

The demonstration of a rise in titre of antibodies in paired sera to a virus during the course of a disease is a strong evidence of its etiology. For this, a sample is collected early in the course (acute phase) of the disease and the 'convalescent' sample collected 10-14 days later. Examination of a single sample of serum for antibodies may not be meaningful except when IgM specific tests are done. The generally used serological tests are hemagglutination inhibition (HI), CFT, neutralisation tests, Immunofluorescence, RIA and ELISA.

5. Molecular Techniques

Molecular techniques detect viral genetic material. They are very sensitive and specific.

(a) Polymerase Chain Reaction (PCR)

By using this technique, viral nucleic acid sequence can be amplified at least 1,00,000 fold in just a few hours. Thus viral DNA extracted from a very small number of virions or infected cells (in picogram quantities) can be amplified to the point where it can readily be identified using labelled DNA probes or restriction fragment length polymorphism (RFLP). For the detection of viral RNA, it is first converted into DNA by reverse transcriptase. PCR can be used for the diagnosis of infections caused by human immunodeficiency virus, human T cell lymphotropic virus-1 (HTLV-1), cytomegalovirus, human papilloma viruses, herpes simplex viruses, hepatitis B virus, hepatitis C virus, hepatitis D virus, hepatitis E virus, rubella virus, Epstein-Barr virus, Varicella-zoster virus, human herpes viruses 6 and 7, paravovirus B19, enteroviruses, Coxsackieviruses, echoviruses, rhinoviruses, measles virus and rotavirus.

(b) Hybridization and Molecular Probes

Labelled DNA or RNA probe complementary to a specific region within the viral genome is used indifferent hybridization tests. For example, *in situ* hybridization for detecting viral nucleic acid in fixed biopsy specimens, Southern-blot and Northern-blot hybridization for detection of DNA and RNA, respectively in the serum and body fluids. After hybridization, the labelled probes, which are either radioisotope labelled or enzyme labelled can be detected by autoradiography and immunofluorescence or enzyme immunoassay, respectively.

PROPHYLAXIS OF VIRAL DISEASES (VIRAL VACCINES)

Prolonged and effective immunity is a characteristic feature of most viral infections. Viral vaccines also confer solid protection and are, in general, more effective than bacterial vaccines. Viral vaccines may be live or killed. Live vaccines are more effective than killed vaccines.

Killed-Virus Vaccines

Killed-virus vaccines have been prepared by inactivating viruses with heat, phenol or formalin. Killed vaccines have the advantages of stability and safety and can be given in combination as polyvalent vaccines. There is also no danger of spread of the virus from the vaccine. The disadvantages are the immunity conferred is often brief and must be boosted with multiple injections, the local immunity and cell mediated immunity are not induced.

Attenuated Live-virus Vaccines

Live-virus vaccines have been developed by attenuating strains (yellow fever vaccine), from temperature sensitive (t_s) mutants (influenza vaccine), by recombination (influenza vaccine) or by plaque selection (sabin vaccine for poliomyelitis).

Attenuated live-virus vaccines have the advantage of acting like natural infection *i.e.,* they multiply in the host and tend to stimulate long-lasting antibody mediated and cell mediated immune responses and to induce antibody production and resistance at the portal of entry (local immunity). Some of them can be given as combined vaccines (MMR vaccine).

The disadvantages of attenuated live-virus vaccines include the risk, however remote, of reversion to virulence, the vaccine may be contaminated with potentially dangerous (oncogenic) viruses; interference by preexisting viruses may sometimes prevent a good immune response and live-virus vaccines are usually heat labile and should be preserved under strict refrigeration.

Passive Immunization

Passive immunity is conferred by administering antibodies formed in another host. Passive immunization with human gammaglobulin, convalescent serum or specific immunoglobulin gives temporary protection against many viral diseases such as measles, mumps and infectious hepatitis. Combined active and passive immunization is an established method for the prevention of rabies.

Subunit Vaccines

They are prepared by splitting the virus with detergents or other chemicals and incorporating the relevant antigens in the vaccine.

Recombinant vaccines

Vaccines are produced by cloning the desired antigen in bacteria or yeast by genetic engineering, e.g., hepatitis B vaccine, rabies vaccine.

Table 81.2 Viral Vaccines

Disease	*Type of vaccine*	*Mode of preparation*
Poliomyelitis	Live	Avirulent strains grown in monkey kidney cell culture
	Killed	Virulent strains grown in monkey kidney cell culture, formalin-killed
Rabies	Killed (Semple type)	Fixed virus grown in sheep brain and inactivated by phenol or beta propiolactone
	Killed	Virus grown in cell culture and inactivated with beta propiolactone
Yellow fever	Live (17D)	Attenuated virus grown in chick embryos and lyophilised
Japanese encephalitis	Killed	Virus grown in mouse brain and inactivated by formalin
Varicella	Live	Attenuated virus grown in chick embryo fibroblast culture
Mumps	Live	Attenuated virus grown in human diploid cell culture
Influenza	Killed (subunit)	Virus disintegrated with sodium deoxycholate
	Live (attenuated)	Virus attenuated by serial passage in eggs
	Live (mutant)	*ts* mutants which are avirulent
	Live (recombinant)	recombinants with surface antigens of new strains and growth characters of established strains
Measles	Live	Attenuated virus grown in tissue culture
Rubella	Live	Attenuated virus grown in tissue culture
Hepatitis B	Cloned subunit	HBsAg cloned in yeast

ANTIVIRAL CHEMOTHERAPY

Antiviral drugs specifically inhibit one or more steps of virus replication such as adsorption, penetration, uncoating, viral nucleic acid synthesis as well as viral protein synthesis, without causing unacceptable side effects. Commonly used antiviral drugs to treat viral diseases are amantadine and rimantadine (Influenza A virus), ribavirin (respiratory syncytial virus), idoxuridine and trifluridine (topical treatment of herpetic keratitis), vidarabine and acyclovir (systemic treatment of herpes simplex and varicella-zoster viruses) ganciclovir (cytomegalovirus), and retrovir (human immunodeficiency virus).

Limitations of antiviral drugs include a narrow antiviral spectrum, ineffectiveness against the latent virus, development of drug-resistant mutants, and side effects. To overcome these limitations of current antiviral drugs, more effective compounds are being developed that allow greater inhibition of viruses, greater selectivity for virus-specific functions, and fewer side effects and avoid induction of resistant mutants.

Table 81.3 Major Antiviral Drugs used for of Viral Infections

Drug	*Viral spectrum*
VIRAL POLYMERASE INHIBITORS	
Acyclovir	Herpes simplex, Varicella-zoster
Cidofovir	Cytomegalovirus, Herpes simplex
Foscarnet	Herpes viruses, HIV-1, HBV
Ganciclovir	Cytomegalovirus
Valacyclovir	Herpes viruses
Vidarabine	Herpes viruses, Vaccinia, HBV
HIV PROTEASE INHIBITORS	
Indinavir	HIV-1, HIV-2
Ritonavir	HIV-1, HIV-2
Saquinavir	HIV-1, HIV-2
REVERSE TRANSCRIPTASE INHIBITORS	
Lamivudine	HIV-1, HIV-2, HBV
Nevirapine	HIV-1
Stavudine	HIV-1, HIV-2
Zidovudine (azidothymidine, AZT)	HIV-1, HIV-2, HBV
Zalcitabine (dideoxycytidine, ddc)	HIV-1, HIV-2, HBV
Didanosine (dideoxyinosine, ddl)	HIV-1, HIV-2
BLOCKING OF VIRAL UNCOATING	
Amantadine	Influenza virus A
BLOCKING OF CAPPING OF mRNA	
Ribavirin	Respiratory syncytial virus, Influenza viruses A and B, Lassa fever

INTERFERONS (IFNs)

Interferons are host-coded proteins of the large cytokine family that inhibit viral replication. They are produced by intact animals or cultured cells in response to viral infection (or viral infected cells) or other inducers. They are body's first line of defense against viral infection and modulate humoral and cell mediated immunity.

Interferons were first discovered by Isaacs and Lindeman (1957). They found that virus-infected cells can elaborate a protein substance called interferon, which, when added to normal cells in culture, protects them from viral infection.

Interferons are a group of glycoproteins that do not have direct action on viruses. They are species specific. Their activity is not virus specific. Interferon induced by one virus is effective against many other viruses. Their production can be increased by increasing the temperature up to 40°C and decreased by steroids and increased oxygen tension. They are sensitive to the action of proteolytic enzymes but resist destruction by nucleases and lipases. They are resistant to heat at 56°C for up to one hour. They are non-dialysable. Interferon production is also induced by bacterial endotoxins, and certain synthetic polycarboxylic acids, apart from viral infections.

Interferons are classified into three antigenically and chemically distinct types—alpha (α), beta (β) and gamma (γ) interferons.

Alpha interferons (IFN-α) are produced by leucocytes being coded by atleast 15 genes in the human genome. There are 20 subtypes of alpha interferon. They are resistant to low pH.

Beta interferon (IFN-β) is produced by fibroblasts and epithelial cells and are coded by one or a few genes. They are resistant to low pH (stable at pH 2.0). It has only one subtype.

Gamma interferon (IFN-γ) is produced by T lymphocytes and Natural Killer (NK) cells coded one or a few genes. It is not stable at low pH. IFN-γ is not produced in response to most viruses but is induced by mitogen stimulation. It has only one subtype. It is a lymphokine with immunoregulatory functions.

Mechanism of Action

Interferons when elaborated by virus-infected cells, bind to cell surface receptors with INF-α and IFN-β sharing a common receptor and IFN-γ recognizing its own specific receptor. This binding triggers tyrosine phosphorylation and activation of transcription factor subunits in the cytoplasm, which then translocate into the nucleus and mediate transcription. This results in the synthesis of several enzymes which may be responsible for the development of antiviral state. These enzymes RNase L (an endoribonuclease), 2-5A synthetase (2′, 5′-oligoadenylate synthetase) and protein kinase, subsequently block viral reproduction by inhibiting the translation of viral mRNA into viral protein.

Interferons can be synthesized in large amounts by recombinant technology by cloning genes into bacteria or yeasts.

Biological Effects

1. Interferons induce resistance to viral infections. They have therapeutic value particularly in Hepatitis C and herpes keratitis.
2. They induce resistance to intracellular parasitic infections such as malaria and toxoplasmosis. They also possess antimicrobial effect on chlamydial infections.
3. They inhibit growth of tumor cells by inhibiting protein and DNA synthesis that inhibits cell growth and differentiation.

4. They increase expression of MHC antigens.
5. They increase cytotoxic effects of natural killer (NK) cells, killer (K) cells and T lymphocytes.
6. They activate macrophages for cytocidal activity.
7. They activate suppressor T cell and suppression of delayed type hypersensitivity (DTH).
8. They modulate antibody formation.

QUESTIONS

Essay Questions

1. Describe the lab diagnosis of viral infections.
2. Give an account of viral vaccines.

Short Notes

1. Interferons.
2. Biological effects of interferon.
3. Mention the uses of interferon.
4. Antiviral agents.
5. Name any four live attenuated viral vaccines.
6. Subunit vaccines.

82

Parvoviruses

- ***Structure***
- ***Classification***
- ***Replication***
- ***Pathogenesis***
- ***Epidemiology***
- ***Laboratory diagnosis***
- ***Prevention and control***
- ***Treatment***

STRUCTURE

Parvoviruses are nonenveloped, icosahedral particles, 18 to 26 nm in diameter (Fig. 82.1). The genome is linear, single-stranded, either positive or negative sense DNA. Virions contain two or three capsid proteins (VP-1 and VP-2).

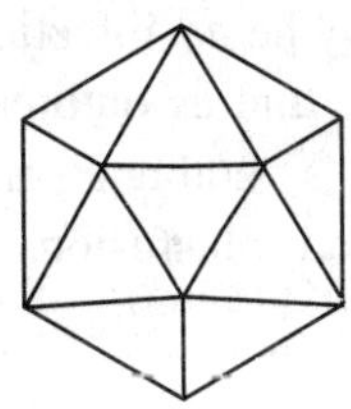

Fig. 82.1 Parvovirus

CLASSIFICATION

Parvoviruses are included under family parvoviridae, which contains two subfamilies: the parvovirinae, which infect vertebrates, and the Densovirinae which infect insects. The parvovirinae comprise tnree genera— *Parvovirus, Erythrovirus* and *Dependovirus*. Human **parvovirus B19** is the only member of the *Erythrovirus* genus. *Dependovirus* contains defective virions and depend on a helper virus, such as an adenovirus, for replication, and are known as "**adenoassociated viruses**".

REPLICATION

Replication takes place in the nucleus of dividing cells (mitotically active). Human parvovirus B19 has a tropisim for erythroid progenitor cells. The virus attaches to erythrocyte P antigen and viral DNA is translocated to the nucleus. The single-stranded DNA genome forms an intermediate double-stranded form, by a cellular DNA polymerase; which replicates to form progeny positive and negative single-stranded DNA that are packaged separately within newly synthesized capsids. The release of progeny virus is by host cell lysis.

PATHOGENESIS

Human parvovirus B19 has been implicated as the causative agent of several diseases. B19 virus is transmitted most commonly via the respiratory route. Other routes of transmission are transplacental and via blood transfusion. It is the cause of erythema infectiosum, polyarthralgia-arthritis syndrome, aplastic crises and hydrops fetalis.

The virus replicates in erythroid precursor cells in the bone marrow, leading to erythroid aplasia. Aplastic anemia develops in patients with underlying hemolytic anemia.

The incubation period is usually 4–14 days but may extend to 20 days. Erythema infectiosum and arthralgia develop 17 to 18 days after the acquisition of the virus and at the time of appearance of specific antibody. Erythema infectiosum is most common in children and characterised by fever and rash, which has a typical "**slapped cheek appearance**". It is also known as "fifth disease", as it was fifth in the old list of six exanthemas of children.

In women, disease late in pregnancy can cause spontaneous abortion and edematous anemic stillbirth, a condition known as hydrops fetalis due to vertical transmission from mother to fetus.

B19 virus may establish persistent infections and cause chronic suppression of bone marrow and chronic anemia in immunodeficiencies, malignancies and organ transplants.

EPIDEMIOLOGY

The B19 virus widespread and the erythema infectiosum is found worldwide. Infections can occur throughout the year, in all age groups, and as outbreaks or sporadic cases. Infections are most commonly seen in childhood and may occur as outbreaks in schools. Infection is transmitted through respiratory tract and sometimes through blood transfusion. Specific IgM and IgG antibodies develop in response to infection.

LABORATORY DIAGNOSIS

B19 virus is not cultivable in cell cultures.

1. B19 virus DNA can be detected in serum, blood cells, tissue samples and respiratory secretions by PCR and nucleic acid hybridisation tests.
2. Detection of B19 IgM antibody is indicative of recent infection. B19 IgM antibody persists for 2–3 months after the onset of symptoms. Anti-B19 antibody is detected by counter-current immunoelectrophoresis or immune electron microscopy, although the most widely used tests are IgM and IgG capture radioimmunoassays or enzyme immunoassays.
3. B19 antigen can be detected in serum by RIA, and enzyme immunoassays and counter-immunoelectrophoresis.

PREVENTION AND CONTROL

Infection control practices should be followed to prevent transmission of B19 virus to health care workers from patients. Most cases are asymptomatic, when viral shedding is maximal, and therefore control of infection is difficult.

TREATMENT

There is no specific antiviral therapy or vaccine for B19 infection. Patients with aplastic crisis require erythrocyte transfusion support until the bone marrow recovers.

QUESTIONS

Short Notes

1. Parvoviruses.
2. Parvovirus B19 or Erythrovirus.
3. Erythema infectiosum of fifth disease.

83

Papovaviruses

- *Introduction*
- *Papillomaviruses—Structure, Classification, Pathogenesis, Epidemiology, Laboratory diagnosis, Prophylaxis, Treatment*
- *Polyomaviruses—Structure, Classification, Pathogenesis, Epidemiology, Lab. diagnosis, Treatment and Prophylaxis.*

INTRODUCTION

The term "**papovavirus**" was derived from the first two letters of the names of three members of this group: human **papillomavirus**, mouse **polyomavirus**, and **simian vacuolating virus (SV_{40})**. The papovaviruses, are oncogenic and belong to the family "Papovaviridae". Based on physicochemical, biologic and molecular criteria, the papovaviridae family is split in two families, namely papillomaviridae including genus *Papillomavirus* and Polyomaviridae consisting of genus *Polyomavirus*.

Papillomaviruses are biologically distinguished from the related polyomaviruses by their differentiated state of host cells for replication, the induction of tumors in natural hosts, the presence of virus particles in some tumor tissues and the maintenance of viral DNA as episomal copies in some transformed cells.

Table 83.1 Important Characteristics of Papovaviruses

Characteristics	*Papillomavirus*	*Polyomavirus*
Virion		
Capsid	Icosahedral, nonenveloped	Icosahedral, nonenveloped
Size	55 nm diameter	45 nm diameter
Genome		
Type	DNA	DNA
Structure	Double-stranded, circular	Double-stranded, circular
Coding information	On one strand	On both strands
Oncogenic Potential		
Tumors in natural hosts	Yes	No

Result of natural infection	Benign wart	Inapparent (subclinical)
Target tissue	Surface epithelia	Internal organs
Transform cells in vitro	Rarely	Yes
Persistence of infectious in tumors	Sometimes	No
Individual members		
Infect humans	Human papillomavirus more than 70 types	JC, BK viruses
Important animal isolates	Papillomavirus from cows and rabbits	Polyomavirus (mouse), SV_{40} (monkey)

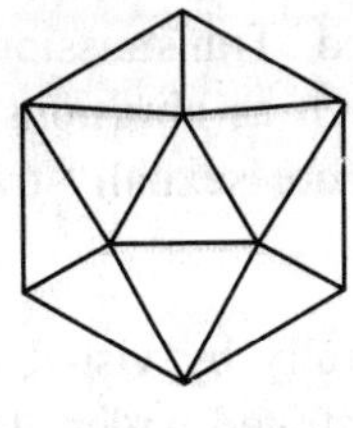

Fig. 83.1 Papovavirus

PAPILLOMAVIRUSES

Structure

Papillomaviruses are small, 55 nm in diameter, nonenveloped, icosahedral viruses. The capsid possesses 72 capsomers. The genome is double-stranded, covalently closed, circular DNA. It replicates and assembles in the host cell nucleus. The organization of papillomavirus genome is complex. (Fig. 83.1).

Classification

Over 70 types (species) of human papillomaviruses (HPVs) are identified based on differences in their DNA base sequences by DNA hybridisation assays.

Pathogenesis

Papillomaviruses are highly tropic for epithelial cells of the skin and mucus membranes and induce hyperplastic epithelial lesions (**warts or papillomas**) in their host species. The clinical spectrum may range from simple warts to malignancies. Wart can occur on any part of the body, including both skin and mucosal surfaces.

Cutaneous Warts

These warts may be classified as common warts (**Verruca vulgaris**) on fingers and hands, plantar warts on sole of foot, flat warts on arms, face and knee. Common warts are most frequently associated with HPV 1–4, 5 and 7 types. Another type of skin lesion that spreads to many body sites, called epidermodysplasia verruciformis is seen in persons with genetic predisposition for multiple warts. These lesions may give rise to squamous cell carcinomas, several years after initial appearance of the original warts, especially in areas of skin exposed to sunlight.

Mucosal Warts

HPV produces anogenital warts (**Condyloma acuminata**) and cervical cancer. Genital warts are moist, soft, pedunculated and found on the external genitalia is usually due to types 6 and 11, and acquired by sexual contact. Cofactors such as tobacco smoke and coinfection with herpes simplex virus are involved in the development of cancer.

Mucosal surfaces of respiratory tract (laryngeal papillomas), oral cavity (warts on buccal mucosa) and the conjunctiva may be involved giving rise to benign papillomas. Laryngeal papillomas in children are caused by HPV 6 and 11. It is believed that the infection is acquired during passage through the birth canal of a mother with genital warts. Larynegal papillomas are benign tumors on vocal cords.

Epidemiology

Papillomaviruses are widely distributed. Transmission occurs by contact. Cutaneous warts are transmitted via epithelial surface lesions such as abrasions. The infection occurs and maintained in the basal layers of the skin. Genital warts are sexually transmitted.

Laboratory Diagnosis

Diagnosis of cutaneous warts is generally by visual inspection. HPVs cannot be cultivated *in vitro* in tissue cultures. They can be demonstrated under electron microscope in wart tissue sections. Nucleic acid hybridisation is used to detect viral DNA in tissue samples. Typing is also done by DNA hybridisation reactions using defined, tissue-specific nucleic acid probes.

Prophylaxis

Sterilization of instruments after examination of patients with HPV infection and health education of public to prevent sexual transmission are important control measures.

Treatment

Most warts regress spontaneously. Treatment of warts generally involves the surgical removal or destruction of the wart tissue by electrosurgery, cryosurgery with liquid nitrogen or solid CO_2, laser vaporization, application of cytotoxic chemicals such as podophyllin, trichloroacetic acid or cidofovir and by administration of interferon.

POLYOMAVIRUSES

The name "polyoma" means many (poly-) tumor (-oma). The polyomaviruses possess the capacity to transform normal cells in culture and to induce tumors in species other than those in which they are normally found in nature. However, polyomaviruses have not yet been shown to cause tumors in humans.

Structure

Polyomaviruses are nonenveloped icosahedral, 45 nm diameter (smaller than papillomaviruses) particles with three capsid proteins (Fig. 83.1). They contain a circular, double-stranded DNA. The genome contains a limited amount of genetic information (6 or 7 genes) and consists of two or three replicative genes (tumor antigens) encoded on one strand and three structural genes (capsid antigens) encoded on the other strand.

Classification

Human and animal polyomaviruses are antigenically distinct; only one serotype is known for each virus. The prototype is SV_{40} virus. Classification is based on structure of the virus particle. Polyomaviruses include mouse polyomavirus. Simian vacuolating (SV_{40}) virus of monkeys, **BK virus** and **JC virus**.

Epidemiology

The human polyomaviruses, BK and JC viruses are transmitted by droplets from the upper respiratory tract of infected persons, and possibly through contact with their urine. Infections usually occur in childhood. BK and JC viruses are widely distributed in human populations and specific antibody has been demonstrated in 70–80% adult sera. Both viruses spread from the upper respiratory tract to kidneys where they establish persistent infections in an inactive state in the tubular epithelium of healthy individuals and may reactivate in immunosuppressed hosts or by renal transplantation or during normal pregnancies.

Pathogenesis

Mouse polyomavirus causes several different types of tumors following injection into newborn mice or hamsters. But tumors do not develop as a result of natural infection among young mice.

Simian vacuolating (SV_{40}) virus replicates in cells of their natural host-monkey. It causes tumors in experimentally inoculated newborn hamsters and rodents. Tumor induction in their natural host (rhesus monkey) has not been observed.

JC polyomavirus is isolated from the brains of patients with progressive multifocal leukoencephalopathy (PML). The virus was designated by the initials of the person from whom it was isolated. The JC virus grows only in human fetal glial cell cultures.

BK polyomavirus was isolated from the urine of a renal transplant recipient and was named after his initials. The BK virus differs from the JC virus in being able to grow in a wide range of primary and continuous cell lines.

Laboratory diagnosis

Identification of BK virus in the urine or JC virus in the PML lesions in the brain tissue by DNA hybridisation are the most sensitive and specific technique for the diagnosis of these infections. Because most people have antibodies to these viruses, serological techniques are not generally useful in the diagnosis of acute infections.

Treatment and prophylaxis

No successful, specific antiviral therapy is available. Because the infection with JC and BK viruses is nearly universal and asymptomatic and PML represents reactivation of latent virus, there are no viable preventive measures at present.

QUESTIONS

Short Notes

1. Papovavirus.
2. Human papillomavirus.
3. Genital warts or condylomata accuminata.

84

Adenoviruses

- *Introduction*
- *Structure*
- *Resistance*
- *Cultivation*
- *Pathogensis*
- *Epidemiology*
- *Lab. diagnosis*
- *Prophylaxis*
- *Treatment*

INTRODUCTION

Adenoviruses were first discovered during screening of throat washings and cultures of adenoids and tonsils, performed in the search for the common cold virus. They are now recognized as a large group of related viruses commonly infecting humans, animals and birds. Adenoviruses belong to family **adenoviridae**, which includes two important genera: one that infects birds (*Aviadenovirus*) and another that infects mammals (***Mastadenovirus***). Human adenoviruses are divided into six groups (A–F) on the basis of their physical, chemical and biologic properties and consists of at least 47 distinct antigenic types.

Table 84.1 Human Adenovirus Types

Group	*Serotypes*
A	12, 18, 31
B	3, 7, 11, 14, 16, 21, 34, 35
C	1, 2, 5, 6
D	8–10, 13, 15, 17, 19, 20, 22–30, 32, 33–36, 36-39, 42–47
E	4
F	40, 41

Structure

Adenoviruses are nonenveloped, icosahedral viruses containing double-stranded linear DNA. The capsid is composed of 252 capsomers arranged as an icosahedron with 20 triangular facets and 12 vertices. Of these 252 capsomers, 240 have six neighbours and are called hexons, while 12 capsomers at the vertices have five neighbours and are called pentons. The pentons are composed of a penton base structure from which projects a glycoprotein fiber, consisting of a rod like portion with a knob attached at the distal end. (Fig. 84.1). The viruses replicate and assemble in the nucleus of host cell.

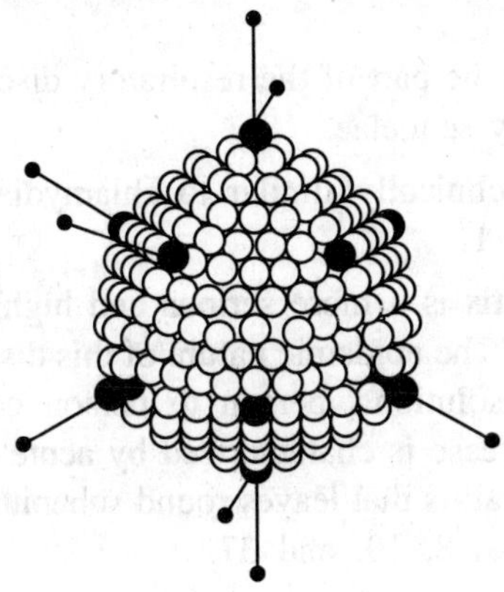

Fig. 84.1 Adenovirus

Resistance

Adenoviruses remain viable for about a week at 37°C. They are readily inactivated at 50°C. They resist ether and bile salts.

Cultivation

Human adenoviruses can be grown on monolayers of HeLa, HEp-2, KB and human embryonic kidney cells. Cytopathic effects may take several days and consists of cell rounding, clustering of swollen cells into grape like bunches. Infected cells show **basophilic intranuclear inclusions** in stained preparations.

Pathogenesis

The adenoviruses infect and replicate well in epithelial cells the respiratory tract, eye, gastrointestinal tract, urinary bladder and liver. The disease symptoms are related primarily to the killing of these cells. They usually do not spread beyond the regional lymph nodes and systemic infections are rare. Most adenovirus infections are asymptomatic. A single serotype may cause different clinical diseases and more than one type may cause the same clinical illness.

1. Respiratory Tract Diseases

Acute febrile pharyngitis. Most common among infants and young children, characterized by cough, sorethroat, nasal congestion and fever. Some of these cases are difficult to distinguish from other mild viral respiratory infections. This condition is mainly caused by group G adenoviruses.

Pharyngoconjunctival fever. Symptoms are similar to those of acute febrile pharyngitis, but conjunctivitis is also present. This condition is more prevalent in children, and occurs both sporadically, and in outbreaks, often within family groups or in groups using the same swimming facility ("Swimming pool conjunctivitis"). Group B adenoviruses, mainly types 3, 7 and 14 are most commonly involved.

Acute respiratory disease. Occurs primarily in epidemics among new military recruits under conditions of fatigue and crowding. The syndrome is characterized by pharyngitis, fever, cough and malaise. The disease is caused by types 4 and 7 and occasionally by type 3.

Pneumonia is a complication of respiratory syndromes described above. Adenovirus types 3 and 7 are particularly associated with this adenoviral pneumonia, which has a mortality rate of 8–10% in infants.

2. Ocular Diseases

Mild ocular involvement may be part of the respiratory diseases caused by adenoviruses. These infections usually heal without any sequelae.

Follicular conjunctivitis is clinically similar to chlamydial conjunctivitis and is self-limited, usually caused by types 3, 4 and 11.

Epidemic keratoconjunctivitis is a more serious and highly contagious disease, in which the corneal epithelium is also involved. The epidemic nature of this disease arises in part from transmission via shared towels or ophthalmic solutions, person to person contact, or by improperly sterilized opthalmologic instruments. The disease is characterized by acute conjunctivitis with enlarged, tender preauricular nodes, followed by keratitis that leaves round subepithelial opacities in the cornea, lasting several years. It is caused by types 8, 19, and 37.

3. Gastrointestinal Diseases

Most of the human adenoviruses replicate in intestinal cells, and are present in stools. However, these are generally asymptomatic infections. Two serotypes (types 40 and 41) have been associated specifically with infantile gastroenteritis and may account for 5 to 15% of all viral diarrheas in children.

4. Other Less Common Diseases

Types 11 and 21 may cause acute hemorrhagic cystitis in children, especially boys. It is characterized by hematuria, and virus occurs in the urine.

Type 37 occurs in cervical lesions and in male urethritis and may be sexually transmitted.

In Immunocompromised patients, such as those with AIDS and in transplant patients, the common respiratory adenovirus infections have a greater risk of proceeding to serious, often fatal, pneumonia.

Patients with AIDS may suffer adenovirus infections, particularly with type 35.

Epidemiology

Adenoviruses are worldwide in distribution and are present year-round. The site of the clinical syndrome caused by an adenovirus infection is generally related to the mode of virus transmission. Adenoviruses are spread predominantly by the fecal-oral route but may also be transmitted by respiratory droplets or by contaminated fomites. Eye infections are transmitted by direct inoculation of the eye by virus-contaminated hands (hand to eye), ophthalmologic instruments or water bodies in which groups of children swim together.

Laboratory diagnosis

Adenovirus infection is suggested clinically by fever, upper respiratory tract infections, and conjunctivitis; the diagnosis is confirmed by virus isolation and demonstration of a rise in antibody titres.

Clinical specimens such as stool or urine, throat swabs, conjunctival swabs are inoculated into tissue cultures such as HeLa, HEp-2 and KB cell lines and primary human embryonic kidney cell lines and observed for the development of characteristic cytopathic effects–cell rounding, clustering of swollen cells. Isolates can be identified as adenoviruses by CFT or Fluorescent antibody tests to detect group-specific antigens. Specific serotypes can be identified by neutralisation and HI tests.

Virus isolation from the eye, lung, or genital tract is diagnostic of current infection. However, their isolation from throat swabs or fecal samples should be interpreted carefully.

The molecular techniques such as PCR, nucleic acid hybridisation can be used for the diagnosis of adenovirus infections in body fluids or tissue samples.

Adenoviruses can be detected by direct examination of fecal extracts by electron microscopy or ELISA or immunofluorescence.

For serological diagnosis, a rise in titer of antibodies should be demonstrated in paired sera by CFT or neutralisation or hemagglutination inhibition tests.

Prophylaxis

The risk of water-borne outbreaks of conjunctivitis can be controlled by chlorination of swimming pools and waste water. Strict asepsis during eye examination, coupled with adequate sterilization of equipment is essential for the control of epidemic keratoconjunctivitis.

A live, attenuated adenovirus vaccine is used for the protection of military population. The oncogenic capacity of the adenoviruses in experimental animals has inhibited the use of vaccines on a wider scale.

Treatment

No antiviral agents are available for treatment adenovirus infections.

QUESTIONS

Essay Questions:

1. Give an account of adenoviruses.

Short Notes:

1. Adenoviruses.
2. Morphology of Adenoviruses.
3. Adenovirus infections or pathogenicity of adenoviruses.
4. Draw a neat labelled diagram of adenovirus particle.
5. Acute follicular conjunctivitis.
6. Adenovirus keratoconjunctivities.

85

Herpesviruses

INTRODUCTION

There are nearly hundred viruses of the herpes group that infect many different animals. The herpesviruses that commonly infect humans (8 species) include herpes simplex virus types 1 and 2, Varicella-Zoster (VZ) virus, cytomegalovirus, Epstein-Barr virus, human herpes viruses 6 and 7 and Kaposi's sarcoma-associated herpesvirus. All herpesviruses have the ability to establish life-long latent, persistent infections following primary infection of their natural hosts and to undergo periodic reactivation. They are frequently reactivated in immunosuppressed patients. The reactivated infection may be clinically quite different from the disease caused by the primary infection.

Structure and Properties

Herpesviruses are large, enveloped DNA viruses. The enveloped virion measures 150–200 nm and the naked virion about 100 nm. The core consists of a linear, double-stranded DNA, surrounded by a protein coat, called capsid that exhibits icosahedral symmetry and has 162 capsomers. Tightly adherent to the capsid is a layer called the "tegument", which appears to consists of amorphous material. The tegument is loosely surrounded by a lipid envelope, that is derived from the nuclear membrane of the infected cell and contains viral glycoprotein spikes about 8 nm long (Fig. 85.1).

Herpesviruses replicate in the host cell nucleus. They form Cowdry type A intranuclear (Lipschutz) inclusion bodies. Because of the presence of lipid envelope, herpes viruses are susceptible to organic solvents like alcohol, ether, chloroform and bile salts.

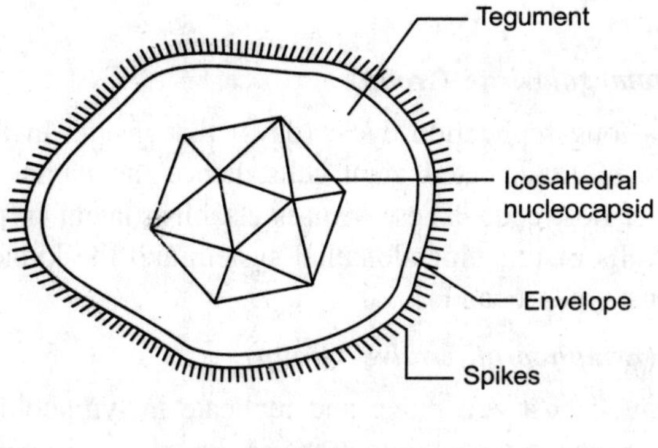

Fig. 85.1 Herpesvirus

Classification

The **herpesviridae** family comprises, enveloped, icosahedral, DNA viruses and divided into three subfamilies based on biologic, physical and genetic properties (Table 85.1).

Table 85.1 Classification of Human Herpesviruses

Subfamily	*Biologic properties*: *Growth cycle*	*Biologic properties*: *Cytopatho-logy*	*Biologic properties*: *Latent cycle*	*Genus*	*Examples*: *Official name*	*Examples*: *Common name*
Alphaher-pesvirinae	Short (hours)	Cytolytic	Neurons	*Simplexvirus*	Human her-pesvirus 1	Herpes simplex viruse type 1
					Human her-pesvirus 2	Herpes simplex virus type 2
				Varicellovirus	Human her-pesvirus 3	Varicella-zoster virus
Bataherpes-virinae	Long (days)	Cytomegalic	Glands, kidneys	*Cytomegalo-virus*	Human her-pesvirus 5	Cytomegalo-virus
		Lymphopro-liferative	Lymphoid tissue	*Roseolovirus*	Human her-pesvirus 6	Human herpes-virus 6
					Human her-pesvirus 7	Human herpes-virus 7
Gammaher-pesvirinae	Variable	Lymphopro-liferative	Lymphoid tissue	*Lymphocry-ptovirus*	Human her-pesvirus 4	Epstein-Barr virus
				Rhadinovirus	Human her-pesvirus 8	Kaposi's sar-coma associa-ted herpes-virus

1. Alphaherpesvirinae (Herpes Simplex Virus Group)

These viruses have a short replication cycle (hours) and a rapid, cytocidal growth cycle. They have the ability to replicate in a wide variety of host cells. They characteristically establish latent infection in sensory nerve ganglia. *e.g.,* **Herpes simplex virus** types 1 and 2 (HSV 1 and 2), **Varicella-Zoster (VZ) virus.**

2. Betaherpesvirinae (Cytomegalovirus Group)

These viruses have a long replication cycle (days) that results in the enlargement of infected cells forming characteristic multinucleated giant cells, hence the name "cytomegalo-". They infect a narrow, restricted range of host cells. These viruses establish latent infections in nonneural tissues such as secretory glands, cells of reticuloendothelial system and the kidneys. *e.g.,* **Cytomegalovirus (CMV)**, human herpesvirus types 6 and 7.

3. Gammaherpesvirinae (Lymphoproliferative Group)

They infect most limited host cell range and replicate in lymphoblastoid cells (specific for B or T lymphocytes). They establish latent infections in lymphoid tissues. *e.g.,* **Epstein-Barr (EB) virus**, human herpes virus type 8 (Kaposi's sarcoma-associated herpes virus).

HERPES SIMPLEX VIRUS (HSV)

Pathogenesis

Herpes simplex viruses are extremely widespread in the human population. There are two distinct herpes simplex viruses, which can be distinguished by restriction enzyme analysis of viral DNA.

1. Type 1 **(HSV-1)**—cause lesions in and around mouth; transmitted by direct contact, droplet spread or kissing.
2. Type 2 **(HSV-2)**—causes genital tract infections; transmitted by sexual contact.

As a general rule, HSV-1 produces "above the waist" and HSV-2 "below the waist" lesions but the rule is not absolute and either can, however, infect and cause similar lesions at the opposite site.

Primary Infection

After inoculation onto the skin or mucus membrane and an incubation period of 4 to 6 days, both HSV-1 and HSV-2 replicate in epithelial cells. Cell lysis and local inflammation occurs, resulting in production of characteristic thin walled, umbilicated vesicles or shallow ulcers containing infectious virus on an erythematous base. Virus then invades local nerve endings and is transported by retrograde axonal flow to dorsal root ganglia, where it replicates and remains latent.

Primary infections are usually mild and occur in persons without antibodies and in most individuals are asymptomatic, but result in antibody production and establishment of latent infections in sensory ganglia.

Latent Infection

The virus resides latently in dorsal root ganglia, in a nonreplicating state, and may lasts for the life time of the host. HSV-1 establishes latent infection in **trigeminal ganglia**, whereas HSV-2 in **sacral** or **lumbar ganglia**—from one to thousands of copies of the viral genome are present as nonintegrated circular molecules of DNA in the nuclei. Expression of HSV genes is shut off in latently infected cells. No virus can be recovered between recurrences at or near the usual site of recurrent lesions.

Reactivation

Several factors such as hormonal changes, fever, damage to the neurons, physical or emotional stress and exposure to UV light are known to induce reactivation of the virus from latent state.

Consequently, the viruses are transported down the axon to the nerve endings at peripheral site and replication proceeds at the skin or mucus membranes. Sensory nerve symptoms such as pain and tingling often precede and accompany the appearance of recurrent lesions. The presence of specific humoral and cell mediated immune responses cannot prevent this recurrence. Many recurrences are asymptomatic, reflected only by viral shedding in secretions. Characteristics lesions are thus produced in some recurrences in the same area as that of the primary lesions.

More than 80% of the human population harbors HSV-1, in a latent form, but only a small portion experience recurrences. Symptomatic recurrent HSV-1 infections are usually manifested as clusters of vesicles at the border of the lips (cold sores, fever blisters, herpes labialis) and heal without scarring in 8-10 days. The frequency of oropharyngeal symptomatic recurrences is quite variable, ranging from none to several per year. Reactivation of HSV-2 genital infections can occur with greater frequency, for example, monthly, and is often asymptomatic, but still results in viral shedding.

Clinical Features

Herpes simplex virus types 1 and 2 may cause several clinical entities, and the infections may be primary or recurrent (Table 85.2).

1. Gingivostomatitis

Mucocutaneous infections are the most common clinical manifestation of HSV-1 and HSV-2. Symptomatic primary infection of HSV-1 involving buccal and gingival mucosa of the mouth occurs most frequently in children below 5 years of age. The incubation period is short, about 3–5 days, (range 2–12 days) and clinical illness lasts 2–3 weeks. HSV-1 gingivostomatitis is characterized by fever, sore throat, pharyngeal edema and erythema followed by development of vesicular or ulcerative lesions on the oral and pharyngeal mucosa. The most striking and common lesion is gingivitis, characterized by swollen, tender gums. Primary infection in adults commonly cause pharyngitis and tonsillitis.

Recurrent disease is characterized by a cluster of vesicles localized at the border of the lip. Intense pain occurs at the outset but fades over 4–5 days. Lesions progress through the pustular and crusting stages and heal without scarring in 8–10 days. The lesions may recur repeatedly and at various intervals, in the same location.

2. Keratoconjunctivitis

The initial infection with HSV-1 may be in the eye, producing severe keratoconjunctivitis. Recurrent lesions of the eye are common and appear as dendritic keratitis or corneal ulcers or vesicles on the eyelids. Recurrent keratitis may progress to deep stromal involvement and may result in deep stromal involvement and may result in permanent opacification and blindness.

3. Genital Herpes

It is usually caused by HSV-2. The disease is characterized by vesiculoulcerative lesions of the penis of the male or the cervix, vulva, vagina and perineum of the female. The lesions are very painful and may be associated with fever, malaise, dysuria and inguinal lymphadenopathy. **Recurrent genital herpes** is common and mild. A limited number of vesicles appear and heal in about ten day.

4. Cutaneous Infections

Eczema herpeticum is a primary infection with HSV-1 seen in children suffering from eczema. The disease is characterized by extensive vesicular eruption of the skin over much of the body and high fever. Skin infections are often severe and life threatening in persons with eczema or burns. Localized lesions caused by HSV-1 or HSV-2 may occur in abrasions (traumatic herpes). These lesions seen on the fingers of dentists and hospital personnel is known as herpetic whitlow and on the bodies of wrestlers, herpes gladiatorum and constitutes an occupational hazard.

Table 85.2 Comparison of Herpes Simplex Virus Type 1 and Type 2

Characteristics	*HSV-1*	*HSV-2*
Site of latency	Trigeminal ganglia	Sacral ganglia
Age of primary infection	Young Children	Young adults
Transmission	Contact (often saliva)	Sexual
Clinical features		
Primary infection:		
Gingivostomatitis	+	–
Pharyngotonsillitis	+	–
Keratoconjunctivitis	+	–
Neonatal infections	±	+
Recurrent infection:		
Cold sores, fever blisters	+	–
Keratitis	+	–
Primary or recurrent infection:		
Cutaneous herpes		
Skin above the waist	+	–
Skin below the waist	–	+
Hands or arms	+	+
Herpetic whitlow	+	+
Eczema herpeticum	+	–
Genital herpes	±	+
Herpes encephalitis	+	–
Herpes meningitis	±	+

5. Encephalitis

Herpes simplex encephalitis is characterized by hemorrhagic necrosis of the temporal lobe. Clinical manifestations include headache, fever, altered consciousness and abnormalities of speech and behaviour. Pleocytosis is present in the CSF. Though the disease is caused by both the types, HSV-1 primary or recurrent infections are common. The virus can reach the temporal lobe by ascending neural pathways, such as the trigeminal tracts or the olfactory nerves. The disease carries a high mortality rate, and those who survive often have residual neurologic defects.

6. Neonatal Herpes

HSV infection of the newborn may be acquired *in utero*, during birth or after birth. About 75% neonatal herpes infections are caused by HSV-2. The disease can be acquired postnatally and may be due to either HSV-1 or HSV-2. Sources of infection include family members and hospital personnel who are shedding virus. The manifestations of neonatal herpes are of three categories: (1) Lesions localized to the skin, eye and mouth (2) encephalitis, and (3) disseminated infection involving multiple organs and can produce intravascular coagulation, hemorrhagic pneumonitis, encephalitis and cutaneous lesions.

Transplacental infection of the fetus with HSV may cause congenital malformations, but is rare.

7. Infections in Immunocompromised Hosts

Patients immunosuppressed by disease or therapy, transplant recipients and persons with malnutrition are at increased risk of developing HSV infections. Herpes lesions may spread and involve respiratory tract, esophagus and intestinal mucosa. In most cases, the disease reflects reactivation of latent HSV infection.

Laboratory Diagnosis

The diagnosis of HSV infection may be made by microscopy, demonstration of viral antigen, isolation of virus, serological demonstration of antibodies and detection of DNA by molecular methods. Specimens include vesicle fluid, skin swab, saliva, conjunctival fluid, corneal scrapings, genital swabs, brain biopsy and CSF.

Microscopy

Smears (Tzanck smear) are prepared from the lesions, preferably from the base of the vesicles and stained with 1% aqueous solution of toluidine blue for fifteen seconds. The presence of multinucleated giant cells and homogenously stained "ground glass" chromatin (Tzanck cells) under light microscope constitute a positive smear. Intranuclear type A inclusion bodies may be seen in Giemsa stained smears. Viral particles may also be demonstrated under electron microscope.

Demonstration of Virus Antigen

The HSV antigen may be demonstrated in smears or sections from lesions, or brain biopsy material by the fluorescent antibody technique.

Isolation of Virus

Vesicle fluid, CSF, saliva, throat washings etc., are inoculated on to primary human embryonic kidney, human amnion, rabbit kidney cells, diploid human lung, vero or HeLa cell lines. The appearance of typical cytopathic effects in 2–3 days suggests the presence of HSV. Then the virus is identified by neutralisation test or immunofluorescence staining with specific antiserum. Typing of HSV-1 and 2 may be done by using specific antisera or by nucleic acid hybridisation or restriction endonuclease analysis of viral DNA.

Intracerebral inoculation into mice and rabbits leads to encephalitis. Corneal scarification produces keratoconjunctivitis in rabbits.

Inoculation on to chorioallantoic membrane of embryonated eggs produces characteristic "pock" lesions, which are small (diameter less than 0.5 mm), white, shiny, and nonnecrotic.

Serology

Antibodies appear in 4–7 days after primary infection, and reach a peak in 2–4 weeks. The antibodies persists with minor fluctuations for the life of the host. The antibodies in patient serum can be measured by neutralisation, CFT, ELISA, RIA or immunofluorescence.

Molecular Methods

The viral DNA in clinical materials can be demonstrated by nucleic acid hybridisation and after amplification by polymerase chain reaction (PCR).

Prophylaxis

Vaccine is not currently available. Newborns and persons with eczema should be protected from exposure to persons with active herpetic lesions. Genital herpes can be prevented by safe sexual practices.

Treatment

Acyclovir (acycloguanosine) is selectively effective against HSV and acts by inhibiting viral DNA synthesis only after initially being phosphorylated by the HSV thymidine kinase. It is the drug of choice for any primary HSV infection, but is especially important in treating herpes encephalitis, neonatal herpes and disseminated infections in immunocompromised patients. Topical, oral and intravenous formulations are all useful against primary infections. Vidarabine (adenine arabinoside) is also effective against neonatal herpes and HSV encephalitis. However, it is more toxic than acyclovir. Topically applied idoxuridine (5-iodo-2-deoxyuridine), trifluridine (trifluorothymidine), vidarabine and acyclovir can be used for treatment of herpetic keratitis. HSV may develop resistance to these drugs due to mutations in the viral thymidine kinase and DNA polymerase genes.

VARICELLA-ZOSTER VIRUS (VZV)

Properties

Varicella-zoster virus is morphologically identical to HSV. It has biologic and genetic similarities to HSV and is classified along with the HSVs in the alphaherpesvirinae subfamily. VZV has not been propagated in laboratory animals or embryonated eggs. However, the virus can be grown in human embryonic tissue, human fibroblasts, human amnion or HeLa cell lines and produces typical intranuclear inclusion bodies. Cytopathic effects are similar to HSV and spread slowly than HSV. Infectious virus remains cell-associated and does not appear freely in the tissue culture fluids.

Pathogenesis

VZV causes varicella (chicken pox) and zoster (shingles). Primary infection with VZV causes chicken pox, mainly in children, whereas the reactivation of the latent virus causes herpes zoster, in adults and immunocompromised individuals. Contact with zoster or chickenpox patient may lead only to chickenpox, but not zoster.

Varicella (Chickenpox)

It is a mild, highly contagious disease, mainly of children, characterized by a generalized vesicular eruption of the skin and mucus membranes. The disease may be severe in adults and immunocompromised individuals.

The disease spreads by air-borne droplets and sometimes by contact with skin eruptions. The route of infection is the mucosa of the upper respiratory tract or the conjunctiva, followed by spread to the regional lymph nodes. The virus enters the blood stream and replicates in cells of the liver and spleen, and are disseminated throughout the body by infected mononuclear leucocytes. Endothelial cells of the capillaries, and ultimately skin epithelial cells, become infected, resulting in the characteristic, virus-containing vesicles of chickenpox, which appear from 14 to 21 days after exposure. The infected individual is contagious from one to two days before the appearance of the exanthema.

Swelling of epithelial cells, ballooning degeneration and the accumulation of tissue fluids result in vesicle formation. Eosinophilic inclusion bodies are found in the nuclei of infected cells. Multinuclear giant cells are common. At the time of primary infection, VZV may establish latency in dorsal root ganglia.

Zoster (Shingles)

It is a sporadic, incapcitating disease of adults or immunocompromised individuals that is characterized by a rash limited in distribution to the skin supplied by a single sensory ganglion. The lesions are similar to those of varicella. There is also an acute inflammation of the sensory nerves and ganglia.

When the latent VZV is reactivated, probably due to waning immunity, it undergoes replication, travels down the nerve to the skin causing intense inflammation and pain and induces vesicle formation. The likelihood of reactivation increases with age and depressed CMI, probably due to depletion of VZV-specific cytotoxic T cells.

Clinical Features

Varicella

The incubation period is 14 to 21 days. Fever, malaise, headache are the earliest symptoms, soon followed by the rash, first on the trunk and then on the face and spreads to the extremities, and buccal and pharyngeal mucosa in the mouth. The lesions of chicken pox are initially vesicles, which become pustular, crusted and then scabbed prior to healing. Successive new lesions continue to appear over a period of 2–4 days. Healing occurs without scarring.

Complications are rare in normal children. The most common complication in adults and immunocompromised patients is varicella pneumonia, but fulminant hepatic failure and encephalitis may also result. In neonatal varicella, the infection is contracted from the mother just before or just after birth but without sufficient maternal antibody.

Zoster

Herpes zoster results from reactivation of the latent virus. The disease usually starts with severe pain in the area of skin or mucosa supplied by sensory nerves and ganglia. Within a few days after onset, a crop of vesicles appears over the skin supplied by the affected nerves. The eruption is usually unilateral; the trunk, head and neck are most commonly involved. Commonly zoster involves ophthalmic branch of the **trigeminal nerve**. In patients with localized zoster and no underlying disease, healing takes place in 10 to 21 days depending upon the age and immune status of the patient. Sometimes debilitating post herpetic neuralgia and abnormal sensory phenomena may occur, which may last as long as several months. In immunocompromised patients, or cancer patients, there is a risk of pneumonia, hepatitis and encephalitis, as well as the extension of the skin lesions outside the area innervated by nerves. Ramsay Hunt syndrome is a rare form of zoster affecting the facial nerve, with eruption on tympanic membrane, external auditory canal and facial palsy.

Laboratory Diagnosis

The specimens collected are scrapings or swabs of the base of vesicles or veside fluid. In stained smears, multinucleated giant cells can be demonstrated under light microscopy. The virus particle in the specimen can be detected under electron microscope. Intracellular viral antigens can be demonstrated by immunofluorescence. Virus can be isolated from vesicle fluid using cultures of human cells in 3–7 days, although cytopathic effects sometimes develop more slowly. Isolates are identified by immunofluorescence with specific antisera.

Prophylaxis

A **live attenuated varicella vaccine** is now used as one of the routine childhood vaccines. The vaccine is also indicated for nonimmune adults those who are at risk of exposure to chickenpox patients. Susceptible persons can be protected by administration of varicella-zoster immune globulin (VZIG). It must be given before disease develops. It has no effect on the occurrence of zoster.

Treatment

Several antiviral drugs are effective against varicella, including acyclovir, valacyclovir, vidarabine and leucocyte interferon.

CYTOMEGALOVIRUS (CMV)

Properties

Cytomegaloviruses, formerly known as **salivary gland viruses**, are a group of ubiquitous herpes viruses of humans, and included under betaherpesvirinae subfamily. Their replication cycle is significantly longer, and infected cells typically are greatly enlarged and multinucleated, thus the name "cytomegalo-". There is only one recognized human species of cytomegalovirus, but there are many distinct strains that can be distinguished by antigenic differences as well as by restriction fragment analysis of their genomes.

Cytomegaloviruses are species-specific and cell type-specific. They are the largest viruses among herpesviruses, measuring 150–200 nm in size. Human cytomegalovirus replicates *in vitro* only but slowly in human fibroblast cell culture, although epithelial cells are affected *in vivo*. CMV produces a characteristic cytopathic effect. Perinuclear cytoplasmic inclusions form in addition to the intranuclear inclusions typical of herpesviruses, giving an owl's eye appearance. Multinucleated giant cells are seen. Inclusion-bearing **cytomegalic cells** can be demonstrated in samples from infected persons.

Epidemiology and Pathogenesis

CMV infections are among the most prevalent viral infections worldwide and present throughout the year. Humans are the only known host for CMV.

Transmission requires close person-to-person contact. Initial infection commonly occurs during childhood. New infections are usually asymptomatic. Virus may be shed in all body fluids including tears, saliva, urine, semen, breast milk, and cervical secretions and is carried in circulating leucocytes. Oral and respiratory spread are common routes of transmission. In adults the virus can also be transmitted: (1) by sexual means, because it is present in semen and vaginal secretions (2) by organ transplants, and (3) by blood transfusions. Since virus is present in milk, neonates may be infected by this route. CMV can also cross the placenta and infect a fetus in utero. Latency is established in secretory (salivary) glands and kidneys. As a result, large quantities of asymptomatic virus shedding occurs over prolonged periods of time.

Clinical Features

CMV infection can result in one of three distinct clinical syndromes: infectious mononucleosis, congenital and perinatal infections and infections of immunocompromised patients.

1. Primary CMV infection of adults may result in infectious mononucleosis syndrome that is clinically similar to that caused by Epstein-Barr (EB) virus. The symptoms persistent fever, muscle pain, lymphadenopathy, elevated levels of abnormal lymphocytes and liver enzymes

are characteristic. CMV mononucleosis can be differentiated by the absence of heterophile antibodies that are present in EB virus mononucleosis. CMV mononucleosis is a mild disease, and complications are rare. Subclinical hepatitis is common.

2. CMV is the most common intrauterine viral infection. However, there is a great variation in incidence of fetal infection and severity of disease, depending on whether the mother is experiencing a primary or recurrent infection. In women with first CMV infection during pregnancy (antibodies are not yet produced against CMV), 30 to 50 percent of fetuses will be infected, and ten percent of these will be symptomatic. The disease is very severe when infection occurs during the first trimester. The disease is referred to as **cytomegalic inclusion disease**. This **congenital infection** may result in death of the fetus *in utero* to various degrees of damage to liver, spleen, reticuloendothelial system and central nervous system. The latter is a common cause of hearing loss and mental retardation. Even in infants who are asymptomatic at birth, hearing deficits and ocular damage (*e.g.,* chorioretinitis) may appear later and continue to progress during the first few years of life. Whether symptomatic or not, congenitally and perinatally infected infants may continue to excrete virus for years after birth, thus serving as an important reservoir. Reactivation of virus shedding in a women with antibodies against CMV gives rise to lower rate of fetal infection and rarely do symptoms or sequelae occur.
3. The third clinical manifestation is CMV infection in severely immunocompromised individuals. In contrast to symptomatic congenital CMV and CMV mononucleosis, which are most commonly manifestations of primary CMV infection, immunocompromised hosts may suffer life-threatening disease from either primary or reactivated CMV infection. Destruction of gastrointestinal tract tissues (esophagitis, enterocolitis, gastritis), pneumonia, retinitis, encephalitis and dementia are common features. Interstitial pneumonia is the leading cause of death in bone marrow transplant recipients. CMV often causes disseminated disease in AIDS patients; gastroenteritis and chorioretinitis are common, the latter may lead to progressive blindness.

Laboratory Diagnosis

Diagnosis is done by

1. demonstration of cytomegalic cells with inclusion bodies in the centrifuged deposits of urine, salvia, cervical secretions, semen, blood and breast milk.
2. demonstration of virus under electron microscope.
3. detection of viral antigen by immunofluorescence.
4. Throat washings, urine and other body fluids or biopsy materials may be inoculated into human fibroblast cell cultures. Cytopathic effects appear slowly in one to two weeks, consisting of small foci of swollen, translucent cells with large intranuclear inclusions. Cell degeneration progresses slowly and the virus remains cell-associated.
5. Antibody detection by serological tests such as CFT, IHA, immunofluorescence, neutralisation, RIA and ELISA.

   Primary and recurrent infections can be distinguished by demonstrating IgG seroconversion or the presence of CMV-specific IgM. Primary CMV infection can be identified in normal hosts by virus isolation coupled with IgM seroconversion.
6. Direct demonstration of viral DNA by hybridisation or restriction enzyme analysis.

Treatment and Prevention

Ganciclovir, cidofovir and foscarnet (phosphonoformic acid) are used for the treatment of CMV infections in immunocompromised patients.

Specific control measures and vaccines are not available. Isolation of newborns with generalized cytomegalic inclusion disease from other newborn is advisable.

EPSTEIN-BARR VIRUS (EBV)

Pathogenesis

EBV discovery in association with the childhood disease Burkitt's lymphoma led to its recognition as the first human virus clearly related to a malignancy. EBV is a ubiquitous herpesvirus that is the causative agent of acute infectious mononucleosis, nasopharyngeal carcinoma, Burkitt's lymphoma and other lymphoproliferative disorders in immunodeficient individuals.

Infectious Mononucleosis (Glandular Fever)

EBV is commonly transmitted by intimate oral contact (kissing) by saliva. The initial site of virus replication appears to be epithelial cells of the oropharynx and salivary glands, following which the progeny viruses infect **B lymphocytes** by binding to viral **receptor CR2 or CD21**, which is also the receptor for C3d component of complement. In contrast to herpesviruses some genes of EBV induce cell multiplication and immortalization, rather than cell death. Thus infection induces polyclonal B cell proliferation and an accompanying nonspecific increase into IgM, IgG and IgA. Autoantibodies are typical of the disease. The IgM class contains "**heterophile antibodies**" that reacts with antigens on sheep and horse RBC. These antibodies are the basis for the classic diagnostic heterophile agglutination test for EBV-infectious mononucleosis, known as Paul-Bunnel test.

Primary infections usually occur in childhood and are asymptomatic resulting in permanent immunity to infectious mononucleosis but fifty percent of those infected later in life (adolescence, young adulthood) develop the disease. Many people shed virus for weeks to months after infection. During the first week of the primary infection, ten to twenty percent of circulating B cells contain EBV genomes, and express the early proteins. Within weeks, an active cytotoxic T cell response to the EBV antigens expressed by the infected B cells results in a rapid decrease of infected B cells to less than one percent. It is the cytotoxic T cell response that constitutes the characteristic "**atypical lymphocytosis**" of infectious mononucleosis.

EBV can remain latent in B cells, with several molecules of its circular DNA present in the cytoplasm as well as copies of its genome integrated into host DNA. Reactivation results in initiation of the viral lytic cycle, with progeny viruses infecting epithelial elis of oropharynx. Reactivations are usually clinically inapparent, but may be serious in immunosuppressed individuals.

The disease appears after an incubation period of four to seven weeks and symptoms include headache, malaise, fatigue, sore throat, fever, lymphadenopathy, splenomegaly. Some patients develop hepatitis. Rash may occur in small percentage of cases.

Chronic EBV Infections

A few patients may develop a severe syndrome following EBV infection that includes pneumonitis, hepatitis and hematogic abnormalities. There is a prolonged, relapsing course, sometimes ending in death. EBV has been proposed as causative agent of "**chronic fatigue syndrome**".

Burkitt's Lymphoma

EBV causes Burkitt's lymphoma, a tumor of the jaw in African children and young adults. Malaria and AIDS are known risk factors for development of Burkitt's lymphoma. The cells of Burkitt's lymphoma contain characteristic chromosome translocations. The break points of these translocations are such that *c-myc* protooncogene on chromosome eight is constitutively activated.

Nasopharyngeal Carcinoma

This cancer of epithelial cells of nasopharynx is common in males of Chinese origin. It differs from Burkitt's lymphoma that there is no characteristic chromosomal alteration, and the cells involved are epithelial in origin. EB virus DNA is regularly found in nasopharyngeal carcinoma cells, and patients have high levels of antibodies to EBV.

Infections in Immunodeficient Hosts

EBV may induce lymphoproliferative diseases or B cell lymphomas that may be fatal in immunocompromised patients, such as transplant recipients and AIDS cases. Lymphomas are often multiclonal and do not show the Burkitt's lymphoma-like chromosome abnormalities. AIDS patients are susceptible to several EBV lesions including diffuse polyclonal lymphomas, lymphocytic interstitial pneumonitis, and **hairy oral leukoplakia** (wart-like growth) or tongue. Not all Burkitt's lymphomas occuring in AIDS patients are associated with EBV.

Laboratory Diagnosis

(*i*) Atypical lymphocytes (cytotoxic T cells) characterised by basophilic vacuolated cytoplasm and kidney shaped nuclei showing a lattice of fenestrated chromatin can be observed in the blood smear of a patient with infectious mononucleosis.

(*ii*) EBV DNA can be detected in patient materials by nucleic acid hybridisation and PCR.

(*iii*) Viral antigens can be demonstrated directly in lymphoid tissues, in nasopharyngeal carcinomas, and sometimes in peripheral blood cells by immunofluorescence. During the acute phase of infection, about 1% of circulating lymphocytes will contain EBV markers; after recovery from infection, about one in one million B lymphocytes will carry the virus.

(*iv*) Demonstration of EBV-specific antibodies: The most common serological tests to demonstrate antibodies to EBV (IgM antibody to viral capsid antigen) are indirect immunofluorescence and ELISA. It is a reliable indication of primary infection.

The classic serological test is **Paul-Bunnel test** often used to diagnose EBV infection. It is a **heterophile agglutination test**. In the course of infectious mononucleosis, most patients develop heterophile antibodies that agglutinate sheep and horse RBC. Inactivated patient serum in doubling dilutions is mixed with equal volumes of a 1% suspension of sheep RBC and incubated at 37° for 4 hrs and examined for agglutination. An agglutination titre of 100 or above is suggestive of infectious mononucleosis. However, these heterophile antibodies may also occur in normal serum and after serum therapy. Infectious mononucleosis antibodies may be differentiated by adsorption tests with guinea pig kidney cells and ox red cells. The heterophile antibody (**Forssman antibody**) induced by serum therapy (administration of horse serum) is adsorbed by guinea pig kidney and ox RBC. Normal heterophile antibodies are adsorbed by guinea pig kidney, but not by ox red cells. Infectious mononucleosis antibody is adsorbed by ox RBC but not guinea pig kidney cells. (Table 85.3). There is a comparable horse erythrocyte agglutination test, a slide agglutination test employing sensitised horse erythrocytes. The Paul-Bunnel antibodies appear early during the course of infectious mononucleosis and disappears within about two months.

Table 85.3 Differential Adsorption Test for Paul-Bunnel Antibody

	Adsorption on	
	Guinea pig kidney	*OX red cells*
Normal serum	Adsorbed	Not adsorbed
Antibodies after serum therapy	Adsorbed	Adsorbed
Infectious mononucleosis	Not adsorbed	Adsorbed

(*v*) **Virus isolation.** EBV can be isolated from saliva, peripheral blood or lymphoid tissues inoculated on to normal human lymphocytes, usually obtained from umbilical cord blood. If the specimen contains EBV, it induces immortalization of lymphocytes to produce a lymphoblastoid cell line.

Treatment and Prevention

Acyclovir reduces EBV shedding from the oropharynx and has been used successfully in the treatment of oral hairy leukoplakia. Although acyclovir inhibits EBV replication, none of the antiherpes drugs including acyclovir has no effect on the symptoms of infectious mononucleosis and is of no proved benefit in the treatment of EBV-associated lymphomas. No vaccine for prevention of EBV infection is currently available.

HUMAN HERPES VIRUS 6 (HHV-6)

HHV-6 classified as a member of betaherpesvirinae, and closely similar to human cytomegalovirus. The virus replicates in salivary glands and are secreted into saliva, and transmission is through oral secretions. The virus also infect peripheral blood lymphocytes, particularly in immature T cells. Other cell types that support viral replication are B cells and cells of glial, fibroblastoid and megakaryocyte origin. HHV-6 infection of lymphoid cells induces a number of significant cell responses, including the synthesis of the CD_4 glycoprotein.

Infections with HHV-6 typically occur in early infancy. The primary infection causes exanthem subitum (roseola infantum, or "sixth disease"), the mild childhood disease characterised by high fever and skin rash. The primary infection in adults is rare, and may result in prolonged lymphadenopathy—a mononucleosis like syndrome, hepatitis and other lymphoproliferative diseases.

Latently infected cells are found among the peripheral blood lymphocytes. Recurrent infections occur in AIDS and immunosuppression for organ transplantation. Reactivation of latent HHV-6 (frequently together with CMV) is associated with sometimes—fatal interstitial pneumonitis, fever, hepatitis and encephalitis, as well as with transplant rejection.

The ability of HHV-6 to induce expression of CD4 in cells not normally expressing it has the consequence of extending the range of cells infectible by HIV. HHV-6 transactivates transcription of HIV, thereby increases the rate of cell death in coinfected cells. Moreover, extensive disseminated HHV-6 infection frequently occurs in terminal AIDS patients. All these facts suggests that HHV-6 may be an important factor in accelerating the progression from early HIV infection to terminal AIDS. The most common clinical syndrome associated with HHV-6 in AIDS patients is encephalitis.

HHV-6 can be isolated from peripheral blood lymphocytes in early febrile stage of the illness by cocultivation with cord blood lymphocytes.

PCR has been used to demonstrate HHV-6 DNA in the CSF of patients with neurologic disease, and in serum of patients undergoing post transplant reactivation of a latent infection. Serologically, there is a cross reaction between HHV-6 and HHV-7 and CMV. Virus antigen can be detected in infected cells by immunofluorescence using monoclonal antibodies.

Because of its genetic relationship with CMV, HHV-6 is in general inhibited by the same drugs. In AIDS patients, treatment of the HIV infection appears to reduce the amount of HHV-6 as well. No vaccine is available. Although there is considerable cross reaction between HHV-6 and HHV-7, there is no cross-immunity between them.

HUMAN HERPES VIRUS 7 (HHV-7)

HHV-7 was first isolated from activated T cells from peripheral blood lymphocytes of a healthy individual. HHV-7 is immunologically distinct from HHV-6, though they share some homology at the DNA level. There are also some genetic similarities with CMV.

HHV-7 is an ubiquitous agent, with most infections occuring in childhood, transmitted through saliva. HHV-7 has been recovered frequently from saliva of healthy individuals. It may cause roseola infantum, identical to that of caused by HHV-6, and in some cases, coinfection may occur with both HHV-6 and HHV-7.

HHV-7 shares with HIV, the same CD_4 receptor on T cells and could therefore contribute to a further depletion of CD_4 T cells in HIV infected persons.

HUMAN HERPES VIRUS 8 (HHV-8)

HHV-8 infection is not as common as other herpesvirus infections in the normal healthy population. It has been detected in over 90% of Kaposi's sarcomas. Hence it is also called "**Kaposi's sarcoma-associated herpes virus (KSHV**). It appears to be lymphotropic and is more closely related to EB virus and herpes virus saimiri than to other known herpes viruses. The viral genome contains several genes related to cellular genes involved in cell proliferation and host responses. These include genes for several cytokines, cytokine receptors and growth factors, which may contribute to viral pathogenesis.

The primary method for detection of HHV-8 is by DNA hybridization following PCR amplification. Antibody status can be evaluated by means of an immunofluorescence test with nuclei from HHV-8 latently infected lymphoma cell line, or ELISA, using one or more virion peptides as the antigen. Antibodies to the HHV-8 antigens are found at increased levels in same population that are at risk for HIV infection, leading to the conclusion that the virus can be sexually transmitted.

CERCOPITHECINE HERPESVIRUS 1 (Old names—Herpesvirus simiae and B virus)

The virus was first isolated from the brain of a laboratory worker who developed a fatal ascending myelitis following the bite by a healthy monkey. It came to be known as the "B" virus from the initials of this patient. B virus is a typical herpesvirus that infects old world monkeys (rhesus, cynomolgus and macaque monkeys), similar to HSV infections of humans; the infections usually being asymptomatic, with the establishment of latent infections in infected hosts. The virus is currently designated cercopithecine herpesvirus 1, replacing the older name Herpes virus simiae.

The virus grows well in monkey kidney, rabbit kidney and human cell cultures, as well as in chick embryos. The growth cycle is short, the virus levels being maximum within 24 hrs. Cytopathic effect is similar to that of HSV consisting of cell fusion into multinuceated giant cells and intranuclear inclusions form.

Virus infections in rhesus monkeys is asymptomatic and vesicular lesions of the oropharynx may occur resembling HSV lesions. Many rhesus monkeys carry latent B virus infections that may be reactivated by conditions of stress. The virus may be present in saliva, conjunctival and vesicular fluids.

Transmission of virus to humans is limited. The infections that do occur carry a high mortality rate. B virus disease of humans is an acute, usually fatal ascending myelitis and encephalomyelitis. The human infection results from a monkey bite. The virus enters through skin and produces vesicles and the necrosis at the site of bite. From here the virus reaches CNS through peripheral nerves. About a week later, motor and sensory abnormalities occur, followed by acute ascending paralysis, involvement of respiratory center and death. Virus can be recovered from the brain and spinal cord of fatal cases. Animal workers and persons handling monkeys are at risk of acquiring B virus infection. Since the infection by the respiratory route is possible, persons having intimate contact with animal workers are also at some risk.

There is no specific treatment once the disease is manifested. However, acylovir is recommended immediately after exposure. An experimental inactivated B virus vaccine has been tested in monkeys, but is not available for use in humans.

QUESTIONS

Essay Questions:

1. Mention herpesviruses of medical importance. Describe briefly herpes simplex virus.
2. Enumerate DNA viruses. Describe herpesviruses.
3. List the human herpesiviruses. Discuss briefly their role as opportunistic pathogens and add a note on laboratory diagnosis.

Short Notes.

1. Herpes simplex virus.
2. Herpes simplex infections in man (or) pathogenicity of HSV.
3. Laboratory diagnosis of Herpes simplex infections in man.
4. Varicella or chickenpox.
5. Herpes zoster or etiology and pathogenesis of herpes zoster.
6. V-Z virus (Varicella-Zoster).
7. Cytomegalovirus or Salivary gland virus or cytomegalic inclusion disease or clinical manifestations of cytomegalovirus.
8. Epstein-Barr virus (or) EB virus (or) Describe the etiology and laboratory diagnosis of infectious mononucleosis.
9. Infectious mononucleosis.
10. Paul-Bunnel test or principle of Paul-Bunnel test.
11. Cytomegalovirus inclusions.
12. Mention the complications of intrauterine infections due to cytomegalovirus.
13. Describe the lesions caused by herpes simplex virus and their laboratory diagnosis.
14. Tzanck's smear.
15. Fever blister.

86

Poxviruses

- *Introduction*
- *Classification*
- *Structure*
- *Replication*
- *Smallpox—Vaccinia nad Variola Viruses, Cultivation, Control and eradication of smallpox, Pathogenesis and clinical features, Laboratory diagnosis, Differential diagnosis, Prophylaxis, Treatment, Smallpox as a biological weapon*
- *Monkeypox*
- *Cowpox*
- *Orf Virus*
- *Molluscum contagiosum Virus*
- *Yatapoxvirus—Tanapox, Yaba Monkey tumor virus*

INTRODUCTION

The poxviruses are large, genetically complex viruses with no obvious symmetry and widely distributed in nature. This group includes variola virus, the cause of smallpox, the first infectious disease to be declared eradicated (1977) from the earth.

Currently, the vaccine poxviruses, known as vaccinia virus is being used as a vector for carrying immunizing genes as live-virus vaccines for a variety of viral discases of humans and animals.

CLASSIFICATION

Based on host range, the family **Poxviridae** is divided into two subfamilies: **chordopoxvirinae**, the poxviruses of vertebrates, and Entomopoxvirinae, the poxviruses of insects. The vertebrate poxviruses fall into eight genera—***Orthopoxvirus***, *Parapoxvirus, Molluscipoxvirus, Yatapoxvirus, Capripoxvirus* (sheeppox, goatpox, lumpy skin disease viruses), *Leporipoxvirus* (myxoma and fibromas in rabbits, hares, squirrels), *Avipoxvirus* (fowlpox, pigeonpox, canarypox, turkeypox) and *Suipoxvirus* (swinepox). Poxviruses causing diseases are enumerated in Table 86.1.

Table 86.1 Poxviruses Causing Diseases in Humans

Genus	*Virus*	*Primary host*	*Disease*
Orthopoxvirus	Variola	Humans	Smallpox (now extinct)
	Vaccinia	Humans	Localized lesion, used for smallpox vaccination

	Buffalopox	• Buffaloes	Human infections rare; localized disease
	Monkeypox	Monkeys	Human infections rare; generalized disease
	Cowpox	Cows	Human infections rare; localized ulcerating lesion
Parapoxvirus	Orf	Sheep	Human infections rare; localized lesion
	Pseudocowpox	Cows	
	Bovine popular stomatitis	cows	
Malluscipox-virus	Molluscum contagioum	Humans	Benign skin nodules
Yatapoxvirus	Tanapox	Monkeys	Human infections rare; localized lesion
	Yabapox	Monkeys	Human infections very rare and accidental; localized skin tumors

STRUCTURE

Poxviruses are large, measuring about 400 × 230 nm and can be seen by light microscopy. They are brick shaped and possess a complex symmetry that conforms to neither icosahedral nor helical symmetry (Fig. 86.1a). There is an outer lipoprotein envelope, that encloses a core, and two structures of unknown function called **lateral bodies**. The core contains a large genome consisting of a single linear molecule of double-stranded DNA, that often appears as a **binconcave nucleoid** (Fig. 86.1b). On either side of the nucleoid is a lateral body. The virion contains several enzymes. The external surface of virus particle contains ridges. All vertebrate poxviruses share a common nucleoprotein antigen in the inner core.

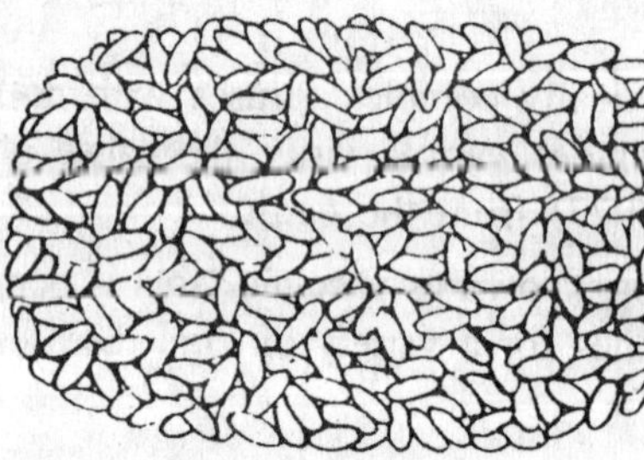

Fig. 86.1 (a) Poxviruses

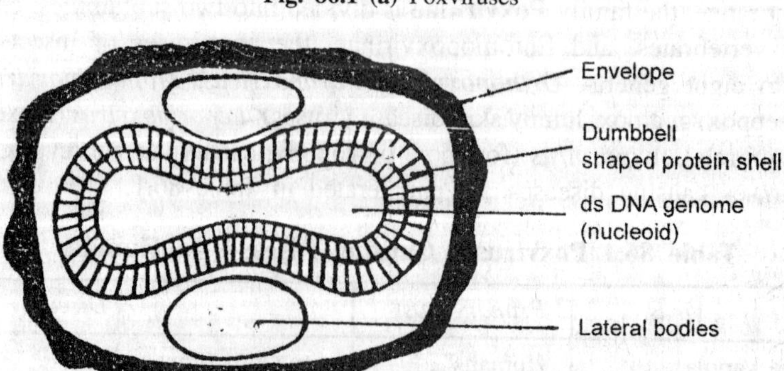

Fig. 86.1 (b) Vaccinia virus

REPLICATION

Poxviruses are unique among DNA viruses in that the entire replication cycle takes place in the cytoplasm of infected cells, the virus providing all of the enzymes (including a viral DNA-dependent RNA polymerase) necessary for replication and gene expression. Final maturation by acquisition of a lipoprotein envelope occurs as the virus buds from the cell. The replication cycle is rapid, and results in early shut-off of all cell macromolecular syntheses, causing death of the cell.

POXVIRUS INFECTIONS—SMALLPOX

Vaccinia and Variola Viruses

Vaccinia virus was used for smallpox vaccination, and is a distinct species of *Orthopoxvirus.* It is an artificial virus and does not occur in nature as such. At some time after Jenner's original use of cowpoxvirus, the vaccine virus underwent some permanent changes and became "vaccinia virus". Vacciniavirus may be the product of genetic recombination, a new species derived from cowpoxvirus or variola virus by serial passage, or the descendant of a now extinct viral genus. Restriction endonuclease maps of the genome of vaccinia virus are distinctly from those of cowpox virus.

Smallpox occurs in two distinct clinical varieties: (*i*) the florid, highly fatal disease, typically seen in Asia, known as **classical smallpox** caused by **variola major**, and (*ii*) The mild, nonfatal disease, typically seen in Latin America, known as alastrim type, caused by **Variola minor**. Variola major and minor are antigenically similar, but differ in certain biological properties. They seem to be stable variants as the disease produced by each always breeds true; alastrim does not lead to smallpox and vice versa.

Cultivation

Both vaccinia and variola viruses grow on the **chorioallantoic membrane** of the 10 to 12 day old chick embryo and produces "**pock**" lesions. Vaccinia pocks are larger, irregular, flat, greyish, necrotic lesions, some of which are hemorrhagic; whereas variola pocks are small, shiny, white, convex, nonnecrotic and nonhemorrhagic. The viruses may also be differentiated by their "ceiling temperatures", the highest temperature above which pocks are not produced. The ceiling temperatures are 41°C for vaccinia, 38°C for variola major and 37.5°C for variola minor.

Variola and vaccinia viruses can be grown in tissue cultures of monkey kidney, HeLa and chick embryo cells. Cytopathic effects are produced by vaccinia in one to two days and more slowly by variola. Eosinophilic inclusion bodies (**Guarnieri bodies**) can be demonstrated in stained preparations. The inclusion bodies consists of aggregations of virus particles in a matrix. Vaccinia but not variola virus produces plaques in chick embryo tissues cultures.

The vaccinia virus can infect a wide range of animals (broad host range) experimentally. Monkeys, cows, sheep, rabbits and mice can be infected by scarification leading to vesicular lesions. The variola virus produces similar lesions only in monkeys (narrow host range). Scarification of rabbit cornea with variola virus leads to keratitis and sections of cornea will show typical Guarnieri bodies. Intranasal instillation of the variola virus in the monkey produces a self-limited attack of smallpox with generalized skin lesions.

Control and Eradication of Smallpox

Smallpox was officially declared eliminated in 1979. The last natural case of variola major detected was Saiban Bibi, a Bangladeshi woman found with smallpox on the Karimganj railway platform in Assam on 24 May, 1975. The last case of variola minor occured in Merca, Somalia, in October 1977. The factors that led to the elimination of smallpox are:

1. The availability of very effective, attenuated vaccine.
2. Antigenically stable and only a single antigenic type existed.
3. The absence of asymptomatic cases or persistent carriers.
4. The absence of an animal reservoir.
5. The emotional effect of this highly fatal, disfiguring disease helping gain public cooperation in the eradication efforts.
6. Long term (life long) immunity conferred by infection.

Pathogenesis and Clinical Features

Smallpox was highly contagious. The most common transmission mode is by oral and nasopharyngeal droplets (air-borne). The dried virus in crusts from skin lesions could survive on the clothes or other materials and result in infection. The virus infects the mucus membranes of the upper respiratory tract and then spreads to regional lymph nodes and small blood vessels in the skin.

The incubation period of smallpox was about 12 days. The onset was usually sudden. One to five days of fever and malaise preceded the appearance of the exanthems, which were popular for one to four days, vesicular for one to four days, and pustular for two to six days, forming crusts that fell off two to four weeks after the first sign of the lesion and leaving pink scars that faded slowly. In each affected area, the lesions were generally found in the same stage of a development (in contrast to chickenpox). Body temperature fell within 24 hours after the rash appeared. Approximately, a third of the infected cases die from bleeding, cardiovascular collapse and secondary infections.

In the preeruptive phase, the disease was not highly infective. By the sixth to ninth days, lesions in the mouth ulcerated and discharged virus. Thus, the disease was highly infectious, early in the disease the virus being originated from lesions in the mouth and upper respiratory tract and spread by respiratory air-borne droplets. Later, pustules broke down and discharged virus into the environment.

Lesions were most abundant on the face and less so on the trunk. In severe cases, the rashes were hemorrhagic. Skin pustules could become contaminated, usually with staphylococci, sometimes leading to bacteremia and sepsis.

Smallpox occurs in two distinct clinical varieties: the florid, highly fatal disease, typically seen in Asia, known as classical smallpox caused by variola major, and the mild, nonfatal disease, typically seen in Latin America, known as alastrim type, caused by Variola minor.

Laboratory Diagnosis

Several tests are available to confirm the clinical diagnosis of smallpox.

Microscopy

Paschen (1906) developed a staining technique for the virus particles and demonstrated the elementary bodies (**paschen bodies**) in smears from smallpox lesions under light microscope.

Electron microscopy of vesicle or scab material is an effective means of rapid diagnosis, poxviruses and herpesviruses are readily distinguished, and the characteristics morphology of parapoxviruses can be recognized.

Rapid diagnosis can be made by the observation of DNA-containing intracytoplasmic inclusion bodies in cells scraped from skin lesions.

Isolation of Virus

The most reliable method is inoculation of vesicular fluid onto the chorioallantoic membrane of chick embryos. Within two to three days, pock lesions are produced on chorioallantoic membrane. Based on pock morphology cases of small pox can be distinguished from vaccinia; vaccinia pocks are large with necrotic centers whereas variola pocks are much smaller. Cowpox and monkeypox viruses produce distinctive hemorrhagic lesions. The parapoxviruses, molluscum contagiosum virus and tanapoxvirus do not grow on chorioallantoic membrane.

The viruses can be grown in cell cultures of monkey kidney, HeLa and chick embryo cells. Eosinophilic inclusions (Guarnieri bodies) can be demonstrated in stained preparations. Immunofluorescence of infected cell cultures will differentiate morphologically similar poxviruses from different genera.

Detection of Virus Antigen

Viral antigen can be detected by gel precipitation in material collected from skin lesions. The test identifies orthopoxviruses as a group.

Demonstration of Antibodies in Patient Serum

Virus isolation is necessary for quick and accurate identification of poxvirus infections. However, antibody assays can be used to confirm a diagnosis. Antibodies appear after the first week of infection and can be detected by hemagglutination inhibition, neutralisation, immunofluorescence, RIA and ELISA tests.

Differential Diagnosis

Smallpox must be differentially diagnosed as it may be confused with chickenpox, pustular acne, meningococcemia, secondary syphilis, drug rashes and other diseases associated with a skin eruption.

Smallpox-like diseases must be identified by restriction enzyme cleavage of viral DNA and the analysis of polypeptides in infected cells demonstrate distinct characteristics for variola, vaccinia, monkeypox and cowpox to ascertain the variola has indeed been eradicated.

Prophylaxis

Smallpox vaccine is a live attenuated vaccinia virus prepared from vesicular lesions (lymph) produced in the skin of calves or sheep, or it can be grown on chick embryos. The final product contains 40% glycerol to stabilize the virus and 0.4% phenol to prevent bacterial contaimination.

The vaccine is administered into the basal layers of epidermis by multiple puncture with a bifurcated needle. Following successful primary vaccination, a vesicle develops at the site in 3–5 days, which becomes pustular, achieving maximum size after 8–10 days. A scab is formed, which separates after 2–3 weeks, leaving a depressed scar, which remains life-long. Smallpox vaccination may carry a small risk of complication such as developing a mild smallpox disease and rarely encephalitis.

Immunization with vaccinia is no longer done routinely, but may be carried out in certain group such as the military and laboratory workers.

Treatment

Vaccinia immune globulin prepared from blood of revaccinated military personnel is recommended for treatment of all complications except postvaccinal encephalitis. The drug methisazone may be beneficial in severe cases of eczema vaccinatum that do not respond to vaccinia immune globulin.

Smallpox as a Biological Weapon

Smallpox is pontentially dangerous biological weapon because it is highly contagious and has a high case fatality rate—more than thirty percent among unvaccinated persons. Since the routine vaccination is stopped, the population susceptible to smallpox infection is increasing each year.

MONKEYPOX INFECTIONS

Monkeypox virus belongs to genus *Orthopoxvirus.* It was first isolated in 1958 from an outbreak of pox disease in captive monkeys. Human infections with this virus were discovered in the early 1970s. This human monkeypox disease occurs as a rare zoonosis in west and central Africa, particularly in Zaire. It is probably acquired by direct contact by handling infected animals. It is not transmitted from person to person. The primary reservoir host may be a rodent.

Clinical symptoms were similar to smallpox. "Cropping" of the rash occured in some patients, posing a diagnostic problem with chickenpox. Pronounced lymphadenopathy occured in most patients, a feature not seen with smallpox or chickenpox. Complications such as pulmonary distress and secondary bacterial infections were common and often serious. Vaccination with vaccinia either protects against monkeypox or lessens the severity of disease.

COWPOX INFECTIONS

Cowpoxvirus belongs to genus *Orthopoxvirus.* The lesions are confined to the teats and udders of cattle. Human infections occur by direct contact during milking, and the lesions in milkers is usually confined to the hands and fingers. They are localized, painful, hemorrhagic ulcers, associated with fever and lymphadenitis.

Cowpoxvirus is similar to vaccinia virus immunologically and in host range. It is also closely related immunologically to variola virus. Edward Jenner observed that those who have had cowpox are immune to smallpox. Cowpox virus produces deep red hemorrhagic lesions on the chorioallantoic membrane of chick embryos.

The natural reservoirs of cowpox are rodents. From these animals the virus may occasionally spread to cattle, humans, cats and various zoo animals. Restriction endonuclease analysis of DNA exhibits distinct differences between variola and cowpox.

Milker's Nodes Virus (paravaccinia) produces skin lesions similar to cowpox, usually painless in cattle. The lesions are small ulcerating nodules. The virus is not related to cowpox and does not grow in eggs. It can be grown in bovine kidney cultures. It resembles the Orf virus morphologically.

ORF VIRUS INFECTIONS

The Orf virus belong to genus *Parapoxvirus*. It causes a disease in sheep and goats and is prevalent worldwide. Orf virus is transmitted to humans by direct contact with an infected animal. It is an occupational disease of sheep and goat handlers. Human infection occurs usually as a single lesion on a finger, hand, or forearm but may appear on the face or neck. Lesions are large nodules, rather painful with surrounding inflamed skin. The disease is also called contagious pustular dermatitis or sore mouth.

MOLLUSCUM CONTAGIOSUM

Molluscum contagiosum is a benign epidermal tumor that occurs only in humans. The causative agent is classified as the sole member of the genus ***Molluscipoxvirus***. The virus is oval or brick shaped, measuring 230×330 nm. The morphology and viral DNA resembles that of vaccinia virus.

The disease is of two types: (*i*) First type is more common among children and spreads by direct or indirect contact (*e.g.,* by barbers, common use of towels, swimming pools). The lesions of this disease are small, pink, wart-like tumors on the face, arms, back and buttocks. They are rarely found on the palms, soles or mucus membranes. The disease occurs throughout the world, in both sporadic and epidemic forms. (*ii*) the second type is common among young adults and is sexually transmitted. It is also seen in some patients with AIDS. The lesions occur in the genital area. Although the typical lesion is an umbiliated papule, lesions may become inflamed or ulcerated and may be confused with those produced by HSV.

The incubation period may be up to six months. Lesions may itch, leading to autoinoculation. The lesions may persists for up to two years but will eventually regress spontaneously. The virus is a poor immunogen and antibodies may not be produced.

The diagnosis of molluscum contagiosum can usually be made clinically. Sections of skin lesions show large, eosinophilic intracytoplasmic inclusions, which displace the nuclei to the margin, known as **molluscum bodies** under light microscope. These molluscum bodies are composed of large number of virus particles embedded in a protein matrix. It can be detected from the material taken from lesions under electron microscope. The virus cannot be grown in animals or tissue cultures.

YATAPOXVIRUS INFECTIONS

Tanapox and Yaba monkey tumor viruses are serologically related to each other but are distinct from all other poxviruses. They are classified in the genus *Yatapoxvirus.* They are morphologically similar to orthopoxviruses. The viruses grow only in cultures of monkey and human, with cytopathic effects. They do not grow on the choriallantoic membrane of embryonated eggs.

Tanapox is a common skin infection in parts of Africa, mainly in Kenya and Zaire. Its natural hosts is probably monkey and the disease spreads from infected animals to humans by contaminated arthropods. Tanapox begins with a fever of 3–4 days alongwith severe headache and prostration. There are usually one or two skin lesions. Pustulation never occurs. Healing occurs in 4–7 weeks.

Yaba monkey tumor poxvirus causes benign tumors (histiocytomas) in monkeys. The tumor regress after about 5 weeks. Monkeys and humans are susceptible to infection. Although animal handlers have become infected, Yaba virus infections of humans are not found naturally in Africa.

QUESTIONS

Short Notes:

1. Enumerate poxviruses and the diseases caused by them.
2. Draw a neat labelled diagram of poxvirus.
3. Variola virus.
4. Vaccinia virus.
5. Smallpox vaccine or complications of small pox vaccine.
6. Molluscum contagiosum or Molluscum bodies.

87

Hepatitis Viruses

- *Introduction*
- *Hepatitis A virus—structure and properties, epidemiology, pathogenesis and clinical features, laboratory diagnosis, prophylaxis, treatment.*
- *Hepatitis B virus—classification, structure and properties, epidemiology, pathogenesis and clinical features, laboratory diagnosis, prophylaxis, treatment.*
- *Hepatitis C virus—structure and properties, epidemiology, clinical features, laboratory diagnosis, prophylaxis, treatment.*
- *Hepatitis D virus—structure and properties, pathogenesis, epidemiology, laboratory diagnosis, prophylaxis.*
- *Hepatitis E virus*
- *Hepatitis G virus*

INTRODUCTION

Viral hepatitis is a systemic infection characterized by inflammation and necrosis, resulting in a clinical illness characterized by fever, gastrointestinal symptoms such as nausea and vomiting, and jaundice. '**Hepatitis viruses**' are those whose pathogenesis specifically involves replication in and destruction of hepatocytes. Thus, the term 'viral hepatitis' refers to primary infection of the liver by any one of 'hepatitis viruses', which currently consists of hepatitis A virus (HAV), hepatitis B virus (HBV), hepatitis C virus (HCV), hepatitis D virus (HDV), hepatitis E virus (HEV) and hepatitis G virus (HGV). HGV has been isolated but has not been characterized enough and is not included. **Hepatitis F virus**, though believed to cause transfusion-associated hepatitis, distinct from type A to E but proved to be a mutant of type B virus and not a separate entity. In addition, there are many viral diseases that involve some degree of liver damage as a secondary effect such as those caused by yellow fever virus, cytomegalovirus, Epstein-Barr virus, herpes simplex virus, rubella virus and enteroviruses. Based on epidemiological and clinical criteria, two types of viral hepatitis had been recognised for long. (*i*) **Type A hepatitis** or **infectious hepatitis (infectious jaundice**). It occurs sporadically or in epidemics, affecting mainly children and young adults, and transmitted by fecal-oral route. (*ii*) **Type B hepatitis** or **serum hepatitis (serum jaundice** or **transfusion hepatitis**). It is transmitted by blood transfusion or serum inoculation (Table 87.1).

Table 87.1 Hepatitis viruses

Feature	*Hepatitis A virus*	*Hepatitis B virus*	*Hepatitis C virus*	*Hepatitis D virus*	*Hepatitis E virus*	*Hepatitis G virus*
Year of identification	1973	1965	1989	1977	1980	1995
Family	Picornaviridae	Hepadnaviridae	Flaviviridae	Unclassified	Caliciviridae	Flaviviridae
Genus	*Hepatovirus*	*Orthohepadnavirus*	*Hepacivirus*	*Deltavirus*	*Unnamed*	*Hepacivirus*
Genome	ssRNA	dsDNA	ssRNA	ssRNA	ssRNA	ssRNA
Genome size	7.5 kb	3.2 kb	9.4 kb	1.7 kb	7.6 kb	9.4 kb
Virion	27 nm, icosahedral	42 nm, spherical	30–60 nm, spherical	36–38 nm, spherical	27–38 nm, icosahedral	?
Envelope	No	Yes (HBsAg)	Yes	yes (HBsAg)	No	?
Stability	Heat- and acid-stable	Acid-stable	Ether- and acid-sensitive	Acid-sensitive	Heat-stable	?
Transmission	Faecal-oral	Parenteral, sexual	Parenteral, sexual	Parenteral, sexual	Faecal-oral	Parenteral, sexual
Vertical transmission						
• Intrauterine	No	Yes	Possible but rare	Possible but rare	Yes	?
• Perinatal	No	Yes	Yes	Yes	Yes	Yes
• Early post-natal infection	Possible but rare	Possible but rare	Possible	?	?	?
Incubation period	2–6 weeks	6 weeks–6 months	6–8 weeks	6 weeks–6 months	2–8 weeks	?
Onset	Acute	Insidious or acute	Insidious	Insidious or acute	Acute	?
Age preference	Children, young adults	Young adults, babies toddlers,	Any age but more common in adults	Any age	Young to middle-age adults	?
Antigens	HAV	HBsAg, HBcAg, HBeAg	HCV	HBsAg, HDAg	HEVAg	?
Antibodies	Anti-HAV	Anti-HBs, Anti-HBc, Anti-HBe	Anti-HCV	Anti-HBs, Anti-HD	Anti-HEV	?
Chronic carrier state	No	5–10%	50%	>50%	No	?
Chronic hepatitis, cirrhosis	No	1–5%	20%	>50%	No	?
Hepatocellular carcinoma	No	Yes	Yes	No	No	?

?, data not yet available.

HEPATITIS A VIRUS (HAV)

Structure and Properties

HAV is a 27–32 nm spherical particle with icosahedral symmetry, containing a linear, single-stranded RNA genome. It is a nonenveloped virus. It was first provisionally classified as **enterovirus 72**. But, based on differences in nucleotide and amino acid sequences, it is assigned to a new separate genus ***Hepatovirus*** of the family **picornaviridae**. Only one serotype is known. There is no antigenic cross reaction with other hepatitis viruses.

It grows poorly in tissue cultures. Various primate cell lines will support growth, though fresh isolates are difficult to adapt and grow.

HAV is resistant to inactivation by heat at 60°C for one hour, 20% ether, acid pH 3.0 and many disinfectants. However, it can be inactivated by boiling for one minute, chlorine (one ppm for thirty minutes) and formalin (1:4000 for 3 days at 37°C) and UV radiation.

Epidemiology

Natural infection with HAV is seen only in humans. HAV is widespread throughout the world. Outbreaks of type A hepatitis are common in families and institutions and among military troops. Overcrowding and poor sanitation favor its spread. The disease is common among children and young adults, but can occur at any age. Recurrent epidemics are common.

HAV is transmitted by ingestion of contaminated food, water or milk, and the virus is shed in the feces (**fecal-oral route**). For example, a common mode of transmission of the virus is through eating uncooked shellfish harvested from sewage-contaminated water (Table 87.2).

Table 87.2 Epidemiologic and Clinical Features of Viral Hepatitis Types A, B and C

	Viral hepatitis type A	*Viral hepatitis type B*	*Viral hepatitis type C*
Incubation period	10–50 days (avg. 25–30)	50–180 days (avg. 60–90)	40–120 days
Principal age distribution	Children,[1] young adults	15–29 years.[2]	Adults.[2]
Seasonal incidence	Throughout the year but tends to peak in autumn.	Throughout the year.	Throughout the year.
Route of infection	Predominantly fecal-oral.	Predominantly parenteral.	Predominantly parenteral.
Occurrence of virus blood	2 weeks before to ≤ 1 week after jaundice.	Months to years.	Months to years.
Stool	2 weeks before to 2 weeks after jaundice.	Absent.	Probably absent.
Urine	Rare.	Absent.	Probably absent.
Saliva, semen	Rare (saliva).	Frequently present.	Unknown.
Clinical and laboratory features Onset	Abrupt.	Insidious.	Insidious.
Fever > 38°C (100.4 °F)	Common.	Less common.	Less common.
Duration of aminotransferase elevation	1–3 weeks.	1–6+ months.	1–6+ months.

contd...

Immunoglobulins (IgM levels)	Elevated.	Normal to slightly elevated.	Normal to slightly elevated.
Complications	Uncommon, no chronicity.	Chronicity in 5–10%.	Chronicity in 50% or more.
Mortality rate (icteric cases)	< 0.5%.	< 1–2%.	0.5–1%.
HBsAg	Absent.	Present.	Absent.
Immunity Homologous	Yes.	Yes.	?
Heterologous	No	No	No.
Duration	Probably lifetime.	Probably lifetime.	?
Gamma globulin (immune globulin USP) prophylaxis	Regularity prevents jaundice.	Prevents jaundice only if gamma globulin is of sufficient potency against HBV.	?

1. Nonicteric hepatitis A is common in children.
2. Among the 15–26 year age group, hepatitis B and C are often associated with drug abuse or promiscuous sexual behaviour. Patients with transfusion-associated HBV or HCV are generally over age 29.

Pathogenesis and Clinical Features

Type A hepatitis is a self-limiting disease with an incubation period of 2–6 weeks. Once in the digestive system, the viruses multiply within the intestinal epithelium and enter blood circulation resulting in viremia, which can last several weeks. The virus reaches the liver through blood circulation. The main site of viral replication is hepatocyte. Viral replication results in severe cytopathology and liver function is significantly impaired. The viruses reproduce in the liver, enter bile and are released into small intestine. This explains why feces are so infectious.

Clinical symptoms last from 2–20 days and include anorexia, general malaise, nausea, diarrhoea, fever and chills. HAV can cause sudden, severe infection of liver of cells, resulting in **jaundice**, characterized by classic yellowing of eyes and skin. Very rarely, a rapid, fatal fulminant hepatitis may occur.

Laboratory Diagnosis

HAV particles can be detected by immune electron microscopy in fecal samples of hepatitis patients. Virus appears early in the disease and disappears within two weeks following the onset of jaundice.

HAV can be detected in the liver, bile, stool and blood by RIA, ELISA, nucleic acid hybridization assays and PCR.

Detection of IgM specific anti-HAV in the blood of an acutely infected patient confirms the diagnosis of hepatitis A. IgM antibodies appear during late incubation period, reaches peak levels in 2–3 weeks and disappears within 3–6 months. It is followed by the appearance of IgG antibody, soon after the onset of the disease and eventually replaces IgM antibody, IgG persists for decades and is a useful indicator of immunity (Fig. 87.1). The methods of choice for measuring HAV antibodies are RIA and ELISA.

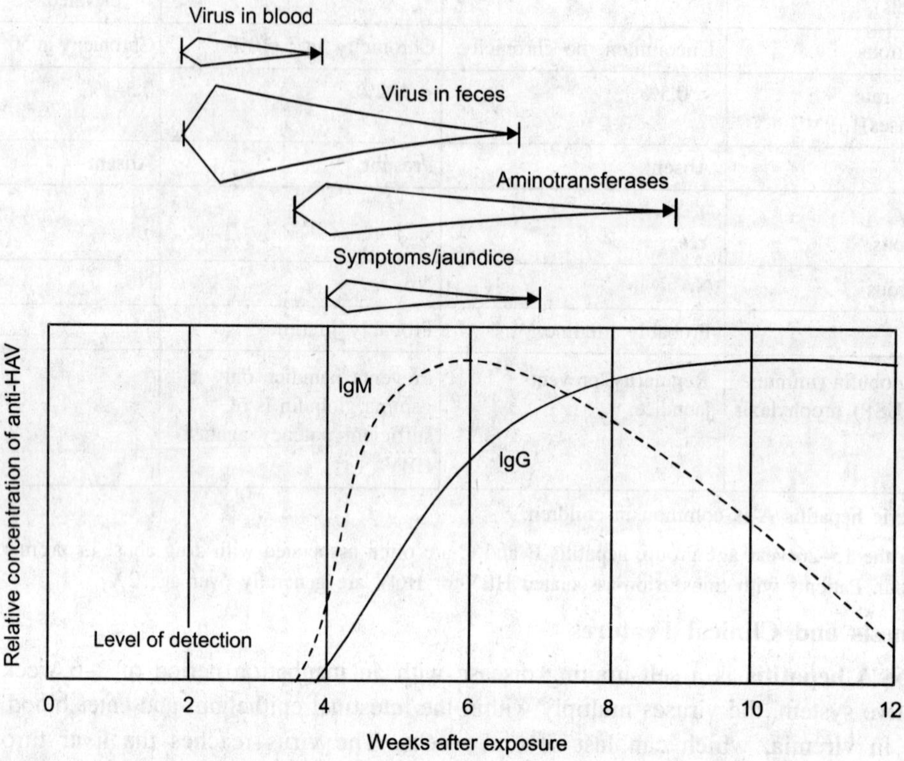

Fig. 87.1. Immunologic and biologic events associated with human infection with hepatitis A virus

Prophylaxis

Control of infection is by simple hygienic measures such as improved sanitary disposal of excreta and prevention of contamination of food and water.

Immune (gamma) globulin (IG) is prepared from large pools of normal adult plasma and confers passive protection in those exposed when given within 1–2 weeks after exposure to hepatitis A. It does not prevent infection but rather makes the infection mild or subclinical and permits active immunity to develop.

A formalin-inactivated (killed) whole virus vaccine made from cell culture-adapted virus is available. The vaccine is safe, effective and recommended for use in persons over two years of age. The vaccine is recommended for high-risk individuals such as travellers going to regions with high prevalence rates of hepatitis A.

Treatment

Treatment for acute hepatitis is largely supportive and directed at allowing hepatocellular damage to resolve and repair.

HEPATITIS B VIRUS (HBV)

Classification

Hepatitis B virus is classified as a member of the family **hepadnaviridae** (hepatotropic DNA viruses) consisting a group of hepatitis–causing viruses with DNA genomes. Each hepadnavirus has a very narrow host range in which it produces both acute infections and chronic, persistent infections. The family hepadnaviridae consists of two genera—***Orthohepadnavirus*** and *Avihepadnavirus*. Hepatitis B virus the only member of the family that infects humans, is classified in the genus *Orthohepadnavirus* along with wood huck and ground squirrel hepatitis viruses. The genus *Avihepadnavirus* contains the Pekin duck and gray heroin hepatitis viruses.

Structure and Properties

The virion of **HBV**, historically referred to as the Dane particle, consists of an icosahedral nucleocapsid enclosed in an envelope.

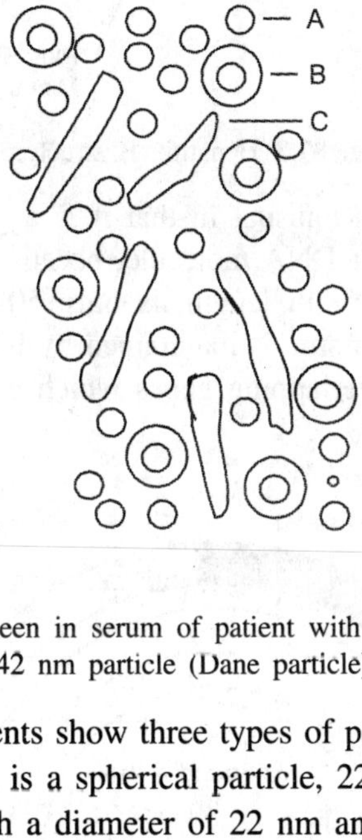

Fig. 87.2 Different types of particles seen in serum of patient with type B hepatitis : A. Spherical 22 nm particle. B. Double shelled 42 nm particle (Dane particle). C. Tubular 22 nm particle

Sera from type B hepatitis patients show three types of particles under the electron microscope (Fig. 87.2). The most abundant form is a spherical particle, 22 nm in diameter. The second type of particle is filamentous or tubular with a diameter of 22 nm and of varying length. These two types of particles are antigenically similar and represent surface subunits of Hepatitis B virus and are known as **Hepatitis B surface antigen (HBsAg)**. It was first observed by Blumberg, in the serum of an Australian patient and was known as **Australia antigen**. The third type of particle is a double walled spherical structure, measuring 42 nm in diameter. This is the complete hepatitis B virus (HBV). It was first described by Dane (1970) and therefore known as **Dane's particle** (Fig. 87.3).

Thus, HBV is a 42 nm DNA virus with an outer envelope and an inner core, 27 nm in diameter, enclosing the viral genome and a DNA polymerase.

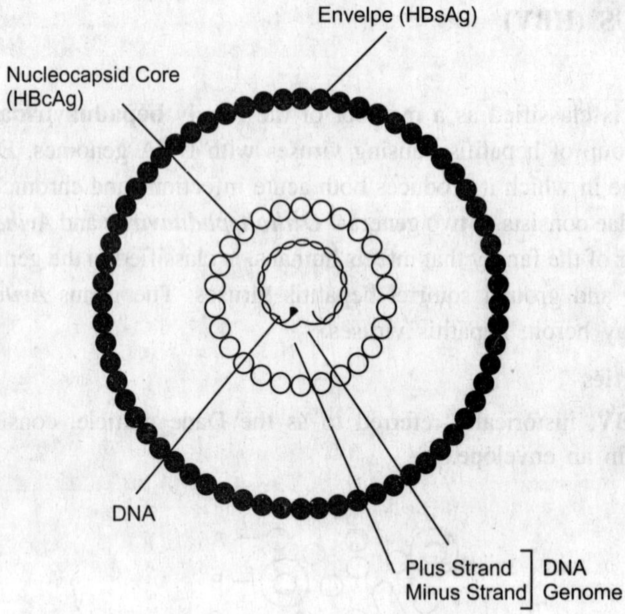

Fig. 87.3 Hepatitis B structure

The short HBV DNA genome is unusual in that it is a partly single-stranded, partly double-stranded, noncovalently closed, circular DNA molecule, because one strand is longer than the other. The short 'plus' strand, which can vary in length, is only 50–80 per cent as long as the 'minus' strand. The circular structure of the genome is maintained by base-pairing of the strands at one end. The genome is organized into four overlapping genes which can code for four proteins (Fig. 87.4, Table 87.3).

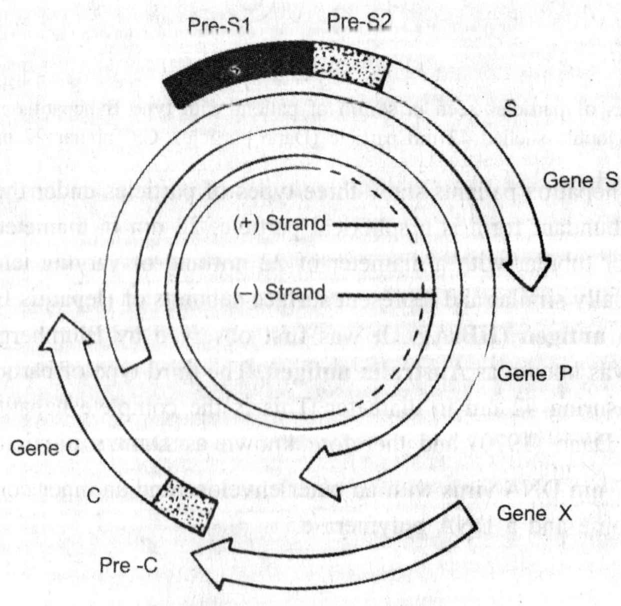

Fig. 87.4 HBV genes and gene products

Table 87.3 HBV genes, Gene Regions and Gene Products

Genes	*Regions*	*Products*
S	S	Major protein (S) ⎤
	S+ Pre-S2	Middle protein (M)⎦ HBsAg
	S+ Pre-S1&S2	Large protein (L)
C	C	HbcAg
	C+ Pre-C	HbeAg
P		DNA polymerase
X		HBxAg

1. The **S gene** codes for the envelope protein, a glycoprotein referred to as the hepatitis B surface antigen (HBsAg). The S gene consists of the S region and two Pre-S region, Pre-S2 and Pre-S1. The protein coded for by the S region is called the S or major protein. When translation begins from the Pre-S2 region, the M or middle protein is formed. When the entire gene from Pre-S1 is translated, the L or large protein results. The L protein is present only in the virion, while the M and S proteins are found in the circulating HBsAg particles also.
2. The **C gene** has two regions, C and pre-C. The C region codes for the core antigen (HBcAg). HBcAg is assembled as the nucleocapsid core particles. It is not secreted and does not circulate in blood. The Pre-C region codes for the protein, HBeAg, a nonparticulate soluble antigen possessing a signal protein which enables it to be secreted and therefore present in circulation.
3. The **P gene** is the largest and comprises 80% of the genome and overlaps all the other genes. It encodes DNA polymerase with three distinct enzymatic functions—DNA polymerase, reverse trnascriptase and RNaseH.
4. The gene *x* encodes a nonstructural, regulatory protein designated the 'x' protein (HBxAg), which has transactivating effects on both viral and some cellular genes.

HBsAg consists of two different antigenic components—the common group reactive antigen "*a*", and two pairs of type specific antigens *d-y* and *w-r*, only one member of each pair being present at a time. HBsAg can thus be divided into four major antigenic subtypes : *adw*, *adr*, *ayw* and *ayr*. The subtypes are not important in immunity, because of the dominant antigen *a* shared by all. They show a distinct geographical distribution. Subtype *ayw* is predominant from West Asia through the Middle East to western and northern India; *adw* is common in Europe, Australia and America; *adr* is prevalent in South and East India and the Far East, *ayr* is very rare.

HBV is present in the blood mainly in the form of HBsAg and to smaller extent as Dane's particles.

HBV replicates within hepatocytes. Viral DNA exists in the hepatocyte nucleus in the free extrachromosomal state or integrated with the cell chromosome. Biologically, HBV is unique in that replication of the DNA genome proceeds via an RNA intermediate which in turn is "reverse transcribed" by a viral enzyme homologous to the retrovirus reverse transcriptase. However, whereas retroviruses package an RNA genome, Hepadnaviridae package a DNA genome.

HBV does not grow in any conventional culture system. However, limited production of the virus and its proteins can be obtained from several cell lines transfected with HBV DNA. HBV genes have been cloned in bacteria and yeasts. The chimpanzee is susceptible to experimental infection.

HBV is relatively heat stable. It is inactivated by heating at 60°C for 10 minutes. Exposure to hypochlorite (10,000 ppm available chlorine) or 2% glutaraldehyde for 10 minutes inactivates infectivity, though HBsAg may not be destroyed.

Epidemiology

Hepatitis B occurs throughout the world. There is no seasonal trend for HBV infection and no high predilection for any age group, although there are definite high-risk groups such as intravenous drug addicts, institutionalized persons, health care personnel, transfusion cases, organ transplant patients, hemodialysis patients and staff, sexually promiscuous persons and neonates born to mothers with hepatitis B. Natural infection is seen only in humans. There is no animal reservoir.

The virus is maintained in the **carriers** whose blood contains circulating virus for long periods, in some even life long. A carrier is a person with detectable HBsAg in blood for more than 6 months. Following infection 5–10 per cent of adults, 30 per cent of children and 90 per cent of neonates become carriers. Carriers are of two types:

1. **Super carriers:** They have high titres of HBsAg, along with HBeAg, DNA polymerase and HBV in circulation. They are highly infectious and minute amounts of carrier sera as little as 0.00001 ml can transmit the infection.
2. **Simple carriers:** They have low titres of HBsAg in blood with negative HBeAg, HBV and DNA polymerase. Simple carriers have low infectivity.

In all populations, males experience a higher rate of chronic HBV infections, a higher rate of progression to **cirrhosis** and a higher rate of **hepatocellular carcinoma**.

Infectious HBV is present in all body fluids of an infected individual. Therefore, blood, semen, saliva, mother's milk etc., serve as sources of infection. Blood of carriers or patients is the most important source of infection and the infection is transmitted by parenteral, perinatal and sexual modes.

1. ***Parenteral transmission:*** HBV is transmitted by blood transfusion, serrum inoculation, needlestick injuries, sharing of syringes and needles particularly among intravenous drug addicts, sharing of razors, tattooing, ear and nose piercing, acupuncture and kissing. Dentists and barbers can infect their clients through the use of contaminated instruments. Transmission of infection may result from accidental inoculation of minute amounts of blood during medical, surgical or dental procedures.
2. ***Perinatal transmission:*** Hepatitis B can be transmitted from an infected mother to the child perinatally. In some parts of the world, such as South East Asia and Japan, perinatal transmission is very common. Almost all infected neonates become carriers, without any clinical illness.
3. ***Sexual transmission:*** HBV can be transmitted by sexual contact, since HBV is present in semen and vaginal secretions. Sexually promiscuous persons and male homosexuals are at very high risk.

Pathogenesis and Clinical Features

Hepatitis B (**serum hepatitis, serum jaundice, transfusion hepatitis**) is of medical and public health importance not only as the cause of acute liver disease, but especially as the cause of chronic, persistent infections that can result in the eventual death of the infected individual due to cirrhosis and liver cancer. Thus, the outcome after infection with HBV varies, ranging from complete recovery to progression to chronic hepatitis and rarely, death due to fulminant disease. In adults, 65–80% infections are inapparent, with 90–95% of all patients recovering completely. In contrast, 80–95% of infants and young children infected with HBV become chronic carriers, and their serum remains positive for HBsAg. Chronic carriers are at high risk of developing hepatocellular carcinoma.

In a majority of individuals, the primary infection is asymptomatic, and resolves as a result of an effective cell mediated immune response. Fully differentiated hepatocytes are the primary cell type infected by HBV. The primary cause of hepatic cell destruction appears to be the cell mediated immune response. The cells involved are HLA-1-restricted cytotoxic T cells, which react specifically with the fragments of nucleocapsid proteins, HBcAg and HBeAg expressed on the surface of infected hepatocytes. This response also contributes to control of the infection by eliminating virus-producing cells. Enhanced natural killer cell activity, as well as production of **alphainterferon**, also contribute to limiting the extent of the infection. Humoral **anti-HBsAg antibody**, which is the neutralizing antibody, does not appear until well into the convalescence period, when it may aid in clearing any remaining circulating free virus. This antibody provides protection against reinfection. On the other hand, it is this same humoral antibody that is thought to be the source of the extrahepatic damage, that is seen in 10–20% of patients, through the formation and deposition of HBsAg—anti HBsAg antibody immune complexes, and the consequent activation of complement.

The incubation period of hepatitis B is 50–180 days, with an average of 60 to 90 days. The course of HBV infection progresses in three phases.

1. ***Preicteric (prodromal) phase:*** Following incubation period, a preicteric (prejaundice) phase occurs lasting several days to a week. This is characterized by mild fever, malaise, anorexia, myalgia and nausea. These symptoms are likely due to the **alphainterferon** synthesis induced by the infection. A minority of patients develop arthralgia, maculopapular rash, **polyarteritis nodosa** and **glomerulonephritis** may be due to deposition of immune complexes.
2. ***Icteric phase:*** The acute, icteric phase then follows, and lasts for one to two months. It is during this phase that dark urine, due to **bilirubinuria**, and **jaundice**, seem as a yellowish coloration of mucus membranes, conjunctivae, and skin are evident. There usually is an enlarged and tender liver as well.
3. ***Convalescent phase:*** In 90–95% of adults, a convalescent period of several more months is followed by complete recovery.

Fulminant hepatitis occasionally develops during acute viral heptatitis, with much more extensive necrosis of the liver. It is fatal in 70–90% of cases, with survival uncommon over the age of 40 years. Fulminant hepatitis is characterized by high fever, abdominal pain and eventual renal dysfunction, coma and seizures. It is not clear why the acute disease takes this course. A more highly virulent strain of HBV, superinfection with HDV or another hepatitis virus (for example, HCV), and/or an uncontrolled immune response by the patient may be responsible for the development of this fulminating hepatitis. In most patients who survive, complete restoration of the hepatic parenchyma and normal liver function is the rule.

Hepatocellular carcinoma, typically appears many years after the primary HBV infection, and the tumor itself is rather slow-growing, and only occasionally metastasizes. Patients with hepatocellular carcinoma exhibit weight loss, right upper quadrant pain, fever and intestinal bleeding. Chronic HBV infection greatly increases the risk of hepatocellular carcinoma. Hepatitis B is second in importance only to tobacco as a known human carcinogen.

Laboratory Diagnosis

The aim of laboratory diagnosis of clinical hepatitis patients are, first, to determine which hepatitis virus is the cause of the illness, and second, for HBV, to distinguish between acute from chronic infections. The diagnosis of hepatitis is made on clinical grounds, coupled with biochemical tests that evaluate liver damage. Elevations of **serum alanine amino transferase** (ALT; formerly SGPT) and **serum aspartate transaminase** (AST; formerly SGOT), bilirubin and the prothrombin time, all contribute to the initial evaluation of the hepatitis. Transaminase values in acute hepatitis range between 500 and 2000 units. ALT values are usually higher than AST. A sharp rise in ALT with a short duration of 3–19 days is more indicative of viral hepatitis A, whereas a gradual rise with prolongation (35–200 days) appears to characterize viral hepatitis B and C infections. Serum bilirubin levels may rise up to 25-fold.

ELISA, RIA and other serologic techniques for detection of viral antigens and antibodies are the primary means used to distinguish between HAV, HBV, HCV and HDV. In addition, demonstration of the presence or absence of specific antiviral antibodies and viral antigens permits differentiating between acute and chronic HBV infections.

Demonstration of HBsAg in the blood is all that necessary for the diagnosis of HBV infection. ELISA, RIA, counterimmunoelectrophoresis, reverse passive latex agglutination and passive hemagglutination tests are used. The simultaneous presence of IgM anti-HBc indicates recent infection and the presence of IgG anti-HBc chronic infection.

HBV infection is unusual in that quantities of virions and virion components in the blood are so great that the time course of their appearance and clearance, along with that of the antibodies directed against them, serve as convenient markers of the stage of the disease, and of the likely future course.

During the incubation period, **HBsAg** and **HBeAg** are the first indicators of HBV infection to appear in the blood. Their presence indicates an active infection, but does not distinguish between acute and chronic infections. HBsAg is the first marker to appear in blood after infection, usually detectable 2–6 weeks in advance of clinical and biochemical (elevation of **transaminases**) evidence of hepatitis and persists throughout the clinical course of the disease but typically disappears sixth month after exposure. When HBsAg is no longer detectable, its antibody, anti-HBs appears and remains for very long periods. **Anti-HBs** is a protective antibody. On the other hand, the continued presence of HBsAg beyond six months and the absence of anti-HBs is an indication that the infection has become chronic (Table 87.4).

Table 87.4 Nomenclature and Definitions of Hepatitis Viruses, Antigens, and Antibodies

Disease	*Component of system*	*Definition*
Hepatitis A	HAV	Hepatitis A virus. Etiologic agent of infectious hepatitis. A picornavirus, the prototype of a new genus, *Hepatovirus*.
	Anti-HAV	Antibody to HAV. Detectable at onset of symptoms; lifetime persistence.
	IgM anti-HAV	IgM class antibody to HAV. Indicates recent infection with hepatitis A; positive up to 4–6 months after infection.
Hepatitis B	HBV	Hepatitis B virus. Etiologic agent of serum hepatitis (long-incubation hepatitis). A hepadnavirus.
	HBsAg	Hepatitis B surface antigen. Surface antigen (s) of HBV detectable in large quantity in serum; several subtypes identified.
	HBeAg	Hepatitis Be antigen. Soluble antigen; associated with HBV replication, with high titers of HBV in serum, and with infectivity of serum.
	HBcAg	Hepatitis B core antigen.
	Anti-HBs	Antibody to HBsAg. Indicates past infection with and immunity to HBV, presence of passive antibody from HBIG, or immune response from HBV vaccine.
	Anti-HBe	Antibody to HBeAg. Presence in serum of HBsAg carrier suggests lower titer of HBV.
	Anti-HBc	Antibody to HBcAg. Indicates infection with HBV at some undefined time in the past.
	IgM anti-HBc	IgM class antibody to HBcAG. Indicates recent infection with HBV; positive for 4–6 months after infection.
Hepatitis C	HCV	Hepatitis C virus, a common etiologic agent of posttransfusion hepatitis. A flavivirus.
	Anti-HCV	Antibody to HCV.
Hepatitis D	HDV	Hepatitis D virus. Etiologic agent of delta hepatitis; causes infection only in presence of HBV.
	HDAg	Delta antigen (delta-Ag). Detectable in early acute HDV infection.
	Anti-HDV	Antibody to delta-Ag (anti-delta). Indicates past or present infection with HDV.
Hepatitis E	HEV	Hepatitis E virus. Enterically transmitted hepatitis virus. Causes large epidemics in Asia and North Africa; fecal-oral or waterborne transmission. Perhaps a calicivirus.
Immune globulins	I G	Immune globulin USP. Contains antibodies to HAV; no antibodies to HBsAg, HCV or HIV.
	HBIG	Hepatitis B immune globulin. Contains high titers of antibodies to HBV.

DNA polymerase activity, HBV DNA and HBeAg, which are representative of the viremic stage of hepatitis B, occur early in the incubation period, concurrently or shortly after the first appearance of HBsAg. Circulating **HBeAg** is an indicator of active intrahepatic viral replication and the presence of DNA polymerase, HBV DNA and virions in the blood reflects high infectivity. The disappearance of HBeAg coincides with the fall of transaminase levels in blood. It is followed by the appearance of anti-HBe. The presence of HBeAg indicates high infectivity and its absence, along with the presence of anti-HBe, indicates low infectivity. As it is invariably present during acute hepatitis, its testing is indicated only in chronic infection and carriers (Table 87.5).

Table 87.5 Interpretation of HBV Serologic Markers in Patiens with Hepatitis B

HBsAg	*HBeAg*	*anti-HBe*	*anti-HB c*		*anti-HBc*	*HBV DNA*	*Interpretation*
			IgM	*IgG*			
+	+	−	−	−	−	+	Incubation period
+	+	−	+	+	−	+	Acute hepatitis B
+	+	−	+	+	−	+	Chronic active hepatitis B or persistent carrier states
+	−	+	−	+	−	−	Asymptomatic carrier state
−	−	−	−	+	+	−	remote HBV infection
−	−	−	−	−	+	−	Immunization without infection

Like HBeAg, **HBV DNA** is also an indicator of viral replication and infectivity. Molecular methods such as DNA : DNA hybridisation and PCR are used for HBV DNA testing. HBV DNA level in blood reflects the degree of viral replication in the liver and so helps to assess the progress of patients with chronic hepatitis under antiviral chemotherapy.

HBcAg is not demonstrable in circulation because it is enclosed within the HBsAg coat, but its antibody, **anti-HBc** appears in serum a week or two after the appearance of HBsAg. It is therefore the earliest antibody marker to be seen in blood, long before anti-HBe or anti-HBs. As anti-HBc remains life long, it serves as a useful indicator of prior infection with HBV, even after all the other viral markers become undetectable. Initially, anti-HBc is predominantly IgM, but after about six months, it is mainly IgG. Selective tests for IgM or IgG anti-HBc therefore enable distinction between acute or chronic infection respectively (Fig. 87.5).

In some individuals with acute infections, HBsAg becomes undetectable before anti-HBs appears. This is referred to as the "**window period**". However, anti-HBc antibody is present.

The presence of anti-HBs without any other serological virus marker indicates immunity following vaccination.

Prophylaxis

General prophylaxis consists use of sterile disposable syringes and needles, screening of blood donors and avoiding promiscuous sex. Healthcare personnel should wear gloves while handling potentially infectious materials. Protective garments should be worn and removed before leaving the work area. Masks and eye protection should be worn whenever splashes or droplets from infectious materials pose a risk. Work surfaces should be decontaminated using a bleaching solution. Disposable syringes and needles should be incinerated. Metal objects and instruments can be disinfected by autoclaving or by exposure to ethylene oxide gas. Laboratory workers should avoid mouth-pipetting, eating, drinking and smoking in the work area.

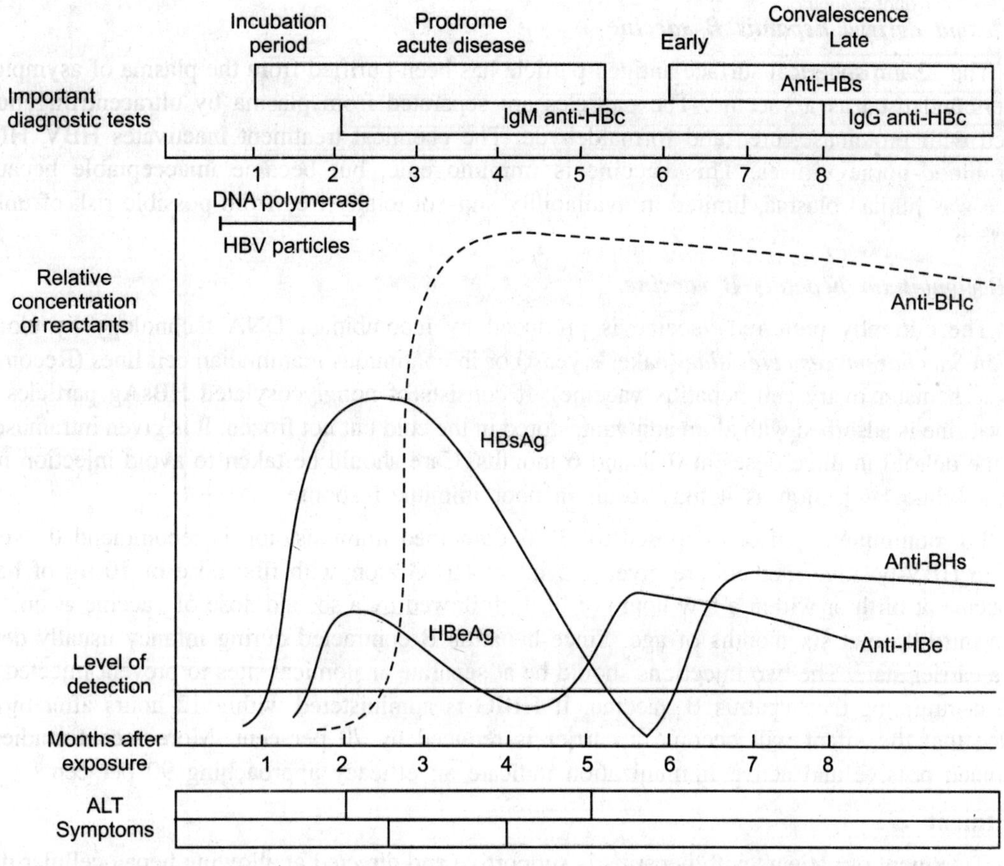

Fig. 87.5 Clinical and serologic events occurring in a patient with acute hepatitis B virus infection

The disease may be prevented by either passive or active immunization.

Passive immunization

Hepatitis B immune globulin (HBIG) is prepared from the pooled plasma of donors having a high titer of anti-HBs antibody. It is administered intramuscularly in a dose of 300–500 IV immediately after exposure, preferably within 48 hrs. as an initial step in preventing infection of individuals accidentally exposed to HBV-contaminated blood by needle-stick or splashed on mucus membranes or conjunctiva. A second dose is given 30 days later. HBIG confers temporary passive immunity. It may not prevent infection, but protects against illness and the carrier state. Therefore passive immunization must be accompanied by a course of active immunization with **hepatitis B vaccine**.

Active immunization

Active immunization with hepatitis B vaccine is recommended by the WHO for all susceptible at risk groups. HBV vaccination is now recommended as one of routine infant immunizations.

Hepatitis B virus has not yet been grown in tissue culture, so other routes have been used to develop vaccines.

(i) Plasma derived hepatitis B vaccine

The 22 nm spherical surface antigen particle has been purified from the plasma of asymptomatic carriers and used as a vaccine. The particles are separated from plasma by ultracentrifugation and treated with proteinase, urea and formaldehyde. The chemical treatment inactivates HBV, HIV and other blood-borne viruses. This vaccine is immunogenic, but became unacceptable because its source was human plasma, limited in availability and not totally free from possible risk of unknown pathogen.

(ii) Recombinant hepatitis B vaccine

The currently preferred vaccine is produced by recombinant DNA technology by cloning S gene in *Saccharomyces cerevisiae* (baker's yeast) or in continuous mammalian cell lines (Recombinant chinese hamster ovary cell hepatitis vaccine). It consists of nonglycosylated HBsAg particles alone. The vaccine is adsorbed with alum adjuvant, stored in the cold but not frozen. It is given intramuscularly into the deltoid in three doses at 0, 1 and 6 months. Care should be taken to avoid injection into fat such as gluteal injection as it may result in poor immune response.

For nonimmune persons exposed to HBV, combined immunisation is recommended. Neonates born to HBV-positive mothers are given 0.5 ml of HBIG alongwith first dose of 10 μg of hepatitis B vaccine at birth or within a few hours of birth, followed by a second dose of vaccine at one month and a third dose at six months of age. Since hepatitis B contracted during infancy usually develops into a carrier state. The two injections should be at separate anatomical sites to prevent injected HBIG from neutralizing the hepatitis B vaccine. If HBIG is administered within 12 hours after birth, the chance that the infant will become a carrier is reduced by 70 per cent. More recent studies with combined passive and active immunization indicate an efficacy approaching 90 per cent.

Treatment

Treatment of patients with hepatitis is supportive and directed at allowing hepatocellular damage to resolve and repair itself. Interferon-alpha is effective in the treatment of chronic viral hepatitis. Several antiviral drugs such as Lamivudine, Ganciclovir, foscarnet and ribavirin have shown some activity against HBV.

HEPATITIS C VIRUS (HCV)

Hepatitis C virus was discovered in 1988 in the course of searching for the cause of non-A, non-B, transfusion associated hepatitis. At that time, HCV accounted for ninety per cent of the cases of **non-A, non-B hepatitis**.

Structure and Properties

It is not possible to grow HCV in tissue cultures and therefore most of what has been learned about the virus and viral proteins has been by the use of recombinant DNA techniques.

HCV is a 50–60 nm virus with a linear, single-stranded (positive sense) RNA genome enclosed within a core and surrounded by an envelope, carrying glycoprotein spikes. HCV is classified as a new genus ***Hepacivirus*** in the family **Flaviviridae.**

HCV displays considerable genetic and antigenic diversity with different genotypes predominating in different parts of the world. The virus undergoes nucleotide sequence variation during chronic infections. Based on differences in nucleotide sequences, HCV has been classified into 11 genotypes and each genotype has several subtypes. This genetic diversity is not correlated with differences in clinical disease, but makes immunisation ineffective. Only a polyvalent vaccine containing several genotypes is likely to be protective.

The virus can be inactivated by exposure to ether, chloroform and other organic solvents and by detergents.

Epidemiology

HCV infections are extensive throughout the world and are seen only in humans. The source of infection is the large number of chronic carriers. HCV is transmitted in somewhat the same way as HBV. The routes of transmission of HCV are through sharing of contaminated needles and syringes, through transfusion of blood and blood products, by occupational needle-stick injuries, by sexual intercourse and by vertical transmission from mother to infant. The latter is not as frequent as for HBV. HCV has been transmitted by commercial intravenous immune globulin preparations. Although HCV was initially identified as a major cause of post transfusion hepatitis, intravenous drug users, transplant recipients, immunocompromised persons and patients on hemodialysis are also at high risk for infection with HCV. Viral replication occurs in the hepatocyte. Destruction of liver cells may result from a direct effect of viral replication and from the host immune response.

Clinical Features

The incubation period for HCV ranges from 5 to 10 weeks, though both shorter (2 weeks) and longer intervals (4 months) have been observed.

The majority of infections with HCV are subclinical, but about 25 per cent of infected individuals present with acute hepatitis including jaundice. Out of these, 85 per cent or more of the acute infections progress to a chronic hepatitis and cirrhosis. Finally, some of these individuals go on to develop hepatocellular carcinoma many years after the primary infection. Thus HCV bears many clinical and epidemiologic similarities to HBV inspite of the distinct molecular differences between the two.

Laboratory Diagnosis

Diagnosis of HCV infection can be established by (*i*) demonstration of antibodies (anti-HCV) by ELISA, that react with a combination of viral proteins, and (*ii*) detection of viral nucleic acid by PCR. Identification of HCV RNA in blood provides more sensitive and specific results within a few days of exposure to HCV.

Prophylaxis

HCV infections can be prevented by screening of blood donors, avoiding use of unsterile needles and syringes etc. The control measures for HIV, HBV and HCV are almost same.

Treatment

Treatment of patients with chronic hepatitis is by interferon-alpha, either alone or in combination with antiviral agents like ribavirin is the method of choice.

HEPATITIS D VIRUS (HDV) (Delta agent or Delta hepatitis Virus)

Structure and Properties

Hepatitis D virus is a defective satellite virus, resembling **viroides** (plant viruses) that is able to replicate only with the help of Hepatitis B viral products. Therefore, HDV is found in nature only as a coinfection with HBV. Its significance lies in the fact that its presence results in more severe acute disease, with a greater risk of fulminant hepatitis, and, in chronically infected patients, a greater risk of **cirrhosis** and **liver cancer**.

HDV is a spherical, 35 to 37 nm particle with a circular, single-stranded RNA genome with negative polarity that codes for one protein, the delta antigen (HDAg), with which the genome is complexed in the virion. In the infectious particle, the nucleoprotein complex is enclosed with an envelope containing HBV-coded HBsAg. (Fig. 87.6) Thus HDV requires HBV to serve as a helper virus for infectious HDV production. The HDV RNA genome is replicated and transcribed in the nucleus by cellular enzymes. This phase of HDV replication is independent of HBV, whose only helper function is to supply HBsAg for the envelope. It is classified in a new genus *Deltavirus*. The RNA genome of the delta agent does not hybridize with the DNA of hepatitis B virus. Only one serotype of **deltavirus** has been recognized.

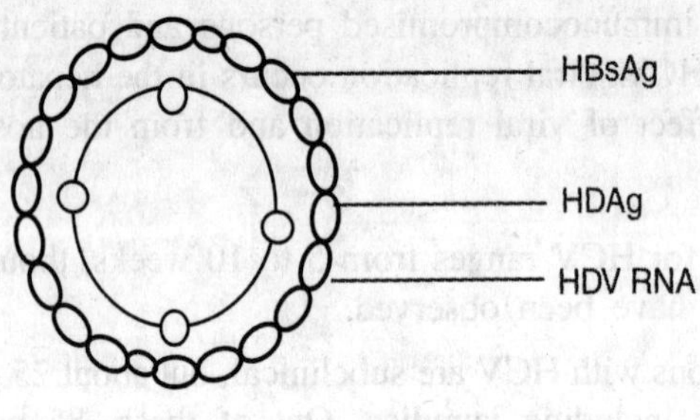

Fig. 87.6 Hepatitis D virus

HDAg is resistant to ethylenediaminetetra acetic acid (EDTA), detergents, ether, nucleases, glycosidases or acid, but partial or complete loss of activity was detected after treatment with alkali, thiocyanate, guanidine hydrochloride, trichloroacetic acid and proteolytic enzymes.

Pathogenesis

Because HDV exists only in association with HBV, it can be transmitted by the same routes: through blood transfusion and vertical transmission from mother to fetus. However, it does not appear to be transmitted sexually as frequently as are HBV or HIV. Pathologically, liver damage is essentially the same as in other viral hepatitis cases, but the presence of HDV results in more extensive and severe damage. Two types of HDV infections are recognized coinfection and superinfection. In coinfection, deltavirus and HBV are transmitted together simultaneously at the same time. Coinfection clinically presents as acute hepatitis B, ranging from mild to fulminant disease. In superinfection, deltavirus infection occurs in a chronically HBV-infected individual. Superinfection usually leads to severe liver damage, fulminant hepatitis after a relatively shorter incubation period.

In the coinfection pattern, antibody to HDAg develops late in the acute phase of infection and may be of low titer. Assays for HDAg or HDV RNA in the serum or for IgM-specific anti-HDV are preferable. All markers of HDV replication disappear during convalescence, even the HDV antibodies may disappear within months to years. However, superinfection by HDV usually results in persistent HDV infection with high levels of both IgM and IgG anti-HD, HDAg and HDV RNA.

Epidemiology

HDV is found throughout the world and infects all age groups. Persons who had received multiple transfusions, intravenous drug abusers, and their close contacts are at high risk. The incubation period varies from 2 to 12 weeks, and may be shorter in superinfection.

Two epidemiologic patterns of HDV infection have been identified. In Mediterranean countries, HDV infection is endemic among persons with hepatitis B and is transmitted by intimate contact. In nonendemic areas, such as the USA and northern Europe, HDV infection is through contact of blood and blood products and is commonly seen in intravenous drug addicts and hemophiliacs.

Laboratory diagnosis

The immunologically based methods used to diagnosis of HBV are also applied to HDV. The delta antigen (HDAg) and IgM antibodies to it in the serum can be detected by immunofluorescence, ELISA, RIA. HDV RNA in serum or liver tissues can be detected by hybridization and PCR.

Prophylaxis

Delta hepatitis can be prevented by immunizing HBV-susceptible persons with hepatitis B vaccine. However, vaccination does not protect hepatitis B carriers from superinfection by HDV. Screening of blood donors for HBsAg automatically limits blood-borne HDV infection.

HEPATITIS E VIRUS (HEV)

HEV is a spherical and nonenveloped virus, 32–34 nm in diameter, with a linear, single-stranded, positive-sense RNA genome. The surface of the virion shows indentation and spikes. It resemble caliciviruses such as the Norwalk virus. It has been provisionally classified in the genus *Hepevirus* under the family caliciviridae. Only one serotype exists.

HEV is a major cause of enterically transmitted, water-borne hepatitis through fecal pollution in developing countries. Hence the name **enterically transmitted NANB (non A, non B) hepatitis**. It often appears as epidemics hence also called epidemic NANB. The largest such epidemic occurred in Delhi during the winter of 1955–56, affecting over 30,000 persons within six weeks. Several outbreaks and sporadic infections have been reported from many parts of the Indian subcontinent, Central and South Asia, North Africa and Central America. The disease is now called **Type E hepatitis** and its causative agent hepatitis E virus (HEV). Type E hepatitis was previously mistaken for hepatitis A because of clinical and epidemiological similarities. It was recognized as a separate entity because of the absence of serological and virological evidence of HAV infection in these cases.

Incubation period of haeptitis E ranges from 2–8 weeks, with an average of 5–6 weeks. It occurs predominantly in young adults. The disease is generally mild and selflimited. The disease is especially severe in pregnant women, in whom death can result from HEV infection. In hepatitis E, when compared to type A hepatitis, bilirubin levels tend to be higher and jaundice deeper and more prolonged. Like hepatitis A, hepatitis E does not progress to chronic hepatitis, cirrhosis, cancer or carrier state.

HEV can be demonstrated by IEM in the bile and feces of patients in the incubation period of acute phase of illness. Experimental infection can be transmitted to many species of primates. *In vitro* cultivation has not been successful so far. HEV RNA can be detected in the feces or in acute phase sera by RT-PCR. Specific tests such as ELISA are available to detect antibodies (IgG and IgM) to HEV by using recombinant and synthetic peptide antigens.

No antiviral treatment or vaccine is currently available. Hepatitis E can be prevented by providing protected water supply and improved sanitation.

HEPATITIS G VIRUS (HGV)

Hepatitis G virus represents a newly discovered virus. It has been proposed that hepatitis C and G should be placed in a separate genus of the family **Flaviviridae** to be called ***Hepacivirus***.

Two flavivirus-like isolates were obtained in 1955 from Tamarin monkeys inoculated with blood from a young surgeon (GB) with acute hepatitis. A similar virus was isolated from another human specimen the same year. These isolates were called GB viruses A, B and C respectively. In 1966, an isolate closely resembling GBV-C was obtained from a patient with chronic hepatitis. This has been called hepatitis G virus (HGV). It has not been grown, but its RNA genome has been cloned. The genome of HGV consists of single-stranded RNA of positive polarity. Its structure resembles that of HCV. The virus is transmitted parenterally through blood transfusion, hemodialysis, sharing syringes and needles among intravenous drug addicts, sexual contact and from mother to child. Since, HGV and HIV are transmitted by same routes, many HIV-infected persons are HGV-coinfected.

HGV is present worldwide. HGV replicates in peripheral blood cells, however, its replication in the liver is not known, with no evidence of liver disease. HGV infection results frequently chronic viremia. It often subsides after several years and anti-HGenv antibody develops.

HGV RNA can be detected in the serum by RT-PCR during viremic phase. Anti-HGenv can be detected in the serum by immunoassays during recovery stage.

HGV infection can be prevented by employing the same measures as for HBV, HCV and HIV.

QUESTIONS

Essay Questions:

1. Name the hepatitis viruses. Describe the structure, general properties, pathogenicity and laboratory diagnosis of hepatitis B virus.
2. Discuss the laboratory diagnosis and prophylaxis of serum jaundice.
3. List the viruses affecting the liver. How are the various markers of hepatitis B virus detected? What is the significance of these markers.
4. Mention the viruses that affect the liver and make a comparison of hepatitis viruses A and B.

Short Notes:

1. Viral hepatitis.
2. Hepatitis A virus (HAV) or Type A hepatitis or infectious hepatitis.
3. Hepatitis B virus or Dane's particle.
4. HBsAg or Australia antigen.
5. Pathogenesis of HBV or Type B hepatitis or serum hepatitis or serum jaundice or transfusion hepatitis.
6. Laboratory diagnosis of type B hepatitis.
7. Prophylaxis of hepatitis B or hepatitis B vaccine.
8. Hepatitis C virus or Type C hepatitis.
9. Hepatitis D virus or Delta agent.
10. Laboratory diagnosis of hepatitis C infections.
11. Enumerate hepatitis viruses.
12. Draw a neat labelled diagram of hepatitis B virus.
13. How is neonate born to hepatitis positive mother protected?
14. Hepatitis B carriers.

88

Picornaviruses

- *Introduction*
- *Classification*
- *Structure*
- *Enteroviruses*
- *Poliovirus*
- *Coxsackieviruses*
- *Echoviruses*
- *Other Enterovirus types*
- *Rhinoviruses*

INTRODUCTION

The family picornaviridae comprises a large number of very small (pico=small), nonenveloped, icosahedral viruses, which contain a single-stranded, nonsegmented, positive-sense RNA genome and four structural proteins.

CLASSIFICATION

The **picornaviridae** family contains five genera: *Enterovirus*, *Rhinovirus*, ***Hepatovirus*** (hepatitis A virus), *Aphthovirus* (foot and mouth disease viruses), and *Cardiovirus* (Table 88.1).

Enteroviruses of human origin include the following:

1. Polioviruses, types 1–3
2. Coxsackieviruses group A, types 1–24 (there is no type 23)
3. Coxsackicviruses group B, types 1–6
4. Echoviruses types 1–34 (there are no types, 10 and 28)
5. Enteroviruses types 68–71.

Since 1969, new enterovirus types have been assigned enterovirus type numbers rather than being subclassified as coxsackieviruses or echoviruses. The vernacular names of the previously identified enteroviruses have been returned. Enteroviruses also exist in many animals, including cattle, pigs, monkeys and mice.

Human rhinoviruses include more than 100 antigenic types. Rhinoviruses of other host species include those of horses and cattle.

Hepatitis A virus was originally classified as enterovirus type 72 but is now assigned to a separate genus. There is also a simian hepatitis A virus.

Table 88.1 Clinical Syndromes of Picornaviruses

Virus	*Disease (Virus types)*
Enteroviruses	
Polioviruses (types 1–3)	Undifferentiated febrile illnesses (1–3)
	Aseptic meningitis (1–3)
	Paralysis and encephalitic diseases (1–3)
Coxsackievirus group A (A1–A22, A24)*	Acute hemorrhagic conjunctivitis (CA24 variant)
	Herpangina (2–6, 8, 10, 22)
	Exanthem (4–6, 9, 16)
	Hand-foot-mouth disease (5, 10, 16)
	Aseptic meningitis (1–2, 4–7, 9, 10, 14, 16, 22)
	Paralysis and encephalitic diseases (occasional 4, 7, 9, 10)
	Hepatitis (4, 9)
	Upper and lower respiratory tract illnesses (9, 10, 16, 21, 24 variant)
	Lymphonodular pharyngitis (10)
	Infantile diarrhea (18, 20–22, 24 variant)
Coxsackievirus group B (B1–B6)	Undifferentiated febrile illnesses (1–6)
	Pleurodynia (1–5)
	Pericarditis, myocarditis (1–5)
	Aseptic meningitis types (1–6)
	Paralysis and encephalitic diseases (1–5)
	Severe systemic infection in infants, meningoencephalitis and myocarditis (1–5)
	Upper and lower respiratory tract illnesses (4, 5)
	Exanthem, heaptitis, diarrhea (5)
Echoviruses (1–9, 11–27, 29–33)*	Aseptic meningitis (many)
	Paralysis and encephalitic diseases (occasional 1, 2, 4, 6, 7, 9, 11, 14–16, 18, 22, 30)
	Exanthem (1–9, 11, 14, 16, 18, 19, 25, 30, 32)
	Hand-foot-mouth disease (19)
	Pericarditis and myocarditis (1, 6, 9, 19, 22)
	Upper and lower respiratory tract illnesses (4, 9, 11, 20, 22, 25)
	Neonatal diarrhea (11, 14, 18, 20, 32)
	Epidemic myalgia (1, 6, 9)
	Hepatitis (4, 9)

(*Contd...*)

New enteroviruses (68–72)	Pneumonia and bronchiolitis (68, 69)
	Acute hemorrhagic conjunctivitis (70)
	Aseptic meningitis, meningoencephalitis, hand-foot-mouth disease (71)
	Hepatitis (72)
Rhinoviruses (1–115)	Upper and lower respiratory tract illnesses (1–115)

* Reclassification of Coxsackivierus A23 as echovirus 9, echovirus 10 as reovirus, echovirus 28 as rhinovirus type 1A, and echovirus 34 as coxsackievirus A24.

Other picornaviruses are foot and mouth disease virus (*Aphthovirus*) of cattle and encephalomyocarditis virus of rodents (*Cardiovirus*).

STRUCTURE

Picornaviruses (pico=small, rna = RNA) small viruses with a diameter 27–30 nm. They are nonenveloped. The virion comprises of a capsid shell of 60 subunits, each of four proteins (VP1-VP4) arranged with icosahedral symmetry around a genome made up of a single-strand positive sense RNA. VP1 protein carries the major antigenic site, which faces outside, for combination with type specific neutralising antibodies (Fig. 88.1).

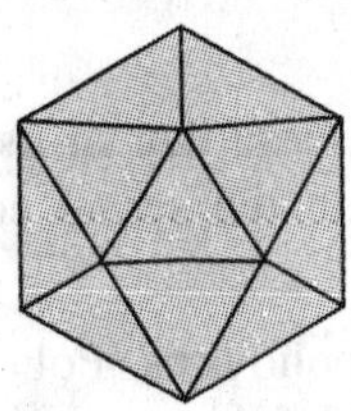

Fig. 88.1 Picornavirus

ENTEROVIRUSES

Poliovirus

General properties

Polioviruses are inactivated when heated at 55°C for 30 minutes, but Mg^{2+} ($MgCl_2$), 1 mol/L prevents this inactivation. Milk or icecream is also protective, but proper pasteurisation inactivates the virus. Whereas purified poliovirus is inactivated by chlorine (0.1 ppm concentration), much higher concentrations of chlorine are required to disinfect sewage containing virus in fecal suspensions and in the presence of other organic matter. Polioviruses are resistant to ether, bile salts, chloroform, detergents and proteolytic enzymes of intestine. All enteroviruses are stable at acid pH (3.0–5.0) for 1 to 3 hours.

Antigenic properties

Poliovirus strains are classified into three serotypes: 1, 2 and 3, based on neutralisation tests. The prototype strains are Brunhilde and Mahoney strains for type 1, Lansing and MEFI for type 2 and Leon and Saukett for type 3. Type 1 is the most common and causes epidemics.

By complement fixation, precipitation or ELISA, two antigens C (C = coreless or capsid or H, heated) and D (D = dense or N, native) are identified. The D antigen is associated with the whole virion containing RNA and is type-specific. The C antigen is empty, noninfectious virus, is less specific and reacts with heterotypic sera. Inactivation of the virus by formalin, heat or UV light liberates C antigen. Thus, the D form can be converted to the C form by heating. Anti-D antibody is protective and therefore the potency of injectable polio vaccine can be measured in terms of D antigen units. Anti-C antibody does not neutralise virus infectivity.

Cultivation and animal susceptibility

The poliovirus grows readily in primary or continuous cell line cultures derived from a variety of human tissues or from monkey kidney, testes or muscle, but not in cells of lower animals. Primary monkey kidney cell lines are widely used for the isolation in the diagnosis and vaccine production. The infected cells round up and become refractile and **pyknotic**. Eosinophilic intranuclear inclusion bodies may be demonstrated in stained preparations. Well formed plaques develop in infected monolayers with agar overlay.

Polioviruses have a restricted host range. Natural infection occurs only in humans. Most strains will infect monkeys when inoculated directly into the brain or spinal cord. Chimpanzees and cynomolgus monkeys can also be infected by the oral route and the infection thus produced is usually asymptomatic, and the animals become intestinal carriers of the virus. Unusual strains have been transmitted to mice or chick embryos. Poliovirus requires a primate-specific membrane receptor for infection, and the absence of this receptor on the surface of nonprimate cells makes them virus-resistant.

Pathogenesis and clinical features

Poliomyelitis is an acute infectious disease that in its serious form affects the central nervous system. The destruction of motor neurons in the spinal cord result in flaccid paralysis. However, most poliovirus infections are subclinical.

Humans are the only natural host of poliovirus. Polioviruses have a tropism for the epithelial cells lining the alimentary tract and for cells of the central nervous system. They attach to a specific receptor on these cells, which in humans is encoded by a gene on chromosome 19. The histocompatibility antigens HLA-3 and HLA-7 are believed to be highly associated with an increased risk of paralysis.

Polioviruses are transmitted by ingestion of contaminated food and water (**fecal-oral route**). Primary replication of poliovirus takes place in the epithelial cells of oropharynx and intestine (**alimentary phase**). From here, the virus spreads to lymphoid tissues—the tonsils and peyer's patches of the ileum and to deep cervical and mesenteric nodes, where it multiplies abundantly (**lymphatic phase**). Subsequently, the virus is carried by the blood stream to various internal organs and regional lymph nodes (**viremic phase**).

The incubation period is usually 7 to 14 days, but it may range from 3 to 35 days.

In most cases, no further virus spread occurs and there is asymptomatic (subclinical or **inapparent infection**) or **minor illness**, characterized by fever, malaise, drowsiness, headache, nausea, vomiting, constipation and sore throat in various combinations. The patients recovers in a few days. This condition is known as **abortive polymyelitis**. This is the most common form of the disease. The diagnosis of abortive poliomyelitis can be made only when the virus is isolated or antibody development is measured.

In addition to the above symptoms and signs, the patient with the nonparalytic form has stiffness and pain in the back and neck. The disease lasts 2 to 10 days, and recovery is rapid and complete. This condition is known as **aseptic meningitis** or **nonparalytic poliomyelitis**.

In a small percentage (1%) of rare cases the disease progresses to neurologic phase, the virus spreads hematogenously to the spinal cord or brain stem or to both. If only scattered nerve cells are destroyed, the patient may develop no visible sign of muscle weakness. More concentrated damage results in paralytic poliomyelitis. The classic presentation of **paralytic poliomyelitis** is flaccid paralysis, most often affecting lower limbs.

Some paralysis is usually irreversible, and residual paralysis remains for life. Paralytic disease is called **spinal poliomyelitis** if the muscles innervated by the motor neurons in the spinal cord are involved, and **bulbar poliomyelitis** if the cranial nerve nuclei or medullary centres are involved. The areas most affected are the lower motor neurons in the anterior horn of the spinal cord, the motor area of the cerebral cortex and the motor nuclei of the cerebral cortex. The lesions feature neuronal necrosis, neurophagia and loss of nerve cells. Areas of neuronal damage show leucocytic inflitration and perivascular cuffing. Bulbar poliomyelitis is serious because it may results in swallowing dysfunction and in cardiac or respiratory failure.

Approximately twenty to thirty percent of patients who partially or fully recover from paralytic poliomyelitis experience a new onset of muscles weakness, pain, atrophy and fatigue after 25 to 35 years after the acute illness. This recrudscence of paralysis and muscle wasting is called postpoliomyelitis syndrome.

Poliomyelitis should be considered in any unimmunized person with the combination of fever, headache, neck and back pain, asymmetric flaccid paralysis without sensory loss and pleocytosis (an increase in the number of lymphocytes in the CSF).

Epidemiology

Humans are the only known reservoir of infection. The patient or asymptomatic carrier is the source of infection. Patients shed the virus in feces for varying periods. No permannent carriers occurs. However, the virus may persist in the environment or sewage for upto six months. Virus shed in throat secretions during the early stage of the disease may also be a source of infection. There is a direct correlation between poor hygiene, poor sanitation, and overcrowding and the acquisition of infection.

Poliomyelitis is worldwide in distribution. In exists year-round in the tropics. In temperate climates, infection occurs mainly during the summer. Warm weather favours the spread of virus by increasing human contacts and the dissemination of virus by extrahuman sources.

Poliomyelitis affects all age groups. In areas with poor sanitation and poor hygiene, most infants are infected relatively early in life and acquire active immunity while still protected by maternal antibodies. The most susceptible are children with less than two years old. In countries with a high polio immunization coverage in their childhood vaccination program, an older age group is the most susceptible group.

In developing countries, poliomyelitis is a disease of infancy **(infantile paralysis)**. In developed countries, before the advent of vaccination, the age distribution shifted so that most patients were over age 5 and 25% were over age 15 years.

In general, infections are asymptomatic or subclinical. The following factors may predispose the incidence of paralysis:

(*i*) Pregnancy carries increased risk of paralysis, probably due to hormonal changes.

(*ii*) Tonsillectomy during the incubation period may predispose to bulbar poliomyelitis.

(*iii*) Severe muscular exertion or trauma during the preparalytic stage increases the risk of paralysis; and

(*iv*) Injections of triple vaccine, particularly alum-containing preparations, may lead to paralysis, involving the inoculated limb. The trauma may lead to virus entry into local nerve fibres, or the segment of spinal cord corresponding to the site may be more susceptible to viral damage due to reactive hyperemia.

Poliovirus type 1 is responsible for most epidemics of paralytic poliomyelitis. Type 3 also causes epidemics to a lesser extent. Type 2 usually causes inapparent infections in the western countries, but in India paralysis due to type 2 is quite common.

Immunity

Immunity in poliomyelitis is type specific. Humoral immunity provided by circulating and secretory antibody is responsible for protection against poliomyelitis. IgM antibodies appear within a week of infection and lasts for about six months. IgG antibodies remain lifelong. Neutralising antibodies in blood generally protects against disease by the same serotype of the virus, but may not prevent infection of intestinal epithelial cells and virus shedding in feces. **Secretory IgA** in the gastrointestinal tract provides **local immunity** preventing intestinal infection and virus shedding. Breast milk containing IgA antibody protects infants from infection. Poliomyelitis tends to be more severe and virus shedding more prolonged in those with impaired humoral immune response.

Laboratory Diagnosis

1. Isolation of virus

The virus may be recovered from stool samples or rectal swabs and from throat swabs taken early in the disease, but not from CSF. Specimens should be kept frozen during transit to the laboratory. Specimens should be processed to destroy bacteria by centrifugation or treatment with ether or addition of antibiotics. Specimens are inoculated onto primary monkey kidney, human amnion, HeLa, HEP-2 or any other human or simian cell lines, incubated and observed. Cytopathogenic effects appear in 3 to 6 days, and consists of cell retraction, increased refractivity, cytoplasmic granularity and nuclear pyknosis. Eosinophilic intranuclear inclusions can be demonstrated in stained smears. The virus isolate is identified and typed by neutralization tests with specific antisera. A wild virulent strain can be differentiated from an attenuated vaccine strain by nucleic acid hybridization and virulence tests in monkeys.

2. Serology

A rise in antibody titre can be demonstrated in paired sera by neutralization or complement fixation tests. During poliovirus infection, complement fixing C (or H) antibodies appear before D (or N) antibodies. Early acute stage sera contain C antibodies only; 1 to 2 weeks later, both antibodies are present; in late convalescent sera, only D antibodies are present. Only first infection with poliovirus produces type-specific complement-fixing antibodies. Subsequent infections with heterotypic polioviruses induce antibodies against the heat-stable group specific antigen shared by all three types of poliovirus.

Prophylaxis

Two types of vaccines are available for active immunization: killed and live attenuated.

(i) Salk's killed polio vaccine

It is a formalin inactivated preparation of the three types of polioviruses grown in monkey kidney tissue culture. Standard virulent strains are used. The three types of polioviruses are grown separately in monkey kidney tissue culture. Viral pools of adequate titre are filtered to remove cell debris and clumps, and inactivated with formalin (1 : 4000) at 37°C for 12 to 15 days. Stringent tests are carried out to ensure complete inactivation and for the absence of any extraneous agents. The three types are then pooled and after further tests for safety and potency are used.

Killed vaccine is given by subcutaneous or intramuscular injection. It is therefore called injectable or inactivated polio vaccine (IPV). Three doses are given with an interval of 4 to 6 weeks between the first and second doses, followed by a booster six months later. First dose should be given to babies after the age of six months to ensure that antibody response is not impaired by residual maternal antibodies.

Killed vaccine induces humoral antibodies (serum neutralizing antibodies) that block the spread of poliovirus to the central nervous system, but does not induce local intestinal immunity, so that virus is still able to multiply in the gut.

(ii) Sabin's live attenuated oral polio vaccine (OPV)

Live attenuated polio vaccine is given orally and is known as oral polio vaccine. It contains live attenuated strains of three serotypes of poliovirus grown in primary monkey kidney or human diploid cell cultures. After tests for neurovirulence, genetic stability, extraneous agents and potency, the vaccine is used in trivalent form or monovalent form in a pleasantly flavored syrup or candy. The vaccine can be stabilized by magnesium chloride so that it can be kept without losing potency for a year at 4°C and for weeks at moderate room temperature of about 25°C. Nonstabilized vaccine must be kept frozen until used.

OPV is given in three doses orally at 6 to 8 week intervals. In the tropics the number of doses may be increased to five. The live polio vaccine multiplies, infects and provides local intestinal immunity. This vaccine mimics wild poliovirus infections by inducing serum neutralizing antibody (IgM and IgG) as well as secretory IgA antibodies in the pharynx and gut. Hence, OPV not only prevents paralytic poliomyelitis but also, can prevent epidemics and has the potential of eradicating poliomyelitis. The main disadvantage of this vaccine is the occurrence of vaccine-associated paralysis. This risk of paralytic poliomyelitis associated with reversion to neurovirulence is exceedingly small, estimated at one case of paralysis for every two to four million doses of trivalent OPV distributed. A potential limiting factor for oral vaccine is **interference**. If the gut of a child is infected with another enterovirus at the time the vaccine is given, the establishment of polio infection and immunity may be blocked. This may be an important problem in tropical regions where enterovirus infections are common.

Live-virus vaccine should not be administered to immunodeficient or immunosuppressed individuals. Only killed-virus vaccine should be used.

Treatment

Specific antiviral agents for the treatment of poliomyelitis are not available. Treatment, therefore, is supportive and symptomatic. Vaccination is the only effective method of preventing poliomyelitis.

COXSACKIEVIRUSES

General properties

Coxsackieviruses are so named because the first isolation was made from Coxsackie village in New York by Daldorf and Sickles (1948). Coxsackieviruses are typical enteroviruses.

Animal susceptibility and cultivation

The characteristic feature of this group is its ability to infect suckling mice but not adult mice. Based on the pathological changes produced in suckling mice, Coxsackieviruses are classified into two groups, A and B. Group A viruses produce a generalised myositis in the skeletal muscles and flaccid paralysis without other observable lesions, leading to death within a week. Group B viruses produce a patchy focal myositis, spastic paralysis, necrosis of the brown fat and often pancreatitis, hepatitis, myocarditis and encephalitis (Table 88.2).

Table 88.2 Coxsackieviruses

	Group A	*Group B*
Pathological changes induced by inoculation into newborn mice	Generalized myositis Flaccid paralysis Death within a week	Patchy focal myositis Spastic paralysis Localized lesions in the liver, pancreas, myocardium, brain and brown fat pads.
Number of serotypes by neutralization tests	23(1–24 except 23)	6(1–6)

Antigenic properties

By neutralisation tests, Group A viruses are classified into 23 serotypes (1–24, except 23) and group B into six (1–6) types. All types in group B share a common complement fixing antigen.

Pathogenesis and clinical features

Like other enteroviruses, coxsackieviruses inhabit the alimentary canal primarily and are spread by the fecal-oral route. They produce a variety illnesses in humans. The incubation period ranges from 2 to 9 days.

1. **Aseptic meningitis:** It is caused by all group B coxsackieviruses and by many group A coxsackieviruses, most commonly A7 and A9.
2. **Herpangina (Vesicular pharyngitis):** The disease presents as small, scattered oral vesicles with red areolae in the posterior oropharynx, tonsils, tongue and palate, which progress to shallow ulcers and heal within a week. There is an abrupt onset of fever and sore throat. It is caused by certain group A coxsackieviruses (2–6, 8, 10). It has nothing to do with herpesviruses, despite the name.
3. **Hand-foot-and-mouth disease:** It is characterized by oral and pharyngeal ulcerations and a vesicular rash of the palms and soles that may spread to the arms and legs. Vesicles heal without crusting, which clinically differentiates them from the vesicles of herpes and poxviruses. It is caused by coxsackieviruses A16, A10 and A5. This disease should not be confused with **foot and mouth disease of cattle**, caused by an unrelated picornavirus that does not infect humans.
4. **Pleurodynia (epidemic myalgia or Bornholm disease):** The disease was first described on the Danish island of Bornholm and characterised by fever and stabbing chest pain on either side or substernally and abdominal pain. The illness is self-limited and recovery is complete. It is caused by group B coxsackieviruses.

5. **Myocarditis and percarditis:** It is caused by group B coxsackieviruses and is fatal in the newborn, or may cause heart damage in older children and adults.
6. **Respiratory infections:** A number of the enteroviruses have been associated with common colds; among these are coxsackieviruses A21, A24, B1 and B3–5.
7. **Type I insulin-dependent diabetes mellitus:** It is sometimes associated with past infection by enteroviruses, especially coxsackieviruses, B3 and B4. The "molecular mimicry" is responsible for virus-induced autoimmune response that destroys pancreatic B cells.
8. **Chronic fatigue syndrome:** It is also called postviral fatigue syndrome and is associated with coxsackie B virus infections.
9. **Generalized disease of infants:** Transplacental and neonatal transmission has been demonstrated with coxsackie B viruses resulting in a serious disseminated disease that may include hepatitis, meningoencephalitis, myocarditis, pericarditis and adrenocortical involvement.
10. **Acute hemorrhagic conjunctivitis:** It is usually caused by enterovirus 70, but may also be caused by coxsackie A 24 virus.

Epidemiology

Coxsackieviruses are worldwide in distribution. Isolations have been made mainly from human feces, pharyngeal swabbings, sewage, and flies. The coxsackieviruses share many properties with polio and echovirsuses. Because of their epidemiologic similarities, various enteroviruses may occur together in nature, even in the same human host or the same specimens of sewage.

Immunity

In humans, neutralizing and complement-fixing antibodies are transferred passively from mother to fetus. Adults have antibodies against more types of coxsackieviruses than do children, which indicates that multiple exposure to these viruses is common and increases with age.

Laboratory Diagnosis

(i) Isolation of virus

The virus is isolated from throat washings during the first few days of illness and from stools during the first few weeks. In coxsackievirus A 21 infections, the virus is abundant in nasal secretions. In aseptic meningitis, the virus can be recovered from CSF and gut. In hemorrhagic conjunctivitis cases, A 24 virus is isolated from conjunctival swabs, throat swabs and feces.

Specimens are inoculated into suckling mice and tissue culture. In tissue cultures a cytopathic-effect appears within 5 to 14 days. In suckling mice, signs of illness appear usually within 3 to 8 days with group A strains and 5 to 14 days with group B strains. The virus is identified by the pathological lesions it produces and by neutralisation tests. Cytopathic effects in tissue cultures resemble those of poliovirus, but develop more slowly, commencing with foci of rounded refractile cells which then lyse and fall off the glass.

Prevention and treatment

There are no vaccines or antiviral drugs currently available for prevention or treatment of coxsackievirus diseases.

ECHOVIRUSES

The echoviruses (enteric, cytopathogenic, human and orphan viruses) are grouped together because they produce cytopathogenic effects in cell cultures but generally are not pathogenic for mice (unlike the coxsackieviruses) and they differ antigenically from the polioviruses. They were first named "orphan viruses" because they could not be associated with any particular disease. Echoviruses are identified by neutralisation tests as serotypes 1–34 (except 10 and 28). They are similar in epidemiology and pathogenesis to other enteroviruses. All echoviruses grow well in the human and simian kidney cell cultures producing cytopathic effects. They infect only humans and are not pathogenic to laboratory animals.

Many echoviruses have been associated with aseptic meningitis. Rashes are common in types 4, 9, 16 ("Boston exanthem disease"), and 18. Rashes are commonest in young children. Occasionally there is conjunctivitis, muscle weakness and spasm (types 6, 9 and others). Infantile diarrhea may be associated with some types occasional cases of paralysis and hepatic necrosis have also been reported.

Like other enteroviruses, echoviruses inhabit the alimentary tract primarily and are spread by the fecal-oral route. Epidemics may occur, especially in summer.

It is not possible in an individual case to diagnose an echovirus infection on clinical grounds. However, in the summer outbreaks of aseptic meningitis and summer epidemics of febrile illness with rash in young children, echoviruses must be considered. The virus is isolated from throat swabs, feces, rectal swabs and CSF by inoculation into monkey kidney tissue cultures. The viral growth is detected by cytopathic effects. The isolate is tested against different pools of antisera against enteroviruses. Serotypes are identified by neutralisation tests.

Certain echoviruses (types 3, 6, 7, 11, 12, 13, 19, 20, 21, 24, 29, 30 and 33) agglutinate human group O erythrocytes. Hemagglutination is followed by elution, rendering the RBC inagglutinable by echo or coxsackieviruses but not by myxoviruses.

Serologic tests are impractical because of the many different viral types. Neutralizing and hemagglutination-inhibiting antibodies are type-specific and may persist for years.

There are no antivirals or vaccines available for the treatment or prevention of any echovirus diseases. Avoidance of contact with patients exhibiting acute febrile illness with rash, is advisable for very young children.

OTHER ENTEROVIRUS TYPES

Four enteroviruses (types 68–71) grow in monkey kidney cultures, and three of them cause human disease.

Enterovirus 68 has been isolated from the respiratory tracts of children with bronchitis or pneumonia.

Enterovirus 70 is the main cause of **acute hemorhagic conjunctivitis**, which occurred in pandemic form in 1969–71 in Africa and Southeast Asia. The disease is most common in adults, with an incubation period of 1 day and a duration of 8 to 10 days. The virus is highly infectious and spreads rapidly under crowded or unhygienic conditions. Acute hemorrhagic conjunctivitis has a sudden onset of subconjunctival hemorrhage ranging from small petechiae to large blotches covering the bulbar conjunctiva. There may also be epithelial keratitis and occasionally lumbar radiculomyelopathy. Complete recovery is the rule. There is no effective treatment.

Enterovirus 71 has been isolated from cases of meningitis, encephalitis and paralysis resembling poliomyelitis. It is one of the main causes central nervous system disease, sometimes fatal, around the world.

RHINOVIRUSES

Rhinoviruses are the **common cold** viruses. These viruses, as well as coronaviruses, adenoviruses, enteroviruses, parainfluenza viruses, and influenza viruses, cause upper respiratory tract infections, including the common cold.

General properties

Rhinoviruses are picornaviruses similar to enteroviruses in size and structure. They differ in two important respects from enteroviruses. First, whereas enteroviruses are acid-stable at pH 3.0, rhinoviruses are acid-labile, with complete inactivation at pH 3.0. Second, rhinoviruses have an optimal temperature of 33°C for replication that is lower than that of enteroviruses (37°C). Rhinoviruses are more thermostable than enteroviruses and may survive for days on fomites. Some serotypes survive for one hour at 50°C.

By neutralisation tests, over 100 serotypes have been identified. Immunity is type-specific. Therefore development of a vaccine is impractical.

Animal susceptibility and cultivation

Rhinoviruses are infectious for humans and chimpanzees only. This have been grown in a number of human cell lines, including human embryonic kidney cells, human embryonic nasal or tracheal epithelium, human diploid cell lines and HeLa cells. They are grown best at 33°C, which is similar to the temperature of the nasopharynx. The cultures are incubated by rolling to provide good oxygenation. The rhinoviruses which grow only in human cells are known as H strains. Some strains grow in both monkey and human cell lines, and are known as M strains.

Pathogenesis and clinical features

The rhinoviruses enter by inhalation of air-borne droplets, invades mucosal tissue by adsorbing to receptors on nasal ciliated epithelial cells. The viruses replicate and are shed, causing spread of infection. The nasal epithelium is damaged and becomes susceptible to secondary bacterial infections such as *Streptococcus pneumoniae* and *Hemophilus influenzae*. Interferon production occurs early and specific antibody appears in nasal secretions, which may facilitate recovery.

The incubation period is short, from 2 to 4 days. Usual symptoms in adults include sneezing, nasal obstruction, nasal discharge and sore throat; other symptoms may include headache, mild cough, malaise and a chilly sensation. There is little or no fever. The nasal and nasopharyngeal mucosa become red and swollen, and the sense of smell becomes less keen. There are no distinctive clinical features to differentiate colds caused rhinoviruses from colds caused by other viruses. Secondary bacterial infection may produce acute otitis media, sinusitis, bronchitis, or pneumonitis, especially in children.

In the adult population, rhinovirus disorders create significant economic losses in terms of lost working hours.

Epidemiology

The disease occurs throughout the world. In temperate zones, its incidence is highest in autumn and spring and in the tropics peak incidence occurs in rainy season. Prevalence rates are lowest in summer.

Common cold is an infectious disease transmitted by inhalation of air-borne droplets (respiratory secretions) expelled from the patients during sneezing and coughing. The fingers of a person with a cold are usually contaminated and transmission to others occurs by hand to hand or hand to object (e.g., doorknob) to hand contamination. Rhinoviruses can survive for hours on contaminated environmental surfaces. Self-inoculation after hand contamination appears to be prime mode of transmission. Infection rates are highest among infants and children and decrease with increasing age.

Laboratory Diagnosis

Rhinoviruses may be isolated from nasal or throat swabs or nasopharyngeal aspirates on human and monkey cell lines, preferably WI-38 and MRC-5 cell lines, incubated at 33°C in roller drums. Viral antigen in nasal secretions can be detected by ELISA. Molecular methods such as PCR can be used to detect virus RNA in nasal secretions.

Treatment and control

No specific prevention method or treatment is available. Since rhinoviruses spread by contaminated hands, washing of hands at appropriate intervals can be a useful preventive measure.

QUESTIONS

Essay Questions:

1. Name the picornaviruses. Describe laboratory diagnosis and prophylaxis of poliomyelitis.
2. Mention enteroviruses of medical importance. Write briefly on morphology, pathogenicity and prophylaxis of polioviruses.
3. Mention the characteristics of picornaviruses. Discuss the prophylaxis of poliomyelitis.
4. Describe the general characteristics of polioviruses. Write briefly on the prophylaxis of poliomyelitis.

Short Notes:

1. Enumerate enteroviruses of medical importance.
2. List four picornaviruses (or) Enumerate picornaviruses.
3. General characters of poliovirus.
4. Pathogenicity of poliovirus.
5. Laboratory diagnosis of poliomyelitis.
6. Prophylaxis of poliovirus infections in man (or) poliovaccines.
7. Killed poliovaccines (or) Salk's vaccine.
8. Live attenuated poliovaccines (or) OPV (or) Sabin's vaccine.
9. Differences between live and killed poliomyelitis vaccines.
10. Classification of picornaviruses.
11. Coxsackievirus.
12. Infections caused by coxsackievirus (or) Name four lesions caused by coxsackievirus.
13. Laboratory diagnosis of coxsackievirus infections.
14. Suckling mice or infant mice.
15. How to differentiate Coxsackie A from Coxsackie B viruses.
16. Echoviruses.
17. Rhinoviruses.
18. Acute hemorrhagic conjunctivitis.
19. Acute viral conjunctivitis.
20. Name four viruses causing aseptic meningitis.

89

Arboviruses

- *Introduction*
- *Togariviruses—Structure and properties, Pathogenesis, Chikungunya, Onyong-nyongvirus, Mayarovirus, Semiliki forest virus, Sindbis virus, Ross river virus, Encephalitis viruses, Laboratory diagnosis.*
- *Flaviviruses—structure and properties; —Mosquito-borne group—Encephalitis viruses (Japanese encephalitis), Yellow fever, Dengue;—tick-borne group-encephalitis viruses, hemorrhagic fevers (KFD);—laboratory diagnosis*
- *Bunyaviruses—structure and properties, Bunyavirus, Phlebivirus, Nairovirus, Hantavirus, Laboratory diagnosis.*
- *Reoviruses—Orbivirus, Coltivirus*
- *Rhabdoviruses—Chandipura virus*
- *Ungrouped arboviruses.*

INTRODUCTION

The **arthropod-borne viruses** or arboviruses are a group of viruses that are transmitted by blood sucking arthropods from one vertebrate host to another. Replication in the vertebrate host produces viremia. The blood-feeding arthropods acquire a life-long infection through the ingestion of blood from a viremic vertebrate. The viruses multiply in the tissues of the arthropod without evidence of disease or damage. The most important arbovirus vectors are mosquitoes followed by ticks. Some arboviruses are maintained in nature by transovarian transmission in arthropods. Thus, arboviruses are maintained in nature by mosquito-vertebrate-mosquito cycles. Almost all arbovirus infections are **zoonoses** except dengue and onyong-nyongvirus. Arboviruses are worldwide in distribution, but are more common in tropical regions. There are more than 450 arboviruses, about 100 are known pathogens for humans. In India, over 40 arboviruses have been detected, of which more than 10 are known to produce human disease.

Arboviruses are classified according to their physical and chemical properties and their antigenic relationships. They are placed among Togaviridae, Flaviviridae, Bunyaviridae, Reoviridae and Rhabdoviridae families (Table 89.1).

A similar ecological group is that of the **rodent borne viruses (roboviruses)** which are maintained in nature by direct transmission from rodent to rodent, without involving arthropod vector. Transmission to humans may occur through many routes by contact with rodent body fluids or excretions. Like arboviruses, roboviruses belong to different taxonomical families, some of them common with arboviruses.

TOGAVIRUSES

Structure and properties

The name Togavirus is derived from "toga", meaning the Roman mantle or cloak, and refers to the viral envelope. Togaviruses are spherical, enveloped viruses with a diameter of 70 nm. The nucleocapsid has 42 capsomers with icosahedral symmetry. The envelope is composed of a lipid bilayer has three or four structural polypeptides, two glycosylated (E1 and E2 glycoproteins). The genome consists a molecule of positive-sense single-stranded RNA. The virus replicates in the cytoplasm of the host cell and is released by budding through host cell membranes. (Fig. 89.1)

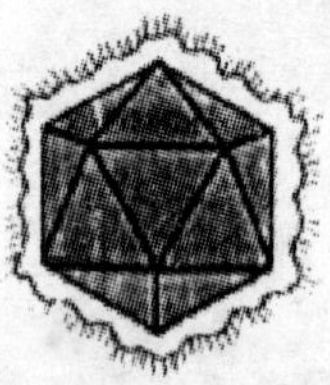

Fig. 89.1 Togavirus

Table 89.1 Some important Arboviruses

Family	*Genus*	*Important species*
Togaviridae	*Alphavirus*	Chikungunya virus, Onyong-nyong virus, Mayaro virus, Semiliki Forest virus, Sindbis virus, Ross River virus, Eastern equine encephalitis virus, Western equine encephalitis virus, Venezuelan equine encephalitis virus
Flaviviridae	*Flavivirus*	Japanese encephalitis virus, Murray valley encephalitis virus, West Nile virus, Ilheus virus, St. Louis encephalitis virus, Yellow fever virus, Dengue virus (types 1, 2, 3 and 4), Russian spring summer encephalitis complex, Louping ill virus, Powassan virus, Kyasanur Forest Disease (KFD) virus, Omsk hemorrhage fever virus
Bunyaviridae	*Bunyavirus*	California encephalitis virus, Oropouche virus, Turlock virus
	Phlebovirus	Sandfly fever virus, Rift valley fever virus
	Nairovirus	Crimean-Congo hemorrhagic fever virus, Nairobi sheep disease virus, Ganjam virus

	Hantavirus	Hantan virus, Seoul virus, Puumala virus, Prospect Hill virus, Sin Nombre virus
Reoviridae	*Orbivirus*	Colorado tick fever virus, African horse sickness virus, Blue tongue virus
Rhabdoviridae	Vesiculovirus	Vesicular stomalitis virus, Chandipura virus

The family Togaviridae has two genera: ***Alphavirus*** (formerly group A arboviruses) and ***Rubivirus***. The genus *Rubivirus* includes **Rubella virus**, which is not arthropod-borne. The genus *Alphavirus* currently comprises 32 species, of which atleast 13 are known to infect humans. All of them are mosquito-borne. All alphaviruses are antigenically related. Because of common antigenic determinants, the virus show cross-reactions in immunodiagnostic techniques such as CFT, RIA, ELISA and Fluorescent-antibody tests. Hemagglutination inhibition tests define seven serogroups of arboviruses. Identification of a specific virus is by neutralisation tests, which is highly specific.

Pathogenesis

Alphaviruses are transmitted to humans, horses and birds through the bite of blood sucking mosquitoes by percutaneous introduction of virus. Viral multiplication takes place in the vascular endothelium, monocytes and macrophages in lymph nodes, bone marrow, spleen and liver followed by viremia. In some cases, the disease may progress to involve target organs causing rash, arthritis, hepatitis, nephritis and encephalitis. Fever is associated with hemorrhagic phase. Skin rash is due to swelling of capillaries, and perivascular edema and hemorrhages are due to thrombocytopenia.

Incubation period of the encephalitis is between 4 and 21 days. There is a sudden onset with severe headache, chills, fever, nausea and vomiting, generalized pain and malaise. Within 24–48 hrs, marked drowsiness develops. Nuchal rigidity is common. Mental confusion, dysarthria, tremors, convulsions and coma develop in severe cases. Inapparent (subclinical) infections are common. Abortive infections simulate aseptic meningitis or nonparalytic poliomyelitis. The pathological features of encephalitis include neuronal necrosis neuronophagia, small hemorrhages with perivascular cuffing and meningeal infiltration–chiefly with monocytes are common.

Chikungunya Virus

Chikungunya virus causes an acute (3 to 7 days) febrile illness with malaise, arthralgia, rash, and arthritis. The virus was first isolated from human patients and ***Aedes aegypti*** mosquitoes during an epidemic in the Newala district of Tanzania in 1952. The name "chikungunya" is derived from the native word for the disease in which the patient lies "**doubled up**" due to **severe joint pains**. Epidemics of chikungunya have occured in many African countries. The virus first appeared in India in 1963, when along with dengue, it caused very extensive epidemics in Kolkata, Chennai and other areas. Chikungunya outbreaks occured at irregular intervals along the east coast of India and in Maharashtra till 1973. Since then the virus has been quiescent. A severe epidemic of chikungunya occured in India during 2005–06.

In India and Southeast Asia, the chikungunya virus has been implicated in the outbreaks of hemorrhagic fever, often in association with dengue viruses.

After an incubation period of 2–4 days, patient develops fever, crippling joint pains, chills, headache, myalgia, backache, rash, lymphadenopathy and conjunctivitis with recovery in 5 to 7 days. The vector is *Aedes aegypti* and *Aedes africanus* mosquitoes. No animal reservoir has been identified. No vaccine is available.

Onyong-nyong Virus

It is closely related to the chikungunya virus antigenically and causes a similar disease. This is transmitted by Anopheles mosquitoes. The virus was first isolated in 1942 in Uganda and is confined to Africa.

Mayaro Virus

The Mayaro virus causes a similar disease in the West Indies and South America and is closely related to chikungunya virus.

Semiliki Forest Virus

This virus was first isolated in 1942 in Uganda from Aedes mosquitoes has not been associated with any clinical illness in humans though neutralising antibodies to the virus have been demonstrated in Africans.

Sindbis Virus

The Sindbis virus, originally isolated from Culex mosquitoes in the Sindbis district of Egypt in 1952, has subsequently been recovered from other parts of Africa, India, Philippines and Australia. In Africa, it is known to be associated with febrile illness. The virus is maintained in enzootic cycles involving a variety of birds and mosquito species of the genera *Culex*, *Aedes* and *Culiseta*.

Ross River Virus

It is associated with epidemic polyarthritis in Australia. Ross river virus is endemic in Australia and has spread in epidemic form to the several islands of the western pacific.

Encephalitis Viruses

Eastern, western and Venezuelan equine encephalitis viruses cause encephalitis in horses and humans. **Eastern equine encephalitis (EEE) virus** is enzootic in fresh water swamps in the eastern USA. It causes sporadic equine and rare human cases; small epidemics may occur. **Western equine encephalitis** (**WEE**) is widespread in the USA and Canada and has been responsible for the outbreak of large epidemics of equine and human disease. Its principal vector, *Culex tarsalis* is a common mosquito especially in irrigated regions. Both EEE and WEE viruses are maintained in natural ecologic cycles involving birds and, principally, bird-feeding mosquitoes. Formalin treated killed vaccines have been developed for EEE and WEE.

Venezuelan equine encephalitis (VEE) exists in South and Central America, Mexico and Florida. VEE viruses have caused massive equine epizootics with associated human epidemics. The disease in humans is influenza-like in about 97% of the patients who develop high fever, headache and severe myalgia. Encephalitis occurs in about 3% cases. The disease was first reported in Venezuela in 1936. The natural cycle of VEE virus involves small mammals and mosquitoes. A live attenuated vaccine for VEE has been developed.

Laboratory Diagnosis

Diagnosis may be established by virus isolation and serology.

(i) Isolation of virus

The causative agent can be isolated from blood during acute phase and CSF, but best specimen is the brain.

The specimen is inoculated in to **suckling mice** (newborn mice) intracerebrally and the viral isolate is identified by neutralisation tests with specific antisera.

The specimens may be inoculated on to cell lines such as Vero, BHK-21 or yolk sac of embryonated eggs. Isolates are identified by hemagglutination inhibition. CFT, immunofluorescence, ELISA or neutralisation tests.

(ii) Serology

Neutralizing and hemagglutination-inhibiting antibodies are detectable within a few days after the onset of illness and for many years. Complement-fixing antibodies appear later. Testing by ELISA for specific IgM is particularly useful in detecting recent infection.

FLAVIVIRUSES

Structure and Properties

The family Flaviviridae is divided into three genera: ***Flavivirus*** (formerly group B arboviruses), ***Hepatitis C virus*** and *Pestivirus*. The viruses in the genus *Pestivirus* (classical swine fever virus and bovine virual diarrhoea virus) are of veterinary interest only.

Flaviviruses are spherical, enveloped viruses with a diameter of 45–60 nm in diameter, somewhat smaller than alphaviruses. The genome comprises a single molecule of positive-sense, single-stranded RNA. The nucleocapsid is surrounded by an encevelope composed of lipid bilayer. It contains three or four structural proteins one is capsid (C) protein, and two are glycosylated (E1 and E2). They are viral hemagglutinins. Viral replication occurs in the cytoplasm and assembly takes place within the endoplasmic reticulum of host cell and release of viral progeny occurs by budding through host cell membrane. The name *Flavivirus* refers to the type species, the yellow fever virus (*flavus*, L = yellow) (Fig. 89.2).

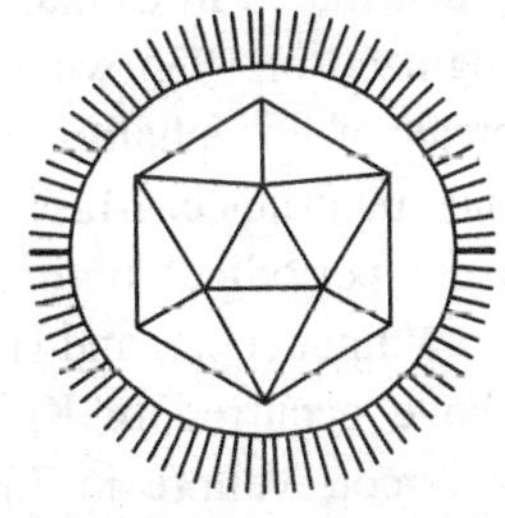

Fig. 89.2 Flavivirus

There are over 60 arthropod-borne flaviviruses, distributed in all parts of the world. They may be discussed under two groups, the mosquito-borne and the tick-borne viruses.

Mosquito-Borne Group

The flaviviruses causing encephalitis, yellow fever, dengue are mosquito-borne.

Encephalitis Viruses

Six members of this group cause encephalitis, each of them limited to a geographic zone.

1. St. Louis encephalitis virus: It is the most important cause of mosquito-borne encephalitis and is widespread in the USA and caused several massive epidemics. The clinical illness ranges from mild febrile illness to frank encephalitis. Wild birds act as the reservoirs and *Culex tarsalis* as the vector. No vaccine is yet available. Therefore St. Louis encephalitis can be prevented by the control of mosquitoes.

2. Ilheus virus: It occurs in South and Central America, maintained in forests by a cycle involving mosquitoes, wild birds and monkeys. Human infections are usually asymptomatic or leads to febrile illness. Encephalitis is rare.

3. West Nile virus: This virus is closely related to St. Louis encephalitis and Murray valley encephalitis viruses. The virus, originally isolated from the West Nile province of Uganda, in 1937, has since been reported from many African countries, Israel, Cyprus, France and India. It causes a dengue-like illness in humans and encephalitis in horses. It is endemic in Egypt, affecting mainly children. The virus is maintained in nature in wild birds by *Culex* mosquitoes. In India, the virus has-been isolated from Culex mosquitoes and from febrile as well as encephalitis patients, from Rajasthan to Karnataka.

4. Murray valley encephalitis virus: This virus was isolated during an epidemic of encephalitis in the Murray River Valley in 1951. It is endemic in Australia and New Guinea. The virus occurs normally in an enzootic cycle involving wild birds and mosquitoes, *Culex annulirostris*. Murray valley encephalitis resembles Japanese encephalitis. Most infections are asymptomatic and a small number of fatalities have been reported mostly from children.

5. Rocio encephalitis virus: It is associated with several outbreaks of encephalitis in Brazil. Wild birds are the vertebrate reservoirs and *Psorophora ferox* and *Aedes scapularis*, the vectors.

6. Japanese encephalitis (JE) virus: Japanese encephalitis virus was first isolated from the brain of a fatal case of encephalitis in Tokyo, Japan. The disease was named Japanese B encephalitis to distinguish it from 'encephalitis A' (encephalitis letharagica, Von Economo's disease) which was then prevalent.

Japanese B encephalitis is widely distributed in China, Korea, Japan, Phillippines and the Indian subcontinent. In India, it was first recognized in 1955 when the virus was isolated from mosquitoes of *Culex* from Vellore during an outbreak of encephalitis in Tamil Nadu. In India it has become a major public health problem of national importance. Most of the cases occur between October and November. From 1976, there have been periodical outbreaks of the disease in various parts of India—Dibrugarh (Assam) in the east Gorakhpur (U.P.) and Haryana in the North, Goa and Maharashtra in the west. In the south outbreaks have occurred in Kolar in Karnataka, Ananthapur, Chittoor, Nellore in A.P. and Tirunelveli, South Arcot, Vellore in Tamil Nadu, in Pondicherry and lately in Kerala.

The JE virus has a complex life cycle, involving Herons and egrets (water birds) as **reservoir hosts** and pigs as **amplifier hosts** and a blood sucking mosquito, ***Culex tritaeniorhynchus***, that breeds in flooded rice fields, marshes, standing water around planted fields.

The disease typically has an abrupt onset with fever, chills, headache and vomiting. After 1–6 days, signs of encephalitis set in with nuchal rigidity, convulsions, altered sensorium and coma and can be fatal in 30% of cases. The fever is high and continuous. There is neutrophil leucocytosis in the peripheral blood and, pleocytosis with normal or raised sugar and a slightly raised protein in the CSF. Convalescence may take many weeks. Residual neurological damage may persist in upto 50 per cent of survivors. However, the large majority of infections are asymptomatic.

Preventive measures include mosquito control and locating piggeries away from human dwellings. A formalin inactivated mouse brain vaccine using the Nakayama strain has been employed successfully for human immunization in Japan, and in small scale, in India also. The immunity produced by this vaccine is short-lived. A live attenuated vaccine has been developed in China from JE strain SA 14-14-2, passed through suckling mice. The vaccine is produced in primary baby hamster kidney cells. Administered in two doses, one year apart, the vaccine has been very effective in preventing clinical disease.

Yellow fever Virus

Yellow fever occurs in Africa and USA. It has not been reported from Asia including India, despite the presence of vector ***Aedes aegypti***. The "yellow" in the yellow fever does not indicate the association of the disease with jaundice, but is derived from the yellow quarantine flag used by the ships during the 17th century to give warning of the presence of this infectious disease, on board.

Two natural cycles of yellow fever are recognized: classic or urban epidemic yellow fever and Sylvan or jungle yellow fever. Urban yellow fever involves person-to-person transmission through the mosquito vector *Aedes aegypti*, which breeds in the accumulations of water that accompany human settlement. Jungle (sylvan) yellow fever is primarily a disease of monkeys and is transmitted from monkey to monkey through forest-dwelling mosquitoes *e.g.*, *Haemagogus* and *Sabethes* in South America and *Aedes africanus* in East Africa. Sylvan yellow fever may also occur when an infected monkey visits a human habitation and is bitten by *Aedes aegypti*, which then transmits the virus to humans.

The virus multiplies in mosquitoes, which remain infectious for life. After the mosquito ingests a virus-containing blood meal, an interval of 12–14 days is required for it to become infectious. This interval is called the extrinisic incubation period.

After an incubation period (intrinsic) of 3–6 days, the disease starts as a fever of acute onset with chills, headache, nausea and vomiting. The pulse is usually slow despite a high body temperature. Jaundice, albuminuria and hemorrhagic manifestations develop and the patient may die of hepatic or renal failure. Histologically, the liver shows cloudy and fatty degeneration and necrosis which is typically midzonal. The necrosed cells coalesce and become hyalinised leading to the formation of characteristic eosinophilic masses known as **Councilman bodies**. Acidophilic intranuclear inclusions (**Torres bodies**) may be seen in the infected liver cells in the early stages.

The control of urban yellow fever can be achieved by eradication of vector mosquitoes. Two very effective vaccines have been developed for human use. The **Dakar vaccine** is a French neurotropic vaccine prepared from infected mouse brain was thermostable, and administered by scarification. But the vaccine carries a high risk of producing encephalitis. Therefore, this was replaced by a nonneurotropic **17 D vaccine**. 17 D vaccine was developed by Theiler (1937) by passaging the Asibi strain serially in mouse embryo and whole chick embryo tissues and then in chick embryo tissue from which the central nervous tissue has been removed. The 17 D vaccine is thermostable and is administered by subcutaneous inoculation. It provides protection for about 10 years. Since yellow fever is absent in India, vaccination is mandatory for travel to or from endemic areas is valid for 10 years beginning 10 days after vaccination. In India, the 17 D vaccine is manufactured at Central Research Institute, Kasauli.

Dengue Virus

Dengue fever, also known as **breakbone fever**, is a mosquito-borne infection characterized by fever, muscle and joint pains, lymphadenopathy and rash. The name "dengue" is derived from the *Swahili ki denga pepo*, meaning a sudden seizure by a demon. The disease used to be called break-bone fever, because it causes severe muscle and joint pains. Dengue fever is clinically similar to the illness caused by chikungunya and onyong-nyong viruses.

Dengue virus is widely distributed throughout the tropics and subtropics. Four types of Dengue virus (DEN) exist : DEN 1, DEN 2, DEN 3 and DEN 4. Considerable cross-reactivity is observed among the different serotypes and recovery from an infection by one type does not provide complete immunity against infection by other types. Thus, one can have as many as four infections in their life, one with each serotype.

Humans and *Aedes* mosquitoes are recognized as reservoir hosts and vectors respectively. Dengue virus is transmitted from person-to-person by ***Aedes aegypti*** mosquitoes. ***Aedes albopictus***, a mosquito of Asian origin is also believed to spread dengue virus. Humans get dengue virus infections from the bite of an infected mosquito. Mosquitoes become infected when they bite infected humans for their blood meal, and later transmit infection to other people they bite. Mosquitoes are infective after a period of 8–14 days (extrinsic incubation period). Once infective, a mosquito remains so probably for the remainder of life (1–3 months or more).

The incidence of dengue has been increasing worldwide over the last few decades and today ranks as the most important vector-borne disease. Most subtropical and tropical regions where *Aedes* mosquitoes exist are potentially endemic areas of this disease. In urban communities, dengue epidemics are explosive and often start during the rainy season, when the vector mosquitoes are abundant. The mosquito has a short flight range, and urban spread of dengue is frequently house-to-house. The mosquito breeds in tropical and subtropical climates in artificial water-holding receptacles around human habitation or around plants close to human dwellings.

In humans, clinical disease begins 2–15 days after an infective mosquito bite. The patient develops fever of sudden onset with headache, chills, malaise, retrobulbar pain, conjunctivitis and severe pain in the back, muscles and joints (break-bone fever). The fever returns to normal after 5–6 days or may subside in about the third day and rise again about 5–8 days after onset (**"saddle-back" form**). A rash may appear on the third or fourth day and last for 24–72 hrs., fading with desquamation. Lymph nodes are frequently enlarged. Leucopenia with a relative lymphocytosis is a regular occurence. Convalescence may take weeks, although complications and death are rare.

Dengue may also occur in more serious forms, with hemorrhagic manifestations. These are known as **dengue hemorrhagic fever** and **dengue shock syndrome**. Dengue hemorrhagic fever may occur in individuals (usually children) with passively acquired (as maternal antibody) or endogenously produced heterologous dengue antibody. Although initial symptoms simulate normal dengue, the patient's condition abruptly worsens. Dengue shock syndrome, characterized by shock and hemoconcentration, may supervene. These altered manifestations of dengue have been observed, often in epidemic form, from South-east Asia, where several dengue serotypes are regularly present. The mortality rate is 1–10%, but may reach 40%. The pathogenesis of this severe syndrome seems to involve preexisting dengue antibody. It is postulated that virus-antibody complexes are formed within a few days of the second dengue infection and that the nonneutralizing enhancing antibodies promote infection of higher numbers of mononuclear cells, followed by the release of vasoactive mediators and procoagulants, leading to the disseminated intravascular coagulation seen in the hemorrhagic fever syndrome.

Conrol depends on antimosquito measures *e.g.*, elimination of breeding places and the use of insecticides. A live attenuated vaccine containing all four serotypes is undergoing clinical trials.

Tick-borne Group

These viruses produce two clinical syndromes, encephalitis and hemorrhagic fevers.

Encephalitis Viruses

1. **Russian spring summer encephalitis (RSSE) virus:** It has been reported from Russia, Eastern Europe and Scandinavia. RSSE is the most serious disease, with high rate of fatality and permanent paralytic sequelae in some survivors. Infection is transmitted by the bite of Ixodid ticks. The virus is transmitted transovarially in ticks so that they can act as vectors as well as reservoir hosts. Wild rodents and migrating birds are other reservoirs. Sometimes infection may be transmitted to sheep or other farm animals. The control of RSSE infection depends on the avoidance of tick bites. A formalin inactivated RSSE vaccine has been found useful.
2. **Louping-ill virus:** Louping-ill virus causes encephalitis in sheep, characterised by a curious "leaping" gait. Human cases that result from contact with these sheep are mild and present as aseptic meningitis. *Ixodes* ticks are the vectors and sheep, rodents, deer and birds acts as vertebrate reservoirs.
3. **Powassan virus:** It was first isolated from the brain of a five year old child, who died of encephalitis in Powassan, Ontario, Canada in 1958. Since then it has caused a number of cases in Canada, USA and Russia. *Ixodes cookei* and *I. marxi* serve as tick vectors. They feed on groundhogs and tree squirrels respectively, which serve as reservoirs.

Hemorrhagic fevers

1. Kyasanur Forest disease (KFD) virus

It causes a hemorrhagic fever that occurs in Karnataka state, India., In 1957, several dead monkeys were noticed in the Kyasanur forest in Shimoga district in Karnataka along with a severe prostrating illness in some of the villagers in the area. A new arbovirus antigenically related to RSSE virus, was isolated by National Institute of virology, Pune, from the patients and dead monkeys. It was named KFD virus after the name of the place from where the first isolations were made.

After an incubation period of 3–7 days, patients develop a sudden onset with fever, headache, conjunctivitis, myalgia and severe prostration. Some cases develop hemorrhages into the skin, mucosa and viscera. The case fatality rate is about 5 to 10%.

Forest birds and small mammals are the reservoir hosts. Infection is transmitted by the bite of **ticks**, the principal vector being ***Haemophysalis spinigera***. These ticks may act as reservoirs because transovarial transmission of virus has been demonstrated in them. As infection in monkeys is fatal, they cannot act as reservoir but only amplifier hosts.

A **killed KFD vaccine** was used in a small field trial and appeared to provide some degree of protection. Though KFD is antigenically related to RSSE virus, the RSSE vaccine cannot confer any protection against KFD.

For many years after its discovery in 1957, the epizootic and epidemic activity of KFD remained confined to the Sagar, Sorab and Shikarpur taluks of Shimoga district, Karnataka. In September 1982, there was an outbreak of epizootic and epidemic of KFD in Belthangadi taluk in South Canara district, Karnataka, due to ecological disturbance caused by destroying an evergreen reserve forest, which is believed to have activated a silent enzootic focus of the virus. The outbreak, known locally as "**monkey fever**".

2. Omsk hemorrhagic fever virus

It was first recognized in Siberia in 1945 as a causative agent of biphasic fever with lymphadenopathy and hemorrhages from mucus membranes. The disease is clinically related to KFD and the virus is closely related to RSSE virus. Water voles or muskrats are the reservoir hosts and *Dermacentor pictus* ticks are the vectors. Omsk hemorrhagic fever occurs in USSR and Rumania.

Laboratory Diagnosis

Diagnosis is by virus isolation and serology. Virus can be isolated by intracerebral inoculation into suckling mice from blood collected in the early stage of dengue fever and yellow fever, from the brain in case of encephalitis, the liver in yellow fever and from the vectors. The viral isolates can be identified by immunofluorescence of the cultured cells, hemagglutination inhibition and neutralization tests.

Neutralizing and hemaglutinating antibodies appear by 5th days in case of yellow fever and by seventh day in case of dengue fever. Paired sera are tested to demonstrate a rise in titre of antibody. Demonstration of IgM antibody by ELISA provides early diagnosis.

BUNYAVIRUSES

Structure and Properties

The family **bunyaviridae** containing over 300 species is the largest group of arboviruses. It contains both arthropod-borne (**arboviruses**) and rodent-borne (**roboviruses**). Bunyaviruses of medical importance fall into four genera—*Bunyavirus*, *Phlebovirus*, *Nairovirus* and *Hantavirus*. Members of the genus *Bunyavirus* are transmitted predominantly by mosquitoes, Nairoviruses by ticks and phleboviruses by sandflies or ticks. The genus *Hantavirus* is non-arthropod-borne but rodent-borne and are maintained in nature by chronic infection of rodents via aerosols formed from their dried excretions.

Bunyaviruses are spherical, enveloped particles, 90 to 100 nm in diameter, with spikes projecting from the surface of the virion. The single-stranded RNA genome is divided into three segments. Therefore, reassortment of RNA segments between closely related viruses is possible. The RNA genome is present in the virions in the form of helical nucleocapsid. The nucleocapsid is surrounded by a lipid-containing envelope. Surface spikes are composed of two glycoproteins that confer properties of neutralization of infectivity and hemagglutination of red blood cells. Virus particles mature by budding into intracytoplasmic vesicles associated with the Golgi system and are liberated from the cell by plasma membrane disruption and by fusion of intracellular vacuoles with the plasma membrane (Fig. 89.3).

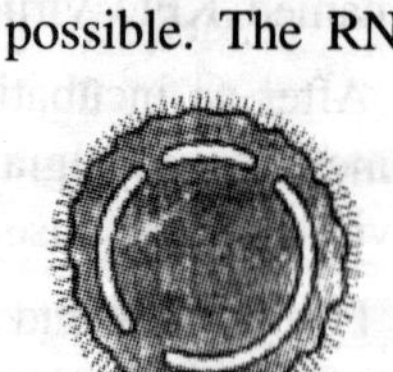

Fig. 89.3 Bunyavirus

Bunyavirus

This genus contains over 150 species, of which only a few cause human infections.

California encephalitis virus

The California encephalitis virus complex comprises 14 antigenically related bunyaviruses, including La Crosse virus. These viruses were originally found in California, but they are endemic in USA. La Crosse encephalitis was first recognized from a fatal case in La Crosse, Wisconsin, in

1960. The vector is woodland mosquito *Aedes triseriatus*, which breeds in tree holes. Small mammals such as squirrels and rabbits are amplifying hosts. The virus is transmitted transovarially in mosquitoes.

The onset of California encephalitis is abrupt, typically with a severe bifrontal headache, fever, sometimes vomiting, lethargy and convulsions. Less frequently there is only aseptic meningitis. Fatalities and neurological sequelae are rare.

Oropouche fever virus

Oropouche virus is a member of Simbu serogroup of bunyaviruses. It is a major cause of nonfatal febrile illness in Brazil, Trinidad and Panama. Large epidemics of fever with aseptic meningitis have been recorded. Oropouche virus is associated with three types of clinical syndromes—fever, fever with rash and meningitis. The incubation period varies from 4 to 8 days. Fever, chills, severe headache, myalgia, arthralgia, dizzines and photophobia are the common clinical manifestations. The disease may be confused with malaria or other febrile conditions. The midge *Culicoides paraensia* is the major vector for oropouche virus. Primates, sloths and wild birds are implicated as vertebrate hosts.

Phlebivirus

The major members of this genus are the sandfly fever and Rift Valley fever viruses.

Sandfly fever virus

Sandfly fever or Phlebotomus fever or Pappataci fever is a mild insect-borne disease with selflimiting nonfatal fever that occurs commonly in countries bordering the Mediterranean Sea and in Russia, Iran, Pakistan, India, Panama, Brazil and Trinidad. The **sandfly** *Phlebotomus papatasii* is the vector. Human and sandflies are believed to be the reservoirs. The bite of sandfly in humans causes small itching papules on the skin that persist for upto five days. There are atleast twenty antigenic types of the virus, but only five appear to cause human disease-Naples, Sicilian, Punta Toro, Chagres, Candiru. The virus is transmitted transovarially in sandflies.

Rift Valley fever virus

It is named after Rift Valley, Kenya, where it was first recognized. Rift Valley fever appears as epizootics in sheep, cattle, camels and goats in Africa. Massive outbreaks have been recognized in South Africa, Kenya, Uganda, Sudan, Egypt and Mauretania. Human cases are usually restricted to veterinarians, butchers, laboratory workers and others in close contact with blood of domestic livestock. Transmission is through aerosolized infected blood and mosquitoes. Epizootics in the Rift Valley arise periodically after heavy rains. There is evidence that the virus is maintained in nature in the dried eggs of *Aedes* mosquitoes that hatch only in very moist conditions.

Nairovirus

The genus is named after the type species Nairobi sheep disease virus.

Nairobi sheep disease virus

Nairobi sheep disease is an acute, hemorrhagic gastroenteritis caused by a ***Nairovirus*** in sheep and goats in East Africa. The virus produces mild febrile illness in shepherds. It is transmitted by *Rhipicephalus* ticks.

Ganjam virus

The Ganjam virus, isolated from ticks collected from sheep and goats in Orissa, India, is closely related to the Nairobi sheep disease virus. The Ganjam virus has also been isolated from humans. Accidental infection in laboratory workers has caused mild febrile illness.

Crimean-Congo hemorrhagic fever virus

The Crimean hemorrhagic fever virus, first isolated in Crimea in 1945, was subsequently found to be identical with the Congo fever virus isolated in 1956 in Congo (Zaire), hence the name Crimean-congo hemorrhagic fever. The disease is endemic in Eastern Europe, Central Asia and many parts of Africa. Cattle, sheep, goats and other domestic animals act as natural reservoirs. It is transmitted by *Hyalomma ticks*. During the acute phase of the disease, the blood of the patient is highly infectious and direct transmission may occur through contact. Antibodies to Crimean-congo hemorrhagic fever virus have been detected in human and animal sera from India. A related virus, Hazara has been isolated in Pakistan. It is also widespread in Iran, Iraq and UAE.

Hantavirus

The *Hantavirus* causes **hamorrhagic fever with renal syndrome (HFRS)**, which is an acute viral infection that causes interstitial nephritis that can lead to acute renal insufficiency and renal failure in severe cases. The disease is also known with other names such as Manchurian epidemic hemorrhagic fever, nephrosonephritis, nephropathia epidemica and rodent-borne nephropathy. This disease was first noticed in the early 1950s when a large number of US soldiers serving in Korea got the infection. But it is prevalent in Russia, Scandinavia and China.

The disease occurs in two forms—the milder nephropathia epidemica, which is prevalent in Scandinavia, characterised by interstitial nephritis generally resolving with a rare fatality, and the more serious epidemic hemorrhagic fever in the Far East with renal insufficiency and renal failure; hemorrhage and shock may occur with a fatality rate of 10%.

The genus contains atleast four species—*Hantaan virus* causing the severe HFRS in the Far East, North Asia and Russia, *Seoul virus* causing a mild disease with worldwide distribution, *Puumala virus* responsible for nephropathia epidemica in Northern and Eastern Europe, and *Prospect Hill virus* isolated from voles in the USA, which has not been associated with any human illness.

Hantavirus species are roboviruses and are natural pathogens rodents. They do not have an arthropod vector. Field mice (*Apodemus agrarius*) is the major host for *Hantaan virus*, domestic Rats (*Rattus rattus* and *Rattus norvegicus*) for *Seoul virus* and voles for Puumala and Prospect Hill viruses. Viremia occurs in infected rodents and the virus is shed in urine, feces and saliva. Transmission from rodent to rodent and rodent to humans is primarily by inhalation of the virus contained in the aerosols formed from their dried excretions.

Hantavirus pulmonary syndrome, a new disease was with severe respiratory illness was identified in USA, in 1993. It was found to be caused by a novel Hantavirus known as Sin Nombre virus which is closely related to Prospect Hill virus. The deer mouse (*Peromyscus maniculatus*) is the reservoir host. The human infection is acquired by inhalation of dust containing rodent excreta, as hantaviruses are shed in saliva, urine and feces of infected rodents. No arthropod vector is involved. The disease is characterized by prodromal fever, myalgia, and other symptoms, including cough, headache and nausea and vomiting, followed by rapidly progressive pulmonary edema.

Preventive measures for hantavirus infections are based on rodent control and avoidance of contact with rodents and rodent excreta.

Laboratory Diagnosis

Bunyavirus illnesses are diagnosed by isolating the virus or by showing a fourfold or greater rise in antibody titer between acute and convalescent phase sera.

The virus can be isolated from blood (or from brain, liver and other organs postmortem) during the viremic phase, but not usually after the third day of the fever. It is propagated by intracerebral inoculation of suckling mice or vertebrate tissue cultures such as vero or BHK-21 cell lines or *Aedes* mosquito cell lines.

The growth of virus in cell cultures can be detected by immunofluorescence and neutralization tests with reference antisera.

Serologic tests used to diagnose bunyavirus infections include the ELISA, CFT, fluorescent antibody test, neutralization and hemagglutination inhibition tests. The CFT, ELISA and fluorescent antibody tests are group reactive; the HI and neutralization tests are type specific. Assessments of IgM may be especially useful in establishing early diagnosis.

REOVIRUSES

Orbivirus

The genus *Orbivirus* of the family **Reoviridae** contains arthropod-borne viruses. They commonly infect insects, and many are transmitted by insects to vertebrates. They differ from other arboviruses in having double-stranded RNA genome.

Orbiviruses are spherical that contain ten segments of double-stranded RNA, exhibit icosahedral symmetry (Fig. 89.4), and have a diameter of 60 to 80 nm. Orbiviruses are sensitive to low pH, in contrast with the general stability of other reoviruses.

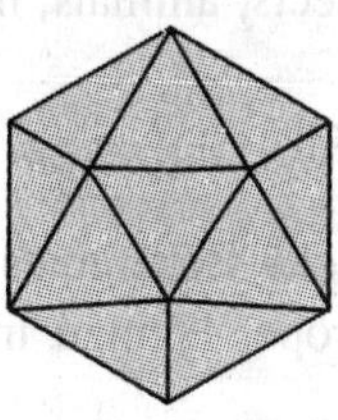

Fig. 89.4 Reovirus

About 100 serotypes are known. None of these viruses cause serious clinical disease in humans, but they may cause mild fevers. Serious animal pathogens include **blue tongue virus of sheep** and **African horse sickness virus**. Antibodies to orbiviruses are found in many vertebrates, including humans.

The African horse sickness virus, transmitted by *Culicoides* causes disease of equines in Africa. In 1959–60 it spread in epizootic waves eastwards to Iran, Afghanistan, Pakistan and India. It caused extensive disease among army horses and mules in India.

Palyam, Kasba, and Vellore viruses belonging to *Orbivirus* have been isolated from mosquitoes in India but their pathogenic significance is not known.

Coltivirus

Coloradotick fever (mountain fever or tick fever) is a mild febrile disease, without rash, that is transmitted by a wood tick *Dermacentor andersoni*. It is caused by a *Coltivirus* of Reoviridae family. It contains a genome of double-stranded RNA with 12 segments.

The incubation period is 4–6 days. The disease has a sudden onset with chilly sensations and myalgia. Symptoms include headache, deep ocular pain, muscle and joint pains, lumbar backache, and nausea and vomiting. The fever is usually diphasic. After the first bout of two days, the patient may feel well. Symptoms and fever then reappear and last 3–4 more days.

During the acute stage, the virus is present in the blood. The virus may be isolated from whole blood in cell culture or suckling mice. Specific neutralizing and complement-fixing antibodies appear in the second week of illness and persist for year. Only one antigenic type is known. As experiment live-virus vaccine has been made.

The disease is prevalent in Colorado, Oregon, Utah, Idaho, Montana and Wyoming. Natural infection occurs in rodents. The tick acts as a reservoir host in which the virus is transmitted transovarially.

RHABDOVIRUSES

Chandipura Virus

It belongs to the genus *vesiculovirus* of Rhabdoviridae family. It was isolated from the blood of patiens during an epidemic of dengue-chikungunya fever in Nagpur in 1967. The virus appears to multiply in sandflies and *Aedes* mosquitoes. Antibodies are common in human sera and animal sera from different parts of India.

UNGROUPED ARBOVIRUSES

Several arboviruses isolated from insects, animals, birds and humans have not yet been assigned to any taxonomic group.

Bhanja Virus

It is isolated from *Haemophysalis* ticks from goats in Ganjam, Orissa. The virus is present in goats in West Africa and South East Europe. Human infections with disease and death have been reported from Yugoslavia.

Wanowri Virus

It is isolated from *Hyalomma* ticks in India and from the brain of a young girl who died after two-day fever in Sri Lanka. The virus is also present in Iran and Egypt.

QUESTIONS

Essay Questions:

1. What are the general properties of arboviruses? List the arboviruses seen in India. Describe the pathogenicity and laboratory diagnosis of dengue virus.
2. Give an account of arboviruses.

Short Notes:

1. Alphavirus
2. Chikungunya
3. Flaviviridae or Flaviviruses
4. Japanese B encephalitis

5. Laboratory diagnosis of Japanese B encephalitis
6. Japanese B encephalitis vaccine (or) prophylaxis against Japanese B encephalitis
7. Yellow fever
8. Yellow fever vaccines
9. 17-D vaccine
10. Dengue fever (or) Break bone fever
11. How is dengue transmitted? What is its important complication?
12. Complications of dengue viruses
13. KFD
14. Bunyaviruses
15. Orbivirus
16. Viral hemorrhagic fevers
17. List the viruses causing acute hemorrhagic fevers.

90

Arenaviruses and Filoviruses

- *Arenaviruses*
  - *— Structure, LCM virus, lassa fever virus, junin virus, machupo virus, guanarito virus, sabia virus, laboratory diagnousis*
- *Filoviruses*
  - *— Structure and general properties,*
  - *— African hemorrhagic fevers (marburg and ebola viruses),*
  - *— Laboratory diagnosis*

ARENAVIRUSES

Structure

Arenaviruses are enveloped, spherical or pleomorphic particles with a diameter of 110 to 130 nm. The viral envelope, which is acquired by budding through the host cell plasma membrane, carries club shaped glycoprotein peplomers about 10 nm long. Sandy-appearing granules resembling ribosomes are found within the virus particles. These particles give arenaviruses their name (arena is Latin for "sand") (Fig. 90.1). These particles are cellular ribosomes incorporated into the virions during assembly. The envelope encloses the helical nucleocapsid segments. The genome consists of two single-stranded RNA molecules/segments, L (large) and S (small), which are unusually ambisense *i.e.*, the 3' half is of negative polarity and the 5' half is positive, which means that coding information is contained in both the genomic and antigenomic viral RNAs. The replication takes place in the cytoplasm of host cell. Arenaviruses do not produce cytopathic effect when replicating in cell cultures.

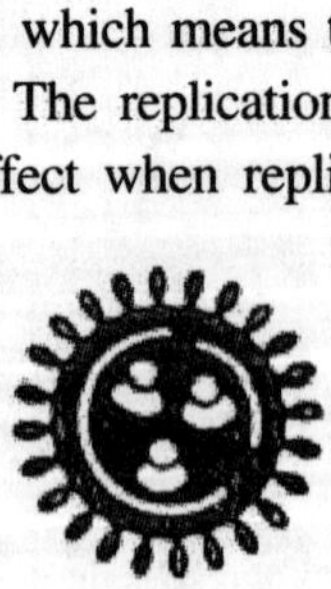

Fig. 90.1 Arenavirus

The family **Arenaviridae** has only one genus *Arenavirus*. These viruses cause chronic infections in rodents. Humans are infected by inhaling contaminated aerosols or by contact with rodent excreta or by eating food contaminated with rodent excreta or by exposure of open wound to infected soil. Several arenaviruses are known to infect the fetus and may cause fetal death in humans. Atleast six arenaviruses are known to cause human disease (Table 90.1).

Table 90.1 Arenaviruses Causing Human Disease

Virus	*Geographic distribution*	*Vertebrate host*	*Human disease*
Lumphocytic choriomeningitis	Worldwide	*Mus musculus*	Influenza-like illness, aseptic meningitis and rarely severe encephalomyelitis.
Lassa	West Africa	*Mastomys natalensis*	Hemorrhagic fever
Junin	Argentina	*Calomys laucha, Calomys musculinus,* and *Akadon azarae*	Argentinian hemorrhagic fever
Machupo	Bolivia	*Calomys callosus*	Bolivian hemorrhagic fever
Guanarito	Venezuela	*Sigmodon spp.*	Venezuelan hemorrhagic fever
Sabia	Brazil		Brazilian hemorrhagic fever

Lymphocytic Choriomeningitis (LCM) Virus

LCM virus is widespread in Europe and America and was discovered in 1933. It is a common human pathogen and may chronically infect mouse or hamster colonies. LCM is an acute disease with aseptic meningitis, a relatively benign infection with little mortality or a mild systemic influenza-like illness. Rarely there is a severe encephalomyelitis or a fatal systemic disease. The incubation period is usually 18–21 days but may be as short as 1–3 days. There may be fever, malaise, generalised muscular aches and pains, weakness, sore throat and cough. The fever lasts for 3–14 days. In the prodromal period or mild systemic form, leukopenia with relative lymphocytosis is frequently present. In the meningitic form, there is pleocytosis in the CSF with a predominance of lymphocytes.

LCM is endemic in mice and other animals (dogs, monkeys, guinea pigs) and is occasionally transmitted to humans. Chronically infected mice excrete the virus in urine and feces and act as a source of infection to contacts. The virus is transmitted vertically to their offspring, which in turn become healthy carriers.

In LCM-infected mice, the immune response may be protective or deleterious. Congenitally or neonatally infected mice do not become acutely ill but carry a lifelong persistent infection. They fail to clear the infection because they were infected before the cellular immune system matured, and the virus is not recognized as foreign. These mice make a strong antibody response leading to hypergammaglobulinemia, that is not able to clear the infection. This leads to circulating antigen-antibody complexes and immune complex disease. The animals exhibit chronic **glomerulonephritis** due to deposition of antigen-antibody complexes. Mice infected as adults may develop a rapidly fatal disease due to a T cell mediated inflammatory response in the brain. A carrier state can be established in adult mice if immunosuppressive treatment is given at the time of infection.

Lassa Fever Virus

Lassa fever was first noticed in 1969 among Americans stationed in the Nigerian village of Lassa. Lassa virus is active in all Western African countries situated between Senegal and Zaire. Lassa virus is extremely virulent and the mortality rate is 36-67%.

The incubation period is 3-16 days. Lassa fever can involve almost all the organ systems, although symptoms may vary in the individual patient. The disease is characterised by very high fever, mouth ulcers, severe muscle aches, skin rash with bleeding (hemorrhages), pneumonia, and heart and kidney damage. Benign, febrile cases do occur. The virus can be isolated from the patient's blood in Vero monkey cell cultures.

A house rat (*Mastomys natalensis*) is the natural reservoir. Rodent excreta acts as a source of infection. The virus is present in the throat, urine and blood of patients and the virus can be transmitted by human to human contact. Nosocomical infections occurred frequently by human contact.

Rodent control is the most important measure in prevention. Meticulous barrier nursing procedures and universal precautions to avoid contact with blood and body fluids can prevent transmission to hospital personnel. The antiviral drug ribavirin is the drug of choice.

South American hemorrhagic fevers

South American arenaviruses are considered to be members of Tacaribe complex, based on serology and phylogenetic studies of viral RNAs. Rodents act as reservoirs and transmission is believed to occur through rodent excreta. The viruses tend to be prevalent in a particular area, limited in their distribution. Most important and serious human pathogens are Junin, Machupo, Guanarito and Sabia viruses.

Junin Virus

It is responsible for Junin hemorrhagic fever prevalent in certain agricultural areas of Argentina; hence, known as Argentine hemorrhagic fever. The disease has a marked seasonal variation, and the infection occurs among workers in maize and wheat fields. The rodent *Calomys musculinus* is the reservoir host. Junin virus produces both humoral and cell-mediated immunodepression, with a mortality rate of 10-15% in untreated patients. Deaths due to **Junin hemorrhagic fever** may be related to an inability to initiate a cell-mediated immune response.

Machupo Virus

It is responsible for **Machupo hemorrhagic fever**, first identified in Bolivia in 1962, and hence known as Bolivian hemorrhagic fever, with a case-fatality rate of 20%. The reservoir host is a rodent *Calomys callosus*. Nosocomial outbreaks have been reported.

Guanarito Virus

It causes **Venezuelan hemorrhagic fever**, first identified in 1990, when a forest land was cleared for small farm use. The clinical disease resembles Argentine hemorrhagic fever.

Sabia Virus

It was first isolated in 1990 from a fatal case of hemorrhagic fever in Brazil. It may induce a clinical disease similar to that of Aregentine hemorrhagic fever.

Laboratory Diagnosis

1. **Isolation of virus.** Arenaviruses can be isolated from blood, CSF, throat washings, pleural fluid, urine and autopsy specimens by inoculation of suckling mice, hamsters and guinea pigs. They can also be isolated by inoculation of Vero and BHK-21 cell cultures. The growth is obtained in 2–3 days and the viral isolate can be identified by indirect immunofluorescence and ELISA.
2. **Detection of viral antigen.** Viral antigen can be demonstrated in the blood and conjunctival cells by indirect immunofluorescence.
3. **Demonstration of antibodies.** Specific IgM antibody or a rising titre of antibody in paired sera can be demonstrated by indirect immunofluorescence during the second week of the illness.

FILOVIRUSES

Structure and General Properties

Filoviruses are pleomorphic viruses with unusual morphology placed in the family Filoviridae. They are generally seen as long filamentous, enveloped particles that may be branched. They are 80–nm in diameter and 800-1000 nm in length. Particles as long as 14,000 nm in length have also been reported. The envelope is composed of lipid bilayer covered with peplomers. The envelope surrounds a helically wound tubular nucleocapsid. The large genome is single-stranded, negative sense RNA and contains seven genes (Fig. 90.2).

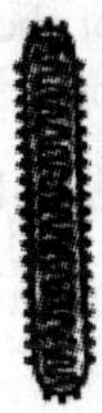

Fig. 90.2 Filovirus

Filoviruses are highly virulent and require maximum biosafety facilities for laboratory work. Filovirus infectivity is destroyed by heating for 30 minutes at 60°C, by UV and gamma radiation, by lipid solvents and by bleach and phenolic disinfectants.

Filoviruses multiply in the cytoplasm of infected cells, forming large inclusion bodies. Progeny virions are released from the plasma membrane by budding. Filoviruses can be grown in Vero cell lines and in many other cell types.

The known Filoviruses are Marburg virus and Ebola virus, which are not related antigenically. The four subtypes of Ebola virus (Zaire, Sudan, Reston, Ivory Coast) share some common epitopes.

African Hemorrhagic Fevers

Marburg virus was initially isolated in Germany and Yugoslavia from laboratory workers who became severely ill while preparing primary cell cultures from African green monkeys (*Cercopithecus aethiops*). Experimentally inoculated monkeys developed a uniformly fatal disease resembling hemorrhagic fever in humans after an incubation period of 4–16 days.

Ebola virus was isolated from patients with hemorrhagic fever in Zaire and the Sudan, in 1976. The virus was named Ebola virus after a river in Zaire.

Marburg and Ebola viruses are highly virulent, with infections usually ending in death. They cause acute diesases characterized by fever, headache, sore throat and muscle pain followed by abdominal pain, vomiting, diarrhea, hiccup, and rash with widespread bleeding into the skin, mucus membranes, visceral organs and the gastrointestinal tract, often leading to shock and death. Very high titers of virus are present in liver, spleen, lymph nodes, lungs and blood. These viruses have the highest mortality rates, often greater than fifty per cent (30-90%) of all the viral hemorrhagic fevers.

Although the natural reservoir for these viruses is unknown, they can be transmitted to humans from infected monkeys and probably other animals or by exposure to blood or other body fluids from an infected patient. Outbreaks of hemorrhagic fever caused by these viruses continue to occur at regular intervals.

There is no specific treatment for infections caused by these viruses. Strict barrier nursing techniques are essential when caring for infected persons.

Laboratory Diagnosis

1. Filoviruses can be identified under electron microscope by their characteristic morphology in the blood and in the cytoplasm of infected cells particularly of liver, lungs and kidneys. A large number of virions can be seen in the damaged hepatocytes and in the bile canaliculi.
2. The virus can be isolated from the blood during the febrile phase, by inoculation of Vero cell lines or MA-104 monkey cell lines. The viral isolate can be identified by electron microscopy or direct immunofluorescence. Because of the hazards of working with Filoviruses, they are studied in only a few reference laboratories around the world.
3. Antiviral antibodies can be demonstrated in patient serum by ELISA.

QUESTIONS

Short Essays:

1. Arenaviruses
2. LCM virus
3. Lassa fever virus
4. South American hemorrhagic fevers
5. Filoviruses
6. African hemorrhagic fevers
7. Marburg virus
8. Ebola virus
9. Lab. diagnosis of Arenavirus infections
10. Hemorrhagic fevers
11. Lab. diagnosis of Filovirus infections.

91

Orthomyxoviruses (Influenza Viruses)

- *Introduction*
- *Structure*
- *Classification*
- *Resistance*
- *Hemagglutinin and hemagglutination*
- *Neuraminidase and Elution*
- *Antigenic structure*
- *Antigenic variations*
- *Cultivation*
- *Pathogenesis*
- *Laboratory diagnosis*
- *Prophylaxis*
- *Treatment*

INTRODUCTION

The term "**myxovirus**" (myxa=mucin) implies an affinity for mucins and denotes a large group of enveloped viruses able to attach to glycoprotein cell surface receptors. Based on fundamental diferences in their structure and their pattern of replication, these myxoviruses are classified into two separate familites—**Orthomyxoviridae** and **Paramyxoviridae** (Table 91.1).

STRUCTURE

All known orthomyxoviruses are influenza viruses. Influenza viruses are spherical, enveloped, pleomorphic particles with 80-120 nm in diameter. The virus core consists of a helical nucleocapsid, in which single stranded negative sense RNA genome is located. The RNA genome is composed of eight distinct segments of RNA. A lipid envelope derived from the cell surrounds the virus particle. Two types of spikes or peplomers which are virus-encoded glycoproteins, the **hemagglutinin (HA)** and the **neuraminidase (NA)**, about 10 nm long project from the surface of the particle. The HA represents about 25% of viral protein and the NA about 5%. These two surface glycoproteins are the important antigens that determines antigenic variation of influenza viruses and host immunity.

Influenza virus particles contain nine different structural proteins. The nucleoprotein (NP) associates with the viral RNA to form a ribonucleoprotein (RNP), 9 nm in diameter that assumes a helical configuration. Three large proteins (PB1, PB2 and PA) are bound to the viral RNP and are responsible for RNA transcription and replication. The matrix (M_1) protein, which forms a shell underneath the viral lipid envelope, is important in particle morphogenesis and is a major component of the virion (about 40%). The M_2 protein is also present as an ion channel in the envelope but at only a few copies per particle.

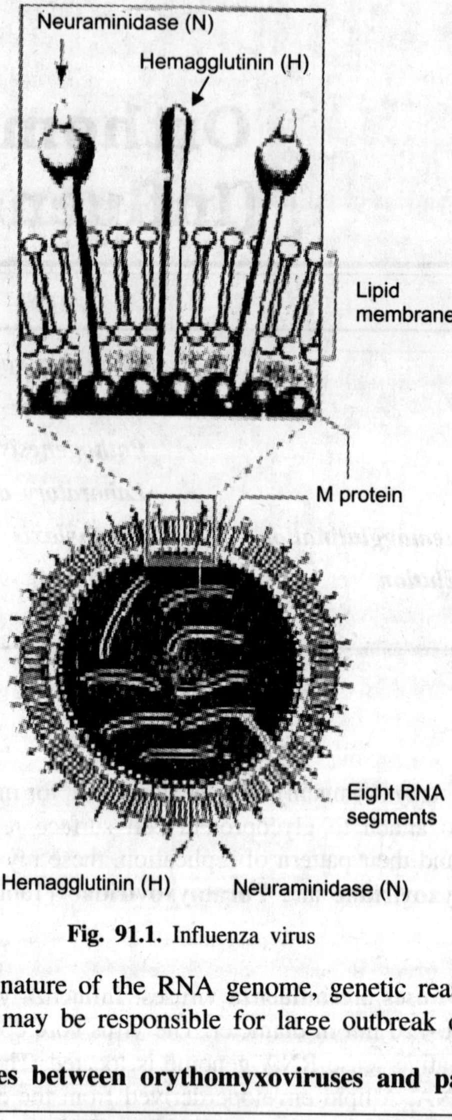

Fig. 91.1. Influenza virus

Because of the segmented nature of the RNA genome, genetic reassortment is very common among influenza viruses, which may be responsible for large outbreak of epidemics.

Table 91.1 Differences between orythomyxoviruses and paramyxoviruses

Property	*Orthomyxoviruses*	*Paramyxoviruses*
Size of virion	80-120 nm	100-300 nm
Shape of virion	Spherical; filamentous in fresh isolates	pleomorphic
Genome	Single stranded RNA in eight pieces	Single stranded RNA in a single piece.

Diameter of ribonucleo-protein helix	9 nm in diameter	18 nm in diameter
RNA is nucleocapsid	RNase-sensitive	RNase-resistant
Site of replication	Nucleus	Cytoplasm
Genetic reassortment	common	absent
Rate of antigenic change	high	low
Effect of Actinomycin D	inhibits multiplication	does not inhibit
Disease caused in humans	Influenza types A, B and C	Parainfluenza 1-4 infections, respiratory syncytial disease, mumps, measles

Influenza virus is unusual among RNA viruses because all of its RNA transcription and replication occur in the nucleus of infected cells. It is the only RNA virus (without a genomic DNA intermediate) that utilized some spliced mRNAs.

CLASSIFICATION

Influenza viruses are classified into three immunological types A, B and C. The family Orthomyxoviridae comprises two genera. *Influenzavirus A, B*, which contains human and animal strains of influenza type A and human strains of type B; and *Influenzavirus* C, which contains influenza type C viruses of humans and swine.

Antigenic differences exhibited by two of internal structural proteins, the nucleocapsid (NP) and matrix (M) proteins, are used to divide influenza viruses into types A, B and C. These proteins possess no cross-reactivity among the three types. Antigenic variations in the surface glycoproteins, HA and NA are used to subtype the viruses. So far, 14 subtypes of HA (H1-H14) and nine subtypes of NA (N1-N9), in many different combinations have been recovered from birds, animals, or humans. Three HA (H1-H3) and two NA (N1, N2) subtypes have been recovered from humans.

The standard nomenclature system for influenza virus isolates includes the foilowing information: type, host of origin, geographic origin, strain number, and year of isolation. Antigenic descriptions of the HA and the NA are given in parentheses for type A. The host of origin is not indicated for human isolates. e.g., A/Hong Kong/03/68 (H3N2), but it is for others, e.g., A/Swine/Iowa/15/30 (H1N1).

RESISTANCE

The virus is inactivated by heating at 50°C for 30 minutes. It remains viable at 0–4°C for weeks. The virus loses infectivity more rapidly at –20°C than at +4°C. The virus survives slow drying and may remain viable on fomites such as blankets for about two weeks. Ether, formaldehyde, phenol, salts of heavy metals and many other chemical disinfectants destroy infectivity. Iodine is highly effective. The virus can be preserved for years at –70°C or by freeze drying.

HEMAGGLUTININ AND HEMAGGLUTINATION

The hemagglutinin (HA) derives its name from its ability to agglutinate RBC. The HA spike on the virus particle is a trimer, composed of three interwined HA1 and HA2 dimers.

Hemagglutination is an important characteristic of influenza viruses. When mixed with a suspension of fowl RBC, the virus is adsorbed on to the mucoprotein receptors on the cell surface. The virus links togethers adjacent RBC producing hemagglutination. The hemagglutinin peplomers on the viral surface are responsible for this activity. When a fixed quantity of RBC are added to a serial dilution of viral suspension, the highest dilution that produces hemagglutination provides **hemagglutination titre**. The test can be carried out in tubes or plastic trays. Erythrocytes, which are not agglutinated settle at the bottom in the form of a button, while the agglutinated cells spread in a shield like pattern. Hemagglutination takes place within a wide range of temperature, from 0°C to 37°C. Influenza viruses vary in their ability to agglutinate RBC of different species. Influenza virus types A and B agglutinate RBC of fowl, human, guinea pig and some other species. Influenza virus type C agglutinate RBC of fowl only, at 4°C.

Hemagglutination provides a convenient method for the detection and titration of the influenza virus in egg and other culture fluids. Hemagglutinin is more resistant to physical and chemical agents than infectivity. Therefore, hemagglutination can be used for the titration of the inactivated influenza virus also, as, for example, in the standardisation of killed influeza virus vaccines.

Hemagglutination can be inhibited by its specific antibody. This is known as "**hemagglutination inhibition (HI)**". It offers a convenient method for the detection and quantitation of the antibody to virus. A disadvantage of this serological test is the presence of nonspecific inhibitors in sera which can be inactivated by the treatment of sera with RDE, trypsin, potassium periodate, Kaolin and CO_2.

The plasma membranes of tissue culture cells in which the virus is multiplying contains hemagglutinins. Therefore, RBC are adsorbed on to the surface of such cells. This is the basis of **hemadsorption**, a technique by which the growth of the influenza virus in cell cultures can be identified.

NEURAMINIDASE AND ELUTION

Hemagglutination is followed after a time by the detachment of the virus from the red cell surface, a process reverse to the hemagglutination, known as **elution** and is caused by the enzyme neuraminidase (N), also known as sialidase present on the viral surface. The enzyme acts by destroying receptors (removes sialic acid from glycoconjugates), hence, it is also known as "receptor destroying enzyme (RDE)". Elution is an enzymatic reaction, which takes place at 37°C, but not at 0°C. Hemagglutination and elution can be used for purifying and concentrating influenza viruses.

Virus particles which have been eluted from RBC are still capable of agglutinating fresh RBC but RBC that are agglutinated by the virus are not susceptible to agglutination by the same strain of the virus. Such RBC may, however, be agglutinated by other myxoviruses. The inability of these RBC to be reagglutinated by the same virus is due to the destruction of the specific receptors by the initial treatment with the virus.

The neuraminidase spike on the virus particle, is a tetramer, composed of four identical monomers. A slender stalk is topped with a box-shaped head. The NA functions at the end of the viral life cycle. It is a sialidase enzyme which facilitates the release of virus particles from infected cell surfaces by removing sialic acid residues from viral glycoproteins. Neuraminidases are also present in bacteria (*Vibrio cholerae*) and in the cells of higher organisms.

ANTIGENIC STRUCTURE

The influenza viruses possess the following antigens—internal antigens—RNP and M proteins, and surface antigens—H and N.

1. Ribonucleoprotein (RNP) Antigen

It is type-specific and based on its nature, influenza viruses are classified into types A, B and C. The RNP antigens of types A, B and C are distinct, but all strains of any one type possess the same antigen. The RNP antigen is stable and does not exhibit any significant antigenic variation. Anti-RNP antibody develops after infection but not following killed vaccines. The RNP antigen is found free in infected tissues and occurs in the supernatant when the virus containing fluid is centrifuged.

2. Matrix (M) Protein

The M protein antigen is also type-specific and distinct for A, B and C types of influenza viruses.

3. Hemagglutinin (H)

Hemagglutinin is a glycoprotein composed of two polypeptides—HA1 and HA2. It is responsible for hemagglutination and hemadsorption. It enables the virus to adsorb on to mucoprotein receptors on RBC as well as on respiratory epithelial cells. Antihemagglutinin antibodies are produced following infection and immunisation and are protective by preventing adsorption of the virus to host cells. The hemagglutinin is a strain specific antigen and is capable of a great variation. Fourteen distinct HA subtypes, named H1 to H14 have been identified in avian influenza viruses, but only three of them have been found in human isolates so far.

4. Neurominidase (N)

Neuraminidase is a glycoprotein enzyme which destroys cell receptors by hydrolytic cleavage. Like hemagglutinin, it is strain-specific, exhibits variation and antineuraminidase antibody is formed following infection and immunisation. It is not effective in protection as the antihemaglutinin antibody. Nine subtypes (N1 to N9) have been identified.

ANTIGENIC VARIATIONS

A unique feature of the influenza virus is its ability to undergo antigenic variation. This is of great importance in the epidemiology of the disease. Antigenic variability is highest in influenza virus type A and less in type B, whereas type C is antigenically stable. Based on the degree of antigenic variation of H and N, two distinct forms of antigenic variations are known.

Antigenic drift

The gradual sequential change in antigenic structure occurring regularly at frequent intervals, is known as antigenic drift. Here, the new antigens, though different from the previous antigens, are yet related to them since antigenic vairation is not complete, so that they react with antisera to the predecessor virus strains, to varying degrees. Antigenic drift is due to mutation and selection, the process being influenced by the presence of antibodies to the predecessor strains in the hosts. Antigenic drift accounts for the periodical epidemics of influenza.

Antigenic shift

It is an abrupt, complete, drastic, discontinuous variation in the antigenic structure, resulting in a novel virus strain unrelated antigenically to predecessor strains. Such changes may involve hemagglutinin, neuraminidase or both. Antibodies to predecessor strains do not neutralise the new variants and can, therefore, spread widely in the population causing major epidemics or pandemics. The changes involved in antigenic shift are due to gene reassortment (recombination). Only type A viruses show antigenic shift.

In addition to above, influenza viruses undergo several other variations.

P-Q-R variation

Influenza virus strains belonging to the same subtype-even strains isolated during the course of a single outbreak-may behave differently in neutralisation tests with antisera. Vander Veen and Mulder called this the P-Q-R variation. Strains in the P phase were neutralised by the homologous antiserum in high titres and by heterologous antiserum in low titres. Strains in the Q phase were neutralised poorly by either homologous or heterologous sera. R phase strains were neutralised by both homologous and heterologous antisera in high titres. The P-Q-R variation appears to be due to the rearrangement of antigenic determinants on the surface of the virion. In the P phase, the dominant antigen is on the surface so that it reacts with the specific antibody with high avidity, while in the Q phase the dominant antigen is apparently buried under the surface and hence inaccessible to the antibody. The P-Q-R phases are interconvertible by passaging the virus in the presence of the appropriate antiserum.

O-D variation

When serially passaged in eggs, influenza virus type A underwent certain changes. Burnett and Bull (1943) called this the O-D variation. The fresh isolate was said to be in the "original" (O) phase and the passaged virus in the "Derived" (D) phase. The O phase virus grew well in the amniotic cavity of chick embryos but only poorly or not at all in the allantoic cavity. It agglutinated mammalian RBC (guinea pig and human) to a high titre and fowl RBC only weakly or not at all. Filamentous forms were common. It was infectious for humans. The D phase virus, on the other hand grew equally well in the amniotic and allantoic cavities and agglutinated fowl RBC as well as or better than mammalian cells, showed no filamentous forms and was relatively avirulent for human beings. The O-D variation was considered a result of mutation.

CULTIVATION

Influenza virus can cause experimental infection in ferrets and mice by intranasal inoculation.

Influenza viruses grow well in the amniotic cavity of 13-day old chick embryos incubated at 33-35°C for 2-3 days. After a few egg passages, the viruses grow well in the allantoic cavity also, except for the type C virus, which does not grow in the allantoic cavity. The influenza virus does not damage chick embryos, which may hatch out normally. Virus growth is detected by the appearance of hemaglutinin in the amniotic and allantoic fluids.

Influenza viruses can be isolated in primary monkey kidney cell cultures and continuous cell lines derived from canine kidney (MDCK) or rhesus monkey kidney (LLC-MK_2). Inoculated cell cultures are incubated in the presence of trypsin, which cleaves and activates the HA so that replicating virus will spread throughout the culture. Cytopathic effects are not prominent and virus growth is detected by hemadsorption or demonstration of HA in the culture fluid.

When passaged serially in eggs, using undiluted infected allantoic fluid as inocula, the progeny virus will show high hemagglutinin titres, but low infectivity. This has been called the **Von Magnus phenomenon** and is due to the formation of incomplete virus particles lacking nucleic acid.

PATHOGENESIS

Influenza virus spreads from person to person by airborne droplets through inhalation or by contact with contaminated hands or fomites. The cells of respiratory epithelium are infected (If virus particles avoid removed by the cough reflex and escape neutralisation by any preexisting specific IgA antibodies or inactivation by nonspecific inhibitors in the mucus secretions) and progeny virions spread to adjacent cells. Viral neuraminidase lowers the viscosity of the mucus film in the respiratory tract, laying bare the cellular surface receptors and promoting the spread of virus containing fluid to the lower portions of the tract. Within a short time, many cells in the respiratory tract are infected and eventually killed and shed. Cytotoxic T cells lyse infected cells.

The incubation period varies from one to four days. Typically, influenza has an acute onset characterized by chills, followed by high fever, headache and dry cough, muscle aches (caused by circulating cytokines), and extreme drowsiness. The disease runs its course in four to five days, after which their is a gradual recovery. Interferon is detectable in respiratory secretions about one day after viral shedding begins. Subclinical infections are common.

Serious complications usually occurs only in the elderly and debilitated, especially those with underlying cardiopulmonary or other chronic disease. Pregnancy has appeared to be a risk factor for lethal complications in some epidemics. The most important complications are—(*i*) pneumonia, croup or middle ear infections in young children. (*ii*) elderly people may develop secondary bacterial pneumonia usually due to *Staphylococcus aureus*, *Streptococcus pneumoniae* and *Haemophilus influenzae*. (*iii*) **Reye's syndrome** is a complication of influenza B, influenza A and chicken pox. Reye's syndrome is an acute encephalopathy of children and adolescents, usually between 2 and 16 years of age. Fatty degeneration of the liver is associated with the syndrome. Aspirin, used to lower virus-induced fever, contributes to the appearance of this syndrome. Therefore, acetaminophen is usually recommended for fevers of unknown origin in children.

LABORATORY DIAGNOSIS

Clinical characteristics of viral respiratory infections can be produced by many different viruses. Consequently, diagnosis of influenza relies on isolation of the virus, detection of viral antigens or viral nucleic acid in the patient's cells or a demonstration of specific antibodies in the patient's serum.

1. Demonstration of the Virus Antigen

Rapid diagnosis of influenza may be made by demonstration of the virus antigen on the surface of the nasopharyngeal cells by immunofluorescence. Detection of viral RNA by reverse transcriptase PCR is extremely sensitive.

2. Isolation of the Virus

Throat swabs, nasal washings or throat garglings are collected using suitable buffered salt solution. If the specimen is not processed immediately, it should be stored at 4°C, or if the delay is long, at –70°C. The specimen should be treated with antibiotics to destroy bacteria.

The specimen is inoculated into the amniotic cavity of 11–13 days old eggs, using atleast six eggs per specimen. After incubation at 35°C for three days, the eggs are chilled and the amniotic and allantoic fluids harvested separately. The fluids are tested for hemagglutination using guinea pig and fowl RBC in parallel, at room temperature and at 4°C. Some strains of the influenza virus type A agglutinate only guinea pig RBC on primary isolation. The type B virus agglutinates RBC of both, while type C strains aglutinate only fowl RBC at 4°C. If no hemagglutination occurs, a blind passage of the chick embryo homogenate into another set of eggs may sometimes lead to the recovery of the virus. The isolate is identified and typed by CFT with antisera to types A, B and C. Subtype identification is made by hemagglutination inhibition test.

Inoculation into primary monkey kidney cells or other suitable continuous cell lines derived from canine kidney (MDCK) or rhesus monkey kidney (LLC–MK) can be done. Inoculated cell cultures are incubated without serum, and in the presence of trypsin. Incubation at 33°C in roller drums is recommended. Virus growth can be identified by hemadsorption with human O group, fowl or guinea pig RBC. Rapid results can be obtained by demonstrating virus antigen in infected cell cultures by immunofluorescence.

3. Serology

Serological diagnosis of influenza is based upon demonstrating a four–fold or higher increase in antibody titre between acute–phase and convalescent phase sera. CFT and HI tests are employed. Human sera often contains nonspecific mucoprotein inhibitors that must be destroyed by treatment with RDE, trypsin or periodate before testing.

Epidemiology

The three types of influenza vary markedly in their epidemiologic patterns. Influenza C causes mild, sporadic respiratory disease and is least significant. Influenza B sometimes causes epidemics, but influenza type A can cause massive epidemics and pandemics.

The incidence of influenza peaks during the winter. Periodic outbreaks appear because of antigenic changes in one or both surface glycoproteins of the virus. All the three types of influenza virus exhibit antigenic drift. However, only influenza A undergoes antigenic shift, perhaps because types B and C are restricted to humans, whereas influenza A viruses are prevalent among animals and birds—ducks, chickens, turkeys, geese; pigs, horses etc. These animal strains are believed to account for antigenic shift, by genetic reassortment of the glycoprotein genes.

Influenza outbreaks occur in waves. Every 10–40 years, when a new subtype of influenza A appears, a pandemic results. This happened in 1918 (Spanish flu–H_1N_1), 1957 (Asian flu–H_2N_2) and 1968 (Hong Kong flu–H_3N_2). The H_1N_1 subtype reemerged in 1977 (Red flu or Russian flu) and has continued to cocirculate with H_3N_2 since then.

School-age children are the predominant vectors of influenza transmission. Crowding in schools favors the aerosol transmission of virus, and children take the virus home to the family.

PROPHYLAXIS

Influenza vaccines are in use and are recommended for the elderly and for people in high-risk groups, such as patients with chronic pulmonary or cardiac disease. The major difficulty in the immunoprophylaxis of influenza is the frequent change in the antigenic structure of the virus. Therefore, the circulating strains worldwide are monitored each season, and the following year's vaccine includes the principal strains recovered during the previous year-usually one type B influenza and two type A influenza strains. Such a trivalent vaccine has been used for the last two decades.

Selected virus strains are grown in embryonated eggs. Virus is harvested from the egg allantoic fluid, purified, concentrated by zonal centrifugation, and inactivated with formalin or betapropiolactone. The quantity of HA is standardized in each vaccine dose (approximately 15 mg of antigen), but the quantity of NA is not standardized, as it is more labile under purification and storage conditions. Each dose of vaccine contains the equivalent of about 10 billion virus particles. Currently available vaccines are either whole virus (WV), subvirion (SV), or surface antigen preparations. The WV vaccine contains intact, inactivated virus; the SV vaccine contains purified virus disrupted with detergents; the surface antigen vaccines contain purified HA and NA glycoproteins. Since vaccine strains are grown in eggs, some egg protein antigens are present in the vaccine and may induce allergic reaction in some individuals. Only surface antigen vaccines are recommended for children under 12 years of age to minimize febrile reactions. The immunity resulting from this inactivated viral vaccine is of short duration for 1–3 years against the homologous virus. The vaccine may produce mild side effects.

The inactivated vaccines do not provide complete protection and fail to induce local immunity, which is especially important in resistance to respiratory pathogens. A live attenuated vaccine has been prepared by using **temperature sensitive (ts) mutants**, which grow at 25°C, but not at 37°C, the temperature of the lower respiratory tract, which replicates in the nasopharynx, which has a cooler temperature (33°C). Live vaccines are administered by intranasally or by aerosol spray. They stimulate the production of local IgA antibodies.

Chemoprophylaxis with the antiviral drugs amantadine and rimantadine which block the viral M_2 protein that functions as an ion channel. These drugs act against type A virus and not against type B which lacks the M_2 protein.

TREATMENT

First generation antiviral agents—amantadine and rimantadine are effective against influenza A. Both drugs stop viral uncoating by inhibition of the viral M_2 membrane protein. These drugs reduce both the duration and the severity of flu symptoms, but only if given early in infection. Given before the onset of symptoms, these drugs can also prevent disease. But their use is limited because they are not effective against influenza B, emergence of drug resistance variants of the virus and neurologic adverse effects (especially for amantadine).

Second generation antiviral agents effective against influenza A and B include Zanamvir and Oseltamivir. They inhibit viral neuraminidase. Zanamvir must be taken by inhalation as nasal spray. Oseltamivir is taken orally.

QUESTIONS

Essay Questions:

1. What are the properties of orthomyxoviruses? Describe the pathogenesis and lab. diagnosis of influenza virus.

Short Notes:

1. Morphology of influenza virus
2. hemagglutinin
3. hemagglutination
4. hemagglutination inhibition or HI test
5. Neuraminidase or RDE
6. Elution
7. Differences between orthomyxo and paramyxoviruses
8. Pathogenesis of influenza virus
9. Reye's syndrome
10. Lab. diagnosis of influenza
11. Antigenic variations of influenza virus
12. Antigenic shift
13. Antigenic drift
14. P-Q-R variation
15. O-D variation
16. Influenza pandemics
17. Influenza vaccines

92

Paramyxoviruses

- *Introduction*
- *Classification*
- *Structure*
- *Parainfluenza viruses*
- *Mumps virus*
- *Measles (Rubeola) virus*
- *Respiratory syncytial virus (RSV)*

INTRODUCTION

The paramyxoviruses include the most important agents of respiratory infections of infants and young children (respiratory syncytial virus and the parainfluenza viruses) as well as the causative agents of two common contagious diseases of childhood (mumps, measles). All members of the paramyxoviridae family initiate infection via the respiratory tract. Replication of the respiratory pathogens is limited to the respiratory epithelia, whereas measles and mumps become disseminated throughout the body and produce generalized disease.

CLASSIFICATION

The **paramyxoviridae** family is divided into two subfamilies—The paramyxovirinae includes three genera : *Paramyxovirus* (parainfluenza virus types 1 and 3), *Rubulavirus* (**mumps virus**, parainfluenza viruses types 2, 4a, 4b) and *Morbilivirus* (measles virus). The second subfamily is pneumovirinae includes the genus *Pneumovirus* (**respiratory syncytial virus**) (Table 92.1). Most of the paramyxoviruses are antigenically stable and consists of a single serotype.

Table 92.1 Members of Family Paramyxoviridae

Subfamily	*Genus*	*Human species*
Paramyxovirinae	*Paramyxovirus*	Parainfluenza virus types 1 and 3.
	Rubulavirus	Parainfluenza virus types 2, 4a, 4b; Mumps virus
	Morbilivirus	Measles virus
Pneumovirinae	*Pneumovirus*	Respiratory syncytial virus (RSV)

STRUCTURE

Paramyxoviruses resemble orthomyxoviruses in morphology, but are larger, 150–300 nm in diameter and more pleomorphic, with filamentous forms ranging in size from 100 to 700 nm. Paramyxoviruses are spherical, enveloped particles that contain a nonsegmented, negative sense, linear, single stranded RNA genome. The helical nucleocapsid is wider than that of orthomyxoviruses, with a diameter of 18 nm. It is surrounded by a lipid envelope which has the matrix (M) protein at its base and two different transmembrane glycoprotein spikes (10 nm long) at the surface. The longer spike is the HN protein, which possesses both hemaglutinin (H) and neuraminidase (N) activity. It is involved in the binding of the virus to the host cell. Measles virus lacks the neuraminidase activity. The second spike is the F (fusion) protein, responsible for fusion of the viral envelope with plasma membrane (Fig. 92.1).

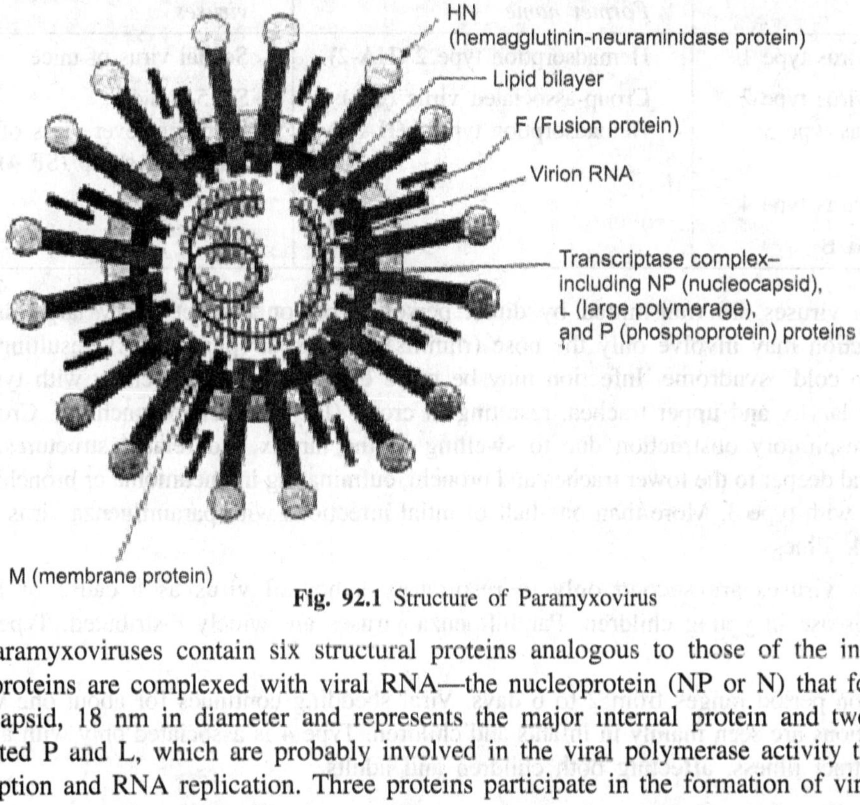

Fig. 92.1 Structure of Paramyxovirus

Paramyxoviruses contain six structural proteins analogous to those of the influenza viruses. Three proteins are complexed with viral RNA—the nucleoprotein (NP or N) that forms the helical nucleocapsid, 18 nm in diameter and represents the major internal protein and two large proteins designated P and L, which are probably involved in the viral polymerase activity that functions in transcription and RNA replication. Three proteins participate in the formation of viral envelope—A matrix (M) protein at its base and two different transmembrane glycoprotein spikes (10 nm long) at the surface. The longer spike is the HN protein, which possesses both hemagglutinin (H) and neuraminidase (N) activity. It is involved in the binding of the virus to the host cell. Measles virus lacks the neuraminidase activity. Hence, referred to as the H protein, rather than HN protein. The second spike is the F (fusion) protein, responsible for fusion of the viral envelope with plasma membrane of the host cells, facilitating virus entry into the cytoplasm where viral replication occurs. It also brings about cell-to-cell fusion, producing large giant cells or syncytia. The F protein also possesses hemolysin activity.

Paramyxoviruses replicate in the cytoplasm of the host cell and the virus matures by budding from the cell surface.

PARAINFLUENZA VIRUSES

The term "parainfluenza" was first coined because infected individuals may present with influenza-like symptoms and like influenza viruses, these viruses have both hemagglutinating and neuraminidase activities. Parainfluenza viruses are ubiquitous and cause common respiratory illnesses in persons of all ages. There are four serotypes of parainfluenza viruses.

Table 92.2 Parainfluenza Virus Types

Current name	Nomenclature of human types *Former name*	Related animal *viruses*
Parainfluenza virus type 1	Hemadsorption type 2 (HA-2)	Sendai virus of mice
Parainfluenza virus type 2	Croup-associated virus (CA)	SV 5 and 41
Parainfluenza virus type 3	Hemadsorption type 1 (HA 1)	Shipping fever virus of cattle and sheep (SF 4)
Parainfluenza virus type 4 Subtypes A and B		

Parainfluenza viruses are transmitted by direct person-to-person contact or by large droplet aerosols. The infection may involve only the nose (rhinitis) and throat (pharyngitis), resulting in a harmless "common cold" syndrome. Infection may be more extensive and, especially with types 1 and 2, involve the larynx and upper trachea, resulting in croup (laryngotracheobranchitis). Croup is characterized by respiratory obstruction due to swelling of the larynx and related structures. The infection may spread deeper to the lower trachea and bronchi, culminating in pneumonia or bronchiolitis or both, especially with type 3. More than one-half of intial infections with parainfluenza virus types 1–3 result in febrile illness.

Parainfluenza viruses are second only to respiratory syncytial virus as a cause of lower respiratory tract disease in young children. Parainfluenza viruses are widely distributed. Type 3 is most prevalent.

The incubation period ranges from 2 to 6 days. Viral shedding continues for about one week. Types 1 to 3 infections are seen mainly in infants and children. Type 4 is associated only with a mild upper respiratory tract illness, affecting both children and adults.

Laboratory diagnosis

Throat swabs, nasal swabs and nasal washes are inoculated into primary human or monkey kidney cell cultures or continuous monkey kidney cell lines (LLC-MK_2) with trypsin. Parainfluenza viruses grow slowly taking 10 days or more and produce very little cytopathic effect. To detect viral growth, hemadsorption using quinea pig RBC is performed. Isolates may be typed by immunofluorescence or hemadsorption inhibition of infected monolayers or by hemagglutination inhibition using virus from the cell culture media.

Viral antigens can be directly detected in exfoliated nasopharyngeal cells by immunofluorescence or ELISA.

Serodiagnosis is by neutralisation, HI, ELISA or CFT by demonstrating a four-fold rise in titer in paired sera.

Treatment and Prevention

Secretory IgA is very important in resistance to parainfluenza virus infections. Therefore, killed vaccines are not protective. An attenuated bovine parainfluenza virus type 3 vaccine is a candidate live-virus vaccine for humans.

The antiviral drug, ribavirin is effective when given by small-particle aerosol as in the treatment of respiratory syncytial virus infections.

MUMPS VIRUS

Mumps (**epidemic parotitis**) is an acute contagious disease commonly affecting children, characterised by nonsuppurative enlargement of one or both parotid glands.

Pathogenesis

Humans are the only natural hosts for mumps virus. The virus is spread by respiratory droplets through inhalation. The virus replicates in the upper respiratory tract and cervical lymph nodes and is disseminated through the blood stream to various organs. The incubation period typically about 18 days but may range from 7 to 25 days. More than one-third of all mumps infections are asymptomatic. The most characteristic feature of symptomatic cases is swelling of the salivary glands.

A prodromal period of malaise and anorexia is followed by rapid enlargement of parotid glands as well as other salivary glands. Gland enlargement is associated with pain and fever. Meningoencephalitis usually occurs 5–7 days after inflammation of the salivary glands, but it may occur simultaneously or in the absence of parotitis and is usually self-limited and resolve without sequelae, although unilateral deafness had been observed. Rare complications of mumps include : (1) self-limited polyarthritis (2) pancreatitis, usually mild, but may rarely severe (3) nephritis (4) thyroiditis, and (5) unilateral nerve deafness.

The testes and ovaries may be affected, especially after puberty. Twenty percent of males over age 13 years develop orchitis, often unilateral. The testes becomes swollen and acutely painful accompanied with fever and chills. It rarely results in sterility.

Mumps virus is antigenically stable and does not exhibit antigenic variation. Individuals who have had the disease develop lifelong immunity.

Laboratory Diagnosis

Typical mumps cases requires no laboratory confirmation but it may be essential with enlargement of the parotids due to suppuration, drug sensitivity, tumors and in meningitis without parotitis.

The virus may be isolated from the saliva within 4–5 days, urine upto two weeks and CSF 8–9 days after the onset of illness. Samples should be inoculated shortly after collection, as mumps virus is thermolabile. Monkey kidney cell cultures or human amnion or HeLa cell lines are used. Cytopathic effects consists of cell rounding and giant cell formation (syncytium). However, virus growth is detected by hemadsorption after two weeks of inoculation and confirmed as mumps virus by hemadsorption-inhibition using specific antiserum.

For rapid diagnosis, mumps virus antigens can be detected as early as 2–3 days after inoculation of cell cultures by immunofluorescence.

Virus isolation can also be made by inoculation into amniotic cavity of six to eight day old embryonated eggs and testing the amniotic fluid for hemagglutinins after 5–6 days. The virus can be identified by hemagglutination inhibition using specific antisera.

Serodiagnosis is based on the demonstration of a rise in titre of antibodies in paired serum samples. CFT and HI tests are used but crossreactions with parainfluenza viruses occur. Therefore, mumps IgM-ELISA is most useful. A positive CFT for antibody to the nucleocapsid protein (S antigen) in the acute phase sera is presumptive evidence of the current infection.

Epidemiology

Mumps occurs worldwide. Cases appear throughout the year. Outbreaks occur where crowding favors dissemination of the virus. The virus is transmitted by direct contact, airborne droplets or fomites contaminated with saliva or urine. Mumps is primarily an infection of children. The disease reaches its highest incidence in children aged 5–15 years. In children under five years of age, mumps may commonly cause upper respiratory tract infection without parotitis.

Prophylaxis

A live attenuated vaccine has been available for many years; this has resulted in a dramatic drop in the number of mumps cases. The Jeryl-Lynn strain of mumps virus attenuated by passage in eggs and grown in chick embryo fibroblast culture is used as the vaccine. The vaccine is recommended for children over one year age and for adolescents and adults who have not had mumps parotitis. It is contraindicated in pregnancy and in patients who are allergic to egg protein or neomycin. A single dose of the vaccine given subcutaneously.

Mumps vaccine is available in monovalent form (mumps only) or in combination with rubella and measles (**MMR**) live virus vaccines. It provides effective protection for atleast ten years.

The mumps immunoglobulin is of no value either for treatment or postexposure prophylaxis.

MEASLES (RUBEOLA) VIRUS

Measles is an acute, highly infectious disease characterized by a maculopapular rash, fever and respiratory symptoms. Complications are common and may be quite serious.

Pathogenesis

Measles virus is transmitted by sneeze-or cough-produced respiratory droplets. The virus is extremely infectious, and almost all infected individuals develop a clinical illness. The cellular receptor for measles virus is the CD46 molecule and the virus replicates initially in the respiratory epithelium and they spreads to various lymphoid tissues. This leads to primary viremia. It disseminates the virus, which then replicates in the reticuloendothelial system, followed by second viremia, which seeds the epithelial surfaces of the body, including the skin, respiratory tract, and conjunctiva, where focal replication occurs. Measles virus can replicate in certain lymphocytes, which aids in dissemination throughout the body. Multinucleated giant cells or **Syncytium** formation (Warthin-Finkeldy cells) with intranuclear inclusions are seen in lymphoid tissues throughout the body. These events occur during incubation period which typically lasts 9–11 days.

Measles is typically a seven to eleven day illness, with a prodromal phase of 2–4 days followed by an eruptive phase of 5–7 days. The prodromal phase is characterized by fever, sneezing, coughing, running nose, redness of the eyes, **Koplik's spots** (small white spots on bright red mucus membranes of the mouth and throat) and lymphopenia. The fever and cough persist until the rash appears and then subside within 1–2 days. The rash, which starts on the head and then spreads progressively to the chest, the trunk, and down the limbs, appears as light pink, discrete maculopapules that coalesce to form blotches, becoming brownish in 5–10 days. The fading rash resolves with desquamation.

Atypical measles is seen occasionally in young adults, who received killed measles virus vaccine during childhood, is characterized by high fever, pneumonitis, edema of the extremities and an unusual rash (raised papules, wheals and tiny hemorrhages in the skin) located predominantly on the extremities. Koplik's spots are absent. Atypical measles may be confused with Rocky mountain spotted fever.

Secondary bacterial infections are common in measles, particularly with betahemolytic streptococci. The most common complications are otitis media, sinusitis, bronchitis, broncheolitis, croup and bronchopneumonia. Giant cell pneumonia may occur in children with immunodeficiencies, which is usually fatal. Postinfectious encephalomyelitis occurs in about 1:1000 cases. It is an autoimmune disease associated with an immune response to myelin protein.

Subacute Sclerosing Panencephalitis (SSPE) is a rare, late complication of measles infection. The disease begins insidiously 5–15 years after a case of measles. It is characterized by progressive mental deterioration, involutntary movements, muscular rigidity and coma. It is invariably fatal. Patients with SSPE exhibit high titres of measles antibody in CSF and serum and defective measles virus in brown cells. With the widespread use of measles vaccine, SSPE has become less common.

Laboratory diagnosis

Typical measles can be diagnosed on clinical grounds. Laboratory diagnosis may be necessary in cases of atypical measles.

1. **Isolation of virus :** Nasopharyngeal swabs, blood, and urinary sediment may be inoculated on to Monkey kidney, primary human embryo kidney and human amnion cell lines. Measles virus grows slowly and takes 7–10 days. Cytopathic effect constitutes appearance of multinucleated giant cells containing both intranuclear and intracytoplasmic, eosinophilic inclusions. Hemadsorption or immunofluorescence can be used to confirm measles antigens in the inoculated cultures.
2. **Detection of antigen :** A simple diagnostic test, which can be used even before the rash appears, is the demonstration of multinucleated giant cells in Giemsa stained smears of nasal secretions. The measles virus antigen can be detected in these cells by immunofluorescence.
3. **Serology :** Demonstration of a rise in titer of antibody between acute and convalescent phase sera or demonstration of measles specific IgM antibody confirms measles infection. ELISA, HI, CFT and neutralisation tests may be used.

Prophylaxis

A highly effective, safe, attenuated live virus vaccine, which has been available for many years, has greatly reduced the incidence of the disease. The vaccine is given in two doses, in the form of **measles-mumps-rubella (MMR) vaccine**, the first at twelve to eighteen months, the second at four to twelve years. Contraindications are immunodeficiency, untreated tuberculosis and pregnancy.

The live attenuated vaccine was developed by passaging Edmonston-Zagreb strain of measles virus, successively through human kidney, amnion cell cultures, chick embryo amnion and finally chick embryo tissue culture. A disadvantage of the vaccine is that it does not induce adequate antibody response in young babies who possess maternal antibodies to measles.

A live attenuated vaccine has been developed which can be given by intranasal aerosol in young babies and gives good protection irrespective of the presence of maternal antibodies.

Treatment

Normal human gamma globulin can be given within six days of exposure in children with immunodeficiency, pregnant women and others at special risk to prevent or modify the disease.

There are no antiviral drugs effective against measles. Secondary bacterial infections can be prevented by antibiotics.

RESPIRATORY SYNCYTIAL VIRUS (RSV)

RSV is the most important cause of lower respiratory tract illness in infants and young children. RSV lacks both hemagglutinin and neuraminidase activities. The viral envelope has two glycoproteins—the G protein by which the virus attaches to host cells and the fusion (F) protein which brings about fusion between viral and host cell membranes and also the fusion of infected cells with adjoining cells resulting in the formation of large **multinucleated giant cells**, known as syncytium, from which the virus gets its name. Its nucleocapsid diameter (13 nm) is less than that of other paramyxoviruses (18 nm).

Pathogenesis

RSV is transmitted via large respiratory droplets by contact with contaminated hands or surfaces. Viral replication occurs initially in epithelial cells of the nasopharynx. Virus may spread to the lower respiratory tract. The incubation period between exposure and onset of illness is 4–5 days. Viral shedding occurs for one to three weeks.

Most RSV infections are symptomatic. The spectrum of respiratory illness ranges from febrile common cold in adults, through febrile broncheolitis with cough and wheezing in infants and older children and pneumonia in infants, to broncheolitis in very young babies. In 25–40% of cases, lower, respiratory tract is involved including broncheolitis and pneumonia. In about one percent, the illness is serious enough to require hospitalization. Most patients recover in 1–2 weeks but those with cardiac defects or immunodeficiency may have protracted illness and high death rates. RSV is an important cause of otitis media in children. A relation between RSV and the sudden death syndrome has been proposed but not proven. Reinfections are common in both children and adults.

Epidemiology

RSV is worldwide in distribution. It causes annual epidemics in the temperate regions during winter and in the tropics during rainy season. It may cause outbreaks of nosocomial infections in nurseries and pediatric hospital wards. Transmission occurs primarily through the hands of hospital staff. RSV infection is most common in children of six weeks to six months of age, with the peak at 2–3 months.

The virus is transmitted by close contact, and through contaminated fingers and fomites. Large droplets of respiratory secretions discharged during coughing and sneezing are more efficient in spreading the virus than fine aerosols.

Laboratory Diagnosis

RSV can be isolated from nasopharyngeal swabs or nasal secretions. The RSV is extremely labile, therefore freezing of the specimen may destroy the virus. Specimens are inoculated into HeLa or HEP-2 cell lines, immediately after collection. The formation of cytopathic effect i.e., multinucleated giant cells with syncytium may take about ten days. RSV does not have a hemagglutinin, therefore hemagglutination and hemadsorption assays cannot be used.

Definitive diagnosis can be made by detection of viral antigens by immunofluorescence on exfoliated cells or ELISA on nasopharyngeal secretions.

Antibodies to RSV can be demonstrated in acute phase sera by immunofluorescence, ELISA, CFT and neutralisation tests.

Porphylaxis

No effective vaccine is available. Prevention consists of practising general hygienic measures.

Treatment

Treatment of RSV infections is primarily by supportive care. Administration of antiviral drug, ribavirin by continuous aerosol has been found beneficial in hospitalized patients, decreasing the duration of the illness and of virus shedding. Administration of immune globulin against RSV may be beneficial.

QUESTIONS

Essay Question:

1. Classify Paramyxoviruses. Describe the structure, pathogenicity, Lab. diagnosis and prophylaxis of measles virus.

Short Notes:

1. Mumps (or) epidemic parotitis (or) mumps virus
2. MMR vaccine
3. Parainfluenza viruses
4. RSV (or) Respiratory syncytial virus
5. Measles or Rubeola or Measles virus
6. SSPE
7. Atypical measles.

93

Rubella Virus

INTRODUCTION

Rubella, also known as **German measles** or 3-day measles is an acute febrile illness characterised by a generalized maculopapular rash and posterior auricular and suboccipital lymphadenopathy that affects children and young adults. It is the mildest, and in most cases, these symptoms may be hardly noticeable, and the infection remains subclinical. The clinical significance of rubella lies not in the primary infection described above, but rather in the fact that when a woman is infected during pregnancy especially in first trimester, there can be severe damage to the developing fetus, including congenital malformations and mental retardation, referred to as **congenital rubella syndrome**.

CLASSIFICATION

Rubella virus, a member of the **Togaviridae** family, is the sole member of the ***Rubivirus*** genus. Although its morphologic features and physicochemical properties place it in the togavirus group, rubella is not transmitted by arthropods, and therefore it is not an arbovirus.

MORPHOLOGY AND PROPERTIES

Rubella virus is pleomorphic, roughly spherical particle, 50–70 nm in diameter, with single stranded RNA genome. It is an enveloped virus. The envelope is composed of lipoprotein and carries hemaglutinin peplomers (Fig. 93.1). It agglutinates goose, pigeon, day-old chick and human RBC at 4°C. Only one serotype is identified.

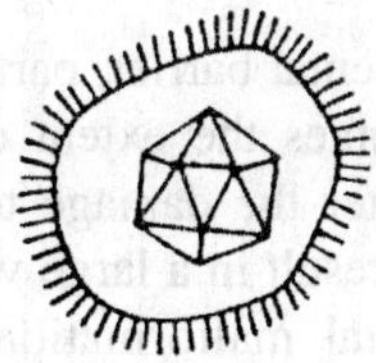

Fig. 93.1 Rubella virus

The virus is inactivated by ether, chloroform, formaldehyde, betapropıolactone and desoxycholate. It can be destroyed by heating at 56°C, but survives for several years at –60°C.

CULTIVATION

The virus can be grown in many primary cell cultures and continuous cell lines, such as rabbit kidney (RK13), baby hamster kidney (BHK 21) and vero, but cytopathic changes develop only in a few cell lines such as RK13. In others, virus growth can be identified by **interference**, using a challenge virus such as ECHO 11.

Experimental infection can be produced in human volunteers and monkeys. A suitable experimental model for the teratogenic effects of rubella is the pregnant rabbit, in which the virus infects the fetus transplacentally, leading to congenital malformations.

PATHOGENICITY

Rubella virus causes postnatal and congenital infections.

Postnatal Rubella

The diesease is transmitted via direct or droplet contact with respiratory secretions. The rubella virus is shed in oropharyngeal secretions and the infection is acquired by inhalation. Initial viral replication occurs in the respiratory tract, followed by multiplication in the cervical lymph nodes, followed by viremic spread to target organs. Rubella begins with malaise and low-grade fever. After an incubation period of 2–3 weeks, patient develops fine, pink, discrete macules of the erythematous rash, which appear first on the face, extends over the trunk and extremities. Posterior auricular and suboccipital lymphadenopathy are present. The illness is of short duration and complete recovery occurs within 3–4 days after appearance of the rash. After the rash appears, the virus remains detectable only in the nasopharynx, where it may persist for several weeks. In about 25% of cases, primary infection is subclinical.

Transient arthralgia and arthritis are commonly seen in women. Rare complications include thrombocytopenic purpura and encephalitis.

Unless an epidemic occurs, the disease is difficult to diagnose clinically, since the rash caused by other viruses is similar.

One attack of the disease confers lifelong immunity, as only one antigenic type of the virus exists. The initial antibody is of IgM type, which do not persist beyond six months. IgG antibodies usually persist for life.

Congenital Rubella Syndrome

Rubella virus can cross the placental barrier, particularly in early pregnancy and infect the fetus. Timing of the fetal infection determines the extent of teratogenic effect. In general, the earlier in pregnancy infection occurs, the greater the damage to the fetus. Infection during the first trimester of pregnancy is most critical. It may result in a large variety of congenital abnormalities or fetal death and spontaneous abortion. Congenital malformations may include deafness, cataract, glaucoma, microphthalmia or retinitis leading to blindness, congenital heart disease especially patent ductus arteriosus, sometimes accompanied by septal defects and pulmonary artery stenosis, microcephaly with mental retardation, thrombocytopenic purpura and hepatosplenomegaly. Birth defects are uncommon if maternal infection occurs after fourth month of pregnancy.

Table 93.1 Common Malformations Associated with Congenital Rubella Syndrome

Type of defect	*Examples*
Ocular defects	Cataracts Microphthalmia Glaucoma Retinitis
Heart defects	Patent ductus arteriosus peripheral pulmonary artery stenosis
Hearing impairment	Cochlear deafness Central auditory imperception
CNS impairment	Mental retardation Encephalitis Psychomotor retardation
Other defects	Intrauterine growth retardation Hepatosplenomegaly Hematologic abnormalities (thrombocytopenia, hemolytic anemia) Hepatitis Pneumonitis

EPIDEMIOLOGY

Rubella is worldwide in distribution. Infection is transmitted by the respiratory route. Congenitally infected infants who shed virus can transmit rubella to susceptible contacts, such as the nurses and physicians caring for them.

LABORATORY DIAGNOSIS

1. Isolation of Virus

Specimens such as nasopharyngeal or throat swabs taken within 3–4 days after symptoms appear and from the throat, urine, CSF or leucocytes of a new-born infant with congenital rubella syndrome can be inoculated on to various tissue culture cell lines on monkey (vero, BSC-1) or rabbit (RK-13, SIRC) origin, or primary African green monkey kidney cultures. Viral growth is identified by interference in primary monkey kidney cells with coxsackievirus A9 or ECHO 11 as challenge virus. Absolute identification of the isolate is by neutralization with referene rubella antibody.

2. Serology

The HI test is the standard serologic test for rubella. However, serum must be pretreated to remove nonspecific inhibitors before testing. ELISA tests are advantageous in that serum pretreatment is not required and they can be adapted to detect specific IgM.

To accurately confirm a recent rubella infection, which is critically important in the case of a pregnant woman, either a rise in antibody titer must be demonstrated between two serum samples taken atleast 10 days apart or rubella-specific IgM must be detected in a single specimen.

PROPHYLAXIS

Live attenuated rubella vaccines are available. The original one HPV77 was prepared in duck embryo cells, it was replaced in 1979 by a second vaccine, RA 27/3, grown in human diploid cells. It produces much higher antibody titers and a more enduring and solid immunity (that lasts for atleast 10 years) than does HPV77, and it is highly effective in preventing subclinical superinfection with wild virus. It may also produce IgA antibody in the respiratory tract and thus interfere with infection by wild virus. This vaccine is given as a single antigen or in combination with measles and mumps vaccines as the **MMR vaccine**. The vaccine virus multiplies in the body and is shed in small amounts, but it does not spread to contacts. Vaccinated children pose no threat to mothers who are susceptible and pregnant. In contrast, nonimmunized children can bring home wild virus and spread it to susceptible family contacts.

The vaccine is safe and causes few side effects in children. There may be mild fever, lymphadenopathy, and a fleeting rash but no permanent residual effects. In adults, the only significant side effect is arthralgia.

Rubella vaccine virus can cross the placenta and infect the fetus. However, it is not teratogenic. Inadvertent administration of the vaccine to a pregnant women may not therefore lead to congenital malformations in the baby.

TREATMENT

Rubella is a mild, self-limited illness, and no specific treatment is given. Laboratory-proved rubella in the first trimester of pregnancy is associated with fetal infection; therapeutic abortion is the only means of avoiding the risk of malformed infants in such cases.

QUESTIONS

Short Notes:

1. Rubella or German measles.
2. Congenital rubella.
3. Rubella vaccine.
4. MMR vaccine.
5. Properties of rubella virus.
6. Pathogenicity of rubella (or) rubella infections.
7. Lab. diagnosis of rubella infections.

94

Coronaviruses

- *Introduction*
- *Structure*
- *Pathogenesis*
- *Epidemiology*
- *Laboratory diagnosis*
- *Treatment and Control*

INTRODUCTION

The family **coronaviridae** comprises two genera *Coronavirus* and *Torovirus*. The toroviruses are widespread in ungulates and appear to be associated with diarrheas. There are two antigenic groups of human coronaviruses, represented by strains 229E and OC43. There is a third distinct antigenic group containing avian infectious bronchitis virus of chickens.

STRUCTURE

Coronaviruses are large, 80–220nm in diameter, spherical and enveloped RNA viruses. The genome contains single stranded, positive sense, unsegmented RNA. It is the largest genome (20–30 kb) among RNA viruses. Isolated genomic RNA is infectious. The helical nucleocapsid is 9-11 nm in diameter. The envelope contains large, widely spaced, club or petal shaped spikes or projections that are 20 nm long. These projections have the appearance of a solar corona, hence the name of the virus (Fig. 94.1) The viral structural proteins include phosphorylated nucleocapsid (N) protein, a membrane (M) glycoprotein that serves as a matrix protein embedded in the envelope lipid bilayer and interacting with the nucleocapsid, and the spike glycoprotein that makes up the petal-shaped peplomers. Some viruses, including human coronavirus OC43, contain a third glycoprotein that causes hemagglutination and has acetylesterase activity.

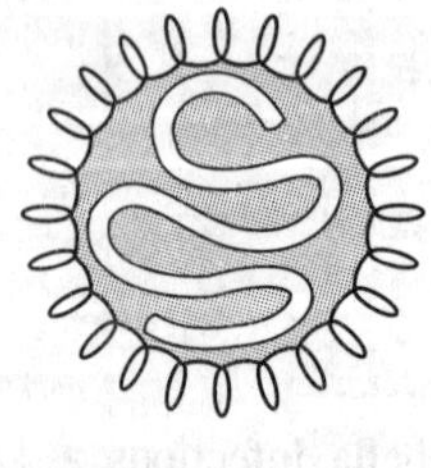

Fig. 94.1 Coronavirus

Human coronaviruses do not grow well in cell cultures. The replication takes place in the cytoplasm of the host cell. Coronaviruses exhibit a high frequency of mutation and RNA recombination during replication, which contributes to the evolution of new virus strains.

PATHOGENESIS

Animal coronaviruses display a tropism for epithelial cells of the respiratory or gastrointestinal tract. Coronavirus infection of tracheal organ cultures *in vitro* results in a slow, patchy destruction of ciliated epithelial cells and the loss of beating cilia. This destructive effect may be related to disease development in vivo.

1. Respiratory Disease

The human coronaviruses produce 'colds', usually afebrile, in adults. The symptoms are similar to those produced by rhinoviruses, typified by nasal discharge and malaise. The incubation period is from 2–5 days, and symptoms usually last about one week. The lower respiratory tract is usually not involved, although pneumonia in military recruits has been attributed to coronavirus infection. Asthmatic children may suffer wheezing attacks, and chronic pulmonary disease in adults may exacerbate respiratory symptoms.

2. Gastrointestinal Disease

Several animal cornaviruses are known that cause acute gastrointestinal infections. Coronavirus like particles have been observed by electron microscopy in feces from both normal persons and patients with enteritis.

3. Neurologic Disease

Some animal coronaviruses cause nervous system disease in animals.

4. Severe Acute Respiratory Syndrome (SARS)

An outbreak of SARS occured in 2003 in china and Hong Kong. A mutant strain of coronavirus of animal origin (cats) has been proved to be causative agent.

EPIDEMIOLOGY

Coronaviruses are found worldwide. They are a second major cause of respiratory illness during some winter months, next only to rhinoviruses. It is estimated that coronaviruses cause 15–30% of all colds.

LABORATORY DIAGNOSIS

1. Isolation of Virus

Human coronaviruses can be cultured in organ cultures of human embryonic trachea.

2. Detection of Antigen

Coronavirus antigens in cells in respiratory secretions or nasopharyngeal aspirates may be detected using the ELISA test. Enteric coronaviruses can be detected by examination of stool samples by electron microscopy. PCR is useful in detecting coronavirus nucleic acid in respiratory secretions and stool samples.

3. Serology

Because of the difficulty of virus isolation, serodiagnosis using acute and convalescent sera is the only practical means of confirming coronavirus infections. CFT, ELISA and hemagglutination tests may be used. Serologic diagriosis of infections with strain 229E is possible using a passive hemagglutination test in which RBC coated with coronavirus antigen are agglutinated by antibody continaing sera.

TREATMENT AND CONTROL

Treatment of common colds is symptomatic. No vaccine or specific drugs are available. Hygienic measures reduce the rate of transmission.

QUESTIONS

Short Notes:

1. Coronaviruses
2. Structure, pathogenicity and lab diagnosis of coronaviruses.

95

Rhabdoviruses

- *Introduction*
- *Structure*
- *Resistance*
- *Replication*
- *Antigenic properties*
- *Cultivation*
- *Pathogenesis*
- *Laboratory diagnosis*
- *Prophylaxis*
- *Epidemiology*
- *Treatment*
- *Vesiculovirus*

INTRODUCTION

The rhabdoviruses are enveloped, bullet shaped viruses containing helical nucleocapsid and are placed in the family **rhabdoviridae** (rhabdos = rod). The Rhabdoviridae members known to infect mammals are divided into two genera : *Lyssavirus* containing rabies virus and *vesiculovirus* containing vesicular stomatitis virus (VSV), a virus of horses and cattle. Other rhabdoviruses infect invertebrates, plants or other vertebrates.

The name ***Lyssavirus*** is derived from *lyssa* meaning rage, a synonym for rabies. Rabies is an acute infection of the central nervous system that is almost always fatal. Rabies is a major public health problem because it is widespread among animal reservoirs, and is transmitted to humans from the bite of a rabid animal.

STRUCTURE

The rhabdoviruses are rod or bullet shaped particles measuring 180×75 nm with one end rounded or conical and the other planar or concave. The particles are surrounded by a lipoprotein envelope with protruding spikes. The spikes (peplomers) are composed of trimers of the viral glycoprotein (G). The spikes may not be present on the planar or concave end of the virion. Beneath the envelope, there is a membrane or matrix (M) protein layer which may be invaginated at the planar end. The membrane may project outwards from the planar end of some virions forming a bleb. Inside the envelope, the core consists of ribonucleocapsid with helical symmetry. The genome is single-stranded, negative sense RNA, that is not infectious. Virions contain an RNA-dependent RNA polymerase (Fig. 95.1).

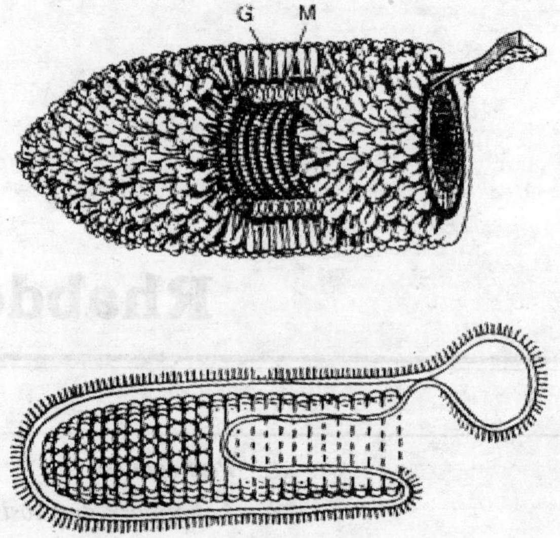

Fig. 95.1 *a, b* Rabies virus G– glycoprotein. spikes, M– Matrix protein

RESISTANCE

Rabies virus is killed rapidly by exposure to UV radiation or sunlight, by heat (one hour at 50° C and five minutes at 60°C), by lipid solvents (ether, 0.1% sodium deoxycholate), by trypsin, by detergents and by extremes of pH. Rabies virus survives storage at 4°C for weeks but is inactivated by CO_2. On dry ice, therefore, it must be stored in glass-sealed vials. The virus is also sensitive to ethanol, iodine, quaternary ammonium compounds, and soaps. It can be preserved at –70°C or by lyophilisation.

REPLICATION

Rabies virus attaches to cells via glycoprotein spikes; the **nicotinic acetyl choline receptor** may serve as a cellular receptor for rabies virus. The ssRNA genome is transcribed by the virion-associated RNA polymerase. The replication and assembly of virions takes place in the cytoplasm of the host cell. The particles acquire an envelope by budding through the plasma membrane.

ANTIGENIC PROPERTIES

There is a single serotype for rabies virus. However, there are strain differences. The surface glycoprotein (G) spikes are important in pathogenesis, virulence and immunity. It is induces neutralising (protective) and hemagglutination-inhibiting (HI) antibodies and stimulates cell mediated immunity. The purified glycoprotein may therefore provide a safe and effective **subunit vaccine**. Rabies virus produces hemagglutination due to glycoprotein spikes, optimally seen with goose RBC at 0–4°C and pH 6.2. HI antibodies develop following infection or immunisation.

The nucleocapsid protein induces complement fixing antibodies, which are not protective. Antiserum prepared against the nucleocapsid antigen is used in diagnostic immunofluorescence tests.

CULTIVATION

1. Animals

All mammals are susceptible to rabies infection. Cattle, cats and foxes are highly susceptible, whereas skunks, opossums and fowl are relatively resistant. Humans and dogs occupy an intermediate position. Pups are more susceptible than adult dogs. Mice are the animals of choice for experimental infection or primary isolation. After intracerebral inoculation, they develop encephalitis and die within 5–30 days.

The freshly isolated rabies virus from natural human or animal infection is termed the ***Street virus***. Following inoculation by any route, it can cause fatal encephalitis in laboratory animals after a long and variable incubation period of about 1–12 weeks. Intracytoplasmic inclusion bodies (**Negri bodies**) can be demonstrated in the brain of animals dying of street virus infection. After several serial intracerebral passages in rabbits, the virus undergoes certain changes and is termed the **"fixed virus"**. The fixed virus is more neurotropic, though it is much less infective by other routes. After intracerebral inoculation, it produces fatal encephalitis after a short and fixed incubation period of 6–7 days. Negri bodies are not demonstrable in the brain of animals dying of fixed virus infection. The fixed virus is used for vaccine production.

2. Chick embryos

Rabies virus can be grown in the yolk sac of chick embryos. Serial passage in chick embryos has led to the development of attenuated vaccine strains like Flury and Kelev. Strains adapted to duck eggs which give high yields of virus have been used for preparation of inactivated vaccines.

3. Tissue culture

The rabies virus can be grown in several primary and continuous cell cultures such as chick embryo fibroblast, baby hamster kidney, mouse neuroblastoma but cytopathic effects are not apparent. The fixed virus strains adapted for growth in human diploid lung fibroblasts, vero monkey kidney cells and chick embryo fibroblast cell cultures are used for the production of rabies vaccines.

PATHOGENESIS

Rabies is primarily a disease of animals and is spread to humans by bites of rabid animals. The virus present in the saliva of the animal is deposited in the wound. Infection can also occur rarely by nonbite exposures such as contamination of an open wound or a mucus membrane via scratches, licks due to contact with saliva of a rabid animal or inhalation of aerosol. The virus multiplies in muscle or connective tissue at the site of inoculation and then enters peripheral nerves at neuromuscular junctions and spreads in the axoplasm towards the central nervous system. The movement of the virus in the axons is passive, at a speed of about 3 mm per hour. The virus multiplies in the brain and may then spread through peripheral nerves to the salivary glands and other tissues. The organ with the highest titres of virus is the submaxillary salvary gland. The virus replicates in the salivary glands and is shed in the saliva. The presence of virus in the saliva and the irritability and aggression brought on by encephalitis ensure the transmission and survival of the virus in nature. Other organs where rabies virus has been found include pancreas, kidney, heart, retina and cornea. The virus is almost invariably present in the cornea and facial skin of patients because of their proximity to the brain, which provides a method for antemortem diagnosis of human rabies. Rabies virus has not been isolated from the blood of infected persons.

Rabies virus produces a specific eosinophilic, intracytoplasmic inclusions, the Negri body, in infected nerve cells. Negri bodies are filled with viral nucleocapsids.

The Rabies disease is an acute, fulminant, fatal encephalitis. Five stages of rabies are recognized in humans: incubation, prodrome, acute neurologic period, coma and death (or rarely recovery).

The incubation period in humans is typically 1–2 months but may be as short as one week or as long as several years (perhaps 6 years or more). It is usually shorter in children and in individuals bitten close to the central nervous system (*e.g.*, the face).

The **prodromal phase**, which lasts from 2 to 10 days, may show nonspecific symptoms such as malaise, anorexia, headache, photophobia, nausea and vomitting, sore throat, and fever. Usually there is an abnormal sensation around the site of infection.

The **acute neurologic phase** begins with signs of CNS dysfunction such as nervousness, apprehension, and hallucinations. General sympathetic overactivity is observed, including larcrimation, pupillary dilatation, and increased salivation and perspiration. Patients exhibit **hydrophobia** (fear of water), since the act of swallowing causes a painful spasm of the throat muscles. The disease is classified as **furious rabies** if hyperactivity (*i.e.* hydrophobia) predominates and as **dumb rabies** if paralysis dominates the clinical picture.

At the end of acute neurologic phase, periods of rapid, irregular breathing begin. Paralysis and the coma phase follow. Death occurs due to respiratory arrest or other complications. Recovery and survival is extremely rare.

LABORATORY DIAGNOSIS

Clinical diagnosis rests on a history of exposure and signs and symptoms charactertic of rabies. Laboratory diagnosis of rabies consists of the following:

1. Demonstration of Negri Bodies

Postmortem, in approximately eighty percent of cases, characteristic Negri bodies may be identified in certain regions of the brain such as hippocampus and spinal chord, which constitutes a definitive diagnosis of rabies. Histologic sections or impression smears of the brain stained by Seller's technique may reveal oval or spherical, 2–10μ in diameter, intracytoplasmic, eosinophilic inclusions with basophilic inner granules, known as Negri bodies.

2. Demonstration of Rabies Antigens

Prior to death (antemortem), the diagnosis can be made by identification of rabies antigens in corneal smears, biopsies of the skin from face or neck or saliva most accurately and rapidly by means of immunofluorescence or immunoperoxidase staining using antirabies monoclonal antibodies. Postmortem, brain smears are used for the detection of rabies antigen.

3. Detection of Nucleic Acids

Reverse transcription-polymerase chain reaction (RT-PCR) can be used to amplify parts of a rabies virus genome from fixed or unflixed brain tissue on postmortem. Sequencing amplified products allows identification of the infecting virus strain. Antemortem, viral RNA can be detected by PCR, dot-blot hybridization assay with cDNA probes on corneal impression smears, saliva or skin biopsy.

4. Virus Isolation

The specimen either brain on postmortem or saliva on antemortem is inoculated intracerebrally into suckling mice. Infection in mice results in flaccid paralysis of legs, encephalitis, and death. The CNS of the inoculated animal is examined for negri bodies and rabies antigen.

For rapid growth (2–4 days) of rabies virus, baby hamster kidney, mouse neuroblastoma, human diploid lung fibroblasts, chick embryo fibroblasts and vero monkey kidney cells may be used. An isolated virus is identified by fluorescent antibody tests with specific antiserum, since no cytopathic effect is observed.

5. Serology

Serum antibodies to rabies can be detected by IF, CFT or neutralization tests. Such antibodies may develop in infected persons or animals during progression of the disease. Antibodies in CSF are produced in rabies infected persons but not in response to vaccination.

PROPHYLAXIS

I. Preexposure Prophylaxis

It is indicated for persons at high risk of contact with rabies virus such as veterinarians, laboratory workers, animal handlers, wildlife workers and travelers to certain foreign areas where rabies is endemic. Three doses of vaccine, 1.0 ml is injected intramuscularly on days 0, 7 and 28 or 0, 28 and 56. A booster dose is recommended after one year and then one every five years.

II. Postexposure Prophylaxis

Once an individual has clinical symptoms of rabies, there is no effective treatment. Therefore postexposure treatment be initiated promptly.

1. Animal bites deposit the virus in wounds

All bites should be thoroughly cleaned with soap and water. After washing the soap away completely, the wound is treated with quaternary ammonium compounds such as cetavlon or tincture of iodine or alcohol (40 to 70 per cent). This is a very important step in the prevention of rabies as soap and quaternary ammonium compounds or iodine destroys the virus effectively. Antitetanus measures and antibiotics may be used to prevent sepsis.

2. Passive immunization

The action of passively administered antibody is to neutralize some of the inoculated virus and lower the concentration of virus in the body by depression of viral replication. It may provide additional time for a vaccine to stimulate active antibody production to prevent entry into the CNS.

Human rabies immunoglobulin (HRIG) 20 IU/Kg body weight or equine rabies immunoglobulin (ERIG) 40 IU/Kg body weight, half the volume injected in the gluteal region and the other half infiltrated at the site of wound. Passive immunization should be given before or simultaneously with the first injection of the vaccine, but not after it.

3. Rabies Vaccines (Active immunization)

Rabies is the only human disease that can be prevented by active immunization after infection, because a long incubation period of the disease allows time for immunity to develop before the onset of symptoms. Rabies vaccines fall into two categories: neural and nonneural.

Neural Vaccines

These vaccines are made from infected sheep, goat or mouse brains, in which virus was inactivated with phenol (at 22°C–**Fermivaccine** or at 37°C–**Semple vaccine**) or betapropiolactone (**BPL Vaccine**). Fermi vaccine contains residual virus, hence not used. The dose schedule of neural vaccines require repeated and painful injections and their potency is low. Moreover, it causes sensitization to nervous tissue leading to neuroparalytic complications.

Infant brain vaccines have been developed to reduce neurological complications, as infant brain does not contain myelin (encephalitogenic factor). Vaccine prepared from suckling mice brain inactivated with UV irradiation, BPL or phenol was widely used in Latin America. Similar vaccines prepared from infant rat brain were used in Russia and from suckling rabbit brain in Netherlands.

NonNeural Vaccines

1. Duck Embryo Vaccine

The fixed rabies virus is grown in embryonated duck eggs and inactivated with betapropiolactone. This vaccine was developed to minimize the problem of postvaccinal encephalitis. But it was discontinued because of´its poor immuogenicity.

2. Human Diploid Cell Vaccine (HDCV)

A fixed rabies virus (Pitman-Moore strain) grown on human diploid cells (WI 38 or MRC5). The virus preparation is concentrated by ultrafiltration and inactivated with betapropiolactone or tri-n-butyl phosphate. It is strongly antigenic and free from nervous tissue and foreign proteins and therefore no serious side effects. Only five doses need by given intramuscularly in the deltoid region in 1.0 ml volumes on days 0, 3, 7, 14, 30 and 90 after exposure. Its only disadvantage is its high cost.

Purified chick embryo cell vaccine (PCEC) and purified vero cell (PVC) vaccines are equally safe and effective and more economical have been developed.

3. Live attenuated Vaccine

Live attenuated viruses adapted to growth in chick embryos (*e.g.* Flury strain) are used for animals but not for humans. Two types of vaccines were developed—the low egg passage (LEP) vaccine at 40–50 egg passage level for immunisation of dogs and the high egg passage (HEP) vaccine at 180 level for cattle and cats. These are not in use now.

4. Recombinant Vaccine

An experimental recombinant viral vaccine consisting of vaccinia virus carrying the rabies susface glycoprotein gene (V-RG) has successfully immunized animals following oral administration. This vaccine may prove valuable in the immunization of both wildlife reservoir species and domestic animals.

EPIDEMIOLOGY

Rabies exists in two epizootic forms Urban (dogs and cats) and sylvatic (wildlife such as jackals, wolves, foxes, mangooses, skunks, and bats). Most cases of human rabies follow dog bites but in endemic areas any animal can transmit the disease. Rabies is worldwide in distribution. A wide variety of wildlife, such as raccoons, skunks, squirrels, foxes and bats provide a reservoir for the rabies virus. Domestic dogs and cats also constitute an important reservoir for rabies virus. Bats present a special problem because they may carry rabies virus while they appear to be healthy, excrete in saliva, and transmit it to other animals, including other bats, and to humans. South American vampire bats may transmit rabies to insectivorous bats living in caves. The latter, in turn may transmit rabies to fruit-eating bats that visit such caves and migrate elsewhere. Bat caves may contain aerosols of rabies virus. Migrating fruit-eating bats are a source of infection for many animals and humans. Bat rabies is largely confined to USA and Canada.

Human to human rabies infection is very vare. Corneal transplants of donors who died with rabies or undiagnosed CNS disease may transmit the infection to recipients.

TREATMENT

There is no successful treatment for rabies. Symptomatic treatment may prolong life, but the outcome is almost always fatal. Prevention of initial exposure is the most important mechanism for controlling human rabies.

VESICULOVIRUS

The viruses of the genus *Vesiculovirus* cause fever, vesicles on the tongue, gums and lips, and exessive salivation in horses, cattle and pigs. Teats of cows may be infected and less commonly lesions may be seen on feet. One of the 35 serotypes of this genus may cause human infection. Man acquires infection by direct contact with vesicle fluid from teat lesions, particularly in milkers and in laboratory workers by aerosol inhalation. After an incubation period of 1–9 days patient develops influenza-like illness, presenting with an acute onset of fever, chills and muscle pain. Symptoms may last for 7–10 days. Diagnosis can be established retrospectively by serological methods.

QUESTIONS

Essay Questions:

1. Describe the general characteristics of rhabdoviridae. Write briefly on the prophylaxis of rabies.
2. Describe the pathogenesis and lab. diagnosis of rabies.
3. Mention the features and classification of rhabdoviruses and discuss the prophylactic measures against rabies.
4. Describe the morphology, pathogenesis, laboratory diagnosis and prophylaxis of rabies.

Short Notes:

1. Morphology of rabies virus.
2. Street virus.
3. Fixed virus.
4. Pathogenesis of rabies.
5. Laboratory diagnosis of rabies.
6. Negri bodies.
7. Prophylaxis against rabies (or) Rabies vaccines for human use.
8. HDCS vaccine.
9. Subunit vaccine.
10. Draw a neat leabelled diagram of rabies virus.
11. Neural vaccines against rabies.
12. Nonneural vaccines used against rabies.
13. Differnces between street virus and fixed virus.

96

Tumor (Oncogenic) Viruses

- *Introduction*
- *Types of tumor viruses*
- *Interactions of tumor viruses with host cells*
- *Oncogenes*
- *Tumor suppressor genes (Antioncognes)*
- *Mechanism of viral oncogenesis*

INTRODUCTION

Viruses that produce tumors in their natural hosts or in experimental animals, or induce malignant transformation of cells on culture, are known as oncogenic viruses. Cellular transformation (**carcinogenesis**) is a multistep process and may be partial or complete, and several genetic changes must occur to convert a normal cell into a malignant one. Intermediate stages have been identified in various systems and designated using terms such as "**immortalization**", "**hyperplasia**" and "proneoplastic."

Cellular **transformation** may be defined as a stable, heritable change in the growth control of cells in culture. The most prominent changes associated with transformed cells include:

1. Alterations in Cell Growth Patterns

Increased growth rate, Growth to higher cell density, decreased requirement for serum growth factors, decreased cell adhesion to a substrate, enhanced ability to grow in semisolid medium and loss of "contact inhibition" which means the transformed cells are no longer inhibited by contact with other cells, as normal cells are, but tend to pile up to form a "focus". Induction of foci provides the basis for quantitative assay for certain tumor viruses.

2. Alterations in Cell Surface

Increased rate of transport of cell nutrients, increased secretion of proteases or protease activators, increased agglutinability by plant lectins, and changes in composition of glycoproteins and glycolipids, sometimes including the presence of virus-encoded proteins.

3. Alterations in Intracellular Components and Biochemical Processes

Increased metabolic rate, inceased glycolysis, altered levels of cyclic nucleotides, activation or repression of certain cellular genes, presence of viral DNA, mRNA and viral coded proteins, and changes in cell cytoskeleton, often resulting in a more rounded cell shape.

4. Tumorigenicity

Production of tumors when transformed cells are injected into appropriate test animals, especially immunologically deficient animals.

TYPES OF TUMOR (ONCOGENIC) VIRUSES

All known tumor viruses either have a DNA genome or generate a DNA provirus after infection of cells. DNA tumor viruses are classified among the papova-, adeno-, herpes-, hepadna- and poxvirus groups.

All **RNA tumor viruses** belong to the retroviridae family. (Fig. 96.1) Retroviruses carry an RNA-directed polymerase (**revese transcriptase**) that constructs a DNA copy (provirus) of the RNA genome of the virus. The DNA provirus becomes integrated into the DNA of the infected host cell and it is from this integrated DNA copy that all proteins of the virus are translated. Among widely studied RNA tumor viruses are those causing avian sarcomas, avian leukoses, mouse leukemias, mouse sarcomas, mouse mammary tumors, feline leukemias, and human T cell leukemia.

Table 96.1 Viruses Associated with Animal Cancers

Virus family	*Virus*	*Associated tumors*
DNA Visuses		
Papovaviridae	Bovine papilloma virus	Dermal and oesophageal Papillomas, and squamous cell carcinoma
	Polyomavirus of rodents	Mouse adenocarcinomas, fibrosarcomas
	Simian virus 40	Sarcoma (rodents)
Herpesviridae	Frog herpesvirus	Renal adenocarcinoma
	Marek's disease virus	Neurolymphomatosis (fowl)
Hepadnaviridae	Woodchuck hepatitis virus	Hepatocellular carcinoma (woodchuck)
Poxviridae	Shope fibroma virus	Fibroma (rabbit)
	Yaba virus	Nodular fibromatous hyperplasia (monkey)
Adenoviridae	Adenovirus types 2, 5, 12	Fibrosarcomas (hamster).
RNA viruses	Mouse mammary tumor virus	Mammary adenocarcinomas,
Retroviridae	Avian leukosis virus	T cell lymphoma
	Rous Sarcoma virus	Various sarcomas, some carcinomas,
	Avian reticuloendothelial virus	Lymphomas and leukemias
	Murine Leukemia and Sarcoma Viruses	Lymphomas and leukemias
		Lymphomas, leukemias and sarcomas
		Lymphosarcomas (mainly T cell)
	Feline Leukemia and sarcoma viruses	myeloid leukemias, fibrosarcomas
	Bovine Leukemia virus	B cell leukemias

Table 96.2 Oncogenic Viruses Associated with Human Cancer

Virus family	*Virus*	*Human cancer*
DNA Viruses		
Papovaviridae	Human papillomavirus	Genital tumors (cervical vulvar, penile cancers), Squamous cell carcinoma
Herpesviridae	Epstein-Barr virus	Nasopharyngeal carcinoma,
	Herpes simplex virus type 2	African Burkitt's lymphoma,
	Cytomegalovirus	B-cell lymphoma, Cervical carcinoma
	Human herpes virus B	Cervical carcinoma, Kaposi's sarcoma
Hepadnaviridae	Hepatitis B virus	Hepatocellular carcinoma
Poxviridae	Molluscipoxvirus	Molluscum contagiosum
RNA Viruses		
Retroviridae	Human T cell leukemia virus-1	Adult T cell leukemia
Flaviviridae	Hepatitis C virus	Hepatocellular carcinoma

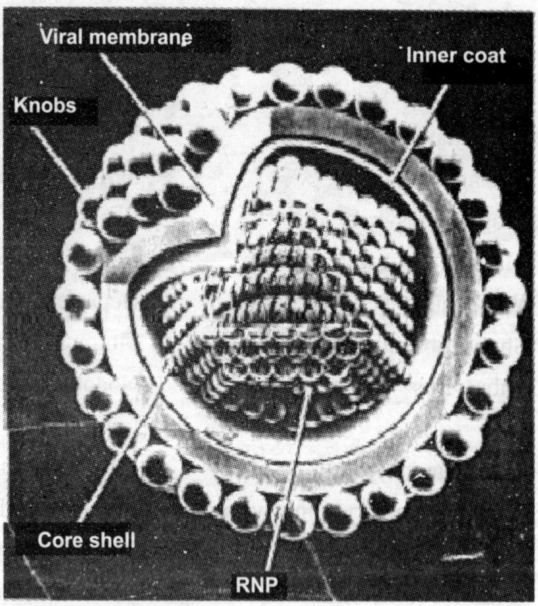

Fig. 96.1 Three dimensional model of a Retrovirus.

DNA tumor viruses replicate in certain cells of their natural hosts but rarely, if over, produce tumors in those hosts conversely, they are unable to replicate in heterologous hosts but can, on occasion, transform them. An example is simian virus SV40 naturally infects rhesus monkeys. The virus replicates in monkey kidney cells but does not transform them. SV40 cannot replicate in rodent cells but can transform them at low efficiency. However RNA tumor viruses can both replicate in and transform homologous cells. Thus, RNA tumor viruses differ from DNA tumor viruses in that the former can transform both permissive and nonpermissive cells.

INTERACTIONS OF TUMOR VIRUSES WITH HOST CELLS

Host cells are either permissive or nonpermissive for replication of a given virus. Permissive cells support viral growth and production of progeny virus; nonpermissive cells do not. Especially with the DNA viruses, permissive cells are not transformed unless the viral replicative cycle that normally results in death of the host cell is blocked in some way; nonpermissive cells may be transformed. Cells that are permissive for one virus may be nonpermissive for another.

ONCOGENES

Oncogene is the general term given to genes that cause cancer. Viral oncogenes (V-onc) are genes which encode proteins triggering transformation of normal cells into cancer cells. Oncogenes are not essential for the replication of the virus and mutants lacking oncognes occur, which replicate normally without being oncognic. Genes closely resembling viral oncogenes are found in normal as well as cancer cells. Oncogenes isolated from cancer cells are called cellular oncognes (C-onc). Similar genes found in normal cells are called proto-oncogenes and they are not of viral origin. On the contrary viral oncogenes appear to be of host cell origin. **Cellular oncogenes** contain introns characteristic of eukaryotic genes, whereas viral oncogenes do not. Apparently viral oncogenes originated at some distant past from protooncogenes by recombination between retroviral and cellular genes.

Protooncogenes are widespread in cells of species ranging from fruit flies to humans and are well conserved in their genomes, suggesting that their functions are essential to normal activities of cells. They have been found to code for proteins involved in regulating cell growth and differentiation. For example, the oncogene *src* is related to tyrosine-specific protein kinases, *sis* to a platelet derived growth factor, and *myc* to DNA-binding proteins, all concerned with normal regulation of normal cell growth.

A widely used method for the study of oncogenes is **transfection**. Certain mouse fibroblast cell lines, such as NIH 3T3, can take up foreign DNA, incorporate them into their genome and express them. This method of gene transfer is called transfection. By this technique, DNA extracted from human tumor cells has been shown to transform 3T3 cells, and such transforming genes have been shown to be identical with cellular protooncogenes.

ANTIONCOGENES (TUMOR SUPPRESSOR GENES)

A new class of genes has been identified in normal human cells, whose function appears to be inhibition of malignant transformation. They have been variously called tumor suppressor genes or antioncogenes or growth suppressor genes. Their prototype is the retinoblastoma (RB) gene, the loss of which is associated with the development of retinoblastoma in children. The P53 gene appears to be a tumor suppressor gene with a wide range of effects. Specific chromosomal deletions, recognised in association with certain types of human cancers may reflect the loss of tumor suppressor genes.

MECHANISM OF VIRAL ONCOGENESIS

Oncogenic viruses are able to transform cells in culture and induce tumors in animals, under natural or experimental conditions. Malignancy is a stable heritable change and is due due to the modification of the host cell genome.

In the case of DNA tumor viruses, the viral DNA (or a portion of it) is integrated with the host cell genome. The viral DNA being incomplete or defective, no infectious virus is produced. However, under its influence, the host cell undergoes malignant transformation.

In general retroviruses induce tumors by two mechanisms-either by introducing a new transforming gene (oncogene) into the cellular genome or by inducing or altering the expression of a preexisting cellular gene. Several molecular mechanisms have been suggested for the conversion of benign protooncogenes to cancer genes. The genes may get overexpressed and the overproduced gene product may lead to abnormal growth.

Recombination between retroviral and cellular genes, promoter insertion, chromosomal translocation, gene amplification and mutation are some of the genetic processes relevant for the conversion of benign protooncogenes to cancer genes.

QUESTIONS

Essay Questions:

1. Enumerate RNA and DNA oncogenic viruses. Write briefly on oncogenic RNA viruses. Add a note on mechanism of oncogenesis.

Short Notes:

1. Retroviruses or oncogenic RNA viruses.
2. Oncogenic Viruses.
3. Mechanism of oncogenesis
4. Reverse transcriptase.
5. Name four viruses associated with malignancy.
6. Oncogenes.
7. tumor suppressor genes or antioncogenes.

97

Reoviruses and Rotaviruses

- *Introduction*
- *Structure*
- *Classification*
- *Rotaviruses—structure, classification, animal susceptibility, cultivation, epidemiology, replication, pathogenesis and clinical features, laboratory diagnosis, prophylaxis, treatment*
- *Reoviruses*

INTRODUCTION

The name 'reovirus' stands for respiratory and enteric orphan virus. Although an orphan virus is typically virus not known to be the cause of any disease, that is no longer the case for reoviruses. Viruses in the family **Reoviridae** are spherical, nonenveloped particles that have an icosahedral structure. The viral geneme consists of ten to twelve segments of double stranded RNA. The virion contain all the enzymes needed to make positive-strand RNA transcripts. Reoviruses replicate completely in the cytoplasm. The single genus in the family that is of medical importance is the genus *Rotavirus*, which causes viral gastroenteritis primarily in infants and young children.

STRUCTURE

The virion measure 60–80 nm in diameter and possess two concentric capsid shells, each of which is icosahedral. Rotaviruses have a triple layered structure. They are nonenveloped. Single shelled virus particles that lack the outer capsid exhibit rough outer edges and are 50–60 nm in diameter. The inner core of the particles is 33–40 nm in diameter. Rotaviruses possess 132 capsomers. The double-shelled particle is the complete infectious form of the virus. The genome-consists of double-stranded RNA in 10–12 discrete segments. The virion core contains several enzymes needed for transcription and capping of viral RNAs. Genetic reassortment occurs readily. Reoviruses are good models for molecular studies of viral pathogenesis.

Reoviruses are unusually stable to heat, to a 3.0–9.0 range of pH, and to lipid solvents, but they are inactivated by 95% ethanol, phenol, and chlorine. Limited treatment with proteolytic enzymes increases infectivity.

CLASSIFICATION

The family Reoviridae is divided into nine general. Four of the genera are able to infect humans and animals. *Orthoreovirus, Rotavirus, Coltivirus,* and *Orbivirus.* Four other genera infect only plants and insects, and one infects fish.

There are atleast three major subgroups and nine serotypes of human rotaviruses. Strains of human and animal origin may fall in the same serotype. Five other serotypes are found only in animals. Only three different serotypes of reovirus are recognized. There are about 100 different orbivirus serotypes. There are two known serotypes for coltiviruses.

Rotaviruses contain 11 genome segments of double stranded RNA, whereas orthoreoviruses and orbiviruses each possess ten segments and coltiviruses have 12 segments.

ROTAVIRUSES

Structure

Rotaviruses are closely related to reoviruses in terms of morphology and strategy of replication. However, Rotaviruses have a characteristic morphology that distinguishes them from other reoviruses, namely, they have the appearance of wheels with spokes radiating from the center (rota, in Latin meaning wheel) and a smooth outer rim. The particles also have a large number of channels connecting the outer surface of the virion to the inner core. It has been suggested that these channels are involved in the import of substrates needed for RNA transcription and the extrusion of newly synthesized RNA transcripts (Fig. 97.1)

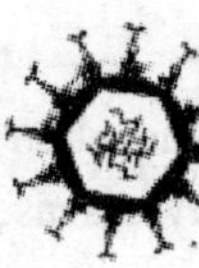

Fig. 97.1 Rotavirus

Classification

Seven major antigenic subgroups or serogroups (A to G) of human rotaviruses have been identified. The viruses usually associated with human gastroenteritis are classified as group A rotaviruses, but antigenically and genomically distinct rotaviruses have also caused diarrheal outbreaks, primarily in adults. This rotavirus is called "adult diarrhea rotavirus". Group B rotaviruses have been implicated in large outbreaks of gastroenteritis in adults in china.

Type-specific antigens, located on the outer capsid differentiate among rotaviruses and are demonstrable by neutralisation tests. Atleast nine (1–9) serotypes have been identified among human rotaviruses, and atleast five more serotypes exist among animal isolates.

Animal Susceptibility

Rotaviruses, found in many mammalian species, often have a fairly broad host range. Most isolates have been recovered from newborn animals with diarrhea.

Cultivation

Rotaviruses does not grow readily in cell cultures. Most group A human rotaviruses can be cultivated if pretreated with the proteolytic enzyme trypsin and if low levels of trypsin are included in the tissue culture medium and rolling of tissue cultures. Trypsin cleaves an outer capsid protein and facilitates uncoating.

Epidemiology

Rotaviruses are the single most important world-wide cause of gastroenteritis in young children. Rotavirus infections account for about fifty percent of cases of acute gastroenteritis in infants and young children under five years of age.

Transmission of rotaviruses is via the fecal-oral route. There is a marked seasonal incidence and rotavirus infections usually predominate during the winter season. Because infectious particles are relatively stable, they can survive for extended periods on various surfaces. Symptomatic infections are most common in children between ages 6 months and 2 years. Nosocomial infections are frequent.

Rotaviruses are ubiquitous. By age 3 years, ninety percent of children have serum antibodies to one or more types. This high prevalence of rotavirus antibodies is maintained in adults, suggesting subclinical reinfections by the virus. Local immune factors, such as secretory IgA or interferon may be important in protection against rotavirus infection.

Pathogenesis and Clinical Features

Following ingestion, rotaviruses infect the epithelial cells of the small intestine (rotaviruses are resistant to acid pH of the stomach), primarily the jejunum. They multiply in the cytoplasm of enterocytes and damage their transport mechanisms. One of the rotavirus-encoded proteins, NSP4, is a viral enterotoxin and induces secretion by triggering a signal transduction pathway. Damaged cells may slough into the lumen of the intestine and release large quantities of virus, which appear in the stool. Viral excretion usually lasts 2–12 days in healthy patients but may be prolonged in those with malnutrition. Diarrhea caused by rotaviruses may be due to impaired sodium and glucose absorption as damaged cells on villi are replaced by nonabsorbing immature crypt cells. It may take 3–8 weeks for normal function to be restored.

The incubation period is usually 1–4 days. Infection can be subclinical or may result in symptoms such as nonbloody, watery diarrhea, fever, abdominal pain, and vomiting leading to dehydration. In infants and children, severe loss of electrolytes and fluids may be fatal unless treated. Patients with milder cases have symptoms for 3–8 days and then recover completely.

Laboratory Diagnosis

Virus in stool is demonstrated by immune electron microscopy, immunodiffusion or ELISA. Dot hybridization using rotavirus-specific cDNA probes may prove convenient. It may be possible to type rotavirus nucleic acid from stool specimens by the polymerase chain reaction (PCR). Several serologic tests can be used to detect a rise in antibody titer, particularly ELISA.

Prophylaxis

Preventions of rotavirus infections requires waste water treatment and improved sanitation measures. Live oral attenuated vaccines derived from animal rotavirus strains (rhesus, bovine) have been shown to be highly efficacious in protecting infants against severe rotavirus gastroenteritis.

Treatment

There is no specific antiviral drug appropriate for treatment of rotavirus infections. The most important clinical intervention is the rapid and efficient replacement of fluids and electrolytes, usually intravenously.

REOVIRUSES

The viruses of this genus are not known to cause human disease. Reoviruses have become an important model system for the study of the pathogenesis of viral infection at the molecular level. Reoviruses are ubiquitous, with a very wide host range. Three distinct but related types of reovirus sharing a common complement fixing antiges have been identified by neutralisation and HI tests. Reoviruses contain a hemagglutinin for human 'O' or bovine erythrocytes.

Reoviruses cause many inapparent infections, because most people have serum antibodies by early adulthood. All three types have been recovered from healthy children, from young children during outbreaks of minor febrile illness, from children with diarrhea or enteritis, and from chimpanzees with epidemic rhinitis. An association of reovirus type 3 with biliary atresia in infants has been suggested.

QUESTIONS

Short Notes:

1. Enumerate the viruses causing diarrhea. Underline the most important of them.
2. Name the viruses causing diarrhea.
3. How is rotaviral diarrhea diagnosed?
4. Rotaviruses.
5. Reoviruses.

98

Calciviruses and Astroviruses

- *Caliciviruses*
- *Norwalk agent*
- *Astroviruses*

CALICIVIRUSES

The family **caliciviridae** camprises small, nonenveloped, spherical virions. They possess single-stranded, positive-sense, nonsegmented RNA genome, surrounded by icosahedral capsid (Fig. 98.1) made up of 90 capsomers and 32 cup shaped (calyx = cup) depressions from which the virus name is derived. This family caliciviridae has a single genus *Calicivirus* (human caliciviruses) and **hepatitis E virus.**

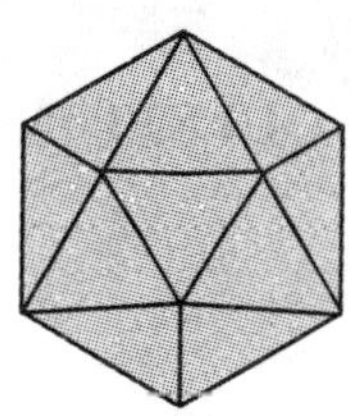

Fig. 98.1 Calicivirus

Caliciviruses are similar to picornaviruses but are slightly larger (27–38 nm) and contain a single major structural protein. In contrast to the picornaviruses, the calicivirus genome contains three open reading frames. There are several serotypes of human caliciviruses, in addition to Norwalk virus, that do not cross react antigenically with known animal strains. Norwalk virus is the prototype human calicivirus. Human caliciviruses seem to be relatively common causes of gastroenteritis in children. A rabbit calicivirus causes rabbit hemorrhagic disease.

NORWALK AGENT

The norwalk agent is classified as a calicivirus. It replicates only in humans in the gastro-intestional tract and is shed in feces. Norwalk virus is a major cause of epidemic acute gastroenteritis, often associated with epidemic outbreaks of water-borne, food-borne and shellfish-associated gastroenteritis, particularly at schools, camps, military bases, prisons and similar settings.

Norwalk agent measures 27 nm with positive sense, single stranded RNA genome. There appear to be atleast four serotypes of Norwalk-like viruses.

Norwalk viral gastroenteritis has an incubation period of 10–48 hours. The symptoms include diarrhea, nausea, vomiting, low-grade fever, abdominal cramps, headache and malaise. Symptoms last 24–48 hours, and the disease is self-limited. Hospitalization is rarely required.

Norwalk virus has a worldwide distribution. Whereas rotavirus antibody develops early in childhood. Norwalk virus antibody is acquired later in life. However, in developing countries, most children have developed norwalk virus antibodies by four years of age.

Virus particles can be demonstrated in stools by immune electron microscopy. RIA and ELISA teste are available for the detection of antiviral antibodies.

Effective handwashing, careful processing of food, purification of drinking water and swimming pool water should reduce the incidence of these infections. Treatment is symptomatic.

ASTROVIRUSES

Astroviruses are small, about 28–30 nm in diameter, spherical virions with a characteristic five or six pointed star-shaped outline. The genome consists of a single, positive-sense, linear, ssRNA molecule. The family **Astroviridae** has only one genus, *Astrovirus,* which has several serotypes. Astroviruses can be isolated in primary human embryonic kidney cells in the presence of trypsin.

Astroviruses have been found in the feces of infants and young children and from calves and lambs with diarrhea. Astroviruses may be shed in extraordinarily large quantities in feces. They are transmitted by fecal-oral route from person to person via contaminated water or food. After an incubation period of 1–4 days, the patient develops watery diarrhea and sometimes vomiting and abdominal discomfort. The disease is selflimited. The virus in the feces can be detected by immune electron microscopy.

QUESTIONS

Short Notes:

1. Caliciviruses
2. Norwalk agent
3. Astroviruses.

99

Slow Virus Infections and Prion Diseases

- *Introduction*
- *Slow Virus Infections—visna, SSPE, PML,*
- *Transmissible spongiform viral*
- *Encephalopathies—scrapie, mink encephalopathy, bovine spongiform encephalopathy, kuru, CJD.*
- *Laboratory diagnosis*
- *Treatment and prevention*

INTRODUCTION

Several animal viruses and unconventional agents produce chronic infections of the central nervous system that result in progressive degenerative changes (Table 99.1).

Table 99.1 Slow and Unconventional Virus Diseases

Disease	*Agent*	*Hosts*	*Incubation period*	*Nature of disease*
Diseases of Humans				
Kuru	Prion	Humans, chimpanzees, monkeys	Months to years	Spongiform encephalopathy
Creutzfeldt-Jakob disease	Prion	Humans, chimpanzees, monkeys	Months to years	Spongiform encephalopathy
Subacute sclerosing panencephalitis	Measles virus variant	Humans	2–20 years	Chronic sclerosing panencephalitis
Progressive multifocal leukoencephalopathy	Papovavirus	Humans	Years	Central nervous system demyelination

Diseases of animals				
Scrapie	Prion	Sheep, goats, mice	Months to years	Spongiform encephalopathy
Transmissible mink encephalopathy	Prion	Mink, other animals	Months	Spongiform encephalopathy
Bovine spongiform encephalopathy	Prion	Cattle	Months to years	Spongiform encephalopathy
Visna	Retrovirus	Sheep	Months to years	Central nervous system demyelination

SLOW VIRUS INFECTIONS

Some chronic degenerative diseases of the central nervous system in humans are caused by 'slow, or 'chronic', persistent viral infections. Slow virus infections have the following characteristics.

1. Long incubation period ranging from months to years.
2. Course of illness lasting for years, with remissions and exacerbations.
3. Predilection for central nervous system.
4. absente of immune response or an immune response that cannot arrest the disease, but may actually contribute to pathogenesis.
5. A genetic predisposition and
6. Invariable fatal termination.

Slow virus infections include visna in sheep, subacute sclerosing panencephalitis (SSPE) and progressive multifocal leukoencephalopathy in humans.

Visna

Visna and **maedi (progressive pneumonia)** viruses are closely, related agents that cause slow infections in sheep. These viruses are classified as Retroviruses, family Retroviridae and subfamily Lentivirinae. They are nononcogenic. These viruses infect all the organs of the body of the infected sheep, but pathologic changes are confined primarily to brain, lungs, and reticuloendothelial system. Inflammatory lesions appear in the central nervous system soon after infection, but there is usually a long incubation period (months to years) before observable neurologic symptoms appear. During the long-term persistent infection, the virus undergoes antigenic variations. Infected animals develop antibodies to the virus, which can be detected in the serum as well as in the CSF of sick animals.

Subacute Sclerosing Panencephalitis (SSPE)

It is a rare, fatal, slowly progressive degenerative (demyelination) disease of the CNS seen among children and young adults, as a delayed sequel to infection with measles infection early in life, usually below two yeas of age. Under electron microscope, large numbers of viral nucleocapsid structures are visible in neurons and glial cells. There is restricted expression of the viral genes (M,F,H) that encode envelope proteins, Therefore, the virus in persistently infected neural cells lacks components essential for the assembly and budding of mature infectious particles. Defective measles virus has been recovered from brains of patients with subacute sclerosing panencephalitis by cocultivation of brain cells with susceptible cells. Such isolates are mutated in one or more viral proteins. Patients with SSPE have high titres of antimeasles antibody in both serum and CSF, but antibody to the M protein is frequently lacking. It appears that reduced efficiency of measles virus transcription in differentiated brain cells is important in maintaining the persistent infection that leads to SSPE.

The course of SSPE is variable and usually starts with a generalized intellectual deterioration, which may last for weeks or months, until definite neurological signs or motor dysfunctions such as dyspraxia, generalized convulsions, aphasia, visual disturbances and mild repetitive simultaneous myoclonc jerks appear. Viral invasion of retina may lead to chorioretinitis, often affecting macular area leading to blindness. Finally, the disease proceeds to progressive cerebral degeneration, leading to coma and death. Disease generally lasts for 1–3 years.

A progressive panencephalitis has also been reported in patients with congenital rubella, which develops in the second decade and consisted of spasticity, ataxia, seizures and progressive decline in intellectual ability.

Progressive Multifocal Leukoencephalopathy (PML)

It is a rare, subacute demyelinating disease with CNS complication found in patients suffering from chronic leukemia, Hodgkin's disease, or lymphosarcoma or in immunosuppressed individuals. It is seen in a significant proportion of patients with AIDS. The disease results from oligodendrocyte infection by a papovavirus known as JC virus. There is progressive deterioration of motor functions, vision and speech. Death occurs in 3–4 months. JC virus, a member of papovaviridae family has been demonstrated by electron microscopy and isolated from brain biopsies of patients.

Transmissible Spongiform Viral Encephalopathies (TSE)

The transmissible spongiform viral encephalopathies are chronic, progressive degenerative diseases of the CNS of humans and animals. The spongiform encephalopathies occuring in humans are designated as Kuru, Creutzfeldt-Jakob disease (CJD), Gerstmann-Straussler syndrome (GSS) and fatal familial insomnia. The most important spongiform encephalopathies of animals are scrapie in sheep, and the bovine spongiform encephalopathy (BSE) in cattle (popularly called 'mad cow disease') and mink.

The causative agents are unconventional viruses, known as prions. They consist of proteinaceous material without nucleic acid. Preparations containing only prion protein (PrP) and no nucleic acid have been found to be infectious. PrP behaves like amyloid. A noninfectious form of PrP is present in normal mammalian brains on the surface of neurons and glial cells, encoded on chromosome 20 in humans. An abnormal isoform of this protein, designated as scrapie isoform of the prion protein (PrP^{SC}) is associated with transmissibility and infectivity. This protein is an altered version of a normal cellular protein (PrP^{c}), differing in conformation. The abnormal isoform PrP^{SC} differs physically from the normal PrP^{C} by its high β-sheet content, its insolubility in detergents, its propensity to aggregate, and its relative resistance to proteolysis. The proliferation and accumulation of PrP^{SC} in the CNS as diffuse deposits and in the form of plaques disrupts the architecture and function in the brain, causing disease.

Prions are unusually resistant to treatment with formaldehyde, β-propiolactone, ethanol, proteases, deoxycholate and ionizing radiation. However, they are sensitive to phenol (90%), household bleach, ether, acetone, urea, strong detergents, iodine and autoclaving.

The diseases caused by these prions possess several distinguishing characteristics.

1. The diseases are confined to CNS.
2. The basic lesion is a progressive vacuolation in neurons, an extensive astroglial hypertrophy and proliferation, and then a spongiform change in the gray matter.
3. Prion protein accumulates within the CNS in the form of amyloid plaques and diffuse deposits.
4. Long incubation periods ranging from months to decades precede the onset of clinical illness and are followed by chronic progressive pathology (weeks to years).
5. The diseases are always fatal, with no known cases of remissions or recoveries.
6. Host shows no inflammatory response.
7. Since prions are not antigenic, host shows no immune response.
8. Interferon production is not elicited.
9. There is no effect on host B or T cell function.
10. Immunosuppression of the host has no effect on pathogenesis of the disease.
11. The prion diseases are infectious, inherited (10 to 15% of cases) and sporadic.

Scrapie

Scrapie is a disease of sheep, usually transmitted vertically from ewe to lamb, and less often by contact. The incubation period is about two to three years. The affected animals are irritable and develop intense pruritus, scraping themselves against trees and rocks, hence the name "scrapie". Scrapie is the prototype prion disease. Emaciation and paralysis set in, leading to death. The disease can be transmitted to sheep, goats, mice, monkeys and other experimental animals by injection of suspensions of brain and spinal cord from affected animals. Different breeds of sheep exhibit marketed genetic differences in susceptibility to infection. Infectivity can be recovered from lymphoid tissues early in infection, but high titres of the agent are found only in the brain, spinal cord and eye, Maximal titres of infectivity are reached in the brain long before neurologic symptoms appear. Extracellular accumulation of protein, known as amyloid plaques develop in the CNS, which stain with Congo red.

Mink Encephalopathy

This disease is caused by an agent that induces neurologic lesions in the gray matter of the brain and clinical disease similar to those of scrapie. It also has a long incubation period in mink that are naturally infected presumably by the oral route. Transmissible mink encephalopathy probably represents a strain of sheep scrapie acquired when mink or mink ranches were fed scrapie-infected carcasses.

Bovine Spongiform encephalopathy (Mad cow disease)

A diesease similar to scrapie, designated bovine spongiform encephalopathy (BSE) or "mad cow disease", emerged in cattle in UK in 1986. This outbreak was traced to the use of cattle feed that contained contaminated bone meal from scrapie-infected sheep carcasses and BSE-infected cattle carcasses processed in a way that failed to destroy the infectivity of the infectious agent. In 1996, a variant form of Creutzfeldt-Jakob disease was recognized in the UK that occured in younger people and had distinctive pathologic characteristics similar to those seen in macaques infected with BSE agent.

Kuru (= tremor)

Kuru occurs only in the eastern highlands of New Guinea. The infectious agent is acquired by consumption of diseased brain tissue in the course of ritualistic cannibalism among the members of a tribe in New Guinea. Since the remains of dead relatives were handled and eaten primarily by women and children, the disease occurs more frequently in women than in men.

The disease had an incubation period of 5–10 years and consists of relentless progressive cerebellar ataxia, tremors, dysarthria and emotional lability without significant dementia, ending fatally. Brain material from patients who died from disease can produce similar disease when injected into chimpanzees, and the serial passage of diseased chimpanzee brain into healthy chimpanzees or rodents transfers the illness. Since cannibalism is outlawed, the disease is disappearing.

Cruetzfeldt-Jakob Disease (CJD)

The CJD is a subacute presenile dementia in humans. If develops gradually, with progressive dementia, ataxia and somnolence, and leads to death in 8–12 months. The histologic lesions resemble those of kuru and scrapie, including the presence of amyloid plaques. The diesease occurs with a frequency of approximately one case per million population per year in the USA and Europe. Most cases occur sporadically and involve persons over 50 years of age. However, the variant form of CJD that may be linked to bovine spongiform encephalopathy has mainly affected people under the age of 30.

CJD has been transmitted accidentally by contaminated growth hormone preparations from human cadaver pituitary glands, by a corneal transplant, and by a cadaveric human duramater grafts used for surgical repair of head injury.

A protein similar to the scrapie PrP^{SC} is present in brain tissue infected with CJD. It has been speculated that the agent of CJD was derived originally from scrapie-infected sheep and transmitted to humans by ingestion of poorly cooked sheep brains.

Gerstmann-Stradussler-Scheinker syndrome (GSS) and fatal familial insomnia (FFI) are two familial forms of CJD.

There are some neuropathologic similarities between CJD and Alzheimer's disease, including the appearance of amyloid plaques. However, the amyloid material the brains of Alzheimer's patients is distinct from that containing PrP^{SC} protein in brain tissue infected with scrapie or CJD.

LABORATORY DIAGNOSIS

A presumplive diagnosis can be made on clinical grounds, but there is some overlap with other dementing illnesses. Routine laboratory tests of serum and CSF are generally normal. The presence of infectious PrP^{sc} in peripheral lymphatic tissue provides specimens for analysis without the need for brain biopsy. Currently, however, the definitive diagnosis of these diseases is by postmortem histopathologic examination of brain sections.

TREATMENT AND PREVENTION

Transmissible spongiform encephalopathies are invariably fatal, and no treatment is currently available that can alter this outcome. The unusually high resistance of the infectivity to most disinfecting agents makes prevention of transmission by the usual infection control procedures ineffective. Current recommendations for decontamination of a CJD brain specimen are autoclaving at 132°C, plus immersion in either undiluted sodium hypochlorite or 1 N sodium hydroxide. With respect to preventing possible transfer of BSE to humans, all animals showing signs of illness are destroyed, and preparation of animal feed from internal organs of potentially infected animals has ceased.

QUESTIONS

Essay Question:

1. Give an account of slow virus infections.

Short Notes:

1. SSPE.
2. Prions.
3. Spongiform viral encephalopathies.
4. Prion specific protein or PrP.

100
Human Immunodeficiency Virus (HIV)

INTRODUCTION

The family **Retroviridae** are distinguished from all other RNA viruses by the presence of an unusual enzyme, **reverse transcriptase**, which convets a single stranded RNA viral genome into double stranded viral DNA. Because these viruses reverse the order of information transfer (RNA serving as a template for DNA synthesis, rather than the almost universal DNA serving as a template for RNA synthesis), they are termed retroviruses (*Retro* is Latin for reversal; Re = reverse; tr = transcriptase). Retroviridae are divided into seven genera on the basis of nucleotide sequence similarity and genome structure. The genera of human importance are shown in the Table 100.1.

Table 100.1 Human Retroviruses

Subfamily	*Genus*	*Virus*	*Disease*
Oncovirinae	*Retrovirus*	H T L V-1 H T L V-2	Adult T cell leukemiallymphoma prevalent in intravenous drug users, not associated with disease
Lentivirinae	*Lentivirus*	H I V-1 H I V-2	A I D S A I D S
Spumavirinae	*Spumavirus*	Human foamy virus	—

Human immunodeficiency virus (HIV), the etiologic agent of AIDS, belongs to ***Lentivirus*** (lenti = slow) genus of the family Retroviridae. Lentiviruses are nononcogenic and can cause neurologic and immunologic diseases. The Lentivirus group includes the causative agents of the slow virus diseases. Visna/maedi in sheep and infectious anemia in goats and horses. Besides HIV, the related animal immunodeficiency viruses are also assigned to this group.

The HIV was formerly known as **Lymphadenopathy associated virus (LAV)** and **human T cell lymphotropic virus-3 (HTLV-3)**. The International committee on virus nomenclature in 1986 decided on the generic name human immunodeficiency virus (HIV) for these viruses.

STRUCTURE

HIV is a spherical, enveloped virus, about 90–120 nm in diameter. The nucleacapsid has an inner cone shaped core and an outer icosahedral capsid. The inner cone shaped core consists two identical copies of linear, positive sense, single stranded RNA associated with reverse transcriptase. The icosahedral capsid is surrounded by a matrix protein followed by a host cell membrane derived lipid bilayer envelope from which virus coded 72 Knob-like glycoprotein peplomers project and the anchoring **transmembrane pedicles** (Fig. 100.1).

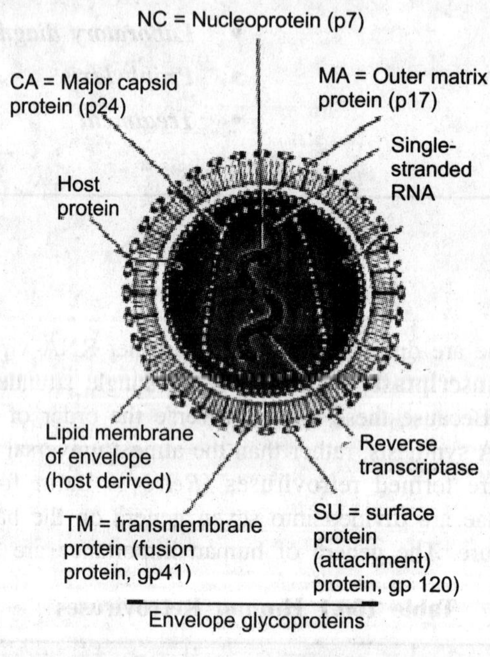

Fig. 100.1 Structure of Human immunodeficiency virus.

HIV GENOME

The genome of HIV contains the three structural genes (*gag, pol and env*) characteristic of all retroviruses, as well as other nonstructural and regulatory genes specic for the virus. The products of these genes act as antigens. Sera of infected persons contain antibodies to them. Detection of these antigens and antibodies is useful in the diagnosis and prognosis of HIV infections.

The *gag* gene codes for CA (capsid protein; P24), MA (matrix protein, P17) and NC (nucleocapsid protein; P9). The *pol* gene codes for reverse transcriptase (RT; P-66, P.51), protease (PR, P11), integrase (IN; P.32), and ribonuclease. The *env* gene codes for surface spike glycoproteins (SU; gp 120) and transmembrane protein (TM; gp41) (Fig. 100.2).

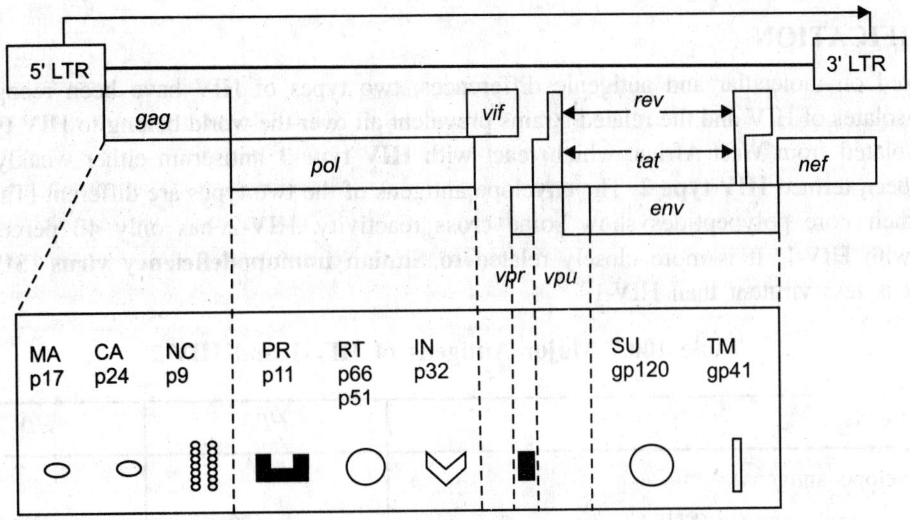

Fig. 100.2 HIV genome

Note: The designation "gp41" refers to the structure of the molecule which is a glycoprotein with an originally determined molecular weight of 41,000. "P24" refers to a protein (nonglycosylated) with a molecular weight of 24,000.

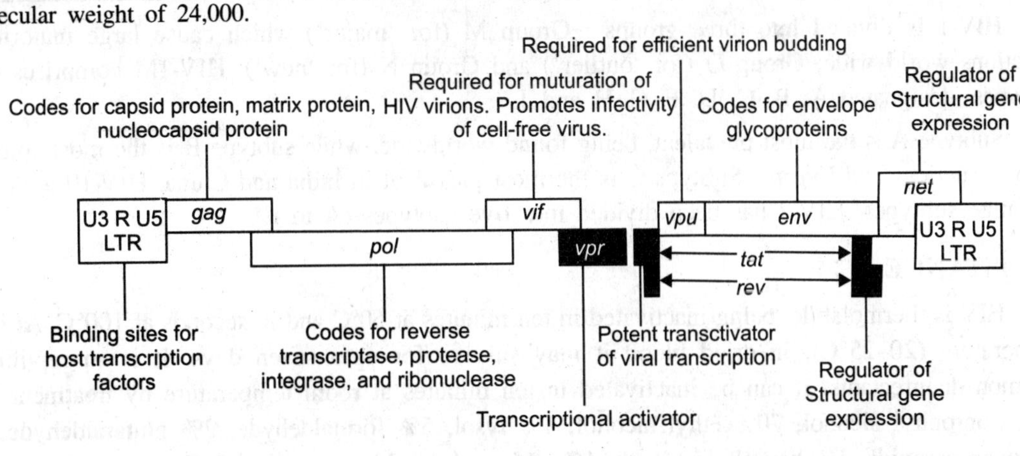

Fig. 100.3 HIV prioviral genome

Genes for additional regulatory and accessory proteins of diverse function are located between the *pol* and *env* genes. At the 5′ end of the viral RNA is a unique sequence, U5, which contains part of the site required for viral integration into the host cell chromosome and also tRNA primer binding site for initiation of reverse transcription. At the 3′ end of the viral RNA is the nucleolide sequence U3, which contain sequences that are important in the control of transcription of the DNA provirus. At either end of the viral genome is a repeated sequence, R, which is involved in reverse transcription. Synthesis of the double stranded DNA provirus. Provirus results in duplication of the R and U sequences, producing two identical repeat units designated long terminal repeats (LTR) (Fig. 100.3).

CLASSIFICATION

Based on molecular and antigenic differences, two types of HIV have been recognized. the original isolates of HIV and the related strains prevalent all over the world belong to HIV type 1. HIV strains isolated from West Africa, which react with **HIV type 1** antiserum either weakly or not at all have been termed **HIV type 2**. The envelope antigens of the two types are different (Table 100.2), though their core polypeptides show some cross reactivity. HIV-2 has only 40 percent genetic identity with HIV-1. It is more closely related **to Simian immunodeficiency virus** (SIV) than to HIV-1. It is less virulent than HIV-1.

Table 100.2 Major Antigens of HIV-1 and HIV-2

Antigens	*HIV-1*	*HIV-2*
1. Envelope antigens		
– Spike antigen (SU)	gp120	gp 140
– Transmembrane pedicle antigen (TM)	gp 41	gp 36
2. Matrix protein antigen (MA)	P 17	P 16
3. Capsid Protein Antigen (CA)	P 24	P26

HIV-1 is divided into three groups : Group M (for 'major') which cause large majority of infections world wide; Group O (for 'outlier') and Group N (for 'new'). HIV-1M comprises eight subtypes, designated A, B, C, D, F, G, H and J.

Subtype A is the most prevalent, being found worldwide, while subtype B is the most common in the Americas and Europe. Subtype C is the most prevalent in India and China. HIV-10 is divided into nine subtypes. HIV-2 has been divided into five subtypes (A to E).

RESISTANCE

HIV is thermolabile, being inactivated in ten minutes at 60ºC and in seconds at 100°C. At room temperature (20–25°C), in dried blood it may survive for upto seven days. It is susceptible to common disinfectants. It can be inactivated in ten minutes at room temperature by treatment with 35% isoprophyl alcohol, 70% ethyl alcohol, 1% lysol, 5% formaldehyde, 2% glutaraldehyde, 3% hydrogen peroxide, 1% household bleach, 1% sodium hypochlorite and 2.5% Tween-20. Because of its lipid envelope, it is highly susceptible to detergents, therefore, standard washing with detergents and hot water are adequate for decontaminating clothes and household utensils. For treatment of contaminated medical instruments, 2% solution of glutaraldehyde is useful.

REPLICATION

HIV attaches via its surface spike, **gp120**, which preferentially binds to **CD4 molecules** on host cells. Thus, the virus infects helper T cells, lymphocytes, monocytes and dendritic cells which contain CD4 protein in their cell membranes. Infection can be blocked by monoclonal antibodies to CD4 and recombinant soluble CD4.

A coreceptor, usually **chemokine receptor** expressed by macrophages and T cells is required for the entry of virus into the cell. Binding to a coreceptor activates the virus transmembrane pedicles (TM protein), triggering fusion between the viral envelope and the cell membrane.

The coreceptor molecule has been identified as **CXCR4** for T cell-tropic HIV strains and **CCR5** for macrophage-tropic strains. The chemokine receptors provide new targets for antiviral therapy (Fig. 100.4 and 100.5).

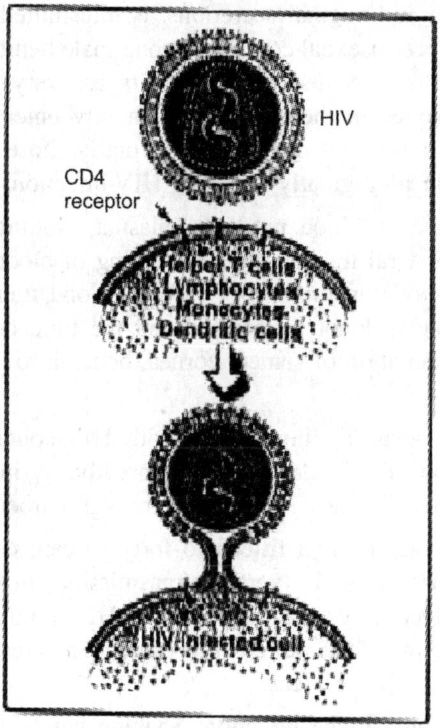

Fig. 100.4 Attachment and entery of HIV

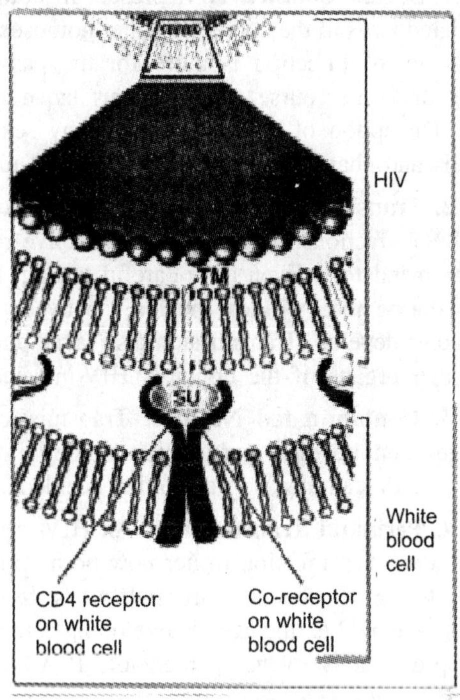

Fig. 100.5 Binding of HIV to the surface of a lymphocyte

After entering the host cell, the HIV RNA is transcribed into DNA by reverse transcriptase (RNA-directed DNA polymerase). This process takes place in the cytoplasm, within the core structure. The viral reverse transcriptase first synthesizes a DNA-RNA hybrid molecule, then its RNAase activity degrades the parental RNA molecule while synthesizing the second strand of DNA. This process results in duplication of the ends to form the long terminal repeats (LTR). The resulting linear molecule of double stranded DNA is the provirus. LTRs at either end of the provirus contain promoter and enhancer sequences that control expression of the viral DNA.

The provirus is transported to the nucleus with the aid of matrix protein (MA). There, viral integrase cleaves the chromosomal DNA randomly and covalently inserts the provirus, which becomes a stable part of the host cell genome, causing a latent infection.

The provirus is transcribed into a full-length mRNA by cell RNA polymerase II, which are translated to produce virion proteins and also genomes of the progeny virus, and are transported to the cytoplasm for viral assembly.

The virion proteins are processed and transported to the plasma membrane by the usual cellular route through Golgi. The genomes and proteins assemble. The naked virion buds out through the host cell membrane, and acquires a lipoprotein envelope, which consists of lipid deiived from the host cell membrane and glycoproteins (TM and SU) which are virus coded.

TRANSMISSION OF HIV

There are four important modes of transmission :

1. Sexual Contact: HIV, present in both semen and vaginal secretions, is transmitted as cell-associated virus in the course of either homosexual or heterosexual contact. Among male hemosexuals, the danger of infection is more for the passive partner because mucosal tears are very frequent during anal intercourse and the virus laden lymphocytes in the semen can directly enter through these. Disruption of mucosal surfaces by sexually transmitted diseases, particularly those such as syphilis and chancroid that result in genital ulceration may greatly facilitate HIV-infection.

2. Transfusions: Transfusion of infectious blood or blood products (plasma, clotting factors or cellular fractions of blood) is an effective route for viral transmission. Screening of blood donors is now mandatory. Even after careful testing, the risk of transmission of HIV by blood transfusions exists during the "**window period**", between the time a donor is infected and the time detectable antibodies develop. Transmission also takes place by donation of semen, cornea, bonemarrow, kidney and other organs, if the donor is HIV-infected.

3. Contaminated Needles: Transmission can occur by inoculation with HIV-contaminated syringes and needles, particularly among intravenous drug addicts who share the syringes and needles. HIV can also be transmitted accidentally by needle stick injuries and through barber's razor.

4. Perinatal Transmission: An HIV-infected woman has a fifteen to forty percent chance of transmitting the infection to her new born, either transplacentally (vertical transmission) *in utero*, or during the birth process or through breast-feeding. Because of the high rates of HIV-1 infection in women of child bearing age in developing countries, perinatally acquired HIV-1 infection is responsible for approximately twenty percent of all AIDS cases in these areas.

Normal social and domestic contact does not transmit the infection. Shaking hands, hugging, putting cheeks together or dry kissing are safe. There has been no confirmed case of transmission through saliva, though the virus may be present in the saliva of infected persons. A salivary protein called secretory leucocyte protease inhibitor has anti-HIV activity. Sharing rooms, bathrooms' and cooking and eating facilities cannot transmit HIV. There is no evidence that mosquitoes, bed bugs or other blood sucking insects can transmit the virus. Infection is not transmitted through air, food, water or fomites.

PATHOGENESIS AND CLINICAL FEATURES

The pathology of HIV disease results from either tissue destruction by the virus itself or the host's response to virus-infected cells. In addition, HIV can induce an immunodeficient state that leads to opportunistic diseases that are rare in the absence of HIV infection. The progression of HIV infection to clinical disease (AIDS) develops in fifty percent of HIV-infected individuals in an average of ten years, and, if untreated, it is uniformly fatal-generally within two years after the onset of clinical symptoms. The stages include the primary infection, dissemination of virus to lymphoid organs (acute phase viremia), clinical latency, elevated HIV expression, clinical disease (AIDS) and death. (Fig. 100.6).

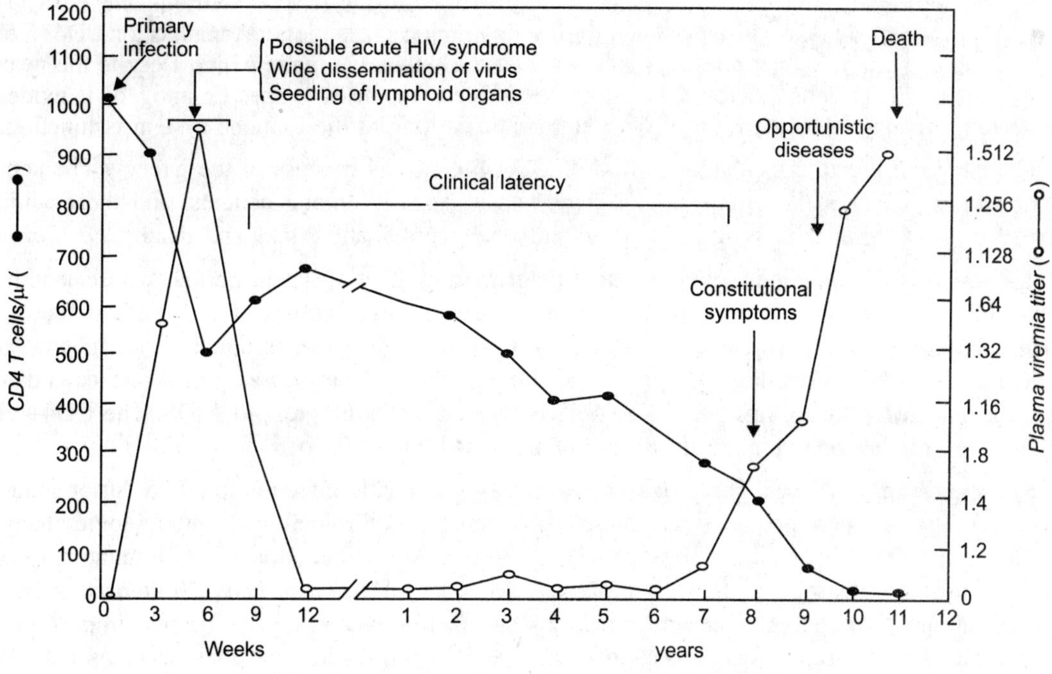

Fig. 100.6 Typical course of HIV infection

1. Initial Infection: After the acquisition of HIV, the initially infected cells are generally macrophages within the genital tract. From this initial localized infection, HIV disseminates via the blood, and the virus may then localize in dendritic cells throughout the lymphoid tissue. From the surface of follicular dendritic cells, HIV can then infect CD4+ lymphocytes moving through the germinal centers of lymph nodes. This process creates a reservoir of chronically HIV-infected cells within the lymphatic tissue of the body.

2. Acute Phase Viremia: Several weeks (generally 3–6 weeks) after the initial infection, one third to two thirds of individuals experience an acute disease syndrome (also referred to as the **primary infection**) similar to infectious mononucleosis. During this period, there is a high level of virus replication occuring in CD4+ cells. Large amounts of virus and capsid protein (CA; P24) are present in the blood, and circulating antibody appears in one to ten weeks after the initial infection (seroconversion). A constant level of virus and virus infected cells is maintained by a combination of replacement of the CD4+ cells killed by HIV infection with cells newly produced in lymphoid organs and the subsequent infection of these new cells with progeny virus. Lymph nodes also become infected during this time; they later serve as the sites of virus persistence during the asymptomatic period.

3. Latent Period: The acute phase viremia is eventually reduced significantly with the appearance of a HIV-specific cytotoxic T-lymphocyte response, followed by a humoral antibody response. A clinically asymptomatic or "latent" period lasting from months to many years (on average about ten years) follows the acute infection. During this latent period, the majority (ninety percent) of HIV proviruses are transcriptionally silent. There are transient peaks of viremia that are often correlated with stimulation of the immune system by infection with other pathogens or by immunization. Although there is continuous loss of those CD4+ cells in which HIV is replicating, active replacement through stem cell multiplication compensates for this loss, and CD4+ count declines only slowly over a period of years. In addition, the host immune response is still sufficiently effective to maintain a relatively stable, low level of virus production. It has been estimated that 10^{11} virions and 10^{9} CD4+ T cells are produced each day. Virus isolated during this period is also less cytopathic for CD4+ cells and replicates more slowly than does that isolated later during symptomatic AIDS. Despite the nearly normal levels of CD4+ cells, however, impairment of T-cell responses to specific antigens is evident. The infection remains relatively clinically asymptomatic as long as the immune system is functional.

The long and variable incubation period of HIV infection is because of the latency. The actual level of virus replication in peripheral blood cells varies greatly among patients, and those with a higher steady-state viral load progress more rapidly to symptomatic AIDS and death.

4. Clinical Complications During The Latent Period: During latent period, whose length is variable, but lasts an average about ten years–there are multiple, nonspecific conditions, such as persistent, generalized lymphadenopathy (swollen lymph nodes), diarrhea, chronic fevers, night sweats, and weight loss. The most common opportunistic infections such as herpes zoster and candidiasis may occur repeatedly during this period, as well as when patients progress to AIDS. The CD4+ cell count remains normal or gradually declines, but is greater than 200 per microlitre.

5. Progression to AIDS: The progression from asymptomatic infection to AIDS is not sudden, but infact occurs as a continuum of clinical states. A number of virologic and immunologic changes occur that affect the rate of this progression. For example, Any stimulation of an immune response causing activation of resting T cells, such as active infection by *Mycobacterium tuberculosis,* activates HIV replication. Other concomitant viral infections-human herpesvirus type 6, herpes simplex virus, cytomegalovirus, EB virus or hepatitis B virus induce HIV expression and may serve as cofactors of AIDS. Not only does this increase the number of infected CD4+ cells, but it also increases the opportunity to create generation of virus mutants, which are highly cytocidal and rapidly multiplying. HIV found in patients with late-stage disease is usually much more virulent and cytopathic than the starins of virus found early in infection. In addition, these variants are often highly syncytium-inducing, promoting fusion between infected and previously uninfected cells. T-cell precursors in the lymphoid organs are also infected and killed, so the capacity to generate new CD4+ cells is gradually lost, so the capacity to generate new CD4+ cells is gradually lost. The capacity to contain the infection is further compromised by the appearance of HIV mutants with altered antigenic specificity, which are not recognized by the existing humoral antibody or cytotoxic T lymphocytes. the result is an inceasingly rapid decline in CD4+ count, accompanied by loss of immune capacity.

The CD4+ (T4) lymphocytes decrease in numbers and T4:T8 (helper: suppressor) cell ratio is reversed. The consequences of CD4+ T cell dysfunction caused by HIV infection are devastating because the CD4+ T lymphocytes plays a critical role in the human immune response. It is responsible directly or indirectly for induction of a wide array of lymphoid and nonlymphoid cell functions such as activation of macrophages, induction of function of cytotoxic T cells, natural killer cells, and B cells, and secretion of a variety of soluble factors that induce growth and differentiation of lymphoid cells and affect hematopoietic cells.

6. End-stage AIDS: Nearly all systems of the body can be affected as a result of HIV infection, either by HIV itself or by severe opportunistic infections. The weakening immune system leads to the development of unusual neoplasms (especially Kaposi's sarcoma).

(a) Spread of HIV to Additional Body Sites

Cell types other than CD4+ lymphocytes can be infected by HIV. Infection of these cells produces some of the additional manifestations of end stage disease. Chief among these are infected cells of the monocyte-macrophage lineage, which are not killed as rapidly as CD4+ T cells and can transport the virus into other organs. Thus, monocyte-macrophage serves as a major reservoir for HIV in the body. Persistence of HIV in monocytes may in part explain the inability of HIV-specific immune response to completely clearly the body of virus. For example, macrophages and monocytes are the HIV-infected cells present in brains of patients with **AIDS encephalopathy** and peripheral neuropathies which typically evolves over a period of one year, with gradual deterioration resulting in severe dementia. This appears to be unrelated CD4+ depletion, but rather to an expanded host range of variant HIV. Galactosylceramide, a common CNS glycolipid, is an alternative receptor for gp120 and may mediate HIV entry into glial cells. Virus may enter the brain through infected macrophages and monocytes and release cytokines that are toxic to neurons as well as chemotactic factors that lead to infiltration of the brain with inflammatory cells. HIV has been found in neurons, oligodendrocytes, and astrocytes.

Infected pulmonary alveolar macrophages may play a role in the **interstitial pneumonitis** seen in certain patients with AIDS. Similarly, the **wasting syndrome** seen in last stages of AIDS is probably related to HIV-infected macrophages induced to produce various cytokines, especially tumor necrosis factor. Virus has also been found in Langerhans cells in the skin, dendritic cells in lymph nodes, and monocytes in bone marrow. The eye is another site affected by HIV infection itself, which produces focal areas of **ischemia** in the retina. HIV infection of blood cell progenitors in the bone narrow leads to the **anemia** seen in most AIDS patients.

(b) Opportunistic Infections in AIDS

The predominant causes of morbidity and mortality among patients with late-stage HIV infection are severe opportunistic infections induced by agents that rarely cause serious disease in immune-competent individuals. Multiple recurrent bouts of infections with fungi, bacteria and viruses occur as the CD4+ cell count declines. For example, the nervous system can be the site of opportunistic infections with *Toxoplasma, Cryptococcus,* JC virus and Mycobacteria. The eye cannot only be infected with HIV, but also with opportunistic agents, the most prominent of which is cytomegalovirus (CMV)—a cause of retinal destruction. The lungs are also primarily affected by opportunistic infections, *Pneumocystis carinii* pneumonia being one of the most common. Mycobacterial infections are also a common problem in the lung; for example, currently thirty percent of AIDS patients die from tuberculosis. Serious gastrointestinal tract illnesses are due to opportunistic pathogens, but these may be in concert with HIV infection. CMV colitis is a common problem, but HIV is often present as well. Protozoal parasitic diseases, as well as infections with gram negative enteric bacteria are the sources of gastrointestinal disorders. The immune deficiency also provides the opportunity for latent herpes virus infections to recur repeatedly or become chronic and spread extensively. Mucocutaneous candidiasis (oral, esophageal or vaginal) is an ongoing problem in AIDS patients as well.

The most common opportunistic infections in AIDS patients include the following :

1. **Protozoa**—*Toxoplasma gondii, Isospora belli, Cryptosporidium Species.*
2. **Fungi**—*Candida albicans, Cryptococcus neoformans, Coccidioides immitis, Histoplasma capsulatum, Pneumocystis carinii* (formerly classified as a protozoan), *Aspergillus* species.
3. **Bacteria**—*Mycobacterium tuberculosis, Mycobacterium avium-intracellulare, Listeria Monocytogenes, Nocardia asteroides, Salmonella species, Streptococcus species.*
4. **Viruses**—Cytomegalovirus, herpes simplex virus, Varicella-zoster virus, adenovirus, JC human papovavirus, hepatitis B virus.
5. **Helminths**—*Strongyloides stercoralis*

(c) Malignancies Associated with AIDS

A number of malignancies commonly arise in HIV-infected patients, as a consequence of immune deficiency. The most characteristic neoplasm present in AIDS patients is **Kaposi sarcoma**, which is 20,000 times more common in AIDS patients than in the general population. Kaposi sarcoma is a vascular tumor thought to be of endothelial origin that appears in skin, mucus membranes, lymph nodes, and visceral organs. Various lymphomas, including those of the CNS, are also common. A new herpesvirus, Kaposi sarcoma-associated herpesvirus or **human herpesvirus types 8 (HHV-8)** may be casually associated with Kaposi sarcoma. In AIDS patients, body cavity lymphomas are also usually associated with HHV-8 infection, whereas many other lymphomas are EBV-associated. The anogenital cancers may arise as a result of coinfections with human papilloma viruses.

With the CD4+ count falling below 200 per microliter and the appearance of increasingly frequent and serious diseases and opportunistic infections ("AIDS-defining illnesses"), the patient is said to have AIDS. AIDS is characterized by a pronounced suppression of the immune system and the development of unusual neoplasms (especially Kaposi's sarcoma) or a wide variety of severe opportunistic infections. The more serious symptoems in adults are often preceded by a prodrome ("diarrhea and dwindling") that can include fatigue, malaise, weight loss, fever, shortness of breath, chronic diarrhea, white patches on the tongue (**hairy leukoplakia**, oral candidiasis), and **lymphadenopathy**. Disease symptoms in the gastrointestinal tract from the esophagus to the colon are a major cause of debility. With no treatment, the interval between primary infection with HIV and the first appearance of clinical disease is usually long in adults, averaging about ten years. Death occurs about two years later.

Pediatric AIDS-acquired from mothers in high risk groups-usually presents with clinical symptoms by two years of age; death follows in another two years. The infected neonate is particularly susceptible to the devastating effects of HIV because the immune system has not developed at the time of primary infection. Clinical findings may include lymphoid interstitial pneumonitis, pneumonia, severe oral candidiasis, encephalopathy, wasting, generalized lymphadenopathy, bacterial sepsis, hepatosplenemegaly, diarrhea and failure to thrive.

The centers for Disease control in Atlanta, USA, have classified the clinical course of HIV infection under various groups.

Table 100.3 Classification of HIV infection and AIDS (Centers for Disease Control, Atlanta, USA)

Group I	— Acute HIV syndrome (seroconversion)	
Group II	— Asymptomatic infection.	
Group III	— Persistent generalized lymphadenopathy	
Group IV	— Other diseases.	
	Subgroup A : Constitutional disease (AIDS-related Complex)	
	Subgroup B: Neurologic diseases	
	Subgroup C: Secondary infectious diseases	
	Subgroup C1	Specified infectious diseases listed in the CDC surveillance definition for AIDS, such as *Pneumocystis carinii* pneumonia, cryptosporidiosis, toxoplasmosis, generalized strongyloidiasis, cryptococcosis, CMV or herpes diseases.
	Subgroup C2 :	Other specified secondary diseases, such as oral hairy Leukoplakia, *Salmonella* bacteremia, nocardiosis, tuberculosis, candidiasis.
	Subgroup D: Secondary cancers, such as kaposi sarcoma, lymphomas.	
	Subgroup E: Other conditions.	

LABORATORY DIAGNOSIS

HIV infection can be detected by virus isolation, demonstration of antiviral antibodies, and measurement of viral nucleic acid or antigens.

1. Virus Isolation

HIV can be cultured from lymphocytes in peripheral blood (and occasionally from plasma, CSF, genital secretions and various organs such as brain and bone narrow). The most sensitive method of isolation is by cocultivation of patient's lymphocytes with uninfected, mitogen-stimulated peripheral blood mononuclear cells in the presence of interleukin-2. Viral growth is detected by testing culture supernatant fluids after about 7–14 days for viral reverse transcriptase activity or for virus-specific antigens (P24). Primary isolates of HIV grow very slowly compared with laboratory-adapted strains. Virus isolation techniques are time-consuming and laborious and therefore not attempted in routine diagnosis.

2. Demonstration of Antibodies to HIV

The majority of individuals seroconvert within two months after viral exposure. Antibodies to viral capsid protein P24 or envelope glycoproteins gp41, gp120 or gp160 are most commonly detected. However, it takes several weeks to months for antibodies to appear after infection, and during part of this period, the individual may be highly infectious. This seronegative infective stage is known as the **window period**. During this window period, infection can be detected by ELISA testing for the P24 antigen in serum, since anti-HIV antibodies are undetectable.

Serological tests for anti-HIV antibodies are of two types-screening and confirmatory tests. The most widely employed screening test is ELISA. HIV-1 ELISA tests detect 40–90% of HIV-2 infections.

A positive test in a serum sample must be confirmed by a repeat test. If the repat ELISA test is reactive, a confirmation test is performed. Confirmation assays have included immunofluorescence and radioimmunoprecipitation, but the most widely used is the Western blot technique, in which antibodies to HIV proteins of specific molecular weights can be detected. For a western blot to be considered positive, at least two bands including p24, gp41 or gp120/gp160 should be present. Other band patterns are interpreted as indeterminate. The major gene products of HIV, detected in various diagnostic tests are listed in Table 100.4.

Demonstration of immune response to HIV is used for diagnosing individuals who may be infected and for screening blood donors to prevent transmission of infection by blood transfusion.

Table 100.4 Major Gene Products of HIV that are Useful in Diagnosis of Infection

Gene product	*Description*
gp160	Precursor of envelope glycoproteins
gp120	Outer envelope glycoprotein (SU)
P66	Reverse transcriptase and RNase H from polymerase gene product.
P55	Precursor of core proteins, polyprotein from *gag* gene
P51	Reverse transcriptase (RT)
gp41	Transmembrane envelope glycoprotein (TM)
P32	Integrase (IN)
P24	Nucleocapsid core protein of virion (CA)
P17	Matrix core protein of virion (MA)

Early diagnosis of HIV infection in infants born to infected mothers can be accomplished using plasma HIV-1 RNA tests. The presence of maternal antibodies makes serologic tests uninformative.

3. Detection of Viral Nucleic Acid or Antigens

Amplification of viral RNA or DNA proviruses by the RT-PCR and branched chain DNA (bDNA) is the most sensitive method for early detection of virus in blood or tissue specimens. Recent adaptation of the technique to obtain quantitative estimates of viral load i.e., amount of viral RNA per milliliter of blood plasma, now permit evaluation of the stage of the disease, effectiveness of a drug regimen, and prognosis.

Low levels of circulating HIV-1 P24 antigen can be detected in the plasma by ELISA soon after infection. The antigen often becomes undetectable after antibodies develop and may reappear late in the course of infection, indicating a poor prognosis. The test can be used to detect antigen in supernatant fluids from virus-infected tissue culture cells.

4. The following parameters help to establish the diagnosis of HIV infection.

(*i*) Leucopenia, lymphocyte count usually below 2000 mm^3.

(*ii*) Absolute CD4+T cell count will be usually less than 200 mm^3. T4 : T8 cell ratio is reversed.

(*iii*) Platelet count shows thrombocytopeneia.

(*iv*) Diminished CMI as indicated by skin tests.

(*v*) Lymph node biopsy showing profound abnormalities.

PROPHYLAXIS

Health education concerning methods for preventing transmission of HIV and identification of sources and elimination of high risk activities are currently the primary means of preventing spread of the virus. Screening of the blood supply has nearly eliminated transmission by blood transfusion. Infected persons should refrain from donating blood, plasma, body organs, other tissues or sperm. HIV infected women should be advised against pregnancy. Perinatal transmission can be reduced by nearly seventy percent with Zidovudine (AZT) therapy of the pregnant women, followed by several weeks of AZT to the newborn. HIV-infected mothers should avoid breast feeding. It is recommended that physicians screen for HIV infection in all adolescents and adults at increased risk of HIV infection.

No specific vaccine is available. The high mutability, diverse antigenic types and subtypes, long latency and persistence in infected cells as provirus pose serious problems in the development of vaccines. The lack of a suitable experimental animal is another constraint. An ideal vaccine should not only prevent infection but also have therapeutic application in asymptomatic seropositives. Several possible strategies have been explored for vaccine production. These include immunisation with (a) modified whole virus, (b) subunits, based on envelope glycoproteins expressed in animal cells, bacteria, viruses—or as synthetic epitopes on adjuvant carriers, and (c) target cell protection by monoclonal antibodies to CD4 and by recombinant soluble CD4.

TREATMENT

Because of the progressive nature of the disease, it is the HIV infection that is treated as the clinical problem, rather than focussing on the end stage—AIDS alone. Virtually every step in the HIV replication cycle is a potential target for an antiviral drug, but only those directed against reverse transcriptase, viral prolease, and viral fusion have been used successfully. Used early in the infection, a combination of three different drugs administered together can reduce the plasma viral load to undetectable levels, atleast temporarily. All such multiple-drug therapies are commonly referred to as "**highly active antiretroviral therapy**" or HAART. Incidence of opportunistic infections in AIDS patients is decreasing in response to widespread use of aggressive multidrug treatment:

Table 100.5 Currently available Drugs for HIV Infection

1.	Nucleoside and nucleotide analog reverse transcriptase inhibitor	Abacavir Didanosine Emtricitabine Lamivudine Stavudine Tenofovir Zalcitabine Zidovudine

2.	Nonnucleoside reverse transcriptase inhibitors	Delavirdine Efavirenz Nevirapine
3.	Protease inhibitors	Amprenavir Atazanavir Indinavir Lopinavir Nelfinavir Ritonavir Saquinavir

For multiple-drug therapy, a combination of either two nucleoside and nucleotide analog reverse transcriptase inhibitors plus one protease inhibitor or two nucleoside and nucleotide analog reverse transcriptase inhibitors plus one nonnucleoside reverse transcriptase inhibitor are employed.

Zidovudine when administered to HIV-1 infected pregnant women during the second and third trimesters of pregnancy, followed by the administration to infants during the first six weeks of life, reduces risk of maternal-infant transmission of HIV-1 from approximately twenty three percent to eight percent.

QUESTIONS

Essay Questions:

1. Describe the structure, pathogenicity and laboratory diagnosis of human immunodeficiency virus.
2. Enumerate retroviruses and discuss about human immunodefeciency virus.

Short Notes:

1. Draw a neat labelled diagram of HIV and label its parts.
2. Prophylaxis against AIDS.
3. Draw a neat diagram of HIV and mention the routes of spread of HIV infection.
4. Mention the antigens of HIV.
5. List four opportunistic infections in AIDS.
6. Name four parasites that occur in AIDS patient.
7. Mention the routes of transmission of HIV.
8. Window period in HIV.
9. List three peptides of HIV-I used for the serodiagnosis.

101

Bacteriophages

- *Introduction*
- *Morphology*
- *Life cycle—virulent or lytic cycle.*
  —temperate or lysogenic cycle.
- *Phage typing.*

INTRODUCTION

A bacteriophage (phage) is a virus that replicates inside of a bacterial cell and consists of a piece of nucleic acid encapsulated in a protective protein coat. Depending on the phage, the nucleic acid can be DNA or RNA, double-stranded or single-stranded, and can have a size from about 3000 bases (3 genes) to about 2,00,000 bases (200 genes).

Phages (phage = to eat) occur widely in nature in close association with bacteria. They can be readily isolated from feces, sewage and other natural sources of mixed bacterial growth. The presence of phages in some natural waters suggests that they may have a role in the control of bacterial populations in such environments. Phages play an important role in the transmission of genetic information between bacteria by the process of transduction. Phages have been used as cloning vectors in genetic engineering.

MORPHOLOGY

Bacteriophages that infect *E.coli* are known as **T even phages** (T2, T4, T6). They serve as prototypes to study the properties of phages. T even phages are tadpole shaped, with a hexagonal head and cylindrical tail. The head consists of a tightly packed core of nucleic acid (dsDNA) surrounded by a protein coat or capsid. The size of the head varies in different phages from 28 nm to 100 nm. The tail is composed of a hollow core, a contractile sheath surrounding the core and a terminal base plate which has six prongs and six tail fibres attached to it (Fig. 101.1). Some phages T1, T5 and lambda of *E.coli* do not possess a contractile sheath. Some phages may be nontailed icosahedral (*e.g.* $\phi \times 174$) or filamentous (*e.g.,* M13).

LIFE CYCLE

Depending upon the nature of relationship to the host bacterium, the life cycle of phages is of two types. (*i*) virulent or lytic cycle, and (*ii*) temperate or lysogenic cycle.

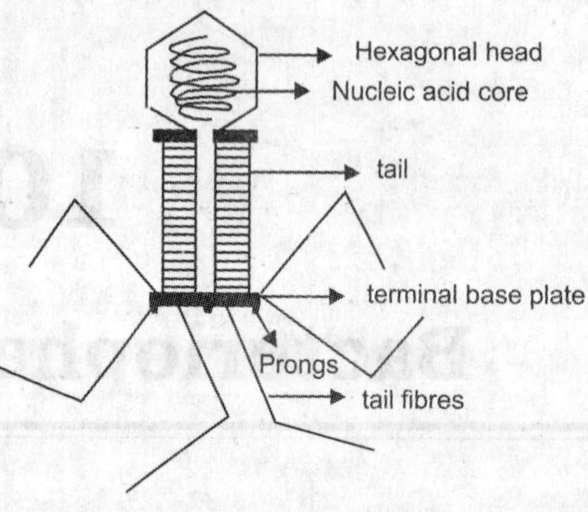

Fig. 101.1 Bacteriophage structure

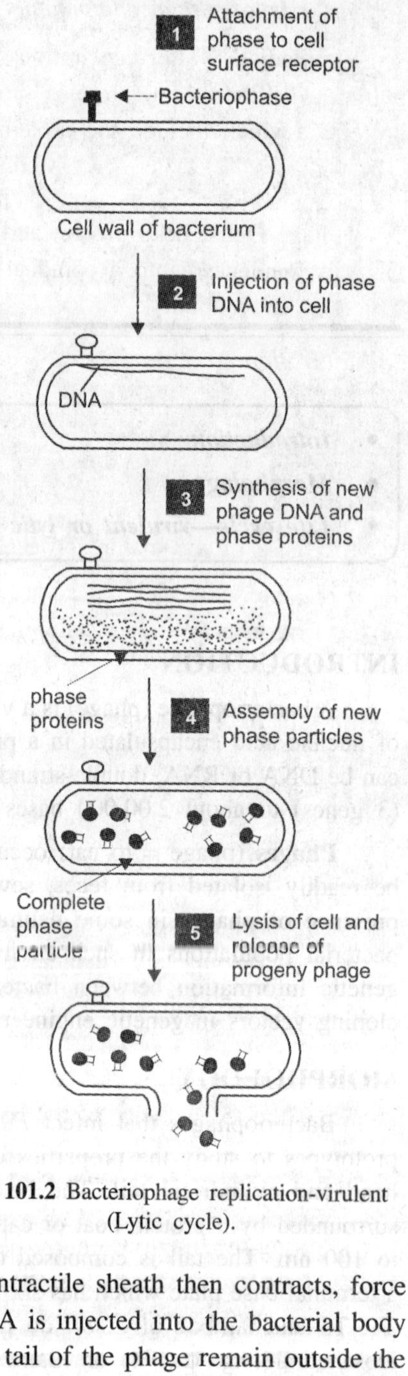

Fig. 101.2 Bacteriophage replication-virulent (Lytic cycle).

Virulent or Lytic Cycle

Infection of a bacterium with a virulent phage results in the death of the host cell by lysis, with release of newly replicated phage particles. Under optimal conditions, a bacterial cell infected with only one phage particle can produce hundreds of progeny phage in twenty minutes. Generally, phage that attack one bacterial species do not attack other bacterial species, which forms the basis of phage typing.

Replication of a virulent phage comprise the following stages: (Fig. 101.2).

1. Adsorption

Phage particles attach to the specific receptors on the host cell by its tail by random collision. Adsorption is a specific process and depends on the presence of complimentary chemical groups on the receptor sites of the bacterial surface and on the terminal base plate of the phage. The infection of a bacterium by the naked phage nucleic acid is known as **transfection**.

2. Penetration

The process of penetration resembles injection through a syringe. Six tail fibres make contact with the host cell surface and firmly attach the terminal base plate to it. The contractile sheath then contracts, force the hollow core to pierce through the cell wall. The phage DNA is injected into the bacterial body through the hollow core. After penetration, the empty head and tail of the phage remain outside the bacterium as the shell or "ghost". Penetration may be facilitated by the presence of **lysozyme**, present in the phage tail, which produces a hole in the bacterial cell wall. The contractile sheath acts like a muscle and derives its energy from ATP present in the phage tail.

3. Synthesis of phage components

Immediately after penetration of the phage nucleic acid, the synthesis of the phage components is initiated. First, "early proteins" appear, which are the enzymes necessary for the synthesis of "late proteins", which include the protein subunits of the phage head and tail.

4. Assembly

Phage DNA, head protein and tail protein are synthesized separately in the bacterial cell. The DNA is condensed into a compact polyhedron and "packaged" into the head and, finally the tail structures are added.

5. Maturation

This assembly of the phage components into the mature infective phage particle is known as maturation.

6. Release

Release of the mature progeny phages typically occurs by lysis of the bacteral cell.

The interval between the entry of the phage nucleic acid into the bacterial cell and the appearance of the first infectious intracellular phage particle is known as the **eclipse phase**. It represents the time required for the synthesis of the phage components and their assembly into mature phage particles.

Temperate or Lysogenic Cycle

Temperate phage enter into a symbiotic relationship with their host cells without lysing them. Following entry into the host cell, the temperate phage DNA becomes integrated with the bacterial chromosome. This integrated phage DNA is known as ***prophage***. The prophages behaves like a segment of the host chromosome and replicates synchronously with it.

This phenomenon is called lysogeny and a bacterium that carries a prophage within its genome is called *lysogenic bacterium.* (Fig. 101.3).

The prophage confers certain new properties on the lysogenic bacterium. This is known as lysogenic conversion or phage conversion. An example is toxin production by the diphtheria bacillus, which is determined by the presence in it of the **prophage beta**. The elimination of the prophage abolishes the toxigenicity of the bacillus.

A lysogenic bacterium is resistant to reinfection by the same or related phages. This is known as superinfection immunity.

During the multiplication of lysogenic bacteria, the prophage may become 'excised' which may initiate lytic cycle. This is known as spontaneous induction of prophage. All lysogenic bacteria in a population can be induced to shift to the lytic cycle by exposure to certain physical and chemical agents such as UV rays, hydrogen peroxide and nitrogen mustard.

PHAGE TYPING

The specificity of phage-bacterium interaction is made use in the identification and typing of bacteria in the epidemiological studies. Phage typing is used for intraspecies typing of bacteria during outbreaks of infections caused by *Staphylococcus aureus*, *Salmonella typhi*, *Vibrio cholerae* and *Bacillus anthracis.*

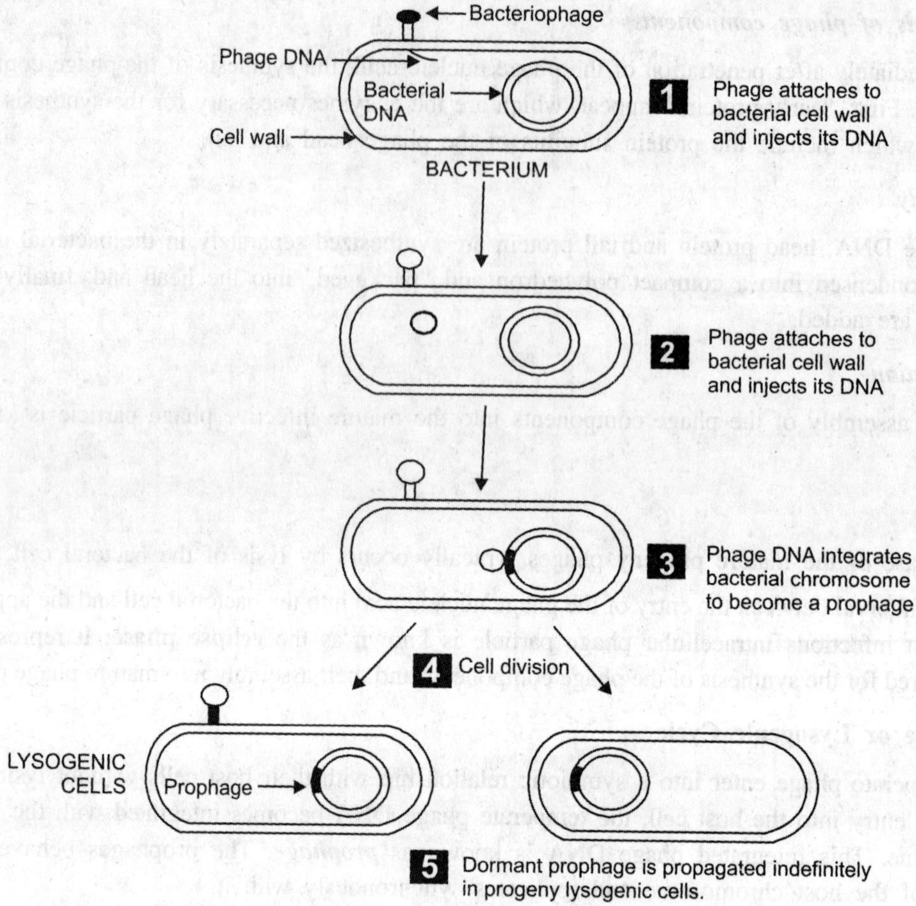

Fig. 101.3 Lysogenic cycle-The integration of phage DNA into the bacterial chromosome

The strain to be typed is inoculated on a plate of nutrient agar to produce a lawn (carpet) culture. After drying, the phages are applied over marked squares in a fixed dose (routine test dose). After overnight incubation, the culture will be observed to be lysed by some phages but not by others. The phage type of the strain is expressed by the designation of the phages that lyse it. Area of lysis caused by phage is known as **plaque**.

QUESTIONS

Essay Question:

1. What are bacteriophages? Describe their life cycle. Add a note on their importance in bacterial genetics.
2. Give an account of bacteriophages.

Short Notes:

1. Bacteriophage
2. Morphology of bacteriophage
3. Life cycle of bacteriophage
4. Lysogeny
5. Phage typing
6. Prophage
7. Draw a neat diagram of bacteriophage and label it.
8. Transfection.

PART-V

MEDICAL MYCOLOGY

102

Introduction to Medical Mycology

- *Introduction to fungi*
- *Classification of fungi*
- *Fungus infections (mycoses)*
- *Laboratory diagnosis of mycoses*
- *Treatment of mycoses*

INTRODUCTION TO FUNGI

The branch of biology, which deals with the study of fungi, is known as Mycology (mykes = mushroom). Medical Mycology is the study of epidemiology, ecology, pathogenesis, diagnosis and treatment of fungal diseases in human beings.

The fungi are a diverse group of heterotrophic organisms that exist as saprophytes, commensals or parasites. Most of them are found on decaying vegetative material and in the soil. They are devoid of chlorophyll and reproduce by means of conidia or spores produced asexually or sexually. Fungi are eukaryotic protists that differ from bacteria and other prokaryotes in many ways.

(*i*) They possess rigid cell walls containing chitin, mannan and other polysaccharides.

(*ii*) The cytoplasmic membrane contains sterols.

(*iii*) They possess true nuclei with nuclear membrane and paired chromosomes.

(*iv*) They possess cell organelles such as mitochondria, golgi bodies, endoplasmic reticulum etc.

(*v*) They divide asexually, sexually or by both processes.

(*vi*) They may be unicellular or multicellular.

The simplest type of fungus is the unicellular budding yeast. Elongation of the cell produces a tubular, thread like structure called **hypha**. They grow by apical extension, forming an interwoven, tangled mass of hyphae called **mycelium**. The hypha is a structural unit of mycelium. Fungi which form mycelia are called molds or filamentous fungi. Hyphae may be septate or nonseptate. The septa, when present, have holes through which free flow of cytoplasmic material can take place. When hyphae are nonseptate, they are multinucleated and are known as coenocytic. In a growing colony of filamentous fungus, the mycelium can be divided into vegetative mycelium which grows into the substrate and the aerial mycelium which projects from the surface.

CLASSIFICATION OF FUNGI

Morphological Classification of Fungi

Based on morphology, fungi can be divided into four groups.

1. **Yeasts**—They are unicellular fungi which occur as spherical or ellipsoidal cells and reproduce by budding. On culture, they form smooth, creamy colonies. Most of the yeasts are nonpathogenic *e.g.*, *Saccharomyces cerevisiae*; but a few are pathogenic *e.g.*, *Cryptococcus neoformans*.
2. **Yeast-like fungi**—These fungi grow partly as yeast and partly as elongated cells resembling hyphae, known as *pseudomycelium*. These fungi reproduce by budding but the buds fail to get separated and elongation takes place forming pseudohyphae *e.g.*, *Candida* species, *Malassezia*.
3. **Molds or filamentous fungi**—They form true mycelia and reproduce by the formation of different types of spores. These spores germinate to form vegetative hyphae, which may be septate or aseptate. e.g., Dermatophytes, *Aspergillus*, *Penicillium*, *Mucor* and *Rhizopus*.
4. **Dimorphic fungi**—These fungi have two types of morphology at different temperatures i.e. yeast forms at body temperature, 37°C (in tissue lesions and in cultures at 37°C) and mycelial form at room temperature, 25°C (in soil and in cultures at 25°C). Most of the true pathogenic fungi are dimorphic in nature e.g., *Histoplasma capsulatum*, *Sporothrix schenkii*, *Blastomyces dermatitidis*, *Coccidioides immitis*, *Paracoccidioides brasiliensis* and *Penicillium marneffei*.

Systematic classification of fungi

Systematic classification is based on the formation of sexual spores; fungi have been divided into four classes.

1. **Zygomycetes (phycomycetes, lower fungi)**—The mycelia are usually nonseptate and form nonmotile, endogenous asexual spores known as **sporangiospores**, produced in indefinite numbers within a swollen sac-like structures called **sporangia**. The sexual fusion results in the formation of a resting, thick-walled cell, known as **zygospore**. e.g., *Mucor*, *Rhizopus*.
2. **Ascomycetes**—Sexual fusion of fungi results in a sac or **Ascus** containing the meiotic products as four to eight spores called as **ascospores**. The mycelia are septate and produce exogenous, asexual spores called **"conidia"**. e.g., *Penicillium*, *Aspergillus*.
3. **Basidiomycetes**—Sexual fusion results in the formation of characteristic club-shaped organs called as **"basidia"**. The basidia are usually aseptate structures with four tiny projections called sterigmata and each sterigma bears haploid meiospore, called "**basidiospore**". The mycelium is septate, branched and produces exogenous asexual spores called **"conidia"** at the tips of hyphae *e.g.*, *Schizophyllum*, *Coprinus*.
4. **Deuteromycetes (Fungi imperfecti)**—It is an artificial group of fungi in which the sexual process has not yet been observed and the fungi are temporarily placed. The mycelia are septate and branched and produce exogenous, asexual spores called **conidia**, which are borne either by budding or on a specialized conidiophore or in a pycnidium. e.g., Dermatophytes.

FUNGUS INFECTIONS (MYCOSES)

According to the site of primary involvement, the fungal diseases of man can be classified into several types.

(i) Superficial mycoses—They involve the outermost layer of skin and its appendages like hair and nail. They can be subdivided into two types :

(*a*) **Surface mycoses**—Fungi infect nonliving surface tissues of skin, hair and nail and cannot induce any immune response e.g. Pityriasis (Tinea) versicolor, Tinea nigra and Piedra.

(*b*) **cutaneous mycoses**—Fungi infect living tissues of skin, hair and nail and can elicit immune response. e.g., Dermatophytes.

(ii) Deep mycoses—Deep mycotic infections may be classified as those that affect subcutaneous tissues and those that involve the internal organs (systemic mycoses).

(*a*) **Subcutaneous mycoses**—They are slowly progressive, chronic granulomatous infections of skin and subcutaneous tissues with involvemnt of underlying fasciae and bone, usually affecting the extremities e.g., Mycetoma, Sporotrichosis, Chromoblastomycosis, Phaeohyphomycosis, Rhinosporidiasis and Lobomycosis.

(*b*) **Systemic mycoses**—These diseases involve the internal organs like lungs, brain due to dissemination through blood. The causative fungi are usually dimorphic, which are endemic in certain parts of America. e.g., Histoplasmosis, Blastomycosis, Coccidioidomycosis and paracoccidioidomycosis.

(iii) Opportunistic mycoses—These diseases are produced by nonpathogenic fungi or contaminants in persons whose immunological defense mechanisms are weakened by endogenous causes like cancer, leukemia, AIDS or exogenous causes like immunosuppressive therapy, aggressive use of drugs and corticosteroids. e.g., Candidiasis, Cryptococcosis, Pneumocystosis, Aspergillosis, Zygomycosis (mucormycosis), Penicilliosis marneffei.

(iv) Miscellaneous mycoses—These diseases include that could not be grouped under any of the above disease groups e.g., allergic diseases, mycotoxicoses, mycetisms, oculomycosis and otomycosis.

LABORATORY DIAGNOSIS OF FUNGAL DISEASES

Specimens for the diagnosis of mycoses include skin scrapings, hair stubs, nail clippings, blood, CSF, sputum, bronchial lavage specimens, pus, biopsy tissues, urine, corneal scrapings, oral scrapings and vaginal scrapings etc., depending on the site of involvement. The fungal etiology of diseases can be established by following methods.

1. Direct Microscopic examination

The direct demonstration of fungi in clinical specimens is very important in the diagnosis of mycoses.

(*a*) **Wet mounts—10% KOH mount**—Specimens such as skin, hair and nail should be mounted under coverslip in 10% KOH on a slide, and allowed to stand for 30 min. to bring about "clearing".

The alkali digests tissue materials, exposing the fungal filaments. Warming over a low flame hastens the digestion of Keratin. The detection of fungus in nails may be possible only after clearing with 20% KOH for overnight or one day (Fig. 102.1).

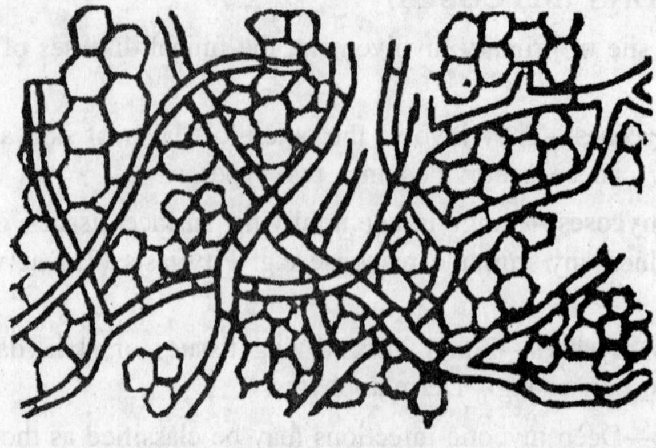

Fig. 102.1. Fungal filaments (hyphae) in skin scrapings in KOH wet mount partially digested epithelial cells form the background

Calcofluor (Blankophor) white wet mount is a sensitive procedure for the visualization of morphology of fungi. A drop of calcofluor white (0.1%) solution can be added to 10% KOH preparation. Calcofluor white is an industrial textile brightener, which nonspecifically binds to chitin and other polysaccharides of the fungal cell wall.

Fungal filaments exhibit fluorescence blue-white or apple-green, depending on the combination of filters used under UV illumination. Calcofluor white fluorescence occurs maximally at an excitation wavelength of 440 nm and fluorescenc blue-white. Since calcofluor white is a nonspecific stain, the actual fungal filaments must be seen before a positive preparation is reported. The presence of KOH in the solution dissolves human cellular elements and debris; this allows for easier visualization of fungal elements.

In the wet mounts under low and high power microscope, yeast cells with or without pseudohyphae, septate hyphae, nonseptate hyphae, spherules, arthrospores or any of the fungal form is visible.

Arthrospores are vegetative spores. The septa in the hypha form chains of small cuboidal or rectangular cells with slightly thickened wall that disarticulate at maturity. The arthrospore production is a characteristic feature of the parasitic phase of dermatophytes and the mycelial phase of *Coccidioides immitis*.

(*b*) **Histopathology**—The hematoxylin and eosin (H & E) staining, Periodic Acid-Schiff (PAS) stain, Gomori's Methanamine Silver (GMS) stains and Gridley stains are widely used for demonstrating fungi in tissues. Masson-Fontana stain is specifically used for the demonstration of phaeoid fungi in tissues.

Periodic Acid-Schiff (PAS) Stain

The principle of PAS stain is that polysaccharides of fungi are oxidized by periodic acid to form aldehyde groups that yield red colored compounds with Schiff's fuchsin sulphite. The proteins and nucleic acids remain unstained. The fungi stain magenta or red.

For PAS staining, following stain solutions are required :

(*i*) 5% aqueous periodic acid

(*ii*) Schiff's reagent

Basic fuchsin 1 gm

Distilled water	200 ml
Potassium/sodium metabisulfite	2 gm
conc. HCl	2 ml
Decolorizing charcoal	2 gm.

The staining is carried out by preparing the smear and fixing it through air drying. The slide is then immersed in 5% periodic acid for 5 minutes followed by 15 minutes in Schiff's reagent. Then the slide is rinsed in water for 5 to 10 minutes and air dried and examined under microscope.

(*c*) **Fluorescent-antibody staining** may be used to detect fungal antigens in clinical material such as pus, blood, CSF, tissue impression smears and in paraffin sections of formalin fixed tissue.

(*d*) **Negative staining** of India ink or nigrosin preparations can be used for the demonstration of capsule of *Cryptococcus neoformans*.

2. Fungal culture

The commonest culture media used in Medical Mycology is Sabouraud's dextrose agar (SDA) with a pH of 5.4. The ingredients of this medium are as follows :

Peptone	10 gm
Dextrose	40 gm
Agar	20 gm
Distilled water	1000 ml
Chloramphenicol	50 mg (0.05 gm)
or (Gentamicin	20 mg)
Cycloheximide	400 mg (0.4 gm)
pH	5.4

Autoclave at 121°C for 15 min.

The acidic pH and high content of sugar makes medium more selective for the isolation of pathogenic fungi Medium can be made further selective by adding antibiotics like chloramphenicol or gentamicin to prevent bacterial contamination and cycloheximide to prevent fungal contamination. Fungal growth is noted by big flowery colonies or pigmented colonies.

Czapek-Dox (CD) agar, Brain-heart infusion agar, blood agar, Cornmeal agar may also be employed for the isolation of fungi.

Growth on the medium is identified based on colony morphology (macroscopic appearance), microscopic morphology and other relevant tests. The colony morphology is studied based on following growth characteristics :

(*i*) rate of growth

(*ii*) color and morphology of the colony on the obverse

(*iii*) pigmentation on the reverse

Lactophenol cotton blue (LPCB) teased mounts

Microscopic examination of culture is done by removing a portion of aerial mycelium with a spud and placed on a glass slide into two or three drops of lactophenol cotton blue and mycelial mass is gently teased with a pair of teasing needles and a coverslip is placed over it. The mount was first observed under low power and then under high power microscope, for presence of hyphae (septate or nonseptate), special hyphal structures such as spiral hyphae, localised swellings formed by tightly twisted hyphae resembling tennis racquets (racquet hyphae) and numerous short branches appearing at the ends of hyphae (favic chandelier). The morphology of asexual spores or **conidia** is of diagnostic importance. They may be small, unicellular "microconidia" or large, unicellular or multicellular "macroconidia". The type of spore formation is distinctive for different fungi. **'Blastospores'** are formed by budding in yeasts. **Chlamydospores** are thick walled, vegetative resting spores formed by rounding up and thickening of hyphal segments (Fig. 102.2).

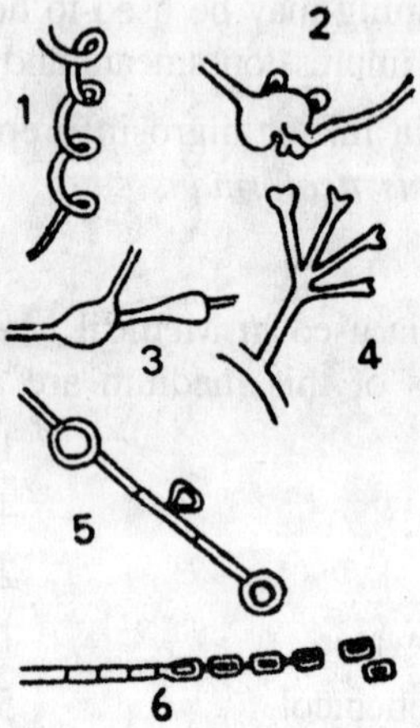

Fig. 102.2. Mycelial forms and asexual spores of fungi
1. Spiral hypha. 2. Nodular organ. 3. Racquet mycelium. 4. Favic chandelier. 5. Chlamydospores. 6. Arthrospores.

This lactophenol cotton blue wet mount can be preserved for few months by sealing the edge of the coverslip with nail polish. The LPCB stain solution contains lactic acid (act as a preservative), phenol (disinfectant) and cotton blue for staining.

Slide Culture

Slide culture technique is used to examine fungal growth in its original form without disturbing the spore arrangement.

A piece of filter paper cut according to the shape of the petriplate is placed inside a sterile petri-plate. A 'V' or 'U' tube is placed on filter paper. A clean glass slide is placed on the 'V' tube perpendicularly and one to two coverslips are placed inside the plate. Petridish was closed with the lid, wrapped with paper and sterilized in hot air oven.

Blocks (1×2 cms) of Sabouraud's dextrose agar with chloramphenicol and cycloheximide, poured into a petriplate to a depth of 4 mm are cut using sterile scalpel blade. One such block is transferred on to the glass slide supported on V-tube in a petri plate. Corners of the agar block is inoculated with the fungal colony. A coverslip is flamed and placed on the surface of agar block using sterile forceps. Little amount of sterile distilled water is added to filter paper and closed with lid and incubated at room temperature. After each day or two, the slide is taken out of petridish and examined under microscope without disturbing the coverslip. When sporulation is well evident, coverslip is carefully removed from the agar block and placed on a drop of lactophenol cotton blue stain taken on a separate glass slide and examined under the microscope.

TREATMENT OF FUNGAL DISEASES

Several antifungal agents are used for the treatment of mycoses, which are listed herebelow :

(i) Antifungal antibiotics

(a) Polyenes—Amphotericin-B, Nystatin, Natamycin, Hamycin.

(b) Others—Griseofulvin.

(ii) Synthetic antifungal agents

(a) Thiocarbamates—Tolnaftate, Tolciclat, Naftifine.

(b) Allylamines—Terbinafine, Bifonazole

(c) Azoles— Clotrimazole, Itraconazole, Miconazole, oxiconazole, Fenticonazole, Tioconazole, Butoconazole, Econazole, Fluconazole, Ketoconazole, Omoconazole, Sulconazole, Tercanazole.

(iii) Miscellaneous antifungal agents

Flucytosine, Ciclopiroxolamine, Amorolfine, Whitfield's ointment, potassium iodide, Selenium sulfide, Undecylenic acid, Haloprogin, Triacetin, Sulphonamides, Gention violet paint.

Antifungal Drug Resistance

Some of the fungi associated with diseases do not respond to the antifungal treatment due to the development of drug resistance. This type of difficulty was being faced in bacterial or parasitic infections but now it has cropped up in fungal diseases as well. Therefore, the antifungal susceptibility testing is performed to provide information that allows the physician to select an appropriate antifungal agent useful for treating a particular fungal infection.

In vitro susceptibility testing of antifungal agents is becoming increasingly important. The US National Committee for Clinical Laboratory Standards (NCCLS) has released the approved version (M 27-A) of standardized broth macrodilution and microdilution methods for the antifungal susceptibility testing of yeasts in 1997. The NCCLS has also proposed the antifungal susceptibility testing of conidia forming filamentous fungi in 1998 which can be performed as per the M38-P document on a similar pattern as that of yeasts.

QUESTIONS

Essay Question

1. Describe the laboratory diagnosis of fungal diseases.

Short Notes

1. Hyphae
2. Mycelium
3. Classification of medically important fungi
4. Morphological classification of fungi
5. Classification of fungi based on sexual spores
6. Arthrospores or Arthroconidia
7. Chlamydospores
8. 10% KOH mount
9. Lactophenol cotton blue stain
10. Sabouraud's dextrose agar
11. PAS
12. Slide culture for fungus
13. Mention four antifungal agents
14. Lab. diagnosis of mycoses
15. Antifungal drug resistance

103

Superficial mycoses

- *Pityriasis versicolor*
- *Tinea nigra*
- *Piedra*
- *Dermatophytoses*

PITYRIASIS VERSICOLOR

It is a chronic, usually asymptomatic, mild, recurrent superficial fungal infection of stratum corneum, characterised by multiple, well defined, non-inflammatory, macular lesions with fine scaling which are discrete or confluent. The lesions may appear hypopigmented or hyperpigmented. In pityriasis versicolor, although any part of the body may be involved but neck, upper part of trunk, face and upper aspects of are the most commonly affected sites.

The disease is world-wide in distribution, but commonly prevalent in tropics and young adults. Excessive sweating is one of the significant predisposing factor.

The disease is caused by lipophilic, yeast-like fungus, called *Malassezia furfur* (*Pityrosporum orbiculare*). It is a normal commensal of skin.

Diagnosis is established by microscopic examination of skin scrapings under 10% KOH wet mount. Clusters of round yeast cells, 2 to 7 μm in size, with occasional buddings are observed. The hyphae are blunt, short and stout that may be curved and infrequently branched. The characteristic "banana and grapes" or "spaghetti and meat balls" forms are diagnostic (Fig. 103.1).

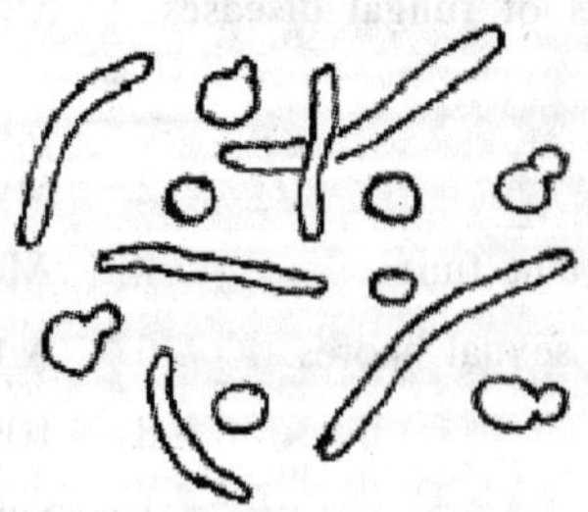

Fig. 103.1 *Malassezia furfur*

Skin scrapings can also be obtained by applying a piece of scotch tape with its adhesive side down followed by pressing the tape firmly to recover the scales.

The fungus can be isolated by inoculating skin scrapings on Sabouraud dextrose agar containing chloramphenicol and cycloheximide. The surface of the medium is overlaid by a thin layer of olive oil. Creamy colonies develop within 5-7 days at 37°C. Lactophenol cotton blue wet mount of the colonies shows budding yeast cells. Hyphae are rarely seen.

Most of the patients of pityriasis versicolor seek medical advice for cosmetic reasons.

TINEA NIGRA

It is a superficial fungal infection of skin characterized by brown to black, deeply pigmented, non-scaly, macular lesions usually affecting the skin of palms and that of soles. It is an asymptomatic infection of stratum corneum, caused by a phaeoid (dematiaceous) fungus, *Hortaea werneckii*. The causative fungus is also known by its synonyms like *Cladosporium werneckii* or *Exophiala werneckii*.

The disease is world-wide and more common among young people.

The epidermal scrapings under 10% KOH wet mount shows brown, septate, branching hyphae and budding yeast cells (Fig. 103.2). Colonies on Sabouraud dextrose agar appear within a week at 25 to 30°C and no growth is seen at 37°C. Initially colonies are brown but later become black colored.

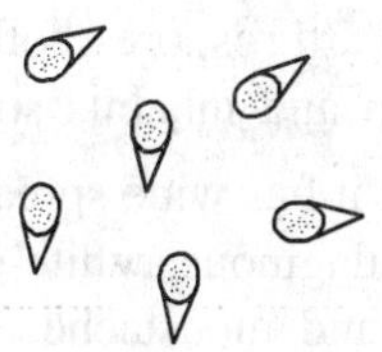

Fig. 103.2 Yeast-like cells of *Hortaea werneckii*

PIEDRA

It is a superficial fungal infection of hair shaft characterized by development of firm, irregular nodules of fungal elements cemented to the hair. There are two types of piedra

(*i*) Black piedra caused by *Piedraia hortae*

(*ii*) White piedra caused by *Trichosporon* species.

Black piedra

It is a nodular type of infection of hair shaft and is caused by a phaeoid fungus ***Piedraia hortae***, an ascomycetous fungi. The disease is also known as "tinea nodosa". It occurs in tropical and subtropical areas of Africa, Asia and Latin America. It is characterized by the formation of discrete, black, gritty hard nodules mainly on the hair of scalp (Fig. 103.3).

The diagnosis is established by microscopic examination of a crushed brittle nodule in 10% KOH wet mount. There are dark colored, septate hyphae around the surface of hair with round to oval asci containing 2-8 hyaline, curved, fusiform aseptate ascospores that bear one or more whip-like appendages at both ends. Many septations in thick-walled hyphae give appearance of arthrospores.

On Sabouraud dextrose agar with chloramphenicol and glycerin and without actidione at 25°C, the culture shows slow growing, dark brown to black, velvety colonies, heaped up at the centre with a flat periphery; with reddish-brown diffusible pigment on agar. The microscopic examination of colonies in lactophenol cotton blue teased mount reveals dark colored hyphae.

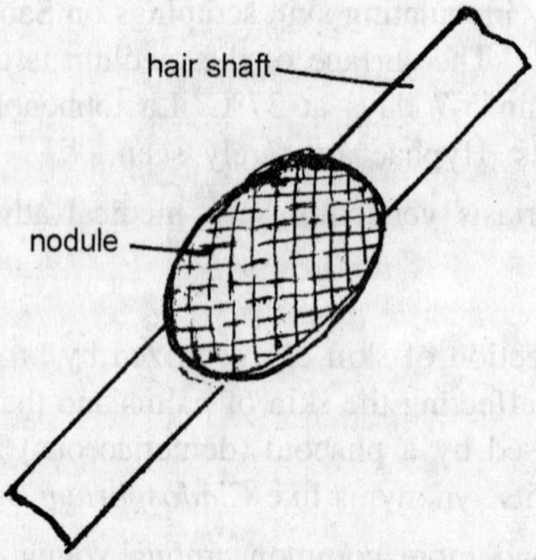

Fig. 103.3 Black piedra-*Piedraia hortae* showing nodules on the hair shaft

White piedra

It is a superficial fungal infection of hair shaft characterized by soft, greyish-white nodules, caused by a yeast-like fungus, *Trichosporon beigelii*, formerly known as *Trichosporon cutaneum*. The fungus is present as branched hyphae and arthrospores both within and around the hair. Trichosporon beigelii is present as normal flora of skin and inhabits soil.

Although white piedra is uncommon it has wide spread distribution in South America and Japan. The disease is characterized by soft, mucilaginous, white-greyish or light brown nodules on the hair shafts of genital area, pubic area, beard and moustache. The fungi grow inward and through shaft to form nodular swellings spaced irregularly along the axis. The hair is weakened at these points hence may easily break. The growth occurs as a collarette around hair shaft and consists of mycelia that fragment into arthrospores (Fig. 103.4).

Under direct microscopic examination of epilated hair, the fungus is seen as hyphae and rectangular arthrospores within and around hair. In this disease, there is no fluorescence under the wood's lamp examination. On Sabouraud dextrose agar with chloramphenicol at 37°C, it forms moist, cream colored, soft, wrinkled colonies. Microscopic examination in lactophenol cotton blue mount reveals septate hyphae that rapidly fragment into arthrospores.

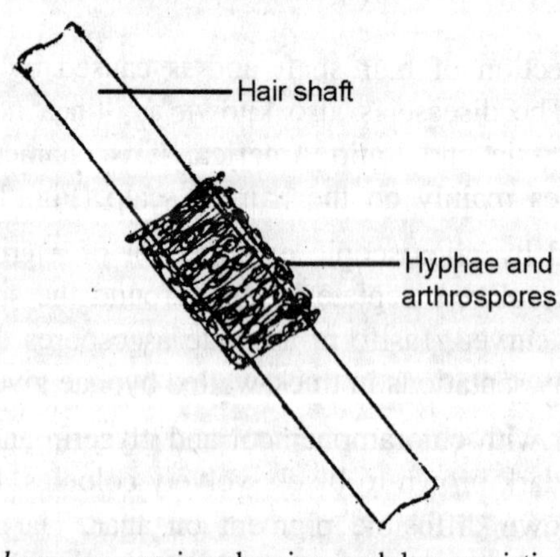

Fig. 103.4 White piedra-*Trichosporon* species showing nodules consisting of hyphae and arthrospores

DERMATOPHYTOSES

Dermatophytoses are the most common types of cutaneous fungal infections seen in man and animals affecting skin, hair and nails. These are caused by a group of filamentous fungi, closely related to each other taxonomically, morphologically, physiologically and antigenically; which have the capacity to invade keratinized tissues of skin and its appendages and are collectively known as "**dermatophytes**". Other frequently used terms like "**tinea**" and "**ringworm**" infections are synonyms of dermatophytoses. The infections caused by nondermatophytic fungi involving the skin are called as "**dermatomycoses**" whereas involving hair and nail are called "piedra" and "**onychomycosis**" respectively.

The dermatophytes are assigned to three main genera namely *Trichophyton, Microsporum* and *Epidermophyton*. All these three fungi belong to Division Deuteromycetes, Class Hyphomycetes, Order Moniliales and family Moniliaceae. Dermatophytoses are caused by 42 species of dermatophytes (*Trichophyton*-24, *Microsporum*-16 and *Epidermophyton*-2). All these fungi reproduce asexually and atleast for some, their sexual states are also reported. The terms anamorph (asexual) and teleomorph (sexual) is often used to describe the taxonomic status of the organism. The teleomorphic states of dermatophytes, genus ***Arthroderma*** is placed in the family Arthrodermataceae of the order Onygenales in class plectomycetes of Division Ascomycota.

In lesions, dermatophytes appear as hyphae and arthrospores. In cultures on Sabouraud's dextrose agar, they form characteristic colonies consisting of septate hyphae and two types of asexual spores, microconidia and macroconidia. The three genera are differentiated by their conidial morphology.

Trichophyton

The colonies are powdery, velvety or waxy with pigmentation characteristic of a particular species. They produce **microconidia** abundantly that may be globose or pyriform and are borne singly along the sides of the hyphae or in grape like clusters. **Macroconidia** are sparse, if present they are elongated, smooth-walled, pencil shaped with blunt ends.

Examples of pathogenic *Trichophyton* species include *T. rubrum*, *T. mentagrophytes*, *T. violaceum*, *T. tonsurans*, *T. schoenleinii*, *T. verrucosum*, *T. concentricum*, *T. equinum*, *T. simii*, *T. soudanense*, *T. gourvillii*, *T. megninii*.

T. rubrum is the commonest species infecting man. It produces clavate, tear drop shaped microconidia along the sides of the hyphae, abundantly. The colonies of *T. rubrum* develop cherry red color pigmentation on the reverse.

The colonies of *T. mentagrophytes* range from granular to powdery and usually exhibit abundant grape-like clusters of subspherical microconidia on terminal branches. The granular form of *T. mentagrophytes* is world-wide in distribution. The spiral hyphae are frequent in *T. mentagrophytes*.

Microsporum

The colonies arc cottony, velvety or powdery, with white to brown pigmentation. The macroconidia are predominant which are large, rough-walled, multicellular, spindle-shaped and are formed at the ends of hyphae. Microconidia are scanty; if present they are usually arranged along the sides of hyphae. Examples of pathogenic Microsporum species are : *M. audouinii, M. gypseum, M. canis, M. nanum, M. ferrugineum, M. equinum, M. fulvum, M. persicolor, M. gallinae, M. vanbreuseghemii, M. racemosum, M. praecox* etc.

M. gypseum colonies grow rapidly producing a flat, spreading, powdery surface that is cinnamon-buff to brown which consists of abundant macroconidia. They are boat-shaped, rough walled with

4-6 septa. M. audouinii rarely forms conidia in the culture but many thick walled chlamydospores (chlamydoconidia) may be present. On rice grain medium *M. audouinii* does not grow, while other *Microsporum* species grow rapidly. *M. canis* forms numerous thick-walled, 8-15 celled macroconidia with curved or hooked spiny tips. A lemon-yellow or yellow-orange pigment develops on the reverse of the colony.

Epidermophyton

Colonies are powdery and greenish-brown (khaki-colored). Microconidia are not produced. Macroconidia are abundant and multicellular (one to nine celled) smooth, thin walled, pear or club-shaped arranged in clusters. *e.g.*, *E. floccosum*, *E. stockdaleae.*

Table 103.1 Distribution of Conidia of Dermatophytes (Fig. 103.5)

Dermatophytes	*Microconidia*	*Macroconidia*
Trichophyton	Abundant (except *T. schoenleinii*)	rare, thin walled, smooth, elongated
Microsporum	rare	abundant, thick-walled rough, spindle shaped (except *M. audouinii*)
Epidermophyton	absent	abundant, smooth walled, pear or club-shaped, arranged in clusters

Ecologically, depending on their natural habitat dermatophytes may be classified as anthropophilic, zoophilic and geophilic species.

Anthropophilic dermatophytes

The fungal species exclusively affecting humans are known as "anthropophilic". They are transmitted by comb, hairbrushes, caps, fallen hairs, desquamated epithelium, swimming pools, showers, towels, etc. The migration of labour, troops movement, emigration and travel play important role in spreading of these fungi *e.g.*, *T. rubrum*, *T. mentagrophytes*, *T. violaceum*, *T. schoenleinii*, *T. tonsurans*, *T. concentricum*, *T. megninii*, *T. soudanense*, *M. audouinii*, *M. ferrugineum* and *E. floccosum*.

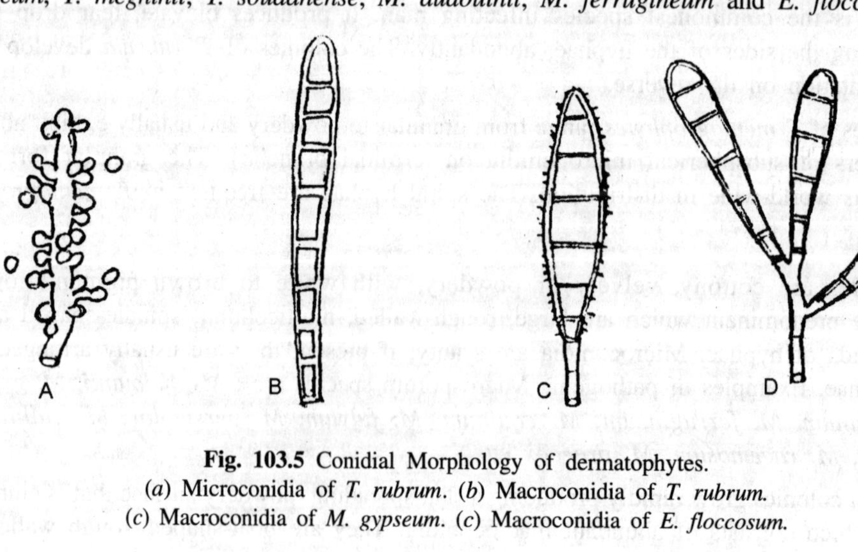

Fig. 103.5 Conidial Morphology of dermatophytes.
(*a*) Microconidia of *T. rubrum*. (*b*) Macroconidia of *T. rubrum*.
(*c*) Macroconidia of *M. gypseum*. (*c*) Macroconidia of *E. floccosum*.

Zoophilic dermatophytes

They inhabit domestic and wild animals such as birds. Human infections are usually acquired by direct contact with animals. Certain zoophilic species may be isolated from soil and fur of apparently healthy animals *e.g., T. verrucosum, T. equinum, T. mentagrophytes, T. simii, M. canis, M. equinum, M. gallinae*.

Geophilic dermatophytes

The natural habitat of these species is the soil. They occur as saprophytes of keratinaceous material in soil. Exposure to soil is the main source of infection for humans and animals *e.g., T. ajelloi, T. terrestre, M. gypseum, M. nanum, M. cookie, M. persicolor, M. amazonicum, M. fulvum, M. racemosum, M. praecox*.

PATHOGENICITY

The dermatophytes grow only within dead, keratinized tissue. The fungi produce keratinolytic proteases, which provides means of entry into living cells. Fungal metabolic products diffuse through the Malphigian layer to cause erythema, vesicles and even pustule formation along with pruritus. The hyphae become old, break into arthrospores, which are shed off, leading to central clearing of the lesions. The lesions are circular and spread with an erythematous border with variable degree of scaling and inflammation.

The clinical manifestations of dermatophytosis are also called "tinea" or "ringworm" and are classified depending on the anatomical site involved.

(*i*) **Tinea capitis**—infection of shaft of scalp hairs. The hair break at follicular orifice which creates patches of alopecia with black dots of broken hairs. A severe form of tinea capitis is formation of **"Keroin"**. Keroin is a severely painful inflammatory reaction producing raised, circumscribed boggy mass on scalp with suppuration. Rarely, mycetoma like grains are produced. Keroin is usually caused by zoophilic dermatophytes such as *T. verrucosum, T. mentagrophytes* and *M. canis*.

"Black-dot" ringworm is usually caused by *T. tonsurans* and *T. violaceum*. They attack the hair shaft by endothrix type invasion with abundant sporulation inside the hair and the breakage of hair near the surface of the scalp. This phenomenon results in a "black-dot" appearance within an area of smooth scalp surface.

Favus (Tinea favosa) is usually caused by *T. schoenleinii*. The intense fungal growth within and around the hair follicle produces a waxy, honey comb-like crusts on the scalp. It may lead to alopecia and scarring. Hair invasion is of two types-ectothrix and endothrix (Fig. 103.6).

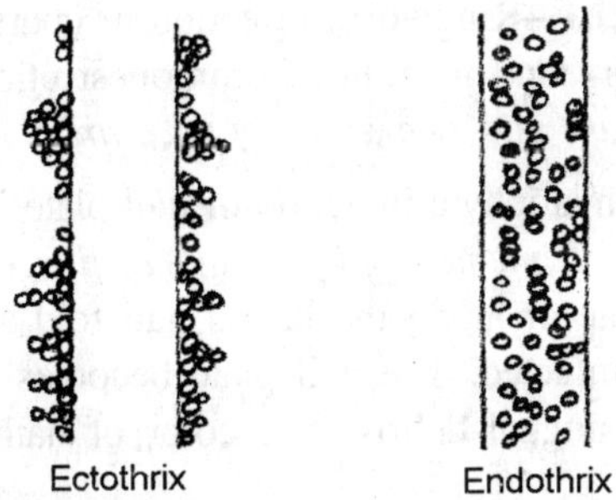

Fig. 103.6 Types of hair infection

(*a*) **Ectothrix infections**—The arthrospores appear as a mosaic sheath around the hair or as chains on the surface of the hair shaft. The cuticle of the hair remains intact. The fungi invade the hair shafts at mid-follicle. As the hair grows out of the follicle the hyphae burst out of the shaft and cover the hair surface with a mass of arthrospores. The infected hair become lustreless, brittle and hair filaments break off at the level of scalp to give an appearance of partial alopecia. *e.g.*, *T. mentagrophytes*, *M. gypseum*, *M. audouinii*, *M. canis*, *T. verrucosum*, *T. rubrum*.

(*b*) **Endothrix infections**—The fungi invade hair follicle and then the hair shaft and forms numerous arthrospores within the hair shaft, which is severely weakened. The cuticle of hair is destroyed. The arthrospores are observed in chains filling inside shortened hair stubs. The infected hair becomes greyish-white, breaks off easily to give "black-dot" appearance. *e.g.*, *T. schoenleinii*, *T. tonsurans*, *T. violaceum*, *T. soudanense*.

T. rubrum that rarely infects hair, has been observed to cause both ectothrix and endothrix infections.

(*iii*) **Tinea corporis**—It refers to the ringworm of glabrous (non-hairy) skin of the body with exception of scalp, hands, feet, nails and groin. The disease is characterized by erythematous-scaly lesions, annular, sharply marginated plaques with raised border which may be single, multiple or confluent. It is the most common type of dermatophytosis in India caused by *T. rubrum*, *T. mentagrophytes*, *T. tonsurans* and any other dermatophyte.

(*iv*) **Tinea cruris (Dhobie's itch, Jock itch)**—The ringworm of inguínale area involving the groin, perianal, perineal areas often involving the upper thigh. The disease is world-wide and is more prevalent in tropical countries. It is more common in men with an underlying predisposing factor such as long-term use of tight-fitting garments. *T. rubrum*, *T. mentagrophytes* and *E. floccosum* are common species causing this infection.

(*v*) **Tinea pedis (Athlete's foot)**—The ringworm infection of feet, toes, interdigital webs and sole. The most common clinical manifestation is intertriginous form associated with maceration, scaling, fissuring and erythema which presents with itching and burning. It is frequently seen among the individuals wearing shoes for long hours and popularly known as Athlete's foot. The warmth and moisture produced by the shoes are the key factors in establishing and maintaining the infection. *T. rubrum*, *T. mentagrophytes* and *E. floccosum* are the common species involved.

(*vi*) **Tinea manuum**—It is the infection of skin of palms, interdigital areas and fingers of hands and lesions present as diffuse hyperkeratotic areas. Most of these cases are caused by *T. rubrum*, *T. mentagrophytes* and *E. floccosum*.

(*vii*) **Tinea barbae (Barber's itch)**—Ringworm infection of coarse hairs of beard and moustache. The lesions are inflammatory and pustular. Commonest etiologic agents are *T. verrucosum*, *T. mentagrophytes*, *T. rubrum* and occasionally *M. canis*.

(*viii*) **Tinea unguium**—It is a dermatophyte infection of nail plates and is largely a disease of adults and is caused by *T. rubrum*, *T. mentagrophytes* and *E. floccosum*. The infection begins under the free edge of the nail plate or along the lateral nail fold and may continue until the entire nail plate and nail bed are infected. The nail plate becomes brittle, thickened and may crack because of piling up of subungual debris. The color of nail is often brown or black.

(*ix*) **Tinea faciei**—This is a dermatophytic infection of glabrous skin of face, excluding beard area. Commonest species associated with this disease are *T. rubrum*, *T. mentagrophytes* and *T. tonsurans*.

(*x*) ***Tinea imbricata***—This is an unusual form of tinea corporis, characterized by polycyclic, concentrically arranged rings of populosquamous patches of scales scattered over and often covering most of the body. It is caused by *T. concentricum* and found in limited geographical areas (Pacific and Fizi islands).

(*xi*) **Tinea gladiatorum**—It is an emerging dermatophyte infection in wrestlers acquired by direct skin-to-skin contact. Most of the lesions are on the arms, trunk or head and neck, corresponding to the areas of contact between the wrestlers. *T. tonsurans* is the commonest isolate.

(*xii*) **"Id" reaction or Dermatophytids**—They are allergic reactions to ringworm and occur in a large variety of clinical forms. The most common location is that a patient with tinea pedis suddenly develops itching and burning of both hands, usually beginning at the sides of fingers near the digital crease. In a few days, vesicles appear that enlarge to bullae and lesions spread to palm. The vesicles are sterile. The reaction may be the result of fungal metabolic products being absorbed from the skin and itching is the only symptom.

LABORATORY DIAGNOSIS

The clinical specimens collected are skin scrapings, nail clippings and hair stubs. The affected part is disinfected with 70% ethyl alcohol. After 1 to 2 minutes, with the help of sterile scalpel blade, scrapings are taken from the active border of the lesions in a sterile glossy paper. In case of nail infections, the superficial part of the nail is scraped away and deeper part of the nail and debris are collected. Infected hair can be selected by examination with Wood's lamp. The affected hairs were epilated with sterile forceps and part of the scalp material is collected in a sterile glossy paper.

Wood's lamp

It is useful in the diagnosis and management of superficial cutaneous fungal infections. Wood's glass consists of barium silicate containing about 9% nickel oxide. It transmits long-wave ultraviolet light with a peak of 365 nm that shows a characteristic fluorescence produced by some microorganisms. The infected hairs show green fluorescence under wood's lamp, particularly in *Microsporum* infections.

Table 103.2 Fluorescence of various Microorganisms under Wood's Lamp

Fluorescence	*Microorganisms*
Bright-green	*Microsporum audouinii*, *M. canis*
Blue-green	*M. ferrugineum*, *M. distortum*
Dull-yellow	*M. gypseum*
Dull-green	*T. schoenleinii*
Golden-yellow	*Malassezia furfur*
Coral-red	*Corynebacterium minutissimum*

Direct Microscopic examination

The specimen is placed on a slide in 10% KOH and covered with a coverslip. It is allowed to stand for 30 min or gently heated to bring about clearing of human cellular elements, so that fungal elements are exposed. In KOH wet mount, the fungus is seen as branching, septate hyphae, which frequently show arthrospores around and through epidermal scales. Demonstration of fungus in nails requires clearing with KOH for overnight. In hair infections, ectothrix and endothrix types may be distinguished. Specimens, particularly nail clippings stained with periodic acid-Schiff stain or Gomori's methanamine silver stains are more useful.

Culture

Specimen is inoculated in duplicate on Sabouraud's dextrose agar with antibiotics and cycloheximide and incubated at 25°C and 37°C. The growth is relatively slow and takes approximately 10 days to three weeks time. Dermatophyte species are identified based on colony morphology, color, pigment production, morphology of microconidia and macroconidia and associated features such as spiral hyphae, racquet hyphae, pectinate bodies, nodular organs and favic chandelier.

Dermatophyte test medium (DTM) is used to isolate and distinguish dermatophytes from the fungal or bacterial contaminants found in cutaneous lesions. It is a selective medium containing antibiotics and antifungal agents and phenol red indicator. It inhibits the growth of most bacteria and fungi, whereas dermatophytes can grow and release alkaline metabolites into the medium; as a result, the color of the medium changes from yellow to red.

In vitro hair perforation test

It is used to differentiate *T. rubrum* from *T. mentagrophytes*. A filter paper disk is placed in the bottom of a petridish, to which a few ml of distilled water is added, then a lock of child's hair are placed into the water and sterilized in an autoclave. Then, a few drops of sterile yeast extract medium is added and the hair strands are inoculated with test fungi and incubated at room temperature. The hair strands are examined microscopically in lactophenol cotton blue at weekly intervals for upto one month, for wedge shaped perforations (Fig. 103.7).

T. mentagrophytes produce hair perforating organs that penetrate hair radially and cause wedge shaped perforations, whereas T. rubrum grow on hair and disintegrate it without making perforations. The test is also used to differentiate *M. canis*, which can penetrate hair from *M. equinum* which cannot penetrate hair.

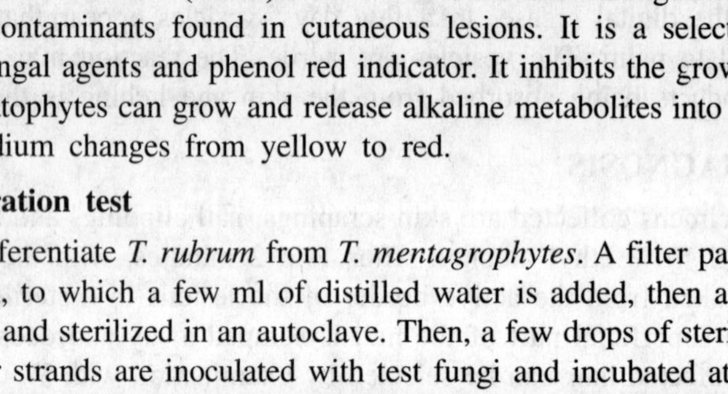

Fig. 103.7 *In vitro* hair perforation test showing wedge shaped perforations.

Urease test on Christensen's agar medium is used to differentiate *T. mentagrophytes*, which can hydrolyze urea and produce pink color; from *T. rubrum*, which is urease negative.

Rice grain test

The test is used to differentiate *M. audouinii* from other *Microsporum* species. On rice grain medium, all *Microsporum* species can grow and form conidia, but *M. audouinii* cannot grow.

Intradermal test with **"trichophytin"** antigen can be used to demonstrate delayed hypersensitivity. The trichophytin is a crude extract from dermatophytes.

QUESTIONS

Essay Question:

1. Describe the morphology, classification, pathogenicity and lab. diagnosis of dermatophytoses. Add a note on "id" reaction.

Short Notes:

1. Pityriasis versicolor
2. Malassezia furfur
3. Tinea nigra
4. Piedra
5. Black piedra
6. White piedra
7. Dermatophytes
8. Mention different species of dermatophytes
9. Trichophyton species
10. *Trichophyton* rubrum
11. *Microsporum*
12. *Microsporum gypseum*
13. *Microsporum canis*
14. *Epidermophyton* or *E. floccosum*
15. Anthropophilic dermatophytes
16. Zoophilic dermatophytes
17. Geophilic dermatophytes
18. Mention the conidia of dermatophytes
19. Ringworm or Tinea
20. Tinea capitis—lab. diagnosis
21. Favus
22. Ectothrix
23. Endothrix
24. Athlete's foot or tinea pedis
25. "Id" reaction or dermatophytids
26. Wood's lamp
27. Lab. diagnosis of dermatophytoses
28. DTM
29. Hair perforation test
30. Rice grain test.

104

Subcutaneous mycoses

- *Sporotrichosis*
- *Mycetema*
- *Chromoblastomycosis*
- *Phaeohyphomycosis*
- *Rhinosporidiosis*
- *Lobomycosis*

SPOROTRICHOSIS (ROSE GARDENER'S DISEASE)

Sporotrichosis is a chronic, pyogranulomatous fungal infection of cutaneous and subcutaneous tissues, which may remain localized or may show lymphatic spread with occasional dissemination to other parts of the body. The disease is characterized by the development of noduloulcerative lesions in skin, subcutaneous tissues and adjacent lymphatics. The lesions are usually found on the exposed parts of body like hands, arms or legs. In addition to its commonest lymphocutaneous form, it can present as fixed cutaneous and mucocutaneous sporotrichosis. Rarely, a disseminated form may occur involving skeletal, pulmonary or central nervous systems. The disease was originally described by Schenck (1898).

Sporotrichosis is caused by *Sporothrix schenkii* (*Sporotrichum schenkii*), a dimorphic saprophytic fungus, distributed world-wide. The fungus is widely associated with plants, wood, bark, leaves, thorns, straw, soil and decaying vegetation. The infection is acquired by thorn pricks or minor trauma, where the fungus is inoculated into skin. The disease is recognized as an occupational hazard in rural workers, gardeners and carpenters. The fungus is seen in yeast phase in infected tissues or cultures at 37°C and in mycelial phase in soil and in cultures at room temperature.

Laboratory diagnosis

The specimens collected are pus or exudates aspirated from subcutaneous nodules or swabs from ulcerated lesions.

In direct microscopic examination under 10% KOH wet mount, the organism in tissues appear as cigar shaped bodies of yeast cells; sometimes "**asteroid bodies**" are seen composed of a central fungus cell surrounded by a refractile, eosinophilic material like a halo, called "**Splendore—Hoeppli phenomenon**" which is believed to be due to immune complex deposition around the organisms.

In cultures on Sabouraud's dextrose agar at room temperature shows delicate, septate, branched mycelia, interwined with each other like "twisted ropes". Septate hyphae carry clusters of small conidia in "flower-like pattern" borne on delicate sterigmata (Fig. 104.1).

Rats and mice are highly susceptible and can be infected by intraperitoneal or intratesticular inoculation.

An intradermal test using "**sporotrichin**" can be used to detect delayed hypersensitivity.

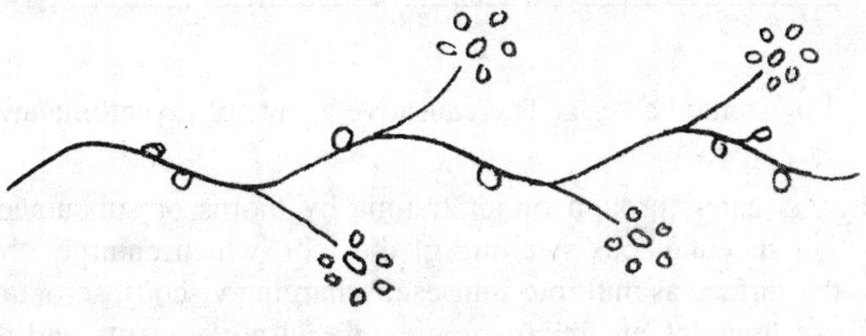

Fig. 104.1 *Sporothrix schenkii.* Culture mount showing branched, septate hyphae with pear shaped conidia in clusters arranged in flower-like pattern

MYCETOMA (MADURAMYCOSIS)

Mycetoma is a slowly progressive, chronic granulomatous infection of skin and subcutaneous tissues with involvement of underlying fasciae and bones usually affecting the extremities. The disease is characterized by a triad of clinical features : (*i*) tumour-like swelling (tumefaction), (*ii*) Multiple draining sinuses, and (*iii*) Presence of grains or granules (Sulphur granules) in sinuses

The sinuses discharge a serous, or purulent fluid particularly following secondary bacterial infections.

The disease was first reported by Gill from Madurai, South India; hence known as "Maduramycosis". It is also commonly known as "**Madura Foot**". The disease is more common in tropics. The disease is named based on the nature of infection, color of grains and cement-like matrix produced in the disease process.

(1) Eumycetoma

Caused by true fungi (Eumycetes). It is of two types, based on the color of grains.

(*a*) Black grain **Eumycetoma**—The causative agents are : *Madurella mycetomatis, Madurella grisea, Exophiala jeanselmei, Curvularia geniculata*

(*b*) White grain **Eumycetoma**—The causative fungi are : *Pseudoallescheria boydii, Aspergillus nidulans, Acremonium falciforme, Fusarium species.*

(2) Actinomycetoma

Caused by Grampositive aerobic filamentous higher bacteria of class **Actinomycetes**. The color and consistency of the grains vary. The causative bacterial agents and the color of their granules is listed herebelow :

Table 104.1 Color of Granules

Bacterial agents	*Color of granules*
Actinomadura madurae	white, yellow
Actinomadura pelletieri	pink to red
Nocardia brasiliensis	yellowish-white
Nocardia caviae	white to yellow

Nocardia asteroides	white to yellow
Nocardiopsis dassonvillei	cream-colored
Streptomyces somaliensis	yellowish-white

(3) Botryomycosis

Caused by several pyogenic bacteria. The causative agents of mycetoma are usually saprophytes, present in soil and thorny vegetation.

The causative agents enter through minor trauma by thorns or subcutaneous inoculation. The disease begins as a small subcutaneous swelling of the foot, which enlarges, burrowing into deeper tissues and tracking to the surface as multiple sinuses discharging viscous, seropurulent fluid containing granules or grains. These granules are microcolonies of causative agents and their demonstration is of diagnostic value. Although mycetoma mainly affects the feet, infections of other parts of the body such as hands, shoulders, buttock and head have been reported. The disease is seen as an occupational hazard among farmers, field workers, carpenters, builders and land workers, particularly those who walk bare-footed.

Sometimes, dermatophytes may form mycelial aggregates in deeper tissues, known as "pseudomycetoma" or "Majocchi's dermatophytic granuloma". It is characterized by formation of yellowish-white pseudograins without any cementing material.

Laboratory diagnosis

The clinical samples are pus, exudates, biopsy containing granules. The granules from the lesions can be collected on a sterile gauze or with the help of a loop. The *sulphur granules* may be demonstrated in pus by shaking it up in a test tube with some saline. On standing, the granules and sediment may be withdrawn with a capillary pipette.

(i) Direct Microscopic Examination

The granules should be washed several times in sterile normal saline. Add a few drops of 10% KOH and granules on a glass slide, place a coverslip, crush the grains gently by applying pressure over coverslip with glass rod or handle of the loop. Leave the mount for few hours and examine under microscope to look for hyphae, septae, pigmentation, chalmydospores and inter-hyphal cement substance.

Actinomycotic grains show thin filaments with a diameter of 0.5 to 1 μm with coccoid or bacillary forms while eumycotic grains show thick, 2 to 6 μm wide interwoven septate hyphae with large swollen cells of 10-15 μm or more at the margin, known as **chlamydospores** (Fig. 104.2).

Gram's stain of pus and crushed grains of actinomycetoma shows Gram-positive, branching, filamentous bacteria. **Modified acid-fast staining** (Kinyoun's method) may be used to demonstrate *Nocardia* species. Special fungal stainings can be done to detect septate hyphae and their arrangement in the cement substance (Fig. 104.3).

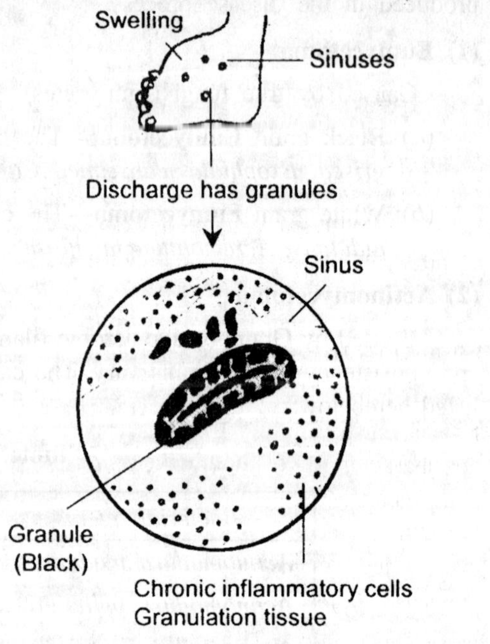

Fig. 104.2 Histopathological section showing Eumycetoma with granulomatous reaction and palisade arrangement of hyphae in cement substance

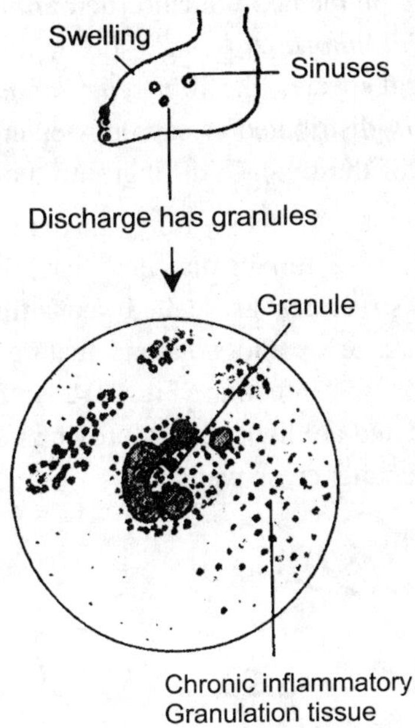

Fig. 104.3 Histopathological section showing Gram positive filamentous bacteria at the margins of grains of actinomycetoma

(ii) Culture

The grains are inoculated on blood agar, brain-heart infusion agar, Lowenstein-Jensen media and Sabouraud's Dextrose agar with antibiotics in duplicate and incubated at 37°C and 25°C.

Botryomycosis

It is a chronic, purulent, granulomatous disease of skin, subcutaneous tissues and visceral organs with the formation of sulphur granules, caused by several bacterial species such as *Staphylococcus aureus, Pseudomonas aeruginosa*, coagulase negative Staphylococci, *E. coli, Proteus vulgaris, Propionibacterium acnes, Streptococcus* sp, *Peptostreptococcus* sp and *Actinobacillus lignieresi.* It is not a fungal disease and resembles mycetoma clinically and histopathologically. It is more common in patients with deficient cell mediated immunity. The sulphur granules are usually white in color.

CHROMOBLASTOMYCOSIS

Chromoblastomycosis is a slowly progressing localized fungal infection of skin and subcutaneous tissues mostly involving exposed parts of the body with no tendency for dissemination. The lesions are characterized by slow developing polymorphic nodular, verrucose, tumoral, plaques and cicatricial skin lesions. The verrucose lesions are frequently ulcerated and may be raised about 1-3 cm above the skin surface with rough irregular surfaces, giving a cauliflower like appearance and hence it is also called **verrucose dermatitis**.

The lower legs are most commonly affected but rarely shoulders, arms, hands, buttocks, ears, chest, face and abdomen may also be involved. The disease is common among rural barefooted workers in tropical and subtropical countries.

The disease is caused by darkly pigmented **phaeoid (dematiaceous) fungi** : *Fonsecaea pedrosoi, Phialophora verrucosa, Cladophialophora carrionii, Fonsecaea compacta* and *Rhinocladiella aquaspersa*. Occasionally other fungal species like *Wangiella dermatitidis* and *Exophiala spinifera* are also involved. These fungi are widely distributed as saprophytes in soil and decaying vegetation. The mode of infection is by inoculation of these phaeoid fungi into the cutaneous tissues through trauma.

The histopathological appearance of these fungi is distinct and consists of dark brown, subglobose, multicellular structures, 5-12 μm in diameter that divide by splitting along the septal planes by transverse septa. These structures are called **sclerotic bodies**, medlar bodies, copper-pennies bodies or muriform cells and are pathognomonic feature of chromoblastomycosis as these are not seen in any other phaeoid fungal infection (Fig. 104.4). The sclerotic bodies are yeast like cells with formation of internal septa and are light yellow-brown in color giving a chestnut appearance. Mature muriform cells have intersecting cross-walls.

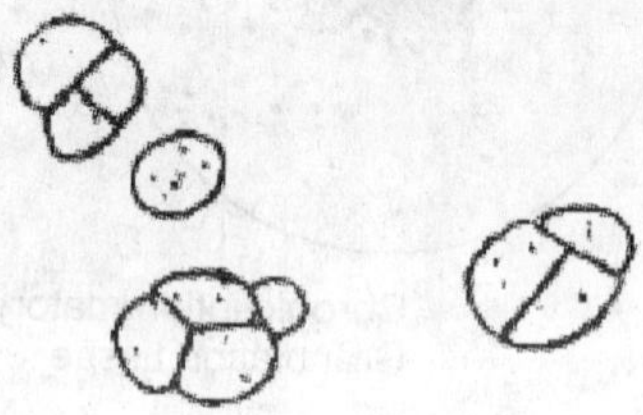

Fig. 104.4 Chromoblastomycosis : KOH mount of lesion showing large septate "sclerotic bodies"

The black dots may be visible on the surface of lesions and represent sites where blood and fungal cells i.e. sclerotic bodies are expelled from the skin through transepidermal elimination which may be sampled for skin scrapings or culture.

The dry, crusty material recovered from the surface of lesions is examined microscopically in 10% KOH wet mount. The biopsy specimen is stained with Hematoxylin and Eosin (H & E) stain, Giemsa stain and Fontana-Masson stain. The presence of characteristic sclerotic bodies are diagnostic.

The specimens are inoculated on to Sabouraud's dextrose agar with actidione and other antibiotics. The identification of causative phaeoid fungus is according to the pattern and type of sporulation.

PHAEOHYPHOMYCOSIS

Phaeohyphomycosis is a subcutaneous and systemic infection, caused by various heterogenous groups of phaeoid (dematiaceous) fungi. These fungi are found in brown, hyaline hyphal form in the tissues and not as thick-walled clusters or muriform cells as seen in chromoblastomycosis.

The most common genera involved in phaeohyphomycosis are *Bipolaris, Curvularia, Exserohilum, Alternaria, Exophiala, Phialophora, Wangiella, Cladophialophora, Cladosporium, Chaetomium* and *Dactylaria*. In addition, *Phialophora parasitica, Curvularia pallescens, Nattrassia mangiferae* have also been rarely reported. The fungi involved are characterized by the brown melanin pigment in the cell walls.

These phaeoid fungi are widely distributed in the nature in soil, decaying vegetation, rotten wood and as plant pathogens. They infect subcutaneous tissues by producing solitary lesions.

Phaeohyphomycosis may be cutaneous or subcutaneous or invasive and cerebral or may affect paranasal sinuses. The disease is common in debilitated and immunodeficients.

The aspirates from the nodules, cysts and drained abscesses are examined in 10% KOH wet mounts. These fungi are usually pigmented and dark brown in color. Sometimes, hyaline hyphae may be seen. Masson-Fontana stain may be used to elicit the presence of melanin in the hyphae. The fungi are seen as short or elongated hyphal forms, irregularly swollen, septate, branched or unbranched, yeast-like cells. Specimens are inoculated on to Sabouraud's dextrose agar with cyloheximide, and incubated at 25°C and 37°C for 4 weeks. The causative fungi are identified by the type and pattern of sporulation.

RHINOSPORIDIOSIS

Rhinosporidiosis is a chronic granulomatous disease of mucus membranes of man and animals, characterized by the development of friable **polyps** in the nose, mouth, eyes, rarely on genitalia and other sites. Hematogenous dissemination is rare. The disease may involve different organs of the body and present as nasal rhinosporidiosis, ocular rhinosporidiosis, cutaneous rhinosporidiosis and miscellaneous manifestations.

The disease is caused by *Rhinosporidium seeberi*. It was thought to be a fungus but on the basis of recent molecular studies it is now considered to be a hydrophilic protistan parasite. It has not been cultivated. The disease is endemic in South India, Sri Lanka, Argentina and Brazil.

The life cycle of *Rhinosporidium seeberi* involves three main stages, which are maturation of trophocyte, development of sporangia and production of endospores.

(*i*) **Trophocyte**—It is a round or oval shaped, measures 6-8 μ with a cell membrane, clear cytoplasm, vesicular nucleus and a nucleolus. It is covered by chitin and lies freely in connective tissue.

(*ii*) **Sporangia**—The trophocyte undergoes mitotic divisions, the cytoplasm condenses, increases in size and the wall becomes thickened by developing into sporangium containing endospores (Fig. 104.5).

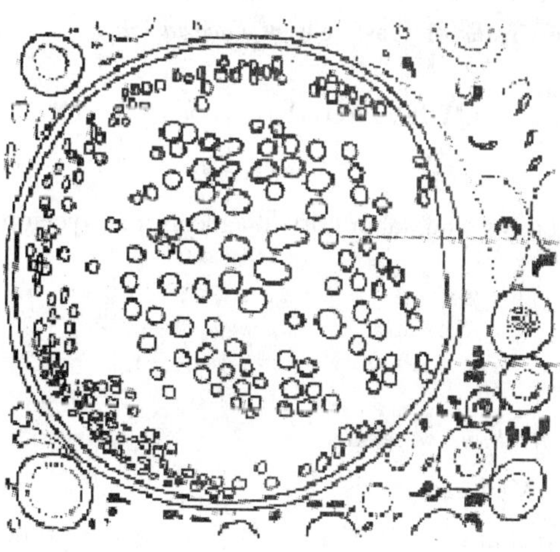

Fig. 104.5 *Rhinosporidium seeberi*. Mature sporangium in the stroma of a lesion

(*iii*) Endospores—Each sporangium may contain 12,000 to 16,000 endospores having a thick outer chitinous wall and inner membranous wall, with a germinal pore situated eccentrically. The endospores may be released either through pore or rupture in the sporangium.

Mode of infection is believed to be frequent bathing or contact with fresh or stagnant water; which may act as a reservoir of infection.

The diagnosis of rhinosporidiosis is by direct microscopy or histopathological examination. A section of **nasal polyp** or biopsy of lesion or nasal washing is stained with hematoxylin and eosin (H & E) shows giant cells, lymphocytic reaction around mature sporangium, filled with endospores. Periodic acid-Schiff and Gomori's methenamine silver stains are also done.

LOBOMYCOSIS

It is a slowly progressing chronic granulomatous fungal infection of skin and subcutaneous tissues. The disease is characterized by presence of macule, papule, keloidal, verrucous, nodular lesions or vegetating crusty plaques and tumors. Infection is acquired by trauma. There is no involvement of internal organs or mucus membranes. The disease is also known as "keloidal blastomycosis" or "Jorge Lobo's disease".

The causative fungus is *Lacazia loboi*, exists only as yeast cells, giving rise to branching chains of **blastoconidia** by budding (Fig. 104.6). It has not been cultured *in vitro*. It does not respond to antifungal agents. The organism is widely distributed in the environment on plants and vegetation.

This rare disease is prevalent in the Latin American countries mainly Brazil, affecting only two mammals, man and dolphins. Surgical excision is employed for treatment.

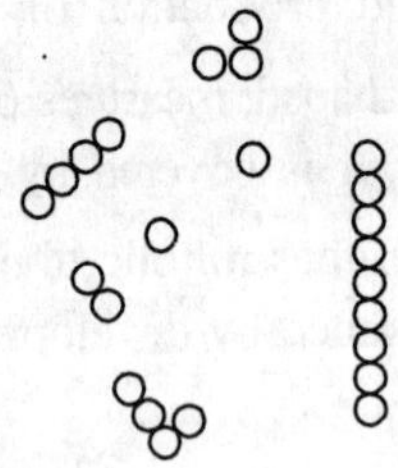

Fig. 104.6 Chains of yeast cells of *Lacazia loboi*

QUESTIONS

Essay Questions:

1. Describe the etiology, pathogenesis and laboratory diagnosis of mycetoma.
2. Describe subcutaneous mycoses.

Short Notes:

1. Sporotrichosis
2. *Sporothrix schenkii* or *Sporotrichum schenkii*
3. Mycetoma or Madura foot or Maduramycosis
4. Eumycotic mycetoma or Eumycetoma
5. Actinomycotic mycetoma
6. Botryomycosis
7. Sulphur granules
8. Granules or grains in mycetoma

9. Laboratory diagnosis of mycetoma
10. Name subcutaneous mycoses and their causative agents
11. Chromoblastomycosis or verrucous dermatitis
12. Sclerotic cells
13. Name the causative agents of chromoblastomycosis
14. Phaeohyphomycosis
15. Describe the morphology, pathogenesis and laboratory diagnosis of *Rhinosporidium seeberi*
16. Rhinosporidiosis
17. *Rhinosporidium seeberi*
18. Laboratory diagnosis of Rhinosporidiosis
19. Lobomycosis or keloidal blastomycosis
20. *Lacazia* loboi

105

Systemic mycoses

- *Dimorphic fungi*
- *Histoplasmosis*
- *Blastomycosis*
- *Coccidioidomycosis*
- *Paracoccidioidomycosis*

Dimorphic Fungi

Dimorphic fungi are those fungi that occur as **yeasts** in host tissues or cultures at 37°C; while in the soil and in cultures at 22°C (room temperature), they appear as **molds** e.g.,

1. *Histoplasma capsulatum* causes histoplasmosis (Darling's disease)
2. *Sporotrichum* (*Sporothrix*) *schenkii* causes sporotrichosis
3. *Blastomyces dermatitidis* causes blastomycosis (North American blastomycosis)
4. *Paracoccidioides brasiliensis* causes paracoccidioidomycosis (South American blastomycosis)

All dimorphic fungi produce systemic infections, except *Sporotrichum schenkii*, which causes subcutaneous infections.

HISTOPLASMOSIS

Histoplasmosis, also known as **Darling's disease**, is an intracellular infection of reticuloendothelial system, caused by ***Histoplasma capsulatum***. The disease is worldwide, but common in USA. The causative fungus is present in soil, rotting trees, particularly in the soil containing bird or bat excreta that has accumulated for several years. This excreta greatly enhances the growth of the fungus in the soil. Infection is acquired by inhalation. Mostly infections are asymptomatic. Some may develop pulmonary disease resembling tuberculosis. It may disseminate and involve reticuloendothelial system with resultant lymphadenopathy, hepatosplenomegaly, fever, anemia with a high rate of fatality. Granulomalous and ulcerative lesions may develop on skin and mucosa.

Diagnosis is made by microscopical examination of stained (H & E staining) smears from blood, bone marrow, scrapings from lesions or biopsies of lymph nodes and also by culture. *Histoplasma capsulatum* is a **dimorphic fungus**. In tissues and in **blood agar** cultures at 37°C the fungus grows in yeast form; In soil and Sabouraud's dextrose agar at room temperature, white mycelial growth appears, with large, thick walled spherical spores with tubercles or finger like projections. The appearance of **tuberculate spores** is diagnostic (Fig. 105.1). Antibody titre increases in progressive disease, can be detected by latex agglutination test, CFT and precipitation tests. Delayed hypersensitivity is developed, which can be detected by using **histoplasmin** antigen. The test is similar to tuberculin test.

African histoplasmosis involves skin, subcutaneous tissues and bones. It is caused by ***Histoplasma duboisii*** and it differs from *H. capsulatum* in forming larger, yeast-like cells.

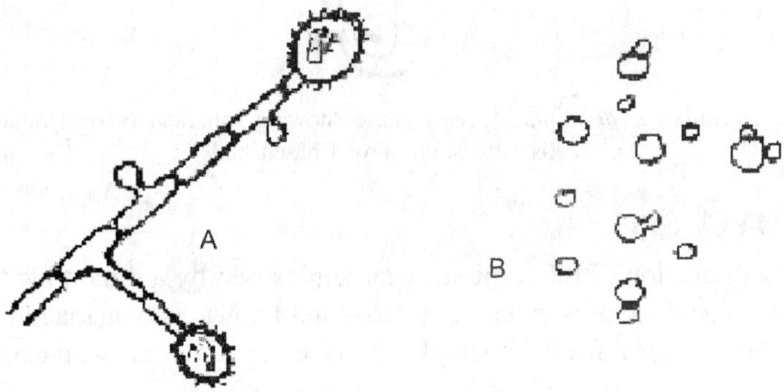

Fig. 105.1 *Histoplasma capsulatum*
(a) Mycelial phase with tuberculate macroconidia and microconidia.
(b) Yeast cells with budding.

BLASTOMYCOSIS (NORTH AMERICAN BLASTOMYCOSIS)

It is an acute or chronic granulomatous and suppurative fungal infection, which can occur in any part of the body but commonly in lungs (**pulmonary blastomycosis**) and skin (**cutaneous blastomycosis**). The disease may disseminate as an opportunistic infection in AIDS, transplant recipients and patients treated with immunosuppressive therapy. The disease may also involve larynx and bones. The disease is known as "North American blastomycosis" or "**Chicago disease**" based on its area of endemicity. The disease was first reported by Casper Gilchrist (1894), hence known as "**Gilchrist's disease**".

The disease is caused by ***Blastomyces dermatitidis***, a **dimorphic fungus**, found as a saprophyte in the soil. The infection is acquired by inhalation of spores from the soil. Primary infection of lungs resembles tuberculosis or histoplasmosis. Fungus may spread from lungs through blood stream and cause multiple abscesses in various parts of the body. Cutaneous disease is usually on the skin of face or other exposed parts of the body. Initial lesion is a papule, around which secondary nodules develop and coalesce, forming large, elevated ulcerative lesions.

Laboratory diagnosis consists of demonstration of the organism in tissues or exudates in 10% KOH wet mounts and by growth on Sabouraud's dextrose agar medium.

Blastomyces dermatitidis is a thermally dimorphic fungus, existing in mycelial sapropic phase with septate hyphae with conidia and sometimes chlamydospores also in soil and in cultures at room temperature. In tissue lesions and in cultures at 37°C, fungus appears as broad-based budding yeast cells, which are large, spherical with thick double contoured walls (Fig. 105.2). The fungus appears in two serotypes AK and K. The former is world-wide, whereas the latter is prevalent in Africa and smaller in size.

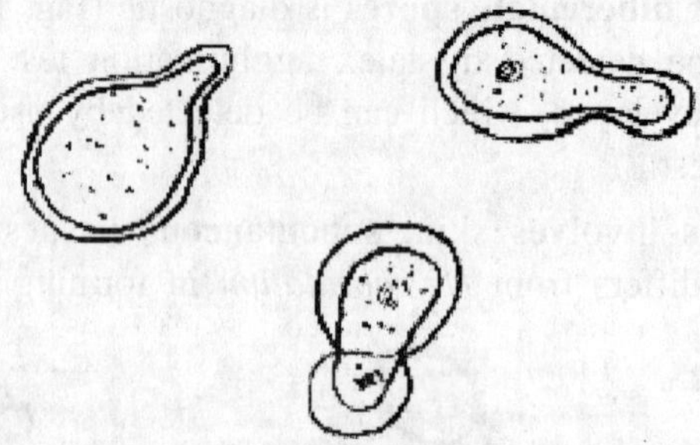

Fig. 105.2 *Blastomyces dermatitidis* yeast phase showing spherical or oval double walled cells with single broad based buds

COCCIDIOIDOMYCOSIS

It is primarily an infection of the respiratory system caused by a dimorphic fungus ***Coccidioides immitis***, found in soil. The disease is endemic in USA and known as San Joaquin valley fever, desert rheumatism, desert fever, valley fever or simply "koksee" in a layman language.

Most of the coccidioidal infections occur in otherwise healthy persons which are subacute and usually self-limiting. In a few cases, the infection produces protracted illness, such as chronic pneumonia or dissemination to the skin, bones, meninges and other body sites. It also occurs as opportunistic infection in AIDS, lymphomas and organ transplant cases.

The infection is acquired by inhalation of air-borne **arthroconidia** from soil. Respiratory infection is usually asymptomatic, leads to delayed hypersensitivity, that can be detected by skin test with **coccidioidin** (similar to tuberculin test). Many cases develop a self-limited influenza like fever, known as **valley fever**. Rarely, some may develop **coccidioidal granuloma**, which is highly fatal.

The causative fungus is dimorphic and exists in two forms. In tissues it exists as a **spherule** filled with **endospores** (Fig. 105.3). The term "*Coccidia*" has been derived from the tissue or parasitic phase resembled protozoa belonging to genus *Coccidia*. The fungus occurs in mycelial phase in soil. Thus the life cycle of *Coccidioides immitis* involves development of hyphae, arthroconidia and spherule. The yeast cell is spherical with a thick doubly refractile wall and filled with endospores. Mycelium consists of hyphae, which fragment into arthrospores, which are highly infectious.

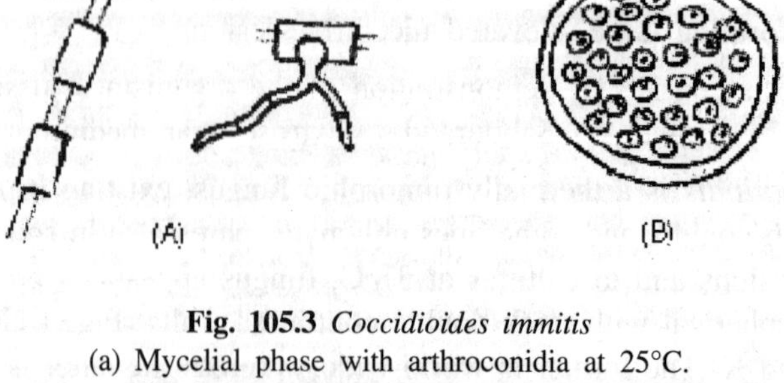

Fig. 105.3 *Coccidioides immitis*

(a) Mycelial phase with arthroconidia at 25°C.

(b) Spherules in tissue phase at 37°C.

PARACOCCIDIOIDOMYCOSIS (SOUTH AMERICAN BLASTOMYCOSIS)

It is an acute or chronic, progressive, granulomatous systemic fungal disease that involves primarily lungs and disseminates to the skin, mucosa, lymph nodes and occasionally internal organs. Ulcerative granulomas are formed in the oral cavity, on the lips, tongue, nasopharynx, conjunctiva, eyelids and on other mucus membrane surfaces.

The causative fungus is *Paracoccidioides brasiliensis*, which is a **dimorphic fungus**. The most important feature is the presence of multi-budding yeast cells, found in the human host and experimental animals *in vivo* and in the cultures incubated at 37°C *in vitro*. Mycelial phase develops at room temperature. The hyphae fragment into **arthrospores** (Fig. 105.4). Infection is due to inhalation of spores released into air.

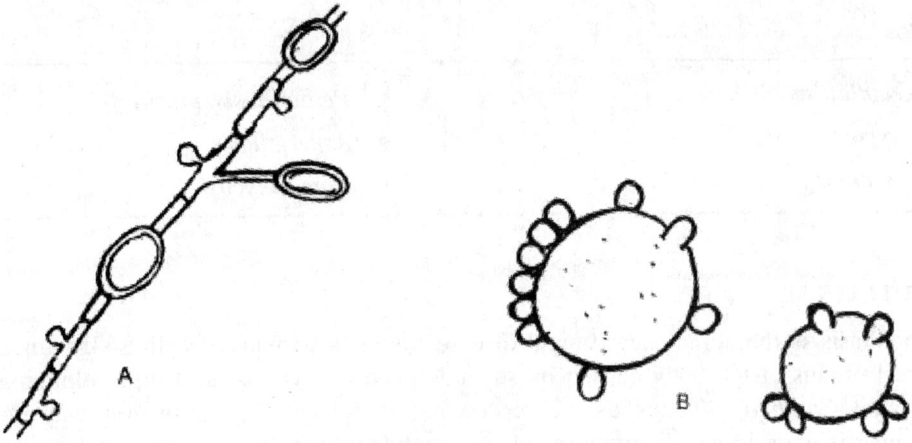

Fig. 105.4 *Paracoccidioides brasiliensis.*
(a) Mycelial phase at 25°C.
(b) Yeast cells with multiple budding in tissues at 37°C.

The diagnosis is based mainly on the demonstration of large, budding yeast cells in the clinical material and detection of a **gp43** antigen or antibody to this antigen. An intradermal test with **paracoccidioidin** may be used to demonstrate delayed hypersensitivity.

QUESTIONS

Essay Question

1. Enumerate dimorphic fungi. Describe the morphology, pathogenicity and lab. diagnosis of dimorphic fungi.

Short Notes

1. Dimorphic fungi
2. Enumerate dimorphic fungi and describe lab. diagnosis of any one of them.
3. Histoplasmosis (or) Darling's disease
4. Histoplasma capsulatum
5. Blastomycosis (or) Blastomyces dermatitidis
6. Coccidioidomycosis (or) Coccidioides immitis
7. Paracoccidioidomycosis (or) Paracoccidioides brasiliensis.

106

Opportunistic mycoses

- *Candidiasis*
- *Cryptococcosis*
- *Pneumocystosis*
- *Penicilliosis marneffei*
- *Aspergillosis*
- *Mucormycosis*

CANDIDIASIS

Candidiasis is the commonest fungal disease found in humans affecting skin, mucosa, nails and internal organs of the body caused by several species of **yeast-like fungi** belonging to genus *Candida* with ***Candida albicans*** as the representative species. The infection may be acute or chronic, superficial or deep. It is found mainly as **secondary infection** or **endogenous opportunistic infection** in individuals with some underlying immunocompromised condition and very rarely as a primary disease.

There are two terms, "**candidosis**" and "**candidiasis**" which are frequently used as synonyms. The nomenclature of the fungus presently known as *Candida albicans* was also designated as *Odium albicans* and *Monilia albicans*. Due to its genus name as *Monilia*, the disease used to be called as "**moniliasis**".

The genus *Candida* consists of over 163 species. Nearly twenty of these species are considered to be pathogenic and most important are *Candida albicans*, *C. tropicalis*, *C. krusei*, *C. glabrata*, *C. kefyr*, *C. guilliermondii*, *C. parapsilosis*, *C. lusitaniae*, *C. dubliniensis* and *C. viswanathii*.

Table 106.1 Differences between Hyphae and Pseudohyphae

Features	*Hyphae*	*Pseudohyphae*
Growth process	Apical elongation	Budding
Terminal cell	longer, cylindrical	shorter, spherical
Cell wall	parallel	constricted at septa
Septa	straight, perpendicular	curved or pinched
Origin of branches	No constriction, septum not required	constricted and septate

Candida is an oval or spherical shaped budding yeast-like fungus, which forms **pseudohyphae** (Table 106.1). The commonest pathogenic species of this genus is *Candida albicans*. Based on the differences between mannan components of cell wall, *Candida albicans* is classified into 2 serotypes A and B.

The *Candida* species are commensals and constitute normal flora of humans. They are found on the skin, in the gastrointestinal tract and female genital tract.

PATHOGENICITY

Candida albicans has several virulence factors contributing to its pathogenicity that include adherence to the epithelial and endothelial cells by adhesin, proteinase production, pseudohyphae formation, phenotypic switching, phospholipase production and antigenic modulation as a result of pseudohyphae formation.

The clinical manifestations of candidiasis may vary from mild, simple lesions to life-threatening systemic infections, which are described below.

(i) Mucosal infections

(*a*) **Oral thrush**—most common form of disease characterized by creamy white patches on tongue or buccal mucosa, which leave a red oozing surface on removal. Common in bottlefed infants and the aged and debilitated.

(*b*) **vaginitis**—Vaginal candidiasis is common in pregnancy, characterized by acidic discharge.

(*c*) **intestinal candidiasis**—occurs as a sequel to frequent oral antibiotic therapy and may present as diarrhea. Oesophagitis and gastritis may be seen (also in HIV infection).

(*d*) **Ocular candidiasis**—keratoconjunctivitis is a complication of long-term use of topical corticosteroids.

(*e*) **Chronic mucocutaneous candidiasis**—It is common in patients with deficient cell-mediated immunity. This condition is a heterogenous group of clinical syndromes characterized by chronic, resistant type of candidiasis of skin, nails and oropharynx.

(ii) Skin and Nail infections

(*a*) **Intertrigo**—It is an inflammatory lesion of the skin folds. The skin lesion is an erythematous, scaly or moist lesion; popular lesions are more prominent. Sites affected are those where skin is macerated by perspiration—groin, perineum, axillae and inframammary folds.

(*b*) **paronychia** and **onychomycosis**—It is an inflammation of nail fold, seen in occupations that lead to frequent immersion of hands in water.

(*c*) **diaper dermatitis** or **napkin candidiasis**—It is characterized by moist, macular erythematous rash in infants; most marked in the intertriginous areas of gluteal crease, perineum and inguinal fold. Maceration and wet diapers are the predisposing factors.

(*d*) **candidal granuloma**—It is commonly found in children. It is described as papules covered with a thick, adherent, yellow-brown crust over face, scalp, fingernails, trunk and legs, which develop into horns or protrusions.

(iii) Systemic infections

Bronchopulmonary candidiasis, urinary tract infections, septicemia, meningitis, endocarditis, arthritis, osteomyelitis, endophthalmitis, and may disseminate into various parts of the body. Immunodeficiency, immunosuppression, diabetes, malignancy are the conditions which can precipitate these infections.

(iv) Allergic diseases

Candids or "id" reactions, eczema, asthma and gastritis are the allergic manifestations seen in candida infections.

Laboratory Diagnosis

The specimens collected from the patients depends upon the site of involvement. Whitish patches from the mucus membranes of mouth, vagina, skin or nails scrapings are collected with the help of sterile swabs.

Microscopy

The specimens are examined under 10% KOH wet mount or normal saline preparations. Gram's staining is performed to see the presence of yeast and pseudohyphae (Fig. 106.1). Calcofluor white stain may be used to highlight the fungal elements. Periodic acid-Schiff stain and Gomori's methanamine silver stains can be used to detect the fungal elements in tissues.

Table 106.2 *Candida* Infections and Predisposing Conditions

Disease	*Predisposing conditions*
Mucosal infections :	
oral thrush	Bottle-fed infants, aged, debilitated
vaginitis	pregnancy
intestinal candidosis	oral antibiotic therapy
ocular candidiasis	topical corticosteroids
chronic mucocutaneous candidiasis	deficient cell mediated immunity
Skin and Nail infections :	
Intertrigo	regions of skin macerated by perspiration
paronychia and onychomycosis	frequent immersion of hands in water
candidal granuloma	immunodeficiency
Systemic infections :	
Bronchopulmonary candidiasis, urinary tract candidiasis, septicemia, meningitis, endocarditis, arthritis, osteomyelitis, endophthalmitis, disseminated candidiasis	Diabetes mellitus, AIDS, immunosuppression, zinc or iron deficiency, malignancy

Culture

The specimens are inoculated on to Sabouraud's dextrose agar with antibiotics and incubated at 25°C and 37°C. The colonies appear in 3-4 days as cream colored, smooth and pasty. The Lactophenol cotton blue mount is prepared from the colonies to examine yeast cells and pseudohyphae. Gram staining should also be performed. In systemic infections blood culture is done in biphasic medium like brain-heart infusion agar-broth.

Candida species can be identified by the color produced on Tetrazolium Reduction Medium (TRM). A new medium called "CHROMagar *Candida*" distinguishes different *Candida* species by color as a result of biochemical reactions.

The identification of *Candida* species and also the differentiation of *Candida albicans* from other species is by growth characteristics, sugar assimilation tests, fermentation tests, germ tube test and chlamydospore formation.

Germ tube test or Reynolds—Braude phenomenon

The *Candida* culture is inoculated into sheep or normal human serum and incubated at 37°C for 2 to 4 hrs. Positive and negative controls may be put up. A drop of suspension is examined on the slide under the microscope. The germ tubes are seen as long tube-like projections extending from the yeast cells. There is no constriction at the point of attachment to the yeast cell as seen in case of pseudohyphae.

Candida albicans and *C. dubliniensis* can form germ tubes within two hours of incubation. The demonstration of the germ tube is also known as "*Reynolds-Braude phenomenon*" (Fig. 106.1c).

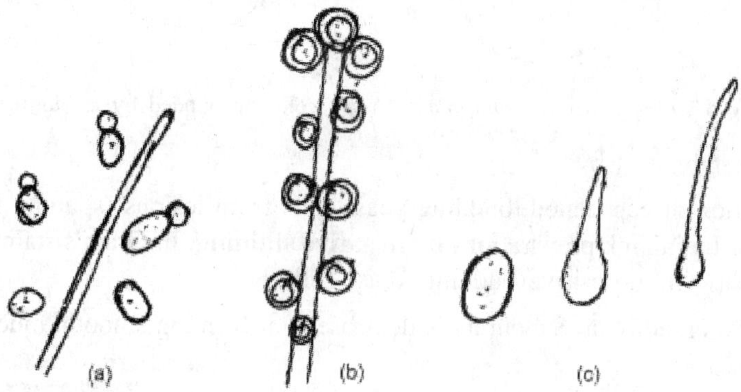

(*a*) **Budding yeast cells with pseudohypha,** (*b*) **Chlamydospores,** (*c*) **Germ tube formation.**

Fig. 106.1 *Candida albicans*

Chlamydospore formation

Candida albicans and *C. dubliniensis* can form chlamydospores on **corn meal agar** or **rice starch** agar when incubated at 25°C. They show the formation of large, highly refractile, thick-walled, terminal chlamydospores after 2 to 3 days of incubation. Chlamydospores are vegetative spores containing stored food (Fig. 106.1b). Corn meal agar medium is prepared from corn meal (ground yellow maize) to which agar is added and dissolved.

Candida albicans can be differentiated from *Candida dubliniensis* by its inability to grow at 42-45°C and formation of light green or blue green color on **CHROMagar**; whereas *C. dubliniensis* can grow at 42-45°C and forms dark green color CHROMagar.

CRYPTOCOCCOSIS

Cryptococcosis is an acute, subacute or chronic fungal disease caused by an encapsulated yeast ***Cryptococcus neoformans***. It is widely prevalent as a soil saprophyte in the environment and abundant in feces of pigeons and other birds.

Infection is acquired by inhalation of small forms or **basidiospores**, sometimes through skin or mucosa. Most infections are asymptomatic. **Pulmonary cryptococcosis** may lead to a mild pneumonitis. It may disseminate through blood stream causing visceral, cutaneous and meningeal disease. Visceral forms simulate TB and cancer clinically. Bones and joints may be involved. Cutaneous cryptococcosis varies from small ulcers to large granulomas. Cryptococcal meningitis is the most important life threatening opportunistic infection in immunodeficiency.

Cryptococcus neoformans is an oval or spherical budding yeast cell with a prominent polysaccharide capsule (Fig. 106.2). Five serological types of Cryptococcal capsule—A, B, C, D and AD have been identified. It has two virulence factors : a polysaccharide **capsule** which inhibits phagocytosis and **phenol oxidase** enzyme which converts phenol compounds to melanin.

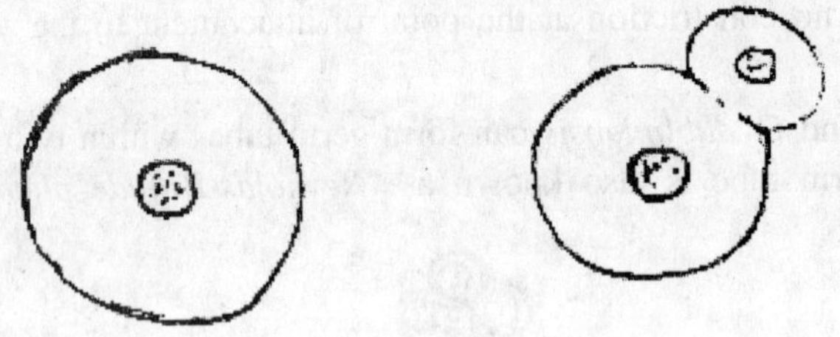

Fig. 106.2 *Cryptococcus neoformans* : Yeast cells surrounded by a wide capsule.

Diagnosis is established by :

(*i*) Demonstration of capsulated, budding yeast cells from lesions (sputum, CSF etc.) with 10% nigrosine or Indian ink preparations by **negative staining**. In Gram's staining, these organisms are visible as Gram-positive budding yeast cells.

(*ii*) Fungus grows readily on Sabouraud's dextrose agar forming smooth, mucoid, cream coloured colonies.

(*iii*) Capsular antigen can be demonstrated from CSF in cryptococcal meningitis, when the CSF is negative by microscopy and culture.

Cryptococcus neoformans can be differentiated from other species of *Cryptococcus* by various tests.

(*i*) *Cryptococcus neoformans* can grow at 37°C, whereas other species grow at room temperature.

(*ii*) *C. neoformans* produces urease enzyme, which hydrolyzes urea; whereas the other species are urease negative.

(*iii*) Pathogenicity test—The suspected clinical specimen or 2 to 4 day old culture is injected into mice either intracerebrally or intravenously into the tail vein or intraperitoneally. *C. neoformans* causes a fatal infection and the inoculated mice dies within 7 to 10 days.

PNEUMOCYSTOSIS

Pneumocystosis is an opportunistic fungal infection of respiratory system leading to interstitial plasma cell pneumonia, so called due to intense plasma cell infiltrate. It is primarily a disease of alveoli caused by a taxonomically unique fungus ***Pneumocystis carinii*** presenting as an **atypical pneumonia**, particularly among malnourished infants and immunocompromised individuals. It is the most common life-threatening **opportunistic infection** in AIDS.

Prior to 1988, *P. carinii* was considered to be a Protozoa belonging to class sporozoa, subclass Coccidia. *P. carinii* now considered to be a fungus and is phylogenetically classified as an ascomycete, due to the following reasons.

1. It can be stained with fungal stains such as methenamine silver stains.
2. It produces chitin at all stages of its life cycle. Several enzymes, including chitinase attack cell wall of *P. carinii* as well as true fungi.
3. The protein synthesis elongation factor (EF3) and thymidylate synthase of *P. carinii* are more homologous to those of ascomycetes.
4. *P. carinii* and fungi have similar cyst wall ultrastructures i.e. mitochondria with lamellar cristae and cyst forms containing intracystic bodies resembling those of ascospores formed by the ascomycetes whereas protozoal mitochondria have vesicular and tubular cristae.
5. The ribosomal RNA studies shows more similarity to fungi than protozoa.
6. There is absence of ergosterol in the cytoplasmic membrane and abundant cholesterol is present and therefore it is resistant to antifungal drugs, which target ergosterol synthesis.

However, *P. carinii* differs from fungi by its inability to grow on fungal culture media and resistance to antifungal drugs. *P. carinii* is susceptible to antiprotozoan agents and can grow on tissue cultures or cell lines.

The life cycle of *P. carinii* in lungs comprises of asexual phase of cell division by an haploid trophozoite stage and sexual phase leading to genesis of a thick-walled reproductive yeast containing eight intracystic bodies. Its life cycle is divided into 3 main stages : trophozoite (vegetative), cystic and sporozoite (Fig. 106.3).

The **trophozoites** are pleomorphic, amoeboid, covered with tubular projections which increase absorptive surface and facilitate attachment to epithelial cells of alveoli. They are covered by thin, flexible, fragile external layer containing β-glucan and glycoprotein. They multiply by binary fission.

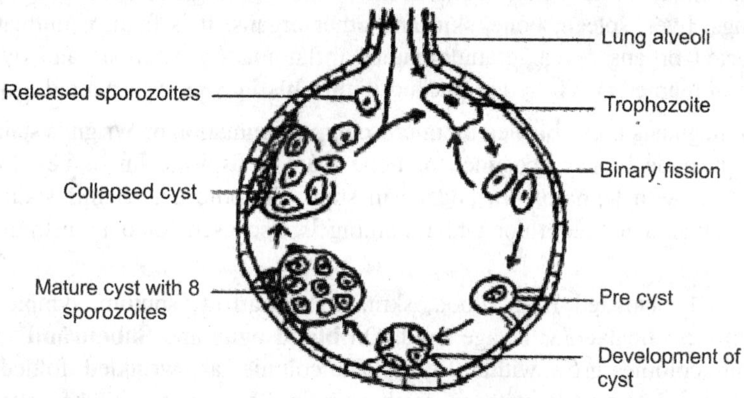

Fig. 106.3 Life cycle of *Pneumocystis carinii* in lung alveolus.

The transition phase between trophozoite and cystic stages is called as precyst (**sporocyst**).

The **cystic stage** is frequently observed in clinical specimens. These are large, oval shaped, thick walled possessing up to 8 intracystic bodies or sporozoites. The **sporozoites** are oval, ameboid, or peach-shaped. They are best demonstrated by Giemsa stain, showing basophilic cytoplasm and reddish-purple nuclei in eosinophilic mass. The sporozoites are extruded through cyst wall and the empty cysts are seen as navicular structures.

The disease is acquired through droplet (**air-borne**) inhalation. The predisposing conditions are cytotoxic and corticosteroid therapy, malignancies like lymphoma, leukemia, Hodgkin's disease and solid tumors; immunosuppression, AIDS, solids organ or bone marrow transplantation. The disease occurs as an **opportunistic infection** predominantly in patients with impaired cell-mediated immunity.

The diagnosis is made by demonstrating the organism in sputum, bronchoalveolar lavage fluid or lung biopsy. **Cysts** can be demonstrated by Giemsa or Methanamine-silver stains. Immunofluorescence is also used to detect both trophozoites and cysts. ELISA can be used to detect *P. carinii* antigen. Molecular methods like PCR can be used to detect *P. carinii* DNA. The foamy eosinophilic exudate and "honey comb" appearance of the lung tissue under hematoxylin and eosin stain confirms the presence of *P. carinii*.

A combination of trimethoprim and sulfamethoxazole is the drug of choice for the first line treatment and prophylaxis of all forms of pneumocystosis.

PENICILLIOSIS MARNEFFEI

Penicillium species occur as saprophytes in the soil and decomposing organic debris. They may cause opprotunistic infections in humans.

Penicillium marneffei is the only **dimorphic fungus** of this genus causing **"penicilliosis marneffei"**, an emerging systemic fungal disease as a secondary and/or **opportunistic infection** in AIDS. The causative organism, ***Penicillium marneffei*** is a thermally dimorphic facultative intracellular fungus and exists as mycelial and yeast-like forms at two different temperatures i.e., 25°C and 37°C, respectively. The yeast form is different morphologically from the yeasts of other dimorphic fungi and divides by fission (**schizogony**) with formation of transverse septum and not by budding.

Penicilliosis marneffei is a progressive, disseminated and potentially fatal fungal infection in the later stages of HIV infection. Clinical manifestations include fever, weight loss, anemia with involvement of lymph nodes, lungs, liver, spleen, bone, skin and other organs. It is fatal, if untreated. Histologic sections of the affected organs reveal granulomatous inflammation, necrosis and oval to elliptical yeast-like cells (3 μ in diameter). These are packed within **histiocytes** or scattered around the tissue.

The laboratory diagnosis is established by microscopic examination of Wright's stained impression smears of skin, lymph node biopsy specimen or bone marrow aspirate. In tissues, the cells having *P. marneffei* are stained with hematoxylin and eosin stain, Periodic acid-Schiff stain and Gomori's methanamine silver stains. The calcofluor white staining is also used for demonstration of the yeast forms.

P. marneffei can be isolated from blood, skin, bone marrow, sputum, lymph nodes, pleural fluid, urine and even bronchoalveolar lavage fluid. On **blood agar** and **Sabouraud's dextrose agar** at 25°C, greyish-white colonies grow within 2 days. The colonies are wrinkled, folded and have red-stained mycelia and sporulate poorly with greenish conidia. The reverse is characteristically bright rose color due to diffusion of a water-soluble brick-red pigment. The fungus contains septate, branched hyphae. The conidiophores are located laterally and terminally. They bear sterigmata (metulae, phialides) in two or three rows which give rise to spherical conidia in chains producing a brush or broom like arrangement (penicillus = brush) (Fig. 106.4).

PCR is highly sensitive for the detection of fungi.

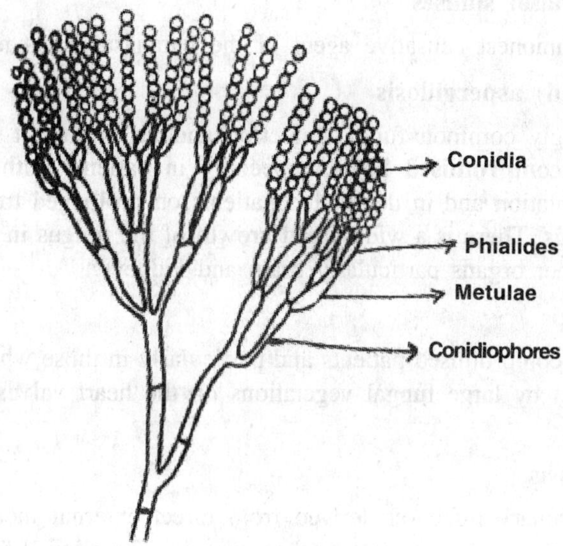

Fig. 106.4 *Penicillium* sp.

ASPERGILLOSIS

Aspergillosis is a systemic fungal infection with tissue invasion or allergic manifestations found in immunocompromised as well as healthy hosts, caused by several species of *Aspergillus*. The infections may be primary or secondary depending on the mode of infection, which vary in severity as well as clinical course.

Aspergillus species are saprobic molds commonly found in the soil and on decaying organic matter worldwide. At present there are more than 185 species, out of which 20 species have been found to cause human infections and three of them are consistently and regularly encountered as etiological agents of 95 per cent of diseases. They are *A. fumigatus*, *A. flavus* and *A. niger*. The other commonly encountered species are *A. terreus*, *A nidulans*, *A oryzae*, *A glaucus* and *A. clavatus*. *A. fumigatus* is the most common species found in human infections. Their spores are ubiquitous in the environment. The human beings are regularly exposed to these spores particularly people working with the decaying vegetation, like **moldy hay** in agriculture, are maximally exposed. The disease process generally follows inhalation of the spores but the fungus may also gain direct entry to the body tissues through wounds or during surgery. The spores of this fungus, particularly of *A. fumigatus* may bypass the upper respiratory tract defenses and reach the alveoli, and commonly encountered as the etiological agent of systemic aspergillosis in man and animals. Aspergillosis occurs as following clinical conditions.

1. Pulmonary Aspergillosis

(*i*) **Allergic aspergillosis**—Asthma or extrinsic allergic alveolitis due to inhalation of spores.

(*ii*) **Allergic bronchopulmonary aspergillosis**—fungus grows within the lumen of bronchioles, which may be occluded by fungus plugs.

(*iii*) **Aspergilloma**—The fungus colonizes in a preexistent pulmonary cavity, such as TB or cystic disease. Fungus grows into large balls called "Aspergilloma". It is also known as **"colonizing aspergillosis"**.

2. Aspergillosis of paranasal sinuses

A. flavus is the commonest causative agent of the paranasal sinus mycosis.

3. Invasive (disseminated) aspergillosis

This is an increasingly common fungal infection and an important cause of morbidity and mortality in the **immunocompromised hosts**, especially in patients with AIDS, leukemia, bone marrow or organ transplantation and in debilitated patients on prolonged treatment with antibiotics, steroids and cytotoxic drugs. There is a widespread growth of the fungus in the lung tissue that may disseminate to involve other organs particularly brain and kidneys.

4. *Aspergillus* Endocarditis

It is seen in immunocompromised patients and particularly in those who have had prior cardiac surgery. It is characterized by large fungal vegetations on the heart valves and high frequency of embolization.

5. Cutaneous Aspergillosis

It can present as primary infection derived from direct external inoculation through contact with objects, external catheter sites, surgical or other traumas. The clinical features includes nodules, papules, plaques and ulcers.

It may be a secondary infection usually on the chest wall in patients with pulmonary aspergillosis and caused by dissemination. The predisposing conditions include immunocompromisation, patients with organ transplant or chronic granulomatous disease, AIDS, patients with burn wounds and autoimmune diseases who receives corticosteroids.

6. Miscellaneous forms of Aspergillosis

Aspergillus species may also cause keratomycosis, otomycosis and onychomycosis.

LABORATORY DIAGNOSIS

The specimens like sputum, bronchoalveolar lavage fluid or biopsy are taken depending on the site of involvement.

Direct microscopic examination of clinical specimens is done in 10% KOH to demonstrate hyaline septate hyphae with characteristic dichotomous branching. The biopsy material is kept in 10% KOH for an overnight at 37°C and examined to see for the septate hyphae. Histopathological examination of biopsy material is done by staining with periodic acid-Schiff or hematoxylin and eosin or Gomori's methanamine silver stains.

The *Aspergillus* species grow easily and relatively quickly on routine mycological as well as bacteriological media. The specimen is inoculated on Sabouraud's dextrose agar with antibiotics and without cycloheximide and incubated at 25°C and 37°C respectively. Colonies appear within 2 days and show velvety to powdery surface. The colonies are colored and may be yellow to green (*A. flavus*), dark green (*A. fumigatus*) or black (*A. niger*). Identification is by growth characteristics and microscopic morphology under lactophenol cotton blue teased mounts. (Fig. 106.5).

(i) *Aspergillus flavus*

The colonies are velvety, yellow to green. The conidiophores are long spiny and rough with a pyriform shaped vesicle at the tip. The **sterigmata** (phialides) are present in single or double rows covering three-fourths or entire circumference of **vesicle** and point out in all directions. The **conidia** are spherical yellowish green.

(ii) *Aspergillus fumigatus*

The colonies are green or dark green colored. The conidiophores are smooth and contain a club shaped vesicle. The sterigmata (phialides) are present in a single row, usually cover upper half of the vesicle, parallel to the axis of the stalk. The conidia are spherical to oval shaped, green colored and found in long chains that tend to sweep towards the central axis.

(iii) *Aspergillus niger*

Colonies are black in color. Microscopically, conidiophores contain globose vesicle with double row of sterigmata (phialides) covering the entire surface. Conidia are spherical and black colored.

(iv) *Aspergillus terreus*

Colonies are cinnamon brown colored. The conidiophores are short, smooth. The sterigmata are compactly columnar and present in two rows on vesicle.

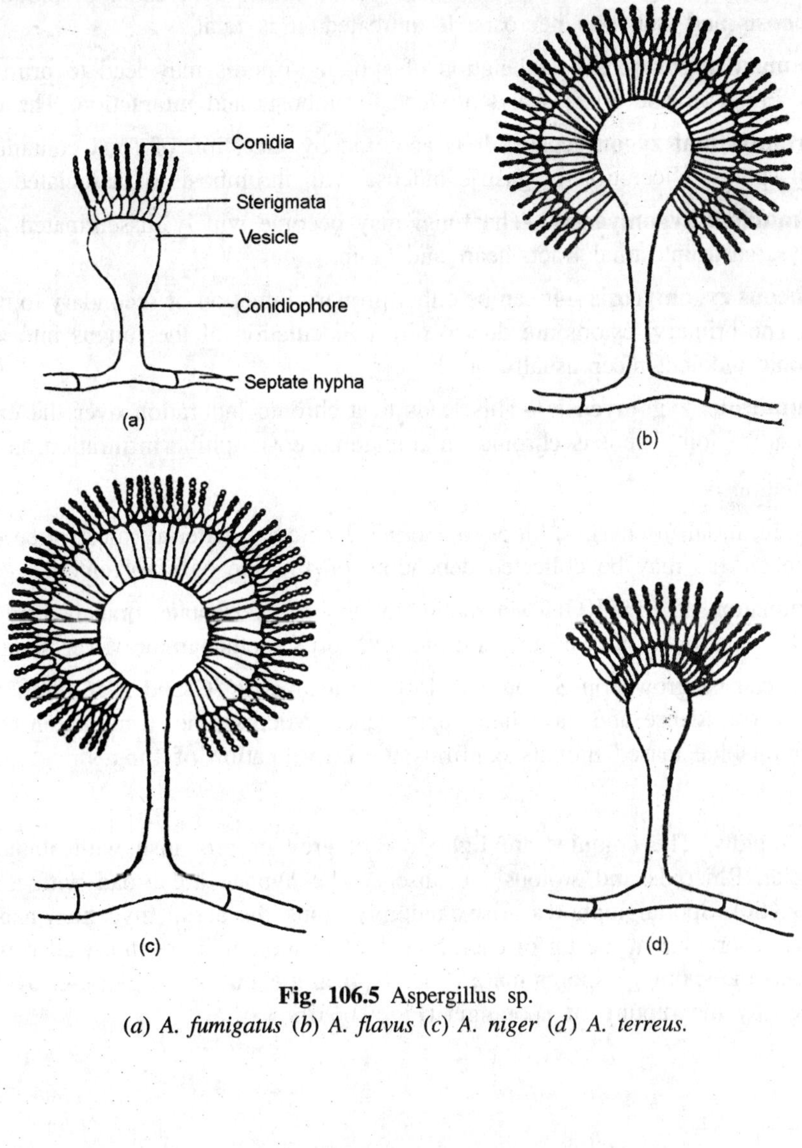

Fig. 106.5 Aspergillus sp.
(*a*) *A. fumigatus* (*b*) *A. flavus* (*c*) *A. niger* (*d*) *A. terreus.*

MUCORMYCOSIS (ZYGOMYCOSIS)

It is an opportunistic invasive infection caused by saprophytic fungi, notably species of ***Mucor***, ***Rhizopus*** and ***Absidia*** of the family Mucoraceae, order Mucorales and class zygomycetes. These fungi are ubiquitous in environment and are common saprophytes of soil, manure, decaying vegetables and fruits. They are frequently encountered as laboratory contaminants. They are essentially **opportunistic fungi**. They replicate in blood vessels with predilection for paranasal sinuses, lungs, gut causing tissue necrosis and suppuration. The major predisposing factors include diabetes mellitus, ketoacidosis, chronic debilitating diseases such as leukemia and lymphoma, starvation, widespread use of broad spectrum antibiotics, corticosteroids, antimetabolites and immunosuppressive drugs and immunodeficiency. The infection is acquired by inhalation of spores. **Zygomycosis** may present in several clinical forms.

1. **Rhinocerebral zygomycosis**—Spores germinate in the nose or upper respiratory tract. Mycelia invade orbit, sinuses and brain, where massive invasion of blood vessels causes thrombosis and ischemic necrosis. If untreated, it is fatal.
2. **Pulmonary zygomycosis**—Inhalation of sporangiospores may lead to primary infection in lungs. Fungi invade arteries and produce thrombosis and infaraction. The disease is fatal.
3. **Gastrointestinal zygomycosis**—It is acquired by ingestion of food contaminated with the fungal spores. Ulceration of gastric mucosa with thrombosis of associated vessels is seen.
4. **Disseminated zygomycosis**—The fungi may become widely disseminated, affecting lungs, kidneys, gastrointestinal tract, heart and brain.
5. **Cutaneous zygomycosis**—It can be either primary infection or secondary to the disseminated form. The primary lesions are due to direct inoculation of the fungus into skin. It leads to a chronic indolent ulcer usually on the leg.
6. **Subcutaneous zygomycosis**—This leads to a chronic induration over the extremities, neck or pelvic region. There is chronic inflammation, eosinophilic infiltration and fibrosis.

Laboratory diagnosis

Pus, sputum, nasal discharges, biopsy material or autopsy material (most often diagnosis made postmortem) specimens may be collected depending on the site of involvement.

The examination of 10% KOH wet mount shows broad, aseptate, branched hyphae. They can be stained with hematoxylin and eosin stain and Gomori's methanamine silver stains.

The fungi can be grown on Sabouraud dextrose agar at 25°C and 37°C with antibiotics. The colonies are floccose, dense and have hairy appearance. Microscopic examination of growth under lactophenol cotton blue teased mounts confirms the identification of fungus.

Mucor

It grows rapidly. The colonies are light to dull grey or brownish with abundant aerial and substrate mycelia. Rhizoids and stolons are absent. The hyphae are broad with thin walls, **non-septate** (coenocytic). Sporangiophores arise randomly along the aerial mycelium and are branched, bearing spherical sporangia at the tip of each branch. The sporangia are thin-walled with columellae becoming dark as the sporangiospores mature. The **sporangiospores** are globose, oval or cylindrical and are released by the rupture of sporangia (Fig. 106.6).

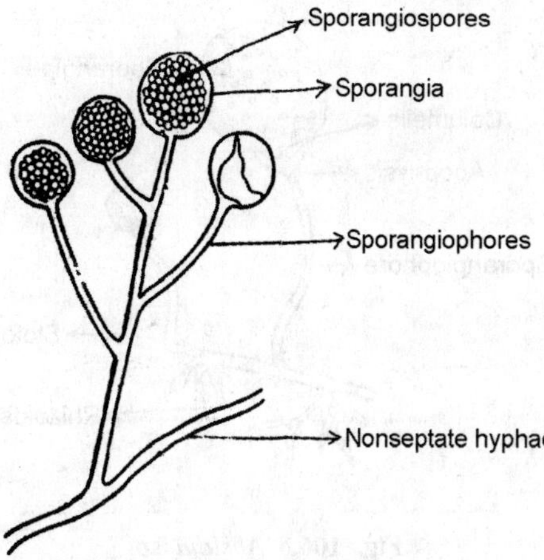

Fig. 106.6 *Mucor* sp.

Rhizopus

The colonies are fast spreading, white to light grey in the beginning but become darker as sporangia mature. The hyphae are broad, non-septate with thin walls, submerged or aerial **stolon** with root-like short branches called **rhizoids**, under the points where sporangiophores develop. The sporangiophores are hyaline to brown, erect, single or in groups of two or three, producing sporangia with columellae at the tip. The **sporangia** are globose, hyaline at first, turning dark brown, grey or black as the **sporangiospores** mature (Fig. 106.7).

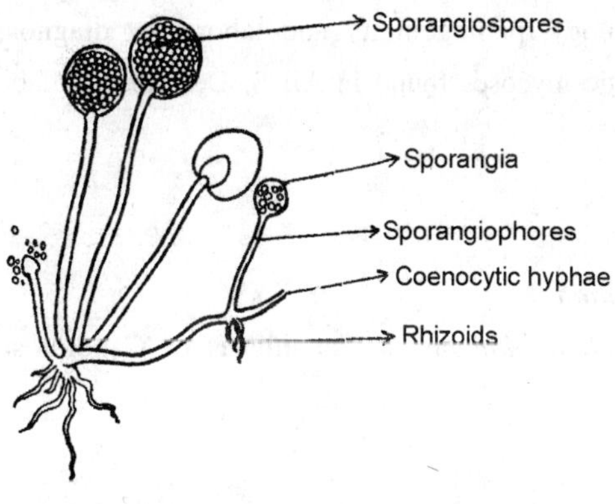

Fig. 106.7 *Rhizopus* sp.

Absidia

They produce many branched, arching stolons, similar to *Rhizopus*. They form rhizoids at nodes that penetrate the substrate. The sporangiophores are internodal in contrast to those of *Rhizopus* that occur at nodes. The sporangiophores gradually expand, forming an apophysis topped by a columella. The prominent **apophysis** helps to differentiate from *Rhizopus* and *Mucor*. The sporangiophores are branched and possess septa so that walls do not collapse which helps in differentiating from other zygomycetes. The columella is hemispherical or elongate, sometimes topped by a spine (Fig. 106.8).

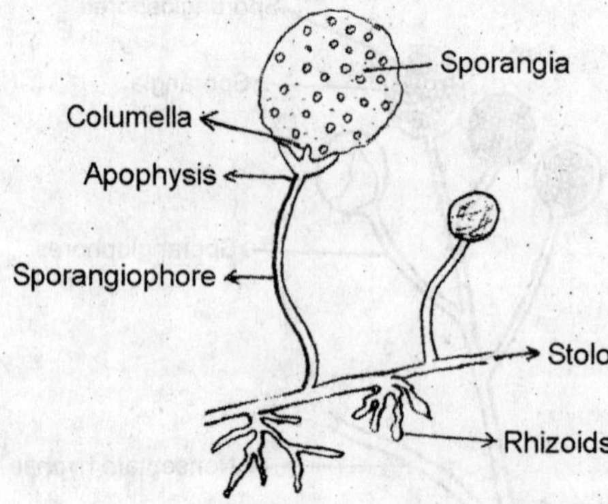

Fig. 106.8 *Absidia* sp.

Zygomycosis is an umbrella term used for diseases caused by many aseptate filamentous fungal species classified under order Mucorales and Entomophthorales of class Zygomycetes under the phylum Zygomycota. Some investigators prefer to call mycoses caused by members belonging to order Mucorales as **mucormycosis** and to order Entomophthorales as entomophthoromycosis or subcutaneous zygomycosis which is further subdivided into two types namely conidiobolomycosis and basidiobolomycosis.

QUESTIONS

Essay Questions:

1. Describe the morphology, pathogenicity and laboratory diagnosis of *Candida albicans*.
2. Enumerate opportunistic mycoses found in AIDS. Describe the laboratory diagnosis of Cryptococcal meningitis.

Short Notes:

1. *Candida albicans*
2. Morphology of *Candida*
3. Pathogenicity of *Candida albicans* or Candidiasis or Candidiosis or Moniliasis
4. Thrush
5. Oral thrush
6. Corn meal agar
7. Chlamydospores
8. Germ tube test or Reynaulds-Braude phenomenon
9. Mention four species of *Candida* of human importance
10. Pseudohyphae or Pseudomycelium
11. Describe the morphology, cultural characters and laboratory diagnosis of *Cryptococcus neoformans*
12. Pathogenicity of *Cryptococcus neoformans* or cryptococcosis
13. Morphology of Cryptococcus neoformans
14. Capsule of *Cryptococcus neoformans*

15. How do you differentiate *Cryptococcus neoformans* from other *Cryptococcus* species
16. Opportunistic systemic mycoses
17. Pneumocystosis
18. *Pneumocystis carinii*
19. *Penicillium marneffei* or Penicilliosis marneffei
20. Aspergillosis
21. Aspergilli or *Asperigillus* species
22. Describe the morphology and cultural characters of *Aspergillus*
23. Opportunistic fungi
24. *Mucor*
25. *Rhizopus*
26. Mucormycosis or Zygomycosis
27. What are the differences between *Mucor* and *Rhizopus*
28. Draw neat labelled diagrams of *Mucor* and *Rhizopus*

107

Miscellaneous mycoses

- *Keratomycosis*
- *Otomycosis*
- *Mycotoxicoses and Mycetismus*

KERATOMYCOSIS (MYCOTIC KERATITIS)

It is an invasive fungal infection of corneal stroma, occurs following injury or trauma caused by a variety of fungal species. Fungal spores colonize the injured tissue and initiate an inflammatory reaction leading to hypopyon, ulcer and endophthalmitis. The causative fungi are saprobic, opportunistic fungi. The predisposing conditions are corneal trauma or widespread use of corticosteroids. The majority of cases of keratomycosis have been caused by *Aspergillus*, *Fusarium* and *Candida* species. Other fungal genera causing keratomycosis are *Curvularia*, *Acremonium*, *Paecilomyces*, *Penicillium*, *Alternaria*, *Fonsecaea*, *Pseudoallescheria*, *Bipolaris* and *Aureobasidium*.

Diagnosis may be made by examination of corneal deep scrapings under 10% KOH wetmount or calcofluor white stain and Gram's stain. The specimens may be cultured on Sabouraud dextrose agar with antibiotics incubated at 25°C and 37°C, on brain heart infusion agar with antibiotics and cycloheximide incubated at 37°C and on blood agar as well. The fungal isolates are identified by their colony characteristics and microscopic appearance in lactophenol cotton blue teased mount and finally by slide cultures.

Fusarium

The colonies are fluffy to cottony. Sometimes diffusable pigment is produced on reverse. The conidiophores are single or grouped into "**sporodochia**", a compact mass of interwoven conidiophores. Conidia are produced singly or in conidial balls, hyaline and unicellular or transversely septate. **Microconidia** are single-celled and often found in chains or balls. **Macroconidia** are oblongate and cylindrical but more often crescent or falciform or bean-shaped (Fig. 107.1).

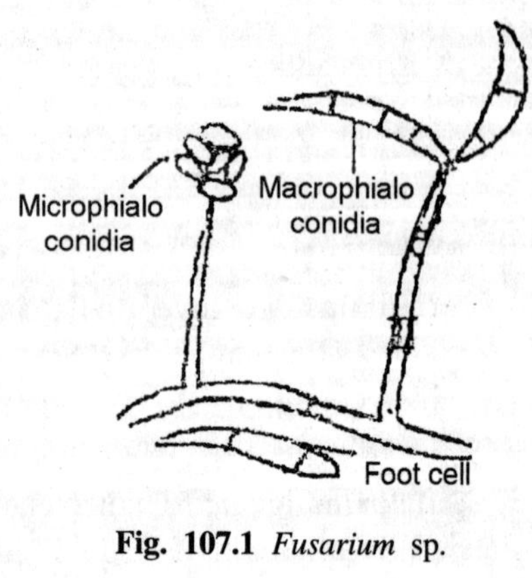

Fig. 107.1 *Fusarium* sp.

OTOMYCOSIS

It is a subacute or chronic superficial fungal infection of external auditory canal. The causative fungi are found as saprophytes in the environment and include

Aspergillus niger, *A. fumigatus*, *A. flavus*, *Penicillium* sp, *Candida albicans*, *C. tropicalis* and *Candida krusei*. The fungi are usually secondary invaders of the tissue rendered susceptible by bacterial infections, physical injury or excessive accumulation of cerumen in the auditory canal. The symptoms are itching, pain and deafness. Secondary bacterial infections caused by *Proteus* and *Pseudomonas* may develop.

The diagnosis is made by microscopy and culture of the pus or debris material taken from external auditory canal. The presence of fungal hyphae is seen in 10% KOH wet mount. The specimens are inoculated on to Sabouraud dextrose agar and the growth can be identified by colony morphology and microscopic morphology under lactophenol cotton blue teased mounts.

MYCOTOXINS AND MYCETISMUS

Certain fungi form poisonous secondary metabolites, known as **Mycotoxins** that can cause intoxication and death in animals and humans consumed alongwith feed/food.

Mycotic poisoning is of 2 types :

(1) Mycetism or Mycetismus—It is caused by ingestion of fungi (containing preformed toxin) e.g., mushroom poisoning. Mycetism may cause gastrointestinal disease, dermatitis or death. The hallucinogenic agents (d-lysergic acid, psilocybin) produced by *Psilocybe* species may cause mycetism.

(2) Mycotoxicosis—The diseases that result due to ingestion of food/feed that contains mycotoxins are known as Mycotoxicoses.

Many fungi such as *Aspergillus*, *Penicillium* and *Fusarium* can elaborate toxins particularly in cereals and oilseed crops e.g., groundnut, peanuts, cotton seed, rice, corn etc. Mycotoxins usually survive cooking.

Table 107.1 Mycotoxins

Toxins of *Aspergillus*	— Aflatoxins B_1, B_2, G_1, G_2, Sterigmatocystin, Ochratoxin, Ascladiol, fumigatin
Toxins of *Penicillium*	— Patulin, penicillic acid, Rubratoxin, penitrem A, citroveridin, citrinin, cyclopiazonic acid, luteoskyrin, Roquefortine
Toxins of *Fusarium*	— Tricothecenes, Alimentary Toxic Aleukia (ALA), Moniliformin, Fumornisins, Zearelenone, Sciepenols
Ergot alkaloids (ergotism)	— Ergosine, Ergometrin, Ergocristine
Other Mycotoxins	— Agaricus toxins Amanitins (mushroom poisoning)

Aflatoxins

Aflatoxins are mycotoxins produced by *Aspergillus flavus*, *A. parasiticus* and *Penicillium puberculum*. The fungi infect food grains such as groundnuts, maize, sorghum, wheat, rice, cotton seed under conditions of improper storage. The most important factors affecting the formation of toxin are moisture and temperature.

Aflatoxins are most potent hepatotoxins, causing liver damage and carcinogenic. The disease produced by aflatoxins is called "**aflatoxicosis**". Aflatoxins are derivatives of furanocoumarin, and although 17 compounds have been identified; B_1, B_2, G_1, and G_2 are commonly occuring. Aflatoxins

M_1 and M_2 are commonly excreted in milk, urine of mammals following the consumption of mycotoxins.

Ochratoxins

They are mainly produced by *Aspergillus* and *Penicillium* sp. Ochratoxins are a group of closely related derivatives of isocoumarin linked to an amino acid L-β-phenyl alanine. Of the 9 toxins, ochratoxin A commonly occurs in nature. It contaminates mainly grains but also found in coffee, beans and peanuts.

Patulin

It is originally isolated as an antibiotic. It is effective against many bacterial species in low concentrations. It is also strongly fungistatic and is toxic to seeds and seedlings of higher plants. Several *Penicillium* sp. and *Aspergillus* sp. produce patulin, which is considered to be a potent human carcinogen.

Tricothecenes

They are produced by several fungi such as *Fusarium*, *Cephalosporium*, *Myrothecium*, *Trichoderma*, *Stachybotrys*.

Zearlenone

It is produced by *Fusarium* sp. found predominantly in maize, though occurs in other cereals also. Over 30 toxins are found. T-2 toxin is a potent inhibitor of eukaryotic protein synthesis and inhibits platelet aggregation. It increases prothrombin time and causes cardiomyopathy.

Alimentary Toxic Aleukia (ATA)

It is produced by *Cladosporium*, *Penicillium*, *Fusarium*, *Mucor*, and *Alternaria*.

Ergotism

Claviceps purpurea produces certain toxic alkaloids, while growing on the fruiting heads of rye which may lead to ergotoxicosis or ergotism in humans and animals. It results in loss of hair, teeth, nails and gangrene.

QUESTIONS

Essay Question

1. Give an account of Mycotoxins

Short Notes

1. Mycotoxins (or) Mycotic poisoning
2. Aflatoxins (or) Aflatoxicosis (or) Mycotoxins of Aspergillus
3. Mention 4 mycotoxins
4. Patulin
5. T-2 toxin
6. Mycotoxicosis and mycetism.
7. Name four fungi causing eye infections
8. Oculomycosis or Mycotic keratitis
9. *Fusarium*
10. Otomycosis
11. Name fungi causing otomycosis and describe laboratory diagnosis of otomycosis

PART-VI

APPLIED AND CLINICAL DIAGNOSTIC MICROBIOLOGY

108

Normal Microbial Flora of The Human Body

INTRODUCTION

The term **"normal microbial flora"** refers to the microbial population that inhabit the internal and external surfaces of healthy normal humans and animals.

The human fetus is sterile under normal conditions, but is exposed to a variety of microorganisms at birth. Microbial colonization of the neonate begins as the child passes through the birth canal and is exposed to the vaginal flora of the mother. The neonate is then exposed to microorganisms in the environment and to those that colonize hospital personnel and other individuals. Within a short time, the infant develops its own indigenous normal microbial flora. The normal flora of any individual undergoes constant change in accordance with changes in life-style and environment. The normal microbial flora is more or less constant for each species and broadly divided into Resident flora and Transient flora.

RESIDENT FLORA

It consists of relatively fixed types of microorganisms constantly found in a given area, at a given age. If disturbed, it promptly re-establishes itself. They prevent colonisation by other microorganisms.

TRANSIENT FLORA

It consists of either nonpathogenic or pathogenic microorganisms that inhabit the skin or mucus membranes for hours, days or weeks. It varies from time to time, derived from the environment, does not establish itself permanently. If the resident flora is disturbed, transient microflora may colonize, proliferate and produce disease.

ROLE OF NORMAL MICROBIAL FLORA

The normal microbial flora plays a very important beneficial role in the human body.

(1) The microbial flora of intestine synthesizes B-complex vitamins and vitamin-K, which may be absorbed. Thus, they supply some nutritional needs of the host.

(2) They prevent or interfere with colonization or invasion of the body by pathogens through bacterial interference.

(3) Normal microflora raises the overall immune status of the host against pathogens having related or shared antigens.

(4) Normal microflora may produce antibiotic like substances called bacteriocins (*e.g.,* colicins, pyocines etc.) which may kill or inhibit the growth of pathogens.

(5) Normal flora may liberate endotoxins, which may activate alternate complement pathway and help the defense mechanisms of the body.

Normal microflora may have some harmful effects.

(1) When host immunity decreases, they may become opportunistic pathogens and cause disease.

(2) Penicillinase producing microorganisms can aggravate infection by conferring drug resistance against antibiotics.

(3) They cause confusion in diagnosis due to their ubiquitous presence in the body, and their morphological similarity with some pathogens.

(4) Certain alpha hemolytic streptococci, that live as commensals in the mouth may cause dental caries.

NORMAL FLORA OF THE SKIN

The human skin is constantly exposed to environment and contains largely transient flora.

The normal resident flora of of the skin differs in different anatomic sites by secretions, habitual wearing of clothing, occupation and environment and proximity to the mucous membranes such as mouth, nose and perineum.

Profuse sweating, washing and bathing cannot eliminate resident flora, whereas transient flora is eliminated from the skin by low pH, fatty acids in sebaceous secretions and the presence of lysozyme.

The normal resident flora of skin includes *Staphylococcus epidermidis* (*albus*), *Staphylococcus aureus*, *Propionibacterium acnes*, Diphtheroids, *Candida* sp, *Pityrosporum* sp.

NORMAL FLORA OF CONJUNCTIVA (EYE)

The conjunctival flora is normally held in check by the mechanical action of blinking, flow of tears, which contain an antibacterial lysozyme.

The normal flora of eye includes *Staphylococcus epidermidis*, *Staphylococcus aureus*, diphtheroids (*Corynebacterium xerosis*), *Neisseria* sp, *Moraxella* sp, *Haemophilus parainfleunzae*.

NORMAL FLORA OF MOUTH AND UPPER RESPIRATORY TRACT

The mouth and upper respiratory tract contains a wide range of microorganisms–*Staph. epidermidis*, *Staph. aureus*, alpha hemolytic Streptococci (viridans streptococci), *Streptococcus pneumoniae*, *Corynebacterium* sp. (diphtheroides), *Neisseria* sp, *Branhamella* sp, *Haemophilus* sp, *Micrococcus* sp.

The lower respiratory tract (trachea, bronchi) do not have a normal flora, because of the efficient mechanical removal of microorganisms by an upward movement of cilia-driven mucus. A few bacteria, which enter alveoli are engulfed by phagocytes.

Viridans Streptococci are the primary microbes in the oral cavity.

The normal flora associated with tongue and buccal mucosa are Viridans Streptococci (*Strept. mitior*, *Strept. salivarius*), *Streptococcus* sp, *Neisseria* sp, *Veillonella* sp, *Actinomyces* sp, *Lactobacillus* sp, Yeasts (*Candida* sp).

The normal flora associated with teeth and gingival crevices are *Bacteroides* sp. *Fusobacterium* sp, alpha hemolytic Streptococci (*Strept. sanguis*, *Strept. mutans*), *Streptococcus* sp, *Actinomyces* sp, *Lactobacillus* sp, *Porphyromonas gingivalis*, *Prevotella* sp, *Spirochetes* (*Treponema denticola*), *Wolinella* sp, *Selenomonas* sp, *Trichomonas tenax*.

The teeth themselves can become areas for microbial adherence. *Streptococcus mutans* is associated with tooth surface and cause **dental caries** (tooth decay). *Streptococcus mutans* produces glucan, a sticky polymer of glucose that acts like a cement and binds the bacterial cells together and to the tooth surface. This glucan is formed in the presence of disaccharide sucrose (the sugar found in confections), through a process catalyzed by an enzyme located on the surface of cocci; which splits sucrose into monosaccharides glucose and fructose. The enzyme then links the glucose molecules together to form glucan, while the fructose is fermented by the Streptococci into Lactic acid. This lactic acid can etch the surface of the teeth, enhancing microbial adherence. Although *Streptococcus mutans* initiates dental caries, other bacteria such as *Lactobacillus* and *Actinomyces* may act as secondary invaders. The aggregation of bacteria and organic matter on the surface of the teeth is termed "**dental plaque**", which contains very high number of bacteria, about 10^8 cells per mg.

NORMAL FLORA OF NOSE, NASOPHARYNX AND ACCESSORY SINUSES

Nares, nasopharynx and accessory sinuses are heavily colonized by bacteria trapped from inhaled air by infiltration through the nasopharynx. The normal flora includes Viridans Streptococci, *Staphylococcus epidermidis*, *Neisseria* sp, *Corynebacterium* sp, *Moraxella lacunata*.

High doses of antibiotics may eradicate normal flora and results in colonization by Gram negative bacilli such as *E.coli*, *Klebsiella*, *Proteus* and *Pseudomonas* sp.

Nasopharynx frequently carries pathogenic bacteria such as *Streptococcus pyogenes*, *Streptococcus pneumoniae*, *Neisseria meningitidis*, *Staphylococcus aureus*, *Bordetella pertussis*, *Haemophilus influenzae* and *Corynebacterium diphtheriae*.

NORMAL FLORA OF THE GASTROINTESTINAL TRACT

Gastrointestinal tract is the most heavily colonized portion of the body.

Stomach consists of *Lactobacillus* sp and yeasts such as *Candida* sp. Administration of cimetidine in peptic ulcer leads to a great increase in microbial flora of the stomach.

Small Intestine consists of Enterococci, Lactobacilli, Corynebacteria, *Candida* sp., *Bacteroides* sp, *E. coli.*

Large intestine or colon has the largest microbial population, around 10^{11} organisms per gram wet weight, which means that about 25% of feces is made up of microorganisms. Over 300 different bacterial species have been isolated from human feces. It has been calculated that an adult excretes 3×10^3 bacterial cells daily through defecation.

There are about 300 times as many anaerobic bacteria as facultatively anaerobic bacteria.

The normal flora of large intestine includes *Escherichia coli*, *Proteus* sp, *Klebsiellae* sp, *Enterobacter* sp, *Bacteroides* sp, *Fusobacterium* sp, *Bifidobacterium* sp, *Eubacterium* sp, *Lactobacillus* sp, *Clostridium* sp, and protozoans such as *Trichomonas hominis*, *Entamoeba histolytica*, *Endolimax* sp and *Iodamoeba* sp.

IMPLANTATION OF LACTOBACILLI

The oral administration of the Gram positive bacterium *Lactobacillus acidophilus* may cure some intestinal disorders. The principle is that ingestion of large numbers of the lactobacilli may result in replacement of undesirable organisms by harmless or beneficial organisms in the intestine. The implantation of Lactobacilli depends on ingestion of large number of the organisms and on supplying lactose that can be readily utilized by the microorganisms. Several commercial products containing lactobacilli are available for therapeutic use.

NORMAL FLORA OF THE UROGENITAL TRACT

The urogential tract is sterile in the upper portions (*i.e.,* upper urethra, urinary bladder, kidneys, testes, ovaries), but it may contain large numbers of microorganisms in the lower urethra, meatus, vagina and vulva. *Staphylococcus epidermidis*, nonhemolytic Streptococci and diphtheroids are predominant in the distal portions of male and female urethras.

Mycobacterium smegmatis, a saprophyte is commonly present in urethral secretions of both males and females.

The vagina of new born is colonized by Lactobacilli due to glycogen deposition in vaginal epithelial cells as a result of estrogen passively transferred from the mother. The pH is acidic due to lactic acid produced by fermentation of glycogen by lactobacilli and may remain for a few days. Once the estrogen is eliminated, the pH becomes neutral or slightly alkaline and remains so till puberty. This causes a change in normal flora to alpha hemolytic Streptococci, nonhemolytic Streptococci, Micrococci, diphtheroids and coliforms.

The adult female genital tract has a very complex normal flora. From puberty to menopause, the pH of vagina becomes acidic 4.4 to 4.6. It is because the estrogen causes glycogen deposition in vaginal epithelial cells. As a result, lactobacilli that are acidophilic colonize vagina and ferment glycogen to produce lactic acid.

The normal adult vaginal flora, often comprises–*Lactobacillus* (Dodderlein's bacilli), *Staphylococcus epidermidis*, Peptococci, Peptostreptococci, *Clostridium* sp, Diphtheroids, *Gardnerella* sp, *Ureaplasma*, Enterococci, *Neisseria* sp, Group B Streptococci (*Strept. agalactiae*), Streptococci and *Candida* sp.

BACTERIA IN BLOOD AND TISSUES

Blood and internal tissues are sterile but there may be a transient bacteremia following brushing teeth, bowel movement and catheterization.

QUESTIONS

Essay Question

1. Describe the normal flora of the human body.

Short Notes

1. Normal flora of genitourinary tract.
2. What is the importance of normal flora?
3. What is the difference between resident and transient flora?
4. Normal flora of intestine.
5. What sites in the body are free from microorganisms?
6. Why is there not a normal flora in the lower respiratory tract.
7. *Lactobacillus acidophilus*.

109

Collection and Transport of Specimens for Laboratory Investigation/Diagnosis

The laboratory diagnosis of infectious diseases begins with the collection of a clinical specimen for examination. The general principles to be followed, while collecting the sample are as follows. (Fig. 109.1).

- Wash hands before and after collection of sample.
- Collect the sample before the administration of antibiotics.
- Strict aseptic techniques must be practiced while collecting the sample.
- Collect the specimen at right time in relation to patient's symptoms.
- The specimen collected must be representative of the infectious process. For example, in a case of pneumonia sputum should be collected but not the saliva.
- The specimen should be collected in an adequate amount.
- The specimen should not be contaminated by organisms from outside source.
- Specimen should be collected in sterile containers and sealed and properly labelled with patient's name, age sex, hospital no., clinical history and treatment given.
- The specimen should be transported immediately without any delay to the laboratory.
- If necessary, transport media may be used for preserving any organisms which may present in the sample.
- The specimens should be immediately processed.

The commonly collected specimens for bacteriological examination are :

Throat swabs, sputum, nasal swabs, ear swabs, eye conjunctival swabs, wound swabs, blood, pus, feces, urine, CSF, aspirations–pleural, ascitic, synovial fluids, vaginal swabs and rectal swabs.

When viral diseases are suspected, several different specimens may be taken in special transport media supplied by virology laboratories. The specimens should be refrigerated at 4°C or should be delivered to the laboratory within one hour. The specimens collected in viral infections are as follows:

CNS diseases – CSF, brain, blood, feces, throat swabs or throat washings.

Respiratory diseases – Sputum, throat swabs or throat washings.

Eye diseases – conjunctival swabs or scrapings.

Skin lesions – Vesicle or pustule fluid in capillary tubes, air-dried slides from scrapings of macules or papules.

For serological tests two blood samples (paired sera) are collected, the first taken as soon as possible after the onset of illness, the second 2-3 weeks later so that antibody titres can be compared to demonstrate a rise. Alternatively, diagnosis may be based on the demonstration of specific IgM antibody in a single, early blood sample.

Specimens collected in fungal diseases include skin scrapings, nails, hair and other specimens in the same way as for bacteriological examination.

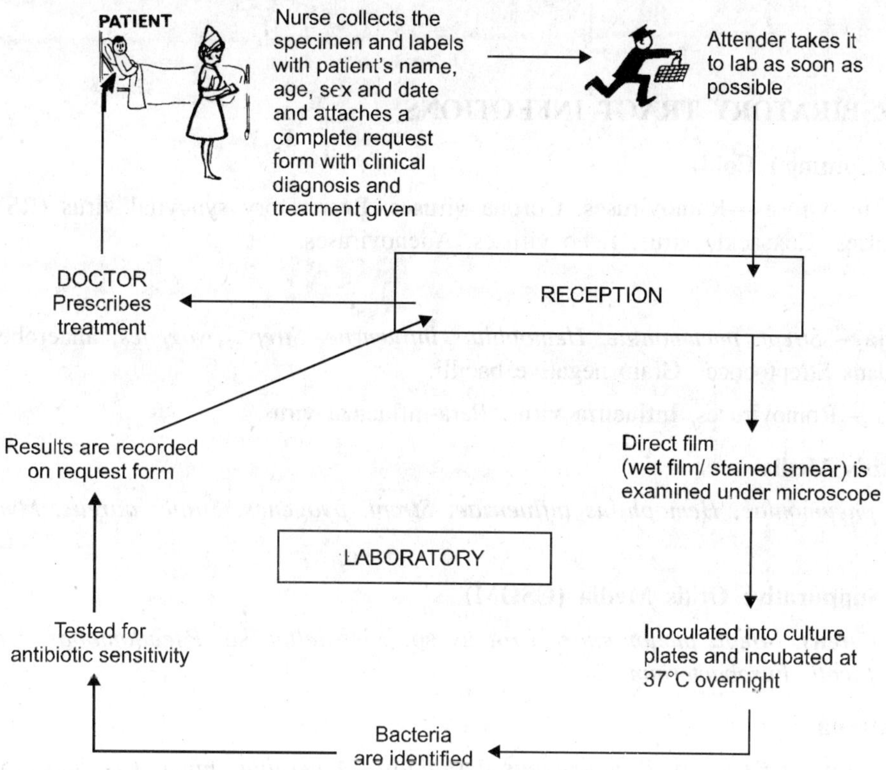

Fig. 109.1 The sequence of laboratory identification of bacteria from infectious material.

110

Respiratory Tract Infections

UPPER RESPIRATORY TRACT INFECTIONS

1. Rhinitis (Common Cold)

Mainly by viruses—Rhinoviruses, Corona viruses, Respiratory syncytial virus (RSV), Para-influenza viruses, Coxsackie virus, Echo viruses, Adenoviruses.

2. Sinusitis

Bacteria – *Strept. pneumoniae*, *Hemophilus influenzae*, *Strept. pyogenes*, anaerobes, *Staph. aureus,* Viridans Streptococci, Gram negative bacilli.

Viruses – Rhinoviruses, Influenza virus, Para-influenza virus.

3. Acute Otitis Media

Strept. pneumoniae, *Hemophilus influenzae*, *Strept. pyogenes*, *Staph. aureus*, *Mycoplasma pneumoniae*.

4. Chronic Suppurative Otitis Media (CSOM)

Staph. aureus, *Strept. pneumoniae*, *Proteus* sp, *Klebsiellae* sp, *Pseudomonas aeruginosa*, *Bacteroides*, *E.coli*, *Fusobacterium*.

5. Otitis Externa

Staph. aureus, *Proteus* sp, *Pseudomonas aeruginosa*, *Aspergillus niger*, *Candida albicans*.

6. Mastoiditis

Same causative agents as acute otitis media; *Pseudomonas aeruginosa*, Gram negative bacilli.

7. Infections of the Oral Cavity

Prevotella (anaerobic Gram negative bacilli), Herpes simplex virus (HSV), *Candida albicans*.

Vincent's Angina– *Borrelia vincentii*, *Fusobacterium*.

Ludwing's Angina– Streptococci, anaerobes.

8. Sore Throat/Pharyngitis/Tonsillitis

Bacteria – *Strept. pyogenes*, Group C Streptococci, Group G Streptococci, *Arcanobacterium hemolyticum*.

Rarely. *Neisseria gonorrhoeae*, *Corynebacterium diphtheriae*, *Mycoplasma pneumoniae*, *Yersinia enterocolitica*.

Viruses – Adenoviruses, Epstein-Barr (EB) virus, Enteroviruses and other viruses that cause common cold.

9. Laryngitis

Strept. pyogenes, *Moraxella catarrhalis*, and viruses that cause common cold.

10. Laryngo Tracheobronchitis (CROUP)

Parainfluenza viruses, Influenza viruses, RSV, Adenoviruses, Rhinoviruses, Enteroviruses and *Mycoplasma pneumoniae*.

11. Epiglottitis

Hemophilus influenzae (type b), *Hemophilus parainfluenzae*, *Strept. pneumoniae*, *Strept. pyogenes, Staph. aureus*.

LOWER RESPIRATORY TRACT INFECTIONS

1. Bronchitis

Bacteria – *Hemophilus influenzae*, *Strept. pneumoniae*, *Moraxella catarrhalis*, *Mycoplasma pneumoniae*, *Staph. aureus*, *Chlamydia* pneumoniae.

Viruses – Parainfluenza virus, Influenza virus, RSV, Adenovirus, Measles virus, Hanta virus.

2. Pneumonia–Community Acquired

Bacteria – *Strept. pneumoniae*, *Hemophilus influenzae*, *Mycoplasma pneumoniae*, *Legionella pneumophila*, *Staph. aureus*, *Strept. pyogenes*, *Moraxella catarrhalis*, *Klebsiella pneumoniae*, *Pseudomonas aeruginosa*, Anaerobes–*Bacteroides*.

Coxiella burnetti (Q fever), *Francisella tularensis* (tularemia), *Myco. tuberculosis* (TB), *Chlamydia psittaci* (psittacosis), *Nocardia* (Nocardiosis).

Viruses – Influenza virus, RSV, Adeno virus, parainfluenza virus, Measles virus, V-Z virus.

Fungi – *Histoplasma, Coccidioides*, *Blastomyces*.

3. Pneumonia–Hospital Acquired

Strept. pneumoniae, *Hemophilus influenzae*, *Klebsiellae* sp, E.coli, *Proteus* sp, *Pseudomonas aeruginosa*, *Acinetobacter*, *Staph.* aureus, oral anaerobes.

4. Pneumonia–HIV-Associated

Pneumocystis carinii, *Cryptococcus neoformans*, *Mycobacterium tuberculosis*, *Mycobacterium avium-intracellulare* complex, *Hemophilus influenzae*, *Strept. pneumoniae*, *Cytomegalovirus*.

5. Whooping Cough

Bordetella pertussis, *Bordetella parapertussis*.

6. Legionnaire's Disease

Legionella pneumophila.

7. Farmer's Lung (Allergic alveolitis)

Type III hypersensitivity, characterized by cough and breathlessness. It is common in farm workers and is due to chronic inhalation of the dust (spores) of moldy hay of thermophilic actinomycetes e.g., *Micropolyspora faeni*, *Thermoactinomyces vulgaris*.

8. Bronchiectasis

Hemophilus influenzae, *Streptococcus pneumoniae*, *Staph. aureus*, anaerobes–*Bacteroides* and anaerobic cocci, *Klebsiella*, *Pseudomonas aeruginosa*, *Aspergillus sp.*

LABORATORY DIAGNOSIS

Specimen Collection

- Throat swab – sore throat, pharyngitis, tonsillitis.
- Sputum – Collected into a sterile, wide mouthed container with a secure lid. The specimen should be coughed. Mucopurulent or purulent sputum should be collected before the start of antibiotics.
- Pleural fluid – in lower respiratory tract infections.
- Blood – for blood cultures.

Microscopy

- Gram's stain – to detect bacteria and pus cells.
- Negative staining – to demonstrate capsules of pneumococci, *Cryptococcus neoformans*.
- Quellung test for pneumococci and *Hemophilus influenzae*.
- ZN stain and Fluorescent stains for AFB.
- 10% KOH wet mount to detect fungi.
- Direct fluorescent antibody (DFA) for *Legionella pneumophila*.

Culture

Specimens are inoculated on to chocolate agar, blood agar and MacConkey agar plates and incubated at 37°C, overnight in an atmosphere of 5% CO_2.

Optochin sensitivity and bile solubility test may be put up for Pneumococci; Bacitracin sensitivity for *Strept. pyogenes* and *Hemophilus* growth factor (X and V) tests are done. Gram negative bacilli are identified by biochemical tests and slide agglutination with specific antisera.

Special media may be used for isolation of specific pathogens.

- Potassium tellurite blood agar for diphtheria bacilli.
- Lowenstein–Jensen (LJ) medium when TB is suspected.
- Mycoplasma agar for *Mycoplasma pneumoniae*.
- Charcoal-yeast extract agar for *Legionella penumophila*.
- Blood cultures should be performed on patients with fever and lower respiratory tract infections.

- Sabouraud's dextrose agar for fungi.
- Antibiotic sensitivity tests may be performed.

Demonstration of antigen (*e.g.*, Pneumococci, *Cryptococcus neoformans*) in sputum, pleural fluid, blood and urine by counter immunoelectrophoresis and is useful when antibiotics have already been started.

Serology – paired sera should be taken to demonstrate specific antibodies against pathogens. CFT, Fluorescent antibody test, Hemagglutination inhibition (influenza), ELISA etc. may be used.

Total and differential WBC count may be useful for differentiating bacterial pneumonias from non-bacterial pneumonias and legionnaire's disease.

111

Meningitis

PURULENT (PYOGENIC) MENINGITIS

It is usually caused by bacteria, characterized by acute inflammatory exudate with large numbers of pus cells (polymorphonuclear cells).

ASEPTIC MENINGITIS

It is usually associated with viral infections and is usually self-limited, characterized by an increase of lymphocytes and other mononuclear cells (pleocytosis) in the CSF (in contrast to pus cells in bacterial meningitis).

ENCEPHALITIS

It is an inflammation of the brain parenchyma and is usually a result of viral infection.

MENINGOENCEPHALITIS

Concomitant meningitis that occurs with encephalitis is known as meningoencephalitis.

BRAIN ABSCESS

Localized collection of pus in a cavity formed by the breakdown of tissue.

CAUSATIVE ORGANISMS

Bacteria – *Neisseria meningitidis*, *Hemophilus influenzae* (usually type b), *Streptococcus pneumoniae*, *Esch. coli*, Group B streptococci, *Listeria monocytogenes*, *Pseudomonas*, *Clostridium welchii*, *Mycobacterium tuberculosis*, *Salmonella*, *Treponema pallidum*, *Leptospira*, *Borrelia burgdorferi*.

Viruses – ECHO viruses, Coxsackie A and B viruses, Poliovirus, Mumps virus, Measles virus, Herpes simplex virus (HSV), Varicella–zoster (VZ) virus. Adenovirus, Arboviruses, Rabies virus, Lymphocytic choriomeningitis (LCM) virus.

Fungi – *Cryptococcus neoformans*, *Candida albicans*, *Histoplasma capsulatum*, *Coccidioides immitis*, *Mucor*, *Aspergillus*.

COLLECTION OF SPECIMEN

CSF is collected by lumbar puncture with careful skin disinfection and using a sterile technique. CSF should be taken in three separate sterile containers or may be divided into three portions. The CSF for serology and for isolation of viruses can be refrigerated, whereas the CSF for isolation of bacteria should not be refrigerated and can be incubated either as such or with an equal volume of glucose broth.

TRANSPORT OF SPECIMEN

CSF specimens should be transported immediately to the laboratory. The CSF should never be refrigerated. If CSF is not rapidly processed, it should be incubated at 35°C or left at room temperature. If there is a delay in transport, the CSF is mixed with equal volume of Glucose broth and transported at room temperature.

EXAMINATION OF CSF

CSF is normally sterile and almost cell free. Visible bacteria or significant rise in cellular content are significant.

PRESSURE AND APPEARANCE

In bacterial meningitis, the CSF will be under pressure. Appearance is cloudy or turbid. In tuberculous meningitis white **'cob-web' clot** is formed on standing.

Cell count. Total WBC count in uncentrifuged CSF is obtained by counting cells manually in a hemocytometer chamber under microscope. Differential count can be obtained by staining a centrifuged CSF deposit.

WET Film. A wet film of CSF can be examined under microscope for pus cells and organisms.

Initial CSF results

Meningitis	Neutrophils per mm^3	Lymphocytes per mm^3	Protein mg%	Glucose	Gram's stain
Viral	–	50–500	60–80	normal	–
Bacterial	500–2000		100–600	Low	Bacteria may be seen
Tuberculous	100–600		80–120	Low	–
Normal CSF	–	1–3	30–45	40–80	–

The CSF specimen from one container or 1st portion of CSF can be centrifuged to obtain sediment (deposit) and supernatant.

Biochemistry. The biochemical estimations of protein and glucose are made from supernatant. A blood sample should be examined for blood glucose, to compare with CSF level.

Detection of antigen – The antigens of causative agents such as meningococcal, pneumococcal, *E.coli* and cryptococcal antigens can be demonstrated in the supernatant by counter immuno-electrophoresis, coagglutination and latex agglutination tests.

Gram's staining. Smears are prepared from centrifuged deposit and stained by Gram's method and examined under microscope to demonstrate bacteria. Meningococci may be seen intracellularly inside the polymorphs.

ZN staining or Fluorescent staining in case of tuberculous meningitis, Negative staining for cryptococcal meningitis may be carried out.

Culture – The CSF specimen from second container or 2nd portion of CSF is inoculated on to chocolate agar and blood agar and incubated overnight at 37°C in 5% CO_2. MacConkey agar may also be used if Enterobacteriaceae organisms are suspected.

Any growth must be regarded as significant until proven otherwise. Some bacteria may require prolonged incubation.

The growth is identified by morphology, biochemical reactions and slide agglutination tests with specific antisera.

The CSF specimen from third container or 3rd portion of CSF may be either incubated as such or after adding an equal volume of glucose broth, overnight at 37°C and inoculated on to chocolate agar and blood agar. This method may yield growth when direct plating fails.

Blood culture should be performed at the same time.

For detection of carriers, nasopharyngeal swabs may be taken for culture.

LABORATORY DIAGNOSIS OF MENINGITIS

Specimen

↓

CSF – Collected under sterile precaution and submitted to laboratory immediately.

GENERAL

1. PHYSICAL:
   - Normal clear
   - Pyogenic – opalescent or turbid
   - Tubercular – Cobweb formation (on standing)
2. CHEMICAL:
   - Protein - increased in pyogenic
   - Glucose - reduced in pyogenic
   - Chloride - reduced in tubercular
3. CYTOLOGICAL
   - Pleocytosis - in all infections
   - PMN leucocytosis - pyogenic
   - Lymphocytosis - Tubercular

MICROBIOLOGICAL

MICROSCOPY

1. Direct
2. Centrifuged sediment

Gram's / Negative / Z–N Staining

CULTURE

- Blood Agar / Chocolate Agar under 10% CO_2. Isolation, Identification by Microscopy and Biochemical tests confirmation by Serology Antibiotic Sensitivity test
- L.J. (Tubercular meningitis)

1. *Neisseria meningitidis* : G-ve intracellular diplococci, growth on BA, Thayer-Martin Agar, Oxidase +ve, fermentation of glucose and maltose, serotyping.
2. *Haemophilus influenzae* : G-ve coccobacilli, growth on chocolate agar, requirement for X and V factors, satellitism, biotyping and serotyping.

Identification of carriers by culture with swabs from posterior nasopharynx by pernasal or West's post nasal swabs.

112

Infective Endocarditis

DEFINITION

Infective endocarditis has been defined as infection of the endocardial lining of the heart, characterized by the production of infective vegetations on the damaged endothelium.

In most cases one or more heart valves (aortic or mitral valve or both) are involved. Replacement valves, especially prosthetic valves are also liable to infection.

Less frequently, it may develop on the mural endocardium or a septal defect.

PREDISPOSING FACTORS

Congenital heart disease, Rheumatic fever, Atherosclerotic aortic valve disease, Prosthetic valve heart surgery, and Drug addiction.

CLASSIFICATION

Infective endocarditis is clinically classified into acute endocarditis and subacute endocarditis.

Infective endocarditis may also be classified as native or prosthetic valve endocarditis depending on the type of valve involved.

Infective endocarditis in intravenous drug addicts constitutes another category.

Acute Infective Endocarditis

It is relatively rare. It is caused by aggressive pathogens–most commonly *Staph. aureus*, but sometimes *Str. pyogenes*, *Str. pneumoniae* or *N. gonorrhoeae*–and presents with high fever, general toxemia and rapidly deteriorating cardiac function due to valve destruction and metastatic lesions are common. It is rapidly fatal unless promptly treated with appropriate antibiotics, and even when the infection is climinated the valves are often so badly damaged as to require immediate replacement.

Subacute Endocarditis

It typically develops insidiously, with low fever, night sweats, weight loss and general ill-health. It usually involves a damaged valve and is caused by the members of the normal flora, typically Viridans Streptococci. It does not produce metastatic lesions and is not very fatal.

The Viridans Streptococci (normal flora of the mouth) can enter the blood from the gums after dental extraction or gingival bleeding. The disease is known as **subacute bacterial endocarditis**.

CAUSATIVE AGENTS OF INFECTIVE ENDOCARDITIS

- Viridans Streptococci
- Enterococci

- *Staphylococcus aureus*
- *Staphylococcus epidermidis*
- HACEK group (*Hemophilus*, *Actinobacillus*, *Cardiobacterium*, *Eikenella*, *Kingella*)
- Diphtheroids
- Coliforms–*E.coli, Klebsiella, Serratia*
- *Pseudomonas*
- *Bacteroides* and fusiform bacilli
- *Coxiella burnetti*
- *Chlamydiae*
- Spirochetes
- *Candida albicans*
- *Aspergillus* sp.

LABORATORY DIAGNOSIS

1. Blood cultures

Atleast 3 sets (aerobic and anaerobic) of blood cultures should be obtained over a period of 3 to 6 hours at 30 to 60 min intervals before the start of antibiotic therapy.

Blood cultures constitute the key confirmatory test.

Blood culture negative endocarditis may be due to

- fastidious bacteria or slow growing bacteria.
- cell wall deficient bacteria.
- previous antibiotic therapy.
- non bacterial causes.
- incorrect clinical diagnosis.
- differential diagnosis–rheumatic fever, vasculitic endocarditis, eosinophilic endocarditis.

2. Echocardiography

It is very helpful in demonstrating cardiac vegetations.

3. Serology

Paired sera are collected from all cases of blood culture negative endocarditis cases and, when culture yield growth of uncertain clinical significance; serological tests can be done to demonstrate antibodies to *Coxiella burnetii*, *Chlamydia psittaci*, *Brucella*, *Candida albicans*, *Aspergillus* usually by CFT.

Immunofluorescent test for antibodies against Viridans Streptococci may be helpful when only an occasional blood culture yields the growth and its significance is uncertain.

113

Blood Stream Infections (Bacteremia, Septicemia)

CAUSATIVE ORGANISMS

Gram Negative bacteria	*Gram Positive bacteria*	*Fungi*
E. Coli *Klebsiellae* sp. *Proteus* sp. *Salmonella* sp. *Hemophilus influenzae* *Pseudomonas aeruginosa* *Enterobacter* *Serratia marcescens* *Bacteroides fragilis* *Neisseria meningitidis*	*Streptococcus pneumoniae* *Staphylococcus aureus* *Streptococcus pyogenes* Group B streptococci Viridans streptococci *Staphylococcus epidermidis* Enterococci *Listeria monocytogenes*	*Candida albicans*

LABORATORY DIGNOSIS

1. Blood cultures – 2 or 3 sets of blood cultures (aerobic and anaerobic) should be performed. (Refer *Salmonella* chapter)
2. Cultures of other infected sites
   - urine and sputum
   - swabs of infected burns, wounds, umbilicus etc.
   - Feces
3. Detection of antigens in serum
   - counter immunoelectrophoresis
   - coagglutination
   - latex agglutination test
   - ELISA
   - Limulate lysate test for detection of endotoxins of Gram negative bacteria.
4. Animal inoculation–to isolate rare pathogens such as *Leptospira*, Rickettsiae and viruses.
5. Serology–to demonstrate a rise in antibody titre against causative organism.

114

Pyrexia of Unknown Origin (PUO)

DEFINITION

PUO is defined as an illness in which persistent fever with a temperature higher than 38.3°C (101°F) on several occasions for a duration of more than three weeks is the predominant clinical feature and remains unexplained after careful clinical examination and routine radiological and laboratory investigations despite one week of inpatient investigations.

CAUSES OF PUO

I—Infections – bacterial, viral, fungal and parasitic

II—Neoplasms – Hodgkin's lymphoma,
- non-hodgkin's lymphoma,
- leukemia
- renal cell carcinoma
- hepatoma
- colon cancer.

III—Collagen vascular diseases
- SLE
- temporal arteritis
- polyarteritis nodosa

IV—Miscellaneous causes–

(A) Granulomatous diseases
- sarcoidosis
- Crohn's disease
- granulomatous hepatitis

(B) Drug induced fevers
- beta lactam antibiotics
- anti-neoplastic drugs

– cardio vascular drugs (*e.g.,* quinidine)

– CNS drugs (*e.g.,* phenytoin)

(C) Pulmonary embolisms

(D) Erythema multiforme

(E) Fictitious fever (psychogenic fever)

(F) Whipple's disease.

Infective Causes of PUO–may be due to non-specific infections or specific infections.

I. *Non-specific causes*. Infection may be caused by many different organisms at an inaccessible site.

– Cryptic abscesses in liver; intraperitoneal, renal, retroperitoneal, para-spinal and pelvic abscesses.
– Osteomyelitis
– Infective endocarditis
– Urinary tract infections
– Sinusitis
– dental abscess
– ear infections
– miscellaneous–prostatitis, cholangitis

II. Specific causes. Specific diseases, each caused by a specific pathogen.

Bacterial diseases — Tuberculosis, Typhoid fever, Brucellosis, Leptospirosis, Relapsing fever, Nocardiosis, Typhus fever, Q fever, Psittacosis, Cat scratch fever.

Viral diseases — Infectious mononucleosis, Cytomegalovirus disease, Hepatitis A or B, Yellow fever, Lassa fever, AIDS

Fungal diseases — Cryptococcosis, Candidiasis, Histoplasmosis, Aspergillosis

Parasitic diseases — hepatic amoebiasis, malaria, kala-azar, Toxoplasmosis, Trypanosomiasis, Pneumocystis, Pneumonia, Filarial infections.

INITIAL SPECIAL INVESTIGATIONS OF PUO

I. HEMATOLOGICAL

1. Hemoglobin and RBC count—Anemia a feature of kala-azar, malaria, endocarditis.
2. WBC count—

   PUS cells—pygenic infections

   Neutropenia—typhoid, malaria, leishmaniasis, SLE, severe drug reactions

   Atypical mononuclear cells—glandular fever

   Eosinophilia—helminths, drug reaction, polyarteritis
3. Thick and thin blood smear—Malarial parasite, *Trypanosoma*, *Leishmania*, *Borrelia*, Filarial worms.
4. ESR > 100 mm/h—TB, collagen diseases neoplasms

II. MICROBIOLOGICAL

1. Blood cultures—multiple blood cultures, not less than three.
2. Blood smears for parasites.
3. Urine microscopy and cultures.
4. Feces microscopy and cultures.
5. Throat swab or sputum cultures.

III. RADIOLOGICAL CHEST X-RAY

Consolidation, empyema, lung abscess, Hilar lymphadenopathy–TB or sarcoidosis.

Laboratory Diagnosis of Enteric Fever and P.U.O.

Isolation and Identification of causative agent by culture

Blood (clot)

Stool, Bile, Urine — Second week onwards → SPECIMEN

5-10 ml. venous blood into 50 ml. Bile broth- Incubate-subculture on MacConkey NLF

Direct plating → BA, CA, DCA, SS, Mac

Enrichment → Subculture

Demonstration of specific antibody

Serum

WIDAL-quantitative estimation of 'O' and 'H' agglutinins in serum. (significant from second week onwards) Doubling dilutions of patients serum in tubes in different rows + constant amount of TO, TH, AH, and BH antigens (killed bacterial suspensions) to different rows-incubation-Titre determination.

Note:

Blood culture-also used in diagnosis of P.U.O. Brucellosis, Septicemia and Pyemia, Bacteriemia in meningitis etc.

Isolation-Morphology

Identification by Biochemical tests

Confirmation by slide agglutination test with specific high titre sera 'O' for grouping 'H' for typing for epidemiology-phage typing.

Interpretation-Titre of 80 and above for 'O' with supportive 'H' agglutinins is significant. Raise in titre in two consecutive tests diagnostic.

Other Serological tests in diagnosis of P.U.O. Brucella agglutination test-Brucellosis/Weilfelix test-Ricketssial fevers/Streptococcus MG and cold agglutination-Primary atypical pneumonia.

CAUSATIVE BACTERIA IN ENTERIC FEVER

1. *Salmonella typhi*-NLF, Motile, fermentation of glucose with acid, without gas indole and urease negative, H_2S +.
2. *Salmonella paratyphi A* : NLF, motile, fermentation of glucose with gas, indole and urease –ve, H_2S –ve.
3. *Salmonella paratyphi B* : NLF, fermentation of glucose with gas, indole and urease –ve, H_2S +++.

Enteric Fever Carriers : Detected by +ve stool or Bile culture or by demonstration of Vi agglutinins in Serum.

115

Bone and Joint Infections

Infection of bones (osteomyelitis or osteitis) and joints (septic or infective arthritis) may occur via the blood stream (hematogenous route) or by direct routes *e.g.,* via a wound.

BONE INFECTIONS (OSTEOMYELITIS)

Acute osteomyelitis is common among children and characterized by the presence of a painful tender bone lesion of acute onset and general systemic symptoms such as pyrexia, tachycardia and polymorphonuclear leucocytosis. It is typically caused by *Staph, aureus*. It presents as a suppurative infection accompanied by edema, vascular congestion and small vessel thrombosis.

Chronic osteomyelitis occurs in adults as well as children characterized by spread of infection into the surrounding soft tissue. The dead bone is separated as a sequestrum. New bone is laid down as a sheath around the sequestrum, known as involucrum. There is usually radiological evidence of osteomyelitis.

CAUSATIVE ORGANISMS

Acute osteomyelitis	*Chronic osteomyelitis*
Staph. aureus (> 90% cases)	*Staph. aureus* (<60% cases)
Strept. pyogenes	*Strept. milleri*
Strept. pneumoniae	*Strept. pneumoniae*
Clostridium welchii	*Actinomyces israelii*
Hemophilus influenzae	Propionibacteria
	Coliforms
	Pseudomonas aeruginosa
	Bacteroides sp.
	Hemophilus sp.
	Salmonella sp.
	Brucella sp.
	Madurella mycetoma
	Cryptococcus neoformans
	Histoplasma duboisii
	Entamoeba histolytica
	Leishmania brasiliensis

LABORATORY DIAGNOSIS

1. Blood cultures.
2. Pus from infected biopsy-cultures, histopathological examination and microscopic examination should be carried out.
3. Radiography and imaging.
4. Serological tests to demonstrate antibodies may be useful when blood cultures are negative in chronic osteomyelitis.

JOINT INFECTIONS (ARTHRITIS)

Septic arthritis is usually blood-borne from an infection site elsewhere in the body, and is most likely to occur in a joint that has suffered trauma, usually caused by *Staph. aureus*.

Reactive arthritis result from hypersensitivity reactions triggered by organisms causing infections elsewhere in the body. It is characterized by inflammation of joints, with pain and swelling and restriction of movement. The fluid aspirated from such a joint is sterile but is often cloudy and its leucocyte content is typical of an inflammatory exudate.

Prosthetic arthritis results from contamination during surgery and commonly caused by *Staph. epidermidis*.

Arthritis may occur following certain sexually transmitted diseases, intestinal infections and as a part of Reiter's syndrome.

CAUSATIVE ORGANISMS

Septic arthritis	*Reactive arthritis*
Staph. aureus (> 80% cases)	*Strept. pyogenes*
Staph. epidermidis	*Neisseria meningitidis*
Strept. pyogenes	*Neisseria gonorrhoeae*
Strept. pneumoniae	*Yersinia enterocolitica*
Hemophilus influenzae	*Shigella dysenteriae*
Neisseria gonorrhoeae	*Salmonella*
Neisseria meningitidis	*Campylobacter jejuni*
Coliforms	*Mycoplasma pneumoniae*
Pseudomonas aeruginosa	*Chlamydia trachomatis*
Bacteroides fragilis	*Hepatitis B virus*
Fusiform bacilli	*Epstein-Barr virus*
Salmonella	
Brucella	
Pasteurella multocida	
Mycobacterium tuberculosis	
Treponema palliduem	

Leptospira icterohemorrhagiae

Borrelia burgdorferi

Rubella

Arbovirus (Onyong-nyong fever)

Enterovirus

Mumps

Parvovirus

LABORATORY DIAGNOSIS

(1) Joint fluid/pus—aspirated from joints.

—usually purulent with a high WBC count mostly polymorphonuclear (>75%) type.

—Gram's stain and/or Acid fast stain of centrifuged deposit may show the causative organism.

—Cultures and antibiotic sensitivity tests are performed.

(2) Blood cultures

(3) Throat swab culture for *Strept. pyogenes* when rheumatic fever is suspected.

(4) Feces culture for intestinal infections.

(5) urethral, cervical and rectal swabs transported in Stuart's medium and cultured for gonococci, when gonococcal arthritis is suspected.

(6) serology to demonstrate antibodies against causative organisms.

(7) detection of CRP.

116

Urinary Tract Infections (UTI)

The laboratory diagnosis of UTI is based on the presence of bacteria (bacteriuria) and pus cells (pyuria in urine).

CAUSATIVE ORGANISMS

Escherichia coli (O serotypes 1, 2, 4, 6, 7, 25 and 50 are common)

Klebsiella

Proteus

Pseudomonas aeruginosa

Streptococcus fecalis (Enterococci)

Staphylococcus saprophyticus

Staphylococcus aureus

Citrobacter

Serratia marcescens

Gardnerella vaginalis

Mycobacterium tuberculosis

Clostridium welchii

Mycoplasma

Chlamydiae (TRIC agents)

Candida albicans

Trichomonas vaginalis

(*Staph. epidermidis* occasionally causes UTI, associated with catheterization, in hospitals).

Collection of Specimen

Urine specimens are frequently contaminated with normal flora from perineum, genitalia and skin. To avoid the risk of contamination during specimen collection, precautions should be taken by prior cleaning of external genitalia and avoiding contact with inside of specimen container.

The urine sample is collected aseptically in a sterile, wide-mouthed container.

(1) Clean catch **midstream specimen of urine** (MSU/MSSU) is the most preferred.

(2) In babies/Infants–

—adhesive collection bags

—suprapubic bladder aspiration (rarely in pregnancy)

(3) In catheterized patients, the urine is collected from the catheter into a syringe and needle before it enters the drainage bag and not from the bag itself.

(4) In pyelonephritis by ureteric cannulation.

(5) If renal tuberculosis is suspected, three consecutive early morning specimens of urine (EMU) should be collected to increase the probability of recovering Mycobacteria.

Transport of Specimen

The urine sample should be transported immediately without any delay, preferably within 2 hrs. for culture. If there is any delay, the spoilage of specimen (or overgrowth of contaminants, if any) can be reduced by

— Refrigeration at 4°C

— using specimen containers with boric acid (the final conc. being 1.8% when urine sample is added), which preserves bacterial count of most urinary bacterial pathogens.

— Dip-slide technique–A slide coated with culture medium on both sides is immersed in freshly voided urine, drained and then sent to Lab in a sterile container for incubation at 37°C.

MICROSCOPIC EXAMINATION OF URINE

Wet Film

The urine sample either directly or a gently centrifuged deposit can be examined as a wet film under high power objective to detect pus cells, RBC, epithelial cells, crystals, casts and bacteria.

WBC count (pus cells) is expressed as cells per ml or cell per high power field (HPF).

Counting Chamber Method

The WBC can be counted in Neubauer chamber (hemocytometer chamber).

Gram's Stain

The presence of pus cells and the morphology of bacteria can be determined by examining a Gram stained smear, if necessary.

Applications of Microscopy

— The presence of pus cells in urine is often considered as indication of UTI.

— presence of casts–glomerulonephritis.

— epithelial cells–suggests contamination.

— pus cells alongwith RBC-hemorrhagic cystitis.

Urine Culture

A standard calibrated loop is dipped vertically into urine and a known volume of urine (0.01 ml) is inoculated on to solid media.

CLED (cystine-lactose-electrolyte deficient) agar

Mac Conkey agar

Blood agar

The plates are incubated aerobically at 37°C, overnight and then examined for number of colonies. For 0.01 ml sample, 100 colonies = 10^5/ml.

Bacterial count greater than 10^5/ml indicates significant bacteriuria.

Bacterial count less than 10^5/ml does not indicate active UTI; but may be found in pyelonephritis, Staphylococcal UTI, chronic recurrent UTI.

Mixed bacterial growth suggests contamination during specimen collection .

Pyuria with no bacterial growth may be due to

— Prior use of antibiotics

— Other source of WBC (e.g., mensturation)

— fastidious, growth factor requiring bacteria

— anaerobic bacteria

— Mycobacteria

Sampling of urine can also be done by means of a small filter paper strip, that transfers a fixed volume of urine on to the agar.

INDIRECT SCREENING TESTS FOR THE PRESUMPTIVE DIAGNOSIS OF UTI

Greiss Test or Nitrate Reductase Test

The presence of nitrite indicates the presence of nitrate reducing bacteria

Catalase Test

Hydrogen peroxide is added to the urine and mixed gently. The formation of air bubbles is a positive test and indicates bacteriuria. However, hematuria also gives a positive test.

Triphenyl Tetrazolium Chloride (TTC) Test

When a few drops of TTC reagent is added to urine and incubated at 37°C for 2-4 hrs, a pink-red precipitate is produced due to the presence of bacteria.

Glucose Test Paper

It is based on the utilization of glucose present in normal urine, by bacteria.

Automated and Semiautomated urine screening systems such as video camera, Remote imaging systems can be used to examine images of urine samples.

Laboratory diagnosis of urinary tract infection (UTI)

SPECIMEN

↓

Mid stream URINE in sterile container

To be Processed within one hour of voiding

MICROSCOPY

1. Wet coverslip preparation of uncentrifuged and well mixed sample. (2 pus cells/Hpf indicative of UTI)
2. Gram's stain of centrifuged sediment.

CULTURE

↓ Inoculation of 0.01 ml. by calibrated loop.

BA
MacConkey
CLED agar

↓

ISOLATION
Colony count

↓

Biochemical reactions for identification of bacteria

↓

Antibiotic sensitivity test is a must for therapy.

> Semiquantitative Estimation of significant bacteriuria : (KASS)
>
> 1000 colonies = 1,00,000 organism/ml of urine
> **Significant of UTI**
>
> 100 - 1000 colonies = 10,000 to 1,00,000 organisms/ ml of Urine.
> **Doubtful Significance**
>
> < 100 colonies = <10,000 organism/ml of urine
> **Not Significant**

117

Sexually Transmitted Diseases (STD)

CAUSATIVE ORGANISMS

Organism	*Disease*
I. Bacterial-	
Treponema pallidum	Syphilis (hard chancre)
Neisseria gonorrhoeae	Gonorrhoea, urethritis, cervicitis, pelvic inflammatory disease (PID), proctitis
Calymmatobacterium granulomatis	Granuloma inguinale (Donovanosis)
Hemophilus ducreyi	Chancroid (soft sore)
Gardnerella vaginalis	non-specific vaginitis.
Ureaplasma urealyticum (T-strains)	non-specific urethritis
Chalmydia trachomatis	Lymphogranuloma venereum (LGV) Nonspecific urethritis, cervicitis, pelvic inflammatory disease (PID), proctitis
II. Viruses-	
Herpes simplex virus (type 1 and 2)	Genital herpes
Human Papilloma virus (HPV)	genital warts (condylomata acuminata)
Pox virus	Molluscum contagiosum
Hepatitis B virus	Type B hepatitis
HIV (type 1 and 2)	AIDS.
III. Fungi-	
Candida albicans	Vaginal thrush, balanitis
IV. Protozoa-	
Trichomonas vaginalis	Vaginitis, urethritis, balanoposthitis
V. Arthropods	
Sarcoptes scabei	Genital scabies
Phthirus pubis	Pediculosis pubis

LABORATORY DIAGNOSIS

Specimens collected are urethral discharge, urethral swabs, cervical swabs, exudates from ulcers.

Specimens for gonococci may be transported to the laboratory in Stuart's medium and for Chlamydiae and Mycoplasmas in a special transport medium.

Microscopy

Smears are examined by

(1) Gram's stain—gonococci within pus cells.

(2) Immunofluorescence—*Chlamydia trachomatis* inclusions.

(3) Wet film of exudate from chancre can be examined under dark field microscope for spirochetes.

(4) 10% KOH wet mount—budding yeast cells.

Culture

Specimens for gonococci may be inoculated on to **Thayer-Martin medium** and incubated under CO_2 at 37°C.

Chlamydia trachomatis requires cell cultures and yolk sac of chick embryo.

Candida albicans grows on Sabouraud's dextrose agar.

Trichomonas vaginalis grows in Diamond's medium.

Serology for Syphilis

Refer chapter on *Treponema pallidum.*

118

Congenital, Perinatal and Neonatal Infections

CAUSATIVE ORGANISMS OF CONGENITAL INFECTIONS

Organism	*Disease*
Treponema pallidum	congenital syphilis
Rubella virus	congenital rubella
Cytomegalovirus	congenital cytomegalic inclusion disease
Toxoplasma gondii	congenital toxoplasmosis
Hepatitis B virus	congenital Hepatitis B
Hepatitis C virus	Congenital Hepatitis C
Herpes simplex virus (Type 2 usually)	neonatal herpes
Varicella-zoster virus	congenital varicella
Parvovirus B 19	anemia, hydrops fetalis
HIV	congential AIDS
Listeria monocytogenes	Listeriosis
Neisseria gonorrhoeae	ophthalmia neonatorum
Chlamydia trachomatis (TRIC agents)	ophthalmia neonatorum and neonatal pneumonia
Candida albicans	neonatal oral thrush
ECHO virus	progressive hepatic failure and clotting abnormalities

TORCH Syndrome

The more common clinical features of congenital infections have been collectively described by the acronym "TORCH" syndrome (*Toxoplasma*, Rubella, Cytomegalovirus, Herpes, while O stands for other).

However, it is important to be aware that infants may not manifest all the features of TORCH syndrome.

Moreover, many of the recently described aetiology of congenital infections *e.g.*, human Parvovirus B19, Echovirus, Varicella-zoster virus do not cause any of the features of TORCH syndrome.

CLINICAL FEATURES OF TORCH SYNDROME

— Low birth weight
— Prematurity
— Cardiac defects
— Ocular lesions–chorioretinitis, cataract, microphthalmia
— CNS defects–microcephaly, hydrocephaly thrombocytopenic purpura
— Jaundice
— Hepatosplenomegaly

CAUSATIVE AGENTS OF PERINATAL AND NEONATAL INFECTIONS

Time of infection	*Route of infection*	*Causative organisms*
Prenatal	Transplacental	*Treponema pallidum* *Listeria monocytogenes* Cytomegalovirus Rubella HIV Parvovirus B 19 Enteroviruses
	Ascending	*E. coli* *Klebsiella* *Group B Streptococci* *Listeria monocytogenes* *Chlamydia trachomatis* genital mycoplasmas
Natal	passing through the birth canal	*E. coli* *Klebsiellae* Group B Streptococci *Listeria monocytogenes* *Neisseria gonorrhoeae* *Chlamydia trachomatis* Cytomegalovirus Herpes simplex virus Enteroviruses Hepatitis B virus HIV
Postnatal	All of the above routes or from the surrounding environment	All the agents listed above In addition— *Staph. aureus* Gram negative bacteria Respiratory syncytial virus

LABORATORY DIAGNOSIS

Serology

(1) Maternal and neonatal serum samples should be tested for antibodies simultaneously, soon after birth and repeated at regular intervals.

In the presence of active congenital infection rising titres during first few months of life can be demonstrated.

When there is no active congenital infection, the infant's antibody titres progressively fall during the first few months of life, compared with the mother's antibody titres, due to the gradual disappearance of maternal antibody from the infant's serum.

(2) Demonstration of raised specific antibodies against Rubella, *Treponema pallidum*, Cytomegalovirus or *Toxoplasma*.

(3) Detection of appropriate antibody on the mother's and infant's sera *e.g.*, antibodies to HIV.

Culture

— Blood cultures

— Swabs of umbilicus, skin, eye or any septic site for culture

— feces for culture

— microscopy and culture of urine and CSF

— pus-Gram's stain

— viruses – CMV (blood, urine, throat swab), HSV (skin lesions, CSF), Varicella-zoster virus (skin lesions), Enteroviruses (stool, CSF), Coxsackie and ECHO viruses (stool) are cultivated in cell cultures, embryonated eggs.

119

Skin Infections

Macule—A circumscribed, flat discoloration of the skin.

Papule—An elevated, solid lesion up to 0.5 cm in diameter. Multiple papules may become confluent and form plaques.

Nodule—A circumscribed, raised, solid lesion greater than 0.5 cm in diameter.

Pustule—A circumscribed collection of leucocytes and fluid that varies in size.

Vesicle—A circumscribed blister like collection of fluid up to 0.5 cm in diameter.

Scales—Excess dead epidermal scales.

Ulcer—A loss of epidermis and dermis

Bulla—A circumscribed lesion of fluid more than 0.5 cm in diameter.

Furuncle (boil)—Abscess that begins as a red nodule in a hair follicle that ultimately becomes painful and full of pus.

Carbuncle—Furuncles that spread more deeply to the dermis and subcutaneous tissues.

Folliculitis—Minor infection of hair follicles; papules or pustules that are pierced by a hair and surrounded with redness.

Erysipelas—Primarily involves the dermis and most superficial parts of the subcutaneous tissue. Lesions are painful, red, swollen, and indurated. Lesion has a marked, well-demarcated, raised border Patients are febrile, and regional lymphadenopathy is present.

Erysipeloid—Purplish-red, non-vesiculated skin lesion with an irregular, raised border. The lesions itch and burn.

Erythrasma—Chronic infection of the keratinized layer of the epidermis. Lesions are dry and scaly.

Impetigo—Erythematous (red) lesions that may be bullous (less common) or nonbullous.

Cellulitis—Diffuse, spreading infections involving the deeper layers of the dermis. Lesions are ill-defined, flat, painful, red and swollen. Patients have fever, chills and regional lymphadenopathy.

Hidradenitis—Chronic infection of obstructed apocrine (sweat) glands in the axillas, genital, or perianal areas with intermittent discharge of often foul smelling pus.

CAUSATIVE AGENTS

Bacteria

Staph aureus, *Strept pyogenes*, other hemolytic Streptococci, anaerobic cocci, *Clostridium* sp., *Corynebacterium diphtheriae*, *Actinomyces israelii*, *Nocardia asteroides*, *Streptomyces*, *Erysipelothrix rhusiopathiae*, *Bacillus anthracis*, *Corynebacterium minutissimum*, coliforms, ***Pseudomonas aeruginosa***, *Neisseria gonorrhoeae*, *Neisseria meningitidis*, *Pasteurella multocida*, ***Francisella tularensis***, ***Bacteroides***, fusiform bacilli, *Burkholderia pseudomallei*, *Burkholderia cepacia*, ***Myco.tuberculosis***, ***Myco.ulcerans***, *Myco.chelonei*, *Myco.balnei*, *Myco.leprae*, *Treponema pallidum*, ***Treponema pertenue***, ***Treponema*** *carateum*, *Borrelia vincenti*, *Borrelia burgdorferi*.

Viruses

Variola and Vaccinia viruses, Molluscum contagiosum, Orf virus, Herpes simplex virus, Varicella-zoster virus, Papova virus, CoxsackieA virus, Echo virus.

Fungi

Candida albicans Malassezia furfur, *Cryptococcus neoformans*, Dermatophytes (*Trichophyton*, *Microsporum*, *Epidermophyton*), *Sporothrix schenkii*, *Histoplama capstulatum*, *Coccidioides immitis*, *Blastomyces dermatitidis*, *Madurella*, *Allescheria*, *Phialophora*.

LABORATORY DIAGNOSIS OF BACTERIAL INFECTIONS

Specimens

Pus, swabs from lesions, serous exudate from ulcers, skin biopsy, skin clippings from ear lobes, nasal septum for leprae bacilli.

Microscopy

(1) Gram's stain reveals causative organisms.

(2) Dark field microscopy for spirochetes.

(3) ZN stain for acid-fast bacilli.

Cultures

Specimens should be cultured on fresh blood agar, chocolate agar and MacConkey agar both aerobically and anaerobically, incubated for 2 days. LJ media is used for Mycobacteria.

Blood cultures should be performed in cases of cellulitis and sepsis.

Serological investigations performed on patients with suspected syphilis, yaws or pinta.

LABORATORY DIAGNOSIS OF VIRAL INFECTIONS

Specimens

Fluid from vesicular lesions, swab of the base of the lesion, biopsy material of nodules, ulcers or papules sent to the laboratory in viral transport medium.

Microscopy

(1) Characteristic inclusions of Pox viruses under light microscope.

(2) demonstration of viruses under EM.

Culrure

Tissue cultures, embryonated eggs are used.

120

Soft Tissue and Wound Infections

CAUSATIVE AGENTS

Staph aureus

Coagulase negative Staphylococci

Strept. pyogenes

Enterococci

Proteus

E. coli

Klebsiella

Pseudomonas aeruginosa

Bacteroides sp.

Prevotella sp.

Anaerobic cocci

Actinomyces israeli

Nocardia sp.

Clostridium perfringens

Clostridium novyi

Clostridium histolyticum

Clostridium septicum

Clostridium bifermentans

Candida sp.

LABORATORY DIAGNOSIS

Specimens

Pus, exudates, necrosed tissue bits, swabs.

Microscopy (1) ***Gram's stain***

(2) ***Gas liquid chromatography*** to detect volatile fatty acids produced by anaerobic bacteria in the pus.

(3) ***Cultures***– Blood agar, chocolate agar, MacConkey agar and Sabouraud's agars are inoculated and incubated aerobically at 37°C overnight.

Blood agar and chocolate agar plates may inoculated and incubated anaerobically overnight.

Tissue specimens may be incubated in RCM broth to recover anaerobic and fastidious pathogens.

Blood cultures may be done if necessary.

The growth is identified by Gram's stain, biochemical tests and slide agglutination tests.

Antibiotic sensitivity tests may be performed on isolates.

Naegler's test may be performed to detect the production of alpha toxin by *Clostridium perfringens*.

LABORATORY DIAGNOSIS OF PYOGENIC INFECTION

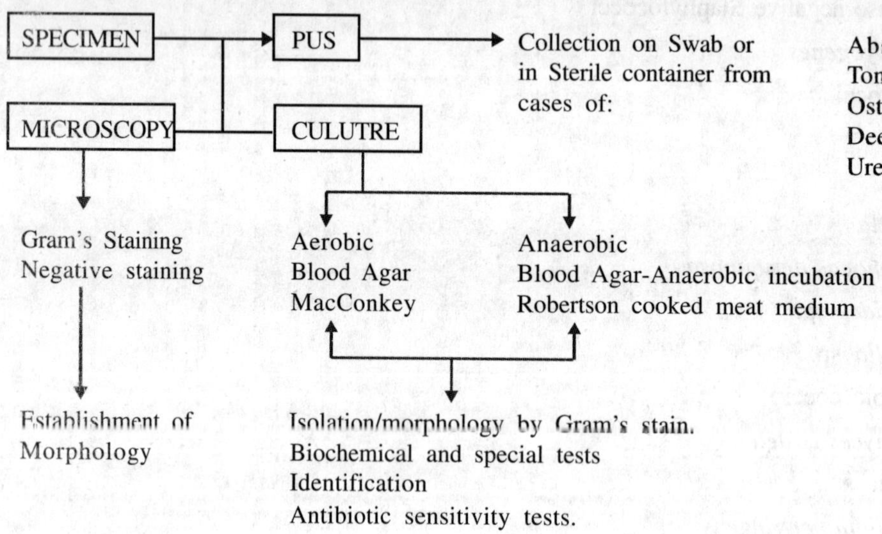

CAUSATIVE BACTERIA AND THEIR IDENTIFICATION

1. *Stahylococcus aureus* : Morphology, aerobic growth, golden yellow pigment production, hemolysis, coagulase activity, fermentation of mannitol, gelatin liquefaction

   (Note : Cases of food poisoning - left over food - selective media (7% Nacl) demonstration of Enterotoxin)

2. *Streptococcus pyogenes* : Morphology, aerobic growth, beta hemolysis, Lancefield's grouping, (ASLO titration – Rheumatic fever and acute glomerulonephritis)

3.	***Streptococcus pneumoniae***	:	Morphology, demonstration of capsule, aerobic growth, Alpha hemolysis, Bile solubility, optochin sensitivity, animal pathogenicity in mice (Note : Isolation from CSF in meningitis)
4.	*Neisseria gonorrhoeae*	:	Morphology, non haemolytic, growth on special media, Oxidase +ve, fermentation tests.
5.	*Pseudomonas* and other Gram –ve bacilli	:	Morphology, growth on MacConkey, Biochemical tests, diffusible pigment production etc.
6.	Anaerobic Bacteria	:	Like *Peptococcus*, *Peptostreptococcus*, *Bacteroides* : Anaerobic growth, morphology, biochemical and other special tests.

121

Acute Diarrhea

DIARRHEA

An increase in frequency, fluidity or volume of bowel movements relative to the usual habits of each individual. In other words, passage of 3 or more motions a day can be taken as diarrhea.

Based on pathogenesis and clinical features, acute diarrhea is classified into

1. Non-inflammatory or secretory diarrhea

It involves the proximal small bowel. The diarrhea is watery, contains little fecal matter, and no leucoytes, RBC and fever.

2. Inflammatory or bloody diarrhea

It involves the colon or the distal small bowel and typically causes dysentery. Feces contain mucus pus cells and RBC. Fever may be present.

3. Invasive or penetrating diarrhea (enteric fever)

It involves the distal small bowel accompanied by signs of systemic infection such as headache, malaise, sore throat and fever.

GASTROENTERITIS

Acute diarrhea associated with vomiting and inflammation.

DYSENTERY

Inflammation of the intestine, especially of the colon, with abdominal pain, tenesmus and frequent stools containing blood and mucus.

TRAVELLER'S DIARRHEA

The diarrheal illness seen in persons from the developed countries within a few days of their visit to one of the developing countries. It results from an encounter with certain viruses, bacteria or protozoa through contaminated food and water.

CAUSATIVE AGENTS

Bacteria

Escherichia coli (ETEC, EPEC, EIEC, EHEC and EAEC), *Vibrio cholerae*, Non-cholera Vibrios (NAG), *Vibrio parahemolyticus*, *Campylobacter jejuni*, *Staph. aureus*, *Salmonella* sp., *Shigella* sp.,

Yersinia enterocolitica, *Bacillus cereus*, *Clostridium welchii*, *Clostridium difficle*, *Clostridium botulinum*, *Aeromonas hydrophila*, *Plesiomonas shigelloides*, *Edwardsiella tarda*.

Viruses

Rotavirus, Norwalk virus, *Adenovirus*, Calicivirus, Coronavirus, Hepatitis A and E viruses.

Parasites

Entamoeba histolytica, *Giardia lamblia*, *Balantidium coli*, *Cryptosporidium*, *Isospora belli*.

Fungi

Candida albicans.

Table 121.1 Mechanism of Pathogenesis

Mechanism	*Examples of microorganisms*
Invasion	*Shigella* sp., EIEC, *Entamoeba histolytica*, *Banatidium coli*, *Plesiomonas shigelloides*, *Yersinia enterocolitica*, *Edwardsiella tarda*.
Adherence (attachment within or close to mucosal cells)	EPEC, *Cryptosporidium parvum*, *Isospora belli*, Rotavirus, Hepatitis A and E, Norwalk virus.
Toxin production	
–Enterotoxin	*Vibrio cholerae*, Noncholera vibrios, *Shigella dysenteriae* type 1, ETEC, *Salmonella* sp, *Clostridium difficle* (toxin A), *Aeromonas*, *Campylobacter jejuni*.
–Cytotoxin	*Shigella* sp., *Clostridium difficle* (toxin B), EHEC.
–Neurotoxin	*Clostridium botulinum*, *Staph. aureus*, *Bacillus cereus*.

LABORATORY DIAGNOSIS

Specimen Collection

The fecal specimens should be collected in a clean, sterile, wide-mouthed card board or plastic containers and delivered to the laboratory within an hour. If stool is unavailable, Rectal swabs may be taken. In parasitic infections, duodenal aspirates may be examined occasionally.

Transport of specimens

If there is a delay of more than 2 hrs in transportation, the specimen or swab should be transported in transport media such as **Cary-Blair medium** or **Sach's buffered glycerol saline**.

Microsocopy

The specimen for microscopy and culture should be taken from an area with blood and mucus.

Wet mount

A direct wet film examination under microscope is useful for detecting motile trophozoites of intestinal protozoan parasites.

Under phase contrast and dark-field microscopy, the **darting motility** and curved forms of *Vibrio cholerae* and *Campylobacter* can be detected.

Simple staining with methylene blue is helpful in detecting pus cells.

Gram's staining can be done for detection of various morphological forms.

Acid fast staining is useful for detection of *Cryptosporidium*, Mycobacteria etc.

Antigen detection

Direct fluorescent–antibody test, enzyme immunoassays, latex agglutination test and DNA probes can be used to detect antigens from fecal samples.

FECAL CULTURES

The specimens should be inoculated on to appropriate culture media. Selective media may be preferred to suppress the growth of commensals. Usually blood agar, MacConkey agar, DCA, Xylose-lysine decarboxylase (XLD) agar, Wilson and Blair's agar and TCBS agar are used. Enrichment media such as Selenite F broth for *Salmonella* sp, and alkaline peptone water for *Vibrio* sp. may be used.

The cultures are incubated at 37°C, for overnight. Some organisms such as *Campylobacter* sp. may require 10% CO_2 and require prolonged (1–2 days) incubation at 43°C.

The growth (colonies) can be identified by Gram's staining, motility tests, biochemical reactions and slide agglutination tests with monovalent and polyvalent antisera. The isolates are subjected to antibiotic sensitivity tests.

DETECTION OF ENTEROTOXINS

Enterotoxins can be detected by various methods.

Labile toxin (LT) is detected by— (1) ligated Rabbit illeal loop test (2) infant Rabbit bowel test (3) tissue culture tests (4) radio immunoassay, and (5) ELISA.

Stable toxin (ST) can be detected by Infant mouse intragastric test and ligated Rabbit illeal loop test.

LABORATORY DIAGNOSIS OF ACUTE DIARRHEA AND BACTERIAL DYSENTERY

DIARRHEA → **SPECIMEN : FECES** ← **DYSENTERY**

DIARRHEA: Loose semisolid or watery faeces

SPECIMEN : FECES IN

1. Sterile container
2. Rectal swab
3. Transport Media

DYSENTERY: Semisolid feces with mucous and blood or only mucous and blood.

MICROSCOPY OF FECES

CHOLERA

1. Darting motility (swarm of gnats) in hanging drop preparation of rice water stool sample.
2. Inhibition of motility with specific titre serum in dark ground microscopy.

BACTERIAL DYSENTERY

Exudative: Loaded pus cells, macrophages, RBC and bacteria reduced or absent.

CULTURE

MacConkey

Isolation Moropholgy LF

↓

Biochemical tests

↓

Identification

↓

Escherichia coli

Serotyping to be established Enteropathogenicity

a) EPEC-'O' group Serotyping
b) ETEC-Rabbit illreal loop test etc.
c) EIEC-Sereny's test

Antibiotic sensitivity test

Enrichment: Alkaline peptone water

→ Mac, TCBS, GTTA

↓

Isolation - characteristic colonial morphology

↓

Biochemical tests

↓

Identification

Biotyping

VP, Hemolysis, chick RBC Agglutination, Polymixin B sensitivity, Phage IV susceptibility-distinguish

El Tor *Vibrio* and Classical *Vibrio*

Serotyping

Inaba, Ogawa, Hikojima

Direct plating / Enrichment

Buffered Glycerol saline (Sach Solution)

↓

Mac, DCA, SS

↓

Isolation - Morphology NLF

↓

Motility and Biochemcial tests

–

Identification

–

Shigella

Mannitol fermentation

Serotyping

Colicine typing

Antibiotic sensitivity test

122

Bacterial Food Poisoning

DEFINITION

Bacterial food poisoning can be defined as an acute diarrhea or acute gastroenteritis due to consumption of food and water contaminated with microorganisms or their products (toxins).

CAUSATIVE AGENTS AND TYPES OF BACTERIAL FOOD POISONING

Based on pathogenesis, food poisoning has been classified into 3 types with different incubation periods.

1. Toxin Type

Where preformed bacterial toxin is ingested with food. The toxin induces diarrhea which is watery with nausea and vomiting. The incubation period is short, 1–6 hrs, since the toxin is already elaborated in the food.

e.g., Staphylococcus aureus, *Bacillus cereus* (emetic form)

2. Infection Type

Infective doses of pathogenic microorganisms are ingested with food. They set up infection in the gut and induce diarrhea. The incubation period is 16–24 hrs (> 16 hrs).

e.g., Salmonella sp. (*S. enteritidis*, *S. typhimurium* etc.)

–*Vibrio cholerae*

–*Vibrio parahemolyticus*

–ETEC

–*Campylobacter jejuni*

–*Shigellae* sp.

3. Intermediate Type

The pathogenic bacteria are ingested with the food, which elaborate the toxin in the gut and induces diarrhea. The incubation period is 8–16 hrs.

e.g., Clostridium welchii (type A)

Clostridium botulinum

E.coli 0 157 : H7 (verotoxigenic *E. coli*)

Bacillus cereus (diarrheal form)

LABORATORY DIAGNOSIS

The specimens collected are :

(*i*) feces

(*ii*) suspected food, and

(*iii*) vomitus

The food sample is macerated in sterile normal saline or ringer's solution and used for smear and culture.

Examination of stained smears of specimens is useful to demonstrate heavy contamination with *Staphylococci*, *Bacillus* cereus and *Clostridium welchii*.

Fluorescent antibody test may be used to detect the suspected organism from the smears prepared from sample.

The specimens are inoculated on to appropriate culture media. Usually blood agar and Mac-Conkey agar are used. But enrichment media and selective media can be used to isolate the causative pathogen. The media are incubated both aerobically and anaerobically at 37°C for 1-2 days. The growth has to be identified by Gram's staining, motility tests, biochemical reactions and slide agglutination tests with appropriate antisera.

Paired serum samples may be useful for serological diagnosis.

In case of death of patient, samples of intestinal contents, spleen, liver and heart blood may be collected.

When food handlers are suspected to be carriers, their nasal swabs or stool samples may be collected.

123

Hospital-Acquired Infections Cross-Infections in Hospitals Nosocomial Infections Hospital Infections

- *Definition*
- *Sources of nosocomial infections*
- *Opportunisitic infections*
- *Transmission of nosocomial infections*
- *Factors contributing to nosocomial infections*
- *Types of nosocomial infections*
- *Causative agents of nosocomial infections*
- *Emergence of drug-resistant microorganisms in hospitals*
- *Lab. diagnosis of Hospital infections*
- *Prevention, control and management of nosocomial infections*
    - *Hand washing*
    - **Asepsis**
- **Antisepsis, disinfection and sterilisation**
- **Hospital environmental sanitation**
- **Hospital personnel**
- **Monitoring**
- **Isolation**
- **Universal blood and bodyfluid precautions**
- **Laundry services**
- **Dietetics services**
- **Instrumental procedures**
- **Hospital building and ward design**
- **Antibiotic policy**
- **Surveillance**
- **Infection control program/policy**

DEFINITION

The term "Nosocomial infections" (nosocomeion = hospital) is applied to infections developing in hospitalised patients, after their admission into the hospital which were not present or in incubation at the time of their admission.

Nosocomial infections may be

(1) Infections acquired outside the hospital which become clinically apparent when the patient is in hospital. *e.g.*, Measles.

(2) Infections acquired and developing within hospitals *e.g.,* wound infections, post-operative infections.

(3) Infections acquired in hospital, which become clinically apparent after the discharge of patients from hospital *e.g.,* infections in babies.

SOURCES OF NOSOCOMIAL INFECTIONS

The "**Reservoirs**" of nosocomial infections can be either living organisms (usually humans, animals or insects) that harbor pathogens; or inanimate objects contaminated with infectious microorganisms, known as "**fomites**".

The sources of nosocomial infection in a patient may be exogenous or endogenous.

1. Exogenous Infections

The source of infection is from external sources, such as (*i*) hospital personnel (*ii*) visitors (*iii*) hospital environment– air conditioners, floors, bed linen, utensils, water taps, sinks, dish mops, food, water, dust, flowers in patient's room, air-borne droplets (*iv*) contaminated medical equipment and fluids, such as – urinary catheters, oral thermometers, intravenous fluids, respiratory equipment, suction apparatus, anesthetic machines. Such infections are usually **Iatrogenic**, that may be induced by diagnostic or therapeutic procedures carried out in the hospital.

2. Endogenous Infections

The source of the most nosocomial infections is endogenous, the pathogen being derived from the patient body itself; caused by bacteria found on the skin and mucus membrane surfaces (*e.g., Staphylococcus aureus*), the intestine (*e.g., E.coli, Streptococcus fecalis*) etc.

OPPORTUNISTIC INFECTIONS

Many of the normal flora may act as opportunistic pathogens, which cause infection and disease, when patient's immunity is compromised. The two important sources of opportunistic infections in hospitals are

(*i*) hands of health care personnel

(*ii*) the skin, mucus membranes, saliva, feces and urine of the patient.

TRANSMISSION OF NOSOCOMIAL INFECTIONS

The transmission of infectious microorganisms from one host to another and the subsequent infection of the new host may occur in a number of ways. Pathogens may escape from Reservoir and transmitted to susceptible persons in a variety of ways; as shown below.

RESERVOIR

Growth and reproduction of pathogen

⇓

Escape Routes of Pathogen
From Reservoir

⇓

Respiratory tract – Oral and nasal droplets expelled from mouth and nose during sneezing, coughing or even talking. These droplets may settle on inanimate objects, which then serve as fomites.

– Gastrointestinal tract

– Genitourinary tract

– fluids exuded from lesions in skin and mucosa and wound infections

⇓

MODE OF TRANSMISSION

Direct contact – hand shaking, coughing, sneezing, kissing, rarely infected animals.

Indirect contact – water, food, milk, air currents, insects, contaminated hands, fomites.

⇓

PORTAL OF ENTRY

Respiratory tract – Air-borne diseases

Gatrointestinal tract – Food-borne and water-borne diseases

Genitourinary tract – Sexually transmitted diseases.

Breaks in skin; wounds and burns – wound and skin infections

Parenteral – inner tissues; – Puncture, injections Insect bite – Arthropod-borne diseases

⇓

SUSCEPTIBLE HOSTS

– New born and geriatric patients

– Ill patients

– Surgical patients

– Wounded and burned patients

– Patients undergoing radiation therapy or chemotherapy

– Patients with invasive devices.

FACTORS CONTRIBUTING TO NOSOCOMIAL INFECTIONS (OR) SUSCEPTIBILITY OF PATIENTS TO INFECTION

Several factors are responsible for frequent occurrence of infections in hospitalized patients.

(1) Many patients, particularly infants and elderly patients may have impaired defense mechanisms due to secondary infections, cancer, surgery, radiation, immunosuppressive agents or procedures and instruments used on the body; making them more vulnerable to infections.

(2) Major invasive procedures, diagnostic or therapeutic, such as invasive devices, arterial and urinary catheters, implants, carried out in hospitals may lead to infections.

(3) Hospital infections are generally more serious and refractory to treatment as the causative agents are resistant to most antibiotics in common use.

(4) Modern methods of treatment such as organ transplantation, implanted prostheses (*e.g.*, heart valves, pace makers, hip joints), dialysis, exchange transfusion have enhanced the risk of hospital infections.

(5) Hospital environment is heavily laden with a wide variety of pathogens. Patients shed them through their bodies. Hospital personnel spread them through their hands and clothing. Bedding, linen and utensils may act as fomites. Equipment may be contaminated. Pathogens are present in hospital dust and air, and sometimes even in antiseptic lotions and ointments. Contamination of hospital food or water may cause outbreaks of infections.

(6) Patient's susceptibility to microorganisms may be increased by clinical conditions and medical procedures which may allow normal flora to be shifted from their normal habitat to some other area of the patient's body and thereby become opportunistic pathogens. For example, *E.coli* from intestine may cause severe infections when transferred to urinary tract. Urinary catheterization can introduce pathogens into the bladder.

Breaking the skin barrier by surgery, biopsy, injection or withdrawal of a blood sample may allow normal skin flora such as *Staphylococcus aureus*, *Staphylococcus epidermidis* to enter tissues and cause infections.

Table 123.1 Factors affecting Patient's Susceptibility to Infection

	Factors	*Examples*
1.	Inadequate cell mediated immunity	Infants very old patients
2.	Health status	Malnutrition Diabetes chronic debilitating diseases Hematological disorders Renal diseases Immunodeficiencies, AIDS
3.	Accidents	Severe debilitation Severe burns Shock
4.	Surgery	Size of wound amount of wound drainage Duration of operation; skill of surgeon. Tissue trauma length of hospitalization foreign bodies – sutures, Catheters prostheses
5.	Therapy	Antibiotics Radiation Steroids immunosuppressive drugs

TYPES OF NOSOCOMIAL INFECTIONS

1. Surgical or Nonsurgical Wound Infections

Some patients may develop surgical site infections and stitch abscesses after the patient is discharged from the hospital. Causative organisms may be *Staphylococcus aureus*; *Streptococcus pyogenes*; Gram negative bacilli – *E. coli*, *Klebsiellae*, *Pseudomonas*, nonsporing anaerobes – *Bacteroides fragilis*; Clostridial infections.

Non-surgical sites of wound infections include injections, cut-downs, umbilical stumps, ulcers and burns. *Pseudomonas aeruginosa* is most important causative agent of burns infections.

2. Urinary Tract Infections

Majority of hospital-acquired urinary tract infections are caused by Gram negative bacilli such as *E.coli*, *Klebsiellae*, *Proteus* and *Pseudomonas*. A few urinary tract infections may be caused by *Staphylococcus* aureus, *Candida* species. The predisposing factors to nosocomial urinary tract infections are old age, female gender, catheterization and other serious underlying diseases.

3. Respiratory Infections

The most common pathogens which cause nosocomial respiratory tract and lung infections (pneumonia) are *Staphylococcus aureus*, *Streptococcus pyogenes*, Gram negative bacilli-*Klebsiella* sp, *Moraxella catarrhalis*.

The risk factors that predispose patients to acquire nosocomial respiratory infections are – coma, old age, chronic pre-existing lung (cardiopulmonary) diseases, chest surgery, intubation (placement of a breathing tube down a patient's throat), attachement to a mechanical ventillator to control breathing, hospitalization in intensive care units, monitoring intracranial pressure in which a catheter inserted through the skill. Sometimes the microorganisms in upper respiratory tract may be coghed up and lodge in lungs instead of being spit out or swallowed.

4. Blood Stream Infections (Bacteremia and Septicemia)

Bacteremia and septicemia may occur as a conseqence of the use of intravenous cannulae as in blood transfusion or intravenous rehydration, phlebitis and cut downs in infants and small children.

The causative organisms may be Gram negative bacilli, *Staphylococcus epidermidis*, *Staphylococcus aureus*, Enterococci, *Candida* sp. etc.

Staphylococcus epidermidis bacteremia is usually associated with implanted artificial heart valves.

The risk factors predisposing to blood stream infections are malnutrition, intravenous cannulae, immunosuppressive therapy, severe preexisting diseases, skin lesions–burns, bedsores and prolonged stay in ICU.

5. Gastrointestinal Infections

Out breaks of Diarrhea, cholera, shigellosis, salmonella gastroenteritis, typhoid fever, Hepatitis type A and Amoebic dysentery etc. can occur in hospitals due to contaminated food and water either from hospital personnel or patients or visitors.

CAUSATIVE AGENTS OF NOSOCOMIAL INFECTIONS

Staphylococcus aureus, *Pseudomonas* and *E.coli* are the most important causative agents of nosocomial infections among bacteria. Most of these strains, that are prevalent in hospital environment are drug resistant.

Viral infections in hospitals are frequently encountered in neonates, infants and immunocompromised patients. Fungal infections are on the rise due to prolonged antibiotic therapy, steroid therapy, immunosuppression, malignancies and Diabetes.

Table 123.2 Commonly Occurring Microorganisms in Hospital Infections

Urinary tract infections	*E.coli, Klebsiella, Proteus, Serratia*, Pseudomonas, fecal Streptococci, *Candida albicans.*
Wound and skin infections	*Staphylococcus aureus*, *E. coli*, *Proteus* sp., *Pseudomonas* fecal Streptococci, Anaerobes–*Bacteroides* *Staphylococcus epidermidis* *Streptococcus pyogenes*
Respiratory infections	*Staphylococcus aureus* *Streptococcus pyogenes* Gram negative bacilli – *Klebsiella* sp, *Pseudomonas.* *Haemophilus influenzae.* *Streptococcus pneumoniae* *Moraxella catarrhalis* Respiratory viruses
Blood stream infections	*Staphylococcus epidermidis* *Staphylococcus aureus* Enterococci Gram negative bacilli *Candida albicans*
Gastro-intestinal infections	*Salmonella*, *Shigella* sp, viruses–Rotavirus.

Most of the infections caused by enterococci, other nonhemolytic streptococci, anaerobic cocci, *Bacteroides* and gasgangrene producing Clostridia are endogenous and self infectious. Group A Streptococci infection is always exogenous, which spreads from person to person (cross infection). Infections by *Staphylococcus* aureus, Group B Streptococci, Enterobacteria (*E.coli, Klebsiella*, *Proteus* etc.) may be acquired either exogenously or endogenously. Infections with *Clostridium tetani*, *Flavobacterium*, *Pseudomonas aeruginos* a *Klebsiella*, *Serratia*, *Enterobacter* are often acquired from environmental sources. HIV and HBV may be acquired from HIV and HBV positive patients by direct inoculation or through contact with broken skin or mucus membrane.

EMERGENCE OF DRUG RESISTANT MICROORGANISMS IN HOSPITALS

The widespread use of antibiotics, chemotherapeutic agents, antiseptics and aseptic techniques in hospitals have produced selective pressures so that sensitive microorganisms die out and those that are resistant multiply, spread and infect patients and become predominant in patients, hospital staff and hospital environment.

In the 1940s and 50s, with the advent of treatment of patients with penicillin and sulfonamides, resistant strains of *Staphylococcus aureus* appeared. Then in the 1970s, treatment of patients with narrow-spectrum cephalosporins and aminoglycosides led to the development and emergence of resistance among Gram negative bacilli – *Klebsiella*, *Enterobacter*, *Serratia*, *Pseudomonas*. During the late 1970s and early 1980s, the use of more potent cephalosporins played a rols in the emergence of antibiotic resistant coagulase negative Staphylococci, Enterococci, **Methicillin–Resistant** *Staphylococcus aureus* (**MRSA**). The 1990s has witnessed the emergence of betalactamase-resistant and vancomycin–resistant enterococci.

After hospitalization, patients normal flora quickly changes and will be replaced by drug-resistant organisms found in hospital environment and spread to other patients, staff and recontaminate hospital environment.

LAB DIAGNOSIS OF HOSPITAL INFECTIONS

For the diagnosis of nosocomial infections the sampling may be done from various possible sources of infection such as – hospital staff. Fomites, water, food, air, equipments, various surfaces, disinfectants, antiseptics, operation theatres, sterilised items (to monitor sterilisation) etc.

Aetiological diagnosis is by routine bacteriological methods like Microscopic examination of stained smear, culture, identification by biochemical tests and antibiotic sensitivity testing. Information about the sensitivity pattern of strains, known as antibiogram is useful as a guide to therapy and may also be used as an epidemiological marker in tracing the source of hospital-acquired infections. Other epidemiological markers used to identify the source of nosocomial infections include biotyping, phage typing, serotyping and bacteriocin typing.

PREVENTION, CONTROL AND MANAGEMENT OF NOSOCOMIAL INFECTIONS

The prevention, control and management of nosocomial infections consists of various measures as described below.

1. Hand Washing

It is a simple procedure where microorganisms are mechanically removed by rubbing soap-lathered hands for atleast ten seconds and rinsing under running water before and after contact with each patient.

All hospital personnel require scrubbing the lower arms and hands with soap and brush for about ten minutes, then rinsing under running water and with an antiseptic. This procedure is called "surgical scrub".

2. Asepsis

Asepsis is the prevention of contact with microorganisms to prevent infections.

"**Medical asepsis**" consists of all practices used to keep hospital personnel, hospital environment and patients free from infectious microorganisms e.g., hand washing, sanitation, isolation of patients etc.

"**Surgical asepsis**" is practiced in the operation theatre and in treatment procedures such as wound dressing, catheterization and intravenous therapy. All surgical instruments, gloves and other items that come in contact with patients are sterilized. The operation theatre environment is sanitized, fumigated. Operation theatre staff should scrub their hands and arms and put on protective clothing such as sterile caps, gowns, masks and gloves. Antiseptics may be used on patient's skin.

	1	0	3	6
	1	1	0	3
	1	1	1	5
	1	1	2	7
	1	1	3	9
	1	2	0	5
	1	2	1	7
	1	2	2	10
	1	2	3	12
	1	3	0	8
	1	3	1	11
	1	3	2	14
	1	3	3	18
	1	3	4	20
	1	4	0	13
	1	4	1	17
	1	4	2	20
	1	4	3	30
	1	4	4	35
	1	4	5	40
	1	5	0	25
	1	5	1	35
	1	5	2	50
	1	5	3	90
	1	5	4	160
	1	5	5	180+

Table 125.1 (b)

Quantity of water	10 ml	1 ml	0.1 ml	
No. of samples of each quantiy tested	5	5	5	
	0	0	0	0
	0	0	1	2
	0	0	2	4
	0	1	0	2
		1	1	4
	0	1	2	6
	0	2	0	4

Number giving positive reaction (acid and gas)			Probable number of coliform bacilli in 100 ml of water
0	2	1	6
0	3	0	6
1	0	0	2
1	0	1	4
1	0	2	6
1	0	3	8
1	1	0	4
1	1	1	6
1	1	2	8
1	2	0	6
1	2	1	8
1	2	2	10
1	3	0	8
1	3	1	10
1	4	0	11
2	0	0	5
2	0	1	7
2	0	2	9
2	0	3	12
2	1	0	7
2	1	1	9
2	1	2	12
2	2	0	9
2	2	1	12
2	2	2	14
2	3	0	12
2	3	1	14
2	4	0	15
3	0	0	8
3	0	1	11
3	0	2	13
3	1	0	11
3	1	1	14
3	1	2	17
3	1	3	20
3	2	0	14
3	2	1	17

	3	2	3	20
	3	3	0	17
	3	3	1	20
	3	4	0	20
	3	4	1	25
	3	5	0	25

Table 125.1 (c)

Quantity of water	10 ml	1 ml	0.1 ml	
No. of samples of each qu̇antiy tested	5	5	5	Probable number of coliform bacilli in 100 ml of water
Number giving positive reaction (acid and gas)	4	0	0	13
	4	0	1	17
	4	0	2	20
	4	0	3	25
	4	1	0	17
	4	1	1	20
	4	1	2	25
	4	2	0	20
	4	2	1	25
	4	2	2	30
	4	3	0	25
	4	3	1	35
	4	3	2	40
	4	4	0	35
	4	4	1	40
	4	4	2	45
	4	5	0	40
	4	5	1	50
	4	5	2	55
	5	0	0	25
	5	0	1	30
	5	0	2	45
	5	0	3	60
	5	0	4	75

	5	1	0	35
	5	1	1	45
	5	1	2	65
	5	1	3	85
	5	1	4	115
	5	2	0	50
	5	2	1	70
	5	2	2	95
	5	2	3	120
	5	2	4	150
	5	2	5	175
	5	3	0	80
	5	3	1	110
	5	3	2	140
	5	3	3	175
	5	3	4	200
	5	3	5	250
	5	4	0	130
	5	4	1	170
	5	4	2	225
	5	4	3	275
	5	4	4	350
	5	4	5	425
	5	5	0	250
	5	5	1	350
	5	5	2	550
	5	5	3	900
	5	5	4	1600
	5	5	5	1800+

False Positive Presumptive Tests

A positive test does not necessarily mean that coliforms are present. Bacteria such as *Pseudomonas maltophila*, *Serratia liquefaciens*, *Hafnia alvei* and *Bacillus* strains may give positive results. False positives occur –

1. due to the presence of aerobic or facultatively anaerobic, spore-forming, gas producing bacteria.
2. due to synergetic fermentation of lactose by gas producing "symbionts", usually when a Gram positive and Gram negative organism growing together.
3. by the presence of oxidase positive bacteria capable of producing gas from lactose.

False positive test can be eliminated by inhibiting the growth non-coliform orgnanisms. This can be achieved by adding triphenylmethane stain in the fermentatiion medium.

Confirmed Test

Fermentation tubes showing any amount of gas are subjected to confirmed test. Gently shake the presumptive positive tubes showing gas and transfer a loopful of culture to the **Brilliant green lactose bile broth (BGLB)** tubes. Incubate all the inoculated tubes at 35°C for 48 hours.

If gas produced – coliform group confirmed.

If no gas produced – test negative – coliform group absent.

All the tubes showing gas production in confirmed test are subjected to the completed test as follows.

Completed Test

Streak the **Eosin-methylene blue (EMB) agar** or **Endo agar** plates with a loopful of culture from positive confirmed test tubes. Invert the plates and incubate at 35°C for 24 hours.

Typical colonies – Nucleated, with or without metallic sheen

Atypical coloneis – Opaque, nonnucleated, mucoid, pink after 24 hrs of incubation

Negative colonies – All other colonies except those described above.

If typical or atypical colonies are present, smears are prepared and Gram's staining is done to confirm the morphological characteristics of coliforms. Colonies are also inoculated into lactose broth fermentation tubes and incubated at 35°C for 48 hrs. The formation of gas in fermentation tubes and demonstration of Gram negative, non-sporulating bacilli constitute completed test for coliform group.

Table 125.2 Differences between *E.coli* and *Enterobacter*

	Indole	*M.R.*	*V.P.*	*Citrate*
E.coli	+	+	–	–
Enterobacter aerogenes	–	–	+	+

Differential Coliform Test or Eijkman Test

The Eijkman test is done to find out whether the coliform bacilli detected in the presumptive test are *E.coli* from human origin or animal origin. Subcultures are made from presumptive positive tubes into **Brilliant green lactose broth (BGLB)** or **lauryl tryptone broth** or **lactose broth** or MacConkey's broth and incubated at 44°C and 37°C in a thermostatically controlled water bath.

The formation of acid and gas at 44°C confirms the presence of *E.coli* of human origin and at 37°C indicates coliform group.

Standard Plate Count (SPC)

Plating is same as for milk examination.

Membrane Filter Method

The bacteriological examination of water by membrane filter method consists of following steps :

1. A sterile filter disk (cellulose acetate membrane filter or millipore) is placed in a filtration unit and sterilized.
2. A known volume of water is drawn through this filter disk into a suction flask. The bacteria are retained on the surface of the membrane filter.
3. The membrane filter disk is placed on the surface of an agar medium in petridish of suitable size and incubated.
4. Upon incubation, colonies develop on the filter disk wherever bacteria were trapped during filtration, and can be easily counted.

This method possesses several distinct advantages :

1. It permits the examination of bacteria from a large volume of water. No dilutions are, therefore, required. Colony count is more accurate and reliable.
2. The filter disk can be transferred to any desired medium. This permits the isolation of any organism on a differential medium.
3. It provides a more rapid examination of water than the standard procedure.
4. It requries much less equipment and, therefore, the examination can be done in the field.

The disadvantage of this method is it cannot be used, if water contains considerable amount of algae, colloidal or other materials which are likely to clog the filter, Secondly, if water samples are heavily contaminated with non-coliforms, the growth of coliforms will be inhibited.

Examination for Fecal Streptococci

Tests for fecal streptococci may be of value when there is a difficulty in interpretation as when presumptive coliforms are present, but *E.coli* are absent or where there is a question concerning the sanitary significance of coliforms isolated from a water sample. In some parts of the world, fecal streptococci, rather than coliforms, are used as indicators of fecal pollution of water. The normal habitat of these organisms is the intestine of humans and animals and they are not found in nature in the absence of fecal contamination. On the other hand, some believe that the coliforms do not always represent fecal pollution because the organisms may persist in soil and water for long periods of time and occasionally multiply outside the human or animal body.

Subcultures from presumptive positive tubes are made into **Glucose azide broth** or **Lactose broth** in which **sodium azide** is incorporated and incubated at 45°C for overnight or prolonged for 48 hrs. The presence of fecal streptococci is indicated by the formation of acid and should be plated on MacConkey agar for confirmation. Fecal streptococci produce characteristic minute pink or red colonies.

Membrane filter method can also be used for the detection of fecal streptococci from water samples.

Bacteriological Standards of Drinking Water

The following standards are laid down by ICMR for treated and untreated water.

Treated water

1. Coliform bacilli should be absent in 100 ml of water sample and the MPN should be less than 10 per 100 ml. This is for 90% samples examined throughout the month.
2. No sample should show an MPN in excess of 10 per 100 ml.
3. An MPN coliform bacteria of 8 to 10 per 100 ml should not occur in consecutive samples.
4. Repeat the sampling at the same point every day until the MPN of coliform bacteria is less than 8 to 10 per 100 ml.

Untreated water

1. Throughout any month none of the samples should show an MPN of coliform bacteria more than 8 to 10 per 100 ml.
2. An MPN of 20 per 100 ml may be permitted occasionally, if *E.coli* is absent.
3. If the MPN of coliform bacteria is consistently 20 or more, water supply should be treated.

Table 125.3 Classificatin of Drinking Water Accoridng to Bacteriological Tests

	Presumptive coliform count per 100 ml	*E.coli count per 100 ml*
Calss 1 Excellent	0	0
Class 2 Satisfactory	1-3	0
Class 3 Suspicious	4-10	0
Class 4 Unsatisfactory	More than 10	0, 1 or more

BACTERIOLOGY OF AIR

Introduction

The microbial population of air is transient and variable. Air is not a medium in which microorganisms grow, but it is a carrier of dust and droplets that may be laden with microorganisms.

Microorganisms may be carried on dust particles, in large droplets that settle out quickly, and in the droplet nuclei, that remain when small liquid droplets evaporate.

Organisms introduced into the air may be transported a few feet or many kilometres. Some air-borne microorganisms die in a matter of seconds; others survive for weeks, months or longer. The fate of air-borne microorganisms depends upon humidity, temperature, sunlight and the size of particles bearing microorganisms and the nature of microorganisms. For example, spores and cysts survive for longer periods in air.

Algae, protozoa, yeasts, molds and bacteria have been isolated from the air near the earth's surface. Whereas bacteria and fungal spores have been found at high altitudes above the earth's surface.

Enumeration of Microorganisms in Air or Sampling Devices for Trapping Microorganisms in Air

There are several methods which require special devices, designed for enumeration of microorganisms in air –

1. Liquid impingement devices
   – Bead bubbler device
   – Lemon's sampler
2. Solid impingement devices
   – Settling plate technique or sedimentation
   – Sieve device
   – Slit sampler
   – Andersen's air sampler
   – Funnel device
3. Filtration
4. Centrifugation
   – Wells air centrifuge
   – Cylindrical sampler
5. Electrostatic precipitation
6. Thermal precipitation.

Impingement in Liquids

The air is drawn through a very small opening or a capillary tube and bubbled through the liquid. The organisms get trapped in the liquid medium. Samples of the liquid are then plated to determine its microbial content.

Bead Bubbler Device* or *Capillary Impinger

It consists of a suction flask containing broth, glass beads and a gas bubbler. The air is drawn through capillary tube and bubbled through the broth so that organisms are trapped in the broth due to mechanical action between glass beads and air bubbles.

Lemon's Device/Apparatus

The lemon sampler consists of a glass folin aeration tube with a bulb at one end perforated by 6 holes. The tube is passed through a two-hole rubber stopper, and the bulb centred near the bottom of the containing test tube. The Kjeldahl trap with square glass baffle is shortened at both ends for convenience, and a slight bend made in the intake so that this may be inserted into the remaining hole of the stopper. A small flow meter measures the rate of air flow entering the upper open end of the folin tube. An air pump is attached to the exhaust end of Kjeldhal trap.

The entire bubbler should be sterilized by autoclaving or rinsing with 70% alcohol and drying. Air drawn in at the rate of 25 to 30 lit. per minute is dispersed through 20 ml of broth containing 2 or 3 drops of olive oil to prevent foaming.

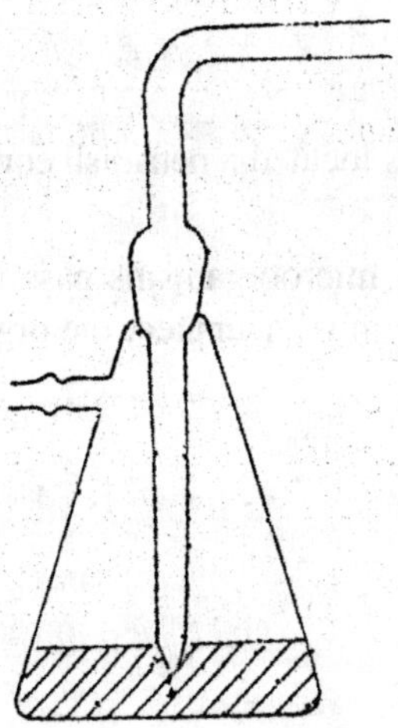

Fig. 125.1 Capillary impinger

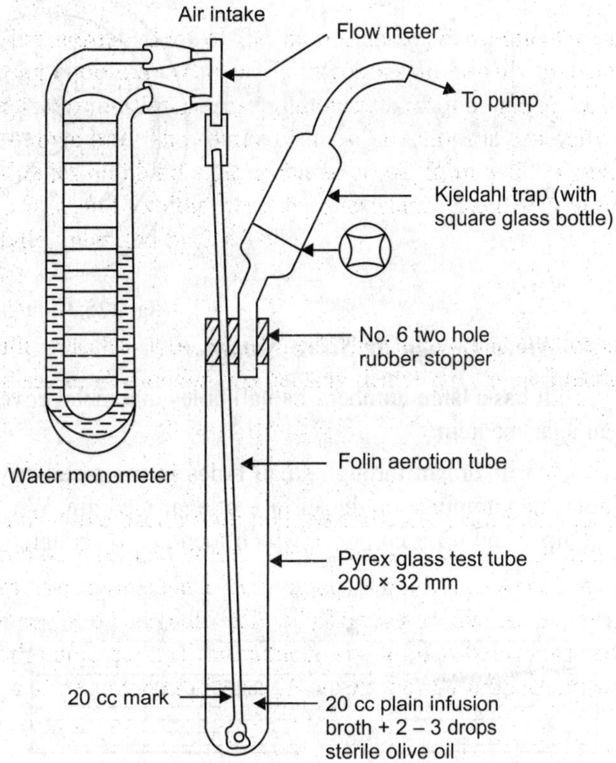

Fig. 125.2 Lemon's device.

Impingement on Solid Surfaces

Settling-Plate Techinque or *Sedimentation*

One technique for the bacteriological sampling of air is simply to expose a petridish containing an agar medium to the air for a designated period of time 30 min to one hour. When the petridish is incubated, microorganisms that have settled on the agar surface grow into colonies. When fastidious pathogens such as streptococci are to be demonstrated blood agar plates can be used.

This method gives a rough approximation of the numbers and kinds of air-borne microorganisms and specially used for bacteriological examination of air in hospital wards and operation theatres. It is one of the simplest procedures used for air examination.

The settling plate technique has certain limitations. It does not indicate the number of organisms present in a given volume of air and is of no value from a quantitative stand point.

Slit Sampler or Slit Device

The air is drawn through a very narrow slit on to a petridish containing agar medium. The slit is approximately the lenght of the petridish. The petridish is rotated mechanically at a particular speed, so that the organisms are evenly distributed on it.

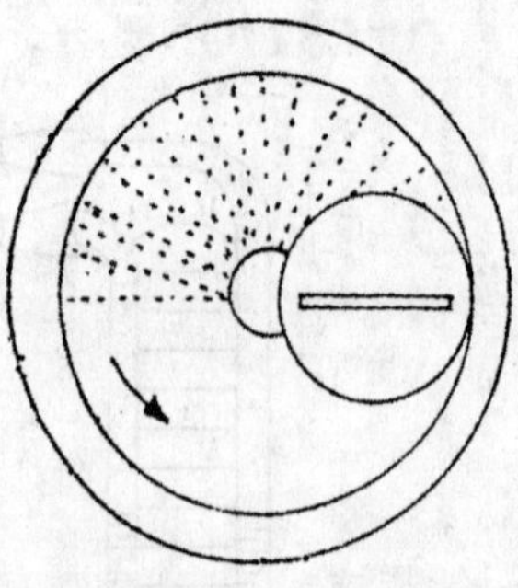

Fig. 125.3 Slit sampler.

Sieve Device or *Sieve Sampler*

It has a large number of small holes in a metal cover, under which is located a petridish containing an agar medium.

Air is drawn through small holes in the metal cover. As air-borne microorganisms pass through holes they impinge on the surface of agar medium. When the agar medium is incubated, the organisms multiply and form colonies, which then can be counted.

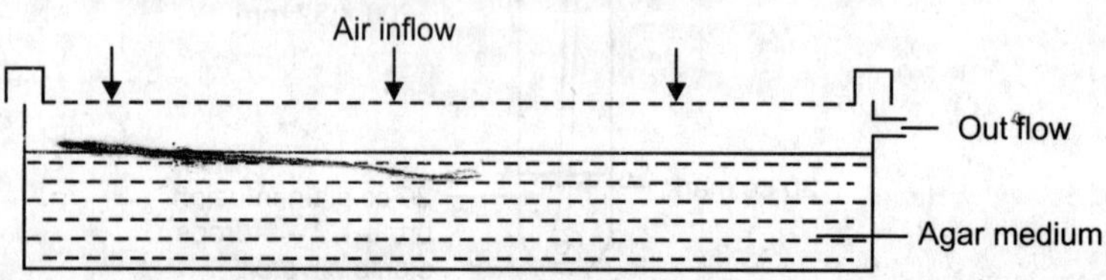

Fig. 125.4 Sieve sampler

Andersen's Air Sampler

In this device, air is drawn through a circular orifice and then through a succession of six circular plates, each perforated with 400 holes. The air passes through the perforations and the particles get impacted on to sterile medium in petridishes. The succession of plates has progressively smaller holes so that the largest particles are impacted on to the first dish and the smallest on the sixth.

Thus, the sampler automatically separates air particles into six aerodynamic sizes which indicate respiratory tract penetration and hazard. It is a device for size grading of air-borne particles on solid culture media, which are incubated and viable count is estimated.

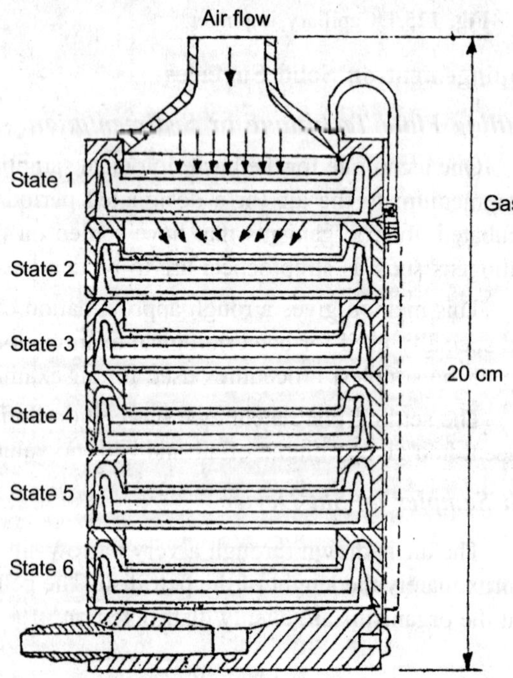

Fig. 125.5 Andersen's air sampler.

QUESTIONS

Essays Type:

1. Describe bacteriological analysis of water.
2. Give an account of bacteriological examination of milk.
3. Describe various sampling devices to trap microorganisms from air.

Short Notes:

1. DMC or Breed's count.
2. Standard plate count or colony count or viable count or pour plate method.
3. Melthylene blue reduction test.
4. Resazurin test.
5. Phosphatase test.
6. Milk ring test.
7. Multiple tube dilution technique.
8. Presumptive coliform count or MPN.
9. Indicators of water pollution.
10. Eijkman test.
11. Membrane filter method.
12. Fecal streptococci as indicators of water pollution.
13. Settling plate technique.
14. Andersen's sampler.

126

Biomedical Waste Management

Biomedical waste or hospital waste is the waste that is generated during the process of patient care.

Safe handling of biomedical waste is a matter of serious concern. Thousands of tonnes of biomedical waste originating from hospitals, nursing homes and clinics in the form of cotton swabs and bandages infected with blood, IV fluid bags, needles, catheters, human tissues and body parts etc. continue to be dumped in open garbage bins on the roads. This improper disposal of waste is one of the prime reasons for the spread of infectious diseases. The Govt. of India has published a Gazette notification on 20th July, 1998, titled Biomedical Waste (handling and management) Rules, making all persons who generate, collect, receive, store, transport, treat, dispose or handle medical waste in any form responsible for handling the medical waste without any adverse effect to human health and environment. It is mandatory for various hospital and health care institutions to implement these rules.

The hospital wastes are segregated preferably at the point of generation into infectious waste and non-infectious waste, which should be collected in appropriate containers.

Infectious wastes include discarded cultures, microbiological wastes, blood and body fluids, contaminated laboratory wastes, used syringes and needles, pathological wastes such as clinical specimens and tissues, bedding and other wastes like bandages and used cotton swabs, and animal carcasses used in laboratory experiments. Chemical waste is also hazardous. Covered containers can be used for segregation of waste. Black plastic bags are used for non-infectious general waste, whereas yellow and red plastic bags are used for infectious waste. Blue or white colored rigid, puncture proof containers are used for syringes, needles, lancets and other invasive instruments. This type of segregation helps in safe handling and transportation of waste and accordingly their treatment.

The treatment of biomedical waste can be done by incineration, autoclaving and chemical treatment.

Incineration is an efficient method for the sterilization and disposal of hazardous infectious hospital waste. Soiled dressings, pathological materials, animal carcasses, infected linen/bedding, sharp needles and other clinical wastes are literally burned to ashes at temperature of 870–980°C in an incinerator by electricity. Plastics such as disposable syringes, rubber catheters, culture plates and specimen containers made of polyvinylchloride (PVC) and polyethylene may emit dense black smoke when incineed. They can be autoclaved before disposal. Toxic air emissions during incineration and heavy metals in ash may constitute health hazard.

Autoclaving is used for microbiological waste, blood and blood products, body fluids and used syringes and needles. Autoclaved material is usually land-filled. Autoclaving is not recommended for pathological waste.

Chemical treatment ensures disinfection. One per cent hypochlorite or any suitable disinfectant may be seud.

Infectious waste after treatment can be disposed of by land-filling or deep burial. Liquid waste can be disposed into sewage drains.

QUESTIONS

Essay Question:

1. Describe the importance and procedures of hospital waste management.

Short Notes:

1. Hospital waste management (or) management of biomedical waste.
2. Incineration.

127

Biological Weapons

Biological weapons or bioweapons are major potential means of mass destruction used in biological warfare. Bioweapons may be defined as microorganisms or their products (toxins that infect and grow in the target host producing a clinical disease that kills or incapacitates the target host. Biological weapons are relatively easy to make. Scientists are busy to design and produce weapons loaded with deadly microbes or their toxins.

The pathogens commonly sued in biological warfare are as follows:

Bacteria:

(*i*) *Bacillus anthracis* (anthrax)

(*ii*) *Yersinia pestis* (plague)

(*iii*) *Francisella tularensis* (tularemia)

(*iv*) *Coxiella burnetii* (Q fever)

(*v*) *Vibrio cholerae* (cholera)

(*vi*) *Clostridium botulinum* (botulism).

Viruses:

(*i*) Variola virus (small pox)

(*ii*) Influenza virus (influenza)

(*iii*) Ebola-influenza hybrid.

Toxins:

(*i*) Botulinum toxin

(*ii*) Aflatoxin

(*iii*) Ricin (a lethal toxin extracted from castor bean)

(*iv*) Saxitoxin (an alkaloid neurotoxin produced by dinoflagellates; when consumed through contaminated food such as shellfish causes paralysis and death).

(*v*) RNAi (Interference RNA tailored to latch on to specific mRNA sequences thus virtually silencing any gene).

Index

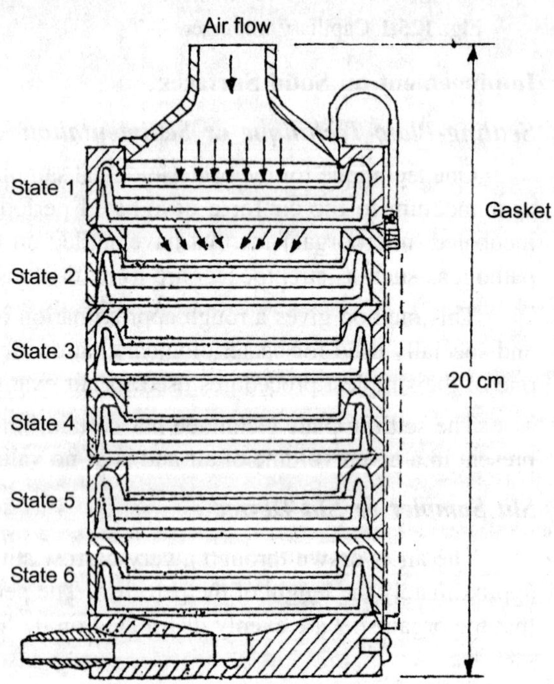

D

I

K

L

T